a LANGE medical book

CURRENT
Diagnosis & Treatment in Orthopedics

SIXTH EDITION

Edited by

Patrick J. McMahon, MD
Chief of Orthopedic Surgery, Veteran Affairs Healthcare System
Clinical Professor, University of Pittsburgh
Pittsburgh, Pennsylvania

Harry B. Skinner, MD, PhD
Professor Emeritus of Orthopedic Surgery
University of California Irvine
Attending Physician
St. Jude Medical Center
Fullerton, California

Mc Graw Hill

New York Chicago San Francisco Athens London Madrid Mexico City
Milan New Delhi Singapore Sydney Toronto

Current Diagnosis & Treatment in Orthopedics, Sixth Edition

1 2 3 4 5 6 7 8 9 LCR 26 25 24 23 22 21

ISBN 978-1-260-13597-8
MHID 1-260-13597-7
ISSN 1081-0056

Notice

Medicine is an ever-changing science. As new research and clinical experience broaden our knowledge, changes in treatment and drug therapy are required. The authors and the publisher of this work have checked with sources believed to be reliable in their efforts to provide information that is complete and generally in accord with the standards accepted at the time of publication. However, in view of the possibility of human error or changes in medical sciences, neither the authors nor the publisher nor any other party who has been involved in the preparation or publication of this work warrants that the information contained herein is in every respect accurate or complete, and they disclaim all responsibility for any errors or omissions or for the results obtained from use of the information contained in this work. Readers are encouraged to confirm the information contained herein with other sources. For example and in particular, readers are advised to check the product information sheet included in the package of each drug they plan to administer to be certain that the information contained in this work is accurate and that changes have not been made in the recommended dose or in the contraindications for administration. This recommendation is of particular importance in connection with new or infrequently used drugs.

This book was set in Minion Pro by KnowledgeWorks Global Ltd..
The editors were Andrew Moyer and Kim J. Davis.
The production supervisor was Catherine H. Saggese.
Project management was provided by Sarika Gupta and Parag Mittal, KnowledgeWorks Global Ltd.

To my son, Thomas, who inspires me with his determination to achieve his best.

Contents

Authors

Sam Akhavan, MD
Director, Orthopaedics Sports Medicine Fellowship
Department of Orthopaedic Sports Surgery
Allegheny General Hospital
Pittsburgh, Pennsylvania
Chapter 4 Sports Medicine: Lower Extremity

Michael S. Bednar, MD
Professor and Chief of Hand Surgery
Department of Orthopaedic Surgery and Rehabilitation
Loyola University Medical Center
Maywood, Illinois
Chapter 11 Hand Surgery

Nicholas M. Bernthal, MD
Ronald Reagan UCLA Medical Center
Orthopaedic Center–Santa Monica
Santa Monica, California
Chapter 6 Musculoskeletal Oncology

Gideon W. Blumstein, MD
Department of Orthopedic Surgery
David Geffen School of Medicine at UCLA
Los Angeles, California
Chapter 6 Musculoskeletal Oncology

Scott D. Boden, MD
Professor and Chair
Department of Orthopaedic Surgery
Emory University School of Medicine
Director, The Emory Orthopaedics & Spine Center
CMO, CQO, Emory University Orthopaedics & Spine Hospital
Atlanta, Georgia
Chapter 5 Disorders, Diseases, and Injuries of the Spine

Patrick Bosch, MD
Albuquerque Orthopedics
UNM Medical Group Inc
2211 Lomas Blvd NE
Albuquerque, NM 87106-2719
Chapter 12 Pediatric Orthopedic Surgery

Zachary D.C. Burke, MD
Resident, Department of Orthopaedic Surgery
David Geffen School of Medicine, UCLA
Los Angeles, California
Chapter 6 Musculoskeletal Oncology

Anthony Davidson, BS
Department of Orthopaedic Surgery
University of Pittsburgh Medical Center
Pittsburgh, Pennsylvania
Chapter 11 Hand Surgery

Patrick DeMeo, MD
Chairperson
Department of Orthopaedic Surgery
Allegheny Health Network
Pittsburgh, Pennsylvania
Chapter 4 Sports Medicine: Lower Extremity

Brett A. Freedman, MD
Department of Orthopedic Surgery
Mayo Clinic
Rochester, Minnesota
Chapter 5 Disorders, Diseases, and Injuries of the Spine

Danielle Greig, MD
Resident
Department of Orthopaedic Surgery
UCLA
Los Angeles, California
Chapter 6 Musculoskeletal Oncology

Kaan S. Irgit, MD
Associate Professor
Department of Orthopaedics and Traumatology
Marmara University School of Medicine
Istanbul, Turkey
Chapter 2 Musculoskeletal Trauma Surgery

Lee D. Kaplan, MD
Chief, Division of Sports Medicine
Associate Professor, Department of Orthopaedics
University of Miami Miller School of Medicine
Director, UHealth Sports Medicine Institute
Petra and Stephen Levin Endowed Chair in Sports Medicine
Medical Director and Head Team Physician
Miami Hurricanes and Miami Marlins
Miami, Florida
Chapter 4 Sports Medicine: Lower Extremity

Connor S. Kasik, DO
Department of Orthopedic Surgery
St. Margaret's Health–Peru
Peru, Illinois
Chapter 4 Sports Medicine: Lower Extremity

Mary Ann E. Keenan, MD
Professor, Orthopaedic Surgery (Retired)
University of Pennsylvania
Philadelphia, Pennsylvania
Consultant, Neuro-Orthopaedics
MossRehab Hospital
Elkins Park, Pennsylvania
Chapter 13 Rehabilitation

Elliott Kim, MD
Spine Surgeon, OrthoVirginia
Alexandria, Virginia
Chapter 5 Disorders, Diseases, and Injuries of the Spine

Kshitij Manchanda, MD
Resident, Department of Orthopaedic Surgery
University of Texas Southwestern Medical Center
Dallas, Texas
Chap 10 Foot and Ankle Surgery

Richard L. McGough, III, MD
Professor of Orthopaedic Surgery, Surgical Oncology, and Rehabilitation Science
Chief, Division of Musculoskeletal Oncology
University of Pittsburgh Medical Center
Pittsburgh, Pennsylvania
Chapter 8 Adult Reconstructive Surgery
Chapter 9 Orthopedic Infections: Basic Principles of Pathogenesis, Diagnosis, and Treatment

Patrick J. McMahon, MD
Chief of Orthopedic Surgery, Veteran Affairs Healthcare System
Clinical Professor, University of Pittsburgh
Pittsburgh, Pennsylvania
Chapter 3 Sports Medicine: Upper Extremity
Chapter 4 Sports Medicine: Lower Extremity
Chapter 8 Adult Reconstructive Surgery
Chapter 13 Rehabilitation

Dimitrios V. Papadopoulos, MD, PhD
Department of Orthopaedic Surgery
University of Pittsburgh Medical Center
Pittsburgh, Pennsylvania
Chapter 11 Hand Surgery

Anton Plakseychuk, MD, PhD
Associate Director
Bone and Joint Center
Magee-Women's Hospital of UPMC
Pittsburgh, Pennsylvania
Chapter 7 Arthritis and Joint Preservation Surgery

George T. Rab, MD
Professor, Department of Orthopaedic Surgery
University of California, Davis
Consultant, Shriners Hospitals for Children, Northern California
Sacramento, California
Chapter 12 Pediatric Orthopedic Surgery

John M. Rhee, MD
Spinal Surgery
Professor, Orthopaedic Surgery and Neurosurgery
Emory University School of Medicine
Atlanta, Georgia
Chapter 5 Disorders, Diseases, and Injuries of the Spine

Steven D.K. Ross, MD
Clinical Professor
Department of Orthopaedic Surgery
University of California, Irvine, College of Medicine
Orange, California
Chapter 10 Foot and Ankle Surgery

Babak Samimi, MD
Samimi Orthopaedic Group
Los Angeles, California
Chapter 2 Musculoskeletal Trauma Surgery

Christopher C. Schmidt, MD
Orthopedic Surgery, Shoulder and Elbow Orthopedic Surgery
University of Pittsburgh Medical Center
Pittsburgh, Pennsylvania
Chapter 11 Hand Surgery

Akash Shah, MD
Resident, Department of Orthopaedic Surgery
UCLA
Los Angeles, California
Chapter 6 Musculoskeletal Oncology

Harry B. Skinner, MD, PhD
Professor Emeritus of Orthopedic Surgery
University of California Irvine
Attending Physician
St. Jude Medical Center
Fullerton, California
Chapter 1 General Considerations in Orthopedic Surgery
Chapter 7 Arthritis and Joint Preservation Surgery

Wade R. Smith, MD, FACS
OrthoONE Trauma at Swedish Medical Center
Englewood, Colorado
Chapter 2 Musculoskeletal Trauma Surgery

Kwesi St. Louis, MD
Arthroplasty Fellow
Department of Orthopedic Surgery
University of California, San Francisco
San Francisco, California
Chapter 9 Orthopedic Infections: Basic Principles of Pathogenesis, Diagnosis, and Treatment

Bobby K.B. Tay, MD
Professor of Orthopaedic Surgery
Vice Chair of Quality and Safety
Department of Orthopaedic Surgery
University of California, San Francisco
San Francisco, California
Chapter 5 Disorders, Diseases, and Injuries of the Spine

Robert Tisherman, MD
University of Pittsburgh Medical Center
Department of Orthopaedic Surgery
Pittsburgh, Pennsylvania
Chapter 7 Arthritis and Joint Preservation Surgery

Jordan A. Weinberg, MD, FACS
Professor and Chair of Surgery
Creighton University School of Medicine–Phoenix Regional Campus
Phoenix, Arizona
Chapter 2 Musculoskeletal Trauma Surgery

Dane K. Wukich, MD
Dr. Charles F. Gregory Distinguished Chair
Professor, Orthopaedic Surgery
UT Southwestern Medical Center
Dallas, Texas
Chapter 10 Foot and Ankle Surgery

Aaron Wynkoop, MD
Department of Orthopaedic Surgery
McLaren-Flint McLaren Regional Medical Center
Flint, Michigan
Chapter 4 Sports Medicine: Lower Extremity

Navid Ziran, MD, FACS
Associate Professor of Surgery
Creighton University School of Medicine–Phoenix Regional Campus
Phoenix, Arizona
Chapter 2 Musculoskeletal Trauma Surgery

Preface

This *Current Diagnosis and Treatment in Orthopedics* is the sixth edition of the Orthopedic Surgery contribution to the Lange Current series of books. Much has changed in orthopedics since the first edition came out, but the goal of this book has not changed. It is intended to fill a need for a ready source of up-to-date information on disorders and diseases treated by orthopedic surgeons and related clinicians. The format in this edition is unchanged from the previous edition: there is emphasis on the major diagnostic features of disease states, the natural history of the disease where appropriate, the workup required for definitive diagnosis, and finally, definitive treatment. The book focuses on orthopedic conditions, deemphasizing the treatment of the patient from a general medical viewpoint, except when it pertains to the orthopedic problem under consideration. Importantly, pathophysiology, epidemiology, and pathology are included when they assist in arriving at a definitive diagnosis or an understanding of the treatment of the disease or condition. In many conditions, such as infection or neoplasm, it is extremely important to understand the pathophysiology because the disease may be encountered at various time points in the progression of the disease.

This edition of *Current Diagnosis and Treatment in Orthopedics* is truly current. The entire book has been updated, including the references, which are recent except when classic articles are necessary to refer back to major advances in understanding or treatment. These selected older references represent landmarks in understanding orthopedic diseases and conditions.

INTENDED AUDIENCE

The unique format of the Lange series textbooks allows readers of many levels of understanding to derive benefit from the information. Students will find that the book encompasses virtually all aspects of orthopedics that they will encounter in classes and as subinterns in major teaching institutions. Residents and house officers can use the book as a ready reference covering the majority of disorders and conditions in emergency and elective orthopedic surgery. Despite its small size, it is truly comprehensive. Because of the organization of the book on a subspecialty basis, review of individual chapters will provide house officers rotating on subspecialty orthopedic services with an excellent basis for further in-depth study.

For emergency room physicians, especially those with medical backgrounds, the text provides an excellent resource in managing orthopedic problems seen on an emergent basis. Similarly, family practice practitioners, pediatricians, general practitioners, internists, physical therapists, and athletic trainers will find the book particularly helpful in the referral decision process and as a resource to explain disorders to patients. Finally, practicing orthopedic surgeons, particularly those in subspecialties of orthopedics, will find the book a helpful resource in reassuring them that their treatment in areas outside their subspecialty interest is current and up-to-date.

ORGANIZATION

The book is structured similarly to the structure of orthopedic surgery. Natural subspecialization has occurred in orthopedic surgery over the years, which has resulted in some overlap in anatomic areas. This has resulted in the book having some overlap and some artificial division of subjects. Because of the primarily subspecialization structure, the reader is encouraged to read entire chapters or, for more discrete topics, go directly to the index for information. For example, the house officer rotating on the pediatric orthopedic service would find reading the pediatric chapter to be a prudent method of developing a baseline knowledge in pediatric orthopedic surgery. Knee problems, however, might be best approached by looking in the sports medicine chapter or in the adult reconstruction chapter, since these areas overlap, mostly in age of patient.

The first chapter introduces aspects of interest in the perioperative care of the orthopedic patient, including social aspects of the patient-physician relationship, and is an outgrowth of the importance of outcomes in orthopedics. Management of orthopedic problems arising from trauma is covered in Chapter 2. New to this edition, because the field of sports medicine has grown so large, we have split this topic into two chapters: Chapters 3 focuses on the upper extremity and Chapter 4 on the lower extremity. Chapter 5 covers all aspects of spine surgery, including infection of the spine, degenerative spinal problems, spinal deformity, and spinal trauma.

Chapter 6 provides comprehensive coverage of tumors in orthopedic surgery, including benign and malignant soft-tissue and hard-tissue tumors. Also new to this edition, because there is so much more information, Chapter 7 on arthritis and joint preservation surgery has been split off from Chapter 8 on adult joint reconstruction. In Chapter 9, infections, with their special implications for orthopedic surgery, are covered. Chapter 10 discusses foot and ankle surgery, and Chapter 11, hand surgery. Chapter 12 covers diseases in orthopedics unique to children. The final chapter, Chapter 13, deals with amputation and all aspects of rehabilitation fundamental to orthopedic surgeons in returning patients to full function.

OUTSTANDING FEATURES

Illustrations have been carefully selected to maximize their benefits in pointing out orthopedic principles and concepts. The effect of changes in imaging technology on optimal diagnostic studies is emphasized, including cost-effectiveness.

Disorders and conditions are explained by diagnoses, and the essentials of diagnosis are listed when helpful. Nonoperative and operative treatments are discussed, as well as the indications for surgery.

Concise, current, and comprehensive treatment of the basic sciences underlying the understanding of orthopedic surgery is provided in individual chapters, where pertinent.

NEW TO THIS EDITION

- Sports medicine has been expanded so that there are now separate chapters on the upper and lower extremity.
- Advances in treatment of back pain, including disk replacement, are included, along with the latest information on reverse shoulder replacement.
- The musculoskeletal tumor chapter includes the latest on molecular biology of neoplasms.
- New materials in orthopedics that are making changes in the way replacement arthroplasty is performed are included.
- The chapter on adult joint reconstruction has been reformatted, and the information on arthritis and joint preservation surgery has been given its own chapter including much on hip conditions amenable to arthroscopic treatments.
- The latest information on important growth factors in orthopedics is elucidated with their current usage.

We are pleased to be able to say, with the concurrence of our coauthors, that these new features added to the information in the previous edition make this edition a significant improvement over the last.

General Considerations in Orthopedic Surgery

1

Harry B. Skinner, MD, PhD

Orthopedic surgery encompasses the entire process of caring for the surgical patient, from diagnostic evaluation to the preoperative evaluation and through the postoperative and rehabilitative period. Although the surgical procedure itself is the key step toward helping the patient, the preliminary and follow-up care can determine whether the surgery is successful.

DIAGNOSTIC WORKUP

History and Physical Exam

Although it may seem obvious, the history and physical exam are still important in the evaluation of the patient. Every office visit is a history and physical exam, whether a new or a return visit. The completeness of the history and physical has assumed new importance in view of the complexities required for compliance with federal regulations. Regulations require that a chief complaint be specified, and this must be clearly defined because it determines the direction for the rest of the history and physical. The history must address the key features of the problem, both to elucidate the medical problem and to cover the subsidiary requirements for billing purposes. The social history and past medical history are similarly important because they change billing codes without necessarily affecting outcome or success of care. The physical again must cover the essentials necessary for diagnosis, and frequently the confirmation of the diagnosis is based on physical exam, but such considerations as skin condition and blood supply must be documented, despite the fact that this process is also part of the surgical evaluation. The next step is imaging and laboratory exams. The most important point here is to use the most cost-effective examination possible while keeping patient safety, satisfaction, and convenience in mind.

Imaging Studies

A. Roentgenography

Roentgenography is still the most cost-effective and most important initial diagnostic test in the orthopedist's armamentarium. Almost every patient should have a radiograph prior to getting a more sophisticated imaging study. Certain situations are obvious; for example, a 68-year-old man with knee pain should have standing, flexed-knee posteroanterior (PA), lateral, and Merchant plain film views taken. If those views show normal joint spaces, consideration of intraarticular pathology, such as a degenerative meniscus tear, can be worked up with magnetic resonance imaging (MRI). The normal views usually ordered are as follows:

1. Neck pain—

No history of trauma, more than 4 weeks' duration.

Younger than 35 years: anteroposterior (AP) lateral, odontoid.

Older than 35 years: obliques.

History of trauma: flexion/extension laterals (obtain on first visit).

2. Thoracic spine pain and tenderness—

Younger than 40 years, no reason to suspect malignancy: AP and lateral (if history of trauma or possibility of osteoporosis on first visit, otherwise at 4 weeks).

Consider cervical (C)-spine as a source of referred pain to thoracic (T)-spine if no tenderness in T-spine.

3. Lumbar (L)-sacral (S)-spine—

Younger than 40 years, no reason to suspect malignancy after 4 weeks' duration of the pain. With significant trauma, at first visit, or possible malignancy (ie, weight loss, malaise, fatigue): AP, lateral.

Add obliques for chronic low back pain (ie, spondylolisthesis).

4. Hips—

AP pelvis, lateral of affected hip.

Consider lumbar-sacral (L-S) series if pain is in the buttock rather than in the groin.

5. Knees—

Older than 40 years or history of meniscectomy: Rosenberg, lateral, and sunrise films. Merchant views are similar to sunrise. The Rosenberg view is a 10-degree down-shot of the PA of the knees while standing at 45 degrees of flexion.

For other knees: AP, lateral, and sunrise.

In children, up to age 16, consider a pelvis film with the complaint of knee pain and negative physical exam referable to the knee.

6. Femur, tibia, humerus, forearm—AP and lateral are indicated for trauma, palpable lesions, or suspected tumors.

7. Ankle—AP lateral and mortise.

8. Foot—AP, lateral, and oblique for routine evaluation.

9. Shoulder—AP of the glenohumeral joint, axillary lateral, acromioclavicular joint, and scapular Y or supraspinatus outlet views.

10. Elbow—AP and lateral (true lateral).

11. Hand/wrist—

Hand: PA and lateral.

Wrist: PA, lateral, and oblique.

For suspected instability: clenched fist PA in radial and ulnar deviation.

Follow-up radiographs are obtained when a change in the radiographic findings is expected. Remember that bone changes occur slowly, so radiographic changes take a comparable length of time. Radiographs are obtained in view of the clinical picture. For example, closed treatment of a distal radius fracture would not be expected to show changes because of healing for a minimum of 2 weeks. However, displacement of the fracture could occur sooner. Hence, radiographs to show displacement might be obtained at 1 week and 2 weeks. If no displacement is observed, the fracture position could be considered stable, and the next films might be obtained at 6 weeks—the earliest time healing might be observed. Similarly, closed treatment of an adult tibia fracture might be followed with radiographs at 2-week intervals, checking for displacement and healing, whereas a tibia fracture treated with an intramedullary rod might be followed at monthly intervals to check for healing.

B. Magnetic Resonance Imaging

This imaging modality is very useful, but like computed tomography (CT), MRI is sometimes too revealing. This method should be reserved for clarifying a particular problem. Frequently in orthopedics, a bony lesion can be localized with a radiograph or bone scan, which then provides a focus for the MRI. MRI is useful for some bony lesions, such as osteonecrosis, tumors, occult and fatigue fractures, and osteomyelitis. It is also helpful in some soft-tissue problems, such as knee meniscus tears and shoulder rotator cuff tears. Distortion of the magnetic field by metallic implants may limit the usefulness of MRI studies of conditions such as total knee or hip replacement or fracture fixation devices. MRI should not be used when the diagnosis can be made with a less expensive test. For example, the use of MRI in knee studies in patients older than 45 years should always be preceded by plain films of the knee, as noted earlier. An MRI of an arthritic knee adds little additional information because the meniscus and anterior cruciate ligament are likely to be damaged from the arthritic process already. However, the MRI can be very helpful in determining soft-tissue extension of tumors or infection.

The advent of new portable MRI units that perform limited studies with more resolution adds a new dimension to their use. These can provide data on the progression of disorders such as rheumatoid arthritis or osteomyelitis in a timely and cost-effective way. The possibility of osteomyelitis in the bones adjacent to ulcers on the foot is easily determined with this test because it shows the changes, typically edema, in the bone with osteomyelitis. A bone scan usually does not have the resolution to distinguish the inflammatory response in the soft tissue from the bony involvement. Osteomyelitis should be treated much differently from a soft-tissue ulcer, which does not affect the bone.

C. Computed Tomography

The CT scan is an extremely important imaging modality for examining bony lesions such as fractures. Frequently, plain films provide some information about the fracture of interest, but the CT scan provides the three-dimensional information that can only otherwise be determined from the integration of the plain films in the surgeon's mind. The CT scan adds significantly to the management of such fractures as tibial plateaus, scapular fractures, ankle fractures, and cervical and lumbar spine fractures, as well as many others. Furthermore, nonunions of fractures, with or without fixation, can be identified and followed with CT scans. Again, if little information can be gained that cannot be already discerned from the plain films, the CT scan only adds expense and patient inconvenience. The spiral CT makes imaging with this modality less expensive and much more rapid. The CT angiogram (CTA) scan is also now the method of choice for determining whether a pulmonary embolus (PE) has occurred. Again, a CT for this indication is easier on the patient, more accurate, and less invasive than angiography.

D. Technetium-99m Bone Scan

The bone scan finds many uses in orthopedic surgery. Keep in mind that the bone scan labels the osteoblast activity with the radioactive tracer, technetium-99; thus, bone formation activity is recorded, and little or no bone resorption activity is noted. Any disorder that results in increased bone formation, therefore, results in a "hot" bone scan. This means that a disorder such as multiple myeloma may not show up on a bone scan because only osteoclastic activity is involved in the majority of lesions. However, boney lesions due to metastasis with osteoblastic activity, such as prostate and often breast, can be identified and monitored for treatment efficacy with bone scans. Bone scans can be helpful in discerning loose joint prostheses, even though the findings are nonspecific. It is very helpful in examining probable benign bone lesions because a cold bone scan largely rules out an aggressive process such as a malignancy. The bone scan is also helpful in diagnosing any disorder of unknown origin when there is pain localized to a particular region. A cold bone scan implies that the problem is a soft-tissue one, whereas a hot bone scan points to a region that may benefit from MRI.

Anand A, Morris MJ, Kaboteh R, et al. Analytic validation of the automated bone scan index as an imaging biomarker to standardize quantitative changes in bone scans of patients with metastatic prostate cancer. *J Nucl Med.* 2016;57(1):41-45. [PMID: 26315832]

Anjum O, Bleeker H, Ohle R. Computed tomography for suspected pulmonary embolism results in a large number of nonsignificant incidental findings and follow-up investigations. *Emerg Radiol.* 2019;26(1):29-35. [PMID: 30238172]

Laboratory Exams

The two most important laboratory exams are for C-reactive protein and the erythrocyte sedimentation rate. These two tests indicate whether an inflammatory process, malignancy, or rheumatologic disorder is a diagnostic consideration. If these tests are negative, systemic causes of a complaint can frequently be ruled out. In that situation, a more localized disorder should be identified. The next most important test is the complete blood count, which provides a general indication of the patient's health, revealing information about anemia, infectious processes, and so on. The next most useful laboratory test for the orthopedic surgeon is the synovial fluid analysis. This test typically should include a culture and sensitivity. If there is any concern about infection, a cell count, differential, protein, and glucose measurement should be performed. The presence of crystals should be investigated because they indicate chondrocalcinosis or gout. Elevated protein and reduced glucose levels suggest infection. For the special case of a possible periprosthetic joint infection, other synovial biomarkers such as alpha-defensin or leukocyte esterase may be beneficial for diagnosis. The final factor that should be considered with any major surgery is the patient's nutritional status, which is evaluated with several tests, including lymphocyte count and levels of prealbumin, albumin, zinc, and serum iron transferrin. In addition, the Mini Nutritional Assessment is a nursing tool to screen elderly individuals at risk of malnutrition.

Higuera CA. Serum erythrocyte sedimentation rate and C-reactive protein level have weaknesses but are the best screening so far. *J Bone Joint Surg.* 2018:100(12):e150.

Wyatt MC, Beswick AD, Kunutsor SK, et al. The alpha-defensin immunoassay and leukocyte esterase colorimetric strip test for the diagnosis of periprosthetic infection. A systematic review and meta-analysis. *J Bone Joint Surg Am.* 2016;98(12):992-1000.

Educating and Informing Patients and Their Families

Surgical procedures in orthopedics have varying degrees of difficulty and importance, ranging from a relatively simple claw toe correction to the performance of a multilevel complex spinal fusion. After the decision to employ surgery as a therapeutic modality is made, it is important to help the patient completely understand what to expect before, during, and after surgery. This process, which the legal profession calls **informed consent**, has the more important purpose of ensuring the patient's cooperation and satisfaction. Informed consent is *not* a signature on a consent form and can only be obtained from a patient who is mentally competent and not coerced.

To comply with the requirements of the legal profession and accrediting organizations, such as The Joint Commission, the surgeon must provide an explanation of the risks, prognosis, alternatives, and complications that might be encountered. The risks should be reviewed in some detail, along with the general risks of typical orthopedic surgical procedures. The risks and the complications that occur in surgery are intimately associated and thus must be dealt with together. The alternatives are sometimes straightforward. For example, a patient with an open fracture has a high risk of infection if not adequately treated with irrigation, debridement, and antibiotics. Thus, in such a situation, any reasonable and prudent person would consent to the procedure. The choice between alternatives can become significantly more subtle, however. For example, it is possible that a choice must be made between two different procedures or between a particular procedure and no procedure. In this situation, the surgeon must consider the psychosocial and physical attributes of the patient so as to assist him or her in making this decision. For example, consider two men, both 75 years of age, with severe degenerative disease in the right knee noted on radiograph. One individual is now at the point where he cannot play golf, a situation that is reducing his physical exercise and a number of his social outlets. The other individual leads a relatively sedentary lifestyle, seldom walks more than a block, and obtains cardiorespiratory exercise by swimming, an activity in which his knee does not bother him. The surgeon should recommend knee replacement to the first individual but not the second. At the same time, both men must be offered the alternatives, which include continued nonsteroidal anti-inflammatory medicine, bracing, sleeping medication, and analgesics.

Patients with active lifestyle are becoming much more concerned about what will happen to them in the postoperative period, including how soon they can safely travel, when they can work, and when they will be fully able to take care of themselves. They are also concerned about what social services are available to help them if they cannot care for themselves fully. The surgeon must be prepared to address these questions and also advise patients with lower extremity or spinal problems about when they will be able to walk. In the same manner, after procedures on the hand or upper extremity, patients must be advised about when they will be able to use the hand. Advising the patient of these situations before surgery can prevent unexpected surprises in the postoperative period.

The patient should also be informed about the range of expectations for ambulation or use of the upper extremity because individuals vary in their response to surgery. For example, patients should be advised that after surgery on the hip or knee, they will need a walker for a few days, move to crutches, and typically be done with the crutches in the range of 2 to 4 weeks. They will use a cane before 6 weeks and be done with the cane before 3 months. Patients' response to surgery is somewhat unpredictable, so conservative estimates on the length of medication use, pain, restricted driving, and so on are prudent. Patients should be cautioned about travel after surgery, particularly with lower extremity injuries, because of the risk of deep venous thrombosis (DVT). In such cases, discourage (for the first 6-12 weeks) plane trips longer than an hour and extended car trips made without stopping approximately every 45 minutes. Anti-inflammatory medication (to reduce platelet adhesion) or anticoagulants should be recommended if such travel is unavoidable.

A. Explaining the Procedures

An essential part of the patient's presurgical preparation and postsurgical cooperation is knowing what to expect at every step in the process. Nuances become important in the process of explaining the surgical procedures and their implications. For example, scheduling a bunion procedure 2 weeks prior to a patient's participation in her daughter's wedding could upset the patient if she fails to realize that she will be unable to wear the shoes she purchased for the event. Similarly, lifestyle considerations can affect the decision-making process in cases of medial gonarthrosis, in which the choice between a unicompartmental knee replacement and a high tibial osteotomy could be influenced by whether the patient plays tennis and holds a physically strenuous job or, alternatively, whether the patient is sedentary and works behind a desk most of the day.

B. Reviewing the Risks and Possible Complications

Reviewing the perioperative risks is important for all patients and optimally should be done well in advance and then repeated closer to the time of surgery. Some patients require more detailed explanations, particularly if their relatives have undergone surgery in the past and had a problem with anesthesia or a complication such as a PE or infection. Based on the patient's responses to explanations, the health care team members need to alter their approach to reach a balance between inadequately informing the patient and inducing unnecessary alarm that could make the patient refuse to undergo a procedure judged to be both beneficial and necessary.

Table 1–1. Rates of death and complications associated with common activities.

Death or Complication	Percentage
Death (from MI after previous MI)	1
Major bleed (7 days, warfarin, INR 2.65)	0.02
GI ulcer/bleed perforation (naproxen 6 months)	1
Paralysis (from epidural)	0.02
Death (frequent flying professor/year)	0.001
Death (automobile/year)	0.016
Earthquake in California/per year	0.00018

GI, gastrointestinal; INR, international normalized ratio; MI, myocardial infarction.

Risk is a poorly understood concept in our culture. Some situations are considered to be higher in risk than they actually are. Some risks are understood better than others. It can help the patient to understand if these risks are put in perspective. The risks can be surprisingly high or low but still disturbing to the patient. For example, many people have moved away from California to avoid an earthquake or refuse to fly commercial aircraft because of the risk, not realizing that the risk of death is 10 to 100 times higher while driving a car (Table 1–1). This lack of understanding of the risk can contribute to significant differences in the perception of liability associated with these activities. For example, the death benefit from a commercial airline accident might reach several million dollars per passenger, whereas death in an automobile accident might have no death benefit at all. Thus, the *perception* of risk is very important and must be clarified in the patient's mind. Similarly, patients can understand and accept having a myocardial infarction (MI) after a major surgery because they can clearly see the strain on the heart from the surgery. However, they are not nearly as understanding of a lower extremity paralysis that can result from the epidural anesthetic for that surgery. The explanation of risks must be individualized for each patient. The patient with a previous MI is clearly different from a healthy 20-year-old (see Table 1–1). Across-the-board rates of problems do not translate into direct risks for the individual patient.

Although all procedures carry some risks, the incidence and type of risks and complications vary with the surgical procedure as well as with the patient's age and general health. Potential problems are listed and discussed here in alphabetical order.

1. Amputation—The potential problem of amputation is seldom of acute concern except in cases of significant trauma. The topic of amputation can frequently be discussed with the risk of infection because ischemia, diabetes, and infection can increase the risk of amputation. Studies are mixed on whether sodium-glucose co-transporter 2 inhibitors, used to treat diabetes, increase the risk of amputation, but perhaps they should be considered in the consent process.

2. Anesthesia—One of the major risks in orthopedic surgery is associated with anesthesia, not because complications of anesthesia are frequent but because they can be devastating. Death occurs at a rate of approximately eight per million hospital surgical discharges. Other complications include, but are not limited to, the following: nerve damage and paraplegia from nerve blocks, headaches from dural leaks following use of spinal anesthetics, aspiration of stomach contents, and cardiac problems, including ischemia and arrhythmias. The surgeon should discuss these problems with the patient only in general terms, allowing the anesthesiologist to provide the most detailed explanations.

3. Arthritis—Virtually any procedure that enters a joint, other than to replace it, has the potential to cause damage to that joint. In some instances, as in an intraarticular fracture, the surgery will likely lessen the risk of arthritis. Even in these instances, the patient should be told that the risk of damage is still real because the joint surface healing will not result in a normal cartilage surface.

4. Blood loss—Patients should be given a reasonably accurate estimate of blood loss as well as the opportunity to donate autologous blood prior to surgery, if transfusion is likely to be necessary. The use of erythropoietin can elevate preoperative hemoglobin (Hgb) levels in selected cases and thereby reduce postoperative homologous blood transfusion needs. The use of erythropoietin is generally accepted by Jehovah's Witness patients, whereas the autologous reinfusion acceptance is variable. Other alternatives include the use of intraoperative blood salvage for reinfusion. Many of these strategies have been obviated by the use of antifibrinolytic drugs such as tranexamic acid and through the recommendations to transfuse at lower Hgb levels. To help minimize blood loss during surgery, the patient's use of nonsteroidal anti-inflammatory drugs (NSAIDs) should be discontinued approximately 2 weeks before surgery. Discontinuation of NSAIDs can significantly compromise comfort and incite rheumatoid flares in many patients who rely on these drugs. To minimize the risk, newer cyclooxygenase-2 (COX-2) inhibitor NSAIDs may be used as a substitute during this period; minimal platelet disorder or bleeding time derangement occurs with these drugs because they do not affect platelet function or inhibit thromboxane A_2, except at high doses.

Due to a host of conditions including DVT, stroke, and atrial fibrillation, patients often present for surgery while being treated with various anticoagulants. Frequently, the patients presenting for elective surgery can be counseled to discontinue NSAIDs or other platelet inhibitors such as clopidogrel or dipyridamole. In cases of urgent surgery, the risk of excessive blood loss must be accepted. Those patients on medications that block the clotting cascade, such as warfarin, dabigatran, edoxaban, rivaroxaban, or apixaban, may need to have their medications reversed to allow surgery to proceed urgently or emergently. Less urgent surgery, such as for a fracture, may allow time for the medication to clear the patient's system and return clotting function to normal. Bridging therapy with heparin (which has a short half-life and can be easily and inexpensively reversed) may be necessary to minimize the risk of stroke or other conditions as the main anticoagulant medication clears the patient's system. It is necessary to know the half-life of these medications in order to plan such therapy or to plan the urgent surgery after washout (Table 1–2).

5. Blood vessel damage—Arterial and venous damage take on greater significance as the size of the vessel increases and the arterial supply becomes more calcified with age and vascular disease. Patients generally understand this, but it must be emphasized where appropriate. Hip and knee replacement puts unusual strains on the femoral and popliteal vessels, from positioning, and may damage calcified arteries.

6. Deep venous thrombosis/pulmonary embolism—Virtually all lower extremity and spine procedures in orthopedics involve some risk of DVT, which should be explained to the patient. As many as 40% to 60% of patients who undergo a relatively high-risk procedure such as total hip arthroplasty develop DVT if not receiving thromboprophylaxis. The risk of PE is much less, however, and is in the range of 0.3% for fatal emboli. This rate of fatal PE is approximately a 10-fold increase over the rate of fatal PE in the US population in men older than 65 years. The risks associated with other procedures may be lower. In any case, the patient should be reassured that prevention procedures commensurate with risk will be undertaken.

7. Fracture—Many procedures in orthopedic surgery carry the risk of a bone fracture. Some procedures, such as uncemented hip replacement, present a higher risk for this complication, but virtually any orthopedic procedure could result in fracture of a bone. The patient must be informed of the risk in relation to the probability of the occurrence of such a problem.

8. Infection—The risk of infection in orthopedic surgery ranges from near zero in procedures such as arthroscopy to several percent in open fracture surgery. The problem of infection should be emphasized in proportion to risk. For example, if a diabetic patient is to undergo knee replacement, he or she should not only be assured that all steps will be taken to prevent infection (eg, administration of prophylactic antibiotics, use of ultrafiltration of air, or ultraviolet lights in the operating room) but should also be told of the various techniques that would be considered if infection occurred. These options include debridement, prosthesis removal, gastrocnemius flap, reinsertion, arthrodesis, and amputation. The common use of external fixation devices for fracture care is accompanied by the frequent problems associated with pin care. The patient and family should be informed about the problems caused by percutaneous devices to prevent the presumption that something has gone wrong. Skin problems are

Table 1–2. Anticoagulant elimination data and monitoring and reversal strategies.[a]

Drug Name	Average Half-Life	Average Washout Time Period	Relevant Coagulation Assay(s)	Reversal Strategies[b]
Warfarin (Coumadin)	40 hours	5 days	Prothrombin time, INR	Vitamin K FFP (15 mL/kg) PCC (Profilnine[c]) :25 units/kg IV; may repeat 1-2 times
Apixaban (Eliquis)	8-15 hours	1-2 days (2 days recommended prior to invasive procedures with moderate to high risk of major bleeding)	Prothrombin time, INR prolonged	FFP (plasma expansion, *not* for reversal) PCC (Profilnine[c]): 25 units/kg IV; may repeat 1-2 times
Dabigatran (Pradaxa)	12-17 hours; longer in renal dysfunction	1-2 days for normal renal function 2-5 days for renal dysfunction	Dilute thrombin time (>65 seconds: excess bleeding risk) aPTT (>2× ULN suggests excess bleeding risk)	Idarucizumab (Praxbind): 2.5 g IVPB every 15 minutes × 2 (5 g total dose); specific for dabigatran *only* FFP (plasma expansion, *not* for reversal) PCC (Profilnine[c]): 25 units/kg IV; may repeat 1-2 times Dialysis
Edoxaban (Savaysa)	10-14 hours; longer in renal dysfunction	1 day for normal renal function 2-5 days for renal dysfunction	Prothrombin time, INR prolonged	FFP (plasma expansion, *not* for reversal) PCC (Profilnine[c]): 25 units/kg IV, may repeat 1-2 times
Rivaroxaban (Xarelto)	5-9 hours; 11-13 hours in renal dysfunction	1 day for normal renal function 2-5 days for renal dysfunction	Prothrombin time, INR prolonged	FFP (plasma expansion, *not* for reversal) PCC (Profilnine[c]): 25 units/kg IV, may repeat 1-2 times
Heparin	1.5 hours	6-12 hours	aPTT, ACT	Protamine
Enoxaparin (Lovenox)	6-7 hours; longer in renal dysfunction	Dose dependent (prophylactic dose or treatment dose) 24 hours Longer in renal dysfunction and/or higher doses	Enoxaparin-specific anti-Xa assay	Protamine
Fondaparinux (Arixtra)	20-40 hours	Dose dependent (prophylactic dose or treatment dose) 48-72 hours Longer in renal dysfunction and/or higher doses	aPTT prolonged	Activated factor VIIa (NovoSeven): 90 μg/kg

[a]Dosing recommendations provided in this document are often based on in vitro laboratory studies. There are limited clinical trials evaluating the efficacy of these agents in reversing non-warfarin based anticoagulation. These recommendations do not replace clinical judgment and thorough patient examination.
[b]For life-threatening bleeding or urgent reversal for invasive procedures.
[c]Factor IX complex.
ACT, activated clotting time; aPTT, activated partial thromboplastin time; FFP, fresh frozen plasma; INR, international normalized ratio; IV, intravenous; IVPB, intravenous piggyback; PCC, prothrombin complex concentrate; ULN, upper limit of normal.
Data from Marty Breen PhD and Martin J. Breen, Pharm.D. and the Pharmacy Department of St. Jude Medical Center.

frequently associated with infection but may arise from other causes, such as adjacent scars compromising the blood supply to a surgical flap. Older patients and individuals who are smokers, have diabetes and/or are obese, or have wounds on the distal lower extremity are at increased risk. In such cases, the patient may be warned that delayed healing or necrosis of the skin edges may occur.

9. Loss of reduction—Although fracture care continues to improve, displacement of hardware or fracture fragments may necessitate a second procedure. The explanation of this risk should be individualized based on the type of fracture. Loss of reduction may contribute to delayed union or nonunion of fractures. These problems may occur despite optimal care by the orthopedic surgeon. Poor vascular supply or smoking can also lead to nonunion. The rate of nonunion is site dependent but is only a few percent.

10. Nerve damage—Certain procedures are associated with nerve damage, although the damage is usually minor. For example, medial parapatellar incisions on the knee cause some numbness from cutting the infrapatellar branch of the saphenous nerve. The patient should be informed in advance if some degree of minor nerve damage is anticipated in association with the particular surgical procedure being pursued, and should also be informed of the risks of unexpected nerve damage that accompany all surgical procedures.

C. Prognosis

The patient's prognosis is intimately related to the procedure. However, certain guidelines may be given. The expected time off work or time away from activities is important to the patient and depends on the patient's occupation, age, and available sick leave. A bank president with more control over her agenda will be able to return to work activities sooner than a day laborer. Driving is an important activity for many people, and limitations placed by a procedure can determine how much postoperative assistance a patient will need. Keep in mind that even though the left lower extremity may be the operated side, allowing the patient to operate a vehicle, sitting in the car for extended periods may predispose the patient to DVT.

The patient should be given reasonable expectations about range of motion, strength, possible disability, and when these should return to normal, if at all. Furthermore, walking or writing ability, ability to use a computer keyboard, and the time to expect to be able to do such activities may be appropriate for some patients. Again, these must be individualized for each patient and determined for each home situation.

D. Keeping the Patient and Family Informed

Immediately before elective surgery, the surgeon can help comfort the patient and family by meeting them in the preoperative area and appearing relaxed, well rested, and positive about the outcome of the surgery. Giving the family a good estimate of the surgery time is important, but they should also be reassured that delays do not necessarily indicate the occurrence of complications that are detrimental to the patient. If the family members wish to be notified about delays, they should be encouraged to leave instructions about where they can be contacted. When surgery is completed and the patient is no longer at risk of untoward accidents such as aspiration during extubation, a member of the surgical team should apprise the family of the outcome. At this time, it is appropriate to emphasize particular concerns to the family, such as the need to continue vigilance for infection in a diabetic patient who has undergone foot surgery.

Cocanour CS. Informed consent: it's more than a signature on a piece of paper. *Am J Surg.* 2017;214(6):993-997. [PMID: 28974311]

Falck-Ytter Y, Francis CW, Johanson NA, et al. Prevention of VTE in orthopedic surgery patients: antithrombotic therapy and prevention of thrombosis, 9th ed: American College of Chest Physicians Evidence-Based Clinical Practice Guidelines. *Chest.* 2012;141(suppl 2):e278S-e325S. [PMID: 22315265]

Giordano NJ, Jansson PS, Young MN, et al. Epidemiology, pathophysiology, stratification, and natural history of pulmonary embolism. *Tech Vasc Interv Radiol.* 2017;20(3):135-140. [PMID: 29029707]

Guohua L, Warner M, Lang BH, et al. Epidemiology of anesthesia-related mortality in the United States, 1999-2005. *Anesthesiology.* 2009;110(4):759-765. [PMID: 19322941]

Johnson BF, Manzo RA, Bergelin RO, Strandness DE Jr. Relationship between changes in the deep venous system and the development of the postthrombotic syndrome after an acute episode of lower limb deep vein thrombosis. A one- to six-year follow-up. *J Vasc Surg.* 1995;21:307-312. [PMID: 7853603]

Mini Nutritional Assessment. Nestlé Nutrition Institute. Accessed October 12, 2020. http://www.mna-elderly.com/forms/MNA_english.pdf.

Nosanchuk JS. Quantitative microbiologic study of blood salvaged by intraoperative membrane filtration. *Arch Pathol Lab Med.* 2001;125:1204-1206. [PMID: 11520273]

Rabinovich A, Kahn SR. The postthrombotic syndrome: current evidence and future challenges. *J Thromb Haemost.* 2017;15(2):230-241. [PMID: 27860129]

Schneider D, Lilienfeld DE. The epidemiology of pulmonary embolism: racial contrasts in incidence and in-hospital case fatality. *J Natl Med Assoc.* 2006;98:1967-1972. [PMID: 17225843]

Sweetland S, Green J, Liu B, et al. Duration of the magnitude of the postoperative risk of venous thromboembolism in middle aged women: prospective cohort study. *BMJ.* 2009;339:b4583. [PMID: 19959589]

Ueda P, Svanström H, Melbye M, et al. Sodium glucose cotransporter 2 inhibitors and risk of serious adverse events: nationwide register based cohort study. *BMJ.* 2018;363:k4365. [PMID:30429124]

Yuan Z, DeFalco FJ, Ryan PB, et al. Risk of lower extremity amputations in people with type 2 diabetes mellitus treated with sodium-glucose co-transporter-2 inhibitors in the USA: a retrospective cohort study. *Diabetes Obes Metab.* 2018;20(3):582-589. [PMID: 28898514]

SURGICAL MANAGEMENT

Preoperative Care

A. The Team Approach

Inclusion of nurses, residents, anesthesiologists, and other members of the surgical team in the planning process can improve the efficiency and therefore affect the outcome of a surgical procedure. Good estimates of the length of the operative procedure and of the patient's anticipated blood loss and muscle relaxation requirements minimize the risks from anesthesia and surgery. Reviewing the site of the operation and assessing the need for any special supplies and equipment, such as prostheses, lasers, or fracture tables, also contribute to efficiency and optimal results. Special care must be exercised by all members of the operative team to prevent "wrong side" surgery. It is now a standard of The Joint Commission to have the surgical team "mark" the surgical site.

B. Preparing and Positioning the Patient

Once the patient is in the operating room, every effort should be made to make him or her comfortable. A calm, efficient, and professional demeanor by everyone involved is necessary both before and after anesthesia is induced. If the anesthesiologist indicates that placement of antithromboembolic hose, intermittent pneumatic compression stockings, or tourniquets will improve efficiency, these can be put in place prior to induction. Placement of arterial lines, central lines, and Foley catheters should be done after the patient is anesthetized, if possible. Location of the operating table must be adjusted to ensure good lighting, optimize the efficiency of the surgeon and staff, and allow for maintenance of surgical sterile techniques.

Positioning of the patient is the responsibility of both the surgeon and the anesthesiologist to facilitate the operation and to ensure the patient's safety. A perfectly executed operation can be marred by a nerve palsy that results from the failure to pad a remote area appropriately. If the patient is placed in the lateral decubitus position, the peroneal nerve at the knee and the brachial plexus of the downside shoulder girdle must be protected. During shoulder surgery, the surgeon must take care to avoid stretching the patient's brachial plexus or cervical nerve roots while attempting to maximize the operative field. Similarly, the patient's shoulder should not be abducted past 90 degrees, and joints with contractures should not be forced into unusual positions. These precautions are particularly necessary in treating rheumatoid patients or older osteoporotic patients. Injury to the extremities and loss of lines can be avoided by careful planning and synchronization when positioning patients into the lateral decubitus position or prone position.

C. Use of Antibiotics

Except in cases in which concern about infection requires unambiguous cultures to be obtained, prophylactic antibiotics have been mandated to be started within 1 hour prior to skin incision by The Joint Commission. A first- or second-generation cephalosporin antibiotic is considered appropriate for orthopedic procedures. The Joint Commission has also mandated that prophylactic antibiotics be stopped within 24 hours of orthopedic surgery.

There is a heightened interest in preventing surgical site infections since Medicare has mandated that the treatment of these infections in total joints is the responsibility of the hospital. Hospitals initially undertook a "screen and treat" protocol where the nares of patients were cultured and subsequently treated, if positive for methicillin-resistant *Staphylococcus aureus*, and patients were advised to shower from the neck down with chlorhexidine gluconate. It has been found to be cost-effective to simply treat all patients with the decolonization protocol, which also decreases the infection rate compared to the "screen and treat" protocol. It is likely that the next step in infection control will be decolonizing operating room staff.

D. Use of a Tourniquet

A tourniquet can be helpful in some procedures and is practically mandatory for others. The decision to use a tourniquet entails a risk/benefit analysis, balancing blood loss and the visualization of the tissues against the potential risks. There has been a shift away from tourniquet use for some procedures. The tourniquet stops the flow of blood to and from an extremity. To achieve this, the pneumatic tourniquet is inflated to a pressure that must be significantly higher than the arterial pressure because the pressure is dissipated in the soft tissue underneath the tourniquet.

1. Tourniquet size and placement—The tourniquet should be wide enough for the extremity while still permitting adequate exposure of the extremity. Particularly in cases involving surgery on muscles that cross the elbow or knee, the tourniquet should be placed as proximal as possible to ensure the muscles have adequate stretch to permit full joint motion. When a tourniquet is used on a large extremity with a great deal of adipose tissue, care must be taken to ensure that the tourniquet does not slip distally, which could result in wrinkles in the tourniquet and localized pressure on the skin.

2. Tourniquet time and pressure—The effects of tourniquets on tissues are a combination of time and pressure on individual structures. Neural and muscle tissue are most sensitive, with deleterious effects arising from direct pressure to structures and from distal ischemia.

Several considerations are involved in the selection of the level of tourniquet pressure. First, the level must be low enough to avoid pressure damage to sensitive neural structures but high enough so the pressure around the arterial supply to the extremity is greater than systolic pressure. Second, if the patient's blood pressure is labile, a margin of safety is usually necessary. The 2009 Association of Perioperative Registered Nurses (AORN) recommendation is to use a graduated increment in pressure above the measured occlusion pressure. Thus, the incremental increases are 40, 60, and 80 mm Hg for occlusion pressures of <130, 131 to 190, and >190 mm Hg, respectively. The measured occlusion pressure is defined as the pressure at which arterial flow to an extremity is stopped. If the tourniquet is on an extremity with a great deal of adipose tissue, higher pressures may be necessary to achieve adequate pressure at the artery to stop blood flow. Tourniquets should be calibrated and can be tested with an independent pressure measurement device or alternatively calibrated by palpation of the pulse and gradual elevation of pressure until the pulse disappears. Complications will arise if tourniquets are used at high pressure for too long. The effects can sometimes be mitigated by using wider cuffs and curved cuffs, which allow for higher and more uniform pressure below the tourniquet. A rule of thumb is that tourniquet pressures should not be elevated for longer than 2 hours, and less time is preferable. In a canine study of the muscle tissue distal to the tourniquet, investigators found that 90-minute tourniquet times with 5 minutes between reinflation minimized the ischemic damage. Concern has been raised regarding the increase of intracranial pressure (as determined by measuring the optic nerve sheath diameter [ONSD]) caused by tourniquet use. Tourniquet times >67 minutes have been shown to increase ONSD to >5 mm after letting down the tourniquet. These findings point to the need for efficiency in performing surgical procedures under tourniquet. After tourniquet release, reflex hyperemia and edema are frequently encountered, making closure more difficult. Exsanguination with an Esmarch bandage prior to tourniquet inflation facilitates emptying of large veins of the thigh and arm, although it is not recommended to use an Esmarch in trauma cases. Careful exsanguination may help prevent DVT, especially when reinflation of the tourniquet is planned.

Barwell J, Anderson G, Hassan A, Rawlings I. The effects of early tourniquet release during total knee arthroplasty: a prospective randomized double-blind study. *J Bone Joint Surg Br.* 1997;79:265-268. [PMID: 9119854]

Besir A, Tugcugil E. Does Tourniquet time or pressure contribute to intracranial pressure increase following tourniquet application? *Med Princ Pract.* 2019;28(1):16-22. [PMID: 30396181]

Classen DC, Evans RS, Pestotnik SL, et al. The timing of prophylactic administration of antibiotics and the risk of surgical wound infection. *N Engl J Med.* 1992;326:281-286. [PMID: 1728731]

Fernandez AH, Monge V, Garcinuno MA. Surgical antibiotic prophylaxis: effect in postoperative infections. *Eur J Epidemiol.* 2001;17:369-374. [PMID: 11767963]

Hargens AR, McClure AG, Skyhar MJ, et al. Local compression patterns beneath pneumatic tourniquets applied to arms and thighs of human cadavers. *J Orthop Res.* 1987;5:247-252. [PMID: 3572594]

Noordin S, McEwen JA, Kragh JF Jr, et al. Current concepts review: surgical tourniquets in orthopaedics. *J Bone Joint Surg Am.* 2009;91A:2958. [PMID: 19952261]

Pedowitz RA, Gershuni DH, Botte MJ, et al. The use of lower tourniquet inflation pressures in extremity surgery facilitated by curved and wide tourniquets and an integrated cuff inflation system. *Clin Orthop Relat Res.* 1993;287:237-244. [PMID: 8448950]

Stambough JB, Nam D, Warren DK, et al. Decreased hospital costs and surgical site infection incidence with a universal decolonization protocol in primary total joint arthroplasty. *J Arthroplasty.* 2017;32(3):728-734. [PMID: 27823845]

Zhou K, Ling T, Wang H, et al. Influence of tourniquet use in primary total knee arthroplasty with drainage: a prospective randomised controlled trial. *J Orthop Surg Res.* 2017;12(1):172. [PMID: 29137681]

Operative Care

The surgical team should make every effort to work efficiently during the period between the administration of anesthesia and the conclusion of the final steps of preoperative preparation, which may take from 10 to 30 minutes or longer. It is in the best interests of the patient to minimize the time between onset of anesthesia and the beginning of surgery.

A. Incision Sites and Approaches

Although the surgical wound "heals side-to-side, not end-to-end," the incorrect placement or the excessive length of a surgical incision for a given procedure only serves to increase surgical trauma to the patient, slow the healing process, and lengthen the rehabilitation period. If there is any doubt about the surgical incision site, roentgenographic examination should be considered. Use of an image intensifier should be considered in obese patients or in patients with previous surgery and retained hardware.

The incision should be made perpendicular to the skin, generally longitudinally, and with a sharp knife. In tumor biopsies, longitudinal incisions are always made. The approach by the surgeon through the subcutaneous fatty layer is variable and depends on the location on the body. In most areas, sharp dissection with a knife through the subcutaneous tissue to the fascial layer is indicated. In the upper extremity and in areas where cutaneous nerves can be troublesome if injured, blunt dissection is used because cutaneous nerves travel in the fatty tissue. Many surgeons prefer blunt dissection with scissors used to spread tissue perpendicular to the wound. Hemostasis is obtained layer by layer. Subcutaneous fat usually is not dissected from the skin because this might devascularize it.

Surgeons must be extremely careful with the skin, making sure to avoid crushing it when forceps are used. The skin should never be clamped, nor should it be excessively stretched. A larger incision is much better for the skin than extreme tension. Care of the soft tissues includes keeping them moist, avoiding excessive retraction, and being especially careful of neurovascular bundles. Nerves suffer damage from both traction and compression. Nerve palsies and paresthesias can spoil an otherwise well-performed operation in the eyes of both the surgeon and the patient. Care of the cartilage includes keeping it moist because drying has a deleterious effect.

Surgical approaches that go through internerve planes, such as between the deltoid and the pectoralis major, should be used to avoid denervation of muscles. The splitting of muscles in the surgical approach should also be avoided because splitting is generally more traumatic and more likely to denervate the muscle. This rule does not always apply in tumor surgery because it is important to keep tumor cells in a single compartment.

B. Orthopedic Instruments and Drains

It is mandatory that tools be sharp at all times because the sharpness enables the surgeon to avoid the excessive pressure that creates problems by plunging into the depths of the wound. When an osteotome or elevator is needed, the concurrent use of a hammer is preferred because achieving exact control is possible by the strength and number of hammer taps, whereas control is difficult to achieve by pushing on an osteotome. With drill points and power saws, the sharpness of the instruments should be maintained to reduce necrosis secondary to heating and to facilitate the operation. Unless using a drill guide, the surgeon should start drilling bone in a perpendicular direction even though the final direction may be at some angle to the direction of the bone. This prevents slipping off the desired bone entry point. Holes in long bones are stress concentration sites. Care should be taken to minimize the likelihood and degree of stress concentration by rounding holes and using drill holes to terminate saw cuts. When holes were made in bone, especially in the lower extremity, the patient should be advised against torsional loading.

Obtaining hemostasis in bone can be troublesome, and the use of microcrystalline collagen or similar material is preferred to bone wax because of the foreign body response. Postoperative bleeding is common from bony surfaces. Despite the past use of drains by surgeons, evidence is accumulating that at least for some operations, such as total hip or total knee replacement, closed wound suction drainage does not change outcomes and is associated with a higher infection rate. If drains are used, they should be secured to prevent accidental removal and should be large enough to prevent clogging by clot formation. Drains are generally removed within 48 hours of surgery unless they are used to eliminate dead space.

C. Closure and Dressing

Wound closure should be done quickly and efficiently to minimize total operative and anesthesia time. It should also be accomplished carefully to avoid damage to the skin. When a previous scar is entered, it is sometimes worthwhile to remove scar tissue from the edge of the skin, as well as from the subcutaneous tissue, to provide a more vascular area for healing. Meticulous subcutaneous wound closure is necessary to avoid tension on the skin in many areas on the extremities. Four-throw square knots are important for knot security, especially when plans call for use of continuous passive motion machines or early motion, which may apply repetitive stress to the wound before it heals. Barbed sutures, while eliminating knots, may not be as strong in maintaining tissue apposition. Tissue adhesives are an advent in wound closure. One study found sutures were significantly better than adhesives for minimizing dehiscence of incisions, although the adhesives generally resulted in a more cosmetic wound.

Dressings should be padded with cotton or gauze to discourage the formation of hematomas. Tape should be avoided when possible because it sometimes causes allergic reactions; also, the combination of wound swelling and shear from the tape can lead to blistering and other problems.

Infected wounds may benefit from negative-pressure wound therapy (NPWT) as an alternative to dressing changes, since wound closure is obviated in most cases. Studies on the efficacy of NPWT are mixed, but the less frequent dressing changes with NPWT are more convenient and less painful overall, and in many cases, the wounds heal more quickly.

Anis HK, Sodhi N, Klika AK, et al. Is operative time a predictor for post-operative infection in primary total knee arthroplasty? *J Arthroplasty.* 2019;34(7S):S331-S336. [PMID: 30545655]

Hazarika S, Bhattacharya R, Bhavikatti M, Dawson M. A comparison of post-op haemoglobin levels and allogeneic blood transfusion rates following total knee arthroplasty without drainage or with reinfusion drains. *Acta Orthop Belg.* 2010;76:74-78. [PMID: 20306968]

Liu Z, Dumville JC, Hinchliffe RJ, et al. Negative pressure wound therapy for treating foot wounds in people with diabetes mellitus. *Cochrane Database Syst Rev.* 2018;10:CD010318. [PMID: 30328611]

Lloris-Carsí JM, Ballester-Álvaro J, Barrios C, et al. Randomized clinical trial of a new cyanoacrylate flexible tissue adhesive (Adhflex) for repairing surgical wounds. *Wound Repair Regen.* 2016;24(3):568-580. [PMID: 26899011]

Minnema B, Vearncombe M, Augustin A, et al. Risk factors for surgical site infections following primary total knee arthroplasty. *Infect Control Hosp Epidemiol.* 2004;25:477-480. [PMID: 15242195]

Monsen C, Acosta S, Mani K, Wann-Hansson C. A randomized study of NPWT closure versus alginate dressings in peri-vascular groin infections: quality of life, pain and cost. *J Wound Care.* 2015;24(6):252-258. [PMID: 2607537]

Ovadia D, Drexler M, Kramer M, et al. Closed wound sub-fascial suction drainage in posterior fusion surgery for adolescent idiopathic scoliosis: a prospective randomize control study. *Spine (Phila Pa 1976).* 2019;44(6):377-383. [PMID: 30299415]

Torcchia AM, Aho HN, Sobol G. A re-exploration of the use of barbed sutures in flexor tendon repairs. *Orthopedics.* 2009;32:10. [PMID: 19824603]

POSTOPERATIVE CARE

Inpatient Care

Postoperative care begins in the postanesthesia room and is the same for both inpatients and outpatients. It is imperative that the orthopedic surgeon takes an active and early role in the treatment of the postoperative patient, including pain management, blood management, and DVT prophylaxis. As soon as practicable, neurologic and vascular evaluation of the operated area should be made. Sensory and motor exam of the pertinent upper or lower extremity nerves should be documented as soon as practical. Early vascular surgery consultation is indicated if pulses are absent or diminished. The wound site should be checked for excessive drainage, and, when appropriate, compartment syndrome should be considered. The general medical condition of the patient, although primarily the concern of the anesthesiologist, should be evaluated to be sure the anesthesiologist is aware of special concerns regarding the individual patient.

During the subsequent postoperative period, orthopedic aspects of care are relatively routine for most procedures. The main responsibility of the orthopedic surgeon is the evaluation of the vascular and neural status of the extremities affected by the surgery, as well as pain control and vigilance for disorders such as DVT or PE. The frequency of postsurgical examinations depends on the clinical setting. Hourly examinations may be necessary in the face of a potential compartment syndrome. Epidural morphine analgesia may significantly mute or alter the pain picture in a compartment syndrome, making accurate clinical evaluation difficult, if not impossible, in the immediate postoperative period.

A. Pain Management

Pain management is a major issue in the United States. There previously was a concern that patients were undermedicated and not achieving adequate pain control. The public embraced this concept, resulting in litigation and disciplinary action by state medical boards for undermedication. Physicians traditionally were seen as being reluctant to prescribe narcotic medication as a result of concerns that they would be disciplined by state medical boards. This concept has led to a major initiative by The Joint Commission to address pain control as a patient "right." The Joint Commission mandates that pain control be a factor in the total evaluation of the patient and pain evaluation be performed as the fifth vital sign. The scale used is the numeric scale from 0 to 10, similar to the visual analog scale, with 0 being no pain and 10 being unbearable pain. Patients typically have no real standards upon which to assign their pain scores, resulting in frequent use of a 10 score, or higher. This scale can be explained to the patient in more understandable terms as follows: 1 to 3 is nuisance pain, 4 to 6 is distracting pain, 7 to 9 is disabling pain, and 10 is worst possible pain. This more functional scale is easier to use by the patient. Acceptable pain levels are defined as ≤4.

The relaxation of the prescription of narcotic medication has led to the opioid crisis and excessive prescription of opioid medications. Drug overdose deaths from prescription narcotics have skyrocketed. This has resulted in the pendulum swinging back in the opposite direction, with legislation to monitor, control, and ultimately, minimize prescription of opioids. Fortunately for surgical patients, other means of controlling pain have become common.

Pain is a very subjective sensation that is an emotional response to the process of nociception: the sum of four separate components beginning with tissue damage, which results in the first component, transduction to a nerve impulse. The next component is transmission to the spinal cord, where the third component occurs: modulation. This modulated signal is then perceived in the cerebral cortex (perception). Pain perception depends on culture, ethnicity, and gender. It is nonlinear, in that a stimulus two times higher does not necessarily result in twice the pain. Pain perception is also based on patient expectations. Studies show that preoperative patient education can reduce patients' pain after major (eg, total knee arthroplasty) orthopedic surgery.

Traditional postoperative pain management included the administration of intravenous (IV) or intramuscular (IM) narcotic analgesics until oral narcotics were able to control the pain. Patient-controlled analgesia became a mainstay because the patient did not have to wait for the nurse and could control his or her medication dosing. In this system, morphine is usually used as the analgesic and is typically administered IV at a rate of 1 mg/h with a patient-controlled additional dose of 1 mg, which can be administered as often as every 10 minutes. Doses can be increased or decreased to tailor the dose to the patient. Dosing at this level can result in depressed respiration in some patients. However, more cautious dosing can result in insufficient pain relief that can stress the heart, leading to myocardial ischemia in some patients. Other problems can result from traditional pain management with narcotics. Patient rehabilitation can be delayed; nausea, vomiting, constipation, hallucinations, disorientation, and urinary retention can result in lengthened hospital stay and patient dissatisfaction.

Alternative postoperative analgesic methods have been used. These include epidural and intrathecal administration of local anesthetics and analgesics on a continuous and one-shot basis. These methods have the potential of providing significant pain relief but must be balanced against the alternatives available and the drawbacks that each presents. The one-shot method of adding morphine to the spinal or epidural anesthetic provides pain relief for a limited time, usually on the order of 12 to 24 hours, although a longer-acting form of morphine (DepoDur) has come on the market for single-injection epidural use, providing pain relief for up to 48 hours. It has the additional problem of limiting additional narcotic analgesia by other routes because overdosing may be possible. Long-term use of continuous epidural or intrathecal analgesia poses the problem of inhibiting rehabilitation. Nurses and physical therapists tend not to mobilize patients with catheters into the spinal canal, and in some hospitals, these patients are mandated to go to the intensive care unit. Nerve blocks and injections into joint cavities are limited by the length of action of the local anesthetic agent. Injection of long-acting agents such as bupivacaine (0.25% or 0.5%) into the soft tissues of a wound diminishes postoperative pain, as do nerve blocks, which must address all nerves to an area to control postoperative pain. Longer-term effects can be achieved by using pumps that provide a continuous anesthetic flow about the nerve or into the joint or body cavity. Ropivacaine is reported to have vasoconstrictive properties and less cardiotoxicity than bupivacaine, although at a higher cost. Studies suggest damage to chondrocytes from exposure to local anesthetics such as lidocaine, bupivacaine, and ropivacaine, with possibly even a single injection. Thus, treatment of postoperative pain with infusions or infusion pumps should be reserved for total joint replacements or tissues remote from and that do not extend into a joint.

In the past, nonnarcotic pharmacologic treatment of acute postoperative pain was largely restricted to ketorolac, which can be administered by the IV or IM route in the patient who is restricted in oral intake. Although ketorolac is an effective analgesic, demonstrated by reduction in the need for morphine, it also increases the perioperative blood loss due to its largely COX-1 activity on platelets. Recently, diclofenac, which has a more balanced COX-1/COX-2 activity, was approved in an injectable formulation. After oral intake is permitted, other NSAIDs can be used for analgesics. The availability of COX-2–selective NSAIDs has opened up the possibility of using these drugs as major analgesics for postoperative pain control, without fear of bleeding problems. These drugs act to reduce the need for narcotics with improved pain relief and decreased narcotic side effects. COX-2–selective drugs that can be administered parenterally, such as parecoxib (prodrug for valdecoxib), are available in Europe, Australia, and China, but not in the United States.

The use of highly specific COX-2 inhibitors as analgesics came into question in the United States with the withdrawal of rofecoxib and valdecoxib from the market because of concern over increased cardiovascular events with long-term use. At this time, other less specific NSAIDs may be considered as alternatives (eg, celecoxib, diclofenac, meloxicam, etodolac) because their effect on platelet function is minimal.

Other analgesics and techniques do not get sufficient recognition for their role in pain control. Acetaminophen is thought to be a central prostaglandin synthase inhibitor and thereby achieves significant relief of pain. It can be tolerated in doses up to 3 g/day, and because it does not act in the same pathway as narcotics, its effect is additive to that of morphine or other narcotics and can reduce the requirement for narcotics. Another analgesic that should be used more often for analgesia is tramadol. This analgesic has very low abuse potential but provides significant analgesia, acting through inhibition of norepinephrine reuptake as well as a weak μ-agonist (similar to morphine) action. Again, this mechanism of action is additive to that of traditional opioids and acetaminophen in its analgesic effect. Glucocorticoids are naturally increased in periods of stress, such as surgery, and should be provided exogenously for patients with suppressed adrenal function. One study showed an increase in cortisol production of 17-fold after total knee arthroplasty, but no such increase after knee arthroscopy. Divided doses of approximately 200 mg of hydrocortisone (8 days of normal production) are typically prescribed for such patients. High doses (20 mg) of dexamethasone (equivalent to 400 mg of hydrocortisone) reduce the early postoperative pain in tonsillectomy patients. Although such doses may reduce postoperative nausea, swelling, and pain, as well as create a feeling of well-being, an increased susceptibility to infection may result from longer-term dosing. Short courses of relatively high doses of glucocorticoids may be beneficial in reducing postoperative pain. Other methods of pain control may be indirect, such as controlling swelling and pain through hemostasis and cold therapy. Hemostasis may be achieved through the use of bone wax on cancellous bone or through the use of fibrin glue. Vasoconstriction from cold therapy can reduce swelling and also have a direct effect on nociceptive transduction.

Periarticular injections of "cocktails" for postoperative analgesia after total joint surgery have demonstrated efficacy in reducing pain. These cocktails are usually composed of four components: a long-acting local anesthetic, such as bupivacaine; a long-acting narcotic, such as morphine; an anti-inflammatory, such as ketorolac; and a steroid, such as methylprednisolone. Various quantities of each component have been tried, but no specific mixture has demonstrated clear superiority. The mixture is injected into the periarticular tissues in a relatively dilute form to carefully infiltrate the entire capsule. Despite the short-acting nature of the component drugs, relatively long-lasting effects of the injections are seen.

A comprehensive approach to pain management can lead to beneficial effects. Multimodal analgesic regimens are suggested using several analgesics that address different points in the nociception process. Combinations of medications can include narcotics, acetaminophen, tramadol, COX-2 inhibitors, and local anesthetics administered through the use of pain pumps. Peripheral nerve blocks and subarachnoid morphine blocks can assist in control of pain in the early postoperative period. Injections of local anesthetics and steroids into the pericapsular tissues can also be helpful. Consideration should be given to administering medications in the preanesthesia room to preempt the pain of surgery. This can also assist in diminishing peripheral sensitization that occurs with tissue damage. In addition to pharmacologic interventions, patient education can reduce preoperative anxiety, reducing pain and increasing satisfaction.

Chu CR, Coyle CH, Chu CT, et al. In vivo effects of a single intra-articular injection of 0.5% bupivacaine on articular cartilage. *J Bone Joint Surg.* 2010;92A:599-608. [PMID: 20194318]

Cohen M, Zuk J, McKay N, et al. Intrathecal morphine versus extended-release epidural morphine for postoperative pain control in pediatric patients undergoing posterior spinal fusion. *Anesth Analg.* 2017;124(6):2030-2037. [PMID: 28448398]

Elmallah RK, Cherian JJ, Pierce TP, et al. New and common perioperative pain management techniques in total knee arthroplasty. *J Knee Surg.* 2016;29(2):169-178. [PMID: 25892004]

Gaffney CJ, Pelt CE, Gililland JM, Peters CL. Perioperative pain management in hip and knee arthroplasty. *Orthop Clin North Am.* 2017;48(4):407-419. [PMID: 28870302]

Grishko V, Xu M, Wilson G, Pearsall AW 4th. Apoptosis and mitochondrial dysfunction in human chondrocytes following exposure to lidocaine, bupivacaine, and ropivacaine. *J Bone Joint Surg.* 2010;92A:609-618. [PMID: 20194319]

Leopold SS, Casnellie MT, Warme WJ, et al. Endogenous cortisol production in response to knee arthroscopy and total knee arthroplasty. *J Bone Joint Surg Am.* 2003;85:2163-2167. [PMID: 14630847]

Schug SA, Parsons B, Li C, et al. The safety profile of parecoxib for the treatment of postoperative pain: a pooled analysis of 28 randomized, double-blind, placebo-controlled clinical trials and a review of over 10 years of postauthorization data. *J Pain Res.* 2017;10:2451-2459. [PMID: 29066931]

Sinatra RS, Torres J, Bustos AM. Pain management after major orthopedic surgery: current strategies and new concepts. *J Am Acad Orthop Surg.* 2002;10:117-129. [PMID: 11929206]

Wall PDH, Parsons NR, Parsons H, et al. A pragmatic randomised controlled trial comparing the efficacy of a femoral nerve block and periarticular infiltration for early pain relief following total knee arthroplasty. *Bone Joint J.* 2017;99-B(7):904-911. [PMID: 28663395]

B. Deep Venous Thrombosis/Pulmonary Embolus

DVT, a potentially life-threatening disorder, frequently accompanies orthopedic surgery. It is much more of a problem for total joint replacements, spine surgery, and lower extremities immobilized after surgery, but can occur without surgery in patients having arthroscopy or cast treatment for fractures or even Achilles tendon ruptures. This is one of the expected risks after surgery and cast treatment. It is such an important issue that since 2006, The Joint Commission has mandated that hospitalized patients be screened and treated to prevent DVT. Venous thromboembolic phenomenon can result in three problems: postphlebitic (or postthrombotic) syndrome, nonfatal PE, and fatal PE. It is necessary to put the risks of PE into appropriate perspective because, contrary to prevailing assumptions in the public and among orthopedic surgeons, PE can occur without surgery (Table 1–3). The risk of having a PE depends on a number of risk factors, including age, weight, genetic clotting disorders, previous DVT, the presence of varicose veins, immobility, smoking, joint replacement, the season of the year, estrogen therapy, and the location. There is an uncertain relationship between DVT and the probability of having a PE. Obviously, one cannot have a PE without having a clot, but determining which clots are likely to break off and become emboli and which ones will cause problems is still an unresolved issue. It is thought that thigh clots are more important than calf clots because of their size and the potential damage they can do. It is generally conceded, however, that DVT is a marker for PE, and that is the surrogate variable used to determine the effectiveness of treatment of PE. A nonfatal PE can cause cor pulmonale, but this is thought to be an unlikely circumstance, and it is speculated that nonfatal PE would result in a residual effect in the range of 0.1% to 0.01% of cases. DVT itself is thought to be a significant problem that results in incompetence of the valves in the deep veins of the calf and thigh. This results in persistent edema, which can progress to brawny edema and ulceration over time. However, many things are thought to cause these changes in addition to DVT. The rate of fatal PE increases with age, although age may simply be a marker for health and activity level. The rate of fatal PE in the general population older than 65 years is in the range of 0.03%, whereas approximate total joint replacement PE rates are typically approximately 0.3%. Thus, there is a 10-fold increase in risk of having a fatal PE with a total hip or knee replacement.

Table 1–3. Meta-analysis summary of rates of complications associated with total hip replacement with the anterior approach or the posterior approach with 90 days of follow-up.

Complication	Anterior (%)	Posterior (%)
Dislocation	2.5	2.0
Fracture	3.9	2.4
Venous thromboembolism	1.1	1.9
Infection	1.4	1.1
Hematoma	1.9	1.9
Reoperation	2.6	1.3

Reprinted with permission, from Miller LE, Gondusky JS, Bhattacharyya S, et al. Does surgical approach affect outcomes in total hip arthroplasty through 90 days of follow-up? A systematic review with meta-analysis. *J Arthroplasty.* 2018;33(4):1296-1302.

Drugs used for chemoprophylaxis of DVT in the United States are administered either orally or by injection. Oral medications include warfarin (the vitamin K inhibitor), factor Xa inhibitors (rivaroxaban, apixaban, and edoxaban), the direct thrombin inhibitor dabigatran, and platelet aggregation inhibitors (aspirin, naproxen, and other NSAIDs). The low-molecular-weight heparins (LMWHs; dalteparin, enoxaparin, and similar drug fondaparinux) are administered parenterally. Each approach has its advantages and disadvantages. The LMWHs do not affect the prothrombin time or the partial thromboplastin time but do affect factor IIa and Xa levels. These do not have to be monitored because the medications are given in standard doses. Sodium warfarin has a slow onset of action, sometimes taking several days to reach therapeutic levels, but its oral route of administration is convenient. However, monitoring of the prothrombin time is necessary to ensure appropriate therapeutic levels. The factor Xa and thrombin inhibitors are given orally in standard doses and require no monitoring. All of the anticoagulants are associated with bleeding problems. Aspirin has been accepted by the American College of Chest Physicians as an acceptable means of venous thromboembolism prophylaxis, in agreement with the American Academy of Orthopedic Surgeons. Proponents of aspirin recommend it because of its low cost and relative safety in terms of bleeding. Mechanical means of preventing DVT include compression hose and intermittent pneumatic compression. These have recently been demonstrated to be as efficacious as chemoprophylaxis when used 18 hours per day.

Generally, for orthopedic indications after high-risk surgery, any of the medications listed earlier are acceptable starting 12 to 24 hours after surgery. Elastic stockings and intermittent pneumatic compression are useful as supplemental protection against DVT. The recommended period is 10 to 14 days, although some physicians in the American College of Chest Physicians suggest extending prophylaxis up to 35 days after major orthopedic surgery. The American College of Chest Physicians recommends against the use of vena cava filters for primary prophylaxis even in in high-risk situations. Table 1–4 lists the current recommendations.

Newer orthopedic literature suggests that aspirin is the drug of choice. However, the choice of prophylactic agent is made by the doctor and the patient and is influenced by their interpretation of the risk of thromboembolism and bleeding problems.

Both warfarin and heparin, either LMWH or regular heparin, have problems that can cause catastrophic side effects in rare cases. Warfarin can cause skin necrosis and venous limb gangrene syndromes unrelated to the operative site. Heparin can induce thrombocytopenia. This is apparently an immunoglobulin G (IgG) antibody formation that occurs 5 to 10 days after starting heparin (including LMWH) and can result in a hypercoagulable state that can result in serious problems of coagulation in unintended areas.

Table 1–4. Recommendations for management of DVT prophylaxis for high-risk orthopedic patients.

Procedure	Grade[a]	Recommendation
THA/TKA	1B	LMWH, fondaparinux, apixaban, dabigatran, rivaroxaban, LDUH, VKA, ASA started 12 or more hours after surgery Or
	1C	Optimal use of intermittent pneumatic compression (18 hours of daily compliance)
Hip fractures	1B	LMWH, fondaparinux, LDUH, VKA, ASA
	1C	IPC
Major trauma, acute SCI	2C	LDUH, LMWH (when safe to use), IPC

ASA, acetylsalicylic acid; DVT, deep vein thrombosis; IPC, intermittent pneumatic compression; LDUH, low-dose unfractionated heparin; LMWH, low-molecular-weight heparin; SCI, spinal cord injury; THA, total hip arthroplasty; TKA, total knee arthroplasty; VKA, vitamin K antagonist.

[a]Grade 1A, clear risk/benefit ratio based on randomized trials without important limitations; grade 1B, same as 1A but with inconsistent results or methodologic flaws; grade 2C, weak recommendation, low-quality or very-low-quality evidence.

Data from Falck-Ytter Y, Francis CW, Johanson NA, et al. Prevention of VTE in orthopedic patients. Antithrombotic Therapy and Prevention of Thrombosis, 9th Edition ACCP Evidence-Based Clinical Practice Guidelines *Chest.* 2012;2(suppl):e278S-e325S; Gould MK, Garcia DA, Wren SM, et al. Prevention of VTE in nonorthopedic surgical patients: Antithrombotic Therapy and Prevention of Thrombosis, 9th ed: American College of Chest Physicians Evidence-Based Clinical Practice Guidelines. *Chest.* 2012;141(2 suppl):e227S-e277S.

1. Diagnosis—DVT is diagnosed with ultrasound in the postsurgical patient with calf swelling or with Homan's sign in the appropriate clinical setting. Several risk factors can be elicited from the history to increase the suspicion of DVT. These include immobilization, lower extremity or pelvic surgery (in the previous 4 weeks), previous history of DVT, and history of cancer. Ultrasound is a reliable, noninvasive screen for DVT of the lower extremity veins and has replaced the venogram as the gold standard for diagnosing DVT. Testing for PE has also evolved. In nonsurgical patients, D-dimer can be helpful in the diagnosis of PE, and the risk of PE continues for weeks after surgery, so there may be a role for it in the late postoperative period. Previously, ventilation/perfusion scans were the standard method, followed by pulmonary angiography, if the probability was intermediate. Now CTA is quite reliable and is the preferred test for diagnosis of PE. Furthermore, evidence from a preliminary study suggests that fibrin monomer discriminates between total hip arthroplasty patients with PE and those without PE. The D-dimer was also higher in PE patients but not significantly until 7 days postoperatively.

Colwell CW, Froimson MI, Mont MA, et al. Thrombosis prevention after total hip arthroplasty: a prospective, randomized trial comparing a mobile compression device with low-molecular-weight heparin. *J Bone Joint Surg Am.* 2010;92A:527-535. [PMID: 20194309]

Falck-Ytter Y, Francis CW, Johanson NA, et al. Prevention of VTE in orthopedic surgery patients: antithrombotic therapy and prevention of thrombosis, 9th ed: American College of Chest Physicians Evidence-Based Clinical Practice Guidelines. *Chest.* 2012;141(suppl 2):e278S-e325S. [PMID: 22315265]

Johnson BF, Manzo RA, Bergelin RO, Strandness DE Jr. Relationship between changes in the deep venous system and the development of post thrombotic syndrome after an acute episode of lower limb deep vein thrombosis: a one- to six-year follow-up. *J Vasc Surg.* 1995;21:307-312. [PMID: 7853603]

Mont MJ, Eurich DT, Russell DB, et al. Post-thrombotic syndrome after total hip arthroplasty is uncommon. *Acta Orthop.* 2008;79:794-799. [PMID: 19085497]

Nazarian RM, Van Cott EM, Zembowicz A, Duncan LM. Warfarin-induced skin necrosis. *J Am Acad Dermatol.* 2009;61: 325-332. [PMID: 19615543]

Rafee A, Herlikar D, Gilbert R, et al. D-dimer in the diagnosis of deep vein thrombosis following total hip and knee replacement: a prospective study. *Ann R Coll Surg Engl.* 2008;90:123-126. [PMID: 18325211]

Shah SS, Satin AM, Mullen JR, et al. Impact of recent guideline changes on aspirin prescribing after knee arthroplasty. *J Orthop Surg Res.* 2016;11(1):123. [PMID: 27765053]

Shiraev TP, Omari A, Rushworth RL. Trends in pulmonary embolism morbidity and mortality in Australia. *Thromb Res.* 2013;132(1):19-25. [PMID: 23725850]

Stevenson M, Scope A, Holmes M, et al. Rivaroxaban for the prevention of venous thromboembolism: a single technology appraisal. *Health Technol Assess.* 2009;13(suppl 3):43. [PMID: 19846028]

Turpie AG, Gallus AS, Hoek JA. A synthetic pentasaccharide for the prevention of deep-vein thrombosis after total hip replacement. *N Engl J Med.* 2001;344:619-625. [PMID: 11228275]

Warkentin TE. Heparin-induced thrombocytopenia. *Curr Opin Crit Care.* 2015;21(6):576-585. [PMID: 26539932]

Outpatient Care

The importance of early mobilization and discharge from hospital for orthopedic surgery patients cannot be overemphasized. There is growing realization that orthopedic surgery patients are not sick, but are basically coming to the hospital for surgery to get their "transmission" or "brakes" fixed (eg, hip replacement, meniscectomy). One study noted that during acute hospitalization, older adults are in bed 83% of the time and in a chair 12% of the time. The longer immobility is extended, the more likely it is that hospital-associated deconditioning (HAD) will occur. HAD is characterized by declines in muscle mass and strength and decreases in cognitive function and activity of daily living performance. Restoring orthopedic patients as close as possible to their presurgery activity level is of utmost importance in minimizing HAD. Early discharge from the hospital puts the patients in an environment that is more conducive to independence and increased activity.

Economic realities today also mandate earlier discharge from the hospital after some procedures and after outpatient surgery for procedures previously done on an inpatient basis. This trend suggests that patients must take more responsibility for their care, and surgeons must provide outpatient access for patients previously treated as inpatients. The indications for discharge have broadened just as the reasons for admission have narrowed. The reasons for keeping a postoperative patient in the acute-care setting are few. The main indications for hospitalization are pain control requiring parenteral narcotics, presence of hemodynamic instability, or a need for frequent physician observation (eg, drains, infection). Even extended administration of IV antibiotic therapy is not an adequate reason for an acute-care stay. Thus, timing of follow-up visits is important to ensure that the patient is not only not unnecessarily inconvenienced but also does not suffer delayed recognition of a complication. In most cases, the first visit should be for wound check or suture removal (10-14 days). Again, economic realities mandate a 90-day follow-up as part of the global surgical fee. Follow-up for a total hip replacement patient might be at 2 weeks, 6 weeks, and 12 weeks after surgery. Longer or shorter intervals may be necessary, depending on how the patient is progressing and how much external support the patient is receiving (physical therapy, home nurse visits, home caregivers, and home environment). Joint replacement patients should be followed up at least yearly on a permanent basis after the first 5 or so years. The American Academy of Orthopedic Surgeons recommends prescription of prophylactic antibiotics for joint replacement patients for procedures such as dental cleaning in which bacteremia may occur as a consensus decision between the surgeon and patient based on limited evidence for and against oral antibiotic prophylaxis.

Long-term follow-up for patients with plates, screws, pins, rods, or other fracture devices is not typically necessary after the healing of the fracture and rehabilitation of the affected muscles and joints. Antibiotic prophylaxis is not necessary for these patients. In cases of painful hardware, removal may be indicated after healing. Removal of hardware in older (>75 years) patients is generally not indicated. In younger (<50 years), active patients, hardware removal may be justified to reduce the stress concentration or stress shielding effects of the metal devices to prevent fracture prophylactically. An adequate period (12 weeks or more, depending on activity) of stress protection, especially in torsion, is indicated to reduce the risk of fracture through defects incurred by the bone during removal of hardware. For a detailed discussion of rehabilitation, see Chapter 13, "Rehabilitation."

Brown CJ, Redden DT, Flood KL, Allman RM. The underrecognized epidemic of low mobility during hospitalization of older adults. *J Am Geriatr Soc.* 2009;57:1660-1665. [PMID: 19682121]

Falvey JR, Mangione KK, Stevens-Lapsley JE. Rethinking hospital-associated deconditioning: proposed paradigm shift. *Phys Ther.* 2015;95:1307-1315. [PMID: 25908526]

Blood Loss and Replacement

A. Criteria for Blood Transfusion

Because blood replacement is a complicated issue, it is fortunate that several issues have been clarified regarding the management of blood replacement for orthopedic procedures. One study reported that the historical blood losses for total hip replacement, total knee replacement, and unicompartmental replacement were 1505, 1322, and 611 mL, respectively, on postoperative day 2. Blood loss for orthopedic procedures will vary with the surgeon, surgical approach, use of a tourniquet, use of a drain, and positioning a limb after surgery. Since the data for that study were generated, the use of tranexamic acid, better surgical techniques (ie, mini-incisions for joint replacement), and a lower "trigger" for transfusing blood have come on the scene.

The American Association of Blood Banks has evaluated the available published data on when to transfuse and published the following clinical guidelines: "transfusion is not indicated until the hemoglobin level is 7 g/dL for hospitalized adult patients who are hemodynamically stable, including critically ill patients." Generally, the decision to transfuse at or slightly above 7 g/dL is based on the physician's clinical assessment as to whether further blood loss is anticipated and/or the patient is symptomatic (ie, postural hypotension, dizziness, or lightheadedness). Numerous other factors, including age, medical condition, cardiac status, estimated blood loss, projected blood loss, availability of blood (autologous, designated donor, or bank), and the patient's perception of risk, are important. Patient involvement in the decision on how to manage blood loss is certainly a good idea. In addition, transfusion should only be done one unit at a time. Blood volume is approximately 7% to 8% of body weight, or approximately 5 L in a 70-kg individual. Normal individuals can be resuscitated from acute blood losses of up to 25% with crystalloid/colloid. Greater blood losses can be tolerated if the euvolemic state is maintained, but transfusion should be considered. The status of the clotting system must be monitored in the acute blood loss phase to prevent accelerated blood loss. Blood loss in the postoperative subacute phase can be managed with volume replacement and evaluation of symptomatology to determine the need for transfusion of red cell mass. Patients at risk of stroke or MI or those with decreased cardiac output may need transfusion at higher Hgb levels. Younger (>50 years), healthier patients may tolerate lower Hgb levels unless they have postural hypotension, tachycardia, dizziness, or fainting.

B. Strategies for Minimizing the Risks Associated With Blood Transfusion

Blood loss is an inevitable part of surgery. With the realization that the banked blood supply is at low risk, but still at risk, of containing infectious agents, strategies to minimize the risk of transmission have been developed.

An obvious method of accomplishing this goal is to reduce blood loss. Anesthetic techniques to reduce mean arterial blood pressure can reduce blood loss by reducing the time of surgery as well as the actual blood loss. The patient must be counseled to avoid antiplatelet drugs in the period prior to surgery. These medications include baby aspirin and clopidogrel but also all of the ubiquitous NSAIDs that are in over-the-counter analgesics, cough and cold remedies, and arthritis medications. In the operative period, topical agents such as bone wax, Gelfoam and similar collagen products, thrombin, tranexamic acid and aminocaproic acid (antifibrinolytics), and fibrin glue should be considered. Tranexamic acid can be administered IV, orally, or locally to help control bleeding. Surgical technique should be efficient and meticulous to reduce time and therefore blood loss. The patient should be positioned to minimize venous pressure and blood loss, such as closing a total knee in flexion or positioning a postoperative total knee in flexion to reduce blood loss.

Presurgical banking of autologous blood by the patient (with or without hematopoietic growth factors), immediate preoperative autodonation by hemodilution, and salvage of the patient's intraoperatively and postoperatively lost blood with infusion of either washed or unwashed red cells can reduce the patient's exposure to the risks of designated donor blood or homologous banked blood. The problems with autologous blood begin with the cost, but there are other issues. Older (>70 years) patients sometimes do not tolerate the anemia from donation. Perhaps the greatest risks are bacterial contamination and clerical error, in which a patient gets a potentially fatal ABO-incompatible unit instead of his or her own. Autologous blood that is not used is discarded and not put into the general blood bank pool.

Preoperative hemodilution has the cost associated with the operating room time to draw off the blood and that of the anesthesiologist in supervising the process.

Despite initial resistance and continued questions about cost-effectiveness by blood bank officials, autologous blood donation has achieved considerable acceptability from patients, physicians, and blood bank administrators. There are disadvantages of autologous donation that counterbalance the obvious advantages of eliminating transfusion-related disease and incompatibility. These are possible bacterial contamination of the blood, perioperative anemia with increased risk of transfusion, administrative error resulting in blood incompatibility from receiving the wrong blood, cost, and wastage of autologous blood that is not used. Blood can be stored for 35 days or can be frozen as a red cell mass for up to 1 year, but loss in viability of the red cells occurs with both storage methods. Use of autologous blood can eliminate the need for banked blood for many, but not all, orthopedic patients.

Some patients have anemia, as demonstrated by their laboratory test results (eg, Hgb level of 10 g/dL and hematocrit level of 30%), which precludes their predonation of blood. The ability of patients to predonate blood and the amount of blood donated can sometimes be increased through the use of recombinant human erythropoietin therapy that can also be used to boost preoperative hematocrit and thereby minimize the effect of surgical blood loss. Injections can be given twice weekly and may result in a higher red cell mass collected and a higher hematocrit level at the time of hospital admission. Although expensive, this therapy can be of benefit to patients, especially those who have blood types that are difficult to match or have religious beliefs that conflict with the practice of receiving blood from others. Erythropoietin is estimated to cost $900 per unit of blood saved, which is more than the cost of autologous blood at $300 to $400 per unit. Furthermore, there may be risks with abnormally high hematocrits. Thus, it is only considered when there is little other choice, such as for surgery on Jehovah's Witnesses who refuse transfusions.

Red blood cells can be salvaged by suction in the operating room or collected via surgical drains in the recovery room. Adequate loss of blood must be present to make these procedures cost-effective. Blood salvage is probably effective (absolute reduction in risk of receiving an allogeneic red cell transfusion of 21%, with a saving of 0.68 units of allogeneic blood per patient) in minimizing perioperative allogeneic transfusion but should be reserved for cases with high expected blood loss (ie, >2 units), patients with low starting Hgbs, and/or Jehovah's Witness patients who will accept intraoperative salvage. The salvaged blood is generally washed to remove cell debris, fat, and bone fragments. Newer filtration techniques permit the transfusion of blood collected from drains without the washing process.

Bezwada HP, Nazarian DG, Henry DH, Booth RE Jr. Preoperative use of recombinant human erythropoietin before total joint arthroplasty. *J Bone Joint Surg Am.* 2003;85:1795-1800. [PMID: 12954840]

Carless PA, Henry DA, Moxey AJ, et al. Cell salvage for minimizing perioperative allogeneic blood transfusion. *Cochrane Database Syst Rev.* 2010,4.CD001888. [PMID: 20393932]

Carson JL, Guyatt G, Heddle NM, et al. Clinical practice guidelines from the AABB; red blood cell transfusion thresholds and storage. *JAMA.* 2016;316(19):2025-2035. [PMID: 27732721]

Magill P, Cunningham EL, Hill JC, et al. Identifying the period of greatest blood loss after lower limb arthroplasty. *Arthroplast Today.* 2018;4(4):499-504. [PMID: 30569010]

Strumper D, Weber EW, Gielen-Wijffels S, et al. Clinical efficacy of postoperative autologous transfusion of filtered shed blood in hip and knee arthroplasty. *Transfusion.* 2004;44:1567-1571. [PMID: 15504161]

Zohar E, Ellis M, Ifrach N, et al. The postoperative blood-sparing efficacy of oral versus intravenous tranexamic acid after total knee replacement. *Anesth Analg.* 2004;99:1679-1683. [PMID: 15562053]

ETHICS IN ORTHOPEDIC SURGERY

Ethics in medicine started with Hippocrates and was codified by Thomas Percival in 1803, with the publication of his Code of Medical Ethics. This was extended by the American Medical Association in 1847 and has undergone several revisions over time. Ethics basically define the standards of conduct of honorable or moral behavior by the physician. Many areas of medical ethics, such as abortion or artificial insemination, have little to do with orthopedics. Although many areas of ethics are more restrictive than the law, litigation and legislation have in some cases become the standard by which orthopedists have to abide, with tighter constraints than ethics alone would place. Although ethics as a field is too broad a subject for a text such as this, certain areas with relevance to orthopedics are addressed here.

Clinical Trials

A particularly difficult ethical area is the clinical research study. Although many of these are now more than adequately controlled by institutional review boards (IRBs), the federal government's Office for Human Research Protections, and sponsors of research, the single practitioner in a small orthopedic group is still at risk of performing human, or even animal, research without appropriate ethical controls. The three main areas for concern are the use of ionizing radiation for exams that are not clinically indicated, the use of patient or third-party-payer funds for exams that are not clinically indicated, and the use of patient data in a manner that does not maintain confidentiality. Certainly, ionizing radiation can be used, even for control subjects, if adequate IRB review and patient/subject consent are obtained. This must be done in a formal manner. However, the use of third-party-payer funds for research or revealing patient confidentiality is never ethical. Performing unindicated studies (laboratory, radiographs) at patient's expense is certainly unethical. In addition, patient confidentiality is fundamental to the doctor–patient relationship. The Health Insurance Portability and Accountability Act (HIPAA) changed the way physicians have to look at confidentiality. Verbal, written, and electronic privacy must be maintained in the office and hospital setting. Patient data have to be closely controlled with care taken regarding personal data assistants, scraps of paper with patient identifiers and data, and roentgenographic images. Photos or slides of football injuries in the public domain may be acceptable for presentation, although in some situations, this may not be true. Certainly, photos or slides of radiographs with patient identifiers for professional presentations or publications cannot be used without written patient permission. The electronic medical record will produce many potential areas that might violate HIPAA regulations, especially with local area networks that permit laptop access in an entire office or building.

The typical orthopedic clinical research study is a retrospective review of a surgeon's cases. This model of research is considered to be of modest value by researchers doing multicenter, randomized, controlled, double-blind studies, but until the funding is found to do this type of study on something as common as knee replacement, retrospective reviews will have to serve as the database for decision making. This is especially true for low-volume procedures. These types of studies raise several issues. The main issues are paying for the study (not through patient or third-party funds), maintaining patient confidentiality, and conflict of interest. The first two issues can be resolved by IRB oversight, and private practitioners are advised to obtain that help from their hospital. Conflict of interest has at least two aspects. Physicians may be consultants or designers of the prosthesis or drug and have a financial interest in the success of the product, and they have ego invested in their surgery; that is, they do not want to look like "bad" surgeons and hence may be hesitant to report poor results. Furthermore, they may be professors and need to demonstrate clinical research publications as part of promotion requirements or simply want to "advertise" their abilities through publication. The latter aspects are implied conflicts of interest but are probably as important as a financial conflict. The potential financial conflict should be disclosed to the patient and to other parties such as the hospital and the journal of publication. Surgeons have an ethical obligation to share medical advances, and presenting surgeons' results with a procedure certainly meets that standard.

New Products

The orthopedic implant industry is similar to other industries in that there is a profit motive that drives innovation. This innovation takes the form of the auto industry: every year there is a new model that makes the previous year's model "old," and every few years, there is big design change that renders the old model obsolete. This is also seen in the trauma and joint replacement product lines. The plates and screws and rods get updated, fancier, and more specific for the individual bone every year. The total knees and total hips undergo changes to address "fringe" issues, such as dislocation for hips and more "natural" motion for knees. Occasionally, in an attempt to keep market share or take market share, companies will come out with a great new "advance," such as metal-on-metal total hip bearing surfaces. Unfortunately, not all changes are improvements or advances, and it is incumbent on the orthopedic surgeon to ethically decide whether he or she has the background, experience, and skill to evaluate and use new changes for the benefit of the patient. If the orthopedic surgeon does not have those abilities, it might be better for the patients to have the new technology evaluated at high-volume centers. Some technology has reached a state where it may take years to evaluate the *potential* benefit to patients. For example, total hip replacement has excellent 15- to 20-year results, which means that it may take >5 years of follow-up to determine if a new technology is even promising, and much longer to show that it is an improvement.

Gifts From Industry

The concept that gifts from industry may affect the choice of medication, prosthesis, and so on, is of concern. Generally, the guidelines recommended by the American Medical Association allow gifts, other remuneration, subsidies for meetings, and so on, if the primary purpose is education or of benefit to the patient. Gifts should be of minimal value and related to the physician's work. The pharmaceutical and orthopedic manufacturers are now self-regulated by industry organizations regarding the type of meetings that they can sponsor. Meetings directly sponsored by the company are only allowed to discuss "label" applications of the drug or device, whereas continuing medical education credit courses, which can only be done through an educational institution, can discuss "off-label" uses of products. Payment for travel costs, lodging, and honoraria to attend such meetings is considered inappropriate unless the physician is performing a service, such as faculty duties or consulting. Although it seems unlikely that a physician would change his or her prescribing practice based on a free meal, the appearance of impropriety is important and should be kept in mind.

Cartwright JC, Hickman SE, Bevan L, Shupert CL. Navigating federalwide assurance requirements when conducting research in community-based care settings. *J Am Geriatr Soc.* 2004;52: 1567-1571. [PMID: 15341563]

Council on Ethical and Judicial Affairs. *Code of Medical Ethics: Current Opinions with Annotations* (2000–2001 edition). American Medical Association; 2000.

Epps CH. Ethical guidelines for orthopedists and industry. *Clin Orthop.* 2003;412:14-20. [PMID: 12838046]

Healy WL Peterson RN. Department of Justice investigation of orthopedic industry. *J Bone Joint Surg.* 2009;91A:1791-1805. [PMID: 19571103]

Laskin RS, Davis JP. The use of a personal digital assistant in orthopaedic surgical practice. *Clin Orthop.* 2004;421:91-98. [PMID: 15123932]

Oyama L, Tannas HS, Moulton S. Desktop and mobile software development for surgical practice. *J Pediatr Surg.* 2002;37: 477-481. [PMID: 11877671]

Pancoast PE, Patrick TB, Mitchell JA. Physician PDA and the HIPAA privacy rule. *J Am Med Inform Assoc.* 2003;10:611-612. [PMID: 14631929]

Musculoskeletal Trauma Surgery

2

Navid Ziran, MD
Kaan S. Irgit, MD
Babak Samimi, MD
Jordan Weinberg, MD
Wade R. Smith, MD

THE HIGH COST OF MUSCULOSKELETAL TRAUMA

Accidents, or unintentional injuries, are the fourth leading cause of death in the United States and the leading cause of death for those aged 1 to 44 years. As of 2015, motor vehicle accidents (MVAs) were the leading cause of death in humans in their first three decades, with 35,000 people killed and 2.3 million injured every year. Globally, approximately 1.3 million humans die every year and over 20 million sustain nonfatal injuries from road traffic accidents. In 2016, road traffic accidents were the eighth leading cause of death and estimated to be the fifth leading cause of death by 2030. The economic impact for MVAs is around $230 billion in the United States and €180 billion in the European Union. The global losses due to road traffic injuries are estimated to be $518 billion and cost governments between 1% and 3% of their gross domestic product.

In 2016, gunshot injuries were the third leading cause of all accidental, or unintentional, injury-related deaths in the United States. There are 60,000 to 80,000 nonfatal gunshot wounds annually in the United States. In 2017, 39,773 persons died from gun-related injuries in the United States, with estimated lifetime medical costs over $2 billion.

In children, trauma is the leading cause of death and disability and accounts for approximately 11 million hospitalizations, 150,000 disabilities, and 15,000 deaths every year in the United States. Although direct costs of pediatric trauma exceed $8 billion per year, indirect costs to families and society are impossible to estimate but are undoubtedly substantial.

With an unprecedented increase in population and life expectancy, age-related musculoskeletal conditions, such as fragility fractures and sports-related ligamentous injuries, are now more common as well. Approximately 1.6 million hip fractures occur worldwide each year. By 2050, this number is expected to increase three- or four-fold. According to the National Osteoporosis Foundation, in 2018, the cost of osteoporosis-related fractures to the health care system was $52 billion. Another national health care issue is opioid abuse, which had an economic burden of approximately $78.5 billion in the United States in 2013. Implementation of new laws at the state and national level are attempting to curb opioid abuse, mortality, and the cost to the health care system.

Both natural and manmade disasters have caused hundreds of thousands of casualties and disabilities over the past 20 years, and the World Health Organization estimates an overall increase over the next two decades. Although true mass casualty situations are rare, the earthquake in Haiti in 2010 left 300,000 individuals injured. These situations require highly organized trauma systems for optimal outcomes.

While considering the cost of musculoskeletal injuries, the effects on the patient, family, and society should also be considered. Health care practitioners should keep in mind that there are direct expenditures for diagnosis, treatment, and rehabilitation as well as indirect economic costs associated with lost labor and diminished productivity. In the current health care climate, the surgeon should not underestimate his or her role in the business of trauma. As in any other business, providing a high-quality, efficient, and cost-effective orthopedic trauma service line is extremely valuable to the hospital system. Surgeons should work side-by-side with hospital administrators to evaluate their own practices and services. Practice habits (eg, costly implants, unnecessary studies) that are not cost-effective should be questioned based on evidence to facilitate a "race to the bottom." These cost-savings can then be reinfused into the orthopedic trauma service line to further streamline care (eg, full-time employees,).

Baerg J, Thirumoorthi A, Hazboun R, Vannix R, Krafft P, Zouros A. Cervical spine injuries in young children: pattern and outcomes in accidental versus inflicted trauma. *J Surg Res.* 2017;219:366-373. [PMID: 29078907]

Koehler RM, Okoroafor UC, Cannada LK. A systematic review of opioid use after extremity trauma in orthopedic surgery. *Injury.* 2018;49(6):1003-1007. [PMID: 29704954]

Maqungo S, Kauta N, Held M, Mazibuko T, Keel MJ, Laubscher M, Ahmad SS. Gunshot injuries to the lower extremities: issues, controversies and algorithm of management. *Injury.* 2020;51(7):1426-1431. [PMID: 32471684]

Mathers CD, Loncar D. Projections of global mortality and burden of disease from 2002 to 2030. *PLoS Med.* 2006;3(11):e442. [PMID: 17132052]

Metcalf KB, Smith EJ, Wetzel RJ, Sontich JK, Ochenjele G. Comparison of clinical outcomes after intramedullary fixation of tibia fractures caused by blunt trauma and civilian gunshot wounds: a retrospective review. *J Orthop Trauma.* 2020;34(6):e208-e213. [PMID: 31764408]

Swaid F, Peleg K, Alfici R, Olsha O, Givon A, Kessel B; Israel Trauma Group. A comparison study of pelvic fractures and associated abdominal injuries between pediatric and adult blunt trauma patients. *J Pediatr Surg.* 2017;52(3):386-389. [PMID: 27817834]

THE FRACTURE HEALING PROCESS

- Fracture healing in humans is still not completely understood.
- Mesenchymal stem cells (MSCs), growth factors, and inflammatory mediators play a temporospatial role.
- Articular cartilage repair remains a difficult problem, but newer techniques are promising.

Bone is a unique tissue among all musculoskeletal tissues because it heals via formation of normal bone, as opposed to scar tissue. The events of fracture healing mimic embryonic development, and the phases of fracture healing include inflammation (duration up to 3-7 days after injury), a reparative phase including soft callus (2 weeks) to hard callus (6+ weeks), and a remodeling phase (months to years after injury).

Fracture healing can also be temporally divided into the following four stages; however, there can be significant overlap:

1. Hematoma formation and inflammation
2. Cartilage formation with subsequent calcification
3. Cartilage removal and bone formation
4. Bone remodeling

An overview of fracture healing is shown in Figure 2–1.

Hematoma Formation and Inflammation

Initially after a fracture, there is an increase in blood flow, hematoma formation, and inflammation. Tumor necrosis factor-α (TNF-α), interleukin (IL)-1, IL-6, IL-11, and IL-18 are all involved to recruit inflammatory cells and promote angiogenesis. Macrophages express TNF-α, which peaks at 24 hours, may recruit other cells, and induces osteoblastic

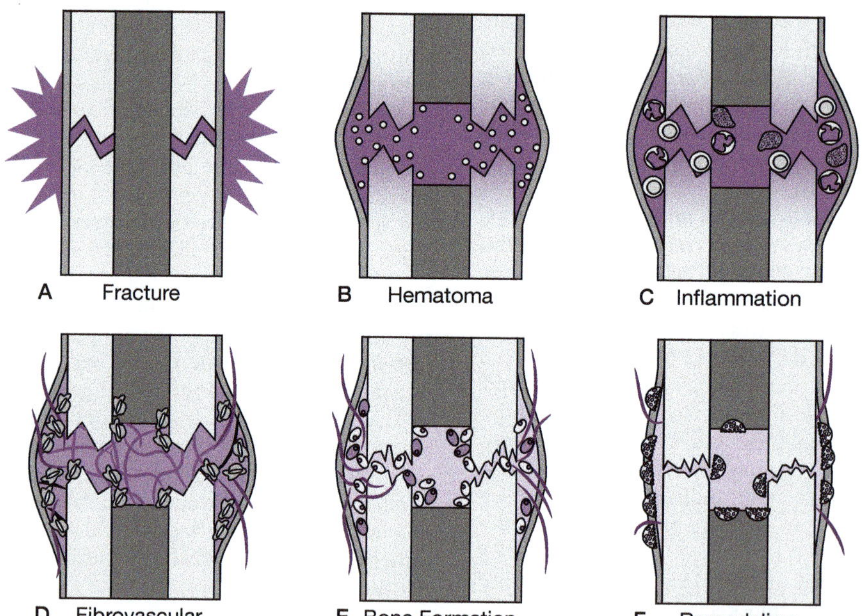

▲ **Figure 2–1.** Fracture healing occurs in separate temporal stages. After fracture (**A**), a hematoma (**B**) forms followed by inflammation (**C**). Mesenchymal stem cell recruitment and expansion from the periosteum and endosteum occur along with vascular ingrowth (**D**). Bone formation (**E**) occurs via both a cartilage intermediate (blue cells) and intramembranous ossification (gray cells). Osteoclast and osteoblasts continue the bone remodeling process for years to restore bone shape and structure (**F**). (Reprinted with permission from Bahney CS, Zondervan RL, Allison P, et al. Cellular biology of fracture healing. J Orthop Res. 2019 Jan;37(1):35-50.)

differentiation of MSCs. The central command orchestrating the initiation of hematoma formation, local inflammation, and tissue regeneration is largely unknown. It is possible that the interplay between the periphery (eg, neural, endocrine) and the central nervous system (CNS) is important to the process. For example, the weight of the pituitary gland begins to increase 30 minutes after fracture and peaks at 2 to 4 hours and 24 hours after fracture. The precise mechanism by which the CNS and/or peripheral nervous system (PNS) initiate the inflammatory process and orchestrate the temporospatial release of growth factors, cell recruitment, and so on has yet to be elucidated.

Cartilage Formation and Calcification

During and after inflammation, MSCs are recruited from the periosteum's cambium layer, the endosteum, surrounding musculature, and systemically. Recruited MSCs differentiate into chondrocytes or osteoblasts depending on the local mechanical environment. Fracture healing can be divided into primary and secondary healing depending on the local mechanical and physiologic factors. In primary healing, the cortex attempts to reestablish itself without the formation of callus (osteonal or haversian healing) via direct woven bone formation. This primary healing occurs when the fracture is anatomically reduced, the blood supply is preserved, and the fracture is rigidly stabilized by internal fixation. Local factors such as high-oxygen tension and high pH also predispose to osteoblast stimulation. Secondary fracture healing results in the formation of callus (cartilage intermediate) and involves the participation of the periosteum and external soft tissues. Low-oxygen tension and low pH favor the MSC differentiation into chondrocytes. This fracture healing response is enhanced by motion and is inhibited by rigid fixation. During secondary bone healing, fractures heal from the periosteum in a centrifugal pattern (ie, radially outward). This increase in the diameter of the fracture callus increases the moment area of inertia, thus improving stability of the healing tissue. Many fractures entail a combination of both primary and secondary fracture healing patterns due to variation in local microscopic mechanical strain. The amount of fracture motion has been demonstrated to affect the differentiation pathway of periosteal progenitor cells in mice. Figure 2–2 demonstrates osteochondral progenitor differentiation into chondrocytes or osteoblasts and the genes involved.

Growth factors and cytokines derived from platelets and other cells are essential for angiogenesis, cellular chemotaxis, proliferation, and differentiation. These growth factors induce MSC differentiation as well as production of type I collagen, type II collagen, and a proteoglycan extracellular matrix (ECM). The transforming growth factor-β (TGF-β) superfamily is critical to the process of matrix production. Bone morphogenetic protein-2 (BMP-2) is important to cell differentiation and/or recruitment during this process. During matrix production, the bony fracture ends are resorbed

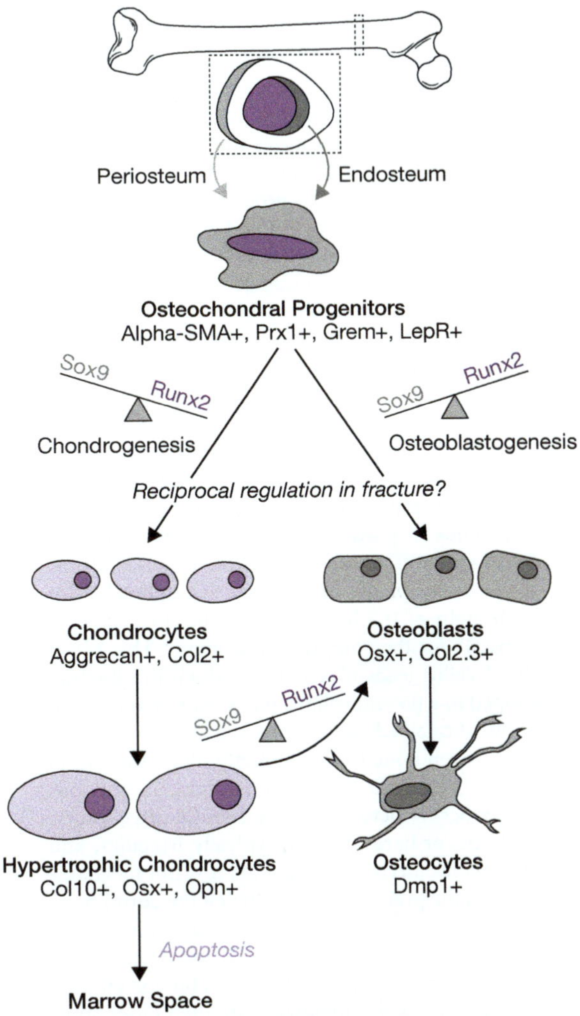

▲ Figure 2–2. Mechanisms of pluripotential stem cell differentiation. After fracture, osteochondral progenitor cells undergo differentiation into either chondrocytes or osteoblasts depending on local mechanical factors. Some of the genes involved in differentiation are shown for each pathway. (Reprinted with permission from Bahney CS, Zondervan RL, Allison P, et al. Cellular biology of fracture healing. J Orthop Res. 2019 Jan;37(1):35-50.)

with a decrease in porosity and stiffness; this change in the fracture ends is frequently visible on radiographs as the fracture edges appear smoother. This "leeching" of local bone serves several purposes. First, it provides a local source of calcium. It also lowers the elastic modulus of the adjacent bone to minimize stress shielding and allows for physiologic mechanotransduction of adjacent healing tissue. Once this matrix has formed with a subsequent increase in mechanical stability, it is now a soft callus and clinically manifested by a decrease in the patient's pain.

Cartilage Resorption and Bone Formation

During this phase, cartilage cells undergo apoptosis, and ECM is removed to allow for vascular invasion. Vascular endothelial growth factor (VEGF) is expressed by osteoblasts and hypertrophic chondrocytes to allow for vascular ingrowth and to transform the ECM into osseous tissue. There are several mediators of this process including macrophage colony-stimulating factor (M-CSF), receptor activator of nuclear factor kappa B ligand (RANKL), osteoprotegerin (OPG), and TNF-α. The Wnt family of molecules has also been demonstrated to play a role in MSC osteoblastic differentiation during this process. It has recently been shown that chondroblasts can transdifferentiate into osteoblasts. In other words, these cells are "plastic" in that they do not need to dedifferentiate and redifferentiate into an osteoblast—they can "jump" cell lineages to perform required functions.

During the transition from soft to hard callus, chondrocytes become hypertrophic and begin to calcify the ECM. This calcium binds to phosphate and forms the nidus for eventual hydroxyapatite crystal formation. Type I collagen binds to the hydroxyapatite; the collagen is responsible for the tensile strength of the bone, whereas the hydroxyapatite is responsible for the compressive strength. This phase of mineralized callus leads to a state in which the fracture site is enveloped in a polymorphous mass of mineralized tissues consisting of calcified cartilage, woven bone made from cartilage, and woven bone formed directly. Bone formation continues until the calcified cartilage is replaced, and this process usually occurs between weeks 2 and 6 after injury. This woven bone, or hard callus, is typically irregular, and although it provides mechanical stability, it is not mechanically as strong as the preinjury bone. During the entire bone formation and remodeling process, osteoclasts are critical to the coupled bone resorption and formation process. The central and peripheral mechanisms responsible for guiding bone regeneration are still unknown. Although older studies suggested that fracture healing is mediated by piezoelectric phenomena, later research demonstrated that streaming potentials may play a more significant role *in vivo*.

Bone Remodeling

After the initial hard callus is formed, the bone continues to remodel as it adapts to local mechanical factors. The hard callus woven bone is typically irregular and provides initial mechanical stability suitable for loading. However, during remodeling, the intramedullary canal is restored, and the woven bone is replaced by lamellar bone arranged in osteonal systems. This remodeling process attempts to restore the Haversian canal system and strengthens the quality of the bone. During this phase, IL-1 and TNF-α have been shown to be highly expressed. The remodeling process begins during hard callus formation but can continue for years as the bone continues to remodel based on local mechanical factors.

Cartilage Healing

Articular cartilage consists of ECM and chondrocytes. The ECM is formed by water (65%-80%), collagen (95% type II), and proteoglycans (chondroitin sulfate and keratan sulfate). Collagen in the ECM provides form and tensile strength. Proteoglycans and water give the cartilage stiffness, resilience, and endurance.

Chondrocytes are sparse in the adult cartilage, which is not a vascularized tissue. Their nutrition comes from the synovial fluid, and adequate circulation of the fluid through the sponge-like cartilage matrix is crucial. The low baseline metabolic rate and small cell-to-matrix ratio of chondrocytes also diminishes the reparative capacity of articular cartilage. Motion of the joint is responsible for most of the circulation. Rigid internal fixation of articular fractures and early weight bearing of immobilized joints allow cyclical compression of the cartilage and circulation of the synovial fluid. If the defect in the cartilage does not go through the calcified plate, the body attempts repair with hyaline cartilage. This regeneration may be seen with superficial articular cartilage lesions. Chondral fissures, flap tears, or chondral defects entail loss of segmental pieces of cartilage and have a limited chondrocytic reparative response. If the calcified plate is violated, as in osteochondral lesions, the subchondral capillaries initiate an inflammatory reaction that fills the defect with granulation tissue and, eventually, fibrocartilage. The quality of this fibrocartilage can be improved by passive or active motion of the joint; however, it does not have the same biomechanical characteristics as the original cartilage.

Current techniques to regenerate cartilage defects include microfracture, osteochondral autologous transplantation/mosaicplasty (OATM), matrix-induced or non–matrix-induced autologous chondrocyte implantation (ACI), and osteochondral allograft (OCA) transplantation. Microfracture involves drilling through the subchondral bone into the marrow to allow for MSCs to regenerate fibrocartilage. OATM entails harvesting cartilage from non–weight-bearing locations, such as the distal femur, and implanting it into the defect; this has demonstrated improved clinical outcomes compared to preoperative conditions. The procedure may be more appropriate for defects less than 2 cm^2 with a known risk of failure between 2 and 4 years. ACI involves harvesting the patient's own cartilage, *ex vivo* expansion, and reimplantation into the defect covered by collagen membrane. Matrix-induced ACI involves embedding the chondrocytes into a matrix prior to reimplantation. OCA transplantation is useful for large osteochondral defects, particularly of the femoral condyles; it involves replacement of the cartilage and subchondral bone defect with a matched allograft containing bone and cartilage. The most cost-effective treatment for different-size cartilage defects remains unknown. Microfracture may be superior for small defects, and matrix-induced ACI has demonstrated greater improvement in functional outcome scores.

Tendon Healing

Tendons are specialized structures that allow muscles to exert their actions on bone. Tendons consist of long bundles of mostly type I collagen scattered with relatively inactive fibrocytes. These cells are nourished by the synovial fluid secreted by the one-cell-thick synovial membrane that covers the tendon (endotenon) and the parietal surface of the sheath (epitenon). The flexor tendons are covered by a richly vascularized adventitia (paratenon). Sharpey's fibers are type I collagen tissue that connect tendons to the periosteum and bone. Tendon healing follows similar phases to bone healing, including inflammation, proliferation, and remodeling. Similar to bone healing, macrophages play a crucial role in regulating the inflammatory response. Growth factors, such as platelet-derived growth factor (PDGF), basic fibroblast growth factor (bFGF), TGF-β, and VEGF, are also involved in the tendon healing process. Rehabilitation strategies play an important role in maintaining mobility while avoiding reinjury/gapping and vary based on the anatomic location.

Muscle Healing

Type 1 fiber, known as slow-twitch, slow oxidative, or red muscle, has a slow speed of contraction and the greatest strength of contraction. It functions aerobically and, therefore, is fatigue resistant. Type 2 fiber, known as fast-twitch or white muscle, is subdivided into two types according to metabolic activity level: fiber that functions by oxidative and glycolytic metabolism (type 2A) and fiber that is largely glycolytic (type 2B). Both subtypes of white fast-twitch muscles are fatigable but have high strength of contraction and high speed of contraction.

Traumatic injury to muscle can occur from a variety of mechanisms, including blunt trauma (muscle contusion), laceration, strains resulting from excessive stretching, or ischemia. Recovery occurs through a process of degeneration and regeneration, with new muscle cells and scar tissue arising from undifferentiated cells. In addition to muscle regeneration, laceration repair requires reinnervation of denervated muscle areas. Muscle contusion frequently results in hematoma. The normal repair process includes an inflammatory reaction, formation of connective tissue, and muscle regeneration. Blunt trauma may result in myositis ossificans, a benign process of ossification within muscle, and may cause decreased function. Orthopedic surgeons should be aware of disuse muscle atrophy due to immobilization and lack of activity.

Nerve Healing

Nerves are cellular structures (neurons) and fibers (axons) that transmit electrical signals to and from the periphery. Efferent neurons transmit signals from the CNS to the PNS. Afferent neurons transmit signals from the PNS to the CNS. Schwann cells encase the nerves in myelin to provide growth factor support (ie, nerve growth factor [NGF]) and insulation. Ionic transmission occurs between the myelin sheaths at the nodes of Ranvier. The transmission of signals corresponds to the degree of myelination; motor neurons fibers are the most heavily myelinated, whereas sensory fibers are unmyelinated.

Multiple nerve fibers combine to form a fascicle surrounded by perineurium. Multiple fascicles are surrounded by epineurium. Nerves fall into patterns of monofascicular, oligofascicular, and polyfascicular structures. The size and distribution of fascicles change as a function of length, reflecting greater or lesser nerve fibers in each fascicle.

Nerve damage may occur through stretching, direct compression (neurapraxia), injury to the axon (axonotmesis), or complete transection of the nerve (neurotmesis). Neurapraxia results in focal segmental demyelination but no damage to axons. Axonal damage from stretching may occur at elongation of 15% or more. Compression of 30 mm Hg may cause paresthesias, and 60 mm Hg may completely block conduction. Examples of neurapraxia include sciatic nerve palsy (most commonly the portion that becomes the deep peroneal nerve) from hip injury/surgery, correction of valgus knee deformity resulting in peroneal nerve palsy, and carpal tunnel syndrome (median nerve). Axonotmesis results in varying degrees of injury to the axon and soft tissue (endoneurium, perineurium, epineurium). Neurotmesis involves complete transection of the nerve and soft tissue with discontinuity. Sunderland also classified nerve injuries from grade I to grade V. Grade I injuries correspond to neurapraxia, grade II to IV injuries correspond to axonotmesis, and grade V injuries correspond to neurotmesis. MacKinnon and Dellon introduced a grade VI that corresponds to a mixed nerve injury that combines the other degrees of injury.

Treatment options include observation for most nerve injuries (neurapraxia, axonotmesis) or surgical repair for primary nerve lacerations (neurotmesis). Nerve grafting with the sural or saphenous nerve can be performed for defects greater than 2.5 cm. Methods to evaluate neural recovery include the physical examination (eg, motor strength, sensation [two-point discrimination], muscle atrophy) and objective evaluation with electromyography (EMG) and nerve conduction velocity (NCV) studies. Neural regeneration typically occurs by reinnervation of the muscle by collateral sprouting or axonal regeneration. For axonal regeneration to occur, there must be an intact anterior horn cell and an endoneural tube. EMG and NCV studies are typically performed at least 4 to 6 weeks after neural injury because the earliest manifestation of axonal denervation is the presence of positive sharp waves and fibrillation potentials. The most important factor that affects nerve recovery after nerve injury is age, with an approximate age of greater than 40 resulting in less recovery potential. The second most important factor is the level of injury, with more distal injuries having a better prognosis. Crush injuries generally have a worse prognosis than lacerations due to the significant soft-tissue damage. Delay of repair (>12-18 months) is also associated with a worse prognosis.

Bahney CS, Zondervan RL, Allison P, et al. Cellular Biology of Fracture Healing. *J Orthop Res.* 2019;37:35-50. [PMID: 30370699]

Chatterjee S, Prasad GC, Udupa KN. Changes in endocrine gland during fracture repair and effect of their ablation. *J Trauma.* 1979;10(9):890-899. [PMID: 5506368]

Einhorn TA, Gerstenfeld LC. Fracture healing: mechanisms and interventions. *Nat Rev Rheumatol.* 2015;11(1):45-54. [PMID: 25266456]

Hagiwara Y, Dyment NA, Jiang X, et al. Fixation stability dictates the differentiation pathway of periosteal progenitor cells in fracture repair. *J Orthop Res.* 2015;33(7):948-956. [PMID: 25639792]

Hsu JD, Robinson RA. Studies on the healing of long-bone fractures in hereditary pituitary insufficient mice. *J Surg Res.* 1969;9: 535-536. [PMID: 5804619]

Lynch TS, Patel RM, Benedick A, Amin NH, Jones MH, Miniaci A. Systematic review of autogenous osteochondral transplant outcomes. *Arthroscopy.* 2015;31(4):746-754. [PMID: 25617008]

Marsell R, Einhorn TA. The biology of fracture healing. *Injury.* 2011;42(6):551-555. [PMID: 21489527]

Medvedeva E, Grebenik EA, Gornostaeva SN, et al. Repair of damaged articular cartilage: current approaches and future directions. *Int J Mol Sci.* 2018;19(8):2366. [PMID: 30103493]

Schrock JB, Kraeutler MJ, Houck DA, McQueen MB, McCarty EC. A cost-effectiveness analysis of surgical treatment modalities for chondral lesions of the knee: microfracture, osteochondral autograft transplantation, and autologous chondrocyte implantation. *Orthop J Sports Med.* 2017;5(5):2325967117704634. [PMID: 28516106]

ORTHOPEDIC ASSESSMENT AND MANAGEMENT OF MULTIPLY INJURED PATIENTS

- The advanced trauma life support system was developed by an orthopedic surgeon in 1978.
- Airway, breathing, and circulation remain the foundation of trauma care.
- Management of the physiologically unstable polytrauma patient continues to change.

A thorough understanding of the pathophysiology of trauma is essential for prompt diagnosis and timely treatment of musculoskeletal injuries. Sound therapeutic principles improve the overall outcome for the patient and optimize the utilization of limited health care resources.

The ABCs of Trauma Care

Prompt recognition of life-threatening injury necessitates a rapid, yet systematic approach. In the severely injured patient, treatment priorities are dictated by the patient's overall condition, with the first goal being to identify and treat immediately life-threatening injuries. Initial assessment consists of four overlapping phases:

1. Primary survey (ABCDE)
2. Resuscitation
3. Secondary survey (head-to-toe evaluation and history)
4. Definitive care

The primary survey is designed to identify life-threatening conditions by adhering to the following sequence:

Airway maintenance (with restriction of cervical spine motion)

Breathing and ventilation

Circulation (with hemorrhage control)

Disability (assessment of neurologic status)

Exposure and environmental control (undress the patient but prevent hypothermia)

A brief overview of the treatment of polytrauma patients, with special emphasis on the orthopedic aspects, follows.

A. Airway

The airway must be assessed first to establish patency. If the patient is able to communicate verbally, the airway is likely patent and not an immediate threat to life. Should this not be the case, rapid assessment for signs of obstruction, foreign bodies, and facial, mandibular, or tracheal/laryngeal fractures must follow. Patients with altered level of consciousness are also at risk for loss of airway patency. Initially, the jaw-thrust or chin-lift maneuver may be used to establish airway patency. However, a definite airway must be established (intubation or surgical airway) if there is any concern regarding the patient's ability to maintain airway patency.

Great care should be taken while assessing the airway. The cervical spine should be carefully protected at all times and not be hyperextended, hyperflexed, or rotated to obtain a patent airway. Any patient with a blunt injury above the clavicle or mechanism of injury consistent with possible spine injury should be considered at risk for cervical spine injury. The cervical spine is protected with a cervical collar. When managing the airway, the cervical collar may be opened to facilitate intubation or a surgical airway while motion of the cervical spine is manually restricted.

B. Breathing

The trauma surgeon should evaluate the patient's chest. Adequate ventilation requires not only airway patency but also adequate pulmonary gas exchange. Remember that the following four conditions, if present, must be addressed emergently:

1. Tension pneumothorax
2. Flail chest with pulmonary contusion
3. Open pneumothorax
4. Massive hemothorax

C. Circulation

Uncontrolled hemorrhage is the principal cause of postinjury preventable death. Postinjury hypotension is considered hypovolemic (and specifically hemorrhagic) in origin until proven otherwise. Level of consciousness, skin color, and pulses are simple to assess and reliably mirror the hemodynamic status of the patient. Major hemorrhage may be a result of intracavitary bleeding into the chest, intraperitoneal abdomen, or retroperitoneum/pelvis, in addition to loss of blood from major wounds of the head/neck, torso, or extremities. The classes of shock (Figure 2–3) are based on numerous parameters including approximate blood loss, heart rate, blood pressure, pulse pressure, respiratory rate, urine output, Glasgow Coma Scale (GCS) score, base deficit, and need for blood products. Specific to orthopedic injuries, fractures of the femur or the pelvis may result in major blood loss, which can severely compromise the survival of the patient. (See sections on pelvic and femoral fractures.)

D. Disability (Neurologic Status)

The GCS (see Chapter 13) should be used to assess neurologic status; it is quick, simple, and predictive of patient outcome. An even simpler way to monitor central neurologic status is to remember the mnemonic AVPU and check whether the patient is *a*lert and oriented, responds to *v*ocal stimuli, responds only to *p*ainful stimuli, or is *u*nresponsive.

E. Exposure and Environmental Control

For a thorough examination of lacerations, contusions, abrasions, swelling, and deformities, the patient should be completely disrobed. This also prevents further displacement of fractures and minimizes the risk of overlooking significant injuries. Hypothermia must be avoided because cardiac function may be affected, especially when there is decreased blood volume. Therefore, immediately following disrobement, the patient must be kept warm via blankets and a warm, closed environment in the emergency department.

F. Care of Patient Before Hospitalization

As a general rule, the following measures should be taken for patients with fractures:

1. The joints above and below fractures should be immobilized, and adequate immobilization of the cervical spine via cervical collar should be obtained to prevent further damage to the neurovascular elements and limit hemorrhage.
2. Splints can be improvised with pillows, blankets, or clothing.
3. Immobilization does not need to be absolutely rigid. Spine boards should be removed as early as feasible during initial assessment to avoid soft-tissue pressure injury from prolonged immobilization on an unforgiving surface.

Parameter	Class I	Class II (mild)	Class III (moderate)	Class IV (severe)
Approximate blood loss	<15%	15%-30%	31%-40%	>40%
Heart rate	↔	↔/↑	↑	↑/↑↑
Blood pressure	↔	↔	↔/↓	↓
Pulse pressure	↔	↓	↓	↓
Respiratory rate	↔	↔	↔/↑	↑
Urine output	↔	↔	↓	↓↓
Glasgow Coma Scale score	↔	↔	↓	↓
Base deficit'	0 to –2 mEq/L	–2 to – 6 mEq/L	–6 to –10 mEq/L	–10 mEq/L or less
Need for blood products	Monitor	Possible	Yes	Massive transfusion protocol

* Base excess is the quantity of base (HCO_3^-, in mEq/L) that is above or below the normal range in the body. A negative number is called a base deficit and indicates metabolic acidosis.

▲ **Figure 2–3. Classifications of shock. For class III or IV shock, damage control orthopedics may be more appropriate treatment than early appropriate care/early total care.** (Reprinted with permission from American College of Surgeons. Advanced Trauma Life Support Manual, 10th ed. American College of Surgeons; 2018.)

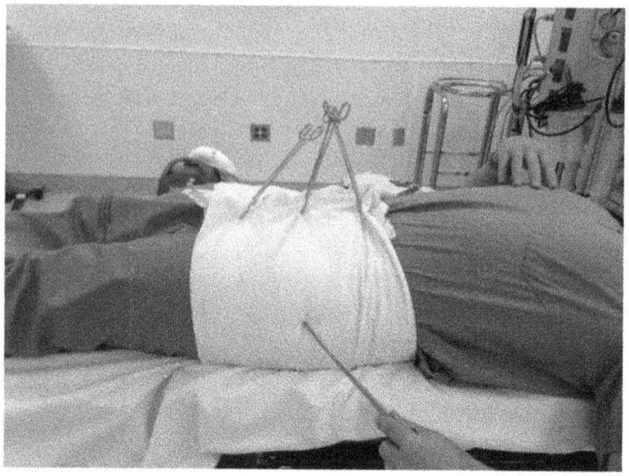

▲ **Figure 2–4.** In patients with a pubic symphyseal dislocation ("open-book" pelvic injury), a sheet can be wrapped around the patient centered on the greater trochanters. The sheet closes down the pelvic volume and may contribute to tamponade.

4. Apply gentle in-line traction to realign the extremity in severe angulation.
5. Overt bleeding should undergo tamponade with dressings and direct pressure.
6. Tourniquets should be avoided unless active extremity bleeding is present and cannot be successfully controlled with application of direct pressure.
7. For patients with a pubic symphyseal dislocation ("open-book" pelvis), a sheet can be placed centered on the greater trochanters to reduce the pelvic displacement and pelvic volume (Figure 2–4).

Orthopedic Examination

A. History

Assess injury mechanism; an adequate assessment of the conditions in which the injury was sustained is crucial. Information from paramedics, relatives, friends, and bystanders should be recorded. Obtain the following information according to injury mechanism:

1. MVA: vehicle speed, direction of impact (eg, T-bone, rear-ended, front-end collision, rollover), patient location in the vehicle, impact location, postimpact location of the patient (if ejection, determine distance), internal and external damage to the vehicle, restraint use and type.
2. Falls: distance of the fall, landing position.
3. Crush: weight of the object, site of the injury, duration of weight application.
4. Explosion: blast magnitude, patient distance from the blast, primary blast injury (force of the blast wave), secondary blast injury (projectiles).
5. Vehicle-pedestrian: type of vehicle, site of collision, speed.

Environmental exposure, comorbidities (eg, diabetes, coronary artery disease), use of steroids, prehospital care, and observations at the accident scene should be determined. Estimated bleeding, open wounds, deformity, motor and sensory function, and delays in extrication or transport are recorded.

B. General Examination

The clinical orthopedic examination requires assessment of the axial skeleton, pelvis, and extremities. The extent of this examination depends on the patient's overall central neurologic status. Unconscious or obtunded patients will not be able to follow commands, and a motor/sensory exam is not possible. Swelling, hematomas, and open wounds are assessed visually in the undressed patient. It is obligatory to palpate the entire spine, pelvis, and each joint. Examination soon after trauma may precede telltale swelling in joint or long bone injuries. In the unresponsive patient, only crepitation and false motion may be discerned. The pelvic examination is of importance if the patient is hemodynamically unstable, given that an open-book fracture may be contributing to hemorrhagic shock. However, forceful manipulation of the pelvis should be avoided in order to prevent aggravation of bleeding. Signs of pelvic injury include blood at the urethral meatus, soft-tissue ecchymosis, and scrotal hematoma, which is possibly a later finding.

C. Neurologic Examination

The neurologic examination of the extremities should be documented to the fullest extent possible, in light of the patient's mental status, because it is central to subsequent decision-making. This examination includes a motor and sensory exam of the upper and lower extremities. Perianal sensation is also important. A normal neurologic examination does not rule out spine injury. Particularly important with spinal cord injury or suspected injury are the reflexes of the anal "wink" and bulbocavernosus muscle. Other spinal reflexes (ie, of the biceps and triceps muscles, of the knee and ankle, and the Babinski reflex) are important in "fine-tuning" the neurologic examination. (These are discussed more fully in Chapter 5.)

D. Muscle Examination

Motor examination can be difficult because of pain or impaired mental status, but even in such cases, useful and relatively complete information can be obtained. One must be sure to evaluate all upper and lower extremity motion.

Hematoma, ecchymosis, and dermabrasions should be noted for the possibility of underlying muscle injury. Muscle strength grading is desirable, but demonstration of a minimum of volitional control, even if only withdrawal to painful stimuli, is important in verifying the presence of intact central sensory-motor integration.

Imaging Studies

Radiologic assessment follows the same general hierarchy as the clinical assessment. The severely injured polytrauma patient requires radiographs of the chest and pelvis to rapidly identify sources of respiratory and circulatory compromise. In the hemodynamically unstable patient, the anteroposterior (AP) pelvis film is sufficient to make immediate treatment decisions. Complementary pelvis films can be obtained later. Intra-abdominal hemorrhage causing hypotension is quickly assessed with bedside ultrasonography (focused assessment sonogram for trauma [FAST]). Radiographic films of the cervical spine performed acutely with a portable x-ray machine have been largely abandoned in favor of computed tomography (CT) imaging once the patient has been stabilized.

Subsequent radiologic evaluation is dependent on clinical findings. Any long bone or joint with a laceration, hematoma, angulation, or swelling and any long bone fracture requires complete radiographic evaluation of the joints proximal and distal to the fracture. At the minimum, two views of the extremities are needed, usually the AP and lateral views. Coordination of more sophisticated studies with other trauma specialties (eg, neurosurgery or urology) is necessary to allow cardiorespiratory monitoring of the patient while efficiently performing these studies.

Evaluation of the Spine

As long as the patient's spine is protected, evaluation of the spine for injury can be deferred, giving priority to management of hemodynamic instability or respiratory compromise. Following that, the presence of spinal injury should be excluded. In the conscious and responsive patient, swelling or tenderness on physical examination of the spine is readily apparent. In the unconscious patient, spine injuries can go undetected, and a careful physical examination must be performed with heavy reliance upon radiographic evaluation.

The primary radiologic modality for imaging the spine is CT with coronal and sagittal reconstructions. When CT is unavailable, essential radiographs for evaluation of the cervical spine include AP, lateral, and open-mouth odontoid views. It is essential to be able to see to the top of T1. If this level is not visualized through these conventional views, the inclusion of oblique and swimmer's views, which is a lateral cervical spine radiograph with the arm abducted and elevated, only slightly improves the sensitivity and, therefore, has been deemed cost-inefficient.

On the open-mouth view, the lateral masses of C1 should line up with the body of C2. The amount of total overhang

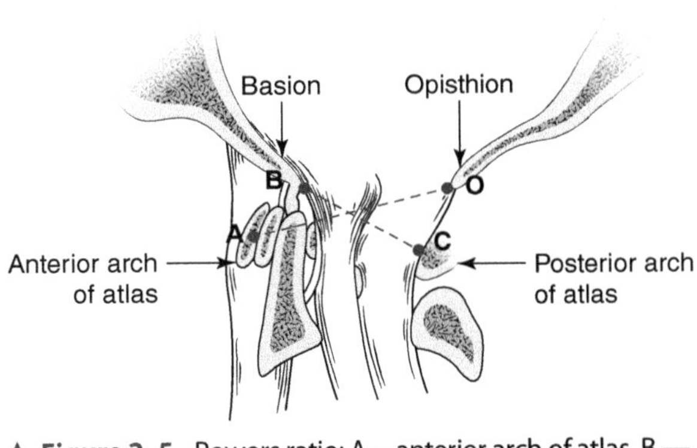

▲ **Figure 2–5.** **Powers ratio: A—anterior arch of atlas, B—basion (anterior margin of foramen magnum), C—anterior portion of posterior arch of atlas, O—opisthion (posterior margin of foramen magnum). The ratio of BC/OA should be approximately 0.77 in the normal population. Anterior atlanto-occipital dislocation is present when the Powers ratio is greater than 1.15.** (Reprinted from Pediatric cervical instability: diagnosis and treatment concepts. Seminars in spine surgery 1996;8(4). Philadelphia: W.B. Saunders Company.)

of C1 over C2 should be less than 7 mm. On the lateral view, the anterior border of the bodies of the cervical segments should be an arc. The distance from the basion to the posterior arch of C1 divided by the distance from the opisthion to the anterior arch of C1 should be less than 1 (Powers ratio) (Figure 2–5). A basion to odontoid tip distance above 10 mm in children and 5 mm in adults indicates craniocervical dislocation, a potentially fatal injury. The posterior border of the anterior arc of C1 should be within 2 to 3 mm of the anterior border of C2. There should be no diastasis of the spinous processes, and the joints and facet joints should all be visible.

In the obtunded patient, x-ray and/or CT radiographic imaging alone is insufficient to completely exclude ligamentous cervical spine injury. The addition of magnetic resonance imaging (MRI) may yield identification of ligamentous injury, but it is often not feasible early in the care of the polytrauma patient. In patients with hemodynamic and/or respiratory compromise, MRI requires extensive time to perform and interferes with the patient's monitoring equipment. MRI is most useful in the patient for whom other imaging modalities are not consistent with the neurologic presentation. In the case of neurologic deficit, careful evaluation of the neurologic status is important, and immediate decompression-stabilization must be considered.

Immediate Management of Musculoskeletal Trauma

The orthopedic injuries in the polytrauma patient are seldom truly emergency situations, except for those involving neural or vascular compromise. For example, fracture-dislocation of the ankle or knee resulting in distal ischemia justifies immediate attempts at reduction to minimize the sequelae of ischemia. A more subtle situation requiring emergent treatment would be dislocation of the hip in which vascular compromise of the femoral head may result. Arterial bleeding from an open fracture should be treated immediately with pressure to minimize blood loss. Other bone and joint injuries, although urgent, may be approached in a more deliberate manner.

Orthopedic surgeons must be aware that management of traumatic skeletal injuries requires consideration of the entire patient as well as the entire extremity.

Complications

Significant postinjury complications are associated with skeletal injury in the setting of polytrauma. The obligatory recumbency necessary for fracture care prior to skeletal fixation puts the patient at risk for pulmonary complications including atelectasis and pneumonia. Venous thromboembolic complications also may occur as a result of the combination of injury and recumbency. In addition, it is understood that the initial physiologic response to injury primes the immune system for an excessive inflammatory response following a second insult, often in the form of fracture fixation (the two-hit model of inflammatory response to injury). This exaggerated inflammatory reaction may result in acute respiratory distress syndrome (ARDS). Fat embolism resulting in respiratory and potentially neurologic compromise may also follow skeletal fixation and intramedullary nailing of femoral shaft fractures in particular. Local complications of traumatic skeletal injury include compartment syndrome and heterotopic ossification.

A. Acute Respiratory Distress Syndrome

ARDS is an acute and diffuse form of pulmonary dysfunction that is associated with a variety of conditions including trauma. Most commonly, ARDS follows high-energy blunt-force trauma, but it may also be seen following resuscitation for hemorrhagic shock from any cause such as penetrating trauma. As stated earlier, ARDS may be a result of the two-hit phenomenon, developing after femoral nailing in patients with associated blunt thoracic trauma. The incidence of ARDS after major trauma is between 5% and 8%, with mortality ranging widely between 3% and 40% of cases.

B. Fat Embolism Syndrome

Fat embolism syndrome (FES) is a potentially severe phenomenon associated with respiratory failure and neurologic impairment as a result of the release of marrow fat into the circulation. Embolism occurs in over 95% of patients after fracture and invariably during reamed nailing of fractures. However, this is a subclinical phenomenon in the majority of patients; only 1% to 5% of patients develop recognizable FES. FES usually develops between 24 and 72 hours after the inciting event and is characterized by the triad of hypoxemia, neurologic impairment, and a petechial rash. Respiratory dysfunction is most common and may be difficult to distinguish from ARDS. Neurologic dysfunction may include depressed level of consciousness, seizures, or focal deficits. The petechial rash is observed in up to 50% of cases and may be the last element of the triad to develop. Treatment is largely supportive, primarily ventilator support, and most patients will have a full recovery, often within days to weeks.

C. Atelectasis

Atelectasis, or localized collapse of alveoli, is a frequent postoperative complication secondary to patient immobilization. Significant hypoxemia may result, and onset may be relatively rapid. Atelectasis may also cause postoperative fevers in early recovery and is often apparent on chest radiographs. Pulmonary toilet from coughing and deep breathing, using incentive spirometry, and, in resistant cases, respiratory therapist–directed positive-pressure treatments usually result in resolution.

D. Pulmonary Embolism and Deep Venous Thrombosis

Pulmonary embolism (PE) is the third most common cause of death in trauma patients who survive after the first day. The trauma patient is at a 13-fold increased risk of venous thromboembolism (VTE). There are several trauma patient risk factors associated with VTE (Table 2–1). Patients at high risk for PE are those with deep vein thrombosis (DVT) in the lower extremities or pelvic veins. Clinically significant PE usually arises from the large veins proximal to the knee. Prevention of DVT reduces the risk of PE. In fact, the initiation of pharmacologic prophylaxis within 24 hours of admission or hemodynamic stability significantly reduces the risk of VTE. Low-molecular-weight heparin is the most commonly prescribed in-hospital prophylactic agent. In patients with relative contraindications to chemical prophylaxis,

Table 2–1. Factors that increase the risk for developing venous thromboembolism (VTE) in trauma patients.

Obesity
Age >55 years
Spinal cord injuries
Major thoracolumbar spinal injuries
Major pelvic and lower extremity trauma
History of prior VTE
Major abdominal surgery
ISS >16
Immobilization in ICU >4 days
Malignancy

ICU, intensive care unit; ISS, Injury Severity Score.

mechanical prophylaxis with lower extremity compression devices is recommended but is not as effective as pharmacologic thromboprophylaxis.

Clinical diagnosis of extremity DVT is confirmed by duplex ultrasonography. Although ultrasonographic screening is employed at many trauma centers, this practice is not supported by most consensus practice guidelines because it has not been demonstrated to improve outcomes. Nonetheless, the diagnosis of DVT necessitates consideration of treatment to prevent a potentially fatal PE. First-line therapy is therapeutic anticoagulation, often with intravenous heparin initially and followed by oral warfarin. In cases where anticoagulation is contraindicated, inferior vena cava filter placement for lower extremity DVT is indicated. Prophylactic placement of a cava filter has not been demonstrated to be effective at PE prevention; however, such filters are often placed in high-risk patients with contraindications to pharmacologic prophylaxis. Please see Chapter 13 for more on antithrombotics.

PE is suspected in the orthopedic patient suffering acute onset of tachypnea and dyspnea in the early postoperative period, within the first days. On physical examination, tachycardia, cyanosis, and pleural friction rub can be noted. Arterial blood gas studies should demonstrate hypoxemia and may also demonstrate hypocapnia, although this is a nonspecific finding. Use of D-dimer is unreliable in the early trauma patient because D-dimer is often elevated from tissue injury; however, D-dimer may be useful later in the recovery period. Definitive diagnosis is best made with CT pulmonary angiography (CTPA). CTPA has become the most efficient imaging modality for diagnosing PE in clinical practice. Sensitivity and specificity are both high, and CTPA may detect alternative causes of hypoxia.

Treatment involves pulmonary support and anticoagulation, similar to DVT. The natural history of treated PE is gradual lysis of the emboli, with the return of flow through the pulmonary arterial tree. The natural history of proximal DVT involves recanalization and arborization to bypass the clot. Patients may suffer from postphlebitic syndrome characterized by chronically painful swelling in the extremity.

E. Compartment Syndrome

The term *compartment syndrome* refers to pathologic developments in a closed space in the body caused by buildup of pressure. Most commonly, such compartments are circumscribed by fascia and incorporate one or more bones. Pressure rises from edema or bleeding within the compartment, further compromising circulation to the contents of the compartment, and can result in muscle necrosis and nerve injury.

Compartment syndrome may result from fracture, soft-tissue injury, vascular injury causing ischemia, or a burn. Failure to redistribute pressure through postural changes results in ischemia of the area under pressure because of collapse of capillaries.

The diagnosis of compartment syndrome must be considered in the postoperative or posttrauma patient who has pain out of proportion to that expected from the inciting injury. As the pain worsens, it can be refractory to narcotic medication. Subsequent to fracture or crush injury, pain with passive stretching of involved muscles is also a subjective finding and must be differentiated from pain arising from the original injury. The involved compartments are firm, and progression can be rapid. The five P's (pulselessness, paresthesia, paresis, pain, and pressure) characteristic of compartment syndrome are helpful but not diagnostic. Pulses are poor indicators of compartment syndrome because they generally remain intact until late. Ultimately, the diagnosis of a compartment syndrome is a clinical one, and the surgeon should have a low threshold to move forward with treatment.

Patients with equivocal clinical findings or those at high risk but without a reliable clinical examination (eg, those who are comatose, have psychiatric problems, or are under the influence of narcotics) should have compartmental pressure measurements.

Intracompartmental pressure within 30 mm Hg or less of the diastolic blood pressure is a potential indication for fasciotomy. Positive clinical findings may justify fasciotomy even despite normal pressures. Late fasciotomy may result in muscle damage or possible necrosis, with resulting risk of infection.

Although compartment syndrome can occur in almost any portion of the body, a high-energy forearm fracture and/or a tibia fracture are at particular risk. The forearm has anterior and posterior compartments, and an extensile volar incision is performed to permit complete release of the anterior compartment, including, if necessary, the carpal tunnel distally and the lacertus fibrosus proximally. Dorsally, a longitudinal incision is used to release the posterior compartment.

In the leg, two incisions are used to release the four compartments of the leg. The anterior compartment is defined medially by the tibia, posteriorly by the interosseous membrane, laterally by the fibula, and anteriorly by the crural fascia. The anterior compartment contains the tibialis anterior, extensor hallucis longus, extensor digitorum longus, and peroneus tertius muscles, as well as the anterior tibial artery/vein and the deep branch of the peroneal nerve. The lateral compartment contains the peroneus brevis and longus muscles and the superficial branch of the peroneal nerve. The superficial posterior compartment contains the gastrocnemius, soleus, plantaris, and popliteus muscles and the sural nerve. The deep posterior compartment is enclosed by the tibia, the interosseous membrane, and the deep transverse fascia, containing the tibialis posterior, flexor hallucis longus, flexor digitorum longus muscles, and posterior tibial and peroneal arteries and the tibial nerve.

The anterior and lateral compartments are decompressed using a longitudinal incision over the anterior intermuscular septum. Posteromedially, a second incision is used to release the superficial and deep posterior compartments. Although single- and limited-incision approaches have been described, these may be unreliable, result in incomplete compartment release, and have a higher incidence of iatrogenic nerve injury in trauma patients.

F. Heterotopic Bone Formation

Clinically significant heterotopic ossification occurs as a consequence of trauma in perhaps 10% of cases and may cause pain or joint motion restriction even to the point of ankylosis. Trauma patients without head injuries frequently manifest heterotopic ossification on radiographs 1 to 2 months following trauma; if the ossification is clinically significant, resection may be indicated when the margins of the bone can be identified on radiographs. This can take up to 3 to 6 months.

Resection is accomplished by removing all of the heterotopic bone. To prevent heterotopic ossification, selected patients may benefit from low-dose radiation (7 Gy) and oral nonsteroidal anti-inflammatory drugs (NSAIDs) for 3 to 6 weeks. Selective NSAIDs such as celecoxib are as effective as traditional NSAIDs such as indomethacin. For acetabular fractures, focused single-dose radiation may be superior to oral indomethacin. Heterotopic bone is a much more common occurrence in patients with head injuries. This is believed to result from release of humeral modulators that have not yet been characterized. There is further discussion of this topic in Chapter 13.

Timing of Fracture Stabilization

The benefit of early fracture stabilization in multiply injured patients has become well established. In the late 20th century, benefits of timely fixation were demonstrated: early mobilization, lower mortality rate, decreased length of stay in the hospital, decreased intensive care requirements, decreased rates of ARDS and pneumonia, decreased risk of fat embolism, and decreased risk of decubitus ulcers. Advocation for early total care (ETC) for polytrauma patients followed. Afterward, it became apparent, however, that certain patients did not do well after ETC, particularly those with head injury or systemic hypotension. Long bone fracture fixation with reamed intramedullary rods, in particular, may cause intraoperative hypotension or an increased release of inflammatory mediators with deleterious results.

As alluded to earlier, the multiply injured patient's immunologic system is stimulated or primed after trauma from the first hit. Subsequent resuscitation, hemorrhage, blood products, hypotension, and surgery, the second event in the two-hit model, may produce an exaggerated systemic inflammatory response syndrome, potentially leading to ARDS or multiple organ failure. Activated neutrophils are the principal effector of the inflammatory response, releasing active oxygen species, which damage the vascular endothelium. Bone marrow contents pushed to the systemic circulation during reaming and nailing can activate neutrophils, leading to systemic inflammatory response syndrome in polytrauma patients, particularly during the first 96 hours after trauma. Damage control orthopedics (DCO) aims to decrease the additional surgical trauma but gain the benefit of early mobilization through early external fixation followed by delayed definitive surgery. For example, conversion of an external fixator to a reamed intramedullary nail has a lower risk of infection if performed within 10 days. Recognition that DCO incurs the need for multiple operations and may incur a higher infection risk led to a return to early definitive care as early appropriate care (EAC). EAC preferentializes definitive femoral fracture fixation over other extremity fractures, which may be splinted and fixed later. This is differentiated from ETC, which advocated early fixation of all fractures. When choosing whether to apply EAC or, perhaps, ETC for some cases, versus DCO, physiologic and hemodynamic stability of the patient should influence this decision. Physiologic markers include venous lactate, base deficit, and arterial blood gas pH. The stable patient may be a good candidate for EAC/ETC; the hemodynamically unstable patient would best be managed by DCO, limiting operative time and blood loss. Patients who meet at least one of the following specific physiologic parameters have less complications: pH greater than 7.25, base excess greater than −5.5 mmol/L, or lactate less than 4.0 mmol/L. Because the timing of orthopedic treatment in the multiply injured patient is controversial and changing, input from the other surgical services, such as general surgery and neurosurgery, is essential. Patients with closed head injuries require the input of neurosurgery regarding suitability for the operating room given the risk of secondary brain injury.

Soft-Tissue Injuries and Traumatic Arthrotomies

Lacerations of the extremities can result in neural or vascular compromise to an extremity and may also cause traumatic arthrotomies. Compromise of the sterility of any joint requires surgical debridement of that joint. For many joints, arthroscopic irrigation and debridement will minimize trauma and improve the return to function. All complete tendon lacerations of the hand, except for those of the palmaris longus, should be repaired. In the foot, extrinsic tendons are repaired to prevent late imbalance or loss of function. Muscle belly injuries generally require surgical debridement because their subfascial location makes simple irrigation difficult. Laceration involving only the muscle belly requires no surgical repair. Frequently, however, muscle belly laceration involves the continuation of the origin or the insertion tendon of the muscle. In this case, optimal function is obtained by reattaching the lacerated ends.

Open Fractures

The Gustilo and Anderson classification, the most popular and generally accepted classification of open fractures, classifies open fractures into three grades, with the third grade divided into three subtypes (Table 2–2). The prevalence

Table 2–2. Gustilo-Anderson classification for open fractures.

Classification	Description
Type I	Puncture wound <1 cm, minimal soft-tissue injury, simple fracture
Type II	Wound 1-10 cm, moderate soft-tissue injury, minimal bony comminution
Type IIIA	Wound usually >10 cm, severe soft-tissue injury, with adequate coverage, comminuted fracture
Type IIIB	Wound usually >10 cm, comminuted fracture with bone exposure, severe soft-tissue injury and periosteal stripping requiring soft-tissue coverage (local vs free flap)
Type IIIC	Associated with vascular injury that requires repair for limb salvage

of wound infection increases with the increase in grade of open injury. Open fractures resulting from natural disasters, highly contaminated injuries, significantly comminuted fractures, and/or fractures from a crush injury are automatically classified as grade III open fractures regardless of the wound size. The degree of soft-tissue injury is not always dictated by the appearance of the skin because some cases have significant muscle and soft-tissue damage despite a benign open wound.

Magnitude of soft-tissue and bony injuries complicates the decision-making between immediate amputation and reconstruction in the lower extremity. Despite the advent of microvascular surgery, prosthetic replacements are a viable alternative to a poorly functioning, insensate lower extremity. Many years of reconstruction to achieve union without infection, multiple operations, inability to return to work, and emotional trauma should be considered in the decision-making of salvage versus amputation.

Treatment of open fractures consists of irrigation and debridement and possible internal versus external fixation. The timing of irrigation and debridement is controversial. Although emergent irrigation and debridement within 6 hours is accepted standard of care, evidence to support this practice is sparse. There is no difference in infection rates in fractures irrigated before or after 6 hours, including those with grade III injuries. The choice of irrigation (pulsed lavage vs gravity flow) remains questionable. The accepted volume of irrigation with 3, 6, and 9 L for grade I, II, and III injuries, respectively, has insufficient supportive evidence; however, the surgeon should use his or her clinical acumen. Antibiotics in the lavage fluid have also demonstrated no benefit in decreasing infection rates. The most important factors to decrease infection risk are the preoperative administration of antibiotics and a meticulous debridement to remove all foreign and necrotic material from the wound. Skin edges should be debrided, as should dead muscle and the surface of any contaminated fat or fascia. Soft-tissue attachments to bone should be maintained whenever possible. Prior to formal debridement, it is appropriate to splint fractures and cover open wounds with sterile wet dressings. Antibiotic therapy is begun immediately, usually with a cephalosporin to cover gram-positive bacteria. Additional coverage for grade III injuries with an aminoglycoside has been suggested. Recent studies have also demonstrated a decreased infection rate in grade III fractures with the use of local antibiotic administration such as antibiotic beads. For grade I and II open fractures, it is recommended to continue antibiotics for 24 hours after wound closure. For grade III fractures, it is recommended to continue antibiotics for 72 hours after injury but no longer than 24 hours after wound closure. Tetanus prophylaxis is administered if needed.

Although it is acceptable practice to leave any wound open, grade I wounds may be closed completely. Following effective operative debridement, grade II wounds may be treated in a similar fashion, with close initial follow-up. Primary closure of grade III wounds may also be performed if there is no undue wound tension, minimal soft-tissue injury, and no significant contamination. Patients with massive wounds should undergo serial irrigation and debridement until the wound is clean.

Flaps and Soft-Tissue Coverage for Open Trauma

Because of extensive soft-tissue damage involved, grade IIIB and IIIC open fractures require aggressive surgical management for wound coverage. These wounds may be treated by regional or free flap reconstruction. With the advent of microsurgical techniques for skin, muscle, and fascia transplantation, the treatment of large soft-tissue trauma has changed, and local rotational flaps, fasciocutaneous flaps, or free tissue transfer can be used successfully. Despite the classical study by Godina favoring immediate free flap reconstruction within the first 48 hours after trauma, controversy still exists regarding the timing for reconstruction. If the patient needs to be stabilized prior to surgery, wound closure for grade IIIB fractures should not be delayed for more than 10 days because doing so significantly increases the risk of infection.

Radical debridement of the zone of injury, similar to the way one would resect a tumor, is required. If radical debridement is not performed, then flap reconstruction should be delayed until soft tissues have healed at the margins and there is no sign of infection. The use of free flaps gives an overall improved outcome by bringing a new source of vascularity to a compromised extremity, preventing infection, and simultaneously providing soft-tissue coverage. Proximal tibia wounds requiring soft-tissue coverage may be amenable to local rotation flaps. Distal tibia fractures with less soft-tissue coverage are often amenable to free flap coverage.

The most common free flaps include fasciocutaneous flaps from the latissimus dorsi, gracilis, serratus anterior, and rectus abdominis muscles. Additionally, there are a host of smaller tissue transfers designed for more specific uses that have advantages in the matching of defect to donor and minimizing problems at the donor site.

Vacuum-assisted closure (VAC) therapy may facilitate wound healing and potentially prevent the need for more complex wound coverage techniques. The VAC system exposes the wound bed to negative pressure in a closed system. The stretching stimulus is transformed into microchemical forces that promote wound healing through increased cell division and proliferation, angiogenesis stimulation, and local increase of growth factors. In addition, edema fluid is removed from the extravascular space, eliminating the extrinsic cause of microcirculatory alteration and improving local blood supply. Although this device does not replace the need for surgical debridement, it may avoid the need for a free tissue transfer in patients with large traumatic wounds. Additional orthopedic indications include the treatment of infected wounds after debridement, war wounds, and fasciotomy closures.

Gunshot Wounds

Gunshot wounds to the musculoskeletal system result in fractures that are often comminuted with related nerve, artery, and tendon involvement. A gunshot wound near a major joint should also be suspected of penetrating the joint. Optimum treatment of fractures caused by gunshots relies upon an appreciation of the kinetic energy of injury, direction, caliber, and distance. Differences between high velocity (>2000 ft/s) and low velocity (<2000 ft/s) are also important. In general, kinetic energy associated with an injury is calculated using the formula, $KE = \frac{1}{2}mv^2$, where m equals mass and v equals velocity. Along with the characteristics of the tissue penetrated, velocity and missile mass are the determinants of resultant type and amount of tissue damage. Velocity is more important than mass; doubling the velocity quadruples the kinetic energy. Shotguns are technically low-velocity weapons, but shotgun injuries are different from single gunshot wounds because typically these injuries are close range, causing extensive bony and soft-tissue damage.

In gunshot and high-velocity missile wounds, tissue damage is caused not only by the bullets but also by the cavitary shock damage it can produce. Shock waves can produce injury in areas that are relatively distant from the direct path of the missile. Cavitation is an important mechanism of tissue damage in high-velocity injuries. For example, hollow-point bullets are designed to mushroom out as they meet tissue resistance. This design causes more soft-tissue cavitary damage while preventing exit through the body. These bullets are routinely used by law enforcement to minimize injury to other individuals from in-and-out bullets. The negative pressure in the cavitary track can also pull in contaminants. Missile wound tracks close to a major vessel may be associated with occult vascular injury despite normal pulses. Doppler ultrasound is indicated when a vascular injury is suspected. A retained bullet or a fragment in the synovial fluid within a joint can cause lead toxicity, provided the bullet or missile contains lead.

The majority of low-velocity gunshot wounds can be managed with local wound care and outpatient treatment. The wound should be left open for drainage. If the fracture requires surgical treatment, antibiotic prophylaxis is recommended. The use of immediate fixation by either internal or external fixator means is controversial. On the one hand, the danger of treatment of these open fractures with foreign material is a deterrent for immediate stabilization. However, in grossly unstable injuries, treatment that would be used for other open fractures appears to be reasonable in selected cases. The use of temporary external fixation as a bridge from the injury to definitive fracture stabilization has become a popular means of initially stabilizing the fracture.

High-velocity ballistic and shotgun injuries require surgical irrigation, appropriate debridement, and at least 24 to 48 hours of intravenous (IV) antibiotic treatment. Vascular injuries should be explored and repaired after prompt fracture stabilization. Distal neurologic deficit alone is not an indication for exploration because it often resolves without surgical intervention and may be due to a blast neuropraxia.

Trauma Patient Scoring Systems

Several classification systems have been developed to facilitate stratification of polytrauma patients according to severity of injury. The classification systems may serve as a guide for both patient treatment and eventual outcomes. The Revised Trauma Score (RTS) was developed to help with patient triage. The scores for systolic blood pressure and respiratory rate are separated into five domains with each assigned a point value from 0 to 4. These scores are added to the GCS to yield an RTS. The GCS is the most accepted score for the clinical assessment of traumatic brain injury. This scale ranges from 3 to 15, with 15 being normal. Evaluation is based on three sections: eye movement, verbal response, and motor response.

The Abbreviated Injury Scale (AIS) divides injuries into nine body regions and stratifies the injuries from minor to fatal on a 6-point scale. These scores take into account life-threatening aspects of injuries, anticipated permanent impairment, treatment, and injury pattern.

The Injury Severity Score (ISS) is the sum of the squares of the highest AIS scores in the three most severely injured body regions, which are chosen from head and neck, chest, abdomen, extremities and pelvic girdle, and external. Multiple-trauma patients are defined as patients with an ISS greater than or equal to 15. The maximum ISS of 75 is considered to be nonsurvivable.

Table 2–3. Mangled Extremity Salvage Score (MESS) variables.

Variables	Score
Skeletal/soft-tissue injury	
Low energy	1
Medium energy	2
High energy	3
Very high energy	4
Limb ischemia	
Pulse reduced or absent but perfusion normal	1[a]
Pulseless, paresthesias, diminished capillary refill	2[a]
Cool, paralyzed, insensate, numb	3[a]
Shock	
Systolic blood pressure always >90 mm Hg	0
Transient hypotension	1
Persistent hypotension	2
Age (years)	
<30	0
30-50	1
>50	2

[a]Score doubled for ischemia >6 hours.

The Mangled Extremity Severity Score (MESS) was developed to help guide the decision on whether or not to attempt limb salvage following major extremity trauma. Factors at the time of injury, which have a bearing on the decision to amputate, include status of the opposite leg, the time of limb ischemia, and the age of the patient (Table 2–3). In the original study, the MESS for salvaged limbs was 3 to 6, and the MESS for amputated limbs was 7 to 12. The MESS was previously used as a predictor of eventual amputation; however, recent studies have shown the MESS and other scoring systems to be not as consistent in predicting the functional outcome for mangled limb patients.

American College of Surgeons. *Advanced Trauma Life Support Manual*, 10th ed. American College of Surgeons; 2018.

Blair JA, Kusnezov N, Fisher T, Prabhakar G, Bader JO, Belmont PJ. Early stabilization of femur fractures in the setting of polytrauma is associated with decreased risk of pulmonary complications and mortality. *J Surg Orthop Adv.* 2019;28(2):137-143. [PMID: 31411960]

Dwyer EP, Moed BR. Venous thromboembolism after hospital discharge in pelvic and acetabular fracture patients treated operatively. *J Orthop Surg (Hong Kong).* 2019;27(1):1-6. [PMID: 30827175]

Firoozabadi R, Alton T, Sagi HC. Heterotopic ossification in acetabular fracture surgery. *J Am Acad Orthop Surg.* 2017;25(2):117-124. [PMID: 28098705]

FLOW Investigators. A trial of wound irrigation in the initial management of open fracture wounds. *N Engl J Med.* 2015;373(27):2629-2641. [PMID: 26448371]

Guerado E, Bertrand ML, Cano JR, Cerván AM, Galán A. Damage control orthopaedics: state of the art. *World J Orthop.* 2019;10(1):1-13. [PMID: 30705836]

Gustilo RB, Anderson JT. Prevention of infection in the treatment of 1025 open fractures of long bones. *J Bone Joint Surg Am.* 1976;58:453. [PMID: 773941]

Halawi MJ, Morwood MP. Acute management of open fractures: an evidence-based review. *Orthopedics.* 2015;38(11):e1025-e1033. [PMID: 26558667]

Mundi R, Chaudry H, Niroopan G, Petrisor B, Bhandari M. Open tibial fractures: updated guidelines for management. *JBJS Rev.* 2015;3(2):e1. [PMID: 27490746]

Sathiyakumar V, Thakore RV, Stinner DJ, Obremsky WT, Ficke JR, Sethi MK. Gunshot-induced fractures of the extremities: a review of antibiotic and debridement practices. *Curr Rev Musculoskeletal Med.* 2015;8:276-289. [PMID: 26047781]

Schmidt AH. Acute compartment syndrome. *Orthop Clin North Am.* 2016;47(3):517-525. [PMID: 27241376]

Weinberg DS, Narayanan AS, Moore TA, Vallier HA. Assessment of resuscitation as measured by markers of metabolic acidosis and features of injury. *J Bone Joint Surg Br.* 2017;99-B(1):122-127. [PMID: 28053267]

Whiting PS, Jahangir AA. Thromboembolic disease after orthopaedic trauma. *Orthop Clin North Am.* 2016;47(2):335-344. [PMID: 26772942]

Whiting PS, White-Dzuro GA, Greenberg SE, et al. Risk factors for deep vein thrombosis following orthopaedic trauma surgery: an analysis of 56,000 patients. *Arch Trauma Res.* 2016;5(1):e32915. [PMID: 27148502]

PRINCIPLES OF FRACTURE FIXATION

- Titanium alloys and stainless steel 316L are the most common materials in fracture implants.
- Improved understanding of fracture mechanics and healing has improved fixation principles.
- Orthobiologics continue to play a larger role in surgical treatment.

Fractures occur when one or more types of stress, in excess of failure strength, are applied to bones. Fractures may occur from axial loading (tension, compression), bending, torsion (a twisting force), or shearing. The type of failure and mechanism of injury may be helpful in determining fracture treatment. Examples of these are shown in Figure 2–6.

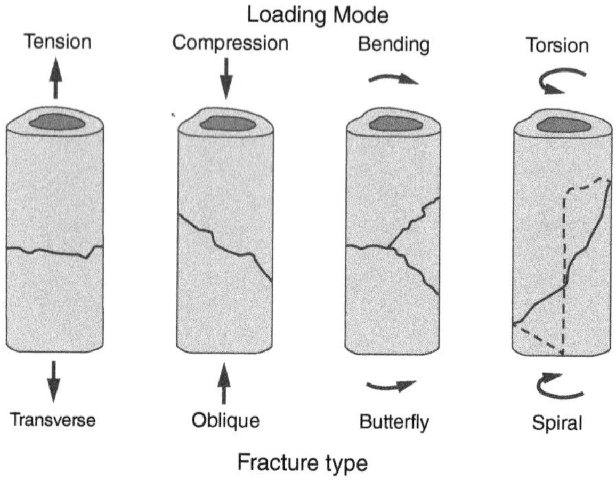

▲ **Figure 2–6. Mechanisms of mechanical failure of bones.** (Reprinted from Browner B, Jupiter J, Krettek C, et al. Skeletal Trauma: Basic Science, Management, and Reconstruction. 2 Vol Set, 4th edition. New York: Elsevier, 2008.)

Biomaterials Used in Fracture Fixation

Operative fracture fixation requires strength and flexibility of the fixation materials. Metal implants made of stainless steel and titanium offer high stiffness and strength and good ductility and are biologically well tolerated. Titanium alloy and stainless steel both may be contoured to fit irregularities without compromising stability. They provide adequate strength and fatigue resistance to permit fracture healing to occur. The elastic modulus of titanium is half that of stainless steel, resulting in half the flexural rigidity in plates of equal size. The modulus measures the material stiffness and its ability to resist deformation when a force is applied. Ductility is the property of a material that undergoes significant plastic deformation before failure. An example of a ductile material is stainless steel.

Biomechanical Principles of Fracture Fixation

Fracture healing requires specific sufficient biologic and mechanical conditions. These conditions are provided by blood supply, inflammatory mediators, hormonal stimuli, and a certain degree of immobilization. By compression of two anatomically reduced fracture fragments, absolute stability can be achieved. A lag screw, compression plate, and a tension band are examples of absolute stability. If there is motion between the fracture fragments, this is called relative stability and promotes indirect bone healing, resulting in callus. Motion should be below strain level of tissue repair. Intramedullary nails, bridge plates, and external fixators are examples of devices that provide relative stability and indirect healing. Frequently, bone healing is a combination of primary and secondary means of healing due to variations in the blood supply and the local mechanical environment.

A. Screws

Screws are the most common and basic form of fixation and function by converting torque, or rotational force, into compression, a linear force. They are used in several ways: lag screws, locking or nonlocked plate screws, and positioning screws. Screws can be used alone or with a plate. Locking screw heads have threads that engage with the threads in the hole of the plate, thus creating a fixed-angle construct. The lag screw technique is a powerful way to compress a fracture and provide stability. This can be achieved by fully or partially threaded screws. An example of a positioning screw is a screw placed between the tibia and fibula in treatment of a syndesmotic injury.

B. Intramedullary Titanium Nails

Intramedullary nails are load-sharing implants that allow circumferential load transmission. The most important point in using an intramedullary nail is the proper entry point. Gentle reaming is superior and safer compared to the unreamed technique. One must pay attention to the general condition of a patient, especially with the multiply injured patient. Reaming and insertion of a femoral nail may exacerbate head/pulmonary injury in the polytrauma patient with preexisting injury. There are many options for the femur, tibia, and humerus nails. We currently recommend that all nails be statically locked. However, the exact number of proximal and distal locking screws for shaft fractures remains controversial. We believe that for shaft fractures with cortical apposition and load transmission, one proximal static screw and one to two distal screws are satisfactory. For shaft fractures with more comminution, less apposition, and less load transmission, one proximal screw and at least two distal screws are preferable.

C. Bone Plate

The placement of a plate on a bone has a significant bearing on its function. Optimal placement of a plate is on the tension side of the bone. A conventional plate and screw system can require substantial surgical exposure for open reduction and internal fixation (ORIF). After reduction of the fracture and/or possible lag screw placement, the plate is applied to the bone and fixed with screws on either side of the fracture. If a lag screw is placed to compress the fracture, the plate is used as a protection plate. The compressive forces acting on the bone-plate interface can compromise the blood supply and hence the healing process. The limited-contact dynamic compression plate (LC-DCP) was developed to reduce the bone-plate contact surface area. During loading, plates typically allow compression opposite the plate.

As mentioned before, locking plates use a system where the screw head threads into the plate hole. Locking the screws into the plate allows the construct to serve as a fixed-angle device. When locking screw/plate constructs fail, either the entire implant backs out or the screws can fail at the head-neck junction. During fixation, the working length of the plate and screws should be kept in mind based on the fracture pattern (eg, longer more flexible plates with fracture comminution). An understanding of fracture mechanics and modulating the flexibility of the implant fixation is important to fracture healing.

D. External Fixation

External fixation is an important treatment modality for musculoskeletal injuries. Five or six mm Schanz screws (pins) are placed above and below the fracture to stabilize it. These pins are attached to an external frame outside the bone and soft-tissue envelope to stabilize fractures. External fixators can be used for temporary or definitive treatment, depending on the patient's physiologic status, the location/type of fracture, and the degree of soft-tissue trauma. In the upper extremity, external fixators play a significant role in treating comminuted distal radius fractures. Factors that affect construct stiffness include: pin diameter, distance between pin/fracture, bone-clamp distance, and number of pins.

For the pelvis, rapidly applied anterior inferior iliac spine or iliac crest external fixation can stabilize the pelvis and close down intrapelvic volume thus facilitating tamponade and reducing blood loss. External fixation of the pelvis is useful in physiologically unstable patients during resuscitation and, in some cases, can provide definitive treatment of pelvic injuries.

For femur and tibia fractures, external fixation provides rapid initial stabilization and can be converted to intramedullary or plate fixation for definitive care once the patient has stabilized.

External fixators are frequently used as provisional treatment for grade III open fractures with segmental bone loss and large soft-tissue injuries of the upper and lower extremity.

Orthobiologics Used in Fracture Fixation

A. Autogenous Bone Grafting

Autologous bone grafting is the gold standard for management of bone defects and nonunions due to a combination of osteogenic (pluripotential cells capable of differentiating into osteoblasts), osteoinductive (factors that induce osteoblast differentiation), and osteoconductive properties (mechanical factors that serves as a scaffold to promote bone formation). Different types of autologous bone grafts have variable properties associated with their structural anatomy. Cancellous grafts are most commonly harvested from the iliac crest. The iliac crest bone graft has been the gold standard of autograft because it is osteogenic, osteoinductive, and osteodconductive; however, it has the potential for donor site morbidity (eg, pain). More recently, the reamer-irrigator-aspirator graft provides larger quantities of autologous bone and is harvested from the femoral and tibial medullary cavities with less morbidity.

B. Osteoconductive Graft Substitutes

Hydroxyapatite and tricalcium phosphate are inorganic structural bone graft substitutes that are primarily osteoconductive. They provide a physical scaffold for bone growth and do not stimulate bone formation. These materials can be injected into fracture sites, such as the distal radius and calcaneus, to provide stabilization from compressive loads. These scaffolds are ideally used in the presence of osteogenic and/or osteoinductive factors.

C. Donor Bone Allografts

Bony allograft is obtained from deceased individuals and is primarily used either as a bone void osteoconductive scaffold and/or for compressive strength (ie, depressed tibial plateau). The greatest concern with using allograft materials is the possibility of viral disease transmission. Several methods may be used to process allograft bone, including low-dose (<20 kGy) irradiation, physical debridement, ultrasonic or pulsatile water washes, ethanol treatment, and antibiotic soaking. Sterilization treatments, such as irradiation and ethylene oxide, are known to compromise the quality to some extent, with ethylene oxide perhaps being worse than irradiation. Freeze-dried bone is convenient for storage at room temperature but must be sterilized secondarily with ethylene oxide. Because ethylene oxide is unable to penetrate into large fragments of bone, secondary sterilization of large structural allografts is safer with radiation. The accepted dosage of gamma radiation is 2.5 mrad, but even this dose may not be sufficient to eradicate the human immunodeficiency virus. Despite these concerns for infection, allograft bone has a safe and effective track record when used appropriately.

D. Osteoinductive Agents

Osteoinductive agents induce differentiation of pluripotential stem cells into osteoblasts. Bone morphogenic proteins (BMPs) are osteoinductive factors and are important components of bone and cartilage repair. With recent advances in molecular biology and recombinant DNA techniques, rhBMP-7 and rhBMP-2 have been used in clinical trials. These proteins can potentially be coupled with an osteoconductive scaffold (ie, collagen matrix) and autogenic blood (ie, hematoma) to stimulate bone healing. Current uses of BMPs include spine fusion and tibial nonunions.

Demineralized bone matrix (DBM) is an osteoinductive and osteoconductive agent containing decalcified bone and growth factors. It is treated to reduce the potential for an immunogenic host reaction and a transmissible infection. The resulting product is a biologic matrix with a variable, non-standardized quantity of growth factors (ie, BMPs). This matrix has the potential to impart a greater osteoinductive effect than standard allograft due to the presence of growth factors.

E. Bone Marrow Aspirate Concentrate

Bone marrow, specifically red marrow, contains two types of adult stem cells: hematopoietic stem cells and MSCs. Recently, autologous bone marrow aspirate has been intensively used in the treatment of various musculoskeletal injuries. Bone marrow aspirate may be harvested from the iliac crest, proximal tibia, distal tibia, or calcaneus; however, the iliac crest has been shown to have a higher concentration of osteoprogenitor cells compared with the distal tibia or calcaneus. Bone marrow aspirate concentrate is used as an adjunct modality for bone healing, hypertrophic nonunions, and cartilage regeneration.

F. Platelet-Rich Plasma

Platelet-rich plasma (PRP) is an autologous concentration of human platelets in a small volume of plasma produced by centrifuging a patient's own blood. Activated platelets release growth factors that stimulate the healing of tissues and positively influence the healing process. PRP has been shown to promote muscle recovery and has demonstrated benefit in select musculoskeletal conditions (eg, epicondylitis). Despite recent advances, however, PRP use in orthopedics remains controversial.

Łapaj Ł, Woźniak W, Wiśniewski T, et al. Breakage of metal hip arthroplasty components: retrieval and structural analysis. *Biomed Mater Eng*. 2019;30(3):297-308. [PMID: 31006657]

Marongiu G, Verona M, Cardoni G, Capone A. Synthetic bone substitutes and mechanical devices for the augmentation of osteoporotic proximal humeral fractures: a systematic review of clinical studies. *J Funct Biomater*. 2020;11(2):E29. [PMID: 32380687]

Schottel PC, Warner SJ. Role of bone marrow aspirate in orthopedic trauma. *Orthop Clin North Am*. 2017;48(3):311-321. [PMID: 28577780]

I. TRAUMA TO THE UPPER EXTREMITY

SHOULDER AND ARM INJURIES

Anatomic and Biomechanical Principles

The humeral shaft extends from the level of the insertion of the pectoralis major muscle proximally to the supracondylar ridge distally. The upper portion of the shaft is cylindrical and then becomes more flattened in an AP direction distally. Medial and lateral intermuscular septae divide the arm into anterior and posterior compartments. In the anterior compartment are the biceps brachii, coracobrachialis, and brachialis muscles, along with the neurovascular bundle coursing along the medial border of the biceps with the brachial artery and vein and the nerves (median, musculocutaneous, and ulnar). In the posterior compartment are the triceps brachii muscle and the radial nerve. Understanding the insertions of the muscle forces around the humerus helps explain the tendency for fractures to displace in predictable patterns based on the influence of these muscles.

The proximal humerus can be separated into the humeral head, the lesser and greater tuberosities, bicipital groove, and proximal humeral shaft. The anatomic neck lies at the junction of the head and the tuberosities. The surgical neck lies below the greater and lesser tuberosities. The major blood supply to the humeral head is through the ascending branch of the anterior humeral circumflex artery, which penetrates the head at the bicipital groove and becomes the arcuate artery. Important structures that lie in the vicinity of the shoulder joint include the axillary nerve, the musculocutaneous nerve, and the brachial plexus and axillary artery, which are anterior to the coracoid process and humeral head. Nerves that innervate muscles around the shoulder include the axillary, suprascapular, subscapular, and musculocutaneous nerves. Fractures of the anatomic neck have a poor prognosis because of complete disruption of the blood supply to the head. Surgical neck fractures are more common, and with these fractures, the blood supply is usually preserved. Within the bicipital groove lies the biceps tendon, which is covered by the transverse humeral ligament. The greater tuberosity provides attachment for the supraspinatus, infraspinatus, and teres minor muscles. The lesser tuberosity is the attachment of the subscapularis muscle. The neck-shaft inclination angle measures an average of 135 degrees, and the humeral head is retroverted an average of about 30 degrees.

The rotator cuff consists of four muscles: the subscapularis, supraspinatus, infraspinatus, and teres minor muscles. The cuff muscles compress the humeral head into the concave glenoid, allowing the deltoid to efficiently elevate the humerus. The infraspinatus and teres minor are the only external rotators, whereas the subscapularis is one of the internal rotators of the humerus. The deltoid and the pectoralis major muscles, along with the rotator cuff, cause predictable displacement of proximal humerus fractures. Additionally, injury to the rotator cuff, independent of bony fractures, needs to be considered when evaluating the shoulder.

Anatomy, biomechanics, and injuries of the clavicle and scapula are discussed in Chapter 3.

A. Nerve Supply

Injuries to the nerves around the shoulders occur with fractures and dislocations. The brachial plexus and axillary artery can also be injured with anterior shoulder dislocations, so neurovascular examination is important. Shoulder dislocations are the most common major joint dislocations and are described in Chapter 3. The radial nerve is commonly injured with humeral shaft fractures, particularly at the junction of the middle and distal third. The Holstein-Lewis fracture is a special spiral fracture that occurs in this location and is discussed in more detail later. Careful evaluation and documentation of radial nerve function is critical. Evaluation should include sensation of the dorsal web space between the thumb and index finger, independent digital extension, and wrist extension.

PROXIMAL HUMERUS FRACTURES

- Second most common fracture of the upper extremity.
- Incidence sharply increases in the elderly.
- The majority of proximal humerus fractures can be treated nonoperatively.

Classification

Neer introduced the concept of proximal humerus parts based on the epiphyseal growth centers that collectively compose the proximal humerus. Parts of the proximal humerus consist of the anatomic neck, surgical neck, greater tuberosity, and lesser tuberosity (Figure 2–7). Parts are considered to be displaced if they are separated by more than 1 cm or angled more than 45 degrees from the normal anatomic position. Other categories include fracture-dislocations and head-splitting injuries. The relationship of the humeral head to the displaced parts in the glenoid, as well as the blood supply, is also taken into consideration.

Clinical Findings

Young individuals sustain these injuries in high-energy accidents, whereas fractures in older patients are usually from lower-energy mechanisms. Clinical presentation is usually with pain, swelling, and ecchymosis. Radiographic evaluation is a cornerstone for diagnosis and planning of treatment. The recommended radiographs are an AP shoulder, AP glehohumeral joint (Grashey view), and either an axillary lateral (if possible) or a scapular-Y view. Other studies such as a CT scan may provide more information for preoperative planning. Rotator cuff injuries can occur with fractures of the tuberosities; however, in most cases, their insertions remain intact on the fractured bone fragments. Because evaluation of the integrity of the rotator cuff may be difficult, an MRI is helpful if there is a high suspicion of soft-tissue injury.

Axillary artery injuries, although uncommon, generally result from fractures or fracture-dislocations in which a medial bone spike injures or penetrates it. The index of suspicion is high if the arm shows significant color differences compared with the uninjured arm. Pulses should be palpated and evaluated by Doppler studies. In late diagnosis, the outcome is determined by the neurologic morbidity, even though the results of acute vascular reconstruction are good. In some cases, collateral circulation around the arm can still provide distal circulation.

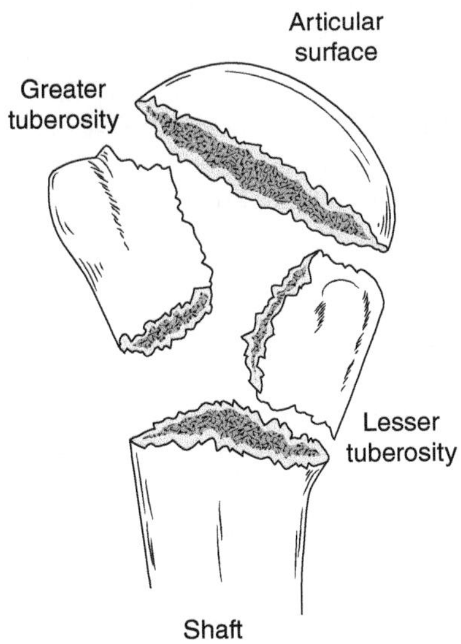

▲ **Figure 2–7.** Different parts of the proximal humerus, per the Neer classification.

Treatment

A. Closed Treatment

Approximately 85% of proximal humerus fractures are minimally displaced or nondisplaced and can be treated nonoperatively with a sling for comfort. More recently, surgical treatment of proximal humerus fractures has not demonstrated cost-efficacy and/or a better functional outcome compared to closed treatment. Low-demand, elderly patients with proximal humerus fractures have similar if not better results with closed treatment compared to surgical treatment. However, other patients (ie, active/younger patients, or those patients with more displaced fractures.) may benefit from surgical treatment of proximal humerus fractures.

The mainstay of closed treatment is initial immobilization and then early motion. After initial pain control, pendulum exercises can begin, along with elbow, wrist, and hand exercises. After 2 weeks, once there is a soft callus, the patient can start pain-free, active-assisted, and passive range of motion. From weeks 4 to 6, the patient can slowly transition from active-assisted/passive range of motion to active-assisted/active motion.

B. Surgical Treatment

Operative treatment of proximal humerus fractures includes closed reduction and percutaneous pinning, intramedullary nails, tension band, ORIF with either conventional plates or locking plates, hemiarthroplasty, and reverse total shoulder arthroplasty. Treatment options will be discussed based on the fracture classification.

C. Two-Part Surgical Neck Fractures

In two-part surgical neck fractures, both tuberosities remain attached to the head, and the rotator cuff, in general, remains intact. The diaphysis is often displaced anteromedially by the pull of the pectoralis major muscle. Reduction may be blocked by interposition of the periosteum, biceps tendon, or deltoid muscle, or by buttonholing of the shaft in the deltoid, pectoralis major, or fascial elements. One attempt at closed reduction is advisable; if this fails, operative intervention is recommended. If, on the other hand, the reduction is successful, percutaneous pinning with fluoroscopy may be an excellent choice for the reducible but unstable fractures. If open reduction is required to remove displaced soft tissues, internal fixation can be accomplished with plate and screw fixation. Locking plates provide angular stability and a favorable bone implant interface for comminuted and osteoporotic fractures. In the osteoporotic patient, wire or suture material for tension banding can be passed through the soft tissues and the rotator cuff, which may be superior to bone for fixation.

Another technique for internal fixation uses intramedullary devices, which can be inserted through a limited deltoid-splitting incision; however, the control of rotational alignment is poor. For elderly (>75 years) or debilitated patients, this may be the best solution to achieve overall alignment with minimal surgical morbidity.

D. Three-Part and Four-Part Fractures

Optimal treatment of three- and four-part fractures of the proximal part of the humerus in patients with poor bone quality is controversial. Although ORIF can provide potential earlier range of motion and pain relief, it has not yielded improved outcomes in the elderly. Complications with ORIF include screw cut-out, avascular necrosis (AVN), and malunion. AVN in three-part proximal humerus fractures has been reported to be as high as 27%. The Atlas Orthogonal (AO) buttress plate has had significant complications, including a high rate of AVN related to degree of soft-tissue dissection, superior placement of the plate with secondary impingement, loss of plate and screw fixation, malunion, and infections. Locking plates have improved fracture stability and healing. Figure 2–8 demonstrates ORIF of a left four-part proximal humerus fracture-dislocation. The inferior screw along the calcar is biomechanically important, and care should be taken to ensure no intraarticular screw placement (ie, check screw position on numerous radiographic views). Screw cut-out is the most common complication. Locking screws are preferable to cortical screws in patients with poor bone to prevent implant failure and re-displacement. Historically, fibular grafts were used to improve screw purchase in the humeral head but have been more recently replaced by calcium-based cements. The use of angular stable plating that allows cement augmentation of the screws is controversial. Intramedullary nail fixation can also be used, but impingement and rod migration in the elderly are potential complications. Fixation of valgus impacted fractures results in a lower rate of AVN if the posteromedial fracture fragment is intact. In the less active or elderly (>75 years) patient, the accepted method of treatment is a hemiarthroplasty with rotator cuff repair or reverse total shoulder arthroplasty. Hemiarthroplasty should be considered in others with head-splitting fractures since either poor bone quality or potential for AVN precludes a satisfactory outcome. Reverse shoulder arthroplasty is preferred for low-demand elderly patients with poor bone and nonreconstructible

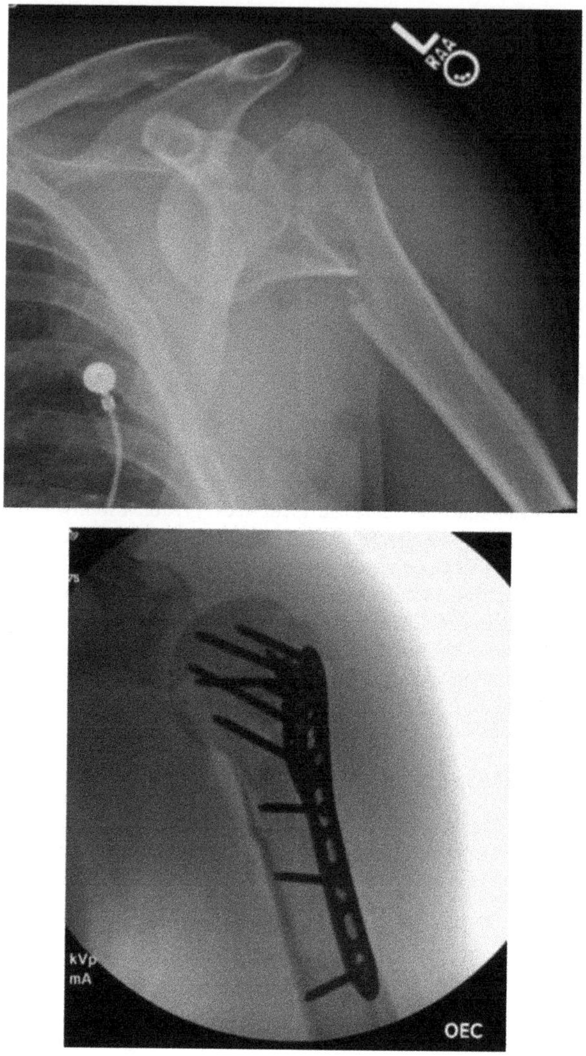

▲ **Figure 2–8.** Pre- and intraoperative anteroposterior radiographs of a left four-part proximal humerus fracture-dislocation.

tuberosities. In younger patients, ORIF may be possible even in comminuted fractures. During ORIF, it is important to ensure repair of the tuberosities to the plate. The age of the patient, the quality of the bone, the fracture pattern, and the amount of comminution are all important considerations in developing a treatment plan. Appropriate prosthesis level and humeral retroversion, as well as the attachment of greater and lesser tuberosities, are critical in achieving a good result. Repair of any rotator cuff defects is important to prevent proximal migration of the humerus and improve shoulder range of motion. Several studies have demonstrated that reverse total shoulder arthroplasty has minimal benefit over nonoperative treatment of three- and four-part proximal humerus fractures in the elderly population. With rehabilitation postoperatively, generally good pain relief can be expected; however, shoulder function may be limited.

E. Two-Part Anatomic Neck Fractures

Two-part anatomic neck fractures are rare, and no single optimal method of management has been established. Closed reduction is difficult because controlling the articular fragment, which is usually rotated and angulated within the joint capsule, is difficult. The fragment can be preserved in a young (<40 years) patient via ORIF with pins or interfragmentary screws. It may be difficult to obtain adequate screw purchase without violating the articular surface. Additionally, the prognosis for head survival is poor because the blood supply is usually completely disrupted. In general, arthroplasty provides the most predictable result in the elderly (>75 years).

F. Two-Part Greater Tuberosity Fractures

Greater tuberosity fractures generally displace posteriorly and superiorly because of traction by the supraspinatus and infraspinatus muscles. This is often associated with anterior glenohumeral dislocation. It is appropriate to attempt closed reduction, which may result in an acceptable position for the greater tuberosity. Neer has reported that displacement of the fragment by more than 1 cm is pathognomonic of a rotator cuff defect. The result of fracture healing in this position is subacromial impingement, with limitation of elevation and external rotation. ORIF is recommended if displacement is greater than 5 mm; some recommend ORIF with greater than 3 mm of displacement in overhead athletes to minimize later impingement syndrome. A variety of methods, including screws, pins, wires, and suture, can be used to repair the greater tuberosity. Treatment of this condition should be directed at bony and rotator cuff repairs. Percutaneous pinning tends to be inadequate for preventing re-displacement of greater tuberosity fractures. Screw fixation may be better, especially in young patients with good bone. Tension-band or nonabsorbable suture techniques can be used for osteoporotic bone.

G. Two-Part Lesser Tuberosity Fractures

If the displaced fragment (usually medially by the subscapularis) is small, closed reduction of this rare injury is satisfactory. This fracture may be associated with posterior dislocation and may be treated by closed reduction in the acute setting. The position of immobilization in this case would be either neutral or slight external rotation to minimize recurrent dislocation. Larger fragments may require internal fixation.

H. Fracture-Dislocations

Fracture-dislocations require reduction of the humeral head, and their management is generally based on the fracture pattern. These injuries usually produce impression defects or head-splitting fractures, with concomitant posterior dislocation. Management is determined by the size of the impression defect and the duration of persistent locked dislocation. Fractures of less than 20% will generally be stable with closed reduction and can be treated with immobilization in external rotation for 6 weeks to restore long-term stability. If the defect is 20% to 50%, however, transfer of the lesser tuberosity with the subscapularis tendon into the defect by open means is indicated.

Ciric D, Mischler D, Qawasmi F, et al. Secondary 50% or perforation risk in plate osteosynthesis of unstable proximal humerus fractures: a biomechanical investigation of the effect of screw length. *J Orthop Res*. 2019;37(12):2625-2633. [PMID: 3135092]

Gallinet D, Cazeneuve JF, Boyer E, et al. Reverse shoulder arthroplasty for recent proximal humerus fractures: outcomes in 422 cases. *Orthop Traumatol Surg Res*. 2019;105(5):805-811. [PMID: 31279769]

Han RJ, Sing DC, Feeley BT, Ma CB, Zhang AL. Proximal humerus fragility fractures: recent trends in nonoperative and operative treatment in the Medicare population. *J Shoulder Elbow Surg*. 2016;25(2):256-261. [PMID: 26440695]

Handoll HH, Keding A, Corbacho B, Brealey SD, Hewitt C, Rangan A. Five-year follow-up results of the PROFHER trial comparing operative and non-operative treatment of adults with a displaced fracture of the proximal humerus. *Bone Joint J*. 2017;99-B(3):383-392. [PMID: 28249980]

Lopiz Y, Alcobía-Díaz B, Galán-Olleros M, García-Fernández C, Picado AL, Marco F. Reverse shoulder arthroplasty versus nonoperative treatment for 3- or 4-part proximal humeral fractures in elderly patients: a prospective randomized controlled trial. *J Shoulder Elbow Surg*. 2019;28(12):2259-2271. [PMID: 31500986]

Nowak LL, Vicente MR, McKee MD, Hall JA, Nauth A, Schemitsch EH. Orthopaedic surgeons' opinions surrounding the management of proximal humerus fractures: an international survey. *Int Orthop*. 2017;41(9):1749-1755. [PMID: 28730322]

Rangan A, Handoll H, Brealey S, et al. Surgical vs nonsurgical treatment of adults with displaced fractures of the proximal humerus: the PROFHER randomized clinical trial. *JAMA*. 2015; 313(10):1037-1047. [PMID: 25756440]

Schliemann B, Wähnert D, Theisen C, et al. How to enhance the stability of locking plate fixation of proximal humerus fractures? An overview of current biomechanical and clinical data. *Injury*. 2015;46(7):1207-1214. [PMID: 25978864]

HUMERAL SHAFT FRACTURES

- Account for 3% to 5% of all fractures.
- Primary radial nerve injury in 4% to 22%.
- Most humeral shaft fractures can be managed nonoperatively.

Fractures of the shaft of the humerus usually result from a direct blow, a fall, an automobile injury, or a crushing injury. Humeral shaft fractures have a bimodal age distribution; young patients sustain this injury with high-energy trauma and elderly patients with low-energy injuries. Missiles from firearms or shell fragments may pierce the arm and cause an open fracture. Other indirect means of injury, such as a fall on an outstretched upper extremity or violent muscle contracture, can cause midshaft fractures.

Classification

Fractures are classified according to whether they are open or closed and according to the level of the fracture in relation to the insertions of the pectoralis major and deltoid muscles. Characteristics of the fracture and associated injuries are also factors. Fractures can be located in the proximal, middle, or distal part of the humerus. They can be classified as spiral, transverse, or comminuted. Holstein-Lewis fracture is a special spiral fracture that occurs at the distal one-third of the humeral shaft. The radial nerve travels adjacent to the posterior aspects of the humerus, and it exits the spiral groove an average of 12.6 cm above the joint. It penetrates through the lateral intermuscular septum into the anterior compartment. Because of the close relationship with the radial nerve, fractures at this level are associated with neuropraxia of the radial nerve, and the incidence of a radial nerve palsy with a Holstein-Lewis fracture is about 22%.

Clinical Findings

Clinical signs and symptoms include a shortened extremity with crepitus and pain at the diaphysis of the humerus. Confirmation should be obtained by radiographs in two planes. Both the shoulder and elbow joints should be thoroughly evaluated, clinically and radiographically, as should the neurovascular status. Radial nerve function should be evaluated and documented.

Treatment

A. Closed Treatment

The majority of closed humeral shaft fractures can achieve union via nonsurgical management due to the excellent vascularity and surrounding soft tissues. Historically, immobilization was provided by shoulder spica casts, hanging arm casts, Thomas arm splints, modified Velpeau dressings, and coaptation splints. The musculature of the upper arm will accommodate 20 degrees of anterior angulation, 30 degrees of varus angulation, and 3 cm of shortening without apparent deformity and functional loss.

Contemporary nonoperative treatment consists of an immobilization period in a coaptation splint with a cuff and collar followed by a functional brace once swelling decreases in about 2 weeks. This technique was initially popularized in 1977 by Sarmiento, and he achieved a 98% union rate in a series of 920 patients with humeral shaft fractures treated in a functional brace. The functional brace is ready-made or custom-made from thermoplastic materials and fixed with Velcro straps that can be adjusted to achieve the appropriate level of compression. Repeat radiographs are checked, and healing is expected in 8 to 12 weeks. Holstein-Lewis fractures can also be treated conservatively without added risk. Closed treatment requires initial weekly radiographic evaluations to ensure the fracture does not displace. Patients with a larger body habitus may develop more varus angulation compared with slimmer patients. Ideally, the vertical position of the arm should be maintained even at night in a cuff and collar and not a sling. Spiral, comminuted, and oblique fractures heal more reliably due to the larger surface area and have potential to consolidate and bridge over a larger zone of injury. These fracture patterns typically tolerate more strain in specific planes than fractures with limited contact area between fragments such as transverse fractures, which may have more difficulty in achieving union because of this and rotational instability.

1. External fixation—External fixation can be used for humeral shaft fractures when there are burns, gunshot wounds, or severe comminuted open injuries with defects of skin, bone, and soft tissue. Other indications include osteomyelitis and infected nonunions. Complications include pin tract infections, nonunion, and neurovascular injury.

B. Open Treatment

Humeral fractures tolerate more deformity than other long bones due to the high degrees of freedom at the shoulder and elbow. However, circumstances may warrant ORIF (Table 2–4). Indications to repair humeral shaft fractures may vary from patient to patient, and include greater than 20 degrees of anterior angulation, greater than 30 degrees of varus/valgus angulation, or greater than 3 cm of shortening. Other factors that are indications for surgery are comminuted and segmental fractures and/or polytrauma. In multiply injured patients, ORIF of the upper extremity can potentially help with mobilization on a platform walker. Recent advances in internal fixation techniques and instrumentation have led to ORIF of more fractures. There are three general methods of internal fixation, described next.

Table 2–4. Indications for surgical treatment of humeral shaft fractures.

Absolute Indications	Relative Indications
Open fracture	Bilateral humerus fractures
Vascular injury requiring repair	Polytrauma with lower extremity fracture
Brachial plexus injury	Pathologic fracture
Ipsilateral forearm fracture (floating elbow)	Segmental fracture
Intraarticular fracture	Neurologic loss after penetrating trauma
	Failure of closed management
	Obesity (predisposes to deformity)
	Radial nerve palsy after manipulation (controversial)

1. Plate fixation—Most midshaft humeral shaft fractures can be treated with 3.5-mm LC-DCP plates via an anterolateral approach (Figure 2–9). These plates have been demonstrated to be strong enough to allow weight bearing. The radial nerve should be identified between the brachialis and brachioradialis distally. For distal fractures, a posterior approach may be more advantageous to expose both the shaft and the elbow. For a posterior approach, the radial nerve should be identified and protected. It exits the spiral groove at an average of 12.6 cm above the joint (Figure 2–10). Biomechanical studies in synthetic and cadaveric models have shown locking screws do not offer benefit in plate fixation of humeral shaft fractures because of the thick humeral cortices.

2. Intramedullary nailing—Intramedullary nails have potential advantages over plates and screws. The intramedullary

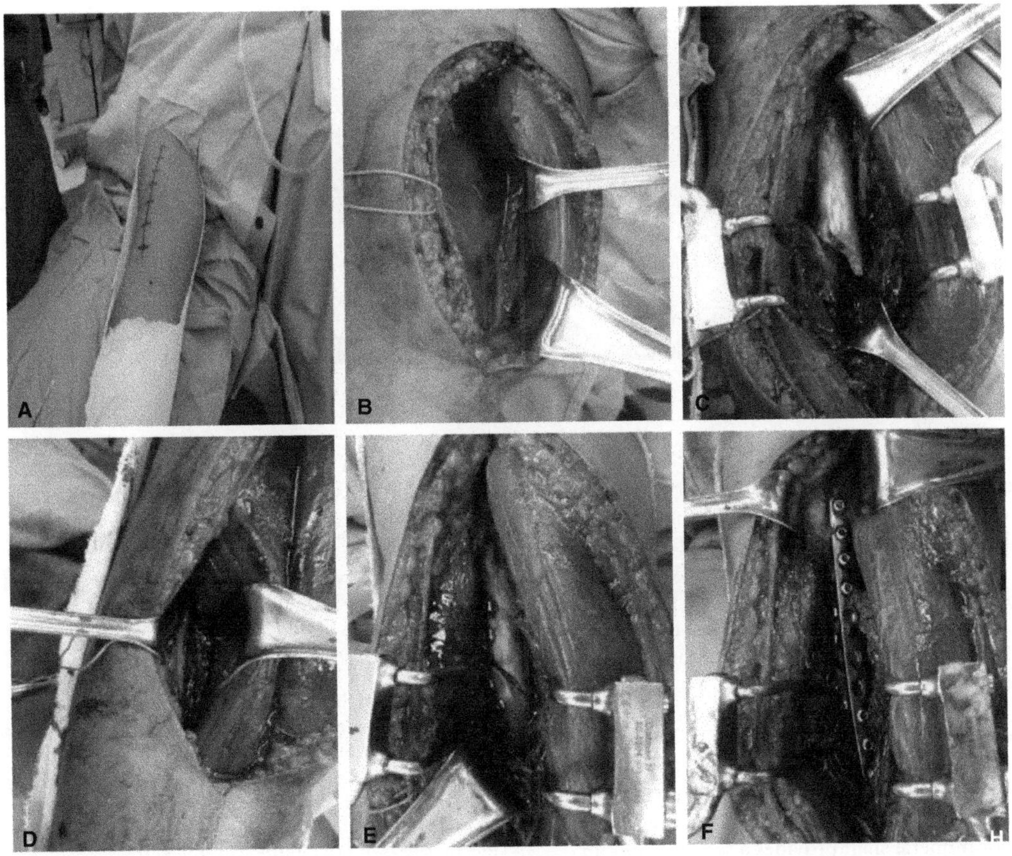

▲ **Figure 2–9.** Anterior approach to the right humerus. **A:** The patient is positioned supine on a hand table. **B:** The biceps is retracted medially to reveal the musculocutaneous nerve. **C:** After the brachialis is split, the fracture is identified. **D:** The radial nerve is identified between the brachialis and brachioradialis. **E:** The fracture is reduced and fixed with 3.5-mm lag screws. **F:** A 4.5-mm narrow limited-contact dynamic compression plate is used as a protection plate due to the patient's larger body habitus. Preoperative (**G** and **H**) and postoperative (**I** and **J**) anteroposterior and lateral radiographs of the right humerus.

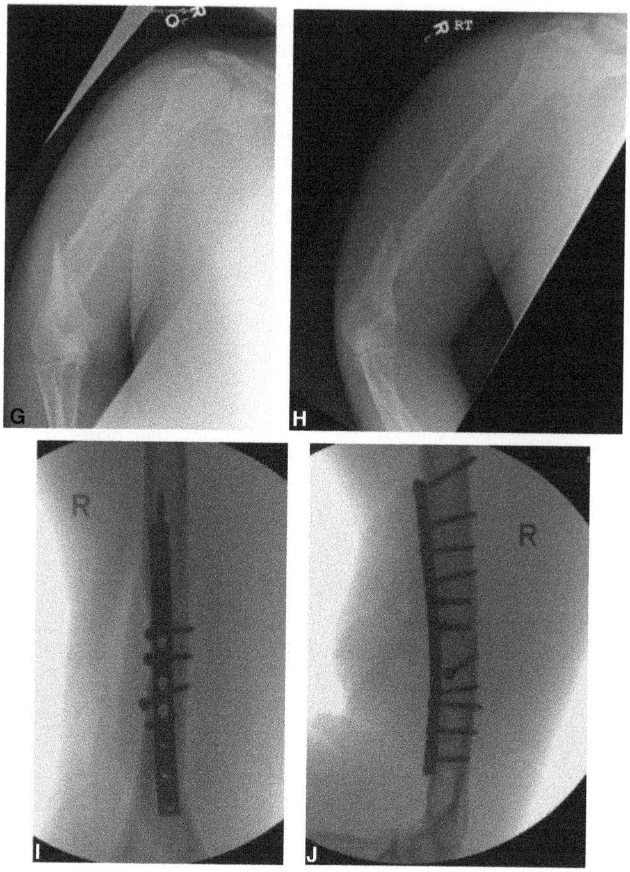

▲ **Figure 2–9.** *(Continued)*

nail is closer to the normal mechanical axis and can act as a load-sharing device if there is cortical contact. Further, there is no soft-tissue and/or periosteal stripping of the fracture. Numerous studies have demonstrated that locked intramedullary humeral nails have similar union rates and functional outcomes to plate fixation. However, there is a significant risk of shoulder complications and reoperation from rotator cuff injury. Retrograde nailing has similar union rates but with a risk of delay in gaining elbow function.

3. Minimally invasive plate osteosynthesis (MIPO)—MIPO is an alternative method for the surgical management of humeral shaft fractures. Using anterior incisions proximally and distally, the plate is inserted percutaneously as a bridge plate. The anterior humeral shaft provides a safe location for plate application. MIPO can be applied to transverse fractures, spiral fractures, segmental fractures, and comminuted fractures with excellent functional results. Shoulder complications are avoided, but the surgeon should be especially careful to avoid injury to the radial nerve.

Given the high rate of spontaneous recovery of radial nerve palsy in closed humeral shaft fractures, early nerve exploration and fracture fixation are not indicated unless there is an open fracture, vascular injury, high-velocity gunshot injury, severe soft-tissue injury, or manipulation-induced secondary radial nerve injury.

Ali E, Griffiths D, Obi N, Tytherleigh-Strong G, Van Rensburg L. Nonoperative treatment of humeral shaft fractures revisited. *J Shoulder Elbow Surg*. 2015;24(2):210-214. [PMID: 25088479]

Hohmann E, Glatt V, Tetsworth K. Minimally invasive plating versus either open reduction and plate fixation or intramedullary nailing of humeral shaft fractures: a systematic review and meta-analysis of randomized controlled trials. *J Shoulder Elbow Surg*. 2016;25(10):1634-1642. [PMID: 27522336]

Kurup H, Hossain M, Andrew JG. Dynamic compression plating versus locked intramedullary nailing for humeral shaft fractures in adults. *Cochrane Database Syst Rev*. 2011;6:CD005959. [PMID: 21678350]

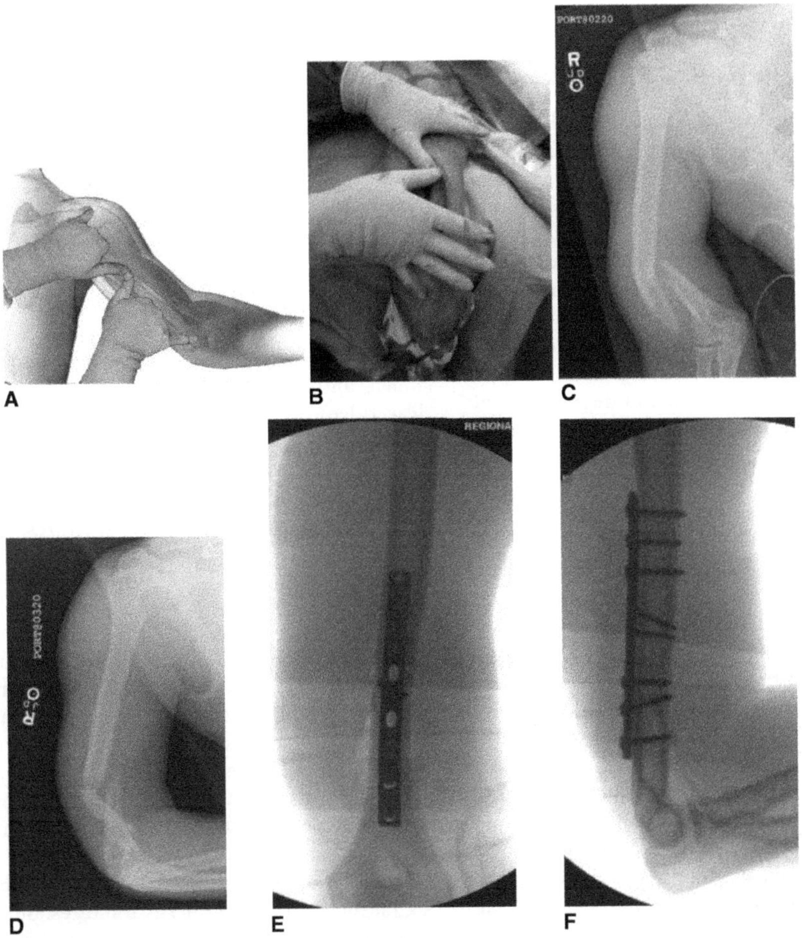

▲ **Figure 2–10.** **A** and **B:** Approximate location of the radial nerve for a posterior approach to the humerus. Preoperative (**C** and **D**) and postoperative (**E** and **F**) anteroposterior and lateral x-rays of a right humerus fracture fixed via a posterior approach. (Figure A: © Bernie Kida, Reprinted with permission.)

Matsunaga FT, Tamaoki MJ, Matsumoto MH, Netto NA, Faloppa F, Belloti JC. Minimally invasive osteosynthesis with a bridge plate versus a functional brace for humeral shaft fractures: a randomized controlled trial. *J Bone Joint Surg Am.* 2017;99(7):583-592. [PMID: 28375891]

Rocchi M, Tarallo L, Mugnai R, Adani R. Humerus shaft fracture complicated by radial nerve palsy: is surgical exploration necessary? *Musculoskelet Surg.* 2016;100(suppl 1):53-60. [PMID: 27900704]

Scaglione M, Fabbri L, Dell'Omo D, Goffi A, Guido G. The role of external fixation in the treatment of humeral shaft fractures: a retrospective case study review on 85 humeral fractures. *Injury.* 2015;46(2):265-269. [PMID: 25530408]

Shields E, Sundem L, Childs S, et al. Factors predicting patient-reported functional outcome scores after humeral shaft fractures. *Injury.* 2015;46(4):693-698. [PMID: 25697858]

Shields E, Sundem L, Childs S, et al. The impact of residual angulation on patient reported functional outcome scores after non-operative treatment for humeral shaft fractures. *Injury.* 2016;47(4):914-918. [PMID: 26754807]

Tetsworth K, Hohmann E, Glatt V. Minimally invasive plate osteosynthesis of humeral shaft fractures: current state of the art. *J Am Acad Orthop Surg.* 2018;26(18):652-661. [PMID: 30113346]

Updegrove GF, Mourad W, Abboud JA. Humeral shaft fractures. *J Shoulder Elbow Surg.* 2018;27(4):e87-e97. [PMID: 29292035]

Wang C, Li J, Li Y, Dai G, Wang M. Is minimally invasive plating osteosynthesis for humeral shaft fracture advantageous compared with the conventional open technique? *J Shoulder Elbow Surg.* 2015;24(11):1741-1748. [PMID: 26480879]

INJURIES AROUND THE ELBOW

Anatomic and Biomechanical Principles

On cross-section, the humerus is circular at the midshaft but flared and flattened at the distal end. The distal humerus consists of an arch formed by two condyles. The lateral condyle serves as part of the ulnatrochlear hinge joint. The medial condyle serves as part of the radiocapitellar joint. The ulnohumeral joint allows the flexion and extension of the joint, and the radiocapitellar joint allows forearm rotation. The proximal ulna, which articulates with the trochlea, contains the olecranon process posteriorly, the coronoid process anteriorly, and the greater sigmoid or semilunar notch. The trochlea has a 300-degree arch of cartilage. The medial column diverges from the humeral shaft at a 45-degree angle, and the lateral column diverges at a 20-degree angle.

The triceps has a broad tendinous insertion into the olecranon posteriorly; anteriorly, the brachialis inserts on the coronoid process and the tuberosity of the ulna. The radial head is stabilized anteriorly and posteriorly by the annular ligament and aligns with the capitellum. The medial epicondyle is the origin of the ulnar collateral ligament and the flexor-pronator group of muscles. The most important portion of the ulnar collateral ligament is the anterior portion that attaches to the coronoid process. The supinator-extensor muscle group attaches to the lateral epicondyle, which is slightly proximal and lateral to the capitellum. Effusions can be discerned by swelling between the lateral epicondyle and the olecranon. The ulnar nerve passes through the cubital tunnel at the medial column of the elbow and must be appropriately assessed following injury. The ulnar nerve enters the anterior forearm by traveling between the two heads of the flexor carpi ulnaris. A complete neurovascular examination of the radial, median, ulnar, and anterior/posterior interosseous nerves should be performed before and after treatment.

DISTAL HUMERUS FRACTURES

- Account for 30% of elbow fractures.
- Intercondylar distal humerus fractures are the most common pattern.
- Surgical treatment is similar to other intraarticular fractures (ie, anatomic reduction and internal fixation).
- Parallel and orthogonal plates have equivalent results.

Distal humerus fractures are among the most challenging fractures treated by the orthopedic surgeon. The usual mechanism of injury is axial loading of the ulna in the trochlear groove. Studies have demonstrated increasing numbers of these injuries in the older (>60 years) population. It is critical to assess the integrity of the medial and lateral columns for repairable bone fragments and the degree of comminution. In addition, the amount of articular displacement may affect the surgical approach (eg, olecranon osteotomy, triceps sparing).

Classification

Distal humerus fractures are classified as supracondylar, distal single column, and distal bicolumnar fractures. Single and bicolumnar fractures are intraarticular fractures and have respective subclassifications. Single column condyle fractures are classified as Milch type I (lateral trochlear ridge intact) and Milch type II (fracture through the lateral trochlear ridge). Bicolumnar distal humerus fractures are classified using the Jupiter classification based on fracture line configuration: high T, low T, Y, H, medial lambda, lateral lambda, and multiplane T. Other intraarticular fractures include capitellum and trochlea fractures.

Treatment

Treatment options for distal humerus fractures include closed management, ORIF, total elbow arthroplasty (TEA), and rarely, elbow arthrodesis. Closed management of distal humerus fractures is reserved for poor surgical candidates, those with limited arm function such as paralysis, and nondisplaced fractures. Casting should be applied in supination for lateral condyle fractures and in pronation for medial condyle fractures.

ORIF is the preferred treatment for displaced intra- and extraarticular distal humerus fractures. Surgical approaches depend on the fracture type. Extraarticular fractures can potentially be reduced and fixed via either a triceps-splitting or triceps-sparing approach because the joint does not need to be visualized. Surgical approaches for intraarticular fractures of the distal humerus include olecranon osteotomy, triceps-reflecting (Bryan-Morrey), triceps-splitting, and triceps-sparing (paratricipital). During the surgical approach, the ulnar nerve should be identified, and care should be taken to avoid excessive traction.

The intraarticular fracture fragments should be anatomically repaired with lag screw fixation across the spindle and bridging the lateral and medial condyles, and the articular surface is then reduced to the metadiaphysis and fixed with small fragment precontoured plates. Figure 2–11 demonstrates orthogonal plating of a right intraarticular distal humerus fracture with an olecranon osteotomy. Results are equivalent with either parallel or orthogonal plates. For larger bone fragments, long columnar screws can also be used; however, care should be taken not to cause rotational malreduction during final tightening of these screws. Surgical complications of distal

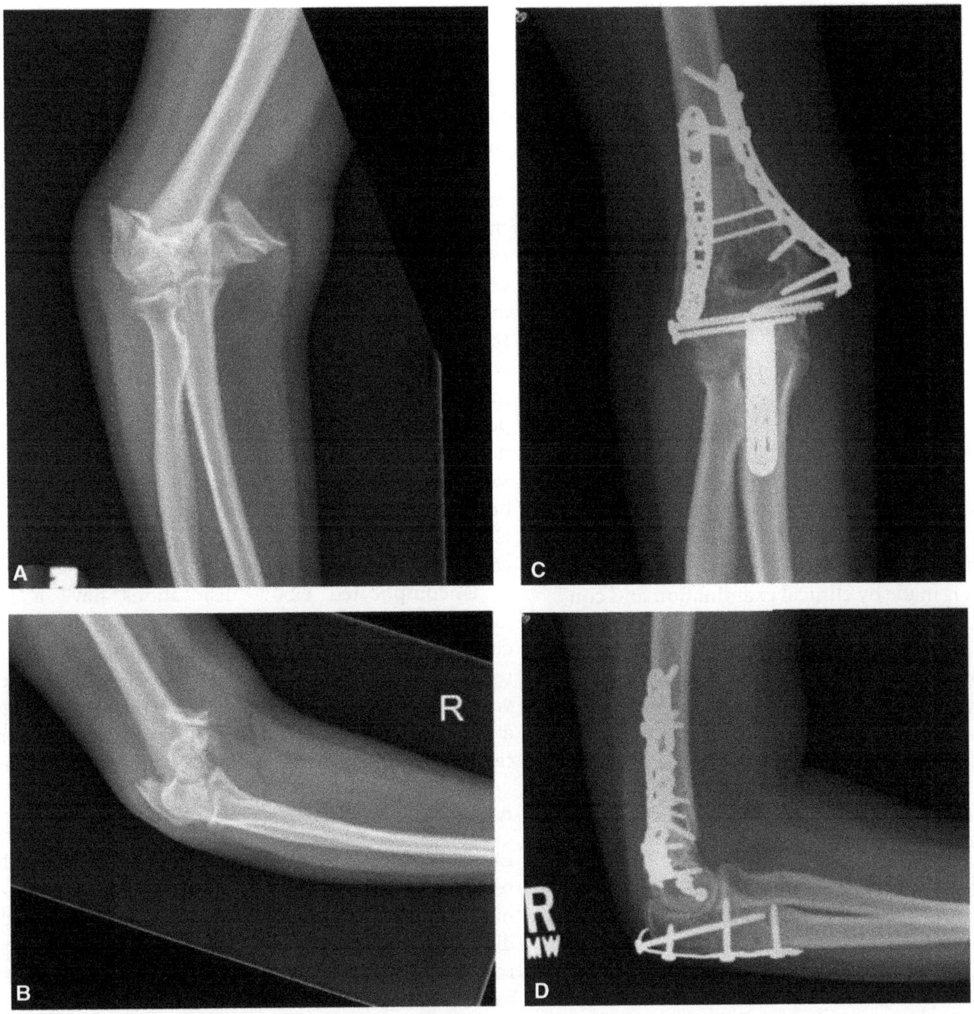

▲ **Figure 2–11.** Preoperative (**A** and **B**) and postoperative radiographs (**C** and **D**) of a right intercondylar distal humerus fracture fixed via a posterior approach to the elbow via an olecranon osteotomy.

humerus fracture include nonunion, malunion, heterotopic ossification, ulnar neuropathy, failure of olecranon osteotomy, and elbow stiffness. Heterotopic ossification is seen in 8% of surgically treated patients; however, routine prophylaxis is not indicated due to the adverse effects of NSAIDs on bone healing.

TEA is generally reserved for distal humerus fractures in the elderly with osteoporotic bone. Newer implant designs have improved over time; however, potential complications remain, including infection and mechanical failure.

Treatment of medial or lateral condyle fractures includes closed management for minimally or nondisplaced fractures. Splinting or casting in supination or pronation can be used for closed treatment of lateral or medial condyle fractures, respectively. Surgical treatment via one of the aforementioned approaches is performed for displaced fractures. Screw-only fixation may be used for fractures with larger bony fragments and adequate bone quality.

Although lateral epicondylar fractures are rare, medial epicondylar fractures are fairly common, especially among children or adolescents. They commonly present as avulsion fractures. Treatment depends on the amount of displacement. If displacement is minimal, then closed reduction is appropriate. A displaced fracture may require percutaneous pinning or open reduction. Elbow instability is not generally a problem; however, irritation of the ulnar nerve can result. If a displaced fracture results in ulnar symptoms or is itself symptomatic, the fragment can be excised at a later date.

ELBOW DISLOCATION

- Posterolateral elbow dislocation is the most common dislocation.
- The second most common major joint dislocation.
- There may be associated fractures and/or soft-tissue injures.

Posterior Elbow Dislocations

Posterolateral dislocations of the elbow are more common than anterior dislocations. They occur via an axially directed force to an extended elbow with the forearm in supination. Both collateral ligaments can be injured, and ligamentous disruption usually progresses from lateral to medial. Diagnosis is made by clinical examination and confirmed by radiographs. The affected extremity is typically shortened, and the elbow is held slightly flexed with inability to flex and extend the elbow. A careful neurovascular examination should be performed and documented. Concomitant injuries of the shoulder and elbow occur in 10% to 15% of cases.

Anterior Elbow Dislocations

Anterior dislocations are relatively rare. Soft-tissue damage is typically severe. Treatment is similar to that for posterior dislocations, except that the method of reduction is reversed.

Medial and Lateral Elbow Dislocations

The radius and ulna may be displaced medially or laterally. Some semblance of joint motion may be present with lateral dislocations, as the ulna may be displaced into the groove between the trochlea and the capitellum. The AP elbow radiograph is diagnostic.

Isolated Ulnar Dislocations

Isolated ulnar dislocations occur when the humerus pivots around the radial head, causing the coronoid process to be displaced posterior to the humerus or the olecranon anterior to the humerus. The more common injury is posterior dislocation, which causes cubitus varus deformity of the forearm. Traction in extension and supination reduces the ulna.

Treatment

Treatment is initiated after documenting the neurovascular examination. A closed reduction should be performed. Traction on the extremity with correction of the initial displacement usually produces reduction with a "clunk." The elbow is put through a flexion-extension and pronation-supination range of motion to evaluate for instability and to ensure that there is no soft-tissue or mechanical blockage. The elbow is generally splinted in 45 to 90 degrees of flexion for patient comfort and to maintain stability. Postreduction radiographs are necessary to confirm reduction and to evaluate for occult fracture. Motion is instituted as soon as possible, generally within 5 to 10 days, to prevent elbow stiffness. Maintenance of reduction is necessary, and radiographs should be taken periodically if any doubt exists. Unstable reductions are rare; however, if encountered, hinged external fixation is necessary. Immobilization for longer periods may be necessary because a stiff but stable elbow is preferable to an unstable elbow. A lateral ulnar collateral ligament injury can be a cause of recurrent instability.

Uncomplicated elbow dislocations have a favorable long-term prognosis. A loss of 5 to 10 degrees of extension compared with the contralateral elbow can be expected. Posterolateral dislocation has been associated with persistent valgus instability in some patients, which is associated with a worse clinical result. If instability is persistent after reduction or there is entrapment of soft tissue, surgery is indicated.

A. Delayed Treatment

Elbow dislocations are best reduced immediately. Late reduction of elbow dislocations is possible with closed techniques weeks from the time of injury; however, they can be difficult to reduce and are best performed in the operating room. Forceful reduction should be avoided because it can cause a fracture. Dislocations left untreated for longer periods generally require open reduction techniques. Improved function with less flexion contracture after open reduction of posterior dislocations is obtained by lengthening the triceps tendon.

B. Elbow Dislocation and Coronoid Fracture

An elbow dislocation and an associated fracture of the coronoid process increase the risk of recurrent and chronic instability. The size of the coronoid fragment dictates the classification: a small marginal fragment (Reagan-Morrey type I), a larger fragment (Reagan-Morrey type II), or a fragment that includes the insertion of the anterior bundle of the ulnar collateral ligament (Reagan-Morrey type III). The decision to fix a coronoid fracture should be based on elbow stability. Even small rim fractures may require surgical fixation if instability is present after repair of associated fractures. When there is greater than 50% loss of the coronoid, fixation is mandatory according to cadaveric studies.

Interfragmentary lag screws can be used to fix a large coronoid fragment.

C. Elbow Dislocation With Radial Head and Coronoid Fractures

An elbow dislocation with an associated radial head and coronoid fracture ("the terrible triad" can be difficult to treat. The most common problems are recurrent and chronic elbow instability, stiffness, posttraumatic arthrosis, and pain. Appropriate treatment should include ORIF of the coronoid fracture and/or repair of the anterior capsule, ORIF or replacement of the radial head, and repair of the lateral collateral ligament complex. Residual instability after treatment is an indication for ulnar collateral ligament repair and/or application of a hinged external fixator.

Atalar AC, Tunalı O, Erşen A, Kapıcıoğlu M, Sağlam Y, Demirhan MS. Biomechanical comparison of orthogonal versus parallel double plating systems in intra-articular distal humerus fractures. *Acta Orthop Traumatol Turc.* 2017;51(1):23-28. [PMID: 27965047]

Dehghan N, Furey M, Schemitsch L, et al. Long-term outcomes of total elbow arthroplasty for distal humeral fracture: results from a prior randomized clinical trial. *J Shoulder Elbow Surg.* 2019;28(11):2198-2204. [PMID: 31445787]

Savvidou OD, Zampeli F, Koutsouradis P, et al. Complications of open reduction and internal fixation of distal humerus fractures. *EFORT Open Rev.* 2018;3(10):558-567. [PMID: 30662764]

Tarassoli P, McCann P, Amirfeyz R. Complex instability of the elbow. *Injury.* 2017;48(3):568-577. [PMID: 24161720]

Taylor PA, Owen JR, Benfield CP, Wayne JS, Boardman ND 3rd. Parallel plating of simulated distal humerus fractures demonstrates increased stiffness relative to orthogonal plating with a distal humerus locking plate system. *J Orthop Trauma.* 2016; 30(4):e118-e122. [PMID: 26529123]

Tunalı O, Erşen A, Pehlivanoğlu T, Bayram S, Atalar AC, Demirhan M. Evaluation of risk factors for stiffness after distal humerus plating. *Int Orthop.* 2018;42(4):921-926. [PMID: 29392385]

Von Keudell A, Kachooei AR, Moradi A, Jupiter JB. Outcome of surgical fixation of lateral column distal humerus fractures. *J Orthop Trauma.* 2016;30(5):245-250. [PMID: 26709815]

Wyrick JD, Dailey SK, Gunzenhaeuser JM, Casstevens EC. Management of complex elbow dislocations: a mechanistic approach. *J Am Acad Orthop Surg.* 2015;23(5):297-306. [PMID: 25911662]

FRACTURES OF THE RADIAL HEAD

- The radial head is a secondary restraint to valgus stability of elbow.
- Most nondisplaced or minimally displaced fractures can be treated closed.
- When there are three or more fracture fragments, radial head replacement may be best.

The radial head is seated in the lesser sigmoid notch of the proximal ulna and has axial contact with the capitellum of the distal humerus. Radial head fractures are generally caused by longitudinal loading from a fall on an outstretched pronated forearm; dislocation of the elbow is another cause.

Clinical Findings

Radial head fractures are the most common fractures of the elbow in adults, and patients have pain in the lateral elbow with forearm rotation. A neurovascular exam should be performed as well as forearm range of motion to evaluate for mechanical block. Aspiration of a joint hematoma with injection of local anesthesia prior to range of motion can be considered if it will change treatment. The interosseous membrane and wrist should also be examined to rule out an Essex-Lopresti lesion (longitudinal disruption of interosseous membrane, distal radioulnar joint injury, and radial head fracture-dislocation).

Classification

Radial head fractures are classified according to the Mason classification: type I are nondisplaced/minimally displaced fractures (<2 mm), type II are displaced fractures greater than 2 mm with possible mechanical block to forearm rotation, type III are comminuted/displaced fractures with mechanical block, and type IV fractures are radial head fractures with an associated elbow dislocation. Radiographs and CT confirm the diagnosis and classification. A fat pad sign on the lateral radiograph may indicate occult minimally displaced fractures.

Treatment

Mason type I fracture are treated closed with range of motion as tolerated. The treatment of type II fractures is controversial. For fractures with near-normal motion, less than 2 mm of step-off, and without associated injury, nonsurgical treatment is indicated. Type II fractures with associated injuries that may compromise elbow stability or fractures with a mechanical block are indications for ORIF. Mason type III fractures are treated with either ORIF, if possible, or radial head arthroplasty. If the fracture is too comminuted (three or more fragments is a good guide), then radial head arthroplasty is the preferred treatment. Figure 2–12 shows pre- and postoperative radiographs of a comminuted right olecranon and radial head fracture.

ORIF can be performed via the Kocher approach between the anconeus and extensor carpi ulnaris. It is sometimes easier to identify this plane more distal in the incision. To avoid injury to the posterior interosseous nerve, the forearm should be maintained in pronation. Small plates and screws can be used to fix radial head fractures. Implants should be placed the on nonarticular safe zone to avoid impingement on the sigmoid fossa of the ulna. The safe zone corresponds to the lateral 90-degree arc with the forearm in neutral rotation.

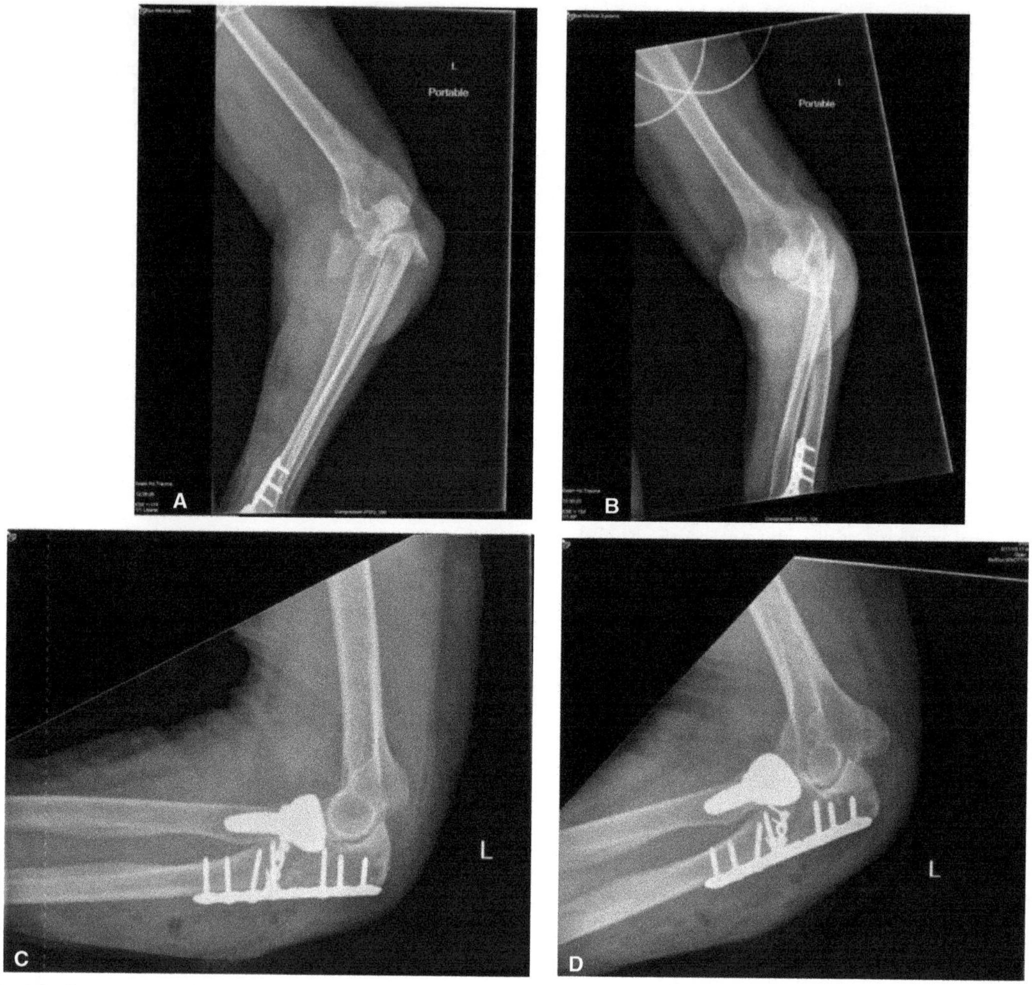

▲ **Figure 2–12.** Preoperative (**A** and **B**) and postoperative (**C** and **D**) right elbow radiographs of a comminuted olecranon and radial head fracture.

If the radial head is replaced, the prosthesis should maintain radial length with satisfactory posterolateral stability of the radiocapitellar joint.

Complications of surgery include implant failure, nonunion, osteonecrosis, and elbow stiffness. Radial head replacement has produced better results than ORIF, and loose implants are generally well tolerated. Radial head excision is a last-resort treatment because it can lead to instability and proximal radial migration.

1. Capitellar Fractures

Capitellar fractures frequently result from the same mechanism that causes radial head fractures. The ulnar collateral ligament, the interosseous ligament, and the distal radioulnar joint may also be injured. Various levels of injury, from cartilage damage to large osteochondral portions of the capitellum, can occur from impaction of the radius against the capitellum. Low-grade radial head fractures create higher-grade cartilage lesions as the intact radial head can cause more damage to the capitellum. Shearing forces can result in two different injuries: an osteochondral injury or complete fracture (type 1 or Hahn-Steinthal), an articular-cartilage-only injury (type 2 or Kocher-Lorenz), a comminuted fracture (type 3), or a fracture line extending into the trochlea (Hahn-Steinthal II). CT reconstructions are useful to further delineate the fracture and for surgical planning. Osteochondral pieces can be overlooked or confused with bone chips from radial head fractures.

▶ Treatment

ORIF via a Kocher approach is indicated for displaced capitellar fractures. Screws should be countersunk below the cartilage. Closed treatment is reserved for nondisplaced or minimally displaced fractures. Early range of motion should be instituted as tolerated.

OLECRANON FRACTURES

- Tension band wire (TBW) fixation is the gold standard treatment for transverse fractures.
- Symptomatic implants are a common complication with TBW techniques.

Olecranon fractures compose approximately 10% of all fractures around the elbow. Fractures of the olecranon commonly result from a fall, a direct blow to the elbow, or an avulsion due to contraction of the triceps.

Clinical Findings

Radiographic evaluation consists of a true lateral radiograph of the elbow. There are numerous classification systems; however, it is generally more useful to classify olecranon fractures based on the location of the fracture line (eg, waist of the olecranon, distal) and the degree of comminution because these factors may play a role in treatment. The Mayo classification delineates three types: Mayo type I, nondisplaced fractures; Mayo type II, displaced fractures, and Mayo type III, unstable fractures; each type is further classified as with or without comminution.

Treatment

Closed treatment is reserved for nondisplaced or minimally displaced (<2 mm) fractures or poor surgical candidates. Patients can be immobilized in a long arm splint in comfortable elbow flexion (60-90 degrees). Displaced transverse or short oblique fractures generally are best treated with ORIF. The optimal method for treating this fracture is either tension band wire (TBW) fixation or tension band plating. The principle behind TBW is to convert tension into fracture compression during elbow motion. There is no difference in patient-reported outcomes between TBW and plate fixation of displaced olecranon fractures, but removal of implants is more common with TBW techniques.

Select comminuted fractures may be treated by selective bony excision or complete excision of the fragment followed by advancement and repair of the triceps. Early protected range of motion exercises can follow all these treatments.

FOREARM FRACTURES

- Accurate reduction of the radius and ulna is critical to preserving function.
- May be associated with wrist (Galeazzi) or elbow (Monteggia) pathology.
- Volkmann ischemia and compartment syndrome are rare but devastating complications.

Forearm fractures occur from either direct or indirect trauma. Indirect trauma includes MVAs, falls, and athletic activities. Associated injuries can include the distal radial ulnar joint (DRUJ) and elbow as well as compartment syndrome.

1. Isolated Fracture of the Ulna (Nightstick Fracture)

Isolated ulna fractures are commonly known as nightstick fractures because they can result from the arm being raised overhead to protect from injury. They may be classified as stable or unstable. Unstable fractures are those that have more than 50% displacement, have more than 10 degrees of angulation, involve the proximal third, or have associated instability at the proximal radioulnar joint or the DRUJ. Nonoperative treatment includes immobilization of the ulna with the elbow and wrist in a cast or a functional brace, and the time to union is approximately 8 weeks. Displaced fractures are treated with 3.5-mm LC-DCP ORIF with six to eight cortices of fixation on either side of the fracture. Nonunion, delayed union, radioulnar synostosis (3%-9%), and neurovascular injury are complications. Loss of forearm rotation and refracture after hardware removal are other important complications.

2. Isolated Radial Shaft Fractures

A fracture anywhere along the length of the radius with or without associated ulnar fracture with injury to the DRUJ is defined as a Galeazzi fracture. Injuries associated with the DRUJ include ulnar styloid fractures, radial shortening greater than 5 mm, and DRUJ dislocation.

ORIF with plate fixation is recommended in adult patients to restore radial bow and ensure reduction of the DRUJ, if involved. After ORIF, the distal radioulnar joint should be carefully inspected. If it is unstable, pinning in a position of stability (usually supination) is required. If it is frankly dislocated and cannot be reduced closed, then open reduction with repair of associated ligaments or removal of interposed soft tissue is indicated.

3. Monteggia Fracture

In 1814, Monteggia of Milan described an injury involving fracture of the proximal third of the ulna, with anterior dislocation of the radial head. This definition was extended by Bado to include the entire spectrum of these fractures with associated radial head dislocations, regardless of the direction of dislocation. They are classified in the following ways:

Type 1: Fracture of the ulnar shaft with anterior angulation and anterior dislocation of the radial head (60% of cases)

Type 2: Fracture of the ulnar shaft with posterior angulation and posterior or posterolateral dislocation of the radial head (15% of cases)

Type 3: Fracture of the ulnar metaphysis, with lateral or anterolateral dislocation of the radial head (20% of cases)

Type 4: Fracture of the ulna and radius at the proximal third, with anterior dislocation of the radial head (5% of cases)

It is important to perform an adequate neurovascular examination at the time of evaluation. Injuries to the anterior and posterior interosseous nerves are most commonly associated with Bado type II and III injuries.

Treatment

Closed reduction is usually satisfactory for children, but ORIF is the treatment of choice for Monteggia lesions in an adult. Optimal results require early diagnosis, anatomic reduction and internal fixation of the fractured ulna, complete reduction of the dislocated radial head, and immobilization for approximately 6 weeks to allow healing with sufficient stability. The radial head can often be completely reduced by closed means once the ulnar fracture is reduced and rigidly fixed. If this is not possible, open reduction is required; attention should be paid to the relationship between the annular ligament, the lateral epicondyle, and the radial head. Entrapment of the soft tissues is the most common reason for inability to obtain closed radial head reduction at the time of ORIF of the ulna.

4. Fractures of Both the Radius and Ulna

Fractures of both the radius and ulna are known as both-bone forearm fractures and usually result from high-energy injuries. These fractures are usually displaced because of the force required to produce such an injury. Careful neurovascular examination and adequate radiographs to show both the wrist and the elbow are mandatory.

Treatment

The treatment of choice for both-bone forearm fractures is ORIF; the volar Henry approach can be used for the radius and the plane between the extensor carpi ulnaris and the flexor carpi ulnaris for the ulna. Anatomic reduction of both bones is critical in order to restore the normal forearm function since the radius rotates "over" the ulna. Technical points to be considered include minimal subperiosteal stripping only of the fracture site. If the fracture configuration allows, 2.4-, 2.7-, or 3.5-mm lag screws can be used followed by 3.5-mm LC-DCP plates to protect this fixation with six cortices proximal and distal to the fracture. Some fracture patterns such as transverse fractures are not amenable to lag screw fixation . In these cases, the plate can be utilized as a reduction tool; these fractures benefit from compression. In general, the plates are applied to the bony surface upon which they fit the best. Figure 2–13 demonstrates postoperative radiographs of a left both-bone forearm fracture with an associated extraarticular distal radius fracture. The recent development and implementation of locked intramedullary nail systems provide an effective alternative to plating. Bone grafting can be used for severely comminuted fractures with significant bone loss. Only the skin is closed to prevent compartment syndrome or Volkmann contracture.

Many recommend plate fixation for Gustilo types I, II, and IIIA open both-bone forearm fractures. Use of an

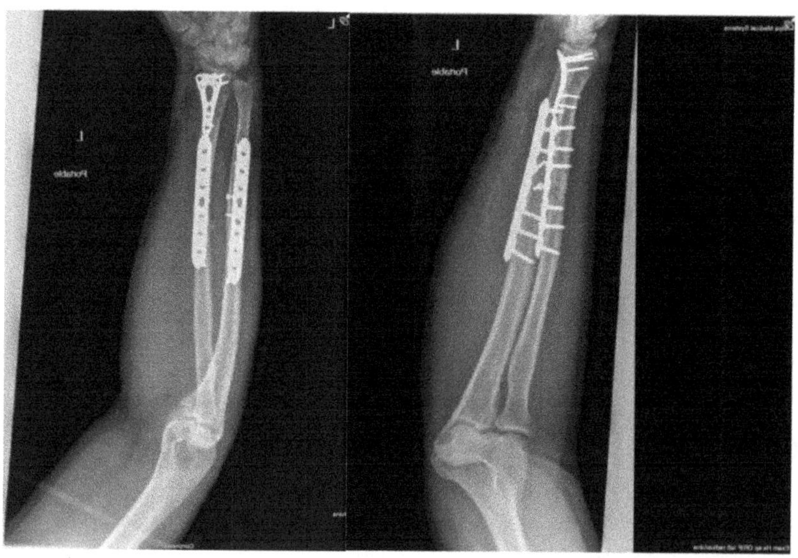

▲ **Figure 2–13.** Postoperative radiographs of a left both-bone forearm fracture with an associated extraarticular distal radius fracture. A long enough distal radius plate was not available to span the extraarticular distal radius and shaft fracture, so a volar distal radius plate and 3.5-mm limited-contact dynamic compression plates were used.

external fixator is a viable alternative if there are severe open wounds with skin and soft-tissue loss, as in Gustilo type IIIB and IIIC injuries.

Adams JE, Sems SA, Steinmann SP. Open treatment of radial head fractures. *JBJS Essent Surg Tech.* 2017;7(4):e35 [PMID: 30233970]

Burkhart KJ, Wegmann K, Müller LP, Gohlke FE. Fractures of the radial head. *Hand Clin.* 2015;31(4):533-546. [PMID: 26498543]

Ditsios KT, Stavridis SI, Christodoulou AG. The effect of haematoma aspiration on intra-articular pressure and pain relief following Mason I radial head fractures. *Injury.* 2011;42(4): 362-365. [PMID: 20932520]

Duckworth AD, Clement ND, McEachan JE, White TO, Court-Brown CM, McQueen MM. Prospective randomised trial of non-operative versus operative management of olecranon fractures in the elderly. *Bone Joint J.* 2017;99-B(7):964-972. [PMID: 28663405]

Duckworth AD, Clement ND, White TO, Court-Brown CM, McQueen MM. Plate versus tension-band wire fixation for olecranon fractures. *J Bone Joint Surg Am.* 2017;99:1261-1273. [PMID: 28763412]

Klausmeyer MA, Mudgal C. Exposure of the forearm and distal radius. *Hand Clin.* 2014;30(4):427-433. [PMID: 25440071]

Ries C, Müller M, Wegmann K, Pfau DB, Müller LP, Burkhart KJ. Is an extension of the safe zone possible without jeopardizing the proximal radioulnar joint when performing a radial head plate osteosynthesis? *J Shoulder Elbow Surg.* 2015;24(10):1627-1634. [PMID: 25940383]

Schulte LM, Meals CG, Neviaser RJ. Management of adult diaphyseal both-bone forearm fractures. *J Am Acad Orthop Surg.* 2014;22(7):437-446. [PMID: 24966250]

FRACTURES AND DISLOCATIONS OF THE DISTAL FOREARM AND WRIST

Anatomic and Biomechanical Principles

The distal radius has three articular components (Figure 2–14): the scaphoid fossa, the lunate fossa, and the sigmoid notch, which articulates with the ulna medially. Between the scaphoid and the lunate fossa is a ridge that corresponds with the scapholunate interval. This entire surface is covered with articular cartilage. The radial styloid is the attachment of the brachioradialis tendon. Also, it is the origin of several important wrist ligaments, including the radial scapholunate and radial lunocapitate ligaments.

The third articular component of the distal radius is the sigmoid notch. This convex structure allows the radius to rotate around the distal ulna. The distal ulna itself has an ulnar styloid, which contains attachments to the triangular fibrocartilage complex (TFCC), including the meniscus homolog, the volar and dorsal ulnar carpal ligaments, and the ulnar collateral ligament at the wrist. The TFCC plays an essential role in the stability of the DRUJ and forearm motion.

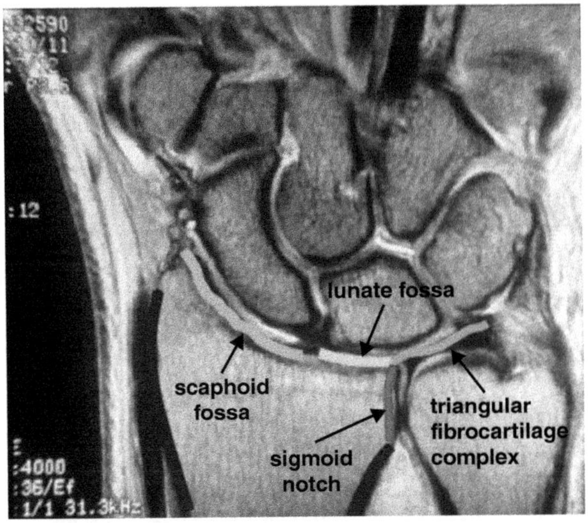

▲ **Figure 2–14.** Coronal T1-weighted magnetic resonance imaging of the right distal radius demonstrating the scaphoid fossa, lunate fossa, sigmoid notch, and triangular fibrocartilage complex.

The concave elliptical distal radius is oriented in the sagittal plane with an average of 11 degrees of volar tilt. In the frontal plane, the average radial inclination is 23 degrees. Distal radial length is measured from the tip of the radial styloid to the ulnar articular surface and averages 13 mm.

In addition to the bony surfaces, the articular cartilage, joint capsule, and wrist ligaments, there are other soft tissues within the distal forearm and wrist. On the dorsal surface, six dorsal compartments contain wrist and digital extensor tendons. On the volar surface reside the contents of the carpal tunnel, with nine flexor tendons and the median nerve. On the ulnar surface, the flexor carpi ulnaris tendon can be palpated near its insertion on the pisiform. The boundaries of the ulnar tunnel, or Guyon's canal, are the volar carpal ligament and transverse carpal ligament, the hook of the hamate radially, and the pisiform ulnarly. Guyon's canal contains the ulnar artery and nerve. The ulnar shaft remains fixed in its rotation at the ulnohumeral joint, and the radius rotates around the ulna in pronation and supination. The radius has a lateral bow that is crucial to the maintenance of full pronation and supination.

The interosseous membrane connects the shafts of the radius and ulna. The central portion is thickened and has been shown to be important in force transmission between the radius and ulna. Origins of flexor and extensor muscles are located along the anterior and posterior surfaces of the radius, ulna, and interosseous membrane.

DISTAL RADIUS AND ULNA INJURIES

- Account for approximately 17.5% of all fractures.
- Most common osteoporotic upper extremity fracture.
- Many distal radius fractures in the elderly can be treated closed with good results.
- Fall on outstretched hand is the most common injury mechanism.
- May be associated with scapholunate and lunotriquetral ligament injury.

1. Distal Radius and Ulna Fractures

In 1814, Abraham Colles described the Colles distal radius fracture as a "silver-fork" deformity. It is characterized by apex volar fracture angulation, dorsal proximal displacement, loss of radial inclination, and radial shortening. In contrast, the Smith fracture, or reverse Colles fracture, is an apex dorsal fracture of the distal radius, with the hand and wrist displaced volarly with respect to the forearm. These fractures may be extraarticular, intraarticular, or a part of a fracture-dislocation involving the wrist. Barton's fracture is an intraarticular fracture-dislocation of the volar rim in which the carpus follows the fracture fragment volarly. The chauffeur's fracture is a radial styloid fracture, described initially in car drivers operating automobiles that required hand cranking to start. When the engine engaged, the crank would "kick back," and the chauffeur's fracture would result. A die-punch fracture is a depressed fracture of the lunate fossa of the articular surface of the distal radius.

Classification

AP, oblique, and lateral radiographs of the wrist are necessary to diagnose distal radius fractures. CT is also beneficial in preoperative planning or ascertaining degree of intraarticular involvement. No one fracture classification system is comprehensive in describing all important variables of distal radius fractures. Classification systems include the Frykman classification, the AO classification, and the OTA fracture classification system. The Frykman classification includes eight types: type 1 is extraarticular, type 2 is extraarticular with ulna styloid fracture, type 3 is intraarticular involving the radiocarpal joint, type 4 is intraarticular with ulna styloid fracture, type 5 is intraarticular with involvement of the DRUJ, type 6 is intraarticular with involvement of the DRUJ with ulna styloid fracture, type 7 is intraarticular involving the radiocarpal joint and the DRUJ, and type 8 is intraarticular involving the radiocarpal joint and the DRUJ with ulna styloid fracture. The AO and OTA classifications are primarily used for research. However, when communicating with other surgeons, most fracture surgeons describe the following characteristics of these fractures because they relate to treatment: intra- or extraarticular, apex volar or dorsal, degree of dorsal comminution, fragments involved, and degree of displacement.

Treatment

Treatment of distal radius fractures is based on the fracture classification and the patient characteristics such as age, comorbidities, and level of activity. In general, younger patients with displaced fractures are best treated by ORIF. Elderly, low-demand individuals have satisfactory outcomes with closed treatment. Successful outcomes correlate with accuracy of articular reduction, restoration of anatomic relationships, and early range of motion. We will further expand on treatment by fracture classification.

A. Extraarticular Nondisplaced or Minimally Displaced Distal Radius Fractures

Extraarticular nondisplaced distal radius fractures can be treated with cast immobilization for 4 to 6 weeks, until fracture healing occurs, followed by mobilization with an off-the-shelf brace. Extreme positions of flexion and ulnar deviation should be avoided due to the risk of carpal tunnel syndrome. In compliant patients with nondisplaced fractures, wrist splints can be considered instead of splint/cast immobilization. Conservative treatment is indicated when radial shortening is less than 5 mm and the dorsal angulation is less than 5 degrees or within 20 degrees of the contralateral distal radius.

Radial length and radial angulation are generally not fully restored with closed reduction techniques. Small amounts of radial shortening can lead to increased load in the lunate fossa, distal ulna, and triangular fibrocartilage. In most low-demand patients, however, this treatment can be successful, and functional wrist motion can be obtained. If shortening is significant, midcarpal instability may occur. Another potential problem is distal radioulnar joint arthrosis and ulnar carpal abutment, which may necessitate later reconstruction. In minimally displaced fractures, a rapid cast conversion to a supportive splint (2 or 3 weeks) and early mobilization can be safely done and may yield improved outcomes.

B. Extraarticular Displaced Distal Radius Fractures

Closed reduction should be attempted in extraarticular displaced fractures. If radial length and volar tilt are restored, then a sugar tong splint or long arm cast can be effective in holding the reduction. A two-point mold should be applied to the splint to maintain the reduction. If the closed reduction is not satisfactory, either closed reduction with external fixation/percutaneous pinning or ORIF can be performed. When the volar cortex is stable, this method is highly successful; however, dorsal comminution is a risk factor for displacement. Loss of reduction is a potential complication in older patients. Figure 2–15 demonstrates volar plate fixation of a displaced extraarticular distal radius fracture.

C. Intraarticular Distal Radius Fractures

The treatment of intraarticular distal radius fractures is to restore the congruity of the articular surface and the

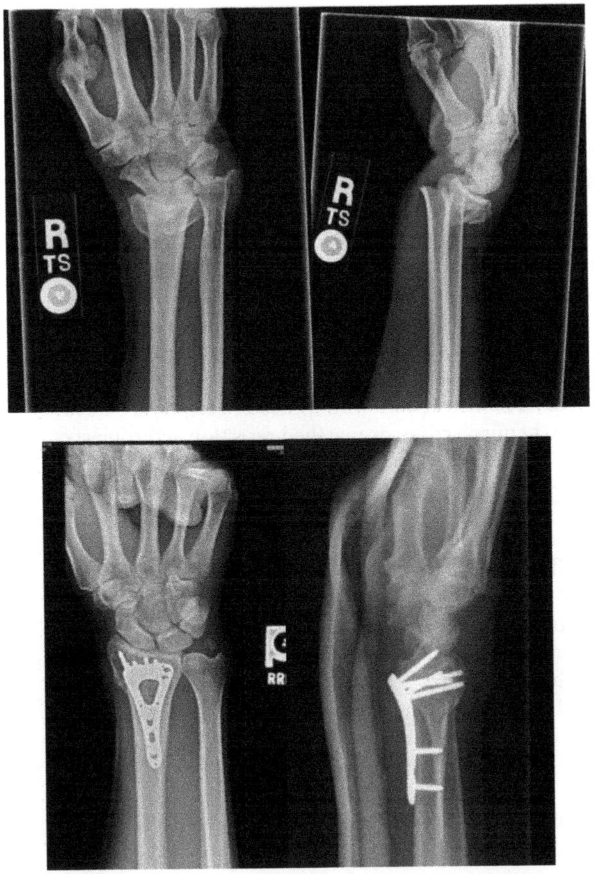

▲ **Figure 2–15.** Pre- and postoperative anteroposterior and lateral radiographs of an extraarticular distal radius fracture fixed with a volar plate.

anatomic axis of the distal radius with ORIF to the preinjury condition. Parameters such as volar tilt of 11 degrees, radial inclination of 22 degrees, and radial height of 11 mm are a good guide but can vary from individual to individual. If there is any confusion regarding accurate parameters, contralateral wrist radiographs are recommended. The goals of surgery should be articular step-off less than 2 mm, radial shortening less than 5 mm, dorsal tilt less than 15 degrees, volar tilt less than 20 degrees, and loss of radial inclination less than 10 degrees.

Fixed or variable-angle locked volar plating systems have revolutionized the management of distal radius fractures because they are strong enough to allow early range of motion after surgery and have resulted in improved long-term results. Newer implants are designed for fragment-specific fixation; however, care should be taken to avoid intraarticular screw placement. Volar and dorsal approaches are the most common surgical approaches.

Indication for dorsal plating include dorsal fracture-dislocations, articular dorsal lip fractures requiring direct reduction, grafting of large defects, and ipsilateral carpal injuries requiring a dorsal approach.

Although it requires a high level of expertise, arthroscopically assisted reduction can be a useful tool for assessing articular reduction, intraarticular step-offs, and associated injuries such as triangular fibrocartilage, scapholunate, and lunotriquetral ligament tears. Some advocate bone grafting in the acute treatment of comminuted fractures.

In case of excessive comminution, such that ORIF will fail to achieve a stable bony construct, use of an external fixator as a distractor and neutralization device is generally indicated. Using fluoroscopy helps with both articular alignment and overall radial length, and minor adjustments can then be effectively done with percutaneous pins.

Complications of distal radius plate fixation are flexor tendon rupture with a volar plate, extensor tendon rupture with a dorsal plate, tendon irritation, carpal tunnel syndrome, loss of reduction, and complex regional pain syndrome.

External fixation has an established track record in treating distal radius fractures that are not amenable to ORIF. With external fixation, there is the additional advantage of not devascularizing bony fragments and not creating the surgical wound. Use of indirect traction on fracture fragments and taking advantage of "ligamentotaxis" via the fixator pins can be effective. With open fractures, an external fixator can facilitate wound care. External fixation is effective in preventing loss of reduction and length in situations where there is significant comminution. Overlengthening should be avoided, and fixation time should not exceed 8 weeks. Complications with external fixation include pin tract infection, superficial radial nerve neuropathy, pin loosening, and stiffness.

2. Distal Radioulnar Joint Dislocation

Approximately 32% to 34% of applied load is transmitted through the DRUJ and ulna, and this load increases during supination. Division of either the volar or dorsal distal radioulnar ligament increases this transmission of load. Even minor disruptions of the anatomic relationships between the distal radius and ulna can result in pain. The DRUJ can be dislocated by a variety of mechanisms, including low- and high-energy trauma. These injuries are associated with disruption of the TFCC, including the articular disk and associated ligaments. There should be a high index of suspicion in diagnosing this lesion because radiographs that are not taken in the perfect lateral orientation will tend to look relatively normal. An MRI is the ideal study for diagnosis. A displaced fracture at the ulnar styloid base indicates a high risk of distal radioulnar instability. In the presence of forearm and elbow fracture-dislocations, further evaluation of the radioulnar joint is mandatory.

▶ Clinical Findings

The amount of DRUJ stability should be carefully assessed and compared with that of the opposite wrist. The patient should position the wrist to reproduce the pain. With the hand pronated, the examiner tries to displace the ulnar head by applying a dorsal to volar load 4 cm proximal to the DRUJ (piano key test). Little resistance to ballottement and volar movement of the ulna head corresponds to a positive piano key test. Subluxation is much more common than anterior or posterior dislocation. Limitation of pronation and supination, or pain associated with such motion, would be expected in such a situation. Palpation of the sixth extensor compartment during resisted pronation is useful to identify any subluxation. The other common cause of distal radioulnar joint problems is rheumatoid arthritis.

Treatment

Dorsal dislocation, or subluxation, should be treated by reduction of the ulnar head into the sigmoid fossa and placement of the forearm in full supination. To maintain reduction, K-wires can be placed across the DRUJ. The arm should be immobilized in supination, which requires a long arm cast or splint. Volar dislocation is relatively rare and is usually stable after reduction. If dorsal or volar dislocation or subluxation of the distal ulna cannot be reduced with manipulation in the outpatient setting, closed treatment can be attempted under anesthesia. If this fails, open reduction and soft-tissue reconstruction may be necessary. If this is performed, a retinacular flap may be used to transpose the extensor carpi ulnaris to a more dorsal position to stabilize the distal ulna, as has been described for Darrach reconstruction of the joint.

3. Malunion of the Distal Radius

Malunion of the distal radius can have a variety of negative consequences. Alteration of the biomechanical function of the wrist may lead to weakness, limitation of wrist and forearm motion, and midcarpal instability. Associated DRUJ arthrosis may be present, as well as ulnocarpal abutment. Rotational deformity is common with angulated malunions. CT scans of both wrists can be used to identify and measure malrotation preoperatively.

Treatment

The treatment for symptomatic distal radius malunions is reconstructive surgery. Such a reconstruction can entail an osteotomy of the radius with iliac crest bone grafting and plate fixation. The DRUJ must be addressed and, depending on the degree of subluxation or arthrosis, may require closed reduction, open reduction, or reconstruction using Darrach or Sauve-Kapandji procedures. In this procedure, instead of distal ulnar resection as in the Darrach procedure, transverse segmental resection of the ulnar metaphysis is followed by creation of an arthrodesis of the distal ulna to the radius, using the resected bone as graft. Forearm rotation occurs through the ulnar metaphyseal pseudoarthrosis. Additionally, restoration of the radial length may be difficult with manipulation alone. Useful adjuncts to achieve restoration of appropriate length and orientation in severe malunion include use of laminar spreaders to distract the proximal and distal fragments of the radius after osteotomy. Alternatively, an external fixator may prove useful in helping to achieve appropriate length after osteotomy.

If the distal radius has started to heal short with significant angular deformity but the fracture is not yet fully healed, osteotomy for early or "nascent" malunion is justified. The advantage of taking down a nascent malunion is that the operation is technically simpler to perform, shortens the time of disability, and leads to better long-term results. Additionally, the DRUJ can be restored more reliably in these early reconstructions than when osteotomy is required for established malunion. The latter often requires adjunctive DRUJ reconstruction with Darrach resection, Sauve-Kapandji, hemiresection, or matched resection arthroplasty.

DISLOCATION OF THE RADIOCARPAL JOINT

Dislocation of the radiocarpal joint is usually accompanied by significant carpal-ligamentous injury or fracture. Treatment of these injuries involves restoration of the bony architecture through immediate closed reduction. If closed reduction is not satisfactory, immediate open reduction should be performed. Associated injuries include transscaphoid perilunate fracture-dislocations or distal radius fracture-dislocations and should be treated with ORIF. Ligamentous repair should be performed at this time. Please see Chapter 10 for more information. Median nerve evaluation is mandatory, and surgical exploration is indicated if a dense neuropathy is present.

Abe Y, Fujii K. Arthroscopic-assisted reduction of intra-articular distal radius fracture. *Hand Clin.* 2017;33(4):659-668. [PMID: 28991578]

Costa ML, Achten J, Rangan A, Lamb SE, Parsons NR. Percutaneous fixation with Kirschner wires versus volar locking-plate fixation in adults with dorsally displaced fracture of distal radius: five-year follow-up of a randomized controlled trial. *Bone Joint J.* 2019; 101-B(8):978-983. [PMID: 31362548]

Gunal I, Ozaksoy D, Altay T, Satoglu IS, Kazimoglu C, Sener M. Scapholunate dissociation associated with distal radius fractures. *Eur J Orthop Surg Traumatol.* 2013;23(8):877-881. [PMID: 23412224]

Krimmer H, Schandl R, Wolters R. Corrective osteotomy after malunited distal radius fractures. *Arch Orthop Trauma Surg.* 2020;140(5):675-680. [PMID: 32193680]

Krustins U, Krustins J, Bringina D, Laurane K, Jumtins A. Comparison of volar locking plates with external fixation and K-wires in arthroscopically assisted intra-articular distal radial fracture fixation. *J Hand Surg Eur Vol.* 2020;45(4):333-338. [PMID: 31594424]

Lafontaine M, Hardy D, Delince P. Stability assessment of distal radius fractures. *Injury.* 1989;20(4):208-210. [PMID: 2592094]

Marcano A, Taormina DP, Karia R, Paksima N, Posner M, Egol KA. Displaced intra-articular fractures involving the volar rim of the distal radius. *J Hand Surg Am.* 2015;40(1):42-48. [PMID: 25446998]

Omokawa S, Abe Y, Imatani J, Moritomo H, Suzuki D, Onishi T. Treatment of intra-articular distal radius fractures. *Hand Clin.* 2017;33(3):529-543. [PMID: 28673629]

Perlus R, Doyon J, Henry P. The use of dorsal distraction plating for severely comminuted distal radius fractures: a review and comparison to volar plate fixation. *Injury.* 2019;50(suppl 1):S50-S55. [PMID: 31040029]

Saving J, Severin Wahlgren S, Olsson K, et al. Non-operative treatment compared with volar locking plate fixation for dorsally displaced distal radial fractures in the elderly: a randomized controlled trial. *J Bone Joint Surg Am.* 2019;101(11):961-969. [PMID: 31169572]

Thorninger R, Madsen ML, Wæver D, Borris LC, Rölfing JHD. Complications of volar locking plating of distal radius fractures in 576 patients with 3.2 years follow-up. *Injury.* 2017;48(6):1104-1109. [PMID: 28336098]

Walenkamp MM, Vos LM, Strackee SD, Goslings JC, Schep NW. The unstable distal radius fracture: how do we define it? A systematic review. *J Wrist Surg.* 2015;4(4):307-316. [PMID: 26649263]

Wu JC, Strickland CD, Chambers JS. Wrist fractures and osteoporosis. *Orthop Clin North Am.* 2019;50(2):211-221. [PMID: 30850079]

II. TRAUMA TO THE LOWER EXTREMITY

PELVIC FRACTURES AND DISLOCATIONS

- Pelvic fractures are potentially life-threatening injuries with high mortality rates.
- Most pelvic ring injuries are caused by MVAs and falls.
- Many pelvic fractures in the elderly can be treated conservatively.
- Pelvic fractures may be associated with bladder injuries, neurologic compromise, and/or sexual dysfunction.

Mechanism of Injury and Classification

Four patterns of injury are responsible for pelvic fractures: anteroposterior compression (APC), lateral compression (LC), vertical shear, or combined mechanism (Figure 2–16).

A type—Stable pelvic ring injuries

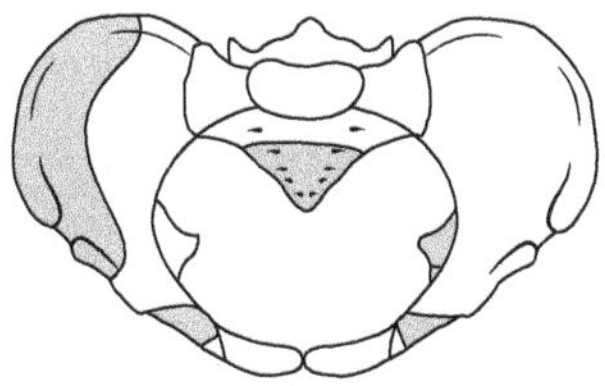

AO/OTA	Tile	Young & Burgess
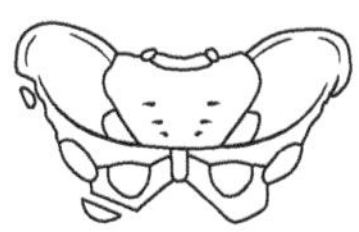 61-A1	A1 Avulsion of the innominate bone	n/d
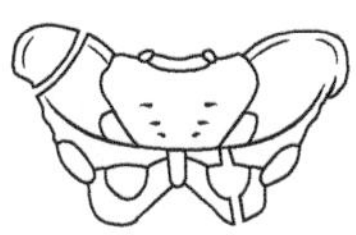 61-A2	A2 Stable iliac wing fracture or stable, minimally displaced pelvic ring fracture	(LC I/APC I)
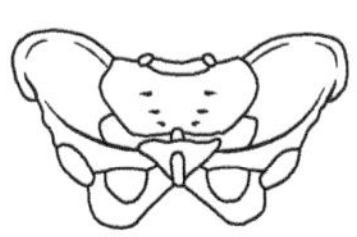 61-A3	A3 Transverse sacrum or coccygeal fracture	n/d

A

▲ **Figure 2–16. A-C:** Different classification systems for pelvic fractures in increasing severity. APC, anteroposterior compression; LC, lateral compression.

A type—Partially stable pelvic injuries
(rotationally unstable)

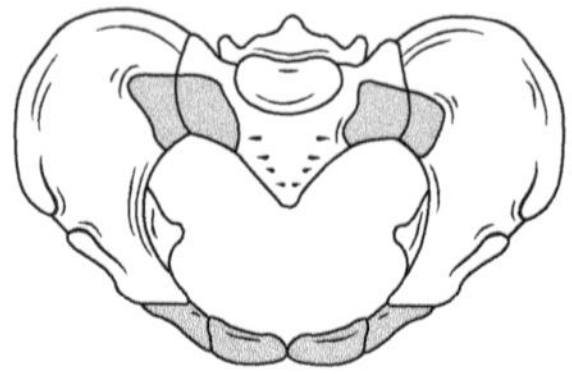

AO/OTA	Tile	Young & Burgess
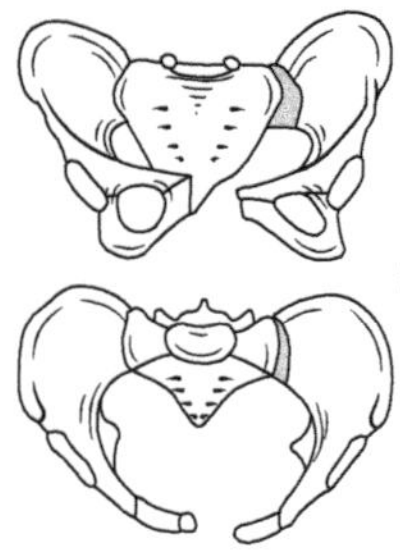 61-B1	**B1** "Open-book" injury - Anterior SI-ligament stretched	**APC I** - Pubic diastasis <2.5 cm **APC II** - Pubic diastasis ≥2.5 cm - Anterior SI-ligament disrupted
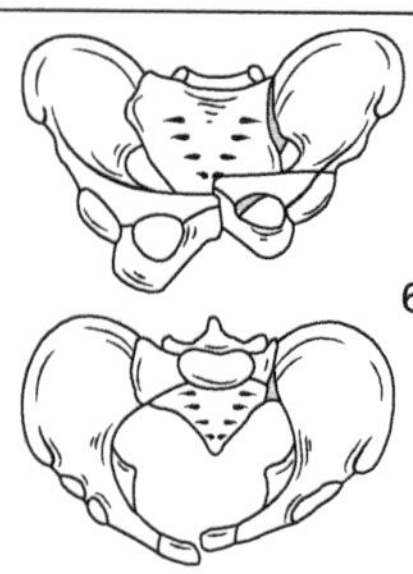 61-B2	**B2** "Lateral compression" injury (B2-2: contralateral "bucket handle" type)	**LC I** - Posterior injury sacral impaction **LC II** - Posterior injury: • Anterior sacral crush (LC IIA) • Iliac wing "crescent" injury (LC IIB)
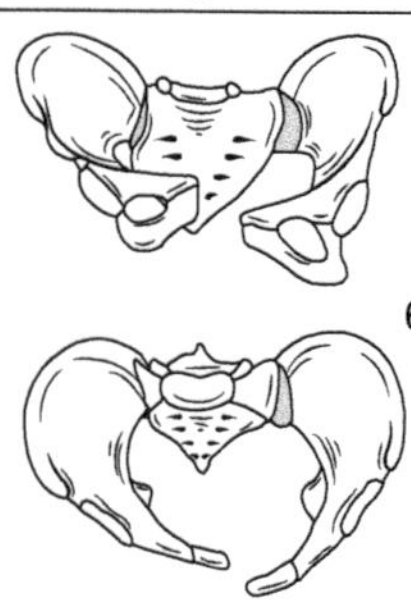 61-B3	**B3** Bilateral "B-type" injuries	**LC III** Unilateral "B1" with contralateral "B2" type injuries ("windswept pelvis")

B

▲ **Figure 2–16.** *(Continued)*

<table>
<tr><td colspan="3">C type—Completely unstable pelvic ring injuries
(rotationally and vertically unstable)</td></tr>
<tr><td colspan="3">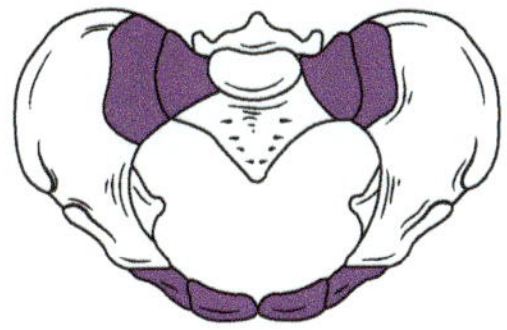</td></tr>
<tr><th>AO/OTA</th><th>Tile</th><th>Young & Burgess</th></tr>
<tr><td>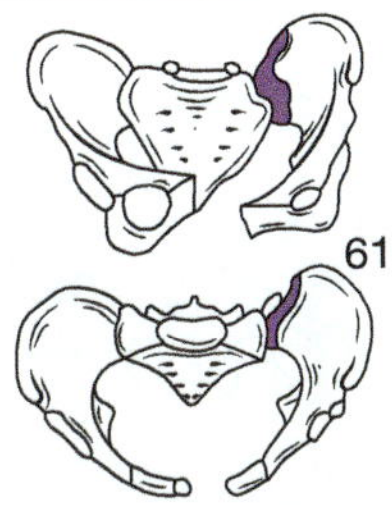
61-C1</td><td>C1
- Unilateral</td><td rowspan="3">APC III
- Pubic diastasis ≥2.5 cm
- Anterior and posterior Si-ligament disruption

VS
(“Vertical shear”)
- APC II with vertical displacement of hemipelvis

CM
(“Combined mechanical”)
Complex fractures with combined elements of APC, LC, and/or VS</td></tr>
<tr><td>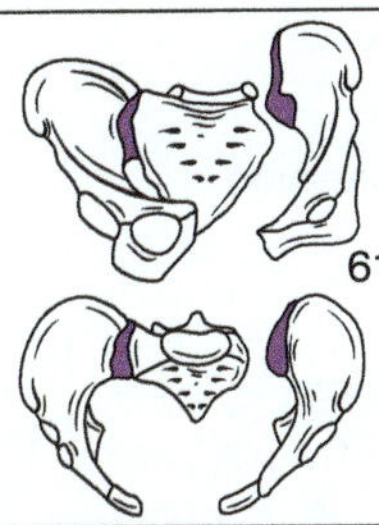
61-C2</td><td>C2
- Bilateral
• One side “B-type”
• One side “C-type”</td></tr>
<tr><td>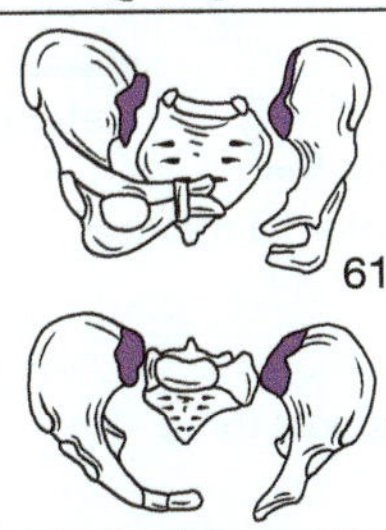
61-C3</td><td>C3
Bilateral “C-type”</td></tr>
</table>

C

▲ **Figure 2–16.** (*Continued*) (© Phil Stahel 2007, Reprinted with permission.)

APC pelvic injuries are due to external rotation forces on the anterior pelvis. This force results in a pubic symphyseal dislocation and disruption of the anterior and/or posterior sacroiliac ligaments, termed a so-called “open-book” pelvis. The energy transmission to the posterior pelvic ring can result in varying degrees of posterior ring disruption from anterior sacroiliac joint widening to a complete sacroiliac joint dislocation. In addition to the pelvic ring injury, there is also an associated soft-tissue disruption to the pelvic floor structures. The APC injury can affect one or both of the hemipelvises. LC pelvic injuries are due to forces from the side of the pelvis. Depending on the force vector and location of impact, this force can create various LC patterns of injury: sacral fractures, sacroiliac fracture-dislocations, ipsilateral rami fractures, or contralateral rami fractures. Because of the compressive force, the sacral fracture is typically impacted, and the rami fractures are horizontal. The sacrospinous and sacrotuberous ligaments remain intact, limiting the instability. These ligaments are responsible for pelvic stability and nutation/counternutation of the sacroiliac joint during activity. In high-energy LC injuries, the ipsilateral hemipelvis is adducted and internally rotated, and the contralateral hemipelvis is externally rotated. The third injury pattern is a vertical shear force vector resulting from fall from height. The force vector is transmitted superiorly from the lower extremity to the affected hemipelvis. This vertical force can result in a pubic symphyseal and sacroiliac joint dislocation with subsequent cranial displacement of the hemipelvis. This injury pattern is most associated with vascular injury and potential physiologic instability. Finally, combined mechanism pelvic injuries are due to a combination of the three aforementioned patterns. This type of injury is common because damaging force vectors to the pelvis are typically multidirectional, resulting in a combined fracture pattern. Figure 2–17 demonstrates the different pelvic injuries based on different force vectors of damage.

Clinical Findings

The physical examination includes inspection of the skin, perineum, and rectum. Closed degloving injuries (Morel-Lavallée) should be identified because their presence can affect treatment. The Morel-Lavallée injury occurs when the subcutaneous tissue and skin of the pelvic flank are sheared from the underlying fascia and muscles. This shearing results in significant ecchymosis, hematoma, and swelling of the pelvic flank. Because the skin is supplied by arteries that arise from the fascial perforating vessels, it can result in impaired vascularity and skin necrosis. Palpation of the pelvic bony landmarks, including posterior palpation of the sacrum and sacroiliac joint, should be done. AP and lateral iliac wing compression maneuvers to assess stability should be performed only once or avoided in hemodynamically unstable patients because they can disrupt initial hematomas and cause bleeding. Male patients with pubic symphyseal dislocation injuries typically have a scrotal hematoma due to disruption of the pelvic floor. This injury causes bleeding that descends down the inguinal canal into the scrotum. Rectovaginal examination is mandatory in all cases to identify open fractures. Bony spikes protruding through the mucosa contaminate the fracture hematoma. Many of these patients have lower urinary tract injuries to the bladder, urethra, and so on, and sexual dysfunction due to the pelvic floor injury is likely underreported. The distal vascular and neurologic status should also be assessed. The most commonly affected nerves include L4 through S1; however, the sacral plexus is at risk in significant injuries.

An initial AP pelvic radiograph, per the Advanced Trauma Life Support (ATLS) protocol, is performed in all suspected pelvic ring injuries. When the patient is hemodynamically stabilized, inlet and outlet views can be performed. Typically, in most trauma centers, patients receive a CT scan of the chest, abdomen, and pelvis prior to the inlet/outlet views. However, a CT scan should never replace the radiographs and instead should be additional. A cystogram can be performed to determine if there is injury to the bladder. In physiologically unstable patients, pelvic angiography with or without embolization may be necessary to treat vascular injuries that are typically branches of the internal iliac artery.

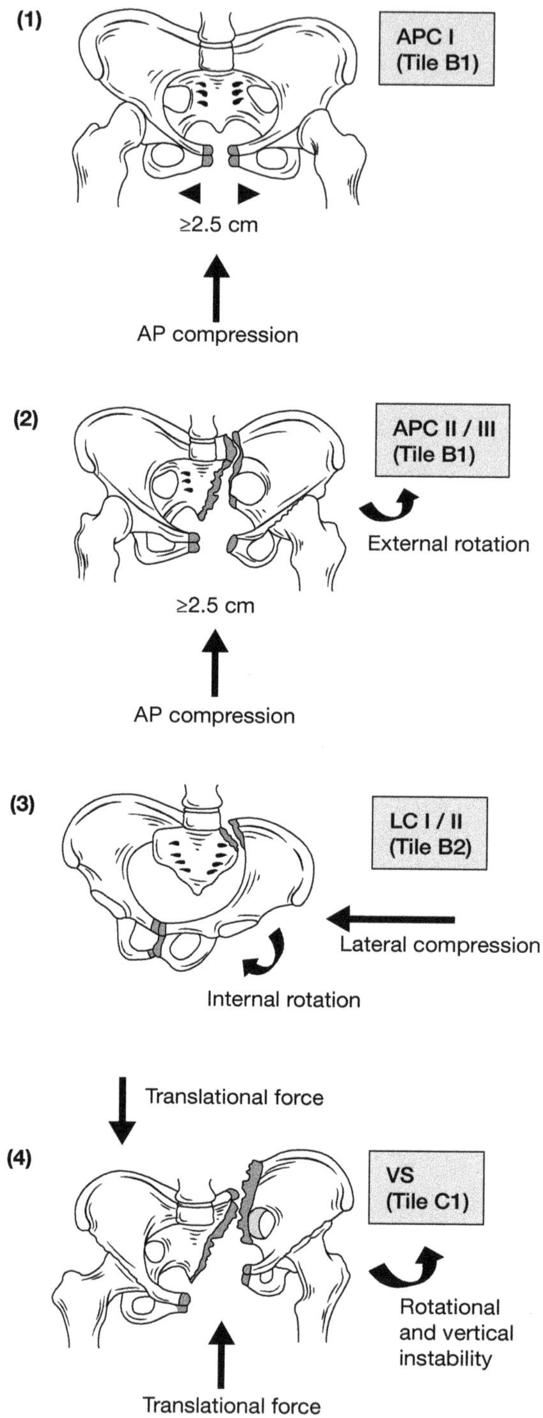

▲ **Figure 2–17.** Different force vectors cause different pelvic injury patterns including anteroposterior compression (APC), lateral compression (LC), and vertical shear (VS). AP, anteroposterior. (© Phil Stahel 2007, Reprinted with permission.)

Treatment

Most pelvis fractures treated by orthopedic surgeons are stable injuries. Low-energy injury patterns are typically managed nonoperatively. On the contrary, management for physiologically unstable pelvic injuries requires a systematic, multidisciplinary approach. In the hemodynamically unstable patient, the ATLS protocol should be followed. Hemorrhage and shock are the primary causes of death due to pelvic fracture. The cornerstones of successful treatment include identification of a significant pelvic injury, rapid resuscitation, hemorrhage control using angiography or pelvic packing, assessment and treatment of associated injuries, and mechanical stabilization in selected cases. Initial resuscitation is started with 2 L of crystalloid, followed by packed blood cells, fresh frozen plasma, and platelets in a 1:1:4 ratios. However, these resuscitation parameters (eg, crystalloid vs packed red blood cells, optimal ratio of packed red blood cells to fresh frozen plasma, etc.) are constantly evolving. A pelvic binder or sheet can be used to stabilize the unstable pelvis temporarily. The sheet or binder should be centered over the greater trochanters (Figure 2–4). After ruling out other sources of bleeding by chest and spine radiography/CT and FAST, an external fixation device such as a pelvic clamp and/or anterior external fixator can be applied. Pelvic packing and/or arterial angiography should be executed according to the protocol of the trauma center. During packing, the sponges should be placed in the space of Retzius over the vesicular venous plexus, the quadrilateral surface, and anterior to the sacroiliac joint/sacrum (Figure 2–18).

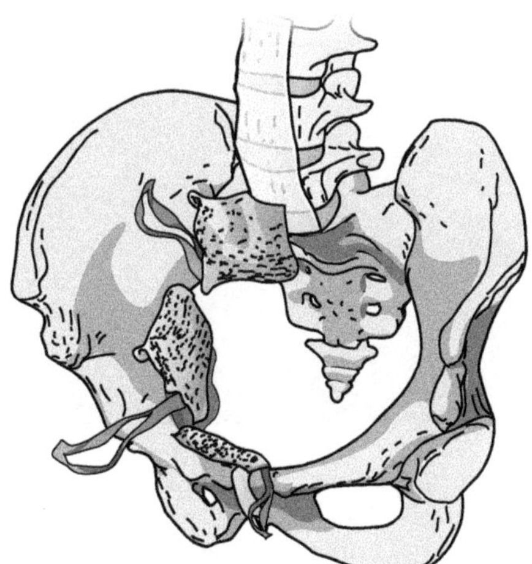

▲ **Figure 2–18.** During pelvic packing, sponges are placed over the anterior sacroiliac joint/sacrum, the quadrilateral surface, and the space of Retzius over the vesicular plexus. Ideally, sponges should be placed where bleeding occurs the most. Note that all the sponges are placed in the true pelvis.

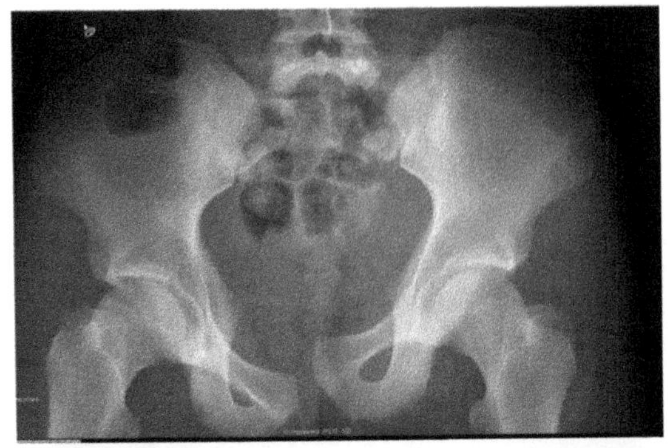

A

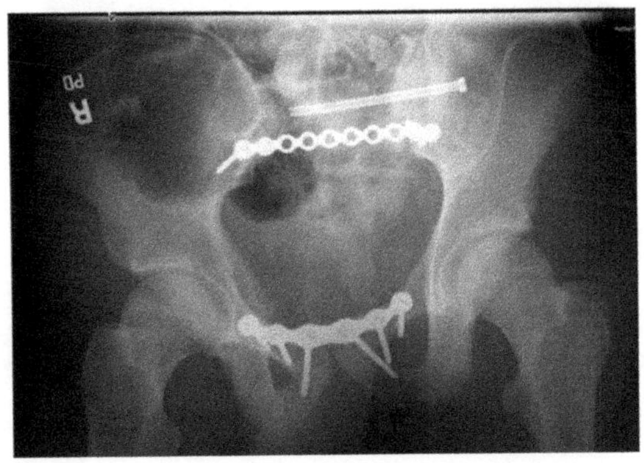

B

▲ **Figure 2–19.** Anteroposterior pelvis radiographs demonstrate (**A**) preoperative and (**B**) postoperative images of a patient who sustained a left sacral fracture and a pubic symphyseal dislocation fixed with a left iliosacral screw, posterior tension band plate, and six-hole symphyseal plate.

Although Figure 2-18 demonstrates 3 sponges on each side of the pelvis, we frequently utilize an initial, indeterminate number of sponges to achieve acute tamponade. In the same operative session, these sponges can are then gently replaced with 3 to 4 sponges per side of the pelvis. The exact number of sponges is not as important as the "space-filling" effect the sponges have on tamponade. If the patient's hemodynamic status stabilizes, the need for definitive versus temporizing mechanical fixation of the pelvis should be determined. Anterior fixation may involve anterior plating of a pubic symphyseal dislocation or external fixation via the anterior inferior iliac spine. Posterior pelvic ring fixation, if necessary, is performed either percutaneously or via ORIF. Methods to fix the posterior pelvic ring include iliosacral/transsacral screws, posterior tension band plating (Figures 2–19 and 2–20), posterior sacroiliac joint fracture-dislocation fixation, and potentially lumbopelvic fixation. There is no evidence that surgical treatment of certain LC1 and LC2 pelvic fractures improves pain, lowers narcotic use, or decreases time to mobilization.

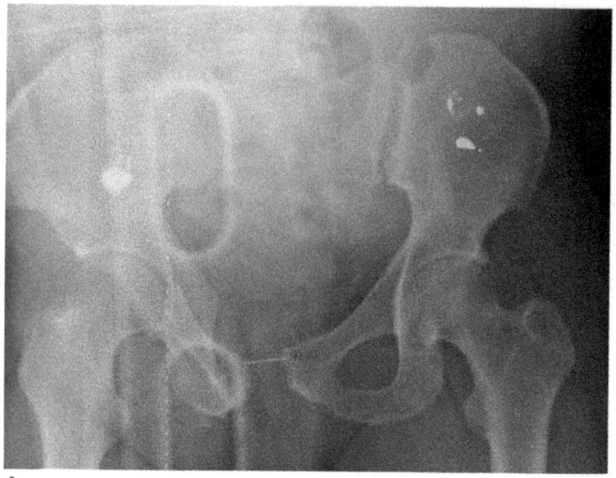

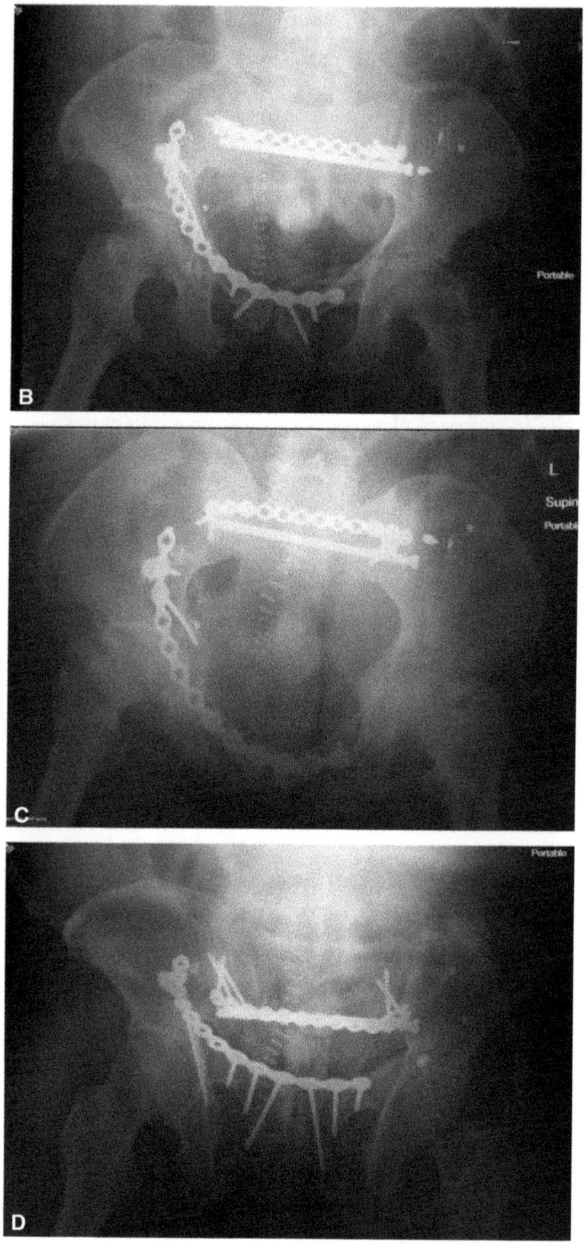

▲ **Figure 2–20. A:** Anteroposterior pelvis radiograph of a patient with a left sacroiliac fracture-dislocation, pubic symphyseal dislocation, and right superior pubic ramus fracture. The patient's pelvis injury was reduced and fixed using table skeletal fixation, an S2 transsacral screw, a posterior tension band plate, and a symphyseal plate spanning to the right internal iliac fossa. **B-D:** Postoperative pelvis radiographs are shown.

In open pelvic fractures, which account for 2% to 4% of all pelvic fractures, early surgical intervention using a multidisciplinary approach should be undertaken. Seventy-two percent of the open pelvic fractures are grade III open wounds and should be appropriately treated. The definitive method of stabilization of open pelvic fractures remains controversial. Internal fixation can be done when no gross contamination is present. Typically, there is compromise of the gastrointestinal/urologic/reproductive systems with potentially gram-negative bacterial contamination. If fecal contamination is present, a diverting colostomy can be performed. Definitive fixation of the pelvis can be performed after a period of antibiotic treatment. If there is a vaginal tear, we have treated these injuries in collaboration with obstetrics/gynecology. The vaginal tear is repaired, the wound is irrigated, and definitive pelvic fixation is performed with gram-negative postoperative antibiotic coverage. Definitive treatment with external fixation of the pelvis is always a potential option for these injuries if there is concern for infection.

A. Associated Injuries

1. Hemorrhage—Approximately 85% of bleeding associated with pelvic ring injuries originates from either the bone or the anterior-posterior pelvic venous plexus. Arterial injuries, as a source of hemorrhage after pelvic ring injuries, occur in approximately 10% to 15% of pelvic fractures. After blunt trauma, the most common pelvic arteries injured are the superior gluteal and internal pudendal arteries. CT scans can be used to detect arterial bleeding before angiography but should be postponed until the patient is hemodynamically stable for transfer. Embolization can be used to halt arterial bleeding. Some centers may have multidisciplinary protocols for managing hemorrhagic, physiologically unstable pelvic ring injuries. For example, pelvic packing against a stable pelvis can help slow down hemorrhage by closing down the pelvic volume and via a direct tamponade effect of the sponges. For continued physiologic instability, angiography and embolization are performed using interventional radiology.

2. Thrombosis—Pelvic fractures increase the risk of VTE events in trauma patients. DVTs not only are seen on distal calf veins, but also occur in pelvic venous plexi. A thrombus in the pelvis is difficult to detect using duplex ultrasound due to the depth of tissue. CT venography can be used to detect pelvic thromboses. Guidelines for prophylaxis are controversial, and one should consider the benefits, risks, and cost of different treatment options. Early administration of low-molecular-weight heparin may decrease the incidence of symptomatic pulmonary emboli. More trauma centers now use intermittent pneumatic compression after trauma and temporary vena cava filters in severely traumatized patients with contradictions to pharmacologic prophylaxis. See Chapter 13 for more on antithrombotics.

3. Neurologic injury—Neurologic injuries are common, and the frequency increases with complexity of the fractures. Up to 40% of unstable pelvic injuries may have neurologic injuries. After unstable vertical shear sacral fractures, the incidence rises to 50%. L5 and S1 are the most commonly affected roots. It is of paramount importance that a thorough neurologic examination is performed and recorded as soon as possible, searching for sensory or motor deficits in the distribution of sciatic, femoral, obturator, pudendal, or superior gluteal nerves. Peripheral nerve injuries have a better prognosis than root injuries. Partial nerve injuries also have a better outcome than complete ones. Most of the lesions are neurapraxias with favorable outcome, but nearly 10% have clinically significant permanent neurologic sequelae. Pelvic ring injuries with neurologic dysfunction are associated with a worse long-term outcome.

Urogenital injuries—Urogenital injuries are common, occurring in as many as 24% of adults with pelvic fractures. Males have twice the urethral injury incidence compared to females because of the longer male urethra. In males, these injuries should be suspected in patients with gross hematuria, blood at the meatus, swelling or hematoma of the perineum or penis, an inability to void, or a "high-riding" prostate upon digital rectal examination.

Additionally, in female patients, vaginal bleeding, labial edema, blood at the meatus, and urinary leak per rectum can be clinical signs of possible urethral injury. Blind insertion of a Foley catheter may cause extension of a partial tear into a complete tear, may increase the extent of a hemorrhage, or may introduce an infectious agent into a previously sterile hematoma, so a retrograde, ascending urethrogram should be obtained. When a partial or complete urethral disruption is diagnosed, urology should be consulted. Treatment frequently entails placement of a suprapubic catheter.

Complications

If anatomic restoration of bony alignment is not achieved, pelvic malunion/nonunion can result. Pelvic malunions/nonunions can result in chronic pain, pain, leg length discrepancy, and sitting and gait abnormalities. The overall nonunion rate is around 3%. Chronic low back pain and sacroiliac pain is frequent, seen in up to 50% at long term follow-up. In addition to VTE, infection and permanent neurologic sequelae mentioned earlier, changes in voiding patterns, altered defecation, and sexual dysfunction are also complications.

1. Fractures of the Acetabulum

- Acetabular fractures can be challenging to reduce and fix.
- Anatomic reduction of the hip joint has the strongest correlation with positive outcome.
- Comminuted fractures of the anterior-posterior wall and/or the acetabular roof result in decreased survivorship of the hip.

The acetabulum results from the closure of the Y or triradiate cartilage and is covered with hyaline cartilage. Fractures of the acetabulum occur via direct impact of the femoral head against the acetabulum. The position of the limb at the time of impact (rotation, flexion, abduction, or adduction) determines the pattern of injury.

Anatomy

The acetabulum is supported by an inverted Y arch of two columns and enhanced by two walls. The posterior wall and posterior column have higher load transmissions, and this corresponds with the bone quality of the columns. The posterior column, namely the sciatic buttress, has much stronger bone than the anterior column. The posterior column begins at the dense bone of the greater sciatic notch and extends distally through the center of the acetabulum to include the ischial spine and ischial tuberosity. The inner surface forms the posterior wall, and the anterior surface forms the posterior articular surface of the acetabulum. The anterior column extends from the iliac crest to the symphysis pubis. The anterior column rotates 90 degrees just above the acetabulum as it descends. The medial part of the anterior column is the true pelvic brim. The quadrilateral plate is the medial structure preventing medial displacement of the femoral head and is a shared structure of the anterior and posterior columns. The acetabular roof comprises an arc of approximately 30 degrees on the AP radiograph and 30 to 40 degrees on the oblique radiographs.

Classification

Letournel has classified acetabular fractures based on the involved columns and/or walls. The fracture patterns have been divided into elementary and associated fracture patterns. Proper fracture classification requires good-quality radiographs. The pelvis, including the acetabulum, is a complex three-dimensional bone, and understanding radiographs is critical to fracture classification, surgical approach, reduction methods, and placement of fixation. Letournel felt that the majority of acetabular fractures can be classified from the AP pelvis view. Two obturator oblique views (Judet views) taken 45 degrees toward and away from the involved side complement the standard AP view of the pelvis. The obturator oblique view is obtained by elevating the fractured hip 45 degrees from the horizontal. This view shows the anterior column as the iliopectineal line and the posterior lip of the acetabulum, and the iliac wing is perpendicular to its broad surface. In this view, the spur sign can be identified in the majority of associated both-column fractures, and it corresponds to the area of the displaced innominate bone above the acetabular roof. The iliac oblique view is obtained by elevating the nonfractured hip 45 degrees and best shows the posterior column and the anterior wall. CT scans also demonstrate loose bodies, marginal impaction, and degree of comminution. The surgeon should attempt to understand the radiographic lines and convert the 2-dimesinoal radiograph to a 3-dimensional mental picture. A thorough understanding of the fracture classification usually translates into the correct surgical approach as well as improved reduction and fixation. These fractures, unlike any other in orthopaedics, require pre-operative mental planning by the surgeon. Drawing the fracture lines on either a 3-D pelvic model or 2-D pelvic paper model is very helpful. The surgeon can then utilize he CT scan to confirm his/her mental picture of the fracture.

Letournel has classified acetabular fractures into 10 different types: five elementary patterns and five associated patterns (Figure 2–21). This is the most widely used classification system, although proper classification can be difficult even for experienced pelvic/acetabular surgeons.

Treatment

The goal of treatment is to attain anatomic reduction of the hip joint because this most strongly correlates with survivorship of the hip. Congruency of the femoral head with the acetabulum is also a positive factor for a good prognosis. Surgical indications include intraarticular displacement of 2 mm or more, femoral head incongruity, marginal impaction, or intraarticular loose bodies. Indications may vary based on the surgeon and/or the patient's physiology/activity level. These injuries are best treated by experienced pelvic and acetabular surgeons. The vast majority of these

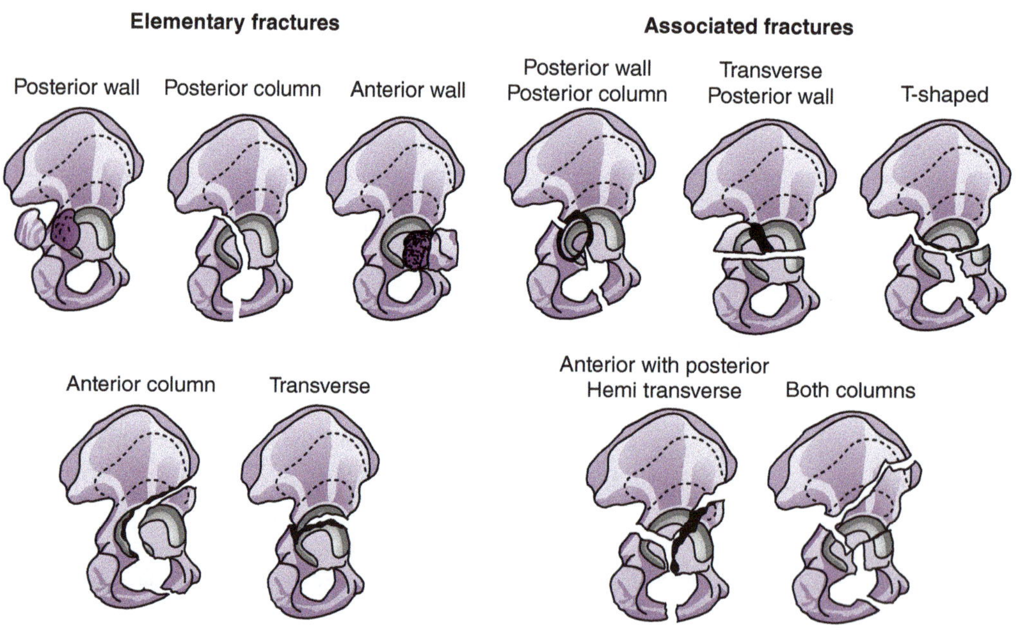

▲ **Figure 2–21. Letournel classification of elementary and associated acetabular fractures.** (Reprinted with permission from Letournel A, Judet R. Fractures of the Acetabulum. 2nd edition. Springer-Verlag, 1993.)

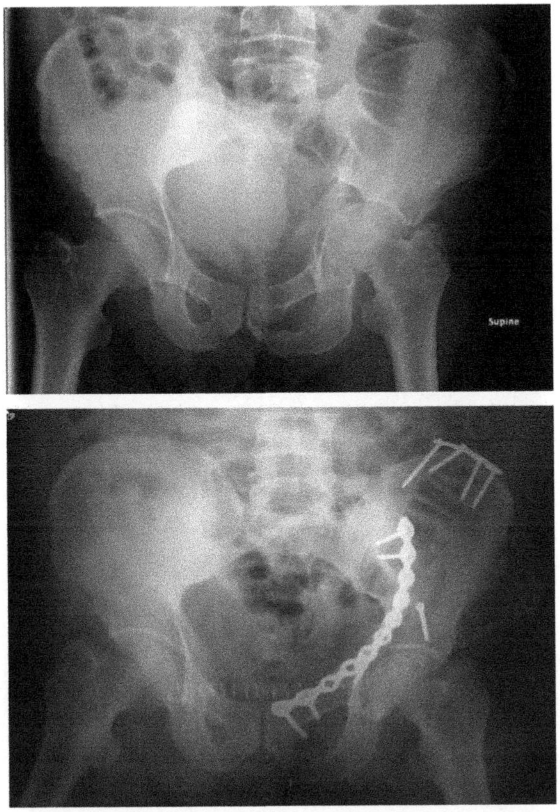

▲ **Figure 2–22.** Pre- and postoperative anteroposterior pelvis radiographs demonstrating surgical fixation of an associated both-column acetabular fracture.

fractures can be treated with the Kocher-Langenbeck and/or the ilioinguinal approach. The ilioinguinal approach allows excellent exposure of the anterior wall for disimpacting the roof and exposure of the quadrilateral surface. An associated both-column acetabular fracture treated by the ilioinguinal approach is shown in Figure 2–22. The modified Stoppa approach can also be used instead of the medial window of the ilioinguinal approach to allow exposure of the pubis or subinguinal exposure of the quadrilateral surface. We have not used the extended iliofemoral approach often; however, its indications are acetabular fractures with involvement of the sciatic buttress/sacroiliac joint, transtectal T-shaped acetabular fractures, and early or late fractures after 3 to 4 weeks that necessitate exposure of the inner and outer aspects of the anterior and posterior columns.

Matta published the largest single-surgeon survivorship study on operative fixation of acetabular fractures, and his 20-year survivorship is shown in Table 2–5. Anterior wall fractures have the lowest 20-year survivorship at 34% because they frequently occur in the elderly with poor bone. This anterior wall/radiographic roof bone is prone to loss of reduction with subsequent joint failure. Because the acetabular roof and posterior wall are the highest regions of load transmission, they are the most prone to failure.

Risks of acetabular surgery include infection, bleeding, iatrogenic nerve injury, vascular injury, heterotopic ossification, blood clots, and posttraumatic arthritis. In Letournel's study of 492 operatively treated acetabular fractures, he reported a sciatic palsy in 6.3%. Extending the hip and flexing the knee with the affected hip in a slight amount of abduction can take tension off the sciatic nerve and lowers the incidence of peroneal nerve palsy. Typically, the patient is non–weight bearing for 8 to 10 weeks, at which time we allow weight bearing as tolerated. Deep acetabular infections are rare; however, they can be treated with irrigation and debridement and placement of biodegradable calcium sulfate antibiotic beads until the fracture is healed. Once the fracture has healed, the implants can be removed. We have not found a benefit to routine radiation and/or NSAIDs for heterotopic ossification prevention. Acetabular nonunions are rare but undergo a standard infection workup and are treated accordingly (eg, revision fixation, bone grafting).

The treatment for elderly patients with poor prognostic acetabular fractures is controversial. Some surgeons recommend limited ORIF with a primary total hip arthroplasty. We perform limited ORIF/percutaneous fixation to minimize operative time and morbidity in these patients. Implants are placed so they will not obstruct a total hip replacement, if necessary. Once the fracture has healed, a total hip replacement is performed.

Complications

Complications inherent to acetabular fractures include posttraumatic degenerative joint disease, heterotopic ossification, femoral head osteonecrosis, DVT, and other complications related to conservative treatment. Surgery is performed to prevent or delay degenerative joint disease but, as mentioned earlier, increases the possibility of complications such as infection, iatrogenic neurovascular injury, and heterotopic ossification.

Cothren CC, Osborn PM, Moore EE, Morgan SJ, Johnson JL, Smith WR. Preperitoneal pelvic packing for hemodynamically unstable pelvic fractures: a paradigm shift. *J Trauma.* 2007;62(4):834-839. [PMID: 17426537]

Hagen J, Castillo R, Dubina A, Gaski G, Manson TT, O'Toole RV. Does surgical stabilization of lateral compression-type pelvic ring fractures decrease patients' pain, reduce narcotic use, and improve mobilization? *Clin Orthop Relat Res.* 2016;474:1422-1429. [PMID: 26304045]

Kaiser SP, Gardner MJ, Liu J, Routt ML, Morshed S. Anatomic determinant of sacral dysmorphism and implications for safe iliosacral screw placement. *J Bone Joint Surg Am.* 2014;96(14):e120. [PMID: 25031382]

Letournel É, Judet R. *Fractures of the Acetabulum.* 2nd ed. Springer-Verlag; 1993.

Slobogean GP, Lefaivre KA, Nicolaou S, O'Brien PJ. A systematic review of thromboprophylaxis for pelvic and acetabular fractures. *J Orthop Trauma.* 2009;23(5):379-384. [PMID: 19390367]

Table 2–5. Two- to twenty-year survivorship of operatively treated acetabular fractures according to fracture type and other characteristics.

	Survivorship (95% Confidence Interval) (%)				
	2 Years	5 Years	10 Years	20 Years	Median Time to Failure
Entire series (n = 816)	91 (90-92)	88 (87-90)	85 (84-87)	79 (76-81)	1.5
Elementary fracture type (n = 241)	91 (89-93)	86 (84-89)	84 (81-87)	73 (68-79)	1.3
Anterior wall (n = 12)	91 (82-100)	68 (53-84)	68 (53-84)	34 (9-59)	2.3
Anterior column (n = 80)	95 (92-97)	92 (88-95)	87 (83-91)	77 (70-85)	3.0
Posterior wall (n = 107)	88 (84-91)	82 (78-86)	81 (77-85)	76 (71-82)	1.2
Posterior column (n = 14)	100	100	100	100	—
Transverse (n = 28)	89 (83-95)	89 (83-95)	89 (83-95)	89 (83-95)	0.3
Associated fracture type (n = 575)	92 (91-93)	89 (88-91)	86 (84-87)	80 (78-83)	1.6
Posterior column, posterior wall (n = 26)	85 (78-92)	85 (78-92)	85 (78-92)	85 (78-92)	0.5
Transverse, posterior wall (n = 143)	89 (86-91)	85 (82-88)	81 (78-85)	74 (68-80)	1.5
T-shaped (n = 96)	89 (85-92)	85 (81-89)	77 (72-81)	74 (65-84)	1.6
Anterior column, posterior hemitransverse (n = 76)	92 (89-95)	92 (89-95)	88 (84-92)	75 (65-84)	1.3
Both columns (n = 234)	96 (94-97)	83 (91-95)	91 (89-93)	87 (83-90)	2.2
Initial displacement					
≥20 mm (n = 226)	86 (84-89)	84 (81-86)	78 (75-81)	68 (63-73)	1.3
≤20 mm (n = 590)	93 (92-95)	90 (89-91)	88 (86-89)	83 (81-85)	1.9
Treatment delay					
<21 days (n = 730)	93 (92-94)	89 (88-91)	86 (85-88)	79 (77-82)	2.0
>21 days (n = 86)	82 (78-86)	80 (75-84)	74 (69-79)	74 (69-79)	0.9
Previous surgery					
Yes (n = 5)	60 (38-82)	30 (6-54)	—	—	0.8
No (n = 811)	92 (91-93)	89 (87-90)	85 (84-87)	79 (77-81)	1.6
Age					
<40 years (n = 386)	96 (95-97)	95 (94-96)	92 (91-94)	87 (84-89)	2.3
40-65 years (n = 318)	88 (86-90)	83 (81-86)	81 (79-83)	74 (71-77)	1.3
>65 years (n = 112)	83 (79-87)	79 (75-83)	70 (65-76)	51 (38-64)	0.8
>75 years (n = 42)	80 (73-87)	74 (66-83)	65 (54-76)	—	0.6

Reprinted with permission from Tannast M, Najibi S, Matta JM. Two to twenty-year survivorship of the hip in 810 patients with operatively treated acetabular fractures. J Bone Joint Surg Am. 2012;94(17):1559-1567.

Tannast M, Najibi S, Matta JM. Two to twenty-year survivorship of the hip in 810 patients with operatively treated acetabular fractures. *J Bone Joint Surg Am.* 2012;94(17):1559-1567. [PMID: 22992846]

Ziran N, Soles GL, Matta JM. Outcomes after surgical treatment of acetabular fractures: a review. *Patient Saf Surg.* 2019;13:16. [PMID: 30923570]

Ziran NM, Smith WR. Management of specific injuries: pelvic fractures. In: Smith WR, Stahel PF, eds. *Management of Musculoskeletal Injuries in the Trauma Patient.* Springer; 2014.

HIP FRACTURES AND DISLOCATIONS

- Globally, 6.3 million hip fractures are estimated by the year 2050.
- Primarily occur in patients over 55 years.
- Almost all hip fractures are treated surgically.
- One-year mortality after femoral neck and intertrochanteric fracture is 14% to 36%.

Anatomic and Biomechanical Principles

The hip joint is the articulation between the acetabulum and the femoral head. The trabecular pattern of the femoral head and neck and that of the acetabulum are oriented to optimally accept the forces crossing the joint. The calcar femorale is the dense bone oriented in the posteromedial portion of the femoral shaft under the lesser trochanter that supports the force transfer from the neck to the shaft.

When standing, the femoral heads support approximately two-thirds of the weight of the body, including the torso, arms, and head, so each hip supports one-third of body weight. During walking and single-limb stance, each hip supports approximately four times the body weight. During single-leg stance, the pelvis tilts in the coronal plane 2 to 6 degrees. To prevent the pelvis from further tilting over, the abductors (gluteus medius and minimus) contract to stabilize the pelvis. During walking, myogenic joint reaction forces can reach up to four times the body weight to stabilize the pelvis. Patients who have weak abductors may lean over the affected musculature during single-limb walking stance, called a compensated Trendelenburg gait. During the swing phase, the muscular compressive forces across the hip joint can be up to 50% of the body weight. The compressive forces with stance phase are due to the gluteus medius, gluteus minimus, and tensor fasciae latae muscles.

1. Femoral Head Fractures

- Rare injuries that may occur in association with hip dislocations or acetabular fractures.
- AVN is a potential complication.

Femoral head fractures are injuries usually associated with hip dislocations or acetabular fractures. They tend to be high-energy injuries and result from MVAs, falls from height, or athletic activities. Hip and pelvis radiographs should be obtained; however, CT is often more informative for treatment planning.

The Pipkin classification is the most widely used system for femoral head fractures:

Pipkin I: fracture below the fovea/ligamentum (non–weight-bearing portion of femoral head)

Pipkin II: fracture above the fovea/ligamentum (weight-bearing portion of femoral head)

Pipkin III: type I or II with an associated femoral neck fracture

Pipkin IV: type I or II with an associated acetabular fracture

Pipkin III fractures have a high rate of AVN and poor outcomes. Pipkin IV fractures tend to be anteroinferior in the head due to the impact against the acetabular fracture. The treatment of femoral head fractures depends on the size of the fragment and fracture displacement. Smaller, nonreparable femoral head fracture fragments can be excised via an anterior approach. Larger fragments can be reduced and fixed via an anterior or posterior approach depending on the presence of associated injuries. Figure 2–23 demonstrates a Pipkin IV femoral head fracture with an associated posterior wall acetabular fracture reduced and fixed via a Kocher-Langenbeck approach. With an anterior approach, the hip can be externally rotated to visualize the femoral head fracture. With either approach, a thorough capsular release facilitates visualization of the femoral head fracture. A Schanz screw can be placed in the intertrochanteric ridge to allow lateral traction on the proximal femur for further visualization. Countersunk 2.4- or 2.7-mm cortical screws or headless screws can be used to fix femoral head fractures. Anatomic reductions or those with less than 1 mm of step-off are associated with better outcomes. AVN depends on the vascular injury from the initial trauma and the duration of hip dislocation, as described earlier in the section on hip dislocation. Comminuted femoral head fractures are best treated with total hip arthroplasty. After fixation of femoral head fractures, patients are typically non–weight bearing for 6 to 8 weeks.

2. Femoral Neck Fractures

Femoral neck fractures occur in the intracapsular region between the trochanters distally and the head proximally. The main arterial blood supply of the femoral neck and head comes from an extracapsular ring of vessels formed by the ascending branch of the lateral circumflex artery anteriorly and medial femoral circumflex artery posteriorly. There is also an intracapsular, subsynovial ring (of Chung) at the articular femoral head margin along the neck. Disruption of this ring of Chung is common with intracapsular, high femoral neck fractures, there is also a vascular contribution from the superior and inferior gluteal arteries proximally, which supply the posterior and posterosuperior hip capsule.

Femoral neck fractures are classified as subcapital, transcervical, and basicervical. Basicervical fractures behave more

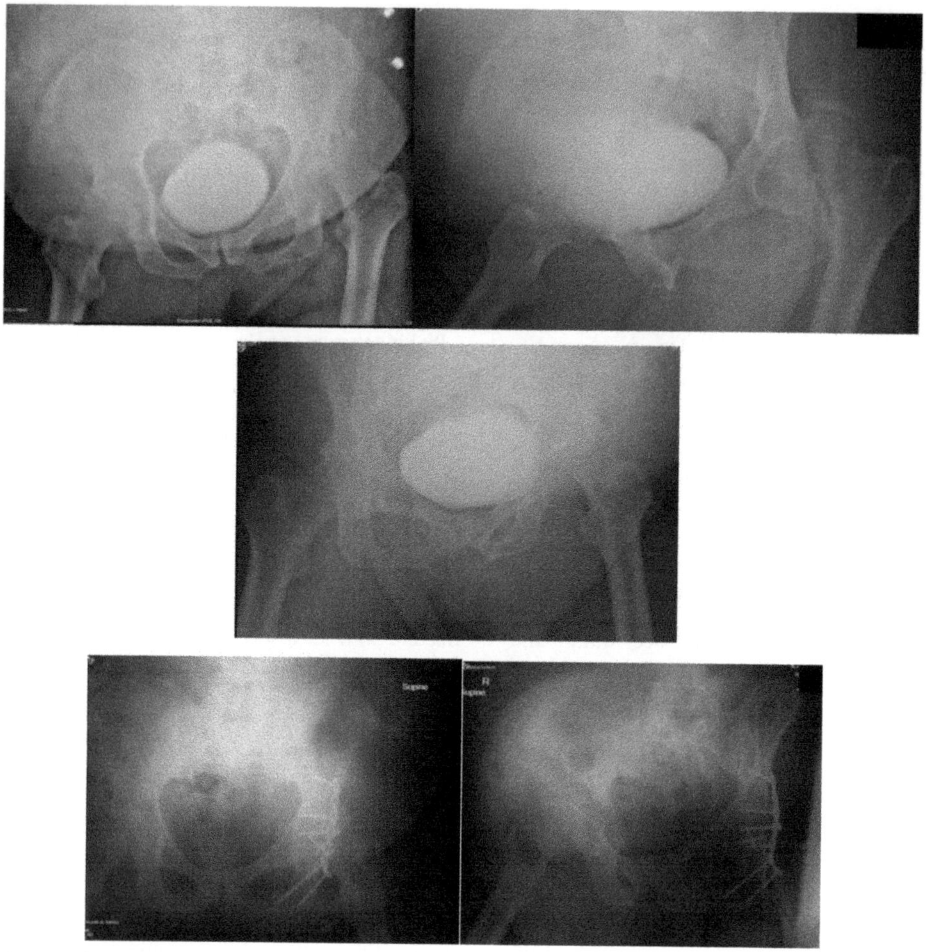

▲ **Figure 2–23.** Pre- and postoperative radiographs of a Pipkin IV left femoral head fracture with associated posterior wall acetabular fracture reduced and fixed via a Kocher-Langenbeck approach.

like an intertrochanteric fracture. These fractures are generally low-energy injuries in the elderly population; however, they can be high-energy injuries at young ages. A typical patient is with a femoral neck fracture is an elderly female who had a falling incident and presents with a painful hip and a shortened and externally rotated extremity. AP and cross-table lateral radiographic views of the involved hip are indicated to diagnose and classify the fracture. Stress fractures of the femoral neck can also occur and should be excluded in young athletes. These and occult nondisplaced fractures can be diagnosed with MRI and/or CT.

Classification

The Garden classification for acute femoral neck fractures is the most widely used:

Type 1: Valgus impaction of the femoral head

Type 2: Complete but nondisplaced

Type 3: Complete fracture displaced less than 50%

Type 4: Complete fracture displaced greater than 50%

This classification is of prognostic value for the incidence of AVN. The higher the Garden classification, the higher is the incidence of AVN. The benefits of either skeletal or skin traction are unclear prior to definitive treatment.

The American Academy of Orthopaedic Surgeons has published evidence-based clinical practice guidelines on the management of hip fractures in the elderly, and factors supported by moderate to strong evidence include the following:

Preoperative regional anesthesia

Hip surgery within 48 hours

Similar outcomes between general or spinal anesthesia

Operative fixation of nondisplaced femoral neck fractures

Arthroplasty for displaced femoral neck fractures

Similar outcomes for unipolar and bipolar hemiarthroplasty

Total hip arthroplasty in properly selected patients with displaced femoral neck fractures

Preferential use of cemented femoral stems

Higher dislocation rate with a posterior approach

VTE prophylaxis should be used

Blood transfusion threshold of no higher than 8 g/dL in asymptomatic postoperative hip fracture patients

Intensive physical therapy after discharge

Nutritional supplementation

Interdisciplinary care program in patients with mild to moderate dementia

Multimodal pain management after hip fracture surgery

Calcium and vitamin D supplementation

Treatment

A. Internal Fixation

Internal fixation of femoral neck fractures is used for nondisplaced fractures, minimally displaced fractures, or fractures in the younger patient. The most widely accepted internal fixation treatments for these fractures are either cannulated screws or a dynamic hip screw. Prior to fixation, a closed reduction is performed with the patient on the fracture table, if necessary. Gentle manipulation is usually sufficient. Rarely, open reduction may be necessary before fixation (ie, young patient with displaced femoral neck fracture). Open reduction, if performed, should be performed via the anterior approach. Care should be taken to avoid injury to the lateral femoral circumflex vessels during the anterior approach. The most accepted method is fixation with three cannulated screws in an inverted-triangle manner with one screw in posteroinferior of the neck. The surgeon should ensure the partial threads of the screw cross the fracture site to allow for compression. The initial screws can be partially-threaded to allow for compression, while the final screw can be fully threaded to prevent further shortening. Fracture collapse with subsequent limb shortening is better tolerated in the elderly. Length-stable fixation (either via a final fully-threaded screw or unloading the extremity until the bone heals) may be an option for younger, more active patients to prevent collapse and limb shortening. There is no benefit to either 6.5-or 7.3-mm screws. For more vertical fractures of the femoral neck (Pauwel's angle of ≥70 degrees), the surgeon can consider a screw directed more perpendicular to the fracture pattern. Care should be taken not to penetrate the femoral head, and the starting point of the screws must be higher than the level of trochanter minor to avoid future fractures. A sliding hip screw/plate construct can also be used for femoral neck fractures and has been found to be beneficial in smokers. The tip-to-apex distance of the lag screw should be less than 25 mm. If the fracture is rotationally unstable, an additional 3.5- or 4.5-mm screw can be inserted superior or posteroinferior in order to control the rotational forces. Because these fractures can collapse, the patients should be informed of the possibility of limb length discrepancy and/or symptomatic implants along the lateral thigh. The patient can usually be mobilized the following day, and weight bearing is allowed according to the bone quality and reduction.

B. Arthroplasty

Arthroplasty is best for displaced fractures (Garden type 3 or 4 fractures) and is most common in the elderly. Overall, total hip replacement seems to be the better alternative in those who are chronologically or physiologically younger, whereas hemiarthroplasty provides sufficient pain and functional outcomes with fewer complications and cost in older individuals. The authors prefer a cemented femoral component to prevent an intra-operative or postoperative fracture. The decision to cement likely depends on numerous factors (bone quality, patient comorbidities, activity level, etc.) and is surgeon- and patient-dependent. Hemiarthroplasty is discussed further in Chapter 8.

Complications

The most common sequelae of femoral neck fractures are loss of reduction with or without implant failure, nonunions or malunions, and AVN of the femoral head. This latter complication can appear as late as 2 years after injury. According to different series, the incidence of AVN for Garden type 1 fractures varies from 0% to 15%, for type 2 fractures 10% to 25%, for type 3 fractures 25% to 50%, and for type 4 fractures 50% to 100%. In patients with poor bone stock (eg, elderly, chronic steroid use, end-stage renal disease), it may be beneficial to delay weight-bearing.

3. Trochanteric Fractures

Lesser Trochanter Fractures

Isolated fracture of the lesser trochanter is rare. When it occurs, it results from avulsion of the iliopsoas. Rarely, a symptomatic nonunion may require fragment fixation or excision.

Greater Trochanter Fractures

Isolated fracture of the greater trochanter may be caused by direct injury or may occur indirectly as a result of avulsion of the gluteus medius and gluteus minimus. It occurs most commonly as a component of an intertrochanteric fracture. If displacement of the isolated fracture fragment is less than 1 cm and there is no tendency to further displacement, as determined by repeated radiographic examinations, treatment may be bed rest until acute pain subsides. As rapidly as symptoms permit, activity can increase gradually to protected weight bearing with limited abduction with crutches. Full weight bearing is permitted as soon as healing is apparent, usually in 6 to 8 weeks. If displacement is greater than 1 cm and/or abductor function is compromised, ORIF may be beneficial. The bone quality in the greater trochanter may be poor, and care should be taken to achieve satisfactory fixation. Potential fixation methods include TBW or fixation with two 3.5-mm lag screws over a washer.

Intertrochanteric Hip Fractures

- Account for 50% of all hip fractures.
- Increased age, female sex, osteoporosis, history of fall, and gait abnormalities are risk factors.

Intertrochanteric hip fractures usually occur along a line between the greater and the lesser trochanter; however, there are variations. They typically occur at a later age than do femoral neck fractures. Because they occur lower in the proximal femur, they are extracapsular and the vascular supply to the femoral head is typically preserved. It usually takes 6 to 8 weeks for these fractures to heal. Nonunions and AVN are uncommon when treated with ORIF.

Clinically, the involved extremity is usually shortened and can be internally or externally rotated. A stable intertrochanteric hip fracture is a fracture line between the greater and lesser trochanter. An unstable intertrochanteric hip fracture includes fractures of the greater and/or lesser trochanter. Other unstable fracture patterns are transverse fractures, fractures with calcar and/or posteromedial comminution, fractures with subtrochanteric extension, and reverse oblique fractures. Figure 2–24 demonstrates intertrochanteric hip fracture classification based on stability.

Treatment

Operative treatment is indicated as soon as the patient is medically able to tolerate surgery. Overall mortality decreases if surgery can be performed within 48 hours. Preoperative traction has moderate supportive evidence in lowering preoperative pain. When surgery is contraindicated, it may be preferable to mobilize the patient as soon as pain permits and accept the eventual malunion or nonunion. Studies have shown that patients treated conservatively have a mortality rate of 70% to 80% in the first year.

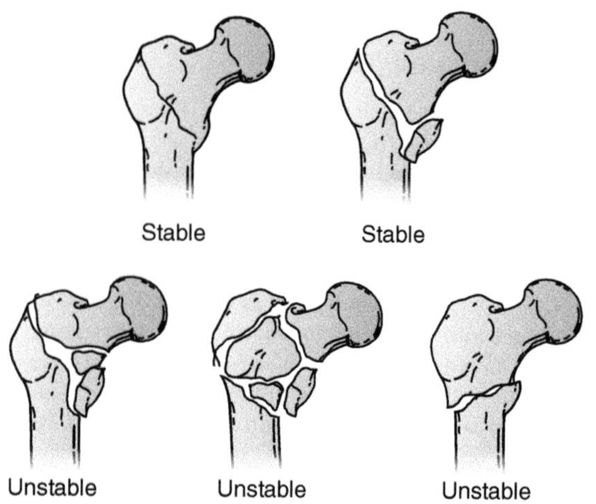

▲ **Figure 2–24.** Classification of intertrochanteric hip fractures based on stable versus unstable. (Adapted from Jensen J. S. Classification of trochanteric fractures. Actaorthop. Scand. 1980; 51:803-810.)

The goal of surgical fixation is to achieve a satisfactory reduction and appropriate fixation so the patient can mobilize quickly. Closed reduction of the fracture is performed on a fracture table. In most cases, gentle traction and/or internal rotation is sufficient to reduce the fracture. In the typical fracture pattern, the fracture proximally disrupts the hip external rotators so the proximal segment may be internally rotated. In these cases, internal rotation of the femoral shaft improves the reduction. However, in low intertrochanteric fractures, where the fracture line is below the insertion of the rotators, the proximal head/neck/trochanter may be externally rotated. In these cases, external rotation and/or abduction of the lower extremity can be beneficial to achieve reduction. In these particular cases, a sliding hip screw may be beneficial because the implant is easier to place than a cephalomedullary nail.

During reduction of intertrochanteric hip fractures, it is important to achieve an excellent reduction of the calcar; if there is residual deformity, valgus is preferred over varus. Implant choices include a sliding hip screw or a short versus long cephalomedullary nail. Both methods of fixation are satisfactory and used according to surgeon preference, although cephalomedullary nails have gained popularity. There is decreased blood loss with cephalomedullary nails compared to sliding hip screws; however, cephalomedullary nails are more expensive. As mentioned earlier, tip-to-apex distance of the sliding hip screw should be less than 25 mm. The choice between a helical blade or lag screw in the femoral head is controversial. Regardless, we try to position the lag screw or helical blade inferior in the head on the anteroposterior radiographic view and either slightly posterior or central position on the lateral view. Because these implants typically cut out superoanteriorly, placement slightly posteroinferiorly results in more bone before cut out can occur. To ensure axial stability, the lateral edge of the screw or blade should be either flush or minimally protruding from the lateral cortex of the femur. If the screw or blade is too short, there is potential for axial instability and displacement of the fracture, especially if there is no distal interlocking screw through the cephalomedullary nail. Dual integrated lag screw designs, those with two screws in the femoral head, have less limb shortening and superior functional outcomes in unstable fracture patterns. The decision to use a long versus short cephalomedullary nail is also surgeon preference because there is no benefit of one over the other for either stable or unstable intertrochanteric hip fractures. With long femoral nails, the nail can sometimes abut against the anterior cortex (Figure 2–25). This usually occurs from difference in the radius of curvature of the nail and the femoral shaft.

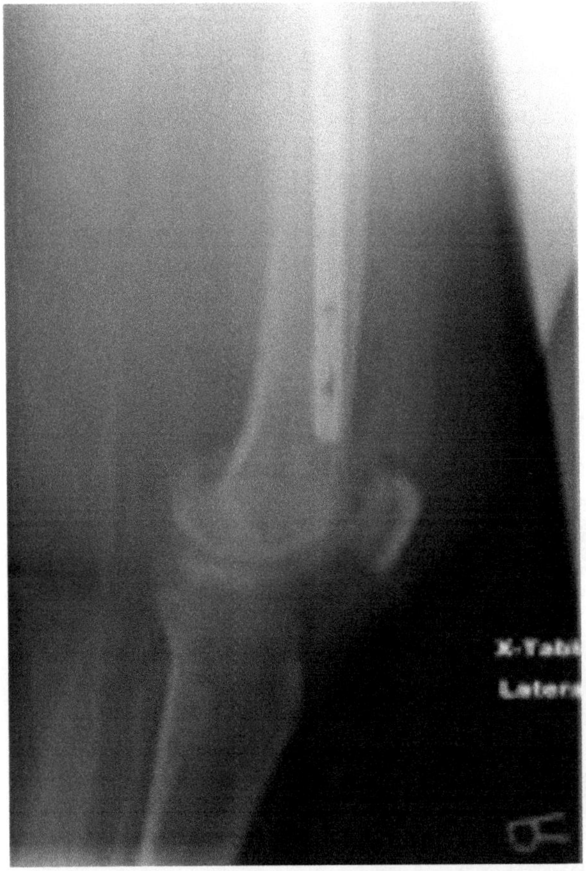

▲ **Figure 2–25.** Long cephalomedullary nails can occasionally abut against the anterior femoral cortex (shown in the lateral distal femur radiograph) usually due to a difference between the radius of curvature of the femur and the nail.

The distal interlocking screw in a cephalomedullary nail improves torsional load-to-failure and torsional stiffness in unstable fractures so it may benefit those with posteromedial comminution, reverse obliquity, and subtrochanteric extension. However, the decision to place a distal interlocking screw is based on surgeon preference and has no benefit in stable fractures. Figure 2–26 demonstrates a right intertrochanteric hip fracture with subtrochanteric extension fixed with a long cephalomedullary nail, cerclage cables, and two distal interlocking screws (not shown). Reverse oblique fractures should be treated as subtrochanteric fractures, and a long cephalomedullary nail is the appropriate implant for this fracture. Finally, calcar replacement arthroplasty may be an option for patients with significant calcar comminution and/or preexisting arthritic changes. Complications of ORIF of intertrochanteric fractures include infection, implant failure, loss of reduction, nonunion, and bursitis/irritation due to lag screw/blade.

4. Subtrochanteric Femur Fractures

- These occur from the lesser trochanter to a point 5 cm distal to it.
- Frequent site of pathologic fracture.

Subtrochanteric fractures occur below the level of the lesser trochanter and are usually the result of high-energy trauma in young to middle-aged adults. They are often comminuted, with distal or proximal extension toward the greater trochanter. The patient usually presents with a swollen painful proximal thigh with or without shortening or malrotation. If the lesser trochanter is intact, the proximal fragment will tend to displace in flexion, external rotation, and abduction because of the unopposed pull of the iliopsoas and abductor muscles. There is a corrleation between bisphosphonate use and l atypical subtrochanteric femur fractures (AFFs). These fractures are typically transverse or short oblique. These fractures may have periosteal ('beaking') or endosteal thickening and may heal slower after surgery. Bisphosphonates should be discontinued.

The Russell and Taylor classification is based on involvement of the piriformis fossa. Type Ia Russell-Taylor fractures do not involve the piriformis fossa, with the lesser trochanter attached to the proximal fragment. Type Ib fractures do not involve the piriformis fossa; however, the lesser trochanter is detached from the proximal fragment. Type II fractures have fracture extension into the piriformis fossa.

For most cases, internal fixation by closed or open methods is best. Earlier implants such as blade plate fixation have largely been replaced with cephalomedullary nails. Temporary skeletal traction is beneficial to maintain length until the definitive surgical procedure.

Fixation can be obtained with either trochanteric ('piriformis') fossa entry or trochanteric entry cephalomedullary nails. The proximal fragment is usually flexed and abducted due to the pull of the iliopsoas the the abductors, respectively. Two ball-spike pushers, one anterior to posterior and another lateral to medial, can be utilized to facilitate reduction. We have found that this maneuver is best performed at the start of the case to also facilitate the starting point on the trochanter. Before or after the nail has been passed, cerclage cables can be used to reduce varus deformity. If the fracture pattern is more transverse and not amenable to cerclage cabling, a laterally placed four- to five-hole 3.5-mm antiglide plate with unicortical locking screws can also be used to prevent later-onset varus deformity. If there is satisfactory cortical contact of the fracture fragments, the authors do not feel the increased mechanical stiffness imposed by a laterally applied antiglide plate interferes with fracture healing. However, if there is concern for excessive construct stiffness, the proximal holes of this laterally-based plate can be left free of screws so it functions as a true antiglide plate. Patients are typically toe-touch weight bearing, although postoperative weight-bearing status varies depending on numerous factors such as surgeon comfort, fracture

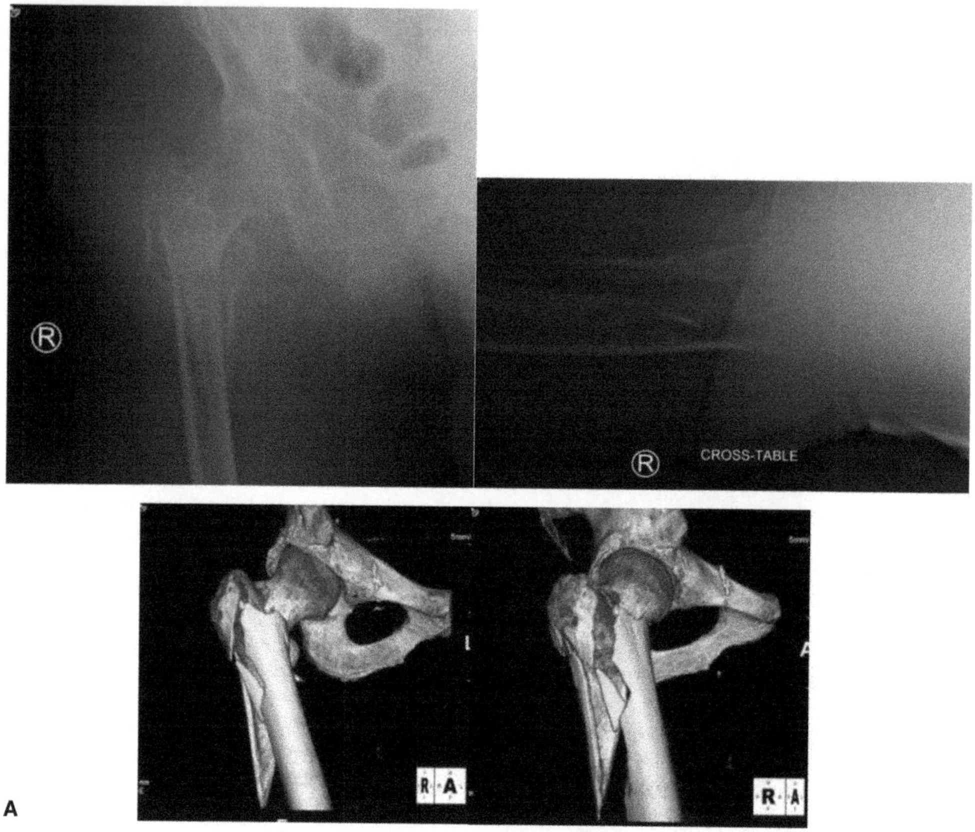

A

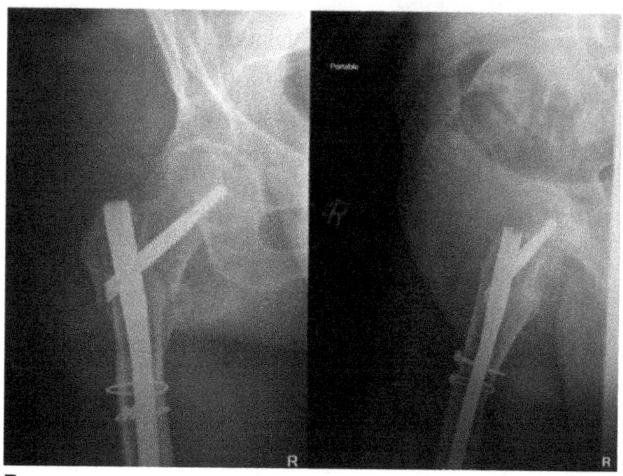

B

▲ **Figure 2–26. A:** Pre- and postoperative radiographs and CT reconstruction of a right intertrochanteric hip fracture with subtrochanteric extension (unstable). **B:** The fracture was reduced and fixed with a long cephalomedullary nail with two cerclage cables and two distal interlocking screws (not shown).

fixation, and bone quality. Union is usually achieved within 8 to 12 weeks; however, it can take longer because these fractures are prone to deformity. Varus deformity and nonunion are the main complications of subtrochanteric femur fractures, but improved reduction techniques and implants have diminished these issues.

Rehabilitation of Hip Fracture Patients

The outcomes of patients after surgical treatment of hip fractures have dramatically changed over the past three decades. The goal of rehabilitation after hip injuries is to return the patient as rapidly as possible to the preinjury functional level. Improvements in biomechanics such as implant designs and surgical techniques have resulted in earlier rehabilitation with more weight bearing. Factors influencing rehabilitation include age, mental status, associated injuries, previous medical status, myocardial function, upper extremity strength, balance, and motivation. For the rare patient treated nonoperatively, rehabilitation focuses on preventing conditions associated with immobilization such as decubitus ulcers, pneumonia, urinary tract infections, DVT, and stiffness. Because the great majority of these injuries are now treated with internal fixation or prosthetic replacement, rehabilitation efforts are focused toward early range of motion, muscle strengthening, and weight bearing. Early full weight bearing as tolerated is encouraged for patients with prosthetic replacements, cemented or not, and for patients with stable fixation of an intertrochanteric fracture to allow compression of the fracture fragments. Partial weight bearing after internal fixation is reserved for those with poor bone quality or if the fracture reduction or implant position is not ideal.

5. Traumatic Dislocation of the Hip Joint

- Usually a result of a high-energy trauma.
- Occurs with or without acetabular fractures.
- Eighty-five percent are posterior dislocations.
- Concomitant femur, knee, and patella fractures are common.

Posterior Hip Dislocation

Usually, the head of the femur is dislocated posterior to the acetabulum when the thigh is flexed. Posterior hip dislocations may occur in a head-on MVA when the knee is driven against the dashboard. Posterior hip dislocation can also be a complication of hip arthroplasty.

The significant clinical findings are shortening, adduction, and internal rotation of the extremity. AP and lateral hip x-rays should be obtained to confirm the diagnosis. If there is a suspected acetabular fracture, Judet views should be done. CT can confirm the position of the femoral head relative to the acetabulum and also demonstrate if there is a fracture. Associated injuries include acetabular fracture, femoral head fracture, and/or sciatic nerve injury. The head of the femur may be displaced through a tear in the posterior hip joint capsule. The short external rotator muscles of the femur are commonly injured. Fracture of the posterior wall of the acetabulum can create instability.

If the acetabulum is not fractured or if the fragment is small, reduction by closed manipulation is indicated. Reduction should be achieved as soon as possible, usually with general anesthesia with maximum muscle relaxation, preferably within the first few hours after injury. Reduction of the hip is performed by applying in-line traction, hip flexion, and internal rotation followed by external rotation (Allis method). An assistant should stabilize the pelvis during this maneuver.

The stability of the reduction is evaluated clinically by ranging the extended hip in abduction and adduction and internal and external rotation. If stable, the same movements are repeated in 90 degrees of hip flexion. The point of re-dislocation is noted, the hip is reduced, and an AP radiograph of the pelvis is obtained. Soft-tissue or bone fragment interposition will be manifested by widening of the joint space as compared to the contralateral side (Figure 2–27). Indications for surgery are irreducible dislocations, nonconcentric reductions, open dislocations, ipsilateral femoral neck fractures, and unstable hip joint especially in the presence of a posterior wall acetabular fracture. CT of

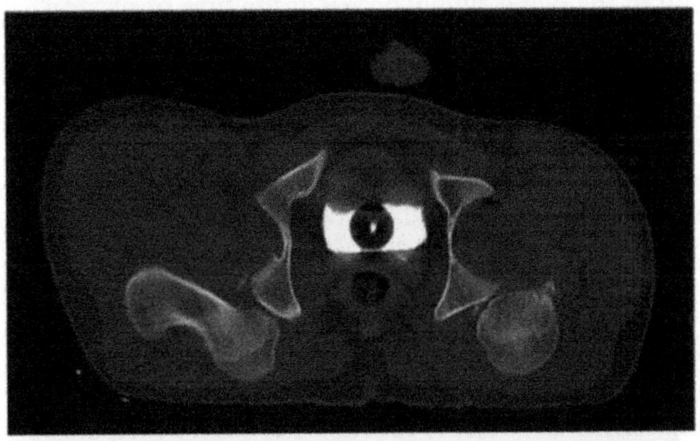

A

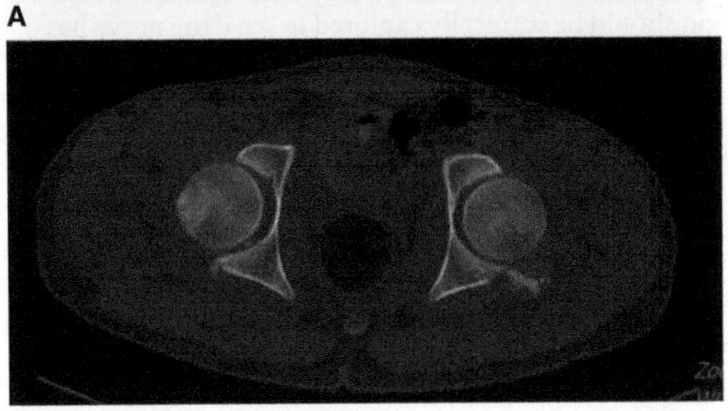

B

▲ **Figure 2–27. A:** Bilateral posterior hip dislocation of a pediatric patient involved in a motor vehicle accident. **B:** After reduction under general anesthesia, eccentric reduction and loose body are observed on the right hip, which may warrant arthroscopy or open arthrotomy.

the hip can diagnose loose bodies in the joint and/or other suspected fractures. Hip arthroscopy may be a safer alternative to arthrotomy for managing loose bodies.

Smaller fractures of the posterior wall can usually be treated conservatively, but larger displaced fragments are not usually successfully reduced by closed methods. If there is any question, a stress test in the operating room to assess hip stability can be done. If the hip is unstable, ORIF of the posterior wall should be performed.

Weight bearing is determined based on the injury. For most injuries, the patient can be weight bearing as tolerated with limitations in hip flexion and internal rotation to prevent re-dislocation. Bracing in abduction is sometimes helpful in uncooperative patients. If there is an associated femoral head fracture or acetabular fracture, weight bearing as tolerated is not allowed for approximately 8 to 10 weeks.

A. Complications

Complications of posterior hip dislocation include AVN of the femoral head, malunion, posttraumatic degenerative joint disease, recurrent dislocation, infection, and sciatic nerve injury. AVN occurs because of disruption of the retinacular arteries and the medial femoral circumflex artery that provide blood to the femoral head. Although the original insult to the blood supply occurs at the time of dislocation, it is better to promptly reduce the hip to prevent further injury. The odds ratio of AVN is 5.6 times greater for hips reduced after 12 hours compared to those reduced before 12 hours. AVN can occur as late as 2 years after the injury. MRI enables early diagnosis, and protected weight bearing is recommended until revascularization has occurred. Sciatic nerve injury occurs in 10% to 20% of patients with posterior hip dislocation, and it is critical to document a motor and sensory exam of the sciatic nerve before and after reduction of the hip. Although usually a neurapraxia, these lesions are permanent in about 20% of patients. The rare patient who is neurologically intact before reduction but has a deficit after reduction should be surgically explored to see if the nerve has been entrapped in the joint.

Anterior Hip Dislocation

- Accounts for 10% to 15% of hip fracture dislocations.
- Occurs when the hip is extended and externally rotated at the time of impact.

Usually, the femoral head remains lateral to the obturator externus muscle but may be found beneath it, known as an obturator dislocation, or under the iliopsoas muscle in contact with the superior pubic ramus, known as a pubic dislocation. The hip is classically extended and externally rotated. The femoral head is palpable anteriorly, below the inguinal flexion crease. AP and transpelvic lateral radiographic views are usually diagnostic; however, CT is increasingly used not only to diagnose the direction of dislocation but also to detect a fracture. Closed reduction, usually under general anesthesia, is generally successful. Postreduction radiographs should be obtained to ensure a concentric reduction with no soft-tissue interposition. The patient can begin weight bearing as tolerated as well as active and passive hip motion, excluding external rotation, abduction, and extension. Bracing in abduction is sometimes helpful in uncooperative patients.

Baldwin PC, Lavender RC, Sanders R, Koval KJ. Controversies in intramedullary fixation for intertrochanteric hip fractures. *J Orthop Trauma.* 2016;30(12):635-641. [PMID: 27437614]

Bernstein J, Ahn J. In brief: fractures in brief: femoral neck fractures. *Clin Orthop Relat Res.* 2010;468:1713-1715. [PMID: 20224957]

Dolatowski FC, Frihagen F, Bartels S, et al. Screw fixation versus hemiarthroplasty for nondisplaced femoral neck fractures in elderly patient. *J Bone Joint Surg Am.* 2019;101:136-144. [PMID: 30653043]

FAITH Investigators. Fracture fixation in the operative management of hip fractures (FAITH): an international, multicentre, randomised trial. *Lancet.* 2017;389(10078):1519-1527. [PMID: 28262269]

Foulk DM, Mullis BH. Hip dislocation: evaluation and management. *J Am Acad Orthop Surg.* 2010;18:199-209. [PMID: 20357229]

Hou Z, Bowen TR, Irgit KS, et al. Treatment of pertrochanteric fractures (OTA 31-A1 and A2): long versus short cephalomedullary nailing. *J Orthop Trauma.* 2013;27(6):318-324. [PMID: 22955331]

Irgit K, Richard RD, Beebe MJ, Bowen TR, Kubiak E, Horwitz DS. Reverse oblique and transverse intertrochanteric femoral fractures treated with the long cephalomedullary nail. *J Orthop Trauma.* 2015;29(9):e299-e304. [PMID: 25909765]

Jiang J, Yang CH, Lin Q, Yun XD, Xia YY. Does arthroplasty provide better outcomes than internal fixation at mid- and long-term followup? A meta-analysis. *Clin Orthop Relat Res.* 2015;473(8):2672-2679. [PMID: 25981713]

Kellam P, Ostrum RF. Systematic review and meta-analysis of avascular necrosis and post-traumatic arthritis after traumatic hip dislocation. *J Orthop Trauma.* 2016;30(1):10-16. [PMID: 26849386]

Roberts KC, Brox WT, Jevsevar DS, Sevarino K. Management of hip fractures in the elderly. *J Am Acad Orthop Surg.* 2015;23(2):131-137. [PMID: 25624365]

Scolaro JA, Marecek G, Firoozabadi R, Krieg JC, Routt MLC. Management and radiographic outcomes of femoral head fractures. *J Orthop Traumatol.* 2017;18(3):235-241. [PMID: 28188487]

Standring S. *Gray's Anatomy: The Anatomical Basis of Clinical Practice.* 41st ed. Elsevier Limited; 2016.

FEMORAL SHAFT FRACTURES

- Usually associated with high-energy mechanisms of injury.
- Closed, static intramedullary nailing is the standard of care.
- Associated orthopedic injuries are common.
- Timing of femoral shaft fixation continues to change in the polytrauma patient.

1. Diaphyseal Fractures

Fractures of the shaft of the femur usually occur as a result of high-energy trauma. Indirect forces, especially torsional stress, are likely to cause spiral fractures that extend proximally or, more commonly, distally into the metaphyseal regions. Most femoral shaft fracture are closed fractures.

Clinical Findings

Clinical findings associated with femur fractures are obvious deformity, pain, hemodynamic and/or physiologic instability, and other associated injuries. Hemorrhagic shock may be present since 1000 to 1500 mL of blood volume can fill the thigh compartments. Radiographs of the hip and knee should be performed in addition to the femur to rule out other injuries. Concomitant ipsilateral femoral neck fractures may occur in up to 9% of patients and must be suspected and evaluated in addition to ipsilateral ligamentous and meniscal injuries of the knee. Injuries to the sciatic nerve and the superficial femoral artery and vein are uncommon but must be recognized promptly.

Classification

The Winquist classification for femur fractures is based on degree of comminution. Type 1 indicates minimal or no comminution at the fracture site. Type 2 is a fracture with comminution leaving at least 50% of the circumference of the two major fragments intact. Type 3 is a fracture with comminution of 50% to 100% of the circumference of the major fragments and for which nonlocked intramedullary nails do not afford stable fixation. Finally, type 4 is a fracture with a completely comminuted segmental pattern with no intrinsic stability. However, describing femur fractures based on location (proximal third, midshaft, or distal third), fracture pattern (transverse, short/long oblique, butterfly, or comminuted), displacement, and/or presence of shortening is usually sufficient.

Treatment

The majority of femur fractures are operatively treated with a statically locked retrograde or antegrade nail. However, a small population of individuals may be too unstable for nailing, in which case external fixation can be done either in the operating room or bedside in intubated patients. Patients with bilateral femur fractures should be approached with caution due to the risk of fat embolism syndrome (FES). A staged approach (external fixation followed by nailing) may be beneficial in these patients to avoid this rare, but significant, complication. Closed treatment is a last resort due to complications such as malunion, nonunion, DVT, ulcers, and pain.

A. Operative Treatment

Prior to operative treatment, it is ideal to have the patient in approximately 20 lb of skeletal traction to maintain length because this can facilitate reduction. Reamed, locked, antegrade intramedullary nailing through the piriformis fossa has been the gold standard for the treatment of femur fractures, but there are newer nails with easier starting spots such as trochanteric entry nails, lateral entry nails, and retrograde nails, which account for the majority of femoral intramedullary nail fixation. Intramedullary fixation of femoral shaft fractures allows early mobilization of the patient within 24 to 48 hours if the fracture fixation is stable, which is of particular benefit to the polytrauma patient. Restoration of length, alignment, and rotation are important considerations.

Open nailing procedures such as those described by Hey Groves resulted in high infection rates. Closed nailing decreases the chance of infection by minimizing bacterial entry into the fracture site and, hence, the intramedullary canal. The patient should be paralyzed to facilitate closed nailing and reduction. Tools such as F-bars, ball-spike pushers, and crutches can be used to manipulate the fracture fragments. Cortical contact at the fracture site is ideal to avoid a large fracture gap and to maintain length. We routinely use one interlocking screw proximal and two distal to the fracture site. Reamed interlocked nailing is recommended for most Gustilo and Anderson grade I, II, and IIIA open fractures. External fixation can be used when there is extensive soft-tissue loss such as grade IIIB and IIIC open fractures. It is also used in the polytrauma patient with a significant chest and head injury that may preclude EAC/ETC. Nonunions are rare, and one should always suspect deep infections when they occur. Infections, leg length discrepancy, and heterotopic ossification are other complications after this procedure. Retrograde nailing has gained popularity due to an easier starting spot and is beneficial in patients with polytrauma, morbid obesity, and pregnancy (Figure 2–28). Caution should be exercised in patients with bilateral femur fractures since early nailing can result in rare, but devastating FES, which has been described earlier. In patients with bilateral femur fractures and polytrauma, it may be beneficial to perform external fixation initially and an intramedullary nail for each extremity later.

Flexible nails do not provide sufficient stability in the adult; however, they are routinely used in children. Plate and screw fixation can also be performed in children but can result in disruption of the fracture hematoma and excessive bleeding, so it requires a subvastus approach with care taken to ligate the venous perforators. External fixation is also an option as treatment for closed femoral shaft fractures in children, and the distal fragment pins should always be inserted with the knee in flexion to avoid quadriceps tenodesis preventing knee flexion.

Attum B, Rodriguez-Buitrago A, Harrison N, et al. Opioid prescribing practices by orthopaedic trauma surgeons after isolated femur fractures. *J Orthop Trauma*. 2018;32(3):e106-e111. [PMID: 29065039]

Brewster J, Grenier G, Taylor BC, et al. Long-term comparison of retrograde and antegrade femoral nailing. *Orthopedics*. 2020;43(4):e278-e282. [PMID: 32324245]

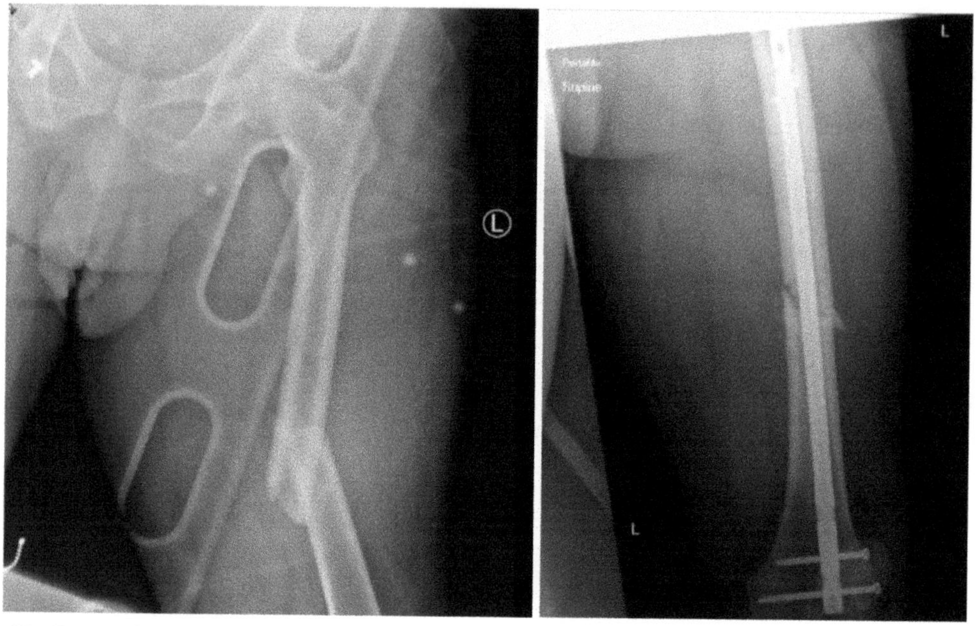

▲ **Figure 2–28.** Pre- and postoperative anteroposterior radiographs of a left femoral shaft fracture treated with a retrograde intramedullary nail.

Brumback RJ, Uwagie-Ero S, Lakatos RP, Poka A, Bathon GH, Burgess AH. Intramedullary nailing of femoral shaft fractures. Part II: fracture-healing with static interlocking fixation. *J Bone Joint Surg Am.* 1988;70(10):1453-1462. [PMID: 3198669]

Byrne JP, Nathens AB, Gomez D, Pincus D, Jenkinson RJ. Timing of femoral shaft fracture fixation following major trauma: a retrospective cohort study of United States trauma centers. *PLoS Med.* 2017;14(7):e1002336. [PMID: 28678793]

Croom WP, Lorenzana DJ, Auran RL, et al. Is contralateral templating reliable for establishing rotational alignment during intramedullary stabilization of femoral shaft fracture? A study of individual bilateral differences in femoral version. *J Orthop Trauma.* 2018;32(2):61-66. [PMID: 28906308]

Hak D, Mauffrey C, Hake M, Hammerberg EM, Stahel PF. Ipsilateral femoral neck and shaft fractures: current diagnostic and treatment strategies. *Orthopedics.* 2015;38(4):247-251. [PMID: 25879185]

Karahan G, Yamak K, Kocoglu T, Altay T, Kayali C. The effect of implant choice on varus angulation and clinical results in the management of subtrochanteric fractures. *J Orthop.* 2020;20: 46-49. [PMID: 32042228]

Lane MK, Nahm NJ, Vallier HA. Morbidity and mortality of bilateral femur fractures. *Orthopedics.* 2015;38(7):e588-e592. [PMID: 26186320]

Lim HS, Kim CK, Park YS, Moon YW, Lim SJ, Kim SM. Factors associated with increased healing time in complete femoral fractures after long-term bisphosphonate therapy. *J Bone Joint Surg Am.* 2016;98(23):1978-1987. [PMID: 27926679]

Scalea TM, Boswell SA, Scott JD, Mitchell KA, Kramer ME, Pollak AN. External fixation as a bridge to intramedullary nailing for patients with multiple injuries and with femur fractures: damage control orthopedics. *J Orthop Trauma.* 2004;18(8 suppl):S2-S10; discussion S10-S12. [PMID: 15472561]

Tazawa R, Minehara H, Matsuura T, et al. Biomechanical evaluation of internal fixation for the treatment of comminuted subtrochanteric femur fractures. *J Orthop Sci.* 2020:S0949-2658(20) 30073-7. [PMID: 32245694]

Tucker WA, Birt MC, Heddings AA, Horton GA. Effect of postoperative nonsteroidal anti-inflammatory drugs on nonunion rates in long bone fractures. *Orthopedics.* 2020;43(4):221-227. [PMID: 32379334]

PATELLA INJURIES

- Largest sesamoid bone in the body.
- Straight leg test is helpful to assess the extensor mechanism.
- Symptomatic implants are a common complication following TBW fixation.

1. Transverse Patellar Fracture

Transverse fractures of the patella (Figure 2–29) are usually the result of an indirect force with the knee in flexion and occur most commonly in the middle. They may be caused by sudden voluntary contraction of the quadriceps muscle or sudden forced flexion of the leg with the quadriceps contracted. Associated tearing of the patella retinaculum occurs depending on the force of the injury. The activity of the quadriceps muscle causes upward displacement of the proximal fragment, the magnitude of which depends on the extent of the retinacular tear.

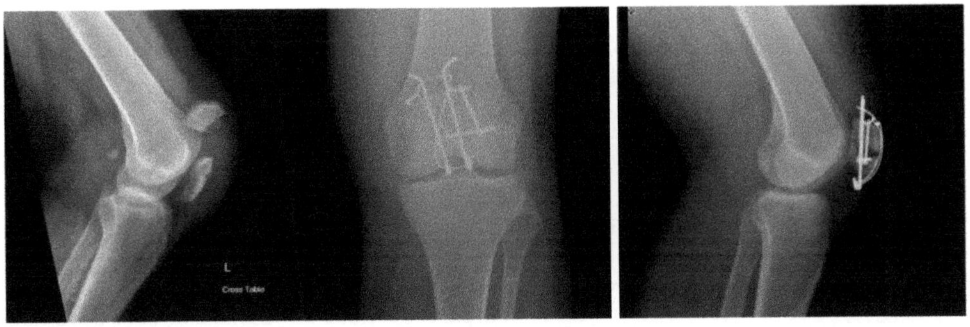

▲ **Figure 2–29.** Pre- and postoperative radiographs of the knee demonstrating reduction and fixation of a transverse patella fracture with comminution. A tension band wire and small screws were used to fix the fracture.

Clinical Findings

Swelling of the anterior knee region is caused by hemarthrosis and hemorrhage into the soft tissues. If displacement is present, the defect in the patella can be palpated, and active extension of the knee is lost. A straight leg raise may be preserved if the medial and lateral patella retinaculum are intact.

Treatment

Nondisplaced fractures can be treated with a walking cylinder cast or brace for 6 to 8 weeks, followed by knee rehabilitation. ORIF is indicated if the fragments are displaced greater than 3 mm or if the articular step-off is greater than 2 mm. The fragments must be accurately repositioned to prevent posttraumatic arthritis of the patellofemoral joint. If the minor fragment is small (no more than 1 cm in length) or severely comminuted, it may be excised and the quadriceps or patellar tendon (depending on which pole of the patella is involved) sutured directly to the major fragment. ORIF of anatomically reduced fragments allows early motion of the knee joint and is best achieved using a figure-of-eight TBW construct over either two longitudinal K-wires or cannulated screws. Symptomatic implant removal is common afterward.

2. Comminuted Patellar Fracture

Comminuted fractures of the patella are usually caused by a direct force. Severe injury may cause extensive destruction of the articular surface of the patellofemoral joint. If comminution is not severe and displacement is insignificant, immobilization for 8 weeks in a cylinder cast is sufficient. Severe comminution can often be treated with small screws, such as 2.7-, 2.4-, and 2.0-mm screws, if the bone fragments are large enough and a circumferential wire around the patella. Rarely, excision of the patella and imbricating the extensor mechanism about the same length of the patella is the only alternative. Excision of the patella can result in decreased strength, pain in the knee, and general restriction of activity. High-energy patella fractures can be complicated by chondromalacia patella and patellofemoral arthritis.

3. Patellar Dislocation

Acute, traumatic dislocation of the patella should be distinguished from chronic, recurrent dislocation because the latter may be associated with another underlying diagnosis. When the patella dislocates, it may be caused by a direct force or activity of the quadriceps with the knee slightly flexed, and the direction is almost always lateral. Spontaneous reduction is apt to occur as the knee is extended. If so, the clinical findings may consist merely of hemarthrosis and localized tenderness over the medial patellofemoral ligament (MPFL). Gross instability of the patella, which can be demonstrated by physical examination, demonstrates pain along the MPFL and apprehension with a lateral-directed force on the patella. Factors such as trochlea dysplasia, patella alta, and excessive femoral anteversion predispose to patella dislocation and are discussed in Chapter 4. MPFL injuries are common, with a complete tear in over 50%, most frequently at the femoral attachment site.

Patella reduction is maintained in a brace or cylinder cast with the knee in extension for 2 to 3 weeks. Isometric quadriceps exercises are encouraged. Physical therapy should be initiated to maximize the strength of the vastus medialis portion of the quadriceps muscle. Dynamic bracing may also be helpful. Operative repair of the injury/pathology is best for chronic, recurrent patella dislocations.

4. Tear of the Quadriceps Tendon

Tears of the quadriceps tendon occur most often in patients over 40 years of age. Apparent tears that are instead avulsions from the patella also occur and may indicate renal osteodystrophy or hyperparathyroidism. Preexisting attritional disease of the quadriceps tendon, whether symptomatic or asymptomatic, may be present, and the causative trauma then may be minor. On physical examination, there is swelling, hemarthrosis, and, with complete tears, inability to extend the knee. Radiographs may demonstrate a bony avulsion from the superior pole of the patella or patella baja. Operative repair is recommended for a complete quadriceps tear. High-tensile-strength suture can be passed through transosseous patella tunnels and tied over a bone bridge. Physical therapy consists of initial immobilization followed by staged knee flexion over time. The rerupture rate is about 2%, and results are worse after delayed repairs.

5. Tear of the Patellar Tendon

The same mechanism that causes tears of the quadriceps tendon, transverse fracture of the patella, or avulsion of the tibial tuberosity may also cause tears of the patellar tendon. The characteristic finding is proximal displacement of the patella or patella alta. Radiographs may demonstrate a bony avulsion from the inferior pole of the patella or patella alta.

Operative treatment is indicated for a complete patella tendon tear, and the tendon is sutured to the patella in a similar fashion as that for the quadriceps tendon. Physical therapy consists of initial immobilization followed by staged knee flexion over time.

Garner MR, Gausden E, Berkes MB, Nguyen JT, Lorich DG. Extensor mechanism injuries of the knee: demographic characteristics and comorbidities from a review of 726 patient records. *J Bone Joint Surg Am.* 2015;97(19):1592-1596. [PMID: 26446967]

Henrichsen JL, Wilhem SK, Siljander MP, Kalma JJ, Karadsheh MS. Treatment of patella fractures. *Orthopaedics.* 2018;41(6): e747-e755. [PMID: 30321439]

Lenihan J, Ramos-Pascual S, Silvestros P, Beak P, Miles AW, Trompeter A. Novel techniques demonstrate superior fixation of simple transverse patella fractures: a biomechanical study. *Injury.* 2020;51(6):1288-1293. [PMID: 32276726]

DISTAL FEMUR FRACTURES

- Account for 7% of all femur fractures.
- Important to distinguish between supracondylar and intraarticular fractures.
- Lower modulus implants may benefit distal femur fracture healing.
- With more total knee arthroplasty in recent years, it is increasingly a periprosthetic fracture.

Distal femur fractures occur in the distal 10 to 15 cm of the femur and are usually due to low-energy mechanisms in the elderly and high-energy mechanisms in younger patients. The distal fragment is usually rotated into extension (apex posterior) from traction by the gastrocnemius muscle. The distal end of the proximal fragment may also perforate the overlying quadriceps muscle and tendon and/or the suprapatellar pouch, causing hemarthrosis. A neurovascular examination should be performed because absence or marked decrease of distal pulses is an indication for immediate reduction. If this fails to restore adequate circulation, a CT arteriogram (CTA) should be obtained immediately and the vascular lesion repaired. Distal femur fractures can occur with other complex injuries around the knee such as proximal tibial fractures ("floating" knee), an open injury, and/or a complete knee dislocation with associated neurovascular injuries.

Distal femur fractures are typically classified as intraarticular or extraarticular. Intraarticular fractures may be intercondylar but may also occur in the coronal plane and involve the posterior condyles (Hoffa fracture).

Treatment

If the fracture is minimally displaced or nondisplaced and the patient is either low demand or not a good surgical candidate, closed treatment is appropriate. A temporary spanning external fixation can be used to stabilize the fracture in polytrauma patients.

Extraarticular fractures can be treated by either retrograde nails or plates and screws. If the fracture is intraarticular, direct reduction and fixation with lag screws is best. Extra-articular fractures may benefit from retrograde nailing however in patients with poor bone, varus/valgus malalignment may occur despite interlocking screws. These fractures are frequently comminuted in the supracondylar region due to poor bone quality, and we prefer titanium plates over stainless steel to prevent stress shielding and subsequent nonunions. Patients are typically non–weight bearing for 8 or more weeks. Resumption of knee range of motion is based on surgeon preference, the quality of fixation, etc. Complications of either surgical or nonsurgical treatment include malunion or nonunion.

INJURIES AROUND THE KNEE

Ligamentous Injuries of the Knee

Diagnosis of ligamentous injuries of the knee is ideally confirmed via a physical examination. However, a thorough physical examination of the acutely injured knee can be difficult due to patient pain and guarding, and radiographs may be of limited benefit. Radiographs can offer a clue to soft-tissue knee injury (ie, avulsion fracture of the lateral tibial plateau associated with disruption of the anterior cruciate ligament [ACL]). MRI is the imaging tool of choice for ligamentous injuries of the knee, with an accuracy rate above 95%. Diagnostic with possible therapeutic arthroscopy is reserved for rare cases when MRI is inconclusive.

1. Medial Collateral Ligament Injury

- Accounts for 40% of all knee ligamentous injuries.
- Commonly occurs in athletes.
- Valgus stress is the most common mechanism.

The medial collateral ligament (MCL) has a superficial and deep component. The superficial component attaches to the posterior aspect of the medial femoral condyle and the metaphysis of the tibia beneath the pes anserinus. It is the primary restraint to valgus stress at the knee at 25 degrees of knee flexion. The deep MCL inserts directly onto the edge of the tibial plateau (meniscotibial ligament) and, due to its meniscal attachments, is commonly associated with medial meniscal tears.

Patients with an MCL injury typically sustain a valgus stress about the knee. The MCL tear may occur at the proximal insertion, mid-substance, or at the tibial insertion site. Physical examination demonstrates tenderness of the medial knee and allows the injury to be graded as follows: grade 1, pain and no valgus laxity at 0 and 30 degrees of flexion; grade 2, pain and valgus laxity at 30 degrees of flexion but stable at 0 degrees; and grade 3, pain and valgus laxity at both 0 and 30 degrees of flexion. Stress radiographs can on rare occasions be useful in confirming the diagnosis and MRI is diagnostic.

Grade 1 and 2 sprains (incomplete) are treated with protective weight bearing in a hinged brace or cast to prevent further injury while healing progresses. Grade 3 sprains (complete) are rarely isolated. A positive valgus stress test at 0 degrees of knee extension may indicate posteromedial capsule or cruciate ligament injury. ACL tear, meniscus tear (medial > lateral), or lateral tibial plateau fractures are commonly associated injuries. Surgery may be indicated if there is a distal avulsion, multiligament injury, or the torn ligament is entrapped in the medial compartment.

2. Lateral (Fibular) Collateral Ligament Injury

- Particularly seen with posterolateral corner injury; isolated lateral collateral ligament injuries are rare.
- Most tears are of the fibular insertion.
- Commonly associated with peroneal nerve injuries and ACL/posterior cruciate ligament (PCL) tears.

The lateral (fibular) collateral ligament (LCL) originates from the lateral femoral condyle and inserts on the fibular head. It is the primary static varus stabilizer of the knee joint. Isolated LCL injuries are extremely rare, and typically, multiple posterolateral corner structures are involved. The posterolateral corner anatomy involves the fibular collateral ligament, popliteus tendon, popliteofibular ligament, posterolateral capsule, biceps femoris tendon, and iliotibial band. Peroneal nerve injuries are commonly associated, and physical examination should include sensory and motor peroneal nerve testing.

Physical examination demonstrates tenderness of the lateral knee, and the injury is graded similarly to MCL injuries but with varus stress. Radiographs, including varus stress radiographs, are useful, and MRI is diagnostic. It is important to make the diagnosis because ACL and PCL reconstructions often fail when there is an unrecognized LCL or posterolateral corner injury (see Chapter 4). When there is an avulsion of the fibular head and this fragment is of sufficient size, internal screw fixation gives excellent results. Nonsurgical repair and reconstructive techniques are all potential treatment options for LCL injuries and based on the severity of injury. Early repair or reconstruction, within 3 weeks, is associated with better outcomes.

3. Anterior Cruciate Ligament Injury

- Commonly associated with meniscal injury.
- Commonly associated with tibial plateau and femoral/tibial shaft fractures.
- Physical therapy/rehabilitation is crucial for a successful outcome.

The ACL originates at the posteromedial aspect of the lateral femoral condyle and inserts near the medial tibial spine. It is composed of the anteromedial (AM) bundle, posterolateral (PL) bundle, and intermediate (IM) bundle. The AM bundle is the primary restraint against anterior tibial translation, and the PL bundle stabilizes the knee near full extension and against rotatory loads. During knee flexion, the AM bundle tightens, and the PL bundles relaxes.

Isolated injuries frequently involve sports with pivoting (eg, football, basketball, soccer, skiing, volleyball), and most injuries have this mechanism, with females having a higher incidence of ACL injury than males. ACL injuries also occur with other trauma. Tibial spine avulsion fractures with associated ACL avulsion are commonly seen in tibial plateau fracture. MCL, PCL, medial/lateral meniscal tears, and cartilage injuries are commonly associated with ACL tears.

Clinical Findings

A patient with an acute isolated ACL tear classically feels a "popping" or snapping sensation in the knee. A moderate effusion and hemarthrosis usually accumulates during the first few hours. The anterior drawer test performed at 90 degrees of knee flexion and the Lachman test performed at 30 degrees are hallmark physical examination findings. The pivot shift maneuver is indicative of a high-grade ACL tear and rotatory instability.

Treatment

Despite the fact that ACL reconstruction does not prevent the risk of degenerative joint disease, ACL tears can cause instability, knee pain, functional impairment, increased risk of meniscal tears, and articular cartilage injury. Although surgical reconstruction is indicated in most instances, functionally stable knees in nonathletic patients can be managed conservatively with rehabilitation and bracing. Patients who remain unacceptably unstable after a trial of conservative treatment can still benefit from delayed reconstructive surgery. When bony avulsions from the femur or tibia are present, surgical repair is indicated because bone-to-bone healing and good long-term results have been demonstrated. Primary repair of the ACL was historically prone to failure, but improvements in techniques for repair are ongoing and promising. The Sherman classification is as follows: type I is an avulsion of the proximal insertion site, type II is a tear close to but not at the proximal insertion site, type III is a tear through the proximal third of the ligament, and type IV is a tear in the ligament mid-substance. Acute repair of type I and II tears has comparable results to reconstruction and is especially relevant to the trauma surgeon who may find ACL tears in concomitant periarticular knee fractures. Repair is performed with high-tensile-strength sutures to either a suture anchor or a button. Arthroscopic reconstruction with patella tendon bone, hamstring or quadriceps tendon autografts, and allografts gives excellent results, but each has its benefits and drawbacks. Anterior knee pain occurs with patella tendon autograft, and residual hamstring or quadriceps weakness may be seen after using hamstring and quadriceps tendon autografts, respectively. If there are any coronal or sagittal plane deformities, such as varus malalignment, they should also be addressed, for example with high tibial osteotomy, before or during ACL reconstruction. Due to the ACL tunnel drilling causing release of bone marrow elements and MSCs, meniscal and cartilage repair is best managed at the time of ACL reconstruction to optimize healing.

4. Posterior Cruciate Ligament Injury

- Typically associated with other derangement (ACL, LCL, MCL, meniscus injuries).
- Primary resistance to posterior tibial translation.

The PCL is a broad thick ligament that extends from the lateral aspect of the medial femoral condyle posteriorly and inserts extraarticularly over the back of the tibial plateau approximately 1 cm below the joint line. It resists posterior translation (gliding) of the tibia under the femoral condyle. It usually ruptures after a posteriorly directed force on the proximal tibia, as is sometimes seen in dashboard injuries during MVAs, or with a direct blow to the anterior tibia.

Clinical Findings

The posterior drawer test will be positive, as will the sag test, which will show posterior sagging of the tibia with the knee flexed to 90 degrees compared with the opposite side. It is crucial to rule out commonly associated posterolateral corner injuries (see Chapter 4). The rupture may be a bony avulsion, as commonly seen on the tibial side, but more often is in the middle substance of the ligament.

Treatment

Although partial and isolated PCL tears can be treated successfully with conservative treatment with rehabilitation and bracing, complete or high-grade symptomatic tears and patients with combined injuries are best managed with surgical stabilization to restore function and joint stability. Primary repair, as seen in ACL tears, can be done for acute avulsions. Arthroscopic PCL reconstruction is best for symptomatic mid-substance and chronic tears.

5. Meniscal Injury

- Most common indication for knee surgery.
- More common in ACL-deficient knees.
- Medial meniscal tears are more common than lateral meniscal tears.
- Tear pattern, localization, and tissue quality are determinants of the management and outcome.
- Meniscus preservation is crucial to prevent early knee arthritis.

The meniscus is a relatively acellular, highly hydrated fibrocartilage that allows a more congruous fit between the convex femoral condyle and the relatively flat tibial plateau. The menisci spread the load more uniformly on the articular cartilage, thus minimizing point contact and wear; therefore, they play a crucial role not only in load bearing but also shock absorption and lubrication of the articular cartilage. Both medial and lateral menisci are attached via meniscocapsular attachments peripherally and at the anterior and posterior horn attachments on the tibia. They are wedge-shaped and thicker at the periphery. The medial meniscus is C-shaped, and the lateral meniscus is more O-shaped. The menisci are vascularized only at the peripheral third, so tears involving the vascularized portion have better repair potential. They are also secondary knee stabilizers and thus more susceptible and important in the ligament-deficient knee.

Clinical Findings

Tears can be secondary to trauma or attrition/degeneration. Tears of the medial meniscus are more common. Degenerative tears in the elderly population occur in the posterior horn of the medial meniscus. Symptoms include pain, swelling, a popping sensation, and occasionally locking and giving way. Physical examination may be significant for medial or lateral joint line pain tenderness and an effusion. Occasionally, grinding or snapping can be felt with tibial torsion and the knee flexed to 90 degrees, known as the McMurray test. Radiographs are of minimal value but may rule out other disorders such as osteoarthritis. MRI is diagnostic and can also detect associated articular cartilage or ligament problems.

Treatment

Initial conservative management with immobilization, protective weight bearing, and exercises can give good results. Small, asymptomatic tears can be followed with observation; however, arthroscopic evaluation and treatment are recommended for recurrent or persistent locking, recurrent effusion, or disabling pain. Partial meniscectomy or repair

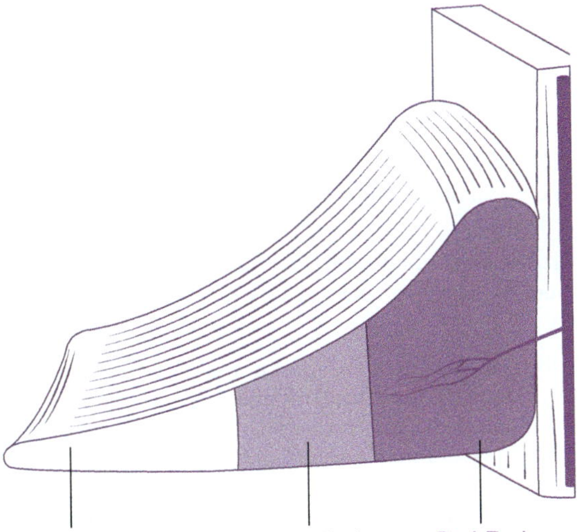

▲ **Figure 2–30.** **Schematic diagram showing the vascular zones of the meniscus. Repairs performed in the red-red zone have a better chance of healing.** (Reprinted with permission from Meniscus Tear: Do I need surgery? Gardiner J. POGO (Physio with a Finish Line), April 20, 2020. https://www.pogophysio.com.au/blog/meniscus-tear-do-i-need-surgery/.)

is indicated depending on the tear pattern, size, and localization. If the tear is in the vascularized portion (red-red zone), repair has the best potential for healing (Figure 2–30). Meniscal repairs in red-red and red-white zones have better outcomes than white-white repairs. Vertical longitudinal tears are the most the commonly repaired meniscus pattern. Unstable, vertical longitudinal tears are called bucket handle tears (Figure 2–31). Resection of such a tear may result in subtotal meniscectomy and higher chance of degenerative joint disease. Acute tears should be reduced and repaired arthroscopically. Radial tears involving the vascularized zone should be repaired with side-to-side sutures. Horizontal tears in young patients that involve the vascularized zone can also be repaired using circumferential sutures. Root tears

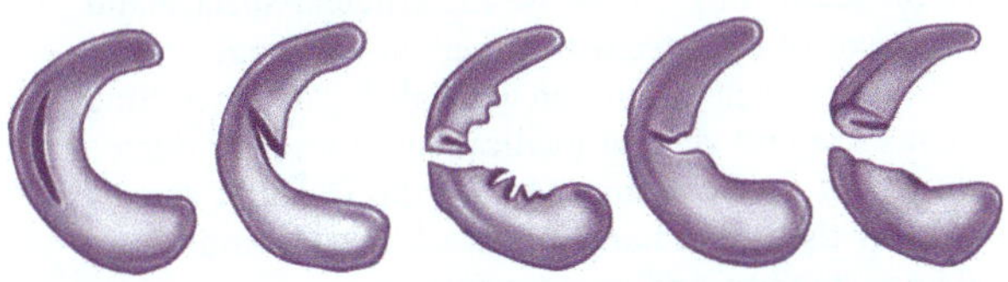

▲ **Figure 2–31.** **Diagram to illustrate the types of meniscal tears.** (Reprinted from Rao AJ, Erickson BJ, Cvetanovich GL, et al: The Meniscus-Deficient Knee: Biomechanics, Evaluation, and Treatment Options. Orthop J Sports Med. 2015;3(10):2325967115611386.)

or radial tears near the meniscal root should also be repaired; otherwise, the entire meniscus is essentially nonfunctional, leading to early degenerative joint disease.

For other meniscal tears such as complex, degenerative, and white-white tears, the affected area should be removed, leaving as much as possible of the healthy meniscus. Meniscus repair is not recommended when there is degenerative joint disease. Meniscal root repair is typically performed via bone tunnels. Meniscal repairs are more successful in patients younger than 45 years of age; however, tissue quality and repair technique are significant factors. If total meniscectomy is performed in young patients with preserved articular cartilage, meniscal transplantation may be indicated. Meniscal transplantation is contraindicated in skeletally immature patients, obese patients, and patients with inflammatory arthritis or moderate or severe degenerative joint disease. Ten-year survival after meniscal transplantation is about 70% with persistent improvement in subjective pain; retears and extrusion are the complications.

6. Chondral and Osteochondral Injuries

- One of the most common knee problems in people over age 40.
- Increased risk with sports participation and ACL-deficient knees.
- Age, defect size, and location are important determinants of management.

The hyaline articular cartilage is avascular and has no intrinsic capability to repair superficial lacerations. Deep injuries involve the bone in the subchondral plate, and extrinsic repair occurs first with a fibrin clot replaced by granulation tissue, which is then transformed to fibrocartilage. Repetitive injury can cause abnormal motion with shearing stresses that can loosen chondral or osteochondral fragments. Compression injuries to the cartilage can lead to posttraumatic chondromalacia.

Clinical Findings

Chondral injuries usually have nonspecific symptoms that mimic meniscal injury. Radiographs will often reveal a loose body if the osteochondral fragment is big enough. Tunnel and patellar tangential radiographic views can be helpful in visualizing fragments. Semi-flexed 45-degree posteroanterior views are most sensitive for early joint space narrowing. Long leg alignment views should be obtained to rule out any malalignment. Although it can miss the delaminating injuries, superficial flap tears, and surface fibrillations, MRI is the best diagnostic tool for articular lesions. Fat-suppressed T2, proton density, and T2 fast spin echo sequences offer improved sensitivity and specificity. However, arthroscopy remains the most accurate diagnostic and gold standard method for diagnosis of symptomatic individuals with mechanical symptoms who fail conservative management.

Treatment

Treatment depends on patient factors such as age, skeletal maturity, activity level, and defect factors such as size, location, containment, and subchondral involvement. Activity modification, physiotherapy, weight loss, and injections can be attempted. Surgical options include debridement, fixation of the osteochondral fragment, microfracture, OATM, and ACI. There is no one best technique for all defects. Selection of the treatment depends on the age of the patient, size of the defect, skeletal maturity, and the presence of adequate subchondral bone. Lesions located on the femoral condyles have the greatest potential for treatment.

7. Knee Dislocation

Traumatic dislocations of the knee are rare injuries that often result from high-energy trauma; however, they can also occur from low-energy injuries in the elderly. They are classified according to the direction of displacement of the tibia (ie, anterior, posterior, lateral, medial, or rotatory). Complete dislocation can occur only after extensive tearing of the supporting ligaments and soft tissues. Injury to the neurovascular structure is common and should be looked for.

Treatment

Knee dislocations require prompt reduction. This is most easily accomplished in the emergency room by applying axial traction on the leg; only rarely can it be done under general anesthesia. The role of angiography is controversial. If pulses and ankle-brachial pressure index are normal, the limb is closely observed. Presence of abnormal foot pulses alone is not sensitive enough to detect a vascular injury needing surgery. An ankle-brachial index should be measured on all patients with suspected knee dislocation, and when less than 0.9, it is abnormal. CTA is best to diagnose a vascular injury and is fast and convenient. Any vascular injury should be repaired as soon as possible; however, injuries may also present in a delayed fashion, more than 48 hours later, due to an intimal tear. Thus, it is important to monitor the vascular status of knee dislocations for up to 72 hours after injury. Ischemia of more than 4 hours correlates with a poor prognosis for salvage of a functional limb. Prophylactic fasciotomies should be performed at the time of vascular repair to prevent compartment syndrome caused by postrevascularization edema.

Most now agree that surgical repair of all ligaments is indicated in relatively young (<50 years old) and active patients. Early reconstructions yield better results. Open dislocations, irreducible dislocations, and popliteal artery damage necessitate immediate surgical treatment. Intensive quadriceps and hamstring rehabilitation is necessary to minimize functional loss. The need for a brace for strenuous activities may be permanent.

PROXIMAL TIBIA FRACTURES

1. Tibial Plateau Fractures

- Tibia plateau fractures represent a spectrum of intraarticular injuries with a wide variety of injury patterns.
- Anatomic reduction is important to prevent posttraumatic arthritis.
- Intraarticular knee joint pathology (eg, meniscal tears, loose bodies) may be associated with tibial plateau fractures.

Proximal tibia plateau fractures account for 1% of all fractures. Lateral tibial plateau fractures account for approximately 60% of all plateau fractures. The impaction injury to the lateral tibia plateau may create a split or void of structural bone loss. These fractures commonly result from axial loading combined with varus and valgus force. Associated meniscal and ligamentous injuries are common. Ninety-one percent of patients have evidence of lateral meniscus pathology, 44% have medial tears (with lateral tears being more common than medial tears), 57% have ACL injuries, and 68% have pathology in the posterolateral corner on MRI. A thorough neurovascular evaluation should be performed.

Classification

The most widely used classification system is the Schatzker classification, which is ordered in degree of energy from low to high: type I, split fracture of the lateral plateau; type II, split depression of the lateral plateau; type III, depression of the lateral plateau; type IV, medial plateau fracture; type V, bicondylar fracture; and type VI, a fracture with metaphyseal-diaphyseal dissociation (Figure 2–32). Proper classification is based on quality radiographs and CT scan. Preoperative MRI is useful for the identification of associated soft-tissue injuries.

Treatment

The goal of treatment is to restore the articular surface and mechanical axis of the knee with either closed or open treatments. The choice will depend on multiple factors, including the patient's age and general medical condition, the degree of displacement and comminution of the fracture, associated local soft-tissue and bony injuries, local skin condition, residual knee stability, and fracture pattern.

Closed treatment with a functional brace is appropriate for minimally displaced fractures with stable ligaments. Varus or valgus laxity at full extension is a poor prognostic sign for closed treatment. An articular step-off of less than 3 mm and/or condylar widening of less than 5 mm and valgus tilt up to 5 degrees can be treated nonoperatively. ORIF

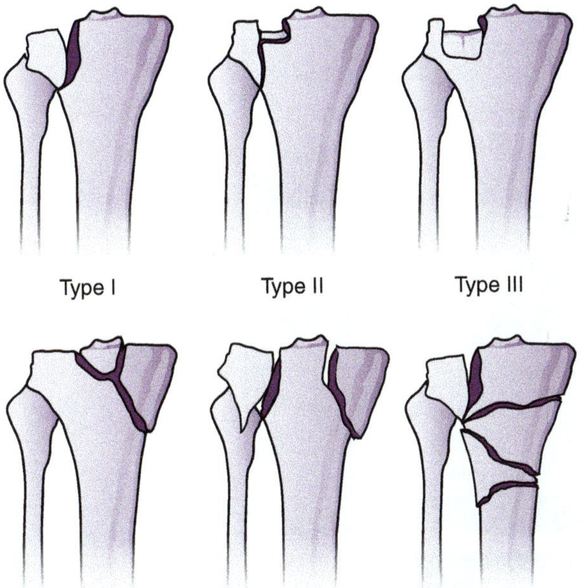

▲ **Figure 2–32.** Schatzker classification of tibial plateau fractures: type I—lateral split, type II—lateral split-depression, type III—lateral depression only, type IV—medial plateau, type V—bicondylar, and type VI—bicondylar with separation of metaphysis from diaphysis. (Reprinted from Ryan Sumpter. EM@3AM: Tibial Plateau Fracture. www.emdocs.net. http://www.emdocs.net/em3am-tibial-plateau-fracture/. Published May 2, 2020. Accessed April 6, 2021.)

is best for medial plateau fractures with any significant displacement due to their propensity for further displacement. Bicondylar fractures with any medial displacement, valgus tilt greater than 5 degrees, or significant articular step-off should be treated with ORIF. Immediate range of motion is usually encouraged with protected weight bearing for 8 to 12 weeks.

Surgery should only be undertaken when the soft tissues allow wound healing. After articular reduction, the fracture is fixed with a buttress plate (usually 3.5 mm). The screws should be within bone and not too long on the medial knee since they can irritate the patient. Fixation should be solid enough to allow knee flexion and extension.

Bicondylar plateau fractures tend to drift into varus and are best treated by first reducing the medial plateau. A small buttress plate can be used to fix the medial plateau and then ORIF of the lateral plateau. Coronal split fracture-dislocations may be associated with a posteriorly dislocated medial tibial plateau and lateral plateau depression (Moore Type I fracture-dislocation) and are best treated with the Lobenhoffer approach. The Lobehhoffer approach is performed with the patient prone. The muscular plane is between the medial gastrocnemius and the pes anserinus. Imaging facilitates exposure, reduction, and fixation of the posteriorly dislocated medial tibial plateau (Figure 2–33), and the lateral tibial plateau fracture can then be address with the patient either prone or supine via a separate approach.

Proximal tibia bone defects (ie, depression) should be grafted with either autograft, allograft, or structural graft substitutes. We prefer cancellous graft. Some fracture patterns (ie, split) with minimal displacement and good bony quality are amenable to percutaneous lag screw fixation.

Arthroscopic-aided fracture reduction has been proposed to be safe and efficacious for Schatzker type I, II, and III injuries. However, extravasation of arthroscopic fluid can cause compartment syndrome. Compartment syndrome should also be suspected in higher-energy Schatzker type IV, V, and VI fractures.

Temporary external fixation with delayed definitive surgery can be performed for unstable fractures.

Complications

Early complications of tibia plateau fractures include infection, wound dehiscence, VTE, compartment syndrome, loss of reduction, hardware failure, and knee stiffness. Late complications include residual instability and posttraumatic degenerative joint disease that may require total knee replacement arthroplasty.

Bedi A, Musahl V, Cowan JB. Management of posterior cruciate ligament injuries: an evidence-based review. *J Am Acad Orthop Surg*. 2016;24(5):277-289. [PMID: 27097125]

Belk JW, Kraeutler MJ, Houck DA, McCarty EC. Knee osteoarthritis after single-bundle versus double-bundle anterior cruciate ligament reconstruction: a systematic review of randomized controlled trials. *Arthroscopy*. 2019;35:996-1003. [PMID: 30733027]

Chahla J, Stone J, Mandelbaum BR. How to manage cartilage injuries? *Arthroscopy*. 2019;35(10):2771-2773. [PMID: 31604490]

Figueroa F, Figueroa D, Calvo R, Vaisman A, Espregueira-Mendes J. Graft choice in combined anterior cruciate ligament and medial collateral ligament reconstruction. *EFORT Open Rev*. 2020;5(4):221-225. [PMID: 32377390]

Grawe B, Schroeder AJ, Kakazu R, Messer MS. Lateral collateral ligament injury about the knee: anatomy, evaluation, and management. *J Am Acad Orthop Surg*. 2018;26(6):e120-e127. [PMID: 29443704]

Hanley J, Westermann R, Cook S, et al. Factors associated with knee stiffness following surgical management of multiligament knee injuries. *J Knee Surg*. 2017;30(6):549-554. [PMID: 27788528]

Irgit KS, Cush G. Tendon transfers for peroneal nerve injuries in the multiple ligament injured knee. *J Knee Surg*. 2012;25(4):327-333. [PMID: 23150160]

Järvelä S, Kiekara T, Suomalainen P, Järvelä T. Double-bundle versus single-bundle anterior cruciate ligament reconstruction: a prospective randomized study with 10-year results. *Am J Sports Med*. 2017;45:2578-2585. [PMID: 28661696]

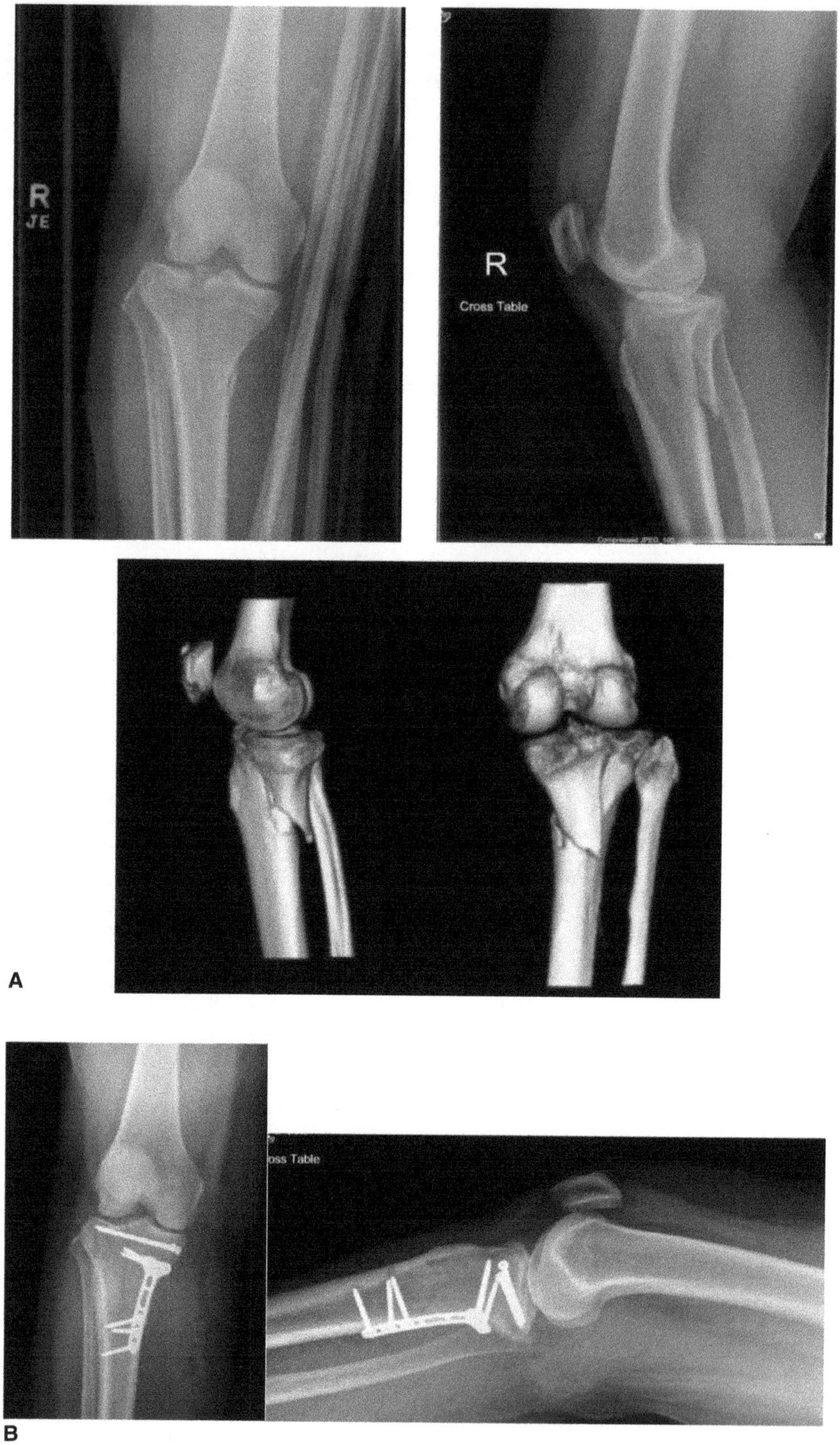

▲ **Figure 2–33.** **A:** Preoperative radiographs and three-dimensional CT reconstruction and postoperative radiographs of a Moore type I right tibial plateau fracture. There is lateral plateau depression and the medial plateau is displaced posteriorly. **B:** The fracture was reduced and fixed via a Lobenhoffer posterior approach.

Kfuri M, Schatzker J. Revisiting the Schatzker classification of tibial plateau fractures. *Injury*. 2018;49(12):2252-2263. [PMID: 30526924]

Klek M, Dhawan A. The role of high tibial osteotomy in ACL reconstruction in knees with coronal and sagittal plane deformity. *Curr Rev Musculoskelet Med.* 2019;12(4):466-471. [PMID: 31760623]

Lai CCH, Ardern CL, Feller JA, Webster KE. Eighty-three per cent of elite athletes return to preinjury sport after anterior cruciate ligament reconstruction: a systematic review with metaanalysis of return to sport rates, graft rupture rates and performance outcomes. *Br J Sports Med.* 2018;52:128. [PMID: 28223305]

Meulenkamp B, Martin R, Desy NM, et al. Incidence, risk factors, and location of articular malreductions of the tibial plateau. *J Orthop Trauma.* 2017;31(3):146-150. [PMID: 27755337]

Mthethwa J, Chikate A. A review of the management of tibial plateau fractures. *Musculoskelet Surg.* 2018;102(2):119-127. [PMID: 29043562]

Paterno MV. Non-operative care of the patient with an ACL-deficient knee. *Curr Rev Musculoskelet Med.* 2017;10:322-327. [PMID: 28756525]

Roth J, Taylor DC. Management of acute isolated medial and posteromedial instability of the knee. *Sports Med Arthrosc Rev.* 2015;23(2):71-76. [PMID: 25932875]

Rothrauff BB, Jorge A, de Sa D, Kay J, Fu FH, Musahl V. Anatomic ACL reconstruction reduces risk of post-traumatic steoarthritis: a systematic review with minimum 10-year follow-up. *Knee Surg Sports Traumatol Arthrosc.* 2020;28(4):1072-1084. [PMID: 31471726]

Stahl D, Serrano-Riera R, Collin K, Griffing R, Defenbaugh B, Sagi HC. Operatively treated meniscal tears associated with tibial plateau fractures: a report on 661 patients. *J Orthop Trauma.* 2015;29(7):322-324. [PMID: 25635356]

Strauss EJ, Day MS, Ryan M, Jazrawi L. Evaluation, treatment, and outcomes of meniscal root tears: a critical analysis review. *JBJS Rev.* 2016;4(8):01874474-201608000-00004. [PMID: 27603272]

Wang J, Wei J, Wang M. The distinct prediction standards for radiological assessments associated with soft tissue injuries in the acute tibial plateau fracture. *Eur J Orthop Surg Traumatol.* 2015;25(5):913-920. [PMID: 25749752]

2. Tibial Tuberosity Fracture

Tibial tuberosity fractures can occur with a violent quadriceps muscle contraction causing avulsion of the tibial tuberosity. When the fracture is complete, the extensor mechanism is disrupted, and active knee extension is impaired. Bracing or cast treatment may be used for nondisplaced fractures; however, screw fixation permits earlier knee motion. ORIF is recommended for all fractures displaced by 5 mm or more.

3. Tibial Eminence (Spine) Fracture

A tibial eminence fracture occurs as an isolated injury or as part of the comminution of a tibial plateau fracture. The isolated type of injury occurs mostly in the pediatric population. Meniscal, capsular, collateral ligament, and osteochondral injuries are seen in up to 40% of patients.

Meyers has classified this lesion into three stages. Nondisplaced type 1 fractures can be treated nonsurgically with a cylinder cast with the knee in extension for 6 weeks. Type 2 fractures are displaced at the anterior margin and can be treated nonoperatively if an anatomic reduction is achieved with a cylinder cast with the knee in extension. Type 3 fractures are displaced and should be surgically fixed with permanent or absorbable sutures, K-wires, or screws. When associated with other fractures of the tibial plateau, the tibial eminence fragment usually maintains its attachment to the ACL, and ORIF resolves knee instability as well.

TIBIA AND FIBULA INJURIES

- Tibia fractures are the most common long bone fracture.
- Open fractures occur with high incidence.
- Intramedullary nails are the standard of surgical care.
- Always evaluate for compartment syndrome.

Anatomy

The tibial diaphysis is straight and triangular in cross-section. The anteromedial border and anterior crest are palpable throughout the entire length of the bone. They are useful landmarks for closed reduction techniques and cast molding. The distal half of the leg has more tendons and less muscle than the proximal half, so soft-tissue coverage and blood supply of the distal tibia are more precarious than in the proximal portion. The tibia and fibula transmit approximately five-sixths and one-sixth of the axial load from the knee to the foot, respectively.

1. Tibia-Fibula Fractures

Fractures of the tibial or fibular diaphysis are the result of direct or indirect trauma. A thorough assessment of the surrounding soft tissues is mandatory. The size of the skin wound does not necessarily correlate with the amount of underlying soft-tissue damage. A 1-cm skin laceration may be associated with extensive muscle and periosteal injury, making the fracture a Gustilo grade III instead of grade I. Closed tibia fractures can be associated with significant soft-tissue injury, including compartment syndrome. In 1982, Tscherne and Oestern classified the soft-tissue injury in ascending order of severity (grades 0 to 3):

Grade 0: Soft-tissue damage is absent or negligible.

Grade 1: There is a superficial abrasion or contusion caused by fragment pressure from within.

Grade 2: A deep contaminated abrasion is present associated with localized skin or muscle contusion from direct trauma. Impending compartment syndrome is included in this category.

Grade 3: The skin is extensively contused or crushed, and muscular damage may be severe. Also, subcutaneous avulsions, compartment syndrome, and rupture of a major blood vessel associated with a closed fracture are additional criteria.

When the fracture is displaced, the clinical diagnosis is usually evident. All compartments should be palpated, and a thorough distal neurovascular examination should be performed. AP and lateral view radiographs are taken of the entire leg, including the knee and ankle joints. Oblique views are sometimes necessary. Fractures of the distal or proximal end of the tibia can be better visualized with a CT scan.

Fibula Diaphysis Fractures

Isolated fibula fractures can be associated with direct or indirect trauma. Indirect trauma can result from an ankle injury (ie, Maisonneuve injury), and the ankle should also be examined. Isolated fibula fractures are usually the result of direct trauma and, if not associated with ankle trauma, are treated conservatively.

Tibia Diaphyseal Fractures

Isolated fractures of the tibial diaphysis are usually the result of torsional stress. There is a tendency for the tibia to displace into varus angulation because of an intact fibula. Fractures of both the tibia and fibula are more unstable, and displacement can recur after reduction. Tibia and fibula fractures at the same level are usually associated with high-energy mechanisms, whereas fractures at different levels usually occur due to torsional injury. The fibular fracture usually heals independently of the reduction achieved. The following reduction criteria are generally accepted for the tibia:

- Cortical apposition of 50% or more of the diameter (both AP and lateral projections)
- Less than 5 degrees of varus or valgus angulation
- Less than 5 degrees of angulation in the AP plane
- Less than 10 degrees of rotation
- Less than 1 cm of shortening

Malunions of the tibia may affect the mechanics of the knee or ankle joint and possibly lead to premature degenerative joint disease. A discussion of the treatment options and associated benefits and surgical risks such as anterior knee pain with intramedullary nailing and those of nonoperative treatment is warranted.

The goal of treatment is to restore tibial length, alignment, and rotation and allow the fracture to heal in an acceptable position. If closed management is chosen, then a closed reduction is best obtained under general anesthesia; however, it can also be done gravity-assisted, such as by the patient hanging his or her leg off the bed. The patient can be immobilized in a well-molded bivalved long leg cast if swelling allows. Radiographs should be performed at 2 weeks to ensure the fracture did not displace to its original position. If radiographs at 6 weeks show acceptable alignment, the patient can be transitioned to a Sarmiento-type fracture brace with increased weight bearing.

If surgical treatment is chosen, a statically locked reamed intramedullary tibial nail is standard of care for most displaced closed and open Gustilo type I to IIIA fractures. Dynamic or static interlocking can be achieved with interlocking screws; however, we prefer to achieve cortical contact by backslapping the distally locked nail, if necessary. Sometimes, due to fracture instability or patient size, closed reduction can be challenging. In these cases, the fracture can be opened, reduced, and fixed with a small provisional 2.7- or 3.5-mm unicortical locking plate. We find that this limited intervention can save time and facilitate a more satisfactory reduction (Figure 2–34). Semi-extended, suprapatellar nailing is an alternative to infrapatellar nailing and useful for proximal one-third tibia fractures. There is no significant benefit of one technique over the other, and they have a similar incidence of anterior knee pain. To prevent deformity, a more posterior and lateral starting spot on the tibia is preferred. As discussed earlier, a small 2.7-mm plate can be used because proximal one-third tibia fractures tend to result in apex anterior malalignment. Blocking screws can also be used to guide the nail more lateral and anterior. ORIF with plates and screws is performed less routinely for tibial shaft fractures; however, it may have utility in comminuted proximal tibia fractures (Figure 2–35). External fixation of the tibia can be performed for significant soft-tissue injuries or in patients with hemodynamic or physiologic instability.

Fracture of the Distal End of the Tibia

- Displaced pilon fractures should be surgically treated in a staged fashion due to the high risk of wound complications.
- Despite improved techniques, posttraumatic degenerative joint disease is a common complication.

Distal fractures of the tibia involving the plafond are also called pilon fractures. As for any intraarticular fracture, the goal of treatment is to restore an anatomic articular surface. Nondisplaced or minimally displaced fractures can be treated closed. Displaced fractures are best treated surgically in a staged fashion. Initial external fixation with or without ORIF of the fibula can be performed acutely to restore provisional length, alignment, and rotation. After the soft-tissue swelling subsides (10-21 days), definitive ORIF can be performed. For fractures with a coronal split and/or a large posterolateral tibia fracture fragment, an initial posterolateral approach can be performed. ORIF of this fragment via a posterolateral approach can facilitate a more accurate

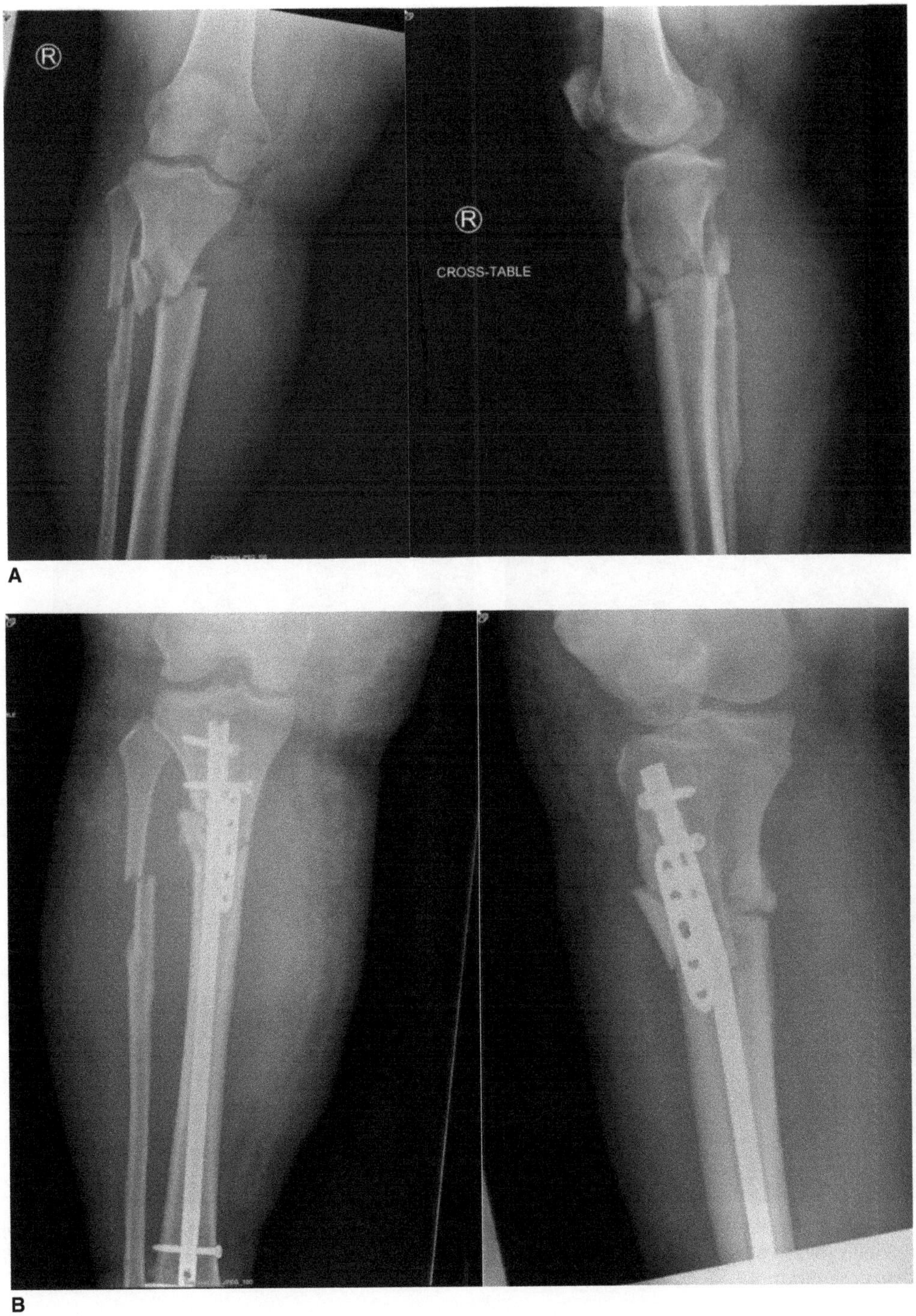

▲ **Figure 2–34.** Preoperative (**A**) and postoperative (**B**) radiographs of a proximal one-third right tibial plateau fracture. The fracture was reduced and provisionally fixed with a 2.7-mm locking plate to prevent displacement of the fracture. After passage of the intramedullary nail, the plate was left in. Plate removal may be beneficial to decrease stiffness of the construct and promote healing.

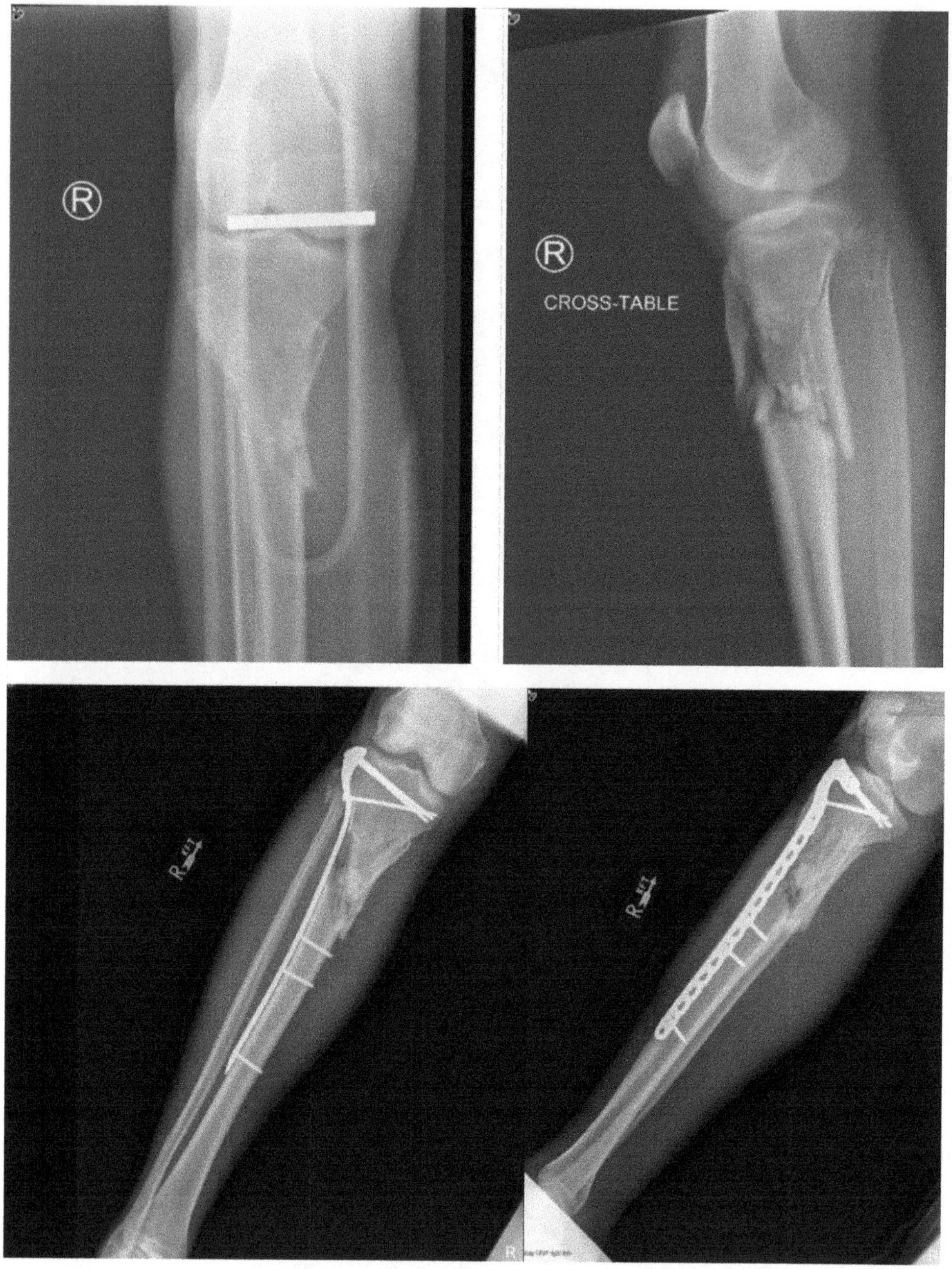

▲ **Figure 2–35.** Pre- and postoperative radiographs of a comminuted proximal one-third tibia plateau fracture with a coronal split. A minimally invasive plate osteosynthesis technique was performed to avoid excessive soft-tissue stripping due to the significant comminution.

reduction of the joint from a subsequent anterior approach (Figure 2–36). In pilon fractures with significant medial comminution, there may be a tendency for the fracture to drift into varus, and a medial plate may then be beneficial. Bone graft can also be added to metaphyseal defects to serve as osteoconductive bone-void fillers. When there is severe articular surface comminution, the soft-tissue risks of ORIF may not be justified. Then, indirect reduction and external fixation is a reasonable option. External fixation can usually restore some length, alignment, and rotation of the distal leg and make an eventual tibiotalar fusion easier should post-traumatic degenerative joint disease occur. Primary ankle fusion is an alternative for severely comminuted fractures, although poor bone can be an obstacle to this.

As discussed earlier, immediate surgery should be avoided due to the risk of wound dehiscence and infection. Fracture healing can take approximately 8 weeks or longer. Postoperative pain, stiffness, and swelling are seen in as many as 25% of patients. Failure of healing occurs in more than 5% of patients.

Complications

Complications after tibia and fibula fractures include infection, malunion, nonunion, degenerative joint disease, and chronic pain.

A. Delayed Union or Nonunion

The tibia, particularly its distal third, is prone to delayed union or nonunion due to lack of soft-tissue coverage. These complications may occur more frequently in high-energy, open, and segmental fractures. On physical examination, patients with a nonunion of the tibia may have pain with palpation of the fracture site 6 months after the injury. Radiographs show the persistence of the fracture line with

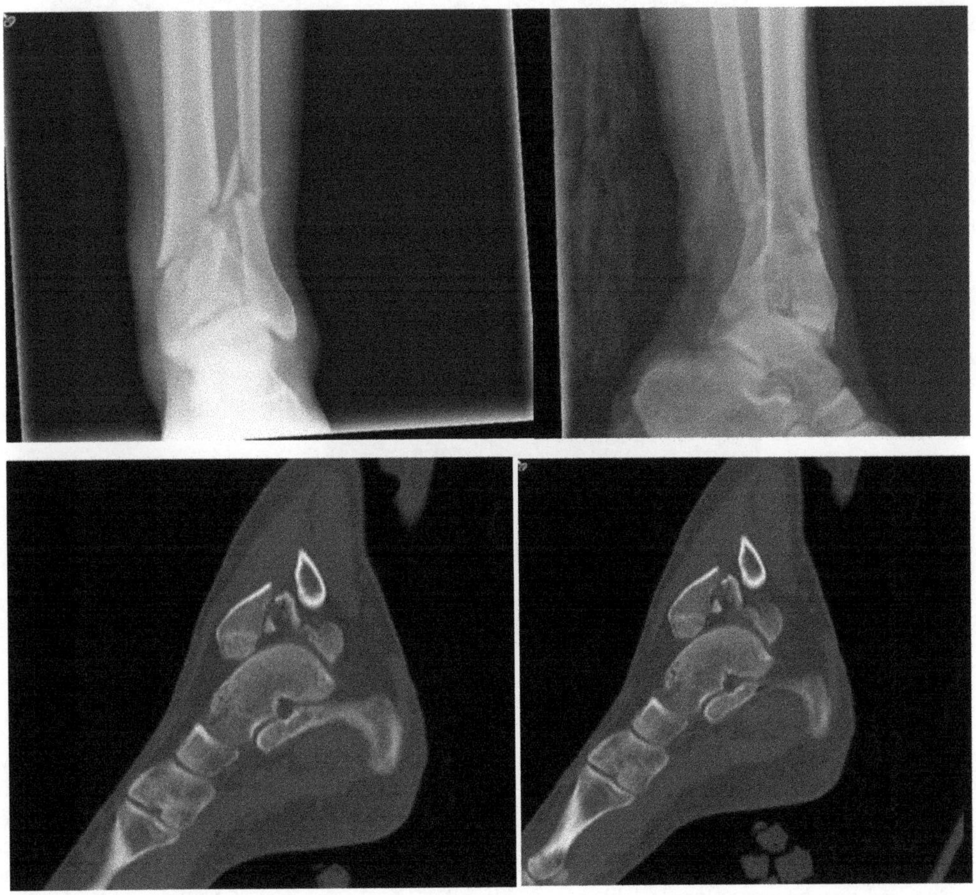

A

▲ **Figure 2–36.** Preoperative radiographs/sagittal CT reconstructions (**A**) and postoperative radiographs (**B**) of a left pilon fracture reduced and fixed via a posterolateral approach followed by an anterior approach. The fibula was reduced and fixed via the posterolateral approach.

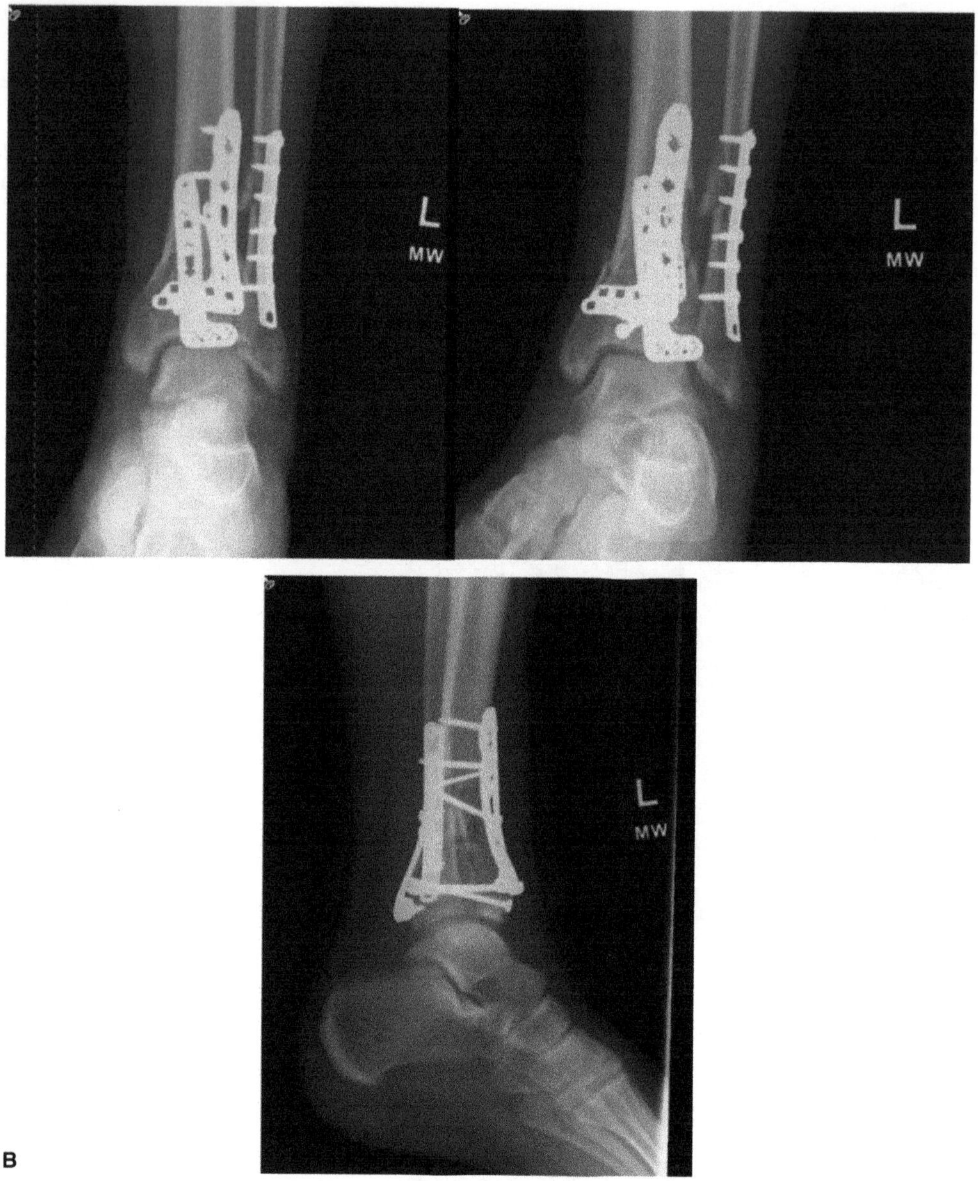

B

▲ **Figure 2–36.** (*Continued*)

or without callus; however, CT scans may be necessary to confirm the diagnosis. Sclerosis and flaring of the bone ends characterize a hypertrophic nonunion, whereas osteopenia and thinning of the fragments are seen in atrophic nonunions. Typically, hypertrophic nonunions benefit from mechanical stabilization, and atrophic nonunions lack blood flow and osteogenicity. However, in reality, many nonunions have characteristics of both types. Treatment is also based on the local soft tissue, location, fracture geometry, and local mechanical factors, so treatment should be tailored to each particular case. It is important to try to understand why the fracture did not heal (eg, too large fracture gap, soft-tissue insult, systemic factors) and attempt to address those issues. Infection should always be ruled out as a possible cause of nonunion, and if suspected, intraoperative cultures should be taken during revision surgery. Nail dynamization may benefit fractures with lack of cortical contact and/or comminuted fractures. Nail exchange may also benefit the nonunion due to the biological effect of reaming as well as the improved mechanical stability with a larger-diameter nail. If the fibula is serving as a fixed strut, an osteotomy can be performed to allow axial motion at the tibia. Central and/or posterolateral bone graft can also be performed for tibial nonunions. Electrical stimulation and low-intensity pulsed ultrasound have some efficacy and may aid in achieving union.

B. Malunion

Malunion may lead to premature degenerative joint disease of the ankle and knee. Corrective osteotomies may be required. When associated with shortening, multiplane correction and lengthening can be achieved with hybrid ring-fixator frames, which allow progressive correction of the deformity.

C. Infection

Infection after open fractures or surgical treatment may be associated with delayed union or nonunion. Perioperative prophylactic antibiotic therapy and adequate debridement and irrigation of open fractures are not always successful in preventing this complication. In open fractures that lack soft-tissue coverage, early soft-tissue coverage with either rotational flaps or free flaps decreases infection rates. Amputation is a treatment of last resort.

D. Complex Regional Pain Syndrome

Complex regional pain syndrome (CRPS) is a rare complication of unknown cause that involves the sympathetic nervous system. It is characterized by pain out of proportion to the original injury, skin changes, cold/heat intolerance, and vasomotor disturbances. There are no established guidelines for its treatment, which includes NSAIDs, bisphosphonates, glucocorticoids, antidepressants, anticonvulsants, vitamin C, physiotherapy, and sympathetic blockade. Suspicion leading to early diagnosis of CRPS and multimodal treatment are beneficial.

Johal H, Bhandari M, Tornetta P 3rd. Cochrane in CORR ®: intramedullary nailing for tibial shaft fractures in adults (review). *Clin Orthop Relat Res.* 2017;475(3):585-591. [PMID: 27995557]

Keating JF, Blachut PA, O'Brien PJ, Court-Brown CM. Reamed nailing of Gustilo grade-IIIB tibial fractures. *J Bone Joint Surg Br.* 2000;82-B:1113. [PMID: 11132268]

Kim JH, Lee DH. Negative pressure wound therapy vs. conventional management in open tibia fractures: systematic review and meta-analysis. *Injury.* 2019;50(10):1764-1772. [PMID: 31047682]

Kostic I, Mitkovic M, Mitkovic M. The diaphyseal aseptic tibial nonunions after failed previous treatment options managed with the reamed intramedullary locking nail. *J Clin Orthop Trauma.* 2019;10(1):182-191. [PMID: 30705557]

Lin CA, Swiontkowski M, Bhandari M, et al. Reaming does not affect functional outcomes after open and closed tibial shaft fractures: the results of a randomized controlled trial. *J Orthop Trauma.* 2016;30(3):142-148. [PMID: 26618662]

Litrenta J, Tornetta P 3rd, Vallier H. Dynamizations and exchanges: success rates and indications. *J Orthop Trauma.* 2015;29(12): 569-573. [PMID: 26595595]

Pincus D, Byrne JP, Nathens AB, et al. Delay in flap coverage past 7 days increases complications for open tibia fractures: a cohort study of 140 North American trauma centers. *J Orthop Trauma.* 2019;33(4):161-168. [PMID: 30893215]

Stella M, Santolini E, Felli L, Santolini F, Horwitz DS. Semi-extended tibial nail insertion using an extra-articular lateral parapatellar approach: a 24-month follow-up prospective cohort study. *J Orthop Trauma.* 2019; doi:10.1097/BOT.0000000000001554. [PMID: 31259804]

Tomás-Hernández J. High-energy pilon fractures management: state of the art. *EFORT Open Rev.* 2017;1(10):354-361. [PMID: 28461913]

Ziran BH, Darowish M, Klatt BA, Agudelo JF, Smith WR. Intramedullary nailing in open tibia fractures: a comparison of two techniques. *Int Orthop.* 2004;28(4):235-238. [PMID: 15160254]

ANKLE FRACTURES AND DISLOCATIONS

- Among the most common injuries.
- Important to recognize associated syndesmotic injuries.

Anatomic and Biomechanical Principles

The ankle joint is limited to one plane of motion: plantarflexion and dorsiflexion in the sagittal plane. Inversion and eversion occur at the subtalar joint, thus providing the lower extremity adaptation to uneven surfaces. The inner and distal articular surfaces of the distal tibia and fibula form the ankle mortise, which is a uniplanar hinge joint. The ankle mortise serves as the roof over the talus. The articular portions of the lateral and medial malleoli serve as constraining buttresses to allow for controlled plantarflexion and dorsiflexion in the ankle mortise. During dorsiflexion, the fibula moves proximally and externally rotates. This geometric configuration of the ankle resists rotation of the talus in the ankle mortise. Further constraint and stability are provided by ligaments and the soft tissue surrounding the ankle. The syndesmotic ligament is composed of four ligaments. The posterior inferior tibiofibular ligament is the thickest and strongest syndesmotic ligament and connects the tibia to the fibula at the level of the tibial plafond. The bony architecture of the mortise also provides some constraint to posterior subluxation of the talus. This is provided by the cup-shaped tibial plafond and the slightly increased width of the talar dome anteriorly as compared with posteriorly.

The distal tibia serves to absorb the compressive loads and stress placed on the ankle. The internal trabecular pattern of the bone helps transmit, diffuse, and resorb the compressive forces. Less activity and old age lead to resorption of cancellous bone, thereby decreasing the compressive resistance of the distal tibia.

Classification

The two most widely used classification schemes for describing ankle fractures are the Lauge-Hansen and Danis-Weber classifications (Figure 2–37). In 1950, Lauge-Hansen described a classification system based on mechanism of injury that includes over 95% of all ankle fractures. Pronation and supination refer to the position of the patient's foot at injury, whereas adduction, abduction, and external rotation refer to the vector of the force that is applied. Thus, four mechanisms of injury were described for ankle fractures: (1) supination adduction, (2) supination-external rotation, (3) pronation abduction, and (4) pronation-external rotation. Lauge-Hansen later added a fifth type of injury, the pronation dorsiflexion injury, in order to include a mechanism for tibial plafond fractures. This fifth type is caused by a compression-type axial loading injury.

The Danis-Weber classification is simpler and is based on anatomy, specifically the location of fibular fracture.

Type A: Fracture in which the fibula is avulsed distal to the joint line. The syndesmotic ligament is left intact, and the medial malleolus is either undamaged or is fractured in a shear-type pattern.

Type B: Spiral fracture of the fibula beginning at or near the level of the joint line and extending in a proximal-posterior direction up the shaft of the fibula. Parts of the syndesmotic ligament complex can be torn, but the large interosseous ligament is usually left intact so that there is no widening of the distal tibiofibular articulation. However, complete syndesmotic disruptions can result from this fracture pattern. The medial malleolus can either be intact or have a transverse avulsion fracture. If the medial malleolus is intact, there can be a tear of the deltoid ligament. An avulsion fracture of the posterior lip of the tibia (posterior malleolus) can also occur.

Type C: Fracture of the fibula proximal to the syndesmotic ligament complex, with consequent disruption of the syndesmosis. Medial malleolar avulsion fracture or deltoid

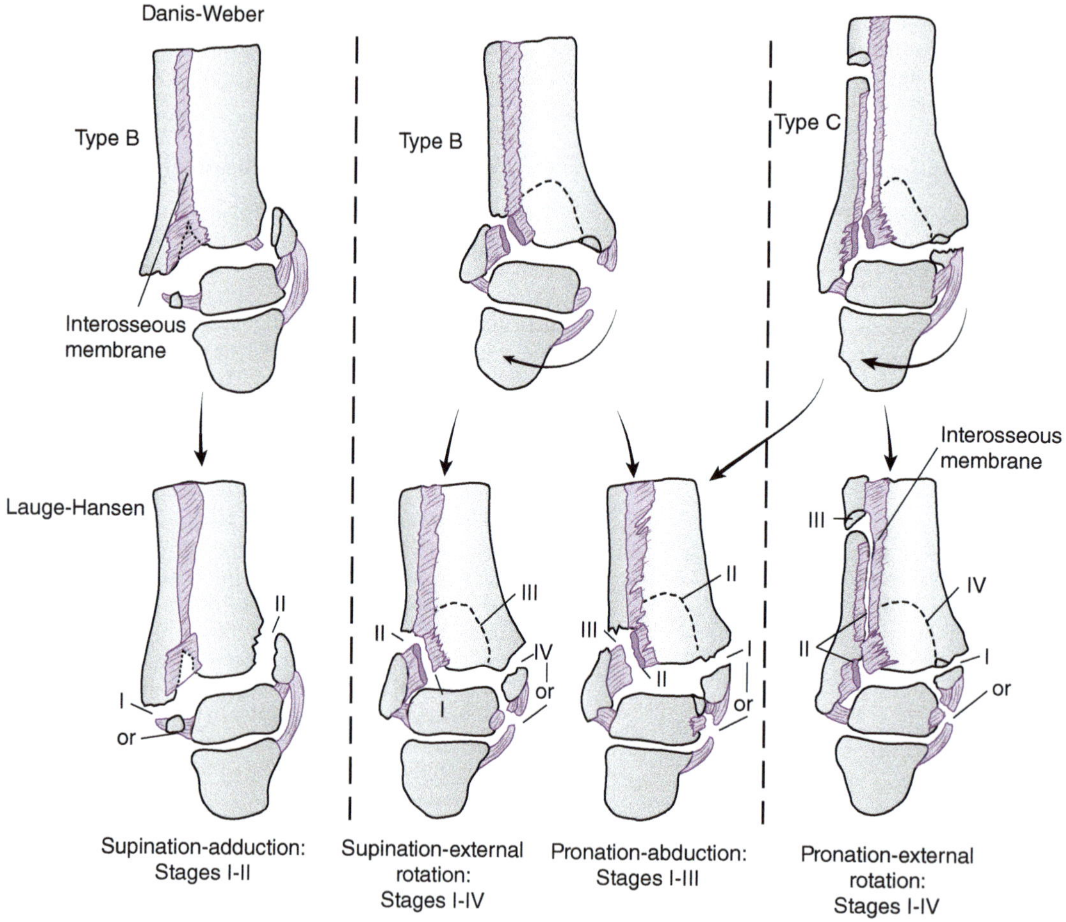

▲ **Figure 2–37. A comparison of the Danis-Weber and Lauge-Hansen ankle fracture classifications.** (Reprinted from Standring, S. Gray's Anatomy: The Anatomical Basis of Clinical Practice: 150 Anniversary Edition. 40th ed. Churchill Livingstone; 2008.)

ligament rupture is also present. Posterior malleolar avulsion fracture can also occur.

Fractures of the ankle are frequently referred to as bimalleolar (fractures of the medial and lateral malleoli) or trimalleolar (fractures of the medial, lateral, and posterior malleoli). Fracture of the lateral malleolus with complete rupture of the deltoid ligament and fracture of the medial malleolus with complete disruption of the syndesmosis and a proximal fibular shaft fracture (Maisonneuve fracture) are also considered bimalleolar fractures on a functional basis.

Treatment

Four criteria should be met for the optimal treatment of ankle fractures: (1) dislocations and fractures should be reduced as soon as possible, (2) all joint surfaces should be restored, (3) the fracture must be held in a reduced position during the period of bony healing, and (4) joint motion should be initiated as early as possible. Outcomes after surgical treatment of ankle fractures are good to excellent; however, articular cartilage damage causes posttraumatic degenerative joint disease. Studies have demonstrated that the ankle has the thinnest articular cartilage but the highest ratio of joint congruence to articular cartilage thickness of any of the large joints. This suggests that loss in congruity of the ankle joint following fracture will be poorly tolerated and lead to posttraumatic degenerative joint disease. Thus, it is important to obtain anatomic reduction of the articular surfaces of the ankle after a fracture. A lateral talar shift of as little as 1 mm will decrease surface contact at the tibiotalar joint by 40%.

If the ankle is dislocated, it should first be reduced, splinted, elevated, and post-reduction x-rays performed. If the ankle is still unstable after reduction, either closed reduction/external fixation or open reduction internal fixation (if soft tissues allow) should be performed. An ankle joint should never be left in a dislocated position. If the fracture is open, the patient should be given appropriate intravenous antibiotics and taken to the operating room on an urgent basis for irrigation and debridement with possible open reduction internal fixation. Open fractures that are clean can undergo ORIF, whereas dirty wounds may require serial I&Ds before definitive surgical treatment. However, the authors' find early weight-bearing after ORIF is best decided on a case-by-case basis.

When performing ORIF of ankle fractures, several principles should be followed. It is important to avoid injury to the superficial peroneal nerve (laterally) and the saphenous vein (medially). Timing of the surgery is dictated by patient comorbidities and the condition of the soft tissue. In the authors' experience, ankle fractures that require surgery are ideally treated immediately, if the soft tissue allows, or in a delayed fashion if the soft tissue is too swollen (ie, fracture blisters, etc.). Extremity elevation is important to help decrease swelling. In the treatment of bimalleolar and trimalleolar fractures, the lateral malleolus should be reduced and fixed first. This has two benefits: (1) it helps to correctly restore the original limb length, and (2) because of the strong ligamentous connections between the lateral malleolus and talus (anterior and posterior talofibular ligaments), initial fixation of the lateral malleolus will correctly position the talus in the mortise. After reducing the distal fibula, if the medial clear space is still wide, it is likely due to 1) interposed deltoid in the joint space or 2) ankle plantarflexion. Since the talus is wider in its anterior portion, dorsiflexion of the ankle will decrease the medial clear space. When performing ORIF of the medial malleolus, it is important to remove any soft tissue or periosteum interposed in the fracture site. It is also preferable to fix the medial malleolus with either two cancellous-type lag screws or by tension banding principles to achieve interfragmentary compression.

The necessity for fixation of the posterior malleolar fragment has changed in recent years. Conflicting data exist regarding the biomechanical influence of posterior malleolar fractures on ankle joint stability and contact pressures, especially in terms of fragment size. It was previously recommended that if the fragment size is greater than 25% to 33% of the articular surface, then it should be reduced and fixed; however, this is controversial. Frequently, when the distal fibula is well reduced, the posterior malleolus reduction is also improved. The posterolateral approach to the tibia has gained much popularity and allows for good visualization of the posterolateral malleolar fragment and distal fibula if ORIF is required. Posterior to anterior lag screws or compression screws are stronger than anterior to posterior screws. Isolated nondisplaced posterior malleolar fractures can be treated with a cast.

Syndesmotic injuries of the ankle occur during external rotation and hyperdorsiflexion. On radiographs, the tibiofibular clear space is normally less than 6 mm, and when it is greater, this is the most reliable indicator of a syndesmotic injury. Intraoperatively, the surgeon can either pull the fibula laterally and assess anterior-posterior stability (gross instability and motion are evidence of syndesmotic disruption) or dorsiflex and externally rotate the foot under fluoroscopy and see if it reveals syndesmotic widening. Syndesmotic malreduction is common, and anatomic reduction is the most important determinant of clinical outcome. The need for routine syndesmotic screw removal remains controversial but may improve functional range of motion. Figure 2–38 demonstrates pre- and postoperative radiographs of a bimalleolar ankle fracture with a syndesmotic injury.

Following surgery, the limb is placed in a bulky sterile dressing with plaster splints from the ball of the foot to the proximal calf to allow for wound healing. The ankle is kept in neutral position to prevent equinus deformity, and the extremity is elevated. After the sutures are removed at 2 weeks, the surgeon must decide whether to begin early mobilization of the ankle joint. If the patient is reliable and stable fixation was achieved, then early range of motion may be initiated, keeping the patient on crutches and not allowing weight bearing. If there is a question about patient reliability or stability of fixation, the limb can be placed in a short leg cast for added protection. Outcomes are improved with

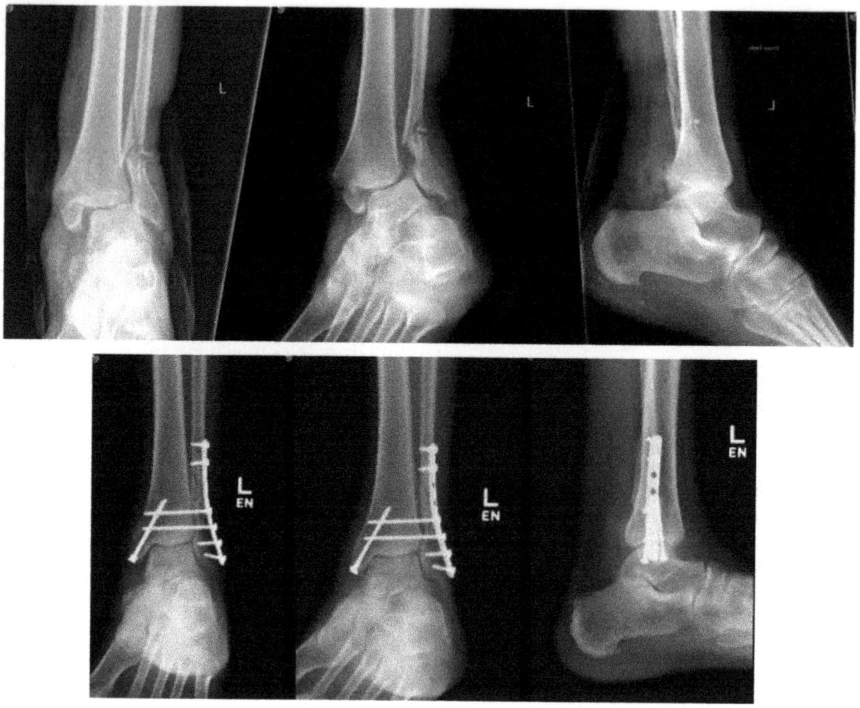

▲ **Figure 2–38.** Preoperative and 4-month postoperative left ankle radiographs of a bimalleolar ankle fracture with a syndesmotic injury reduced and fixed with plates and screws.

early weight bearing after ORIF of unstable ankle fractures with no increase in complications and similar return to work as those treated with non–weight bearing. If patients are immobilized and non–weight bearing, they are allowed to be weight bearing as tolerated and sent to physical therapy after 6 weeks. Physical therapy often helps promote ankle motion, strengthening, and ankle proprioception.

Aiyer AA, Zachwieja EC, Lawrie CM, Kaplan JRM. Management of isolated lateral malleolus fractures. *J Am Acad Orthop Surg.* 2019;27(2):50-59. [PMID: 30278012]

Blom RP, Meijer DT, de Muinck Keizer RO. Posterior malleolar fracture morphology determines outcome in rotational type ankle fractures. *Injury.* 2019;50(7):1392-1397. [PMID: 31176480]

Dehghan N, McKee MD, Jenkinson RJ, et al. Early weightbearing and range of motion versus non-weightbearing and immobilization after open reduction and internal fixation of unstable ankle fractures: a randomized controlled trial. *J Orthop Trauma.* 2016;30(7):345-352.

Fisher N, Atanda A, Swensen S, Egol KA. Repair of bimalleolar ankle fracture. *J Orthop Trauma.* 2017;31(suppl 3):S14-S15. [PMID: 28697074]

Greaser MC. Foot and ankle stress fractures in athletes. *Orthop Clin North Am.* 2016;47(4):809-822. [PMID: 27637667]

Kortekangas T, Haapasalo H, Flinkkilä T. Three week versus six week immobilisation for stable Weber B type ankle fractures: randomised, multicentre, non-inferiority clinical trial. *BMJ.* 2019;364:k5432. [PMID: 30674451]

Kwon JY, Cronin P, Velasco B, Chiodo C. Evaluation and significance of mortise instability in supination external rotation fibula fractures: a review article. *Foot Ankle Int.* 2018;39(7):865-873. [PMID: 29652191]

Lampridis V, Gougoulias N, Sakellariou A. Stability in ankle fractures: diagnosis and treatment. *EFORT Open Rev.* 2018;3(5): 294-303. [PMID: 29951269]

Moore JA Jr, Shank JR, Morgan SJ, Smith WR. Syndesmosis fixation: a comparison of three and four cortices of screw fixation without hardware removal. *Foot Ankle Int.* 2006;27(8):567-572. [PMID: 1691920]

Ræder BW, Figved W, Madsen JE, Frihagen F, Jacobsen SB, Andersen MR. Better outcome for suture button compared with single syndesmotic screw for syndesmosis injury: five-year results of a randomized controlled trial. *Bone Joint J.* 2020; 102-B(2):212-219. [PMID: 32009435]

Rammelt S, Boszczyk A. Computed tomography in the diagnosis and treatment of ankle fractures: a critical analysis review. *JBJS Rev.* 2018;6(12):e7. [PMID: 30562210]

Tenenbaum S, Shazar N, Bruck N, Bariteau J. Posterior malleolus fractures. *Orthop Clin North Am.* 2017;48(1):81-89. [PMID: 27886685]

Tornetta P. Competence of the deltoid ligament in bimalleolar ankle fractures after medial malleolar fixation. *J Bone Joint Surg.* 2000;82-A:843. [PMID: 10859104]

Van Heest TJ, Lafferty PM. Injuries to the ankle syndesmosis. *J Bone Joint Surg Am.* 2014;96:603-613. [PMID: 24695928]

Welck MJ, Hayes T, Pastides P, Khan W, Rudge B. Stress fractures of the foot and ankle. *Injury*. 2017;48(8):1722-1726. [PMID: 26412591]

FOOT INJURIES

Anatomic and Biomechanical Principles

The foot is a highly specialized structure comprised of 28 bones and 57 articulations. In combination with muscles and ligaments, it permits walking, running, jumping, and accommodation of irregular surfaces with a minimal expense of energy.

Embryologically, the foot develops from proximal to distal into three functional segments: the tarsus, metatarsus, and phalanges. Anatomically, the foot is divided into the hindfoot (talus and calcaneus), the midfoot (navicular, cuboid, and three cuneiforms), and the forefoot (five metatarsals and 14 phalanges).

Bones, ligaments, and muscles of the foot comprise the three arches of the foot: medial longitudinal, lateral longitudinal, and anterior transverse. The ligaments involved in the longitudinal arches are the short/long plantar and calcaneonavicular ligaments. The arch anatomy functions as a spring, absorbing shock and returning energy to facilitate walking and running. The first and fifth rays form the edges of the spring during loading. The plantar aspect of the foot is divided into four layers, each containing different muscles and tendons, from superficial to deep.

HINDFOOT

1. Calcaneus Fractures

- The most common tarsal fracture.
- Approximately 60% to 75% of calcaneal fractures are intraarticular.
- Seventeen percent of calcaneal fractures are open.
- Wound dehiscence and infection are the most common acute postoperative complications.
- Posttraumatic arthritis remains a long-term complication.

The most common mechanism of calcaneal fractures is an axial load, which drives the talus into the calcaneus. Ten percent of calcaneal fractures are associated with compression fractures of the thoracic or lumbar spine, and 5% are bilateral. More than 70% of calcaneal fractures are intraarticular, involving the subtalar joint, mostly caused by a fall from height. Most of these injuries occur in individuals involved in labor. Long-term surgical outcomes are controversial due to heterogeneity in studies; however, higher-energy mechanisms may be associated with a poorer prognosis. Posttraumatic subtalar arthritis with associated pain is the most common long-term sequela of both operatively and nonoperatively treated intraarticular calcaneal fractures. Wound dehiscence and infection are short-term complications associated with extensile-based surgical approaches to the calcaneus.

Clinical Findings

Pain is usually significant but may be masked by associated injuries. Swelling, deformity, and blistering of the hindfoot skin occur frequently during the first 36 hours as a result of the severe damage to surrounding soft tissues. The heel pad in particular is a highly specialized fatty structure that acts as a hydraulic cushion. Major disruptions of the heel pad lead to persistent pain and deformity and can produce poor functional results despite adequate bony healing.

A. Imaging Studies

Radiographs include three views: AP, lateral, and axial projection (Harris view). The Harris view provides information about the sustentaculum tali, the lateral wall, and presence of hindfoot varus/valgus. Disruption of Bohler's angle (Figure 2–39) can be determined from a lateral radiograph. Oblique or Broden's views are also useful to demonstrate subtalar joint incongruity. CT scanning will further delineate fracture patterns and occult injuries.

B. Classification

Various classification systems for calcaneus fractures have been advocated. In general, calcaneus fractures can be divided into intraarticular and extraarticular fractures. Intraarticular fractures are associated with worse outcomes than extraarticular fractures. Sanders has developed a classification system for intraarticular fractures based on semicoronal CT images (Figure 2–40). The system is based on the number of intraarticular posterior facet fragments. This

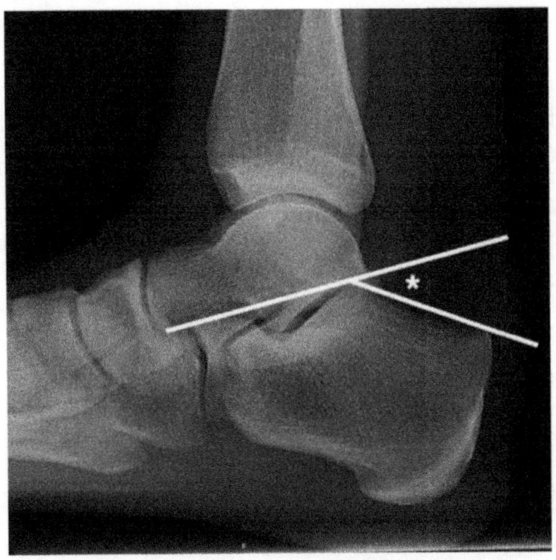

▲ **Figure 2–39.** Lateral x-ray of a right calcaneus demonstrating a normal Bohler's angle (indicated by the *). An angle less than 20 degrees is indicative of a calcaneal fracture with posterior facet collapse.

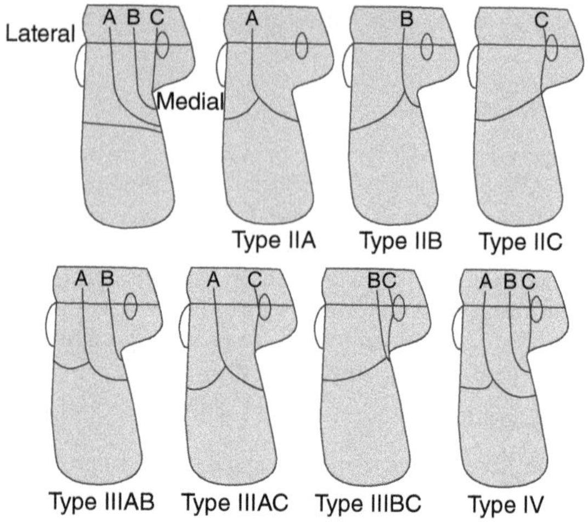

▲ **Figure 2–40. Sanders CT classification of calcaneus fractures. The classification is based off a semicoronal CT of the calcaneus. The number refers to the number of fracture fragments at the widest portion of the posterior facet, and the letters correspond to the position of the fracture lines (A is lateral, B is middle, and C is medial).** (Adapted from Sanders R: Intra-articular fractures of the calcaneus: Present state of the art. J Orthop Trauma. 1992;6:252-265.)

classification has been found to be useful in both treatment and prognosis. Type I fractures are nondisplaced articular fractures. Type II fractures are two-part fractures of the posterior facet and are divided into A, B, and C based on the location of the fracture line. Type III fractures are three-part fractures with a centrally depressed fragment, also divided into A, B, and C. Type IV fractures are four-part articular fractures with extensive comminution. After a minimum of 10 years, type III fractures are four times more likely to require an arthrodesis than type II fractures.

The Essex-Lopresti classification for calcaneal fractures describes the joint depression-type and the tongue-type fractures (Figure 2–41):

1. Tongue-type fractures: This fracture pattern splits the tuberosity in the axial plane and involves the subtalar joint. The pull of the Achilles tendon displaces the dorsal fragment cranially.
2. Joint depression fracture: This fracture pattern creates a separate fragment of the posterior facet with joint incongruity.

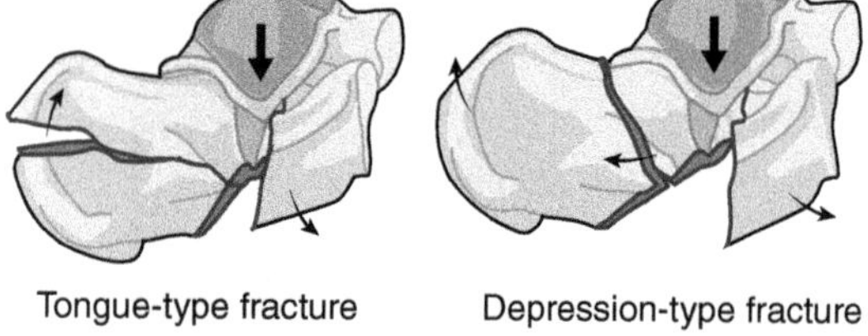

▲ **Figure 2–41. Essex-Lopresti classification of calcaneal fractures.** (Reprinted with permission from Essex-Lopresti P. The mechanism, reduction technique, and results in fractures of the os calcis, 1951-52. Br J Surg. 1952 Mar;39(157):395-419.)

Treatment

Treatment of displaced intraarticular fractures remains controversial. Surgical techniques are evolving for the treatment of calcaneal fractures. And, in skilled hands, surgical treatment of calcaneal fractures demonstrates decrease incidence of post-traumatic subtalar arthritis with an increase in complications. Currently, there is insufficient evidence demonstrating superiority of surgical treatment over nonsurgical treatment. Heavy smoking, severe peripheral vascular disease, and poorly controlled diabetes are relative contraindications for surgery. The extent of varus displacement in the axial plane (Harris view) may guide operative management more than the extent of joint depression in the posterior facet.

Early closed manipulation of displaced intraarticular fractures can restore the anatomic configuration of the heel region and prevent skin breakdown (Figure 2–42), and percutaneous fixation may then be performed. This is particularly successful for noncomminuted tongue-type fracture patterns. An axial pin is inserted in the tongue fragment, which is then disimpacted and reduced. The pin is then pushed further to stabilize the fracture (Essex-Lopresti technique).

For displaced intraarticular calcaneal fractures, ORIF with plates and screws, with or without bone grafting, has been the standard of surgical care. The aim of ORIF is to restore the articular surface of the subtalar joint, restore Böhler's angle, improve varus deformity, and reduce lateral wall blow-out. Figure 2–43 demonstrates a Sanders type II right calcaneal fracture with joint depression reduced and fixed via an extensile lateral approach approximately 2 weeks after injury.

Immediate surgery of calcaneal fractures is associated with a high incidence of wound healing complications. Therefore, a 10- to 14-day delay (ie, visualization of skin wrinkles) to surgical fixation is recommended to decrease the risk of wound breakdown and infection. Two common surgical approaches are the sinus tarsi and extensile lateral approaches. The sinus tarsi approach may have a lower incidence of wound healing problems compared to the extensile approach. Few advocate primary subtalar arthrodesis for severely comminuted (Sanders type IV) fractures.

Fractures of the sustentaculum are rare injuries that are usually caused by a high-energy trauma. This fracture should be suspected in the patient with a history of an eversion injury and pain below the medial malleolus. The injury is diagnosed by CT scan. Displaced sustentaculum fractures may require ORIF through a medial approach.

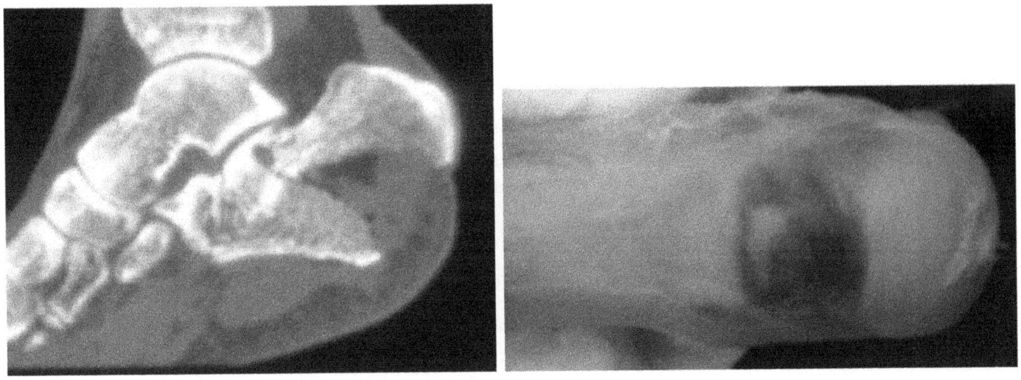

▲ **Figure 2–42.** Sagittal CT reconstruction and photograph of a tongue-type calcaneal fracture. Due to potential skin compromise, these fractures may require immediate reduction and fixation.

Fractures of the anterior process of the calcaneus are usually caused by forced inversion of the foot, and they must be differentiated from midtarsal and ankle sprains. The firmly attached bifurcate ligament avulses a bony flake from the anterior process. Maximal tenderness and swelling occur midway between the tip of the lateral malleolus and the base of the fifth metatarsal. A lateral oblique radiograph will demonstrate the fracture line. Treatment is usually conservative for minimally displaced fractures.

Complications

The most significant short-term complication from surgically treated calcaneal fractures is postoperative wound breakdown and infection. Posttraumatic degenerative joint disease is a long-term complication requiring subtalar fusion or triple arthrodesis. Other complications include compartment syndrome, nerve entrapment syndromes (medial or lateral plantar branches and sural nerve, either from

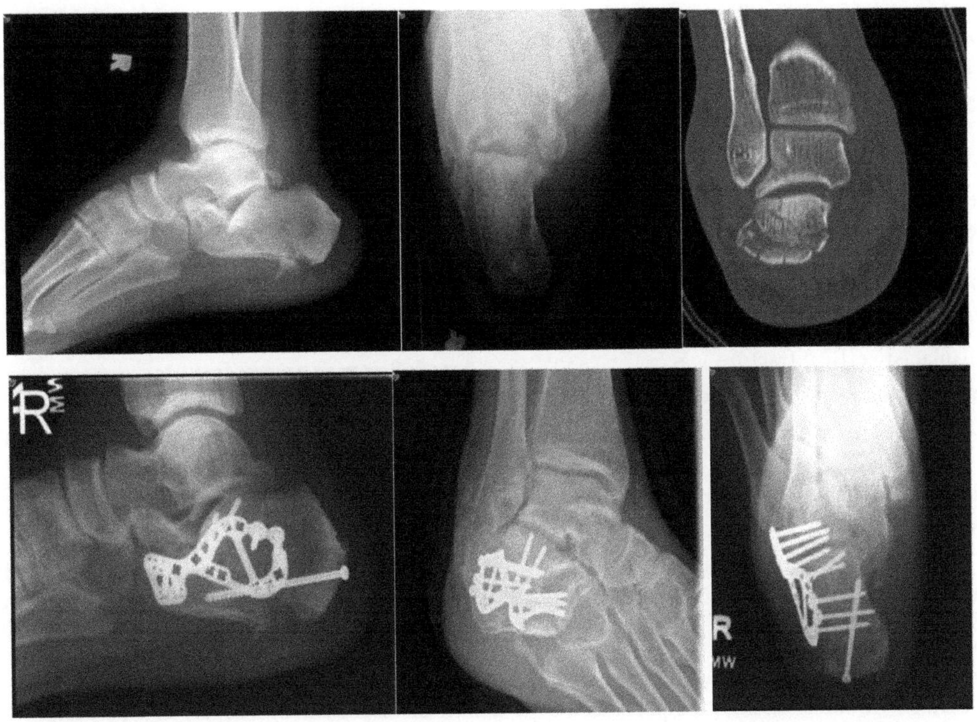

▲ **Figure 2–43.** Pre- and postoperative radiographs and CT scans of a Sanders type II right calcaneal fracture with joint depression. The fracture was fixed after approximately 2 weeks via an extensile lateral approach.

posttraumatic or postsurgical scarring), peroneal tendon injury, calcaneofibular impingement, heel pad pain, exostosis, and malunion. Compartment syndrome occurs in 10% of patients and should be evaluated with physical examination.

2. Talus Fractures

- Second in frequency among all tarsal fractures after calcaneus fractures.
- Sixty percent of talus covered with articular cartilage and has no muscular attachments.
- AVN still a concern despite improved surgical techniques.

Fractures of the talus commonly occur either through the body or the neck. Talar neck fractures represent almost 50% of all talus fractures. The blood supply to the talus is composed of the posterior tibial artery via the deltoid artery and artery of the tarsal canal (47%), the anterior tibial artery (36%), and the perforating peroneal artery (16%) that enters the talar neck area and is tenuous. The major blood supply enters posterior to the talar neck; thus, fractures that do not extend posteriorly into the body may have a lower risk of vascular compromise. The deltoid artery supplies blood to the talar body in the majority of cases. Fractures and dislocations may disrupt the vascularity to the talus and cause delayed healing and/or AVN. The talus has no muscle attachments and transmits body weight from the tibia down to the calcaneus and toward the navicular. The subtalar joint axis of motion is inversion and eversion and facilitates walking on uneven ground.

Talar Neck Fractures

The most common mechanism of a talar neck fracture is hyperdorsiflexion with an axial load causing impingement between the talar neck and tibia. The most widely used classification for talar neck fractures was described by Hawkins in 1970 and added to by Canale and Kelly in 1978.

Type 1: Nondisplaced vertical fracture

Type 2: Displaced fracture and subtalar dislocation

Type 3: Displaced fracture and subtalar and tibiotalar dislocation

Type 4: Displaced fracture with subtalar, tibiotalar, and talonavicular dislocation

The Hawkins classification has prognostic value for AVN of the talus. Current reported incidence of AVN based on the Hawkins classification is 5.7% with type 1, 18.4% with type 2, 44.7% with type 3, and 12.1% with type 4 fractures. These rates are lower than the initial report by Hawkins. The incidence of AVN based on Hawkins classification paper is: 0% for type 1, 42% for type 2, 91% type 3, and 52% for type 4 (per Canale and Kelly, 1978). However, newer imaging modalities and improvements in surgical treatment may account for this discrepancy. Radiographs and CT scans should be performed to visualize degree of displacement, step-off, and presence of dislocation.

Treatment of talar neck fractures is directed toward anatomic reduction and minimizing complications. Type 1 fractures are usually treated nonoperatively with a non–weight-bearing short leg splint or cast for 6 to 8 weeks. All displaced fractures (types 2-4) are treated operatively. In select type 2 cases, a closed reduction can be performed; if the fracture is also reduced satisfactorily, then closed management can be considered. Anteromedial and anterolateral surgical approaches can be performed, and usually fracture comminution is located dorsally and medially. Fixation can be performed with 3.5-mm or smaller titanium screws (either anteroposterior or posteroanterior) and/or plates (Figure 2–44). The patient remains non–weight bearing for approximately 6 to 8 weeks or until a subchondral lucency is visualized in the dome of the talus known as Hawkins sign, an indicator of talus vascularity. The absence of the Hawkins sign does not predict the occurrence of AVN in histologic and MRI-based studies.

Complications of surgical treatment of talar neck fractures include AVN, infection, delayed union, nonunion, malunion, and degenerative joint disease of the tibiotalar and subtalar joints.

Talar Body Fractures

Talar body fractures occur due to high-energy trauma with the hindfoot either in supination or pronation. Lateral process talus fractures result from forced dorsiflexion, axial loading, and inversion with external rotation. Associated fractures of the malleoli, talar neck, and calcaneus may also occur. Sneppen classification distinguishes five types:

Type 1: Osteochondral fracture

Type 2: Coronal, sagittal, or horizontal fracture

Type 3: Posterior process fracture

Type 4: Lateral process fracture

Type 5: Crush fracture of the body

Treatment of talar body fractures is based on restoring joint integrity of both the tibiotalar and subtalar joints. Minimally displaced fractures can be treated closed. AP, mortise, lateral, and Broden (ankle internally rotated 45 degrees) radiographic views aid in quantifying articular surface involvement and displacement. CT scans are recommended in all talar body fractures to assess comminution and associated fractures.

Surgery may be indicated in fractures with greater than 2 mm of displacement. Surgery can be performed via the same approaches as talar neck fractures (anteromedial

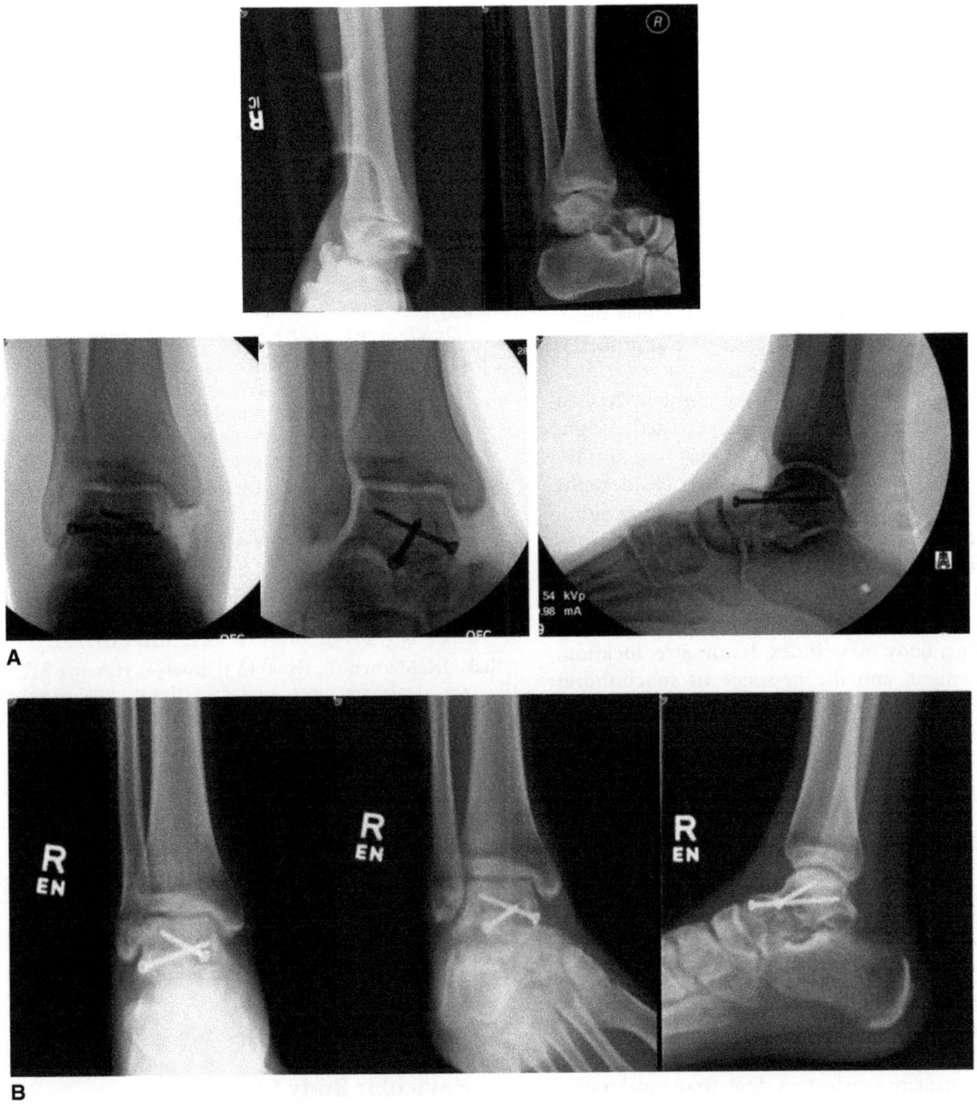

▲ **Figure 2–44.** Preoperative and intraoperative (**A**) and 3-month postoperative (**B**) radiographs of a right Hawkins type 2 talar neck fracture reduced and fixed with titanium screws.

and/or anterolateral) based on the location of the fracture. A medial malleolar osteotomy may be necessary for exposure. Fixation is usually achieved with 3.5-mm or smaller titanium screws.

Complications of talar body fracture management are similar to those of talar neck fractures: AVN, posttraumatic degenerative joint disease (subtalar and/or talonavicular), malunion, and pain. Patients with posttraumatic degenerative joint disease may benefit from arthrodesis (subtalar, tibiotalar, and/or talonavicular).

Osteochondral Fractures of the Talar Dome

Any chronic pain after ankle sprain should raise the suspicion of an osteochondral lesion. A history of trauma may not always be present. Initial radiographic evaluation often does not demonstrate these lesions because only 50%

of osteochondral lesions can be detected via radiographs. MRI is helpful as well but is not as sensitive and specific as arthroscopy.

Classical staging performed by Berndt and Harty is based on the appearance on radiographs:

Stage 1: Localized compression

Stage 2: Incomplete separation of the fragment

Stage 3: Completely detached but nondisplaced fragment

Stage 4: Completely detached, displaced fracture

A cyst around the osteochondral lesion is a bad prognostic factor and may suggest a more aggressive approach is needed than debridement and microfracture.

Symptomatic stage 1, 2, and 3 lesions are initially treated conservatively with immobilization and restricted weight bearing. Only 50% of osteochondral lesions may heal nonoperatively. Healing can be monitored with either radiographs or MRI, the latter being more accurate. Osteochondral lesions that fail nonoperative treatment and all stage 4 lesions require surgical treatment. If the fragment can be repaired, reduction and fixation is recommended. For unrepairable fragments, excision with or without microfracture drilling is recommended. Age, body mass index, lesion size, location, duration, displacement, and the presence of subchondral cysts all may help guide treatment. Treatments discussed earlier for knee osteochondral lesions may be helpful for talar osteochondral lesions as well. Degenerative joint disease of the tibiotalar joint is a frequent long-term complication.

Subtalar Dislocation

Subtalar dislocation is the simultaneous dislocation of the talocalcaneal and talonavicular joints without a talar neck fracture. Inversion injuries result in medial dislocations (85%), whereas eversion injuries result in lateral dislocations (15%). Anterior and posterior dislocations are rare.

Prompt closed reduction under sedation is usually successful. Immobilization in a non–weight-bearing short leg cast for 6 weeks is usually satisfactory. Soft-tissue interposition, particularly of the posterior tibial tendon, may prevent closed reduction, in which case open reduction is indicated.

Extrusion of the Talus

Extrusion of the talus usually results from high-energy trauma. Most dislocations are open (70%), and they can occur with or without fracture. Aggressive debridement, salvage of the extruded talus, and open reduction are recommended. Complications include AVN, persistent pain, and infection, and tibiocalcaneal fusion may be necessary.

Halvorson JJ, Winter SB, Teasdall RD, Scott AT. Talar neck fractures: a systematic review of the literature. *J Foot Ankle Surg.* 2013;52:56-61. [PMID: 23153783]

Hawkins LG. Fractures of the neck of the talus. *J Bone Joint Surg Am.* 1970;52:991-1002. [PMID: 5479485]

Jordan RK, Bafna KR, Liu J, Ebraheim NA. Complications of talar neck fractures by Hawkins classification: a systematic review. *J Foot Ankle Surg.* 2017;56(4):817-821. [PMID: 28633784]

Kanatlı U, Eren A, Eren TK, Vural A. Treatment of osteochondral lesions of the talus with cell-free polymer-based scaffold in single-step arthroscopic surgery. *Arthrosc Tech.* 2017;6(5): e1727-e1734.

Mehta CR, An VVG, Phan K, Sivakumar B, Kanawati AJ, Suthersan M. Extensile lateral versus sinus tarsi approach for displaced, intra-articular calcaneal fractures: a meta-analysis. *J Orthop Surg Res.* 2018;13(1):243. [PMID: 30249288]

Sharr PJ, Mangupli MM, Winson IG, Buckley RE. Current management options for displaced intra-articular calcaneal fractures: non-operative, ORIF, minimally invasive reduction and fixation or primary ORIF and subtalar arthrodesis. A contemporary review. *Foot Ankle Surg.* 2016;22(1):1-8. [PMID: 26869492]

Smyth NA, Zachwieja EC, Buller LT, Miranda AD, Steinlauf SD. Surgical approaches to the calcaneus and the sural nerve: there is no safe zone. *Foot Ankle Surg.* 2018;24(6):517-520. [PMID: 29409272]

Spierings KE, Min M, Nooijen LE, Swords MP, Schepers T. Managing the open calcaneal fracture: a systematic review. *Foot Ankle Surg.* 2019;25(6):707-713. [PMID: 30467055]

Stake IK, Madsen JE, Hvaal K, Johnsen E, Husebye EE. Surgically treated talar fractures. A retrospective study of 50 patients. *Foot Ankle Surg.* 2016;22(2):85-90. [PMID: 27301726]

Vallier HA. Fractures of the talus: state of the art. *J Orthop Trauma.* 2015;29(9):385-392. [PMID: 26299809.]

Wei N, Zhou Y, Chang W, Zhang Y, Chen W. Displaced intra-articular calcaneal fractures: classification and treatment. *Orthopedics.* 2017;40(6):e921-e929. [PMID: 29116324]

Whitaker C, Turvey B, Illical EM. Current concepts in talar neck fracture management. *Curr Rev Musculoskelet Med.* 2018; 11(3):456-474.

MIDFOOT

Navicular Body Fractures

Navicular body fractures occur either centrally in a horizontal plane or, more rarely, in a vertical plane. They are occasionally characterized by impaction. CT scanning is more reliable than radiographs to detect the fractures. Noncomminuted fractures with displacement of the dorsal fragment can be reduced. Closed manipulation by strong traction on the forefoot and simultaneous digital pressure over the displaced fragment can restore normal position. If a tendency to redisplace is apparent, this can be counteracted by temporary fixation with a K-wire or screw. Non–weight-bearing immobilization in a cast or splint is required for a minimum of 6 weeks. Comminuted and impacted navicular fractures cannot be anatomically reduced in a closed manner. Fragments that involve greater than 25% of the bone benefit from ORIF to prevent dorsal subluxation.

Navicular Avulsion Fractures

Avulsion fractures of the tarsal navicular may occur as a result of a severe midtarsal sprain and can be treated in a closed fashion. Avulsion fractures of the tuberosity near the insertion of the posterior tibialis tendon are uncommon and must be differentiated from an accessory navicular or os tibiale externum. Dorsal lip avulsions may also occur.

Navicular Stress Fractures

The navicular is also a frequent site of fatigue fracture in runners. CT, radionuclide imaging, or MRI is often necessary to make the diagnosis. Six to ten weeks in a non–weight-bearing short leg cast is usually required for fracture healing.

Cuneiform and Cuboid Body Fractures

Because of their relatively protected position in the midtarsus, isolated fractures of the cuboid and cuneiform bones are rarely encountered. Avulsion fractures may occur as a component of severe midtarsal sprains. Extensive fractures usually occur in association with other injuries of the foot and often are caused by severe crushing. A "nutcracker" fracture is a compression fracture of the cuboid and, when associated with lateral column shortening, can be treated by lateral column lengthening, ORIF, and bone grafting.

Midtarsal Dislocations

Midtarsal dislocation through the naviculocuneiform and calcaneocuboid joints, or more proximally through the talonavicular and calcaneocuboid joints (Chopart's joint), may occur as a result of a twisting injury to the forefoot. Fractures of varying extent of adjacent bones are frequently associated. When acute treatment is administered, closed reduction by traction on the forefoot and manipulation is generally effective. If reduction is unstable and displacement tends to recur upon release of traction, stabilization for 4 weeks by percutaneous K-wires is recommended.

FOREFOOT

Tarsometatarsal (Lisfranc) Dislocations

Lisfranc injuries have traditionally been associated with high-energy trauma such as MVAs and industrial accidents but may also be a result of athletic activity. These injuries are often overlooked after an athletic injury or in a polytrauma patient, so a high index of suspicion is necessary for proper diagnosis.

The base of the second metatarsal is recessed proximally to the base of the other metatarsals in a cleft between the first and third cuneiforms, thus "locking" the joint. Whereas primary stabilization is provided by bone, the strong ligamentous attachments provide substantial stability to the Lisfranc joint. The ligaments are divided into plantar, dorsal, and interosseous components; the plantar ligament is the strongest. Injury to this tarsometatarsal complex may occur due to purely ligamentous injury or fracture-dislocation. The mechanism is due to a rotational force and axial load through a hyperplantarflexed forefoot.

Diagnosis is confirmed with weight-bearing foot radiographs because non–weight-bearing radiographs may not demonstrate the injury. On the AP view, the medial base of the second metatarsal should line up with the medial border of the middle cuneiform and there should be no widening of the interval between the first and second ray. On the lateral view, there may be dorsal displacement of the first or second metatarsal on the midfoot. On the oblique view, the medial aspect of the fourth metatarsal should line up with the medial cuboid. For more subtle or purely ligamentous injuries, MRI may be more sensitive. Three commonly occurring patterns of this injury are identified: total incongruity, partial incongruity, and divergent.

Nondisplaced Lisfranc injury can be treated in non–weight-bearing immobilization for 6 weeks. Fractures displaced greater than 2 mm, as compared to the opposite foot, are best treated with ORIF utilizing either screws or plates/screws. Immobilization is recommended for 6 weeks, followed by progressive weight bearing. Primary arthrodesis is another option but is more expensive and has a higher complication rate than ORIF. However, ORIF has a higher rate of implant removal (43.6%) compared to arthrodesis (18.4%).

Complications of Lisfranc injuries include posttraumatic degenerative joint disease, which is higher in nonoperative treatment. Other complications are CRPS, symptomatic implants, and loss of reduction.

Metatarsal Shaft Fractures

Nondisplaced fractures of the metatarsal shafts usually occur from direct trauma. Displacement is rarely significant when the first and fifth metatarsals are not involved because they act as internal splints. Most of these fractures can be treated closed with a hard-soled shoe or boot with partial weight bearing. For displaced fractures of the shaft, either closed or open reduction with K-wires or small plates and screws can be performed. Residual apex dorsal displacement of the metatarsal shaft may cause prominence of the metatarsal head on the plantar surface. This concentrated local pressure may produce a painful skin callus. Residual apex plantar angulation of the first metatarsal will transfer weight to the heads of the second and third metatarsals. If there are numerous displaced metatarsal fractures, closed versus open reduction can be performed.

Metatarsal Head and Neck Fractures

Fractures of the metatarsal neck usually occur from direct trauma to the foot, and the vast majority of these injuries can be treated closed in a hard-soled shoe or boot. Apex dorsal displacement is common and should be reduced to avoid reactive skin callus formation from pressure on the plantar skin. Intraarticular fractures of the metatarsal heads are rare. Even when they heal in a displaced position, some remodeling occurs, and the functional outcome is surprisingly good. The indications for open reduction with or without internal fixation remain controversial. K-wires can be used for fixation if surgery is necessary.

Fracture of the Base of the Fifth Metatarsal

Fractures of the base of the fifth metatarsal are the most common of all metatarsal fractures. Three distinct patterns occur: (1) an avulsion fracture of the tuberosity that may, on rare occasions, involve the joint between the cuboid and the fifth metatarsal; (2) a fracture at the metadiaphyseal junction up to 1.5 cm distal to the tuberosity (ie, Jones fracture); and (3) a transverse fracture of the proximal metatarsal diaphysis.

Avulsion fractures of the base of the fifth metatarsal usually occur after an adduction injury to the forefoot. The peroneus brevis muscle may pull and displace the fractured fragment proximally. A hard-soled shoe, cast brace, or elastic wrapping for 3 to 6 weeks can be used for treatment. Symptomatic nonunions, displacement greater than 2 mm, and/or greater than 30% involvement of the cubometatarsal joint may be indications for surgery. Symptomatic, small fragments can be excised.

Nondisplaced Jones fractures are best treated in a non–weight-bearing cast for 6 to 8 weeks. ORIF of Jones fractures is recommended for a displaced fracture and/or a high-performance athlete. Surgical fixation can be performed either with intramedullary screw fixation or plate and screws. This anatomic area is a vascular watershed region and prone to nonunion (15%-30%). Proximal diaphyseal fractures or "chronic Jones fractures" are likely secondary to fatigue failure and can be treated with a non–weight-bearing short leg cast for 6 weeks.

If a nonunion occurs and there is no evidence of bone healing at 12 weeks, internal fixation and bone grafting are recommended. Refracture may occur in 33% of the Jones fractures treated conservatively.

Fractures and Dislocations of the Phalanges of the Toes

Fractures of the phalanges of the toes are most commonly caused by a direct force such as a crush injury. Barefoot walking in the house is a potential risk factor. Spiral or oblique fractures of the shaft of the proximal phalanges of the lesser toes may occur as a result of an indirect twisting injury. Fractures of the foot phalanges can generally be treated in closed fashion with a hard-soled shoe or boot. If the great toe proximal phalanx is displaced or intraarticular, ORIF may be considered. Phalangeal fractures can be treated by binding the involved toe to the adjacent uninjured toe (buddy taping). Dislocation of the metatarsophalangeal joints and dislocation of the proximal interphalangeal joints usually can be reduced by closed manipulation. These dislocations are rarely isolated and usually occur in combination with other injuries to the forefoot.

Fracture of the Sesamoids of the Great Toe

Fractures of the sesamoid bones of the great toe are rare but may occur as a result of a crushing injury. These injuries must be differentiated from a bipartite sesamoid by comparing radiographs of the contralateral uninvolved foot. Nondisplaced fractures require no treatment other than a hard-soled shoe or metatarsal bar. Displaced fractures may require immobilization in a walking boot or cast, with the toe strapped in flexion. Displaced fractures can be treated with ORIF. Persistent delay of bone healing may cause disabling pain arising from arthritis of the articulation between the sesamoid and the head of the first metatarsal. If nonoperative treatment has failed, excision of the sesamoid may be necessary; however, this should be a last resort treatment.

Stress Fractures

Stress fractures of the metatarsals are also known as fatigue fractures and are commonly seen in young, active adults involved in vigorous, repetitive exercises. Stress fractures occur when damage from cyclical loading of a bone overwhelms its physiologic capacity for repair. A high longitudinal arch and excessive forefoot varus are intrinsic precipitating factors for stress fractures of the forefoot. Stress fractures can also occur in the calcaneus. Pain is worse with ambulation, and patients frequently are point tender over the involved area. If radiographs do not demonstrate fracture, an MRI is helpful. Treatment entails immobilization and unloading the lower extremity to allow the bone to heal. Because of the high risk of displacement and nonunion, early surgical management is proposed for high-risk stress fractures in the elite athlete.

Alcelik I, Fenton C, Hannant G, Abdelrahim M, Jowett C, Budgen A, Stanley J. Asystematic review and meta-analysis of the treatment of acute Lisfranc injuries: open reduction and internal fixation versus primary arthrodesis. *Foot Ankle Surg.* 2020;26(3):299-307. [PMID: 31103276]

Barnds B, Tucker W, Morris B. Cost comparison and complication rate of Lisfranc injuries treated with open reduction internal fixation versus primary arthrodesis. *Injury.* 2018;49(12):2318-2321. [PMID: 30314633]

Bowes J, Buckley R. Fifth metatarsal fractures and current treatment. *World J Orthop.* 2016;7(12):793-800. [PMID: 28032031]

Brin YS, Nyska M, Kish B. Lisfranc injury repair with the TightRope device: a short-term case series. *Foot Ankle Int.* 2010;31:624-627. [PMID: 20663431]

Bucknam RB, Scanaliato JP, Kusnezov NA, Heida KA Jr, Dunn JC, Orr JD. Return to weightbearing and high-impact activities following jones fracture intramedullary screw fixation. *Foot Ankle Int.* 2020;41(4):379-386. [PMID: 31904264]

Buda M, Kink S, Stavenuiter R, et al. Reoperation rate differences between open reduction internal fixation and primary arthrodesis of Lisfranc injuries. *Foot Ankle Int.* 2018;39(9):1089-1096. [PMID: 29812959]

Clements JR, Dijour F, Leong W. Surgical management navicular and cuboid fractures. *Clin Podiatr Med Surg.* 2018;35(2): 145-159. [PMID: 29482786]

Duplantier NL, Mitchell RJ, Zambrano S, et al. A biomechanical comparison of fifth metatarsal Jones fracture fixation methods. *Am J Sports Med.* 2018;46(5):1220-1227. [PMID: 29466679]

Engelmann EWM, Rammelt S, Schepers T. Fractures of the cuboid bone: a critical analysis review. *JBJS Rev.* 2020;8(4):e0173. [PMID: 32304497]

Ponkilainen VT, Laine HJ, Mäenpää HM, Mattila VM, Haapasalo HH. Incidence and characteristics of midfoot injuries. *Foot Ankle Int.* 2019;40(1):105-112. [PMID: 30269512]

Porter DA. Fifth metatarsal Jones fractures in the athlete. *Foot Ankle Int.* 2018;39(2):250-258. [PMID: 29228800]

Saxena A, Behan SA, Valerio DL, Frosch DL. Navicular stress fracture outcomes in athletes: analysis of 62 injuries. *J Foot Ankle Surg.* 2017;56(5):943-948. [PMID: 28842101]

Torg JS, Moyer J, Gaughan JP, Boden BP. Management of tarsal navicular stress fractures: conservative versus surgical treatment: a meta-analysis. *Am J Sports Med.* 2010;38(5):1048-1053. [PMID: 20197494]

Waverly BJ, Sorensen MD, Sorensen TK. Early weightbearing protocol in operative fixation of acute Jones fractures. *J Foot Ankle Surg.* 2018;57(3):489-493. [PMID: 29685559]

3 Sports Medicine: Upper Extremity

Patrick J. McMahon, MD

SHOULDER INJURIES

The shoulder is the third-most commonly injured joint during athletic activities, after the knee and the ankle. Sports-related injuries of the shoulder may result from a direct traumatic event or repetitive overuse. Any activity that requires arm motion, particularly overhead arm motion such as throwing, may stress the shoulder, resulting in injury. The glenohumeral joint of the shoulder is mobile partly from minimal containment of the humeral head by the shallow and smaller glenoid fossa. The trade-off for this mobility is less structural restraint to undesirable and potentially damaging movements. Thus, a fine balance must be struck to maintain full range of shoulder motion and normal glenohumeral joint stability.

Anatomy

A. The Bony Articulation of the Glenohumeral Joint

The glenohumeral joint is a modified ball-and-socket joint. The glenoid fossa is a shallow inverted, comma-shaped, articular surface one-fourth the size of the humeral head. The articular surface of the humeral head is retroverted approximately 30 degrees relative to the transverse axis of the elbow. Because the scapula is oriented anterolaterally about 30 degrees on the thorax, relative to the coronal plane of the body, the orientation of the glenoid fossa matches the humeral head retroversion so that with the arm relaxed at the side, the arm is positioned for activities in front of the body. With shoulder motion, the scapula also moves so that the glenoid accommodates changing humeral head positions. As a result, the humeral head is centered in the glenoid throughout most shoulder motions. When this centered position is disturbed, instability may result.

B. The Clavicle and Its Articulations

The clavicle articulates medially with the sternum at the sternoclavicular joint and laterally with the acromion of the scapula at the acromioclavicular joint. The clavicle rotates on its long axis and acts as a strut, serving as the only bone connecting the appendicular upper extremity to the axial skeleton.

C. The Glenohumeral Joint Capsule, Ligaments, and Labrum

The thin redundant joint capsule has almost twice the surface area of the humeral head to allow large range of joint motion. Different regions of the joint capsule provide stability at different joint positions. With the arm at the side, the superior portion of the capsule is taut and the inferior portion is lax. With overhead elevation, this relationship reverses.

The superior capsule forms a thick band called the coracohumeral ligament originating from the base of the coracoid and inserting on the anterior part of the greater tuberosity and superior part of the lesser tuberosity of the humerus. The capsule is uniformly thin and translucent anterior and posterior to the coracohumeral ligament. There are also folds or thickenings visible on the inside of the capsule with the shoulder at the side, which have been termed glenohumeral ligaments. Traditionally, the capsule has been described as being composed of the superior, middle, and inferior glenohumeral ligaments (Figure 3–1), the capsuloligamentous structures. While use of the term “ligament” is generally accepted, it needs some clarification. Ligaments are soft-tissue structures that connect bones. They are most commonly bandlike with parallel collagen fibers running between their insertion sites and have clearly defined edges, such as the medial collateral ligament of the knee. The glenohumeral capsule as a whole may be considered a sheet-like ligament connecting the humerus and the scapula. The collagen fibers are not organized in a parallel fashion, the margins of the folds are indistinct, and functional study does not indicate it to have band-like properties. This may be a reason that the ligaments of the anterior capsule have been described with variable prevalence; different authors have had varying success in identifying them. Also, with the shoulder in

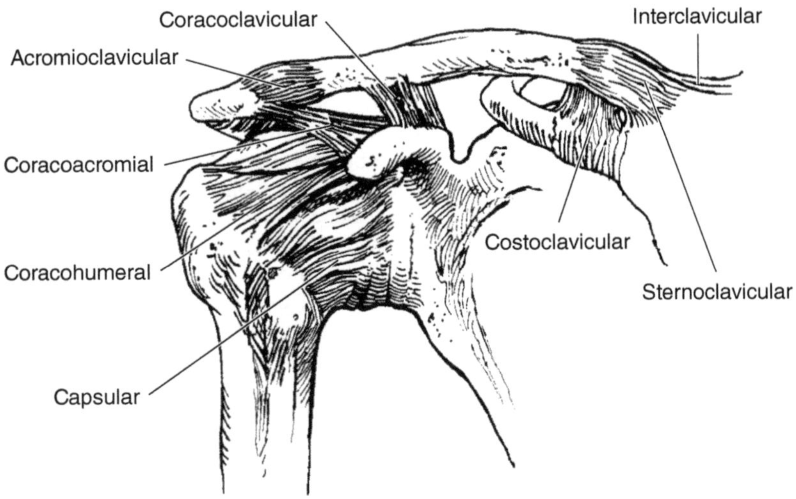

▲ **Figure 3–1.** Ligaments about the shoulder girdle.

combined abduction and external rotation, even the most consistently reported fold in the anteroinferior capsule, the anterior band of the inferior glenohumeral ligament, is often indistinct. While terminology may be currently causing confusion in anatomic, biomechanical, and clinical studies, there is little doubt that different regions of the capsule have differing roles in joint function, and this understanding has resulted in improved outcomes for shoulder injuries.

The capsule inserts into the glenoid bone and onto the glenoid labrum. The glenoid labrum acts not only as an attachment site for the capsuloligamentous structures but also as an extension of the articular cavity. Its presence deepens the glenoid socket by nearly 50%, and the triangular cross-section of the labrum acts as a chock-block to help prevent subluxation.

D. The Scapulothoracic Articulation

Movement of the concave surface of the anterior scapula articulating with the convex posterolateral thorax accounts for part of shoulder motion. In the resting position, the scapula overlays the second through the seventh ribs, and during full shoulder elevation, movement of the scapula accounts for about one-third of the motion. The scapula is attached to the rest of the skeleton by the clavicle; there are no normal osseous or ligamentous connections between the scapula and the thorax. The gliding surface of the scapulothoracic articulation is formed between the subscapularis muscle, the serratus anterior muscle, and the thorax with bursae. The major bursae between the subscapularis and the serratus anterior muscles and between the serratus anterior muscle and the thorax can be injured and result in crepitus and pain. Movement of the scapula is precise in orienting the glenoid fossa for optimal glenohumeral joint instability. Abnormalities of scapulothoracic motion such as scapular winging and dyskinesias can result in pain, weakness, and loss of shoulder motion.

E. The Shoulder Musculature

The 17 muscles around the shoulder may be divided into four functional groups: glenohumeral, thoracohumeral, scapulothoracic, and those that cross both the shoulder and elbow. The other muscular attachment to the scapula is the inferior belly of the omohyoid muscle.

1. Glenohumeral muscles—Four muscles compose the rotator cuff: the supraspinatus, subscapularis, infraspinatus, and teres minor. The supraspinatus has its origin on the posterosuperior scapula, superior to the scapular spine. It passes under the acromion, through the supraspinatus fossa, and inserts on the greater tuberosity with an extended attachment of fibrocartilage. Its attachment is just posterior to the attachment of the coracohumeral ligament. The supraspinatus is active during the entire arc of scapular plane abduction; paralysis of the suprascapular nerve results in an approximately 50% loss of abduction torque. The infraspinatus and the teres minor muscles originate on the posterior scapula, inferior to the scapular spine, and insert on the posterior aspect of the greater tuberosity. Despite their origin below the scapular spine, their tendinous insertions are not separate from the supraspinatus tendon. These muscles function together to externally rotate and extend the humerus. Both account for approximately 80% of external rotation strength in the adducted position. The infraspinatus is more active with the arm at the side, and the teres minor with the elevated shoulder. Medial to the posterior ridge of the greater tuberosity, a palpable landmark of the posterior shoulder, is the interval between the infraspinatus and the teres minor. The subscapularis muscle arises from the anterior scapula and is the only muscle to insert on the lesser tuberosity, just inferior to the coracohumeral ligament. The subscapularis is the sole anterior component of the rotator cuff and functions to internally rotate and flex the humerus. The tendinous insertion of the subscapularis is continuous with the anterior capsule so that both provide anterior glenohumeral stability.

The deltoid is the largest of the glenohumeral muscles. It covers the proximal humerus on a path from its tripennate origin at the clavicle, acromion, and scapular spine to its insertion midway on the humerus at the deltoid tubercle. Abduction of the joint results from activity of the anterior and middle portions. The anterior portion is also a forward flexor. The posterior portion does not abduct the joint, but instead adducts and extends the humerus. The deltoid is active throughout the entire arc of glenohumeral abduction; paralysis of the deltoid results in a 50% loss of abduction torque. The deltoid muscle can fully abduct the glenohumeral joint with the supraspinatus muscle inactive.

The teres major muscle originates from the inferior angle of the scapula and inserts on the medial lip of the bicipital groove of the humerus, posterior to the insertion of the latissimus dorsi. The axillary nerve and the posterior humeral circumflex artery pass inferior to the subscapularis muscle and the inferior glenohumeral joint capsule, and then inferior to the teres minor muscle through the quadrilateral space also bordered by the teres major, the triceps, and the humerus. The teres major muscle contracts with the latissimus dorsi muscle, and the two muscles function as a unit in humeral extension, internal rotation, and adduction.

2. Thoracohumeral muscles—The pectoralis major and the latissimus dorsi muscles are powerful movers of the shoulder and, hence, contribute to the joint force that in turn usually stabilizes the glenohumeral joint. The pectoralis major muscle arises as a broad sheet of two distinct heads from the clavicle, and the lowermost fibers of the sternal head insert most proximally on the humerus.

Muscles that have origin on the thorax contribute to glenohumeral stability but may have roles in instability as well. When the shoulder is forced back in the apprehension position of combined abduction and external rotation, the lowermost fibers of the sternal head of the pectoralis major muscle are stretched to an extreme and may then pull the humeral head out of the glenoid.

3. Scapulothoracic muscles—The levator scapulae, rhomboid major and minor, trapezius, and serratus anterior muscles move the scapula during shoulder motion.

4. Biceps brachii muscle—Both heads of the biceps brachii muscle have their origin on the scapula. The short head originates from the coracoid and, with the coracobrachialis muscle, forms the conjoined tendon. The long head of the biceps has its origin just superior to the articular margin of the glenoid from the posterosuperior labrum and the supraglenoid tubercle and is inside the synovial sheath of the glenohumeral joint. It traverses the glenohumeral joint, passing over the anterior aspect of the humeral head to the bicipital groove where it exits the joint under the transverse humeral ligament.

Its origin on the scapula and insertion of the radius leaves the long head of the biceps brachii muscle with potential for function at both the shoulder and the elbow. Its function at the elbow has been well established to include both flexion and supination. Long considered a depressor of the humeral head, the role of the active biceps has been recently questioned as electromyographic studies have shown that there was little or no activity of the biceps when elbow motion was controlled. This does not preclude a passive role or an active role associated with elbow motion, as tension in the tendon may then contribute to glenohumeral joint stability.

5. Long head of the triceps brachii—The long head of the triceps brachii has its origin from the inferior surface of the glenoid. It is a landmark for dissection under the glenoid in reverse total shoulder arthroplasty, and ossification of the muscle origin after this dissection occasionally occurs. Its role in glenohumeral stability is uncertain, but like the biceps brachii, it may have a passive role or an active role associated with elbow motion.

F. The Neurovascular Supply

The axillary artery traverses the axilla, extending from the outer border of the first rib to the lower border of the teres minor muscle, forming the brachial artery. The axillary artery lies deep to the pectoralis muscle but is crossed in its midregion by the pectoralis minor tendon, just before the tendon inserts on the coracoid process. The axillary vein travels with the axillary artery, and branches of the axillary artery supply most of the shoulder girdle. The brachial plexus consists of the ventral rami of the fifth through eighth cervical nerves and the first thoracic nerve. This network of nerve fibers begins with the joining of the ventral rami proximally in the neck and continues anteriorly and distally, crossing into the axillary region obliquely underneath the clavicle at about the junction area of the distal one-third and proximal two-thirds. Clavicular fractures in this area have the potential of injuring the brachial plexus. The plexus then lies inferior to the coracoid process, where its cords form the peripheral nerves that continue down the arm. Muscles of the shoulder girdle are supplied by the nerves arising at all levels of the brachial plexus. An exception is the trapezius muscle that is innervated by the spinal accessory nerve that can be found lateral to the levator scapulae muscle adjacent to the superomedial angle of the scapula.

Grob K, Monahan RH, Manestar M, Filgueira L, Zdravkovic V. The posterior ridge of the greater tuberosity of the humerus: a suitable landmark for the posterior approach to the shoulder joint? *J Shoulder Elbow Surg*. 2018;27(4):635-640. [PMID: 29305099]

History and Physical Examination

A. General Approach

History of shoulder complaints includes age, the time or duration of injury, the mechanism of injury, arm dominance, location, intensity, aggravating and alleviating factors, radiation of discomfort, physical activity level, and occupation. Previous responses to treatments will help to characterize their efficacy and establish a pattern of progression. The physical examination begins with both shoulders being fully exposed. While some of the provocative tests are best done in the supine position, patients should first be examined in the upright position. The skin and then the surface anatomy are checked for asymmetry, atrophy, or external lesions. The supraspinatus and infraspinatus fossae are especially important to examine for atrophy. The area of pain should be pointed out by the patient prior to the physician manipulating the shoulder to avoid hurting the patient unnecessarily. A thorough neurovascular examination of the upper extremity should be performed.

B. Shoulder Range of Motion

1. Types of movement—Many terms may be used to describe movements of the shoulder joint (Figure 3–2). Elevation is motion between the thorax and arm, regardless of the plane. Beginning with the arm at the side, flexion is anterior elevation in the sagittal plane of the body, and extension is posterior elevation in the sagittal plane of the body. Abduction is elevation of the arm in the coronal plane of the body, and adduction is lowering of the arm in the coronal plane of the body. Internal rotation is when the arm rotates medially, inward toward the body, and external rotation is when the arm rotates laterally or outward from the body. Horizontal adduction occurs when the arm at 90 degrees of elevation moves forward and medially toward the center of the body, and horizontal abduction occurs when the arm at 90 degrees of elevation moves outward, away from the body.

2. Evaluation of movement and strength—Range of motion of the injured shoulder should be evaluated in comparison with the opposite shoulder and done both passively and actively. The scapula should be inspected for any changes in synchrony, such as scapular winging, elevation of the scapula, and dyskinesias manifested as any other irregular or asymmetric movements. Information may be gained on loss of glenohumeral flexibility and instability resulting from muscle, tendon, and capsuloligamentous abnormalities. Loss of flexibility has many causes but most often occurs from contracture of the glenohumeral joint capsule. Sudden pain or clicking may indicate an intraarticular problem. Strength is best tested near the end range of motion where subtle weakness is best assessed. For example, test internal rotation strength with the arm behind the back near the limit of full

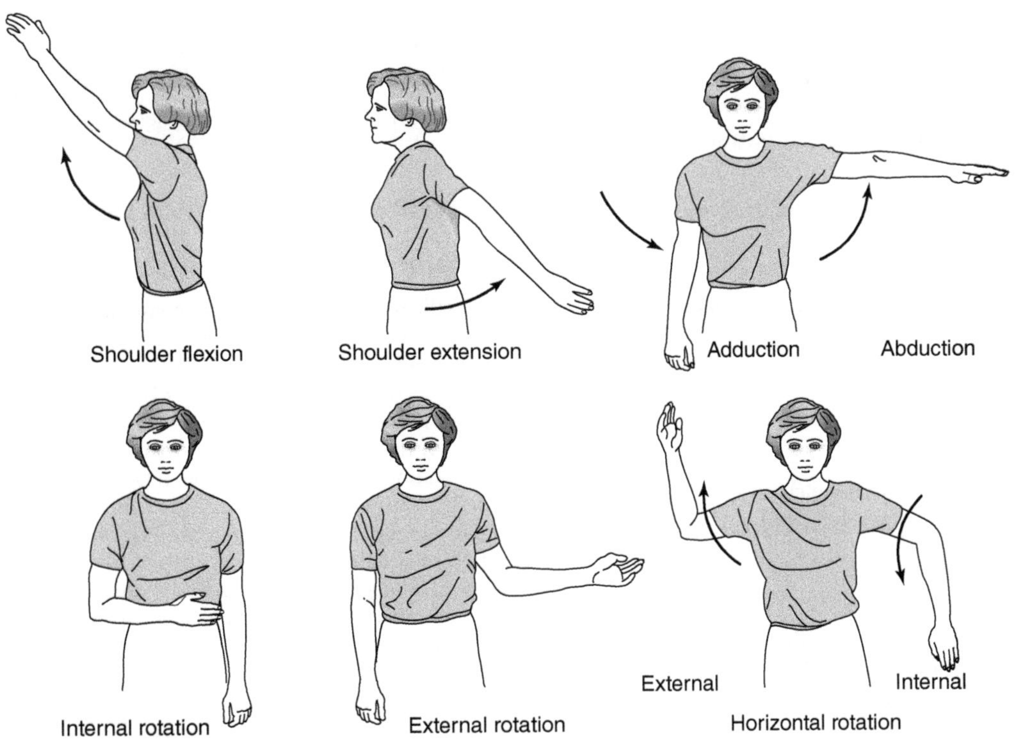

▲ **Figure 3–2.** Descriptions of shoulder motion.

internal rotation and external strength with the arm near the limit of full external rotation.

3. Provocative tests—Specific tests are then performed that aid in making the correct diagnosis. The specific tests for instability, impingement syndrome, bicipital tendonitis, and superior capsulolabral/biceps anchor lesions are discussed later with their diagnoses.

Imaging and Other Studies

Many radiologic views are available to evaluate shoulder injuries. An initial radiographic evaluation of the shoulder should consist of an anteroposterior (AP) view of the glenohumeral joint in both internal and external rotation and an axillary lateral view. Additional plain radiographic views depend on the underlying pathology. A supraspinatus outlet view is helpful in evaluation of acromion and rotator cuff injuries, and an acromioclavicular (ie, Zanca) view is helpful with acromioclavicular joint injuries. Magnetic resonance imaging (MRI) may be indicated in evaluation of rotator cuff and biceps disorders recalcitrant to conservative treatment and also shows the muscles and articular surfaces. A magnetic resonance arthrogram may be useful in detecting labral pathology. Computed tomography (CT) scans can be helpful after fracture and in evaluating scapula pathology. Ultrasonography is also useful in diagnosis of rotator cuff and biceps tendon injuries. Electromyographic examination can be useful in identifying shoulder pain of neurologic origin.

Arthroscopic Evaluation

A. Indications for Arthroscopic Evaluation of Shoulder Injuries

Indications for arthroscopic examination of the shoulder include the following:

1. Impingement syndrome, including subacromial bursitis, rotator cuff tendonitis, and rotator cuff tears
2. Acromioclavicular joint osteoarthritis
3. Loose bodies
4. Chronic synovitis
5. Glenohumeral instability
6. Superior capsulolabral/biceps anchor (ie, SLAP) lesions
7. Adhesive capsulitis (ie, frozen shoulder)

B. Technique

With the patient either in the lateral decubitus or the beach chair position, the arthroscope is inserted into the posterior shoulder. With visualization of the glenohumeral joint, an anterior portal immediately lateral to the coracoid allows additional inflow and the surgeon to insert surgical instruments. Additional portals may be used; for example, an additional anterior portal inferior to the first may be used for instability repair. The arthroscope is then removed from the joint and placed into the subacromial bursa. A portal lateral to the acromion allows instruments to be inserted for subacromial decompression and rotator cuff repair.

C. Steps in Evaluation

Examination of shoulder range of motion and stability with the patient under anesthesia is helpful in the diagnosis and treatment of shoulder injuries. This should be performed in the operating room prior to arthroscopy. The steps in basic arthroscopic examination should then include the following:

1. Glenohumeral articular surfaces
2. Rotator cuff from inside the joint
3. Labrum including the biceps anchor
4. Anterior, inferior, and posterior capsule
5. Rotator cuff from outside the joint, the subacromial space
6. Acromion
7. Acromioclavicular joint

Humphries A, Cirovic S, Bull AM, Hearnden A, Shaheen AF. Assessment of the glenohumeral joint's active and passive axial rotational range. *J Shoulder Elbow Surg.* 2015;24(12):1974-1981. [PMID: 26410346]

Johnson CD, Nijst BKJF, Eagle SR, et al. Evaluation of shoulder strength and kinematics as risk factors for shoulder injury in United States special forces personnel. *Orthop J Sports Med.* 2019;7(3):2325967119831272. [PMID: 30891463]

SHOULDER TENDON AND MUSCLE INJURY

Rotator Cuff Tendon Injuries

Injury to the rotator cuff is the most common cause of shoulder pain and disability. Symptoms include shoulder pain, weakness, and decreased range of motion, and although pain does not correlate with severity of disease, weakness and decreased range of motion are more common with severe rotator cuff tendon tears than subacromial bursitis or rotator cuff tendinosis. Symptoms are often worsened by activity, especially with overhead activity. Night pain is also common, and many patients complain of awakening after rolling onto the affected shoulder.

Any prolonged repetitive activity involving overhead motion such as tennis, pitching, golf, or swimming may cause rotator cuff injury, but the onset is without any inciting event about one-half of the time. Injury, whether repetitive or acute, can produce a continuous vicious cycle (Figure 3–3). Blood supply to this tendon is precarious, thus decreasing its capacity for healing.

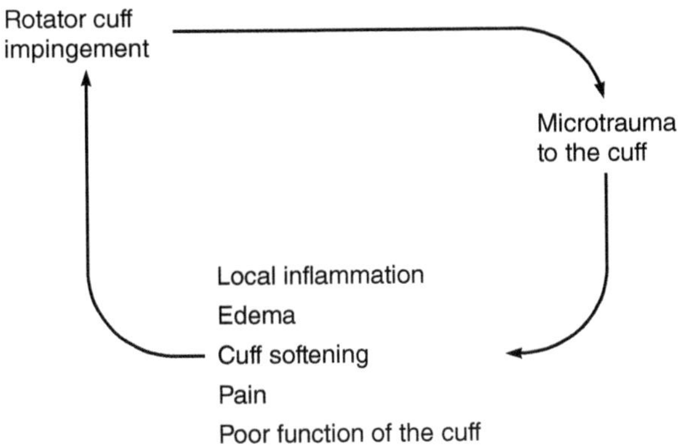

▲ **Figure 3–3.** The cycle of injury and reinjury resulting from rotator cuff impingement.

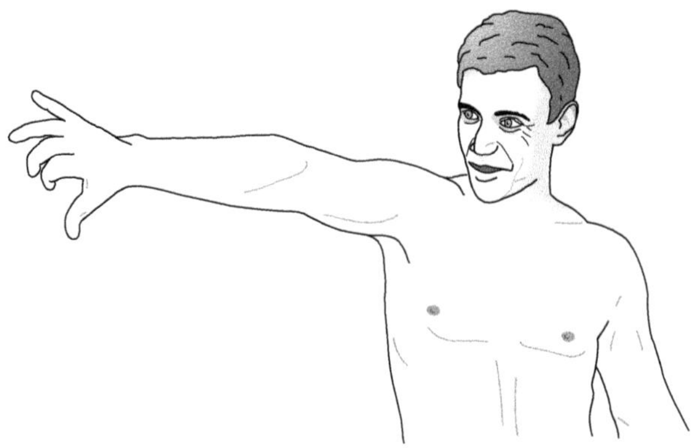

▲ **Figure 3–4.** Evaluating for impingement of the supraspinatus tendon with the "empty can" test.

1. Subacromial Bursitis and Rotator Cuff Tendinosis

Essentials of Diagnosis

- *Mild or moderate pain with overhead shoulder motion.*
- *Occasional night pain.*
- *Normal range of motion or mild limitation from the shoulder pain.*
- *No weakness or mild weakness from the shoulder pain.*
- *Positive impingement signs.*
- *No muscle atrophy.*
- *Pain is significantly diminished with a subacromial lidocaine injection.*

Prevention

Limiting repetitive overhead activities and maintenance of good rotator cuff strength are keys to prevention. Additionally, overall conditioning and stretching and strengthening with careful attention to technique can be helpful in minimizing many of the injuries from overuse.

Clinical Findings

Bursitis of the shoulder refers to an inflammation of the subacromial bursa. It is usually present with rotator cuff tendinosis, and the two entities are similar. There is pain with activities involving overhead motion, and there is usually no pain or only mild pain with the arm at the side.

Of the four rotator cuff muscles, the supraspinatus tendon is most often initially involved. Rotator cuff tendinosis also results from impingement syndrome, which is irritation of the rotator cuff tendons as they pass through the subacromial space and is characterized by pain with activity involving overhead motion. The patient may occasionally be awakened by pain at night.

Active range of shoulder motion is usually normal but may be limited by pain. There is no atrophy of the shoulder muscles, and manual muscle testing is usually normal but may demonstrate mild weakness from pain. Passively, when the internally rotated shoulder is moved into forward flexion, the patient will experience discomfort. This is called the Neer impingement sign (Figure 3–4). For the Hawkins impingement sign, the shoulder is forward flexed or abducted to 90 degrees and then internally rotated. Pain with impingement signs diminishes with the Neer impingement test (10 mL of lidocaine is injected into the subacromial space), and if limited, there is also increase in strength and range of motion.

Radiographic views of the subacromial space such as the supraspinatus outlet view may show a spur on the undersurface of the acromion, causing narrowing of the subacromial space. In recent years, advances in imaging methods such as ultrasonography and MRI have aided in the diagnosis of subacromial bursitis, rotator cuff tendinosis, and rotator cuff tendon tears (Figure 3–5).

Treatment

Treatment starts with conservative measures such as activity modification, physical therapy, and oral nonsteroidal anti-inflammatory drugs (NSAIDs). Only with normal function of the rotator cuff tendons will glenohumeral mechanics be improved and the symptoms cease. If this treatment fails, a subacromial injection of corticosteroids may be helpful. Most patients respond well to these nonoperative treatments.

Surgical intervention is indicated if symptoms do not resolve after a few months of such treatment. Then, acromioplasty, also called subacromial decompression, which is shaving the undersurface of the acromion, usually results in relief of symptoms. An exception is the young athlete with glenohumeral instability and secondary tendinosis. In this case, the instability should be treated first, and the rotator cuff tendinosis will then resolve. This procedure can be done arthroscopically to decrease postoperative discomfort and

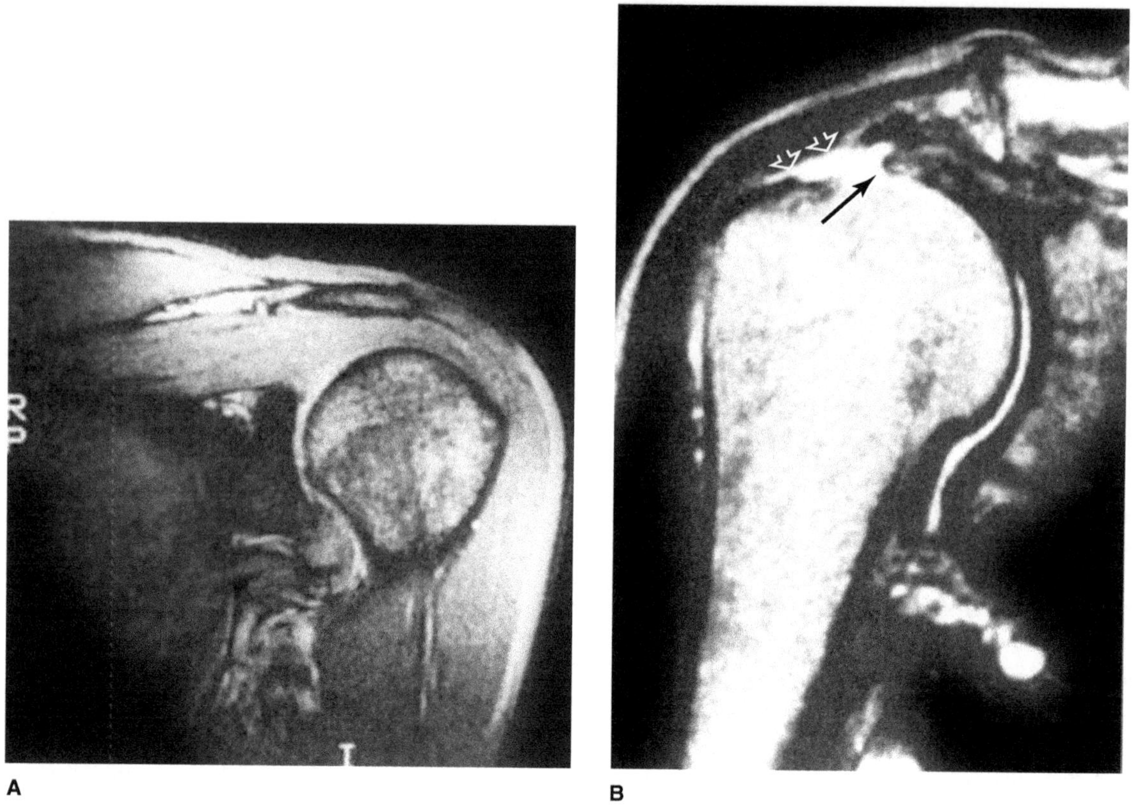

▲ **Figure 3–5.** Magnetic resonance imaging demonstrating (**A**) normal shoulder anatomy and (**B**) cystic changes at the greater tuberosity with rotator cuff tear (*arrow*).

minimize complications such as infection, stiffness, and deltoid muscle rupture from the acromion. Those who require surgical treatment are usually able to return to pain-free activities.

2. Rotator Cuff Tendon Tear

Essentials of Diagnosis

- *Moderate or severe pain with activity involving overhead motion.*
- *Persistent night pain.*
- *Diminished range of motion with moderate and severe tears.*
- *Weakness with moderate and severe tears.*
- *Positive impingement signs.*
- *Atrophy of rotator cuff muscles with severe tears.*
- *Pain is significantly diminished with a subacromial lidocaine injection.*

Prevention

Limiting repetitive overhead activities and maintenance of good rotator cuff strength are keys to prevention. Maintenance of overall body conditioning with regular stretching and strengthening of the rotator cuff and scapular stabilizing muscles can help prevent rotator cuff injuries.

Clinical Findings

A rotator cuff tendon tear is characterized by pain with activity involving overhead motion. However, the patient is often awakened at night with pain as well. Those with a chronic rotator cuff tear may experience a gradual loss of strength. Pain may be persistent, occurring even when the arm is at the side. Active range of shoulder motion may be limited, and if the tear is severe, there will be atrophy of the shoulder muscles. Manual muscle testing may demonstrate weakness, especially with external rotation. The Neer and Hawkins impingement signs are positive, and the pain diminishes with a subacromial injection of lidocaine. Radiographic evaluation is similar to that for subacromial bursitis and rotator cuff tendinosis.

Treatment

Radiographic evaluation and treatment are similar to subacromial bursitis management. Unlike acute tears, chronic rotator cuff tears often present insidiously, with slow progression from subacromial bursitis to rotator cuff tendinosis and eventual tendon tear. Differentiating severe rotator cuff tendinosis from partial or small full-thickness chronic rotator cuff tears may be difficult.

There are two important considerations in treating an individual with a rotator cuff tear—the current symptoms and the risk of the tear progressing. Although the lesion location and size are helpful in describing a rotator cuff tear, symptoms do not correlate with these factors alone. Some individuals are able to cope with the symptoms of a rotator cuff tear, and some may be completely asymptomatic. The severity of symptoms is influenced by a number of other factors, including pain tolerance, the acute or chronic nature of the injury, the age and activity level of the individual, superior migration of the humeral head, shoulder muscle strength, muscle atrophy, fatty changes in the muscle, arthritis, and workman's compensation status.

Rest, rehabilitation, and taking NSAIDs, sometimes for as long as 4 to 9 months, may relieve symptoms. Range-of-motion and strengthening exercises are recommended, unless they cause significant discomfort. Strengthening the other shoulder muscles may increase the individual's ability to cope with the rotator cuff tear. Avoidance of activities that exacerbate the symptoms, such as activities involving overhead motion, is also recommended. Symptoms of pain, weakness, or decreased range of motion that persist after a nonoperative treatment program indicate the need for surgical intervention.

Because rotator cuff tears may progress in size over time, immediate repair may be warranted in some at-risk individuals. Both epidemiologic and imaging studies of the general population indicate a high incidence of partial-thickness rotator cuff tears at younger ages and full-thickness rotator cuff tears at older ages. The increasing prevalence of rotator cuff injuries in older individuals may be the best evidence that rotator cuff tears progress in severity. Specifically, about 25% of individuals over 60 years of age have a tear, and in those over 80 years of age, there is a full-thickness rotator cuff tear in about 50% of individuals. The risk of a rotator cuff tear progressing to a more severe tear is thought to be higher in young, active individuals, partly because they have many more years to sustain an injury.

The thin degenerated tissue of a chronic rotator cuff tear makes surgical repair more difficult than repair of an acute tear. The repair can be accomplished with either an arthroscopic or an open technique. For years, surgical decompression was routine with rotator cuff repair, but results are similar whether or not it is done. The arthroscopic technique yields results comparable to the open technique.

Some severe tears may be impossible to repair. This includes many of the tears that are large to massive in size, involving two or more rotator cuff tendons; when the humeral head is positioned superior, against the acromion; and when there is meaningful atrophy of the rotator cuff muscles or fatty changes. Debridement of the rotator cuff and the subacromial spurs may diminish pain in such instances. Reconstruction of the superior capsule including the coracohumeral ligament with a graft may increase range of motion and strength by diminishing abnormal glenohumeral joint mechanics.

Rehabilitation after a repair lasts from 3 to 6 months with gradual exercise progression needed to diminish pain and restore normal, or near-normal, function. This varies with the size of the tear that was repaired and the quality and type of surgery performed. Typically, soon after the procedure, the patient begins simple motion exercises that do not damage the repair such as pendulum exercises, along with elbow, wrist, and hand exercises. At 6 weeks, low-intensity active strengthening exercises against gravity are begun. Three months after surgery, strengthening can progress as tolerated. The goals are to restore normal strength with a functional, pain-free range of motion.

Prognosis

The prognosis following a rotator cuff tear depends on many factors, as described earlier. About 80% of all rotator cuff tears heal. There are few specific criteria governing return to activities and sports following rotator cuff injuries. Determining factors must be individualized, considering the nature and treatment of the rotator cuff injury as well as the desired activity and sport. Patients must be pain-free and have attained full range of motion with near full strength prior to returning to activities and their sport to minimize reinjury. Typically, it takes 6 to 12 months for return to activities, work, or sports after a rotator cuff tear, and generally, the smaller the tear, the better is the prognosis.

3. Partial-Thickness Rotator Cuff Tendon Tear

A partial articular-sided tendon avulsion is much more common than a bursal-sided tear of the rotator cuff. As with other rotator cuff injuries, symptoms may resolve with appropriate physical therapy and analgesics. Yet, some individuals with a partial-thickness tear have persistent or recurrent symptoms. If a conservative program of exercises and gradual return to activity do not lead to steady improvement, then further diagnostic evaluation with ultrasonography, MRI, or arthroscopy may be helpful. Whereas repair of the partial-thickness rotator cuff tear may be best in some, debridement of the abnormal cuff may diminish or relieve symptoms in others.

Involvement of greater than 50% of the tendon thickness is generally used as an indication for repair. Repair necessitates a rehabilitation program similar to that described earlier for full-thickness rotator cuff tears. Following debridement, immediate resumption of range-of-motion and muscle-strengthening exercises begins. Typically, it requires 3 to 4 months for an individual to return to normal activities and as long as 12 months for an overhead-throwing athlete like a pitcher to return to baseball following arthroscopic debridement of a partial-thickness rotator cuff tear.

4. Cuff "Arthropathy"

Severe rotator cuff tears may lead to the humeral head being positioned superior against the undersurface of the acromion. Because of the tear of the rotator cuff, the humeral head no longer stays centered on the glenoid and the pull of the deltoid is unopposed. Over time, the humeral head and the glenoid wear from the abnormal contact. Many individuals have severe shoulder dysfunction, sometimes described as pseudoparalysis. They are able to move their shoulder only the smallest amounts. Interestingly, others are able to lift their arms and complain only of pain and weakness. This is a difficulty in caring for rotator cuff injuries. Symptoms may not correlate with the severity; some are able to cope with the injury, while others cannot. Nonoperative treatment including rehabilitation, NSAIDs, and steroid injection is usually effective in diminishing symptoms. In the elderly, shoulder hemiarthroplasty diminishes pain but improves function mildly. Reverse total shoulder replacement results in more pain relief, and improvement in function is possible. However, complications such as dislocation, heterotopic bone, and acromion fractures occur, so it is reserved for the elderly.

Altintas B, Anderson N, Dornan GJ, Boykin RE, Logan C, Millett PJ. Return to sport after arthroscopic rotator cuff repair: is there a difference between the recreational and the competitive athlete? *Am J Sports Med.* 2020;48(1):252-261. [PMID: 30855979]

Castricini R, La Camera F, De Gori M, et al. Functional outcomes and repair integrity after arthroscopic repair of partial articular supraspinatus tendon avulsion. *Arch Orthop Trauma Surg.* 2019;139(3):369-375. [PMID: 30269221]

Chalmers PN, Beck L, Miller M, et al. Acromial morphology is not associated with rotator cuff tearing or repair healing. *J Shoulder Elbow Surg.* 2020;29(11):2229-2239. [PMID: 32417045]

Collin P, Kempf JF, Molé D, Meyer N, et al. Ten-year multicenter clinical and MRI evaluation of isolated supraspinatus repairs. *J Bone Joint Surg Am.* 2017;99(16):1355-1364. [PMID: 28816895]

Diebold G, Lam P, Walton J, Murrell GAC. Relationship between age and rotator cuff retear: a study of 1,600 consecutive rotator cuff repairs. *J Bone Joint Surg Am.* 2017;99(14):1198-1205. [PMID: 28719559]

Witney-Lagen C, Mazis G, Bruguera J, Atoun E, Sforza G, Levy O. Do elderly patients gain as much benefit from arthroscopic rotator cuff repair as their younger peers? *J Shoulder Elbow Surg.* 2019;28(6):1056-1065. [PMID: 30704915]

Zhang Y, Zhai S, Qi C, et al. A comparative study of arthroscopic débridement versus repair for Ellman grade II bursal-side partial-thickness rotator cuff tears. *J Shoulder Elbow Surg.* 2020;29(10):2072-2079. [PMID: 32499197]

GLENOHUMERAL JOINT INSTABILITY

Distinguishing between shoulder laxity and instability is difficult, both because of the wide variability of normal joint laxity and the absence of biomechanical studies defining laxity and instability. In contrast, other joints such as the knee have precise definitions of instability. A Lachman test revealing greater than 5 mm of translation compared to the contralateral side is widely accepted as being associated with an anterior cruciate ligament rupture and resulting knee instability. At the shoulder, instability is often defined as translations that result in symptoms. This imprecise definition of shoulder instability can hamper proper diagnosis.

To make the correct diagnosis, the glenohumeral joint must be tested for anterior, posterior, and inferior instability. Different classifications of glenohumeral joint instability have been proposed, based on various characteristics. TUBS and AMBRI have been used to distinguish the two main types of instability. TUBS is an acronym describing instability caused by a *t*raumatic event, which is *u*nidirectional, is associated with a *B*ankart lesion, and often requires *s*urgical treatment. AMBRI refers to *a*traumatic, *m*ultidirectional instability (MDI) that may be *b*ilateral and is best treated by *r*ehabilitation. In this classification, the etiology of MDI is thought to be enlargement of the capsule from either a genetic or microtraumatic origin. TUBS and AMBRI are of historic interest as clinicians have recognized more types of instability.

FEDS is an acronym describing the four most important characteristics of shoulder instability (*f*requency, *e*tiology, *d*irection, and *s*everity) and can be obtained by history and physical examination. Frequency is classified as solitary, occasional (two to five episodes), or frequent (more than five episodes). Etiology is classified as traumatic or atraumatic. Direction is classified as anterior, inferior, or posterior. Lastly, severity is classified as subluxation or dislocation.

The positive sulcus sign has been used as the diagnostic hallmark for MDI, but we now know that the sulcus sign is sometimes found in shoulders of asymptomatic individuals with increased laxity. Laxity or joint play is a trait of body constitution that differs from one individual to another. Individuals may be loose or tight jointed. A shoulder is hyperlax if the examiner can easily subluxate the humeral head out of the glenoid in the anterior, posterior, and inferior directions without eliciting symptoms. Unfortunately, this makes classification of instability based on etiology, or direction alone, difficult. Instead, classification is best based on the direction of instability that elicits symptoms and the presence or absence of hyperlaxity (Table 3–1).

Table 3–1. Classification of glenohumeral instability based on the direction of instability and the presence or absence of hyperlaxity.

Direction / Laxity	UDI	MDI
Normal laxity	Very common 60%	Very rare 3%
Increased laxity	Common 30%	Rare 7%

Reprinted, with permission, from Gerber C. Observations of the classification of instability. In: Warner JJP, Iannotti JP, Flatow EL, eds. *Complex and Revision Problems in Shoulder Surgery*. Philadelphia: Lippincott-Raven; 1997:9-18. MDI, multidirectional instability; UDI, unidirectional instability.

MDI is best defined as instability in both the anterior and posterior directions, which is most often subluxation rather than dislocation.

Shoulder instability is often associated with a tear of the glenoid labrum. This is the fibrocartilaginous rim around the glenoid fossa that deepens the socket, is a connection for the surrounding capsuloligamentous structures, and provides stability for the humeral head. Glenoid labrum tears may occur from repetitive shoulder motion or acute trauma. In the athlete with repeated anterior subluxation of the shoulder, tears of the anteroinferior labrum may occur and lead to progressive instability. Patients with glenoid labrum injuries may describe their pain as interrupting smooth functioning of the shoulder during their specific activity. A labrum tear may be felt as a "pop" or "click" with motion of the shoulder. MRI arthrogram is useful for detection of these lesions.

Hettrich CM, Cronin KJ, Raynor MB, et al. Epidemiology of the Frequency, Etiology, Direction, and Severity (FEDS) system for classifying glenohumeral instability. *J Shoulder Elbow Surg*. 2019;28(1):95-101. [PMID: 30348544]

Glenohumeral Joint Instability Evaluation

A. Anterior Instability

The apprehension test is performed to assess anterior instability. The test applies an anterior-directed force to the humeral head from the back with the arm in the apprehension position of combined abduction and external rotation (Figure 3–6). A positive test results from the patient's apprehension that the joint will dislocate. This maneuver mimics the position of subluxation, or dislocation, and causes reflex guarding. Conversely, the relocation test is positive if relief is obtained by applying a posterior-directed force to the humeral head (Figure 3–7).

B. Posterior Instability

No single test has high sensitivity and specificity for posterior instability. The Jahnke test, sometimes called the jerk test, is performed by applying a posteriorly directed force to the forward flexed and internally rotated shoulder. There may be pain or apprehension of instability. The shoulder is then moved in horizontal abduction, into the coronal plane, as an anterior-directed force is applied to the humeral head. A clunk occurs as the humeral head reduces from the subluxed position (Figure 3–8). In the Kim test, with the patient in a sitting position and the arm at 90 degrees of abduction, an axial load is applied to the arm through the flexed elbow. Then, while the arm is further elevated and horizontally abducted 45 degrees diagonally upward, an inferior and posterior force is applied to the proximal arm. A sudden onset of posterior shoulder pain indicates a

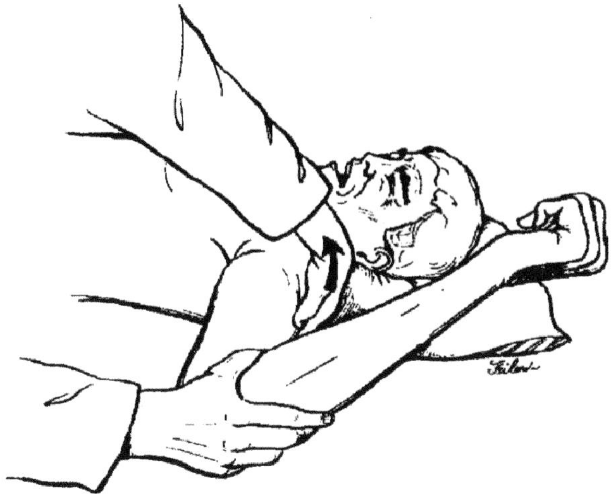

▲ **Figure 3–6.** The apprehension test of combined abduction and external rotation for anterior instability.

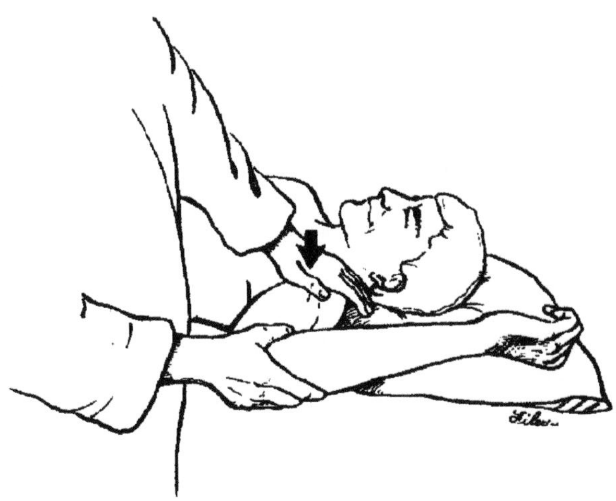

▲ **Figure 3–7.** The relocation test is positive if relief is obtained by applying a posterior-directed force to the humeral head.

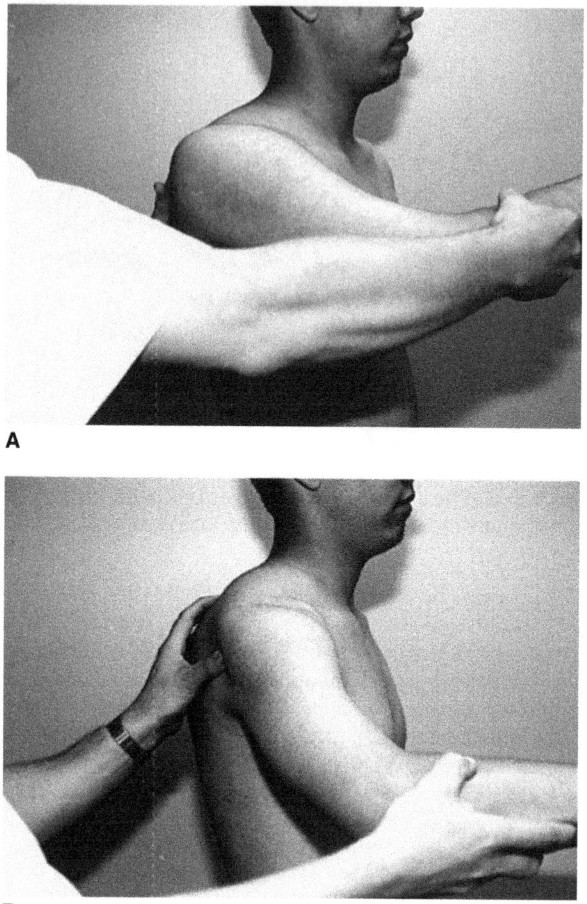

A

B

▲ **Figure 3–8.** The Jahnke test for posterior instability. **A:** A posterior-directed force applied to the forward flexed shoulder (in the upper left column). **B:** The shoulder is then moved into the coronal plane as an anterior-directed force is applied to the humeral head (in the lower left column). A clunk occurs as the humeral head reduces from the subluxed position. (Reprinted, with permission, from Hawkins RJ, Bokor DJ. Clinical evaluation of shoulder problems. In: Rockwood CA, Matsen F III, eds. *The Shoulder.* New York: WB Saunders; 1998.)

positive test result. To perform the circumduction test, the patient is instructed to actively move the shoulder in a large circle starting from a flexed, internally rotated, and cross-body position, then to forward flexion, then to an abducted and externally rotated position, and lastly to the arm at the side. The examiner stands behind the patient and palpates the posterior shoulder. If positive, the joint subluxes in the forward flexed, internally rotated, and cross-body position and reduces as the shoulder is moved from this position.

C. Inferior Instability

The sulcus sign is used to evaluate laxity and inferior instability. The test is performed with the athlete in a sitting position with the arm at the side. The arm is pulled longitudinally inferior. If positive, discomfort or apprehension of instability is experienced as the humeral head translates inferior and the skin just distal to the lateral acromion hollows out (Figure 3–9). Meaningful difference in comparison to the other side is helpful in diagnosis of instability.

GLENOHUMERAL DISLOCATION

When the shoulder is forced beyond the limit of its normal range of motion, the articular surface of the humeral head may translate abnormally on the glenoid to varying degrees (ie, sublux), and they may lose contact with each other

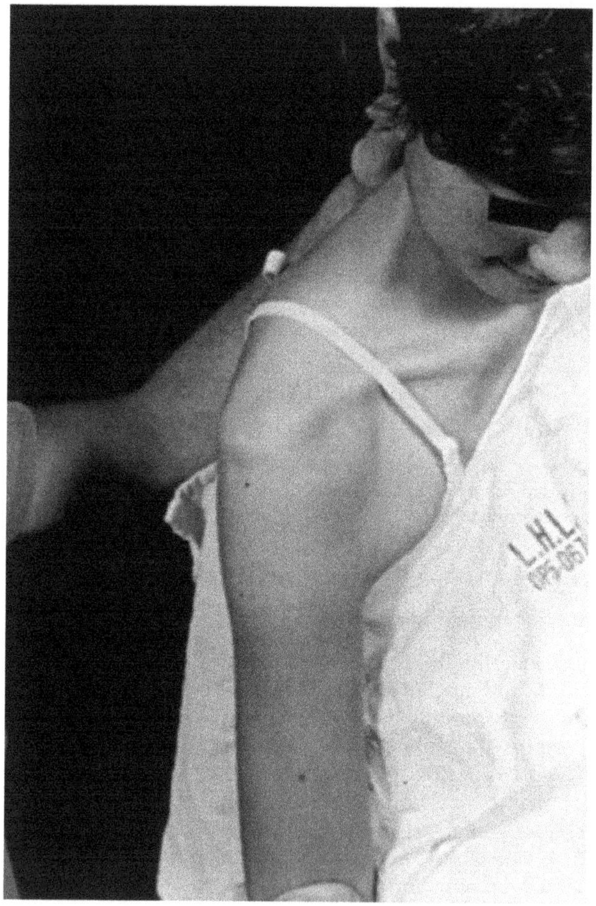

▲ **Figure 3–9.** The sulcus test for inferior instability. (Reprinted, with permission, from Hawkins RJ, Bokor DJ. Clinical evaluation of shoulder problems. In: Rockwood CA, Matsen F III, eds. *The Shoulder*. New York: WB Saunders; 1998.)

(ie, dislocate). The majority of glenohumeral subluxations or dislocations are in the anteroinferior direction.

1. Anterior Dislocation

Essentials of Diagnosis

- *The arm is typically held in slight abduction, and the forearm is held by the opposite hand and is not able to be internally rotated.*
- *There may be a visible dimple under the acromion due to the absence of the humeral head.*
- *The humeral head may be palpable under the coracoid or in the axilla.*
- *AP radiographs show the dislocation, and lateral radiographs will confirm the direction of dislocation and possible associated injuries.*

Prevention

Shoulder dislocations are typically the result of an acute traumatic injury. Therefore, although avoiding injury to the shoulder is the best form of prevention, the risk of dislocation can be minimized by avoiding the vulnerable position and with regular stretching and strengthening.

Clinical Findings

Anterior glenohumeral dislocation occurs from either the shoulder being pushed back into the apprehension position of combined abduction and external rotation, exceeding the normal range of motion, or a direct posterior or posterolateral blow on the shoulder. The anterior capsule is either stretched or torn, usually from its attachment to the anterior glenoid. The head may be displaced into a subcoracoid, subglenoid, or rarely subclavicular or intrathoracic position. Two lesions are typically seen in patients who are young, under about 25 years of age at the first episode, with recurrent anterior dislocations (Figure 3–10). The Bankart lesion is an anteroinferior capsular injury associated with a tear of the glenoid labrum off the anteroinferior glenoid rim. The Bankart lesion may occur with a fracture of the glenoid rim. Such fractures are often small and minimally displaced, and treatment is based on the instability rather than the fracture. The second lesion commonly associated with recurrent anterior dislocations is the Hill-Sachs lesion, a compression fracture of the posterolateral humeral head. It is created by the sharp edge of the anterior glenoid as the humeral head dislocates over it. When large, both the Bankart and the Hill-Sachs lesions predispose to recurrent dislocations when the arm is placed in the apprehension position of combined abduction and external rotation. If the glenoid rim fracture involves more than 20% of the glenoid diameter, the joint becomes prone to recurrent instability, and treatment with open reduction and internal fixation is best. If the fracture is old or the glenoid rim is worn to a similar level, then bone grafting is indicated.

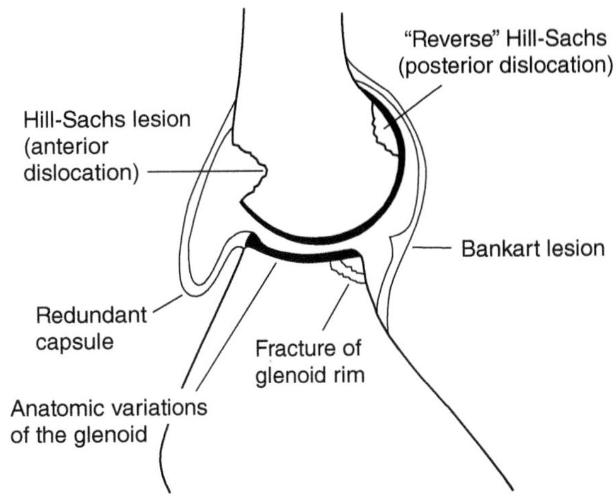

▲ **Figure 3–10.** Anatomic lesions producing shoulder instability.

Other injuries associated with anterior dislocation may occur. These include rotator cuff tears, which occur more commonly in those who dislocate and are over 40 years of age; avulsion of the greater tuberosity from the humerus caused by traction from the rotator cuff; and injury to the axillary nerve, which may be stretched or torn. Loss of axillary nerve function results in denervation of the deltoid and teres minor muscles and loss of sensation over the proximal lateral aspect of the arm. Axillary nerve palsy may also occur during reduction of the dislocation and therefore should be tested both before and after reduction. The deltoid extension lag sign, described in the section on axillary nerve injury, may be the best way to assess function of this nerve. Lastly, the dead arm syndrome may occur after anterior joint instability. For example, a pitcher may report a sudden inability to throw, with the arm going numb and becoming extremely weak after ball release. The symptoms are transient, resolving within a few seconds to minutes.

Those who sustain an anterior shoulder dislocation will try to hold the injured arm in slight abduction with the arm near their side, gripping the forearm with the opposite hand to minimize painful motion. Most people know their shoulder is dislocated and will immediately seek help. On physical examination of an anterior dislocation, the examiner may note a space underneath the acromion where the humeral head should lie and a palpable anterior mass, the humeral head in the anterior axilla. Range of motion is painful, and internal rotation is limited. AP and axillary lateral radiographs will reveal the diagnosis of anterior dislocation.

Treatment

Acute and recurrent anterior glenohumeral dislocations must be distinguished because the first dislocation is the result of severe force so there is increased probability of associated injuries. Subsequent, recurrent dislocations may occur with lesser and lesser force, and reduction may be accomplished with much less effort. Anterior dislocations may be reduced by one of several techniques. Longitudinal traction may be exerted on the affected arm with external rotation, followed by internal rotation of the arm. Care must be taken to avoid direct pressure on the neurovascular structures. Another method is to have the patient lie face down on the table and tie or tape a bucket to the injured arm and slowly fill it with water. This allows the musculature around the shoulder to relax from the force of the weight and effect a spontaneous reduction. After reduction, it is important to do a neurologic evaluation including sensation to light touch and pinprick over the lateral shoulder in the sensory region of the axillary nerve because it is the most commonly injured nerve. An extension lag test is done by passively extending the shoulder and asking the patient to hold the arm in the extended position and, if the axillary nerve is injured, the patient will be unable to do so. Recovery of the nerve can be assessed in the following weeks by noting improving strength with this test. Vascular assessment is done by noting significant color differences compared with the uninjured arm, palpating pulses, and evaluating with Doppler if needed.

Following reduction of an initial dislocation, the shoulder should be immobilized with a sling for 2 to 6 weeks. Emphasis must be placed on strengthening the rotator cuff muscles to compensate for the injured capsuloligamentous structures. When weight training is begun 2 to 3 months after injury, exercises such as military press, fly exercises, deep shoulder dips, and other exercises that put the shoulder in the vulnerable apprehension position of combined abduction and external rotation should be avoided until healing is complete. Before returning to athletics, the patient should have normal range of motion without pain and normal strength in the shoulder. Surgical treatment should be considered if these measures fail to provide the desired results.

Recurrent dislocations can be treated with minimal immobilization until the pain subsides, followed by range-of-motion and muscle-strengthening exercises. Many restraining devices are available to help prevent recurrent dislocations during sporting activities, focusing on keeping the arm from going into the apprehension position of combined abduction and external rotation. These orthotics may be effective, but because they limit the athlete's range of shoulder motion, their use is limited for certain competitive activities.

If an athlete has sustained multiple dislocations and is unresponsive to conservative treatment, surgical reconstruction of the shoulder joint may be indicated. There is a wide variety of repair procedures with either open or arthroscopic techniques. Repair of the labral lesion (ie, Bankart repair) and tightening of the anteroinferior capsule are integral to all of these procedures (Table 3–2), and success is frequent. When present, large Hill-Sachs and bony Bankart lesions should be treated as well.

Table 3–2. Repair of capsule and labrum back to the glenoid rim.

Bankart procedure
duToit procedure
Viek procedure
Eyre-Brook procedure
Moseley procedure
Muscle and capsule plication
Putti-Platt procedure
Symeonides procedure
Muscle and tendon sling procedures
Magnuson-Stack procedure
Bristow-Helfet-Latarjet procedure modifications
Boytchev procedure
Nicola procedure
Gallie-Le Mesurier procedure
Boyd transfer of long head of biceps (for posterior dislocation)
Bone block
Eden-Hybbinette procedure
DeAnquin procedure (through a superior approach to the shoulder)
Osteotomies
Weber (humeral neck)
Saha (humeral shaft)

Following most surgical procedures, aggressive range-of-motion exercises do not start immediately and are usually begun about 3 weeks postoperatively. The goal is to have full abduction and 90 degrees of external rotation by 12 weeks, and at this time, patients may begin strengthening with a variety of weight-training exercises, avoiding exercises that strain the anterior capsule.

Prognosis

Young patients are at a high risk for re-dislocation after a primary traumatic anterior shoulder dislocation if treated conservatively with rehabilitation. Surgical stabilization should be considered. Even after surgical stabilization, patients have up to a 10% chance of re-dislocation, especially if they returning to play in contact sports.

2. Posterior Dislocation

Essentials of Diagnosis

- *The arm is typically held with the hand on the belly and is not able to be externally rotated.*
- *Posterior dislocations can be more difficult to diagnose and treat than anterior dislocations.*

- *AP radiograph may not show the dislocation, but lateral radiographs will confirm the direction of dislocation and associated injuries, if present.*

Prevention

Shoulder dislocations are typically the result of an acute traumatic injury. Therefore, while avoiding injury to the shoulder is the best form of prevention, the risk of dislocation can be minimized by avoiding the vulnerable position and with regular stretching and strengthening.

Clinical Findings

Posterior glenohumeral dislocations result from the posterior capsule being torn, stretched, or torn from the posterior glenoid. Posterior labral avulsion is less common with posterior dislocation than anterior labral avulsion with anterior dislocation. A reverse Hill-Sachs lesion or compression fracture of the anterior humeral head (see Figure 3–10) may appear on the anterior articular surface of the humerus. With a posterior dislocation, there may also be avulsion of the lesser tuberosity from the humerus, caused by traction from the rotator cuff or injury of the rotator cuff. Posterior dislocations are often difficult to diagnose, as the patient may have a normal contour to the shoulder or the deltoid of a well-developed athlete may mask signs of a displaced humeral head. The patient holds the injured shoulder in internal rotation, usually with the hand on the belly, and the examiner cannot externally rotate it. An AP radiograph may appear nearly normal, but the axillary lateral radiograph will reveal the diagnosis of posterior dislocation.

Treatment

Applying longitudinal traction in the line of the arm, with an anterior-directed force to the humeral head, reduces a posterior dislocation. Following reduction, the shoulder is immobilized for 2 to 6 weeks in external rotation and a small amount of abduction. Emphasis must be placed on strengthening the rotator cuff muscles to compensate for the injured capsuloligamentous structures. Weight training is begun 2 to 3 months after injury, avoiding the vulnerable position of forward flexion and internal rotation. Before returning to athletics, the patient should have normal range of motion without pain and normal strength in the shoulder. Surgical treatment should be considered if these measures fail to provide the desired results.

Prognosis

Patients with an acute posterior dislocation are often able to return to their sport following a course of rehabilitation emphasizing range-of-motion and rotator cuff strengthening.

3. Multidirectional Instability

Essentials of Diagnosis

- *Shoulder pain is not specific to a particular shoulder position or often associated with other shoulder injuries.*
- *Evidence of both anterior and posterior instability.*
- *Positive sulcus sign.*
- *MDI is often difficult to diagnose.*
- *Fatigue or paresthesias may be present.*
- *Must be evaluated for hyperlaxity that must then be distinguished from instability.*

Prevention

Multidirectional dislocation most commonly results with minimal trauma but can occur from an acute traumatic injury. While avoiding injury to the shoulder is the best form of prevention, the risk of dislocation can be minimized by avoiding the vulnerable positions and with regular stretching and strengthening.

Clinical Findings

Patients will have instability in both the anterior and posterior directions, which is most often subluxation rather than dislocation. This may result in a painful shoulder, especially if rotator cuff strength decreases. The pain often results from rotator cuff inflammation, likely from attempts to stabilize the humeral head during activity. Patients may complain of vague symptoms, including upper extremity fatigue, discomfort, pain, apprehension, and paresthesias. They may also describe episodes of instability. Physical examination should include tests for anterior, posterior, and inferior instability as described earlier. It should also include evaluation for signs of generalized hyperlaxity, which include hyperextension of the metacarpophalangeal joints, elbows, and knees and the ability to adduct the thumb to the ipsilateral wrist and ability to bend over with the knees straight and touch the floor with the palms of the hands. Generalized hyperlaxity does not necessarily indicate symptomatic instability of the shoulder. MRI can be a useful adjunct to plain radiographs and may reveal an enlarged capsule and labral or rotator cuff pathology.

Treatment and Prognosis

Initial treatment for MDI is nonoperative and leads to successful results in the vast majority of cases. This includes patient education, modification of activity, and a strengthening program for the rotator cuff and scapular stabilizing muscles. When this fails, surgery is often effective in relieving symptoms, but because of differences in classifying MDI, results of treatment vary as well. For those with multidirectional instability classified as instability in both the anterior and posterior directions, about two-thirds of patients, less than that with unidirectional anterior instability, will have relief after surgery.

Bernhardson AS, Murphy CP, Aman ZS, LaPrade RF, Provencher MT. A prospective analysis of patients with anterior versus posterior shoulder instability: a matched cohort examination and surgical outcome analysis of 200 patients. *Am J Sports Med.* 2019;47(3):682-687. [PMID: 30698986]

Best MJ, Tanaka MJ. Multidirectional instability of the shoulder: treatment options and considerations. *Sports Med Arthrosc Rev.* 2018;26(3):113-119. [PMID: 30059445]

Dickens JF, Slaven SE, Cameron KL, et al. Prospective evaluation of glenoid bone loss after first-time and recurrent anterior glenohumeral instability events. *Am J Sports Med.* 2019;47(5): 1082-1089. [PMID: 30943084]

Duchman KR, Hettrich CM, Glass NA, et al. The incidence of glenohumeral bone and cartilage lesions at the time of anterior shoulder stabilization surgery: a comparison of patients undergoing primary and revision surgery. *Am J Sports Med.* 2018;46(10):2449-2456. Erratum in: *Am J Sports Med.* 2018;46(11):NP59. [PMID: 29985051]

Hovelius L, Olofsson A, Sandström B, et al. Nonoperative treatment of primary anterior shoulder dislocation in patients forty years of age and younger. A prospective twenty-five-year follow-up. *J Bone Joint Surg Am.* 2008;90:945. [PMID: 18451384]

Hurley ET, Jamal MS, Ali ZS, Montgomery C, Pauzenberger L, Mullett H. Long-term outcomes of the Latarjet procedure for anterior shoulder instability: a systematic review of studies at 10-year follow-up. *J Shoulder Elbow Surg.* 2019;28(2):e33-e39. [PMID: 30545784]

Shanley E, Thigpen C, Brooks J, et al. Return to sport as an outcome measure for shoulder instability: surprising findings in nonoperative management in a high school athlete population. *Am J Sports Med.* 2019;47(5):1062-1067. [PMID: 30865844]

Sheean AJ, Arner JW, Bradley JP. Posterior glenohumeral instability: diagnosis and management. *Arthroscopy.* 2020;36(10): 2580-2582. [PMID: 32442706]

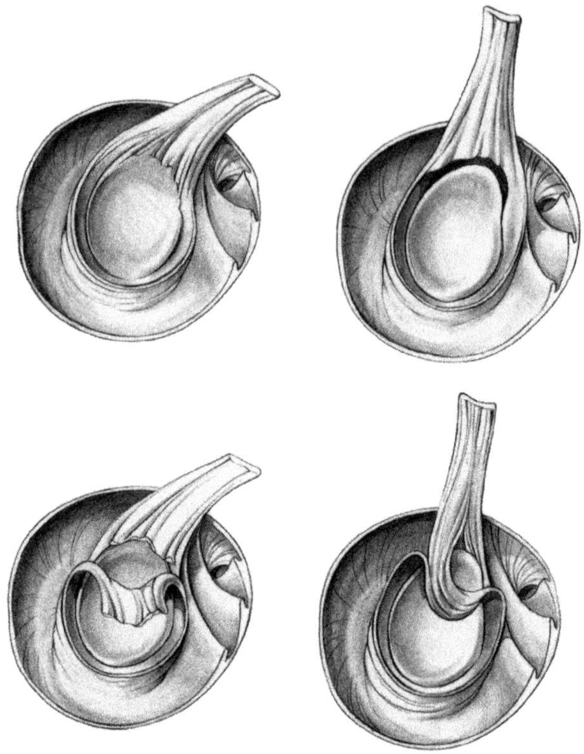

▲ **Figure 3–11.** The original five types of the SLAP lesion include fraying of the superior capsulolabrum (type I), detachment of the superior capsulolabrum and the biceps anchor (type II), bucket handle tearing of the superior capsulolabrum (type III), detachment of the superior capsulolabrum and tearing into the biceps anchor (type IV), and combinations of these (type V). There are now other types.

SLAP LESIONS

SLAP lesions involve the origin of the long head of the biceps brachii (biceps anchor) and the superior capsulolabral structures. The acronym SLAP is for *s*uperior *l*abrum *a*nterior and *p*osterior. A type I lesion is fraying of the superior labrum. Type II lesions are most common, accounting for over 50% of patients with a SLAP lesion, and are detachment of the superior labrum from the glenoid. A type III lesion is a bucket handle tear of the superior labrum with firm attachment of the remainder of the labrum. In a type IV lesion, there is a tear of the superior labrum that extends into the biceps tendon (Figure 3–11).

A type V lesion is an anterior-inferior Bankart lesion that continues superiorly to include the superior labrum. A type VI lesion is a superior labral tear with an unstable flap tear, and a type VII lesion is a superior labral tear that extends anteriorly beneath the middle glenohumeral ligament. A type VIII lesion is a superior labral tear with a posteroinferior labral tear. Lastly, a type IX tear is a circumferential tear of the labrum.

Proposed mechanisms of injury include the arm at the side being pulled down, a fall onto an outstretched arm with the shoulder positioned in abduction and slight forward flexion at the time of the impact, and in overhead athletes, possibly from posteroinferior capsular tightness that results in diminished internal rotation of the abducted shoulder, diagnosed with comparison to the contralateral side. With overhead throwing, posteroinferior capsular tightness results in posterosuperior translation of the humeral head, accompanied by pain in the cocking phase of throwing and demonstrated on clinical examination by pain in the posterior shoulder when placed in the apprehension position of combined abduction and external rotation and a peel-back injury of the superior labrum resulting in the SLAP lesion. Mild anterior shoulder instability results from SLAP lesions and may also occur from these alterations in the glenohumeral joint and aberrations of scapulothoracic motion. However, SLAP lesions may most commonly be found incidentally in elderly individuals undergoing surgical treatment of a rotator cuff tear.

Essentials of Diagnosis

- *Common clinical complaints are shoulder pain, usually anterosuperior in location, that is greater with activities involving overhead motion and a painful "catching" or "popping."*
- *Pain with resisted forward flexion with the shoulder in the internally rotated and slightly adducted position, relieved by externally rotating the shoulder.*
- *MRI arthrography aids in the diagnosis.*

Prevention

Because labral injuries can result from repetitive activity or an acute traumatic event, it is important to maintain good strength and flexibility of the shoulder to minimize these injuries.

Clinical Findings

SLAP lesions cause shoulder pain both from mechanical symptoms and/or mild shoulder instability. Correlating history, physical examination, and MRI arthrography yield best chances of diagnosis. For the active compression test, the internally rotated shoulder is forward flexed to 90 degrees and is then positioned across the body in horizontal abduction about 10 degrees. The test is positive if the patient has pain with resisted forward flexion that is relieved by external rotation of the shoulder.

A complicating factor in making the diagnosis is that the majority of SLAP lesions are associated with other shoulder pathology such as rotator cuff tears, acromioclavicular joint pathology, and instability. Only about a quarter of SLAP lesions are isolated.

Treatment

Definitive diagnosis of SLAP lesions is best made with diagnostic arthroscopy. Treatment can be simplified by noting whether the lesion would contribute to detachment of either the biceps anchor or the labrum from the glenoid bone. Lesions producing meaningful detachment generally require repair. Lesions extending into the biceps tendon or in elderly individuals may require debridement, biceps tenotomy, or tenodesis.

Douglas L, Whitaker J, Nyland J, et al. Return to play and performance perceptions of baseball players after isolated SLAP tear repair. *Orthop J Sports Med.* 2019;7(3):2325967119829486. [PMID: 30873424]

Gilliam BD, Douglas L, Fleisig GS, et al. Return to play and outcomes in baseball players after superior labral anterior-posterior repairs. *Am J Sports Med.* 2018;46(1):109-115. [PMID: 28942657]

Kandeel AA. Type V superior labral anterior-posterior (SLAP) lesion in recurrent anterior glenohumeral instability. *J Shoulder Elbow Surg.* 2020;29(1):95-103. [PMID: 31471245]

Morse KW, Eno JJ, Altchek DW, Dines JS. Injuries of the biceps and superior labral complex in overhead athletes. *Curr Rev Musculoskelet Med.* 2019;12(2):72-79. [PMID: 30848418]

Ren YM, Duan YH, Sun YB, Yang T, Hou WY, Tian MQ. Is arthroscopic repair superior to biceps tenotomy and tenodesis for type II SLAP lesions? A meta-analysis of RCTs and observational studies. *J Orthop Surg Res.* 2019;14(1):48. [PMID: 30760293]

SHOULDER STIFFNESS

Essentials of Diagnosis

- *All ranges of motion of the shoulder are diminished.*
- *Loss of active and passive range of motion.*
- *May be idiopathic or posttraumatic.*
- *Initially painful.*

Prevention

Even those with an idiopathic shoulder etiology likely have some sort of shoulder problem that precedes the shoulder stiffness. Treating the preceding shoulder problem such as rotator cuff tendonitis and initiating gentle range-of-motion and strengthening exercises as soon as possible after the traumatic event are essential to minimizing the likelihood of developing shoulder stiffness.

Clinical Findings

Often called adhesive capsulitis or frozen shoulder, shoulder stiffness is a painful condition characterized by significant restriction in both active and passive range of motion. With shoulder stiffness, the articular surfaces are normal and the joint is stable, yet there is a restriction in range of motion. Stiffness usually results from soft-tissue contracture but can also occur from bone malalignment, bursal adhesions, or a shortened muscle-tendon unit. The restrictions of shoulder motion are global. That is, none of the shoulder planes of motion is spared.

Shoulder stiffness may be separated into idiopathic and posttraumatic etiologies. Idiopathic shoulder stiffness is most common in older individuals, especially women between 40 and 60 years of age. Other factors that predispose to idiopathic shoulder stiffness include cervical, cardiac, pulmonary, neoplastic, neurologic, and personality disorders. Patients with diabetes mellitus are also at a high risk of developing shoulder stiffness, with 10% to 35% of diabetics having restriction of shoulder motion at some time. Diabetics who

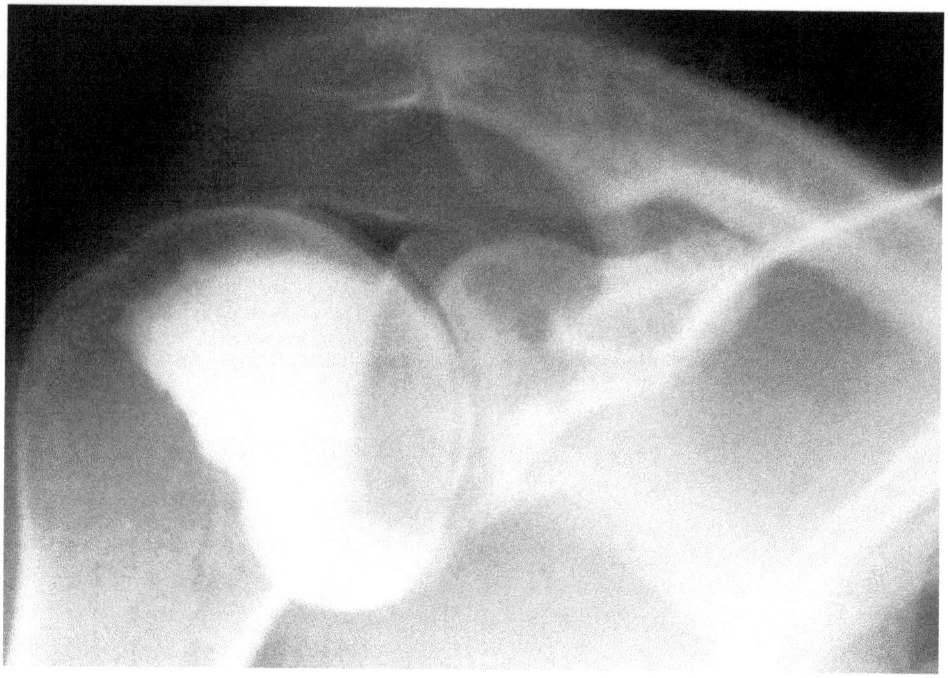

▲ **Figure 3–12.** Adhesive capsulitis of the shoulder. Note the small irregular joint capsule with addition of contrast material.

have been insulin-dependent for many years have the greatest incidence and can have bilateral involvement. Because of this close association, clinicians should ask their patients with shoulder stiffness about symptoms of diabetes; 70% of individuals with shoulder stiffness may have diabetes or a prediabetes condition. The pathophysiology of idiopathic shoulder stiffness remains uncertain, but the pathoanatomy is commonly limited to contracture of the glenohumeral capsule (Figure 3–12). Most prominently involved is the rotator interval, which includes the superior glenohumeral ligament and coracohumeral ligament.

Although all patients can recall some traumatic event that preceded their shoulder stiffness, those with distinct trauma such as a prior fracture, rotator cuff tear, or surgical procedure have a posttraumatic etiology. Stiffness after shoulder surgery is typical and usually resolves with time and appropriate rehabilitation. The shoulder should not be neglected after any surgery about the shoulder girdle. This includes axillary or cervical lymph node dissections, especially when combined with radiation therapy, cardiac catheterization in the axilla, and coronary artery bypass grafting with sternotomy and thoracotomy. All surgeons should be aware that these procedures may result in restricted shoulder motion.

The clinical presentation of idiopathic shoulder stiffness is classically described as having three phases. The first phase is the painful, freezing phase. The pain is typically achy in nature, and sudden jolts or attempts at rapid motion exacerbate the chronic discomfort. The pain may begin at night, and shoulder motion becomes progressively limited. Patients often hold their arm at their side and in internal rotation with the forearm across the belly. They may also be treated for nonspecific shoulder pain with a sling in this position. This inflammatory phase often lasts between 2 and 9 months.

The second phase of progressive stiffness lasts between 3 and 12 months. Stiffness progresses to a point at which shoulder motion is restricted in all planes. Essentially, the shoulder has undergone fibrous arthrodesis. Fortunately, pain progressively decreases from the initial inflammatory phase. With time, patients are able to use the shoulder with little or no pain, within the restricted range of motion, but attempts to exceed this range are accompanied by pain. The patient's symptoms then plateau. Unfortunately, this phase may be persistent, with symptoms lasting for extended periods. In the resolution, or thawing phase, the shoulder range or motion slowly and progressively increases. It can be as short as a month, but typically lasts several months and can last for a few years.

On clinical examination, there is loss of both active and passive range of shoulder motion. Often the first motion to be affected is internal rotation, demonstrated by an inability to bring the arm up the back to the same level as the normal shoulder. MRI reveals decreased rotator interval size, and arthrography demonstrates marked reduction in joint capacity; often the affected shoulder will not take more than a few milliliters of dye, whereas the normal capacity is 20 to 30 mL.

Treatment

Treatment varies, but conservative modalities and progressive range-of-motion exercises are often effective. Range-of-motion exercises for external rotation and abduction will help minimize the length of restriction in motion and dysfunction. Steroid injections can be successfully placed into the glenohumeral joint with an anterior approach and may aid in diminishing pain but probably do not change the course of the disease. Nonoperative treatments are successful for most. Operative treatments of manipulation under anesthesia and arthroscopic capsular release are effective for others

Prognosis

Whether treated nonoperatively or operatively, a return of about 80% shoulder range of motion is usual.

Cho CH, Jin HJ, Kim DH. Comparison of clinical outcomes between idiopathic frozen shoulder and diabetic frozen shoulder after a single ultrasound-guided intra-articular corticosteroid injection. *Diagnostics (Basel).* 2020;10(6):E370. [PMID: 32512719]

Lyhne JM, Jacobsen JR, Hansen SJ, Jensen CM, Deutch SR. Diabetic and non-diabetic patients report equal symptom relief after arthroscopic capsular release of frozen shoulder. *J Clin Orthop Trauma.* 2019;10(2):261-264. [PMID: 30828189]

Redler LH, Dennis ER. Treatment of adhesive capsulitis of the shoulder. *J Am Acad Orthop Surg.* 2019;27(12):e544-e554. [PMID: 30632986]

Shao X, Shi LL, Wang P, Zou F, Wang J. Transcoracoacromial ligament glenohumeral injection technique: accuracy of 116 injections in idiopathic adhesive capsulitis. *Arthroscopy.* 2018;34(8):2337-2344. [PMID: 30078427]

FRACTURES ABOUT THE SHOULDER

1. Clavicle Fracture

The clavicle is one of the most commonly fractured bones in the body, with direct trauma being the usual cause in athletic events (Figure 3–13). Football, wrestling, and ice hockey are the sports most commonly involved in clavicular fractures, which is not surprising because all three are associated with high-speed contact between players.

Essentials of Diagnosis

- *History of injury to the shoulder.*
- *Swelling and ecchymosis overlying the injured clavicle.*
- *Pain and crepitation upon palpation of the fracture site.*
- *Pain and limited range of motion of the arm, specifically in forward flexion and abduction.*
- *Appropriate radiographs will define the location and severity of the fracture.*

Clinical Findings

Despite the proximity of vital structures, clavicular fractures that occur during athletic activities are rarely associated with neurovascular damage, and accompanying soft-tissue disorders are uncommon. However, some neurovascular complications, such as a tear of the subclavian artery or a brachial plexus injury, are serious, although rare. Therefore, when evaluating and treating clavicular fractures, an initial neurovascular examination is very important. Pulses in the distal part of the upper extremity, strength, and sensation must be carefully evaluated.

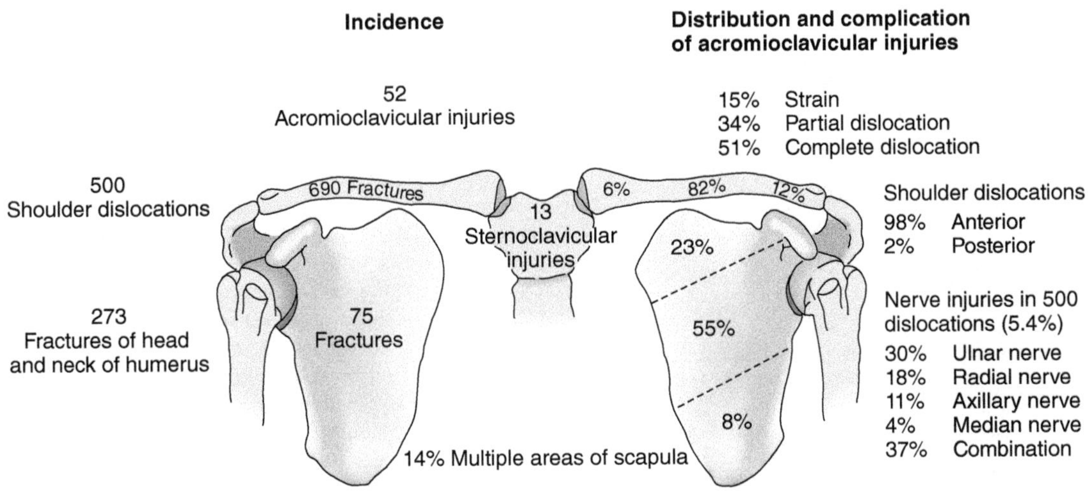

▲ **Figure 3–13.** Analysis of 1603 shoulder girdle injuries, showing the frequency and location of fractures and dislocations.

The patient will usually give a history of falling in the area of the shoulder or receiving a blow to the clavicle and experiencing immediate pain and an inability to raise the arm. Radiography will usually confirm the clinical impression and must show the entire clavicle including the sternal end, the glenohumeral joint, and the upper third of the humerus. Midclavicular fractures account for 80%, distal fractures for 15%, and proximal fractures for 5% of fractures. Most fractures of the shaft of the clavicle heal well.

Because the clavicle fixes the shoulder girdle to the thorax, a fracture through the clavicle causes the shoulder to sag downward and forward. The pull of the sternocleidomastoid muscle may displace the proximal fragment superiorly. These forces tend to hinder the initial reduction and maintenance of reduction. In addition, distal fractures, which are more common in older age groups, may involve tears in the coracoclavicular ligament, which allows the proximal clavicle to ride up superiorly, mimicking an acromioclavicular dislocation. Delayed union is much more common in these distal fractures than in other clavicular fractures.

Treatment

Mid and proximal clavicular fractures are usually treated with a short period of rest and a sling on the affected side to support the extremity. Immobilization is usually discontinued at 3 to 4 weeks, and once the clavicular fracture has healed, range-of-motion and strengthening exercises should begin. Comminuted mid and proximal clavicular fractures with meaningful displacement may be best treated with open reduction and internal fixation. Distal fractures with tears in the coracoclavicular ligament, mimicking an acromioclavicular dislocation, are also best treated with open reduction and internal fixation.

Prognosis

Onset of activity prior to healing may contribute to nonunion or recurrent fracture. Athletes should not be allowed to return to play until shoulder strength and range of motion return to preinjury levels. Generally, no special braces or pads are required when the athlete returns to play.

Guerra E, Previtali D, Tamborini S, Filardo G, Zaffagnini S, Candrian C. Midshaft clavicle fractures: surgery provides better results as compared with nonoperative treatment: a meta-analysis. *Am J Sports Med.* 2019;47(14):3541-3551. [PMID: 30835150]

Lenza M, Buchbinder R, Johnston RV, Ferrari BA, Faloppa F. Surgical versus conservative interventions for treating fractures of the middle third of the clavicle. *Cochrane Database Syst Rev.* 2019;1:CD009363. [PMID: 30666620]

Malik SS, Tahir M, Jordan RW, Malik SS, Saithna A. Is shortening of displaced midshaft clavicle fractures associated with inferior clinical outcomes following nonoperative management? A systematic review. *J Shoulder Elbow Surg.* 2019;28(8):1626-1638. [PMID: 30929954]

Reito A, Launonen A, Paloneva J. Factors explaining heterogeneity in studies comparing surgical and nonsurgical treatment of midshaft clavicle fractures: a meta-regression analysis of randomized controlled trials and high-quality observational studies. *J Shoulder Elbow Surg.* 2020;29(8):1726-1734. [PMID: 32513430]

2. Proximal Humerus Fracture

Essentials of Diagnosis

- *History of trauma to the shoulder.*
- *Swelling and ecchymosis overlying the shoulder that may extend down to the elbow.*
- *Tenderness and crepitation over the fracture site.*
- *Pain with attempted range of motion of the shoulder.*
- *Appropriate radiographs will define the location and severity of the fracture.*

Fractures of the proximal humerus represent approximately 4% to 5% of all fractures. They most often present in elderly osteoporotic patients or in young adolescents with open growth plates. When they occur in an athlete, they are typically the result of a high-energy impact injury or are secondary to an underlying pathologic bone condition.

Clinical Findings

The proximal humerus consists of four major bony components: the humeral head, the greater tuberosity, the lesser tuberosity, and the humeral shaft. Fractures, which can occur between any or all of these regions, are traditionally defined by the location and displacement of the fracture fragments (Figure 3–14). The most common fracture is between shaft and the proximal humerus, and this location is called the surgical neck. The patient with a proximal humerus fracture will usually be able to report the mechanism of injury and will complain of pain, swelling, and an inability to use the shoulder. A physical examination will often reveal loss of the normal contour of the shoulder, tenderness about the shoulder, ecchymosis that may extend down to the elbow, and crepitus with attempted motion. A thorough neurovascular examination is essential, as brachial plexus and axillary nerve injuries have been reported in association with proximal humerus fractures. Because the axillary nerve is the nerve most commonly injured in these cases, sensation to light touch and pinprick over the lateral aspect of the upper arm and deltoid muscle function must be tested. It may not be possible to assess more than whether the deltoid muscle contracts or not. An accurate radiographic evaluation is necessary to confirm the type and severity of the fracture and is essential in determining the treatment plan. AP and lateral views in the plane of the scapula, as well as an axillary view to rule out an associated glenohumeral dislocation, are necessary.

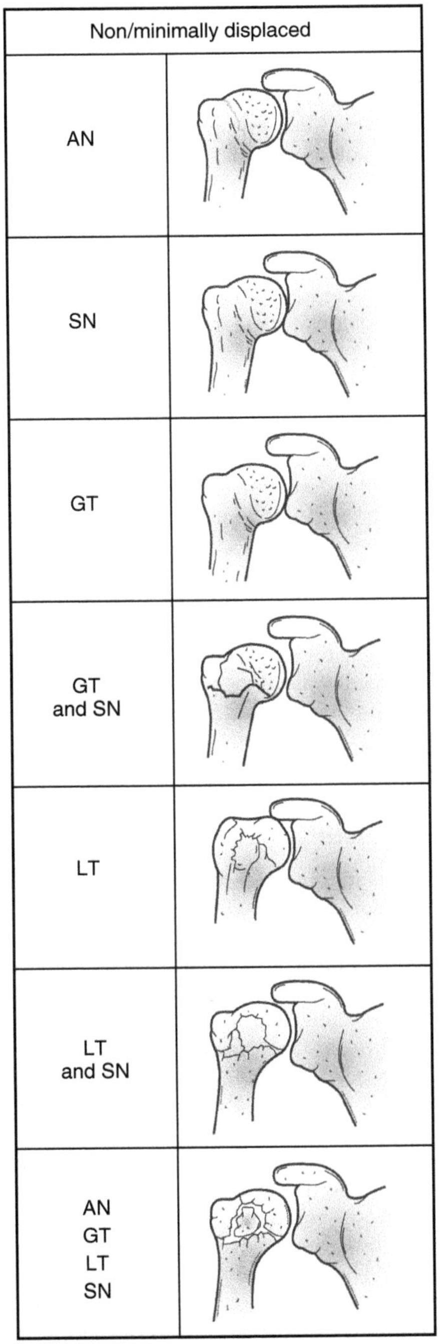

▲ **Figure 3–14.** **Four-part classification for fractures of the proximal humerus. AN, anatomic neck; GT, greater tuberosity; LT, lesser tuberosity; SN, surgical neck.** (Reprinted with permission from Norris TR, Green A. Proximal humerus fractures and fracture-dislocations. In: Browner BD, et al, eds. *Skeletal Trauma: Fractures, Dislocation and Ligamentous Injuries*. New York: Elsevier; 1998.)

Treatment

Most proximal humerus fractures are minimally displaced and can be treated nonoperatively with sling immobilization and early range of motion starting about 2 weeks after the injury. However, about 20% need to be treated operatively because of displacement, angulation, dislocation, activity level, and associated injuries. More displacement can be tolerated at the surgical neck than the greater tuberosity. Surgical options include closed reduction, percutaneous pinning, open reduction with internal fixation, humeral head replacement, and reverse total shoulder arthroplasty.

Prognosis

For minimally displaced fractures, the prognosis is generally good. Loss of motion is the most common complication. It can take 12 to 18 months to attain the maximal result, so range-of-motion exercises should be continued for an extended period of time.

Floyd SB, Campbell J, Chapman CG, Thigpen CA, Kissenberth MJ, Brooks JM. Geographic variation in the treatment of proximal humerus fracture: an update on surgery rates and treatment consensus. *J Orthop Surg Res*. 2019;14(1):22. [PMID: 30665430]

LaMartina J 2nd, Christmas KN, Simon P, et al. Difficulty in decision making in the treatment of displaced proximal humerus fractures: the effect of uncertainty on surgical outcomes. *J Shoulder Elbow Surg*. 2018;27(3):470-477. [PMID: 29433645]

Yang TC, Su YP, Chang MC. The elderly have similar outcomes compared to younger patients after ORIF with locking plate for comminuted proximal humerus fracture. *Acta Orthop Traumatol Turc*. 2019;53(1):1-5. [PMID: 30591240]

3. Proximal Humeral Epiphyseal Fracture

In young athletes, epiphyseal fractures of the proximal humerus may occur. The separate growth centers of the articular surface, greater tuberosity, and lesser tuberosity coalesce at approximately age 7 years, with the remaining growth plates closing between 14 and 21 years of age. Therefore, fracture separations may occur at any age until the growth plates have closed. Fortunately, fractures in this area usually do not arrest growth.

Essentials of Diagnosis

- *History of trauma to the shoulder in children with a peak age of 15 years.*
- *Swelling and ecchymosis overlying the shoulder that may extend down to the elbow.*
- *Tenderness and crepitation over the fracture site.*
- *Pain with attempted range of motion of the shoulder.*
- *Widening of the proximal humeral physis on radiographs.*
- *Appropriate radiographs will define the location and severity of the fracture.*

Clinical Findings

Injury can occur to the shoulder in the growing musculoskeletal system of young athletes engaged in sports that involve overhead throwing. Proximal humerus pain associated with widening of the proximal humerus epiphysis, especially while throwing, has been termed "little league shoulder." Although widening of the proximal humerus epiphysis can be an adaptive change to throwing, when painful, it may represent a fracture resulting from overuse. Acute proximal humerus fracture are seen in children with a peak age of 15 years

Treatment

Cessation of throwing is the first step in treatment. Once pain has resolved, range-of-motion and strengthening exercises can be initiated. Ultimately, throwing can be resumed as long as the patient is pain-free. Those treated early have faster return to sport.

Harada M, Takahara M, Maruyama M, et al. Outcome of conservative treatment for Little League shoulder in young baseball players: factors related to incomplete return to baseball and recurrence of pain. *J Shoulder Elbow Surg.* 2018;27(1):1-9. [PMID: 29054382]

Passaretti D, Candela V, Sessa P, Gumina S. Epidemiology of proximal humeral fractures: a detailed survey of 711 patients in a metropolitan area. *J Shoulder Elbow Surg.* 2017;26(12): 2117-2124. [PMID: 28735839]

4. Scapula Fracture

Scapula fractures are separated into glenoid, scapula body, acromion, and coracoid fractures.

Essentials of Diagnosis

- *History of trauma to the shoulder with acute fracture.*
- *Tenderness over the fracture site.*
- *Pain with attempted range of motion of the shoulder.*
- *Appropriate radiographs and CT scans will define the location and severity of the fracture.*

Glenoid Fracture

The most common glenoid fractures involve either the anterior or posterior glenoid rim, are associated with shoulder dislocation, and are discussed in the section on shoulder instability. Other fractures of the glenoid are much less common and involve the glenoid fossa or the neck. In addition to the usual radiographic views of the shoulder including the scapula (AP, axillary, and Y lateral views), CT scans are helpful in assessment of these fractures. The amount of displacement of intraarticular fractures of the glenoid fossa is important in the decision as to whether they can be treated with nonoperative or operative treatment. If untreated, displaced fractures of the glenoid fossa can lead to persistent pain, chronic instability, osteoarthritis, malunion, and nonunion. Involvement of more than 20% of the glenoid rim is associated with shoulder instability and is the most common indication for surgery. Severe displacement and angulation of other fracture locations are indications for operative treatment, but the amounts are not clearly defined.

Glenoid neck fractures are classified by displacement and angulation. Most can be treated nonoperatively, but when shortened more than 1 cm and angulated more than 40 degrees, surgery is indicated. Like scapula body fractures, they are often associated with other injuries.

Scapula Body Fracture

Scapula body fractures are often high-energy, blunt trauma injuries that occur due to motor vehicle accidents. They are associated with rib and clavicle fractures; injuries to the lungs, head, blood vessels, and spine; and brachial plexus injuries. Scapula body fractures are uncommon, accounting for less than 1% of all fractures. About half of scapula fractures involve the body and spine of the scapula. CT scans are helpful in addition to the usual radiographic views of the shoulder including the scapula. Most can be treated with a short period of immobilization, about 2 weeks in a sling, followed by early immobilization. Severe displacement and angulation are indications for operative treatment, but the amounts are not clearly defined.

Acromion Fracture

Acromion fractures most commonly occur from a fall onto the point of the shoulder. They are classified as type 1, or nondisplaced; type 2, or displaced but not compromising the subacromial space; and type 3, or displaced and compromising the subacromial space. Nondisplaced, acute fractures can be treated nonoperatively with sling immobilization for about 6 weeks followed by progressive range-of-motion and strengthening exercises, but nonunion persists in about half of patients with this treatment. Outcomes are better when the fracture is farther from the base of the acromion. Displaced fractures and those close to the base of the acromion are best treated with open reduction and internal fixation.

Os acromiales most commonly occur from an unfused ossification center but present as if they were nonunions of acromion fractures. They are present in 8% of individuals and are bilateral about 60% of the time. They are usually asymptomatic. Classification is pre-, meso-, meta-, and basi-acromia based on their location. Pre-acromia involve only the anterior acromion, the location of the anterior portion of the deltoid muscle. Meso-acromia also involve the middle portion of the deltoid muscle, meta-acromia also involve the posterior portion of the deltoid muscle, and basi-acromia are at the base of the acromion, at the scapular spine. When loose and painful, pre-acromion can be treated with excision, meso-acromion can be treated with excision or fixation and fusion, and meta- and basi-acromion with fixation and fusion.

Coracoid Fracture

Fractures of the coracoid process are rare; they can occur after coracoclavicular ligament reconstruction or repair and have been reported in skeet shooters and baseball and tennis players. They are identified on radiographs and CT scans. Type I fractures, posterior to the coracoclavicular ligaments, are associated with a wide variety of shoulder injuries including dissociation of the scapula and clavicle, and surgical treatment may be indicated. Type II fractures are anterior to the coracoclavicular ligaments, and conservative treatment, including cessation of activity, usually results in uncomplicated healing after 6 to 8 weeks.

Bi AS, Kane LT, Butler BA, Stover MD. Outcomes following extra-articular fractures of the scapula: a systematic review. *Injury*. 2020;51(3):602-610. [PMID: 32014261]

Edgington J, Antonacci CL, Alberta FG. Nonoperative management of a displaced cartilaginous avulsion fracture of the inferior aspect of the scapula. *JSES Int*. 2020;4(2):280-286. [PMID: 32490414]

Steinmetz RG, Maupin JJ, Johnson EB, et al. Are routine follow-up radiographs necessary for extra-articular scapula body fractures managed conservatively? *J Am Acad Orthop Surg*. 2020:10.5435/JAAOS-D-19-00553. [PMID: 32235240]

GLENOHUMERAL JOINT OSTEOARTHRITIS

Essentials of Diagnosis

- *Constant achy pain in all shoulder positions, even with the arm at the side.*
- *Pain worsened with activity.*
- *Crepitus with motion.*
- *Pain is relieved with lidocaine injection into glenohumeral joint.*

Prevention

It is best to curtail activity once the articular surfaces of the glenohumeral joint have been injured to minimize progression of osteoarthritis. Even rigorous activity in the uninjured shoulder is unlikely to result in osteoarthritis.

Clinical Findings

Achy, persistent pain is the initial symptom of osteoarthritis of the glenohumeral joint and is almost always accompanied by limitation of motion. Most common after the sixth decade, osteoarthritis can present at earlier ages from traumatic or genetic etiologies such as multiple epiphyseal dysplasia and glenoid dysplasia. Pain is exacerbated by activity and often persists for hours after the activity ceases. In mild to moderate cases, the pain diminishes with NSAIDs. Shoulder motion is associated with crepitus, and active and passive range of motion are the same, similar to adhesive capsulitis. Shoulder weakness and mild muscle atrophy are secondary to the pain and disuse of the shoulder that occur when the osteoarthritis is severe.

Radiographs of the shoulder reveal decreased joint space, osteophytes, subchondral sclerosis, and subchondral cysts of the glenohumeral joint. The prominence of these findings is associated with the severity of the disease but is only loosely associated with complaints of pain. Like the hip, knee, and other joints, some have severe pain with mild radiographic findings, whereas others cope well with severe findings. CT scans may help to evaluate abnormalities of the bone such as glenoid retroversion, and MRI may be useful to evaluate soft-tissue injuries such as rotator cuff tears.

Treatment

Rest, rehabilitation, and taking NSAIDs may diminish symptoms in those with mild to moderate osteoarthritis. Range-of-motion and strengthening exercises are recommended as long as they do not exacerbate symptoms, and this is true of most other activities as well. Heavy weight lifting is not recommended. Injection of corticosteroids may relieve symptoms for a period of time, and repeated injections at intervals of a few months are sometimes effective. Individuals with pain, weakness, or decreased range of motion that persists after nonoperative treatment may elect surgical intervention with glenohumeral joint arthroplasty.

Prognosis

Shoulder arthroscopy and debridement diminish pain in those with mild osteoarthritis. Glenohumeral joint arthroplasty is effective in significantly diminishing shoulder pain from severe osteoarthritis when both the humeral head and the glenoid are resurfaced (total joint arthroplasty). Another option is hemiarthroplasty of the humeral head only, which decreases pain, on average, by about two-thirds and obviates glenoid component loosening that is more common over long periods of time than the humeral component loosening. About 90% of total joint arthroplasties will last 10 years, and nearly 80% will last 20 years. Neither procedure yields normal joint function; patients have only partial improvement in strength and range of motion. Return to sports and work as long as it is not heavy labor work is reliable.

Mannava S, Horan MP, Frangiamore SJ, et al. Return to recreational sporting activities following total shoulder arthroplasty. *Orthop J Sports Med*. 2018;6(7):2325967118782672. [PMID: 30046628]

Millett PJ, Fritz EM, Frangiamore SJ, Mannava S. Arthroscopic management of glenohumeral arthritis: a joint preservation approach. *J Am Acad Orthop Surg*. 2018;26(21):745-752. [PMID: 30273222]

Patel RB, Muh S, Okoroha KR, et al. Results of total shoulder arthroplasty in patients aged 55 years or younger versus those older than 55 years: an analysis of 1135 patients with over 2 years of follow-up. *J Shoulder Elbow Surg.* 2019;28(5):861-868. [PMID: 30591214]

Scott EJ, Anthony CA, Rooney P, Lynch TS, Willey MC, Westermann RW. Mobile phone administration of hip-specific patient-reported outcome instruments correlates highly with in-office administration. *J Am Acad Orthop Surg.* 2020;28(1): e41-e46. [PMID: 31860543]

Steinhaus ME, Gowd AK, Hurwit DJ, Lieber AC, Liu JN. Return to work after shoulder arthroplasty: a systematic review and meta-analysis. *J Shoulder Elbow Surg.* 2019;28(5):998-1008. [PMID: 30885548]

Vezeridis PS, Ishmael CR, Jones KJ, Petrigliano FA. Glenohumeral dislocation arthropathy: etiology, diagnosis, and management. *J Am Acad Orthop Surg.* 2019;27(7):227-235. [PMID: 30278009]

ACROMIOCLAVICULAR JOINT INJURY

Essentials of Diagnosis

- *Pain and swelling over the acromioclavicular joint.*
- *May have visible elevation or displacement of the clavicle relative to the acromion (asymmetric to the contralateral shoulder).*
- *Pain with forward elevation of the arm.*
- *Appropriate radiographs can be confirmatory.*

Prevention

Avoiding falls to the tip of the shoulder is the best way to prevent these injuries.

Clinical Findings

Acromioclavicular dislocations or subluxations, commonly referred to as separations, vary in severity depending on the extent of injury to the stabilizing ligaments and capsule. The typical mechanism of injury is a fall resulting in a direct downward blow to the tip of the shoulder. Clinically, pain at the top of the shoulder over the acromioclavicular joint is the predominant symptom, with varying decreases in motion depending on the severity of the injury. The athlete who has sustained this type of injury will typically leave the field holding the arm close to the side.

When checking for instability of the acromioclavicular joint, the examiner should manipulate the midshaft of the clavicle, rather than the acromioclavicular joint to rule out pain from contusion to the acromioclavicular area. For milder acromioclavicular injuries, the patient should put the hand of the affected arm on the opposite shoulder, and the examiner may then gently apply downward pressure at the patient's affected elbow, noting if this maneuver causes pain at the acromioclavicular joint.

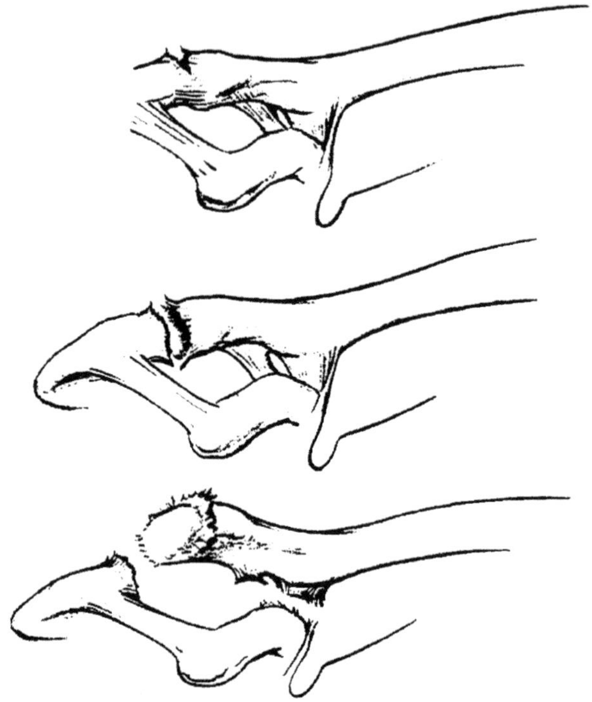

▲ **Figure 3–15.** Grades of acromioclavicular joint separations.

Acromioclavicular joint injuries are divided into six grades, and the first three are the most common (Figure 3–15). Grade I injuries are typically produced by a mild blow causing a partial tear of the acromioclavicular ligament. When the acromioclavicular ligament is completely torn, but the coracoclavicular ligament remains intact, a grade II injury that involves subluxation or partial displacement results. When the force of injury is severe enough to tear the coracoclavicular and acromioclavicular ligaments in addition to the capsule, a grade III injury occurs.

In grade IV injuries, the clavicle is displaced posterior and buttonholed through the fascia of the trapezius muscle. Grade V injuries demonstrate severe inferior displacement of the glenohumeral joint, with the clavicle often 300% superior to the acromion. Lastly, in grade VI injuries, the distal end of the clavicle is locked inferior to the coracoid.

Acromioclavicular joint displacement is often obvious on physical examination, but it is best classified by radiography. An AP radiograph that is aimed 10 degrees cephalad allows visualization of the acromioclavicular joint. A radiograph of the entire upper thorax allows the vertical distance between the coracoid and the clavicle on both the involved and uninvolved sides to be compared. AP radiographs with weights applied to the upper extremities are usually unnecessary. An axillary lateral radiograph is also essential for proper classification.

Treatment

Management of acromioclavicular joint injuries depends on their severity. Grade I and II injuries may be treated with a sling until discomfort dissipates, usually within 2 to 4 weeks. Next a rehabilitation program starts, with the goal of normal range of motion and strength to the upper extremity being restored. Ice and other modalities are used for an acute acromioclavicular injury to reduce soreness and swelling. Pain is the limiting factor in beginning range-of-motion and isometric muscle-strengthening exercises. It should be used as a guide for initiation and progress through rehabilitation. Range-of-motion exercises can be begun rather quickly and strengthening added when pain permits.

Treatment of acute grade III injuries or complete dislocations in athletes is controversial; most believe grade III injuries are best managed nonoperatively, but some advocate operative treatment. Grade IV to VI injuries are best treated with open reduction and internal fixation usually with reconstruction of the coracoclavicular ligament.

Before resuming athletic activities, the patient should have full, painless range of motion, no tenderness on palpation, and sufficient strength.

Prognosis

Athletes who do not need to elevate their arms, such as soccer or football players, tend to return to sports earlier than players engaged in sports that require overhead arm activity, such as tennis, baseball, and swimming.

Gowd AK, Liu JN, Cabarcas BC, et al. Current concepts in the operative management of acromioclavicular dislocations: a systematic review and meta-analysis of operative techniques. *Am J Sports Med.* 2019;47(11):2745-2758. [PMID: 30272997]

Mori D, Yamashita F, Kizaki K, Funakoshi N, Mizuno Y, Kobayashi M. Anatomic coracoclavicular ligament reconstruction for the treatment of acute acromioclavicular joint dislocation: minimum 10-year follow-up. *JB JS Open Access.* 2017;2(3):e0007. [PMID: 30229219]

Nordin JS, Olsson O, Lunsjö K. Acromioclavicular joint dislocations: incidence, injury profile, and patient characteristics from a prospective case series. *JSES Int.* 2020;4(2):246-250. [PMID: 32490410]

STERNOCLAVICULAR JOINT INJURY

In the skeletally mature adult athlete, injury to the sternoclavicular joint usually involves the surrounding soft tissue and capsule tearing, leading to subluxation or dislocation. The mechanism of injury is either a fall or blow to the point of the shoulder, which predisposes the athlete to anterior dislocation, or a direct blow to the clavicle or chest with the shoulder in extension, which predisposes the athlete to posterior dislocation. The injury may range from a symptomatic sprain to a complete sternoclavicular dislocation with disruption of the capsule and its restraining ligaments.

1. Anterior Dislocation

Essentials of Diagnosis

- *A fall or blow to the point of the shoulder.*
- *Painful prominence overlying the proximal end of the clavicle.*
- *Appropriate radiographs or CT scan can be diagnostic.*

Clinical Findings

The most common type of sternoclavicular dislocation is anterior dislocation. This is recognized clinically by an anterior prominence of the proximal clavicle on the involved side. Radiographic documentation of an anterior sternoclavicular dislocation is difficult because the rib, sternum, and clavicle overlap at the joint but may be confirmed by oblique views. A CT scan is very sensitive and should be done if the radiograph appears normal but a dislocation is suspected.

Treatment

Although dislocation of the anterior sternoclavicular joint may cause considerable distress initially, the symptoms usually subside rapidly, with no loss of shoulder function. A variety of surgical and nonsurgical approaches have been advocated, but surgery for anterior dislocations can diminish but often does not resolve the instability and can result in significant complications. Closed treatment modalities vary from using a sling to attempted closed reduction, which may be successful initially but is difficult to maintain.

2. Posterior Dislocation

Essentials of Diagnosis

- *History of trauma to the upper chest wall.*
- *Pain in the region of the proximal end of the clavicle.*
- *Patient may present with hoarseness, dysphagia, or severe respiratory distress.*
- *Appropriate radiographs or CT scan can be diagnostic.*

Clinical Findings

Posterior sternoclavicular dislocation is much less common but is associated with more complications because of the potential for injury to the esophagus, great vessels, and trachea. Presentation ranges from mild to moderate pain at the sternoclavicular joint to hoarseness, dysphagia, shortness of breath, and subcutaneous emphysema from tracheal injury.

Treatment

In most instances, closed reduction of posterior dislocations, if performed early, is successful and stable. To effect reduction, a pillow is placed under the upper back of the supine

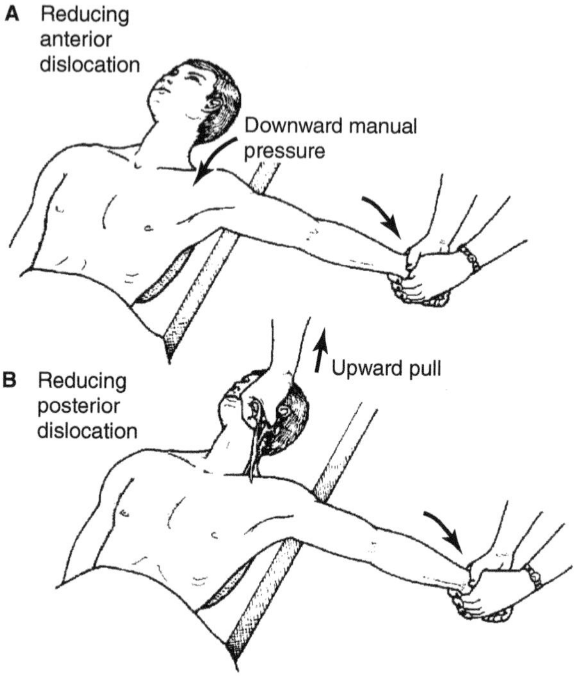

▲ **Figure 3–16.** Method for reducing (**A**) anterior sternoclavicular dislocation and (**B**) posterior sternoclavicular dislocation.

patient, and gentle traction is applied with the shoulder held in 90 degrees of abduction and at maximum extension (Figure 3–16). Severe symptoms and signs necessitate closed reduction under general anesthesia or open reduction.

Usually a sling is used until the joint has healed sufficiently, usually within 2 to 3 weeks, and then range-of-motion exercises may begin. Elevation of the arm should not be attempted until 3 weeks after injury.

3. Medial Clavicular Epiphyseal Fracture

In athletes younger than 25 years of age, sternoclavicular injuries may not result in true dislocations, but rather in fractures through the growth plate of the proximal clavicle. These clavicular epiphyseal fractures may appear clinically as dislocations, particularly if some displacement is present, and may be treated conservatively. Typically, these are not associated with growth deformities, and reduction of the fracture is not needed unless there is severe displacement. Symptomatic treatment for pain will usually suffice. Sometimes an adolescent presents with an enlarging mass at the sternoclavicular joint, accompanied by parents with worries of cancer. A careful history reveals trauma several weeks earlier, and the mass represents the callus of a healing clavicular epiphyseal fracture that can be demonstrated radiographically.

Bakir MS, Unterkofler J, Haralambiev L, et al. Medial injuries of the clavicle: more prevalent than expected? A big data analysis of incidence, age, and gender distribution based on nationwide routine data. *Eur J Trauma Emerg Surg*. 2020:10.1007/s00068-019-01293-0. [PMID: 31960070]

Leonard DA, Segovia NA, Kaur J, Lucas J, Bishop J, Vorhies JS. Posterior sternoclavicular dislocation: do we need "cardiothoracic backup"? Insights from a national sample. *J Orthop Trauma*. 2020;34(2):e67-e71. [PMID: 31764407]

OTHER SHOULDER TENDON AND MUSCLE

BICEPS TENDON INJURIES

1. Bicipital Tendinosis

Essentials of Diagnosis

- *Pain localized to the anterior proximal humerus and shoulder joint.*
- *Pain with resisted forward flexion and supination.*
- *Pain may be relieved by a steroid injection into the sheath of the biceps tendon.*

Prevention

Similar to the prevention of rotator cuff injuries, general conditioning and stretching and strengthening before activities can help minimize injury to the biceps tendon.

Clinical Findings

The long head of the biceps tendon is an intraarticular structure deep in the rotator cuff as the long head of the biceps tendon passes under the acromion to its insertion at the top of the glenoid. The same mechanism that initiates symptoms of impingement syndrome in rotator cuff injuries may inflame the biceps tendon in its subacromial position, causing bicipital tendinosis. Tendinosis may also result from subluxation of the tendon out of its groove in the proximal humerus and can occur under, into, or on top of the subscapular tendon. Subluxation of the biceps tendon is almost always associated with a subscapularis tendon tear. The symptoms of bicipital tendinosis, whether they are the result of impingement or tendon subluxation, are essentially the same. Pain is localized to the proximal humerus and shoulder joint, with resisted supination of the forearm, resisted elbow flexion, and palpation of the tendon at the bicipital groove aggravating the pain. The Yergason test is performed with the elbow flexed to 90 degrees, the forearm pronated, and the arm stabilized against the thorax. Active supination of the forearm and flexion of the elbow, against resistance, elicits pain in the bicipital groove. A positive test can indicate biceps tendonitis and instability of the long head of the biceps tendon in its groove.

Treatment

If the biceps tendinosis is associated with shoulder impingement, then therapy aimed at treating the impingement syndrome will relieve the bicipital tendinosis. If subluxation of the tendon within its groove is the cause of the irritation, conservative therapy includes NSAIDs and restriction of activities, followed by a slow resumption of activities after a period of rest. Strengthening of the muscles that assist the biceps in elbow flexion and forearm supination is also beneficial. Steroid injections into the sheath of the biceps tendon are helpful but may be hazardous if placed into the tendon as tendon rupture can result. Persistent symptoms may warrant tenodesis of the biceps tendon directly into the humerus.

Prognosis

Most recover from biceps tendinosis with nonoperative treatments. Return to work and athletics typically takes 4 to 6 months following a proximal biceps tenodesis after rehabilitation aimed at normal shoulder and elbow range of motion and strength.

2. Biceps Tendon Tears at the Shoulder

Essentials of Diagnosis

- *"Popeye" appearance of the biceps muscle from distal retraction.*
- *May or may not be painful and ecchymotic depending on the chronicity of the injury.*
- *Weakness of elbow flexion and forearm supination.*

Prevention

Similar to the prevention of rotator cuff injuries, general conditioning and stretching and strengthening before activities can help minimize injury to the biceps tendon.

Clinical Findings

The long head of the biceps tendon usually ruptures from its origin, along the intraarticular tendon or at the entrance of the bicipital groove proximally. Diagnosis is usually easy, as the deformity is obvious. The muscle displaces distally, producing a bulging or "Popeye" appearance, and the short head remains intact. Acute rupture of the long head of the biceps tendon can result from forceful flexion of the arm but also can occur over time as small successive tears render the tendon vulnerable to acute rupture, and these are often associated with a rotator cuff tear in middle-aged and older individuals. Tears of the biceps can also occur at the musculotendinous junction and the muscle itself, and rupture of the biceps tendon distally involves both heads and the muscle is displaced proximally. Ecchymosis is common after biceps tendon tears and is located over the biceps muscle.

Treatment

Surgical treatment of proximal ruptures, if indicated, is usually reserved for younger patients and those with persistent pain and cramping with use of the biceps muscle. The proximal end of the tendon is usually found beneath the attachment of the pectoralis major.

Prognosis

Return to work and athletics typically takes 4 to 6 months following a proximal biceps tenodesis after rehabilitation aimed at normal shoulder and elbow range of motion and strength.

McCrum CL, Alluri RK, Batech M, Mirzayan R. Complications of biceps tenodesis based on location, fixation, and indication: a review of 1526 shoulders. *J Shoulder Elbow Surg*. 2019;28(3):461-469. [PMID: 30573431]

McMahon PJ, Speziali A. Outcomes of tenodesis of the long head of the biceps tendon more than three months after rupture. *World J Orthop*. 2016;7(3):188-194. [PMID: 27004167]

PECTORALIS MAJOR RUPTURE

Essentials of Diagnosis

- *Sudden pain.*
- *Ecchymosis and swelling along the pectoralis major muscle.*

Prevention

Similar to the prevention of rotator cuff injuries, general conditioning and stretching and strengthening before activities can help minimize injury to the pectoralis major.

Clinical Findings

Rupture of the pectoralis major tendon is an uncommon injury, usually occurring during bench press exercises in weight lifting and caused by sudden unexpected muscle contraction during pulling or lifting. The athlete usually experiences sudden pain and develops local ecchymosis and swelling. As the swelling subsides, a sulcus and deformity may be visible, and the patient notices weakness of the arm in adduction and internal rotation. MRI is effective in diagnosis of the location of the injury in the muscle, tendon, or insertion into bone.

Treatment

The rupture may be partial or complete, and nonoperative treatment usually results in satisfactory function for the activities of daily life. Surgery may be considered if the athlete wishes to return to heavy weight lifting.

Prognosis

Athletes are permitted to return to contact sports once they have achieved full strength and range of motion, which typically occurs 6 months following a pectoralis major repair.

Marsh NA, Calcei JG, Antosh IJ, Cordasco FA. Isolated tears of the sternocostal head of the pectoralis major muscle: surgical technique, clinical outcomes, and a modification of the Tietjen and Bak classification. *J Shoulder Elbow Surg.* 2020;29(7): 1359-1367. [PMID: 32089403]

SHOULDER NEUROVASCULAR INJURY

1. Brachial Plexus Injury

Essentials of Diagnosis

- *Often preceded by a fall onto the shoulder.*
- *Paresthesias and/or motor loss in the affected extremity that can be transient or permanent.*
- *Electromyography/nerve conduction velocity (EMG/NCV) can help localize the lesion and aid in prognosis.*

Clinical Findings, Treatment, and Prognosis

Brachial plexus injuries are typically caused by a fall on the shoulder, as seen in acromioclavicular joint injuries. Most athletic brachial plexus injuries are mild and do not result in motor loss, and there are only paresthesias, which can resolve in minutes to weeks, although some cases may persist for months or years. EMG/NCV will show changes as early as 3 weeks after the injury, and then a transient slowing of conduction across the plexus or a mild prolongation of nerve latency may be seen. The "burner" or "stinger" is one of the most common brachial plexus injuries encountered in athletes. The key to diagnosis is a short duration of upper extremity paresthesias and shoulder weakness, with pain-free range of motion of the cervical spine. Players may return to competition after shoulder strength and full, pain-free range of motion have returned.

When a severe injury occurs and is chronic, it results in instability of the shoulder demonstrated on a standing radiograph as inferior instability. Arthrodesis is an alternative when muscle paralysis is permanent.

Ahearn BM, Starr HM, Seiler JG. Traumatic brachial plexopathy in athletes: current concepts for diagnosis and management of stingers. *J Am Acad Orthop Surg.* 2019;27(18):677-684. [PMID: 30741724]

2. Long Thoracic Nerve Injury

Essentials of Diagnosis

- *Palsy of the serratus anterior results in medial winging of the scapula.*
- *May be painless, but often there is medial scapula pain.*
- *EMG/NCV can help localize the lesion and aid in prognosis.*

Clinical Findings, Treatment, and Prognosis

Traction, blunt trauma, or iatrogenic surgical injury may cause long thoracic nerve injury, with subsequent serratus anterior paralysis resulting in medial winging of the scapula. That is, the scapula moves medial and the medial border wings away from the thorax. Iatrogenic surgical injury is more commonly a cause of spinal accessory nerve injury, and this results in lateral winging of the scapula. That is, the scapula moves lateral and the medial border wings away from the thorax. These can be differentiated on physical examination by the position of the scapula. Treatment after traction and blunt trauma is usually conservative initially, with rehabilitation during return of function. When paralysis is permanent, pectoralis transfer aids in treatment of long thoracic nerve palsy, and levator scapulae transfer aids in treatment of spinal accessory nerve palsy.

3. Suprascapular Nerve Injury

Essentials of Diagnosis

- *Poorly localized pain and weakness in the posterolateral shoulder.*
- *Weakness and atrophy of the supraspinatus and/or infraspinatus muscles.*
- *MRI may reveal the presence of a cyst in the suprascapular or spinoglenoid notch.*
- *EMG/NCV can help localize the lesion and aid in prognosis.*

Clinical Findings, Treatment, and Prognosis

Entrapment of the suprascapular nerve is often associated with activities such as weight lifting, baseball pitching, volleyball, and backpacking. Traction and repetitive shoulder use are the mechanisms of injury. Compression of the nerve may occur from entrapment at the anterior suprascapular notch of the scapula or at the level of the spinoglenoid notch. The latter occurs in volleyball players and baseball players and is likely caused by rapid overhead acceleration of the arm. Compression is associated with poorly localized pain and weakness in the posterolateral aspect of the shoulder girdle. This may be followed by atrophy of the supraspinatus or infraspinatus muscles. Eventually, there is weakness of forward flexion and external rotation of the shoulder. The diagnosis is confirmed by EMG and nerve conduction studies.

Conservative therapy consists of rest, NSAIDs, and physical therapy designed to increase muscular tone and strength. If this is unsuccessful, then surgical exploration is indicated, which may reveal hypertrophy of the transverse scapular ligament, anomalies of the suprascapular notch, and ganglion cysts. Results of surgery vary with the lesion discovered, but many patients return to full function postoperatively.

4. Musculocutaneous Nerve Injury

Essentials of Diagnosis

- *Weak or absent biceps muscle function with sensory loss in the lateral forearm.*
- *EMG/NCV can help localize the lesion and aid in prognosis.*

Clinical Findings, Treatment, and Prognosis

This nerve is susceptible to direct frontal blows or surgical procedures. Injury is associated with numbness in the lateral forearm to the base of the thumb and weak to absent biceps muscle function. Most injuries seen in sports are transient and respond to conservative treatment in a matter of days to weeks.

5. Axillary Nerve Injury

Essentials of Diagnosis

- *Present following a shoulder dislocation or proximal humerus fracture.*
- *Weakness or absence of deltoid muscle function.*
- *Positive deltoid extension lag sign.*
- *EMG/NCV can help localize the lesion and aid in prognosis.*

Clinical Findings, Treatment, and Prognosis

The mechanism of injury may be trauma by direct blow to the posterior aspect of the shoulder, following dislocation or fracture of the proximal humerus, and following surgery. The axillary nerve can be injured especially during arthroscopic capsular release procedures and is most prone to be injured with release of the anteroinferior capsule. The axillary nerve passes caudal to the glenohumeral joint capsule, and its position relative to the capsule varies with shoulder position; its distance from the capsule diminishes with abduction of the shoulder. With the arm at the side, it courses 1 to 1.5 cm lateral to the anteroinferior glenoid rim at the 5 o'clock position (right shoulder). As the nerve courses posterior, it is located increasing more lateral to the glenoid rim. It is 2 to 2.5 cm from the posteroinferior glenoid rim at the 7 o'clock position (right shoulder). The degree of injury to the nerve varies because the initial presentation may be mild weakness during elevation and abduction of the arm with or without numbness of the lateral arm. The deltoid extension lag sign is indicative of axillary nerve injury. To perform this test, the examiner elevates the arm into a position of near full extension, asks the patient to hold the arm in this position, and then releases the arm. If there is complete deltoid paralysis, the arm will drop. For partial nerve injuries, the magnitude of the angular drop, or lag, is an indicator of deltoid strength. Approximately 25% of all dislocated shoulder injuries are associated with axillary nerve traction injuries, which respond well to rest, physical therapy, and time. If recovery is not complete within 3 to 6 months, surgical intervention is recommended with exploration, using neurolysis or grafting, or both, as necessary. Results of surgery are usually favorable, with sensory recovery occurring before motor recovery.

Didesch JT, Tang P. Anatomy, etiology, and management of scapular winging. *J Hand Surg Am.* 2019;44(4):321-330. [PMID: 30292717]

THORACIC OUTLET SYNDROME

Essentials of Diagnosis

- *Symptoms are often nonspecific; may be neurologic, venous, or arterial; and may include edema, pallor, or coolness as well as paresthesias.*
- *Doppler examination and EMG/NCV studies can assist in the diagnosis.*

Clinical Findings, Treatment, and Prognosis

The symptoms resulting from thoracic outlet compression may be neurologic, venous, or arterial. Obstruction of the subclavian vein may lead to stiffness, edema, and even thrombosis of the limb. Arterial obstruction may be the result of direct compression and manifests with pallor, coolness, and forearm claudication. Doppler examination may reveal changes in arterial and venous flow. EMG/NCV can be helpful in diagnosis.

Nonoperative treatment is recommended for less severe forms of this syndrome, and once the pain subsides, an exercise program to strengthen the core muscles is beneficial. Correcting poor posture and an ongoing maintenance program are mandatory once improvement is reached. Progression of symptoms or failure of nonoperative treatment is an indication for surgery that is often effective at diminishing symptoms.

Balderman J, Abuirqeba AA, Eichaker L, et al. Physical therapy management, surgical treatment, and patient-reported outcomes measures in a prospective observational cohort of patients with neurogenic thoracic outlet syndrome. *J Vasc Surg.* 2019;70(3):832-841. [PMID: 30852035]

Ohman JW, Thompson RW. Thoracic outlet syndrome in the overhead athlete: diagnosis and treatment recommendations. *Curr Rev Musculoskelet Med.* 2020;13(4):457-471. [PMID: 32514995]

ELBOW INJURIES

EPICONDYLITIS

1. Lateral Epicondylitis

Essentials of Diagnosis

- *A history of repetitive activity or overuse.*
- *Pain localized to the lateral elbow that may radiate to the forearm.*
- *Tenderness at the extensor carpi radialis brevis origin, just anterior and distal to the center of the lateral epicondyle.*
- *Normal elbow range of motion.*
- *Usually normal radiographs and rarely (<10%) calcification adjacent to the lateral epicondyle.*

Lateral epicondylitis is commonly known as tennis elbow and involves the tendons of the extensor muscles of the wrist and hand. Patients who perform repetitive wrist extension against resistance (such as the backhand stroke in tennis) are at risk. The pain starts insidiously and worsens gradually and is more bothersome than disabling. Tenderness is located at or just distal to the lateral humeral epicondyle, and pain is produced by extending the wrist against resistance. This is most marked when done with the elbow extended. The tendon of the extensor carpi radialis brevis is the most common site of the lesion. Other causes for lateral elbow pain should be considered, including radiocapitellar arthritis and posterior interosseous nerve compression. Radiographs only rarely reveal soft-tissue calcification near the lateral humeral epicondyle, and MRI is of questionable aid in making the diagnosis.

Treatment includes minimizing inciting activities, using a counterforce brace, and stretching the extensor and supinator muscles by flexing the wrist with the elbow extended. It is often helpful to pronate the forearm. Exercises to strengthen the wrist extensor muscles should be included. A lighter racquet, proper grip size on the racquet, and proper technique can be helpful for tennis players. If these treatments fail, an injection of steroid or platelet-rich plasma into the most tender region is often helpful. Surgical treatment yields satisfactory outcomes in recalcitrant cases, and multiple procedures, including arthroscopic techniques, have been described. Common to all procedures is release of the common extensor origin, and some also repair the tendon to bone after debridement. Ultrasound-guided percutaneous tenotomy may be effective as well. Histologic studies of the afflicted tendon show degenerative changes with angiofibroblastic proliferation. These are thought to be similar to the pathologic changes of the torn rotator cuff, with diminished vascularity, an altered nutritional state, and tearing of the susceptible tendon.

2. Medial Epicondylitis

Essentials of Diagnosis

- *A history of repetitive activity or overuse, often from activities that result in valgus elbow forces, such as occurs with baseball throwing.*
- *Pain localized to the medial elbow that may radiate to the forearm.*
- *Tenderness at the flexor-pronator origin, most commonly of the pronator teres and the flexor carpi ulnaris.*
- *Normal elbow range of motion.*
- *Usually normal radiographs and rarely (<10%) calcification adjacent to the medial epicondyle.*

Medial epicondylitis involves the common flexor pronator origin and is commonly known as golfer's elbow. Treatment is similar to the management of lateral epicondylitis, although with emphasis on the wrist flexors and the forearm pronators. Stretching is done by extending the wrist with the elbow extended. It is often helpful to pronate the forearm. Ulnar nerve compression at the elbow may occur with medial tennis elbow. The common flexor origin is an important medial stabilizer of the elbow, so if surgical treatment is indicated in overhead athletes, the debrided tendon should be reattached rather than released from the medial epicondyle.

Clark T, McRae S, Leiter J, Zhang Y, Dubberley J, MacDonald P. Arthroscopic versus open lateral release for the treatment of lateral epicondylitis: a prospective randomized controlled trial. *Arthroscopy.* 2018;34(12):3177-3184. [PMID: 30509427]

Houck DA, Kraeutler MJ, Thornton LB, McCarty EC, Bravman JT. Treatment of lateral epicondylitis with autologous blood, platelet-rich plasma, or corticosteroid injections: a systematic review of overlapping meta-analyses. *Orthop J Sports Med.* 2019;7(3):2325967119831052. [PMID: 30899764]

Krogh TP, Fredberg U, Ammitzbøll C, Ellingsen T. Clinical value of ultrasonographic assessment in lateral epicondylitis versus asymptomatic healthy controls. *Am J Sports Med.* 2020:363546520921949. [PMID: 32484714]

Kroslak M, Pirapakaran K, Murrell GAC. Counterforce bracing of lateral epicondylitis: a prospective, randomized, double-blinded, placebo-controlled clinical trial. *J Shoulder Elbow Surg.* 2019;28(2):288-295. [PMID: 30658774]

ELBOW INSTABILITY

Rupture of the collateral ligaments of the elbow occurs most commonly from elbow dislocation. This can result from excessive valgus force, and initially, the medial ulnar collateral ligament ruptures. Excessive posterolateral rotatory force may also result in rupture of the lateral ulnar collateral ligament. In either case, the elbow may dislocate, and typically the direction is posterior. Treatment after relocation and brief immobilization consists of active range-of-motion exercises. Recurrent instability is rare; instead, a small loss of elbow extension, usually less than 10 degrees, commonly results.

1. Valgus Instability

Essentials of Diagnosis

- *Sudden or gradual onset of medial elbow pain after throwing.*
- *Pain greatest at late cocking and acceleration phase of throwing.*
- *Maximum tenderness about 1 cm distal to the medial epicondyle.*
- *Provocative maneuvers that place valgus stress on elbow reproduce symptoms.*
- *There may also be ulnar neuropathy and posteromedial elbow impingement, medial epicondylitis, and cubital tunnel syndrome.*

Valgus instability may result from an acute injury or over time from overuse in overhead-throwing sports such as baseball, football, and javelin throwing. With acute medial ulnar collateral ligament rupture, a pop may be felt during a throw. Tenderness is present on the medial side of the elbow, usually just distal to the medial epicondyle. Instability can then be appreciated with the valgus stress test. This is done on the relaxed patient and the elbow slightly flexed about 20 to 30 degrees, as failure to unlock the olecranon from within the olecranon fossa in full extension creates a false sense of stability. Comparison to the contralateral side aids in making the correct diagnosis. If the medial ulnar collateral ligament has been injured but remains intact, then the valgus stress test may elicit pain, but no instability. The "milking maneuver" (Figure 3–17) is a valgus stress applied in about 90 degrees of elbow flexion and will also elicit pain along the medial side of the elbow. Eliciting pain while moving the elbow in a bit of flexion and extension during the milking maneuver, known as the moving milking maneuver, is also effective for diagnosing medial ulnar collateral ligament injuries of the elbow.

An AP radiograph taken while the examiner performs the valgus stress test may also aid in making the diagnosis. Alternatively, gravity can be used to apply the valgus stress and can be done with a small weight of about 1 lb (2.2 kg) applied at the wrist. For this, an AP radiograph of the elbow is taken with the elbow slightly flexed about 20 to 30 degrees as in the valgus stress test. When instability is present, there will be a wider medial opening than on the contralateral normal side. It is important that the patient relaxes. Ultrasound can also be used to assess medial opening and may also be done at 90 degrees of elbow flexion, simulating the milking maneuver. MRI may also be useful, especially an MRI arthrogram, as dye leaking through the ulnar collateral ligament and the T sign of dye extending distal to the ulna articular surface are diagnostic of a tear. MRI arthrograms are also effective in detecting partial ruptures and chronic medial ulnar collateral injuries. Surgical repair may be indicated in overhead-throwing athletes after an acute rupture of their medial ulnar collateral ligament when they still want to continue to participate in their sport. Soccer, basketball players, and other athletes participating in non–overhead-throwing sports may be treated with a program of early active range-of-motion exercises with expectation of full return to their sport. Chronic medial ulnar collateral ligament injuries resulting from overuse are best treated with rehabilitation, NSAIDs, and avoidance of throwing for as long as 3 months. Those with

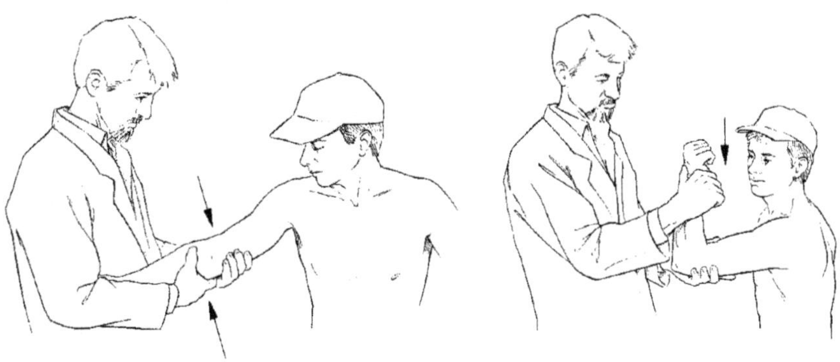

▲ **Figure 3–17. The valgus stress and milking maneuver tests for medial ulnar collateral ligament injury.** (Reprinted, with permission, from Chen FS, Rokito AS, Jobe FW. Medial elbow problems in the overhead-throwing athlete. *J Am Acad Orthop Surg*. 2001;9:102.)

chronic injury commonly also have ulnar neuropathy and/or posteromedial elbow impingement of the medial olecranon on the medial part of the olecranon fossa with osteophytes in these locations. Only those with residual pain and instability after participation in nonoperative program should undergo reconstruction of the anterior band of the medial ulnar collateral ligament. In this surgery, pioneered by Dr Frank Jobe in athletes, a tendon graft, usually the palmaris longus, is used to reconstruct the ligament from the anterior and distal aspect of the medial humeral epicondyle to the sublime tubercle of the ulna. About 90% of athletes are able to return to highly competitive throwing after such surgery.

Foruria AM, Gutiérrez B, Cobos J, Haeni DL, Valencia M, Calvo E. Most coronoid fractures and fracture-dislocations with no radial head involvement can be treated nonsurgically with elbow immobilization. *J Shoulder Elbow Surg.* 2019;28(7):1395-1405. [PMID: 30956143]

Goodman AD, Lemme N, DeFroda SF, Gil JA, Owens BD. Elbow dislocation and subluxation injuries in the national collegiate athletic association, 2009-2010 through 2013-2014. *Orthop J Sports Med.* 2018;6(1):2325967117750105. Erratum in: *Orthop J Sports Med.* 2018;6(2):2325967118764935. [PMID: 29372170]

Griffith TB, Ahmad CS, Gorroochurn P, et al. Comparison of outcomes based on graft type and tunnel configuration for primary ulnar collateral ligament reconstruction in professional baseball pitchers. *Am J Sports Med.* 2019;47(5):1103-1110. [PMID: 30896975]

Marshall NE, Keller R, Limpisvasti O, Schulz B, El Attrache N. Major League Baseball pitching performance after Tommy John surgery and the effect of tear characteristics, technique, and graft type. *Am J Sports Med.* 2019;47(3):713-720. [PMID: 30624958]

Rezaie N, Gupta S, Service BC, Osbahr DC. Elbow dislocation. *Clin Sports Med.* 2020;39(3):637-655. [PMID: 32446580]

2. Posterolateral Rotatory Instability

Essentials of Diagnosis

- *Sudden or gradual onset of lateral elbow pain.*
- *There may be snapping, catching, locking, or a sensation of elbow instability.*
- *A history of tennis elbow surgery.*
- *The provocative maneuver of the posterolateral rotator instability test reproduces symptoms.*

Posterolateral rotatory instability of the elbow may result from a fall on the outstretched arm, surgery of the lateral side of the elbow, or chronic varus stress, as may occur in long-term crutch walkers. The instability covers a spectrum of severity from mild subluxation to recurrent dislocation. Those with mild forms complain of intermittent symptoms on the lateral side of the elbow associated with supination of the forearm such as pain, snapping, or catching. More severe symptoms include locking or sensations of elbow instability. To perform the posterolateral rotatory instability test, a valgus stress is applied to the supinated elbow with the patient supine and the upper extremity over the head (Figure 3–18). Subluxation of the radial head occurs with the elbow in extension and resolves when the elbow is flexed. This maneuver also reproduces the patient's symptoms. A lateral stress radiograph, done while the posterolateral rotatory instability test is performed, may also demonstrate the instability (see Figure 3–18). Treatment for acute injury consists of an elbow brace to hold the forearm in pronation and restrict the terminal 30 degrees of elbow extension for a 6-week period of time. Chronic cases are best treated with reconstruction of the lateral ulnar collateral ligament. Postoperatively, the

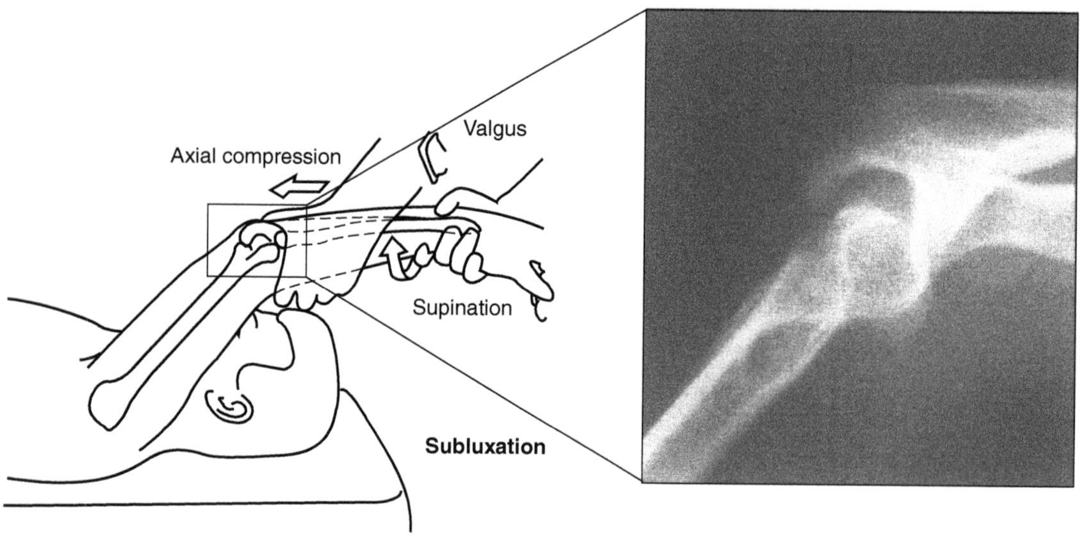

▲ **Figure 3–18.** The posterolateral rotatory instability test reproduces the patient's symptoms. At right is a lateral stress radiograph.

patient is put in the same brace as used for acute posterolateral rotatory instability for 6 to 12 weeks.

Ciccotti MC, Ciccotti MG. Ulnar collateral ligament evaluation and diagnostics. *Clin Sports Med.* 2020;39(3):503-522. [PMID: 32446571]

CUBITAL TUNNEL SYNDROME

Essentials of Diagnosis

- *Medial elbow pain and paresthesias in ring and little fingers.*
- *Positive Tinel sign over cubital tunnel and positive elbow flexion test.*
- *Associated with both medial epicondylitis and medial ulnar collateral ligament injury.*
- *Exacerbated by throwing in baseball players.*

Prevention relies on avoidance of prolonged elbow flexion and, in the overhead athlete, on sound techniques that minimize valgus load on the elbow. Correction of known causes of nerve irritation, including valgus instability of the elbow, may also prevent the syndrome. The cubital tunnel is formed by the medial epicondyle, the elbow joint, and the two heads of the flexor carpi ulnaris. Structures proximal to, within, and distal to the tunnel can cause compression, entrapment, traction, subluxation, or irritation of the ulnar nerve. Proximally, these structures include the arcade of Struthers (not to be confused with the *ligament* of Struthers, which is associated with median neuropathy) and medial head of the triceps. Within the groove, they include the medial epicondyle, the epicondylar groove, anconeus epitrochlearis, the two heads of the flexi carpi ulnaris, and their interconnecting ligament of Osborne. Distally, an offending structure may be the deep flexor-pronator fascia. Regardless of cause or site, the final common pathway of cubital tunnel syndrome is the onset of nerve ischemia and fibrosis.

Initial symptoms may be medial elbow pain with occasional radiation to the medial forearm. Paresthesias may occur in the ulnar two fingers. Athletes will often present with these symptoms before onset of weakness. Mechanical complaints such as snapping may occur with nerve subluxation. Diagnosis is chiefly clinical and relies on two provocative tests: a positive Tinel sign over the nerve and a positive elbow flexion test. This test is performed by placing the elbow in full flexion and the wrist in maximal extension. A test is positive if pain or paresthesias are elicited within 1 minute. Sensory changes can be detected with Semmes-Weinstein monofilament testing and, in more advanced cases, with two-point discrimination tests. Motor deficits often occur late, and athletes usually complain of pain and paresthesias before asymmetric hypothenar atrophy, decreased pinch and grip strength, abducted small finger or Wartenberg sign, Froment sign, and clawing of the ulnar two fingers occur. Motor deficits may not be present, even in late cases, if the intrinsic muscles of the hand receive innervation from the median nerve—the result of an anatomic variant known as the Martin-Gruber anastomosis.

A thorough exam of the neck and proximal upper extremity is performed to eliminate neuropathic etiologies with similar manifestations such as cervical radiculopathy, brachial plexopathy (of the medial cord), and thoracic outlet syndrome.

Plain radiographs including special views such as cubital tunnel view may reveal bony abnormalities causing ulnar nerve compression, and MRI may identify soft-tissue abnormalities having the same effect, but these are rare. EMG and NCV studies will be negative in more than 50% of patients. Slowing of conduction velocities to less than 50 m/s when the elbow is flexed is indicative of disease. Reduction in sensory nerve action potential also confirms early neuropathy.

Treatment of ulnar neuropathy at the cubital tunnel is initially nonoperative with avoidance of elbow flexion, rest, ice, and anti-inflammatory medication. Night-time extension splinting is often quite helpful in reducing symptoms early in the disease process, and daytime splinting at 30 to 45 degrees of elbow flexion, if tolerated, is also helpful. Corticosteroid injections are not recommended due to the superficial position of the nerve. Conservative management will often fail in athletes due to high demands, especially if there is a subluxing ulnar nerve. Surgical indications include failed nonoperative management, muscle atrophy, and severe sensory deficits. Surgery is effective at preventing further nerve injury, and recovery after surgery is uncertain. Several techniques have been used, including simple decompression, medial epicondylectomy, subcutaneous transposition, and submuscular transposition. With each technique, the ulnar nerve should be released at all possible sites of compression, from the ligament of Struthers proximally, through the cubital tunnel, and past the two heads of the flexor carpi ulnaris. Each technique has potential complications and approximately an 85% success rate. After brief postoperative immobilization, passive and then active range of motion is begun, followed by strengthening. Throwing exercises are started by the eighth postoperative week. Complications are uncommon but, in addition to other surgical risks, include injury to the medial antebrachial cutaneous nerve and worsening of symptoms possibly from compromised blood flow to the nerve or perineural scarring. Unrecognized medial elbow pathology will also limit success.

Conservative therapy has excellent results except in high-demand athletes. Results of surgical intervention vary inversely with degree of preoperative nerve involvement. Many patients with good to excellent results return to unrestricted play by 6 months postoperatively. This can be career-ending for a throwing athlete if symptoms are not mild and have been present for a long time prior to treatment.

Frantz LM, Adams JM, Granberry GS, Johnson SM, Hearon BF. Outcomes of ulnar nerve anterior transmuscular transposition and significance of ulnar nerve instability in cubital tunnel syndrome. *J Shoulder Elbow Surg.* 2019;28(6):1120-1129. [PMID: 30770314]

BICEPS TENDON TEARS AT THE ELBOW

Essentials of Diagnosis

- *"Popeye" appearance of the biceps muscle from proximal retraction.*
- *May or may not be painful and ecchymotic depending on the time from injury.*
- *Weakness of elbow flexion and forearm supination.*

Prevention

General conditioning and stretching and strengthening before activities can help minimize injury to the biceps tendon.

Clinical Findings

The long head of the biceps tendon may rupture distally at the insertion into the radial tuberosity, at the myotendinous junction, or within the muscle itself. The muscle mass moves proximally, producing a bulging or "Popeye" appearance to the arm. Rupture of the biceps tendon distally involves both heads. The mechanism is usually a forceful flexion of the arm and is more common in older athletes or following direct trauma. Microtears probably serve to render the tendon vulnerable to an acute tearing event. The amount of ecchymosis after the injury is dependent on the location of the tear, with avascular areas having less ecchymosis and the musculotendinous junction producing quite a noticeable amount of ecchymosis. Diagnosis is usually easily accomplished, as the deformity is obvious.

Treatment

Partial tears of the biceps tendon at the elbow can be initially treated nonoperatively and with surgery if symptoms prevent return to normal activities. In older individuals, nonoperative treatment is an option for complete rupture, although elbow flexion and forearm supination remain weak and supination is more noticeable as they may cope with other elbow flexors. In others, rupture of the distal biceps tendon often warrants surgical repair and is effective in restoring strength of elbow flexion and forearm supination. The tendon is easily found after acute injury, about 6 cm above the elbow joint, and care must be taken to avoid damage to the lateral antebrachial cutaneous nerve. After approximately 3 months, the tendon may be coiled up and scarred, and restoration of normal muscle contour may be difficult. Surgical repair can be been done with a two-incision technique, and the tendon that avulsed is sewed back though holes in the bone or one-incision techniques using anchors.

Prognosis

Athletes are permitted to return to full-contact play once healing is sufficient and they have achieved maximal functional strength and range of elbow motion, which typically occurs 4 to 6 months following a distal biceps repair. Complications include loss of elbow range of motion, rerupture, nerve injuries (sensory injury of the lateral antebrachial nerve or more severe motor injury of the posterior interosseous portion of the radial nerve), heterotopic bone, and synostosis of the radius and ulna.

Bauer TM, Wong JC, Lazarus MD. Is nonoperative management of partial distal biceps tears really successful? *J Shoulder Elbow Surg.* 2018;27(4):720-725. [PMID: 29396100]

Ford SE, Andersen JS, Macknet DM, Connor PM, Loeffler BJ, Gaston RG. Major complications after distal biceps tendon repairs: retrospective cohort analysis of 970 cases. *J Shoulder Elbow Surg.* 2018;27(10):1898-1906. [PMID: 30139681]

Schmidt CC, Brown BT, Schmidt DL, et al. Clinical and functional impairment after nonoperative treatment of distal biceps ruptures. *J Shoulder Elbow Surg.* 2019;28(4):757-764. [PMID: 30595503]

OTHER ELBOW OVERUSE INJURIES

1. Posterior and Posteromedial Elbow Impingement

Essentials of Diagnosis

- *Posterior elbow pain during terminal extension of the throwing arm or posteromedial elbow pain during the acceleration phase of throwing.*
- *Loss of elbow extension and tenderness along the posterior or posteromedial olecranon.*
- *Pain elicited with forced rapid elbow extension in presence of valgus load.*
- *Posterior and posteromedial olecranon osteophyte sometimes visible on plain films.*
- *Associated with valgus extension overload and valgus instability.*

Impingement may result from mechanical abutment of bone and soft tissues in the posterior elbow. This may or may not be associated with injury of the ulnar collateral ligament.

Hyperextension injuries with an intact ulnar collateral ligament occur in gymnasts, football lineman, weightlifters,

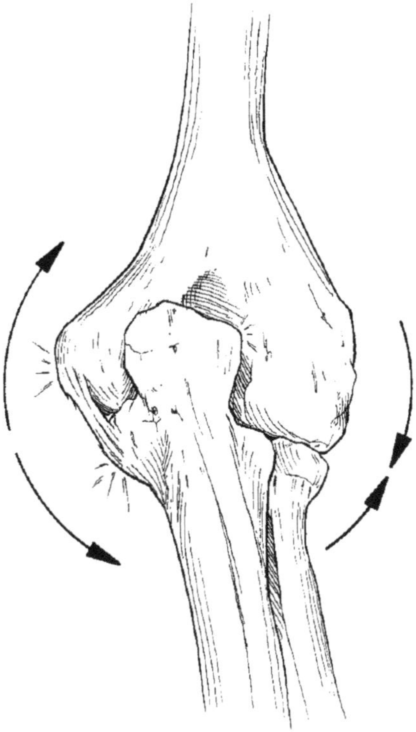

▲ **Figure 3–19.** Mechanism of posteromedial impingement between the medial aspect of the olecranon and the lateral side of the medial wall of the olecranon fossa. (Adapted from Kvitne RS, Jobe FW: Ligamentous and posterior compartment injuries, in Jobe FW [ed]: Techniques in Upper Extremity Sports Injuries. Philadelphia: Mosby-Year Book, 1996.)

and others. The lesion is usually located in the center of the posterior elbow, and the pain is reproduced by forcible extension of the elbow. If there is insufficiency of the ulnar collateral ligament, as is often the case when there is posterior elbow impingement in overhead athletes, the lesion is posteromedial. In this case, the impingement is between the medial aspect of the olecranon and the lateral side of the medial wall of the olecranon fossa (Figure 3–19). Pain may be reproduced with the valgus stress test, as described earlier for valgus instability, but the pain is posteromedial and medial. Radiographs may demonstrate osteophytes of the olecranon fossa.

As with most injuries caused by repetitive trauma, treatment begins with prevention. The number of innings pitched is probably the most important factor relating to injury. If symptoms persist, removal of osteophytes is successful treatment, provided that no ulnar collateral ligament injury is present. Treatment of the valgus instability is also required for a successful outcome.

Koh JL, Zwahlen BA, Altchek DW, Zimmerman TA. Arthroscopic treatment successfully treats posterior elbow impingement in an athletic population. *Knee Surg Sports Traumatol Arthrosc.* 2018;26(1):306-311. [PMID: 28534159]

2. Fatigue Fracture of the Medial Epicondyle

Essentials of Diagnosis

- *Sudden onset of medial epicondyle pain and swelling from throwing.*

In children, fatigue fractures of the medial epicondyle cause pain and swelling. This has been blamed on throwing curve balls, but some studies have shown that a properly thrown curve ball causes no more injuries than the traditional fastball. Prevention or minimization of damage involves several steps. First, it is important to maintain proper conditioning by continuing pitching practice in the off-season or beginning the baseball season in a slow progressive fashion. Second, pain and inflammation should be avoided, and if the elbow becomes painful, the athlete should stop throwing immediately. An accurate pitching count should be kept during a game, and a stopping point should be planned in advance. If the pitcher begins having pain or shows loss of control, pitching should be temporarily terminated, and treatment to decrease the swelling and inflammation should begin. No competitive throwing is allowed until full range of motion returns and no pain or tenderness is associated with throwing.

3. Osteochondritis Dissecans of the Capitellum

Essentials of Diagnosis

- *Gradual onset of lateral elbow pain in overhead athletes and gymnasts.*
- *Catching or locking of the elbow.*
- *Grinding of the lateral elbow.*
- *There may be loss of range of motion, especially if there is an effusion or there are associated loose bodies.*

Osteochondritis dissecans of the capitellum affects pitchers over 10 years of age (Figure 3–20) and gymnasts sometimes at an earlier age. Changes in the radiocapitellar joint are very worrisome because of possible permanent loss of function. Nonoperative treatment of cessation of inciting activities often results in lesion healing in the pediatric population. Many surgical procedures have been described, but if fragmentation occurs, small loose bodies may require excision. Osteochondral transplants have been effective for larger lesions.

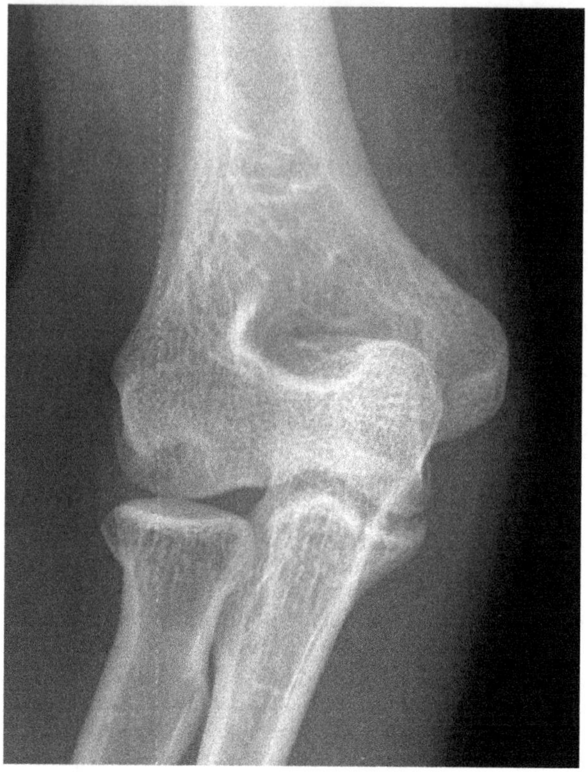

▲ **Figure 3–20.** Anteroposterior view of an elbow with osteochondritis dissecans of the capitellum.

Kessler JI, Jacobs JC Jr, Cannamela PC, Weiss JM, Shea KG. Demographics and epidemiology of osteochondritis dissecans of the elbow among children and adolescents. *Orthop J Sports Med.* 2018;6(12):2325967118815846. [PMID: 30622996]

Niu EL, Tepolt FA, Bae DS, Lebrun DG, Kocher MS. Nonoperative management of stable pediatric osteochondritis dissecans of the capitellum: predictors of treatment success. *J Shoulder Elbow Surg.* 2018;27(11):2030-2037. [PMID: 30340803]

Wang KK, Williams K, Bae DS. Early radiographic healing and functional results after autologous osteochondral grafting for osteochondritis dissecans of the capitellum: introduction of a new magnetic resonance imaging-based scoring system. *Am J Sports Med.* 2020;48(4):966-973. [PMID: 32053395]

Sports Medicine: Lower Extremity

4

Aaron Wynkoop, MD
Connor Kasik, DO
Patrick DeMeo, MD
Sam Akhavan, MD
Lee D. Kaplan, MD
Patrick J. McMahon, MD

KNEE INJURIES

Anatomy

The bones of the knee, the distal femur, the proximal tibia, and the patella depend on supporting ligaments, the joint capsule, and the menisci to provide stability for the joint.

A. Menisci and Joint Capsule

The menisci, or semilunar cartilages, are C-shaped fibrocartilaginous structures that provide shock absorption, allow for increased congruency between joint surfaces, enhance joint stability, and aid in distribution of synovial fluid.

The medial and lateral menisci provide a concave surface with which the convex femoral condyles can articulate. If the menisci are not present, the convex femoral condyles articulate with the relatively flat tibial plateaus, and the joint surfaces are not congruent. This decreases the surface area of contact and increases the pressure on the articular cartilage of the tibia and femur, which may lead to rapid deterioration of the joint surface. The medial meniscus is firmly attached to the joint capsule along its entire peripheral edge. The lateral meniscus is attached to the anterior and posterior capsule, but there is a region posterolaterally where it is not firmly attached (Figure 4–1). This results in the medial meniscus being less mobile than the lateral meniscus and more susceptible to tearing when trapped between the femoral condyle and tibial plateau. The lateral meniscus is larger than the medial meniscus and carries a greater share of the lateral compartment pressure than the medial meniscus carries for the medial compartment.

B. Ligaments

Within the knee, the anterior cruciate ligament (ACL) prevents anterior translation and rotation of the tibia on the femur (Figure 4–2). The posterior cruciate ligament (PCL) prevents posterior subluxation of the tibia on the femur. (Figure 4–3). On the medial side, the medial collateral ligament has superficial and deep portions (Figure 4–4), which stabilize the knee to valgus stresses. The lateral collateral or fibular collateral ligament runs from the lateral femoral condyle to the head of the fibula. It is the main stabilizer against varus stress (Figure 4–5). The lateral collateral ligament is part of the posterolateral "complex" or "corner" of the knee that also resists external rotation. An important component is the popliteofibular ligament, present in 90% of knees, that runs from the tendon of the popliteus muscle to the styloid on the posterior fibular head.

History and Physical Examination

A. General Approach

The history of a knee injury may be obtained by asking the patient the questions listed in Table 4–1. The physical examination begins with observation of the patient's gait. The uninjured knee is then examined for comparison with the injured knee. Note atrophy of any of the muscles. Assess for deformity, crepitus, and any swelling or effusion. A small effusion will cause obliteration of the recesses on the medial and lateral aspects of the patellar tendon; with a larger effusion, there is diffuse swelling of the suprapatellar pouch. Then, a fluid wave can be palpated on the sides of the patella. The knee is palpated to define areas of localized tenderness including the femoral condyles, joint lines, tibial plateaus, quadriceps tendon, patellar tendon, and patellofemoral joint as these may give clues as to a possible osteochondral lesion, meniscus lesion, fracture, or chondrosis, respectively. The joint lines are located at the level of the inferior pole of the patella when the knee is flexed to 90 degrees. Active and then passive range of motion is evaluated. Check for joint hypermobility, meaning the joints move beyond the normal range of motion. Range-of-motion evaluation of the injured knee may also reveal loss of full extension, and it is important to treat this before stiffness ensues. Evaluate strength of the

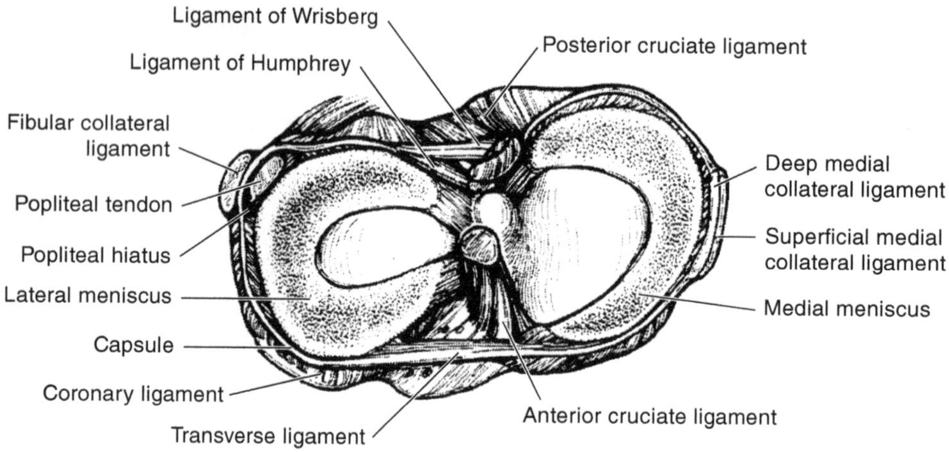

▲ **Figure 4–1. The medial and lateral menisci with their associated intermeniscal ligaments. Note: The lateral meniscus is not attached in the region of the popliteus tendon.** (Reprinted with permission, from Scott WN. *Ligament and Extensor Mechanism Injuries of the Knee: Diagnosis and Treatment*. New York: Mosby-Year Book; 1991.)

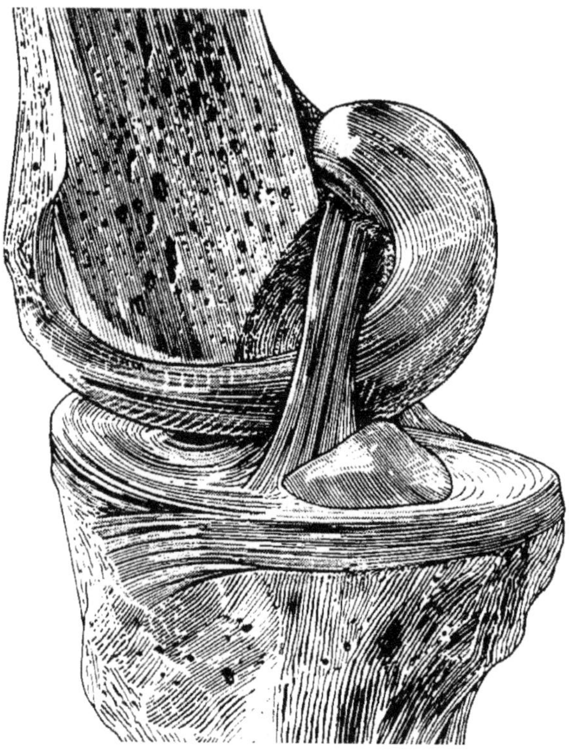

▲ **Figure 4–2. Drawing of the anterior cruciate ligament with the knee in extension, showing the course of the ligament as it passes from the medial aspect of the lateral femoral condyle to the lateral portion of the medial tibial spine.** (Reprinted with permission, from Girgis FG, Marshall JL, Monajem A. The cruciate ligaments of the knee joint: anatomical, functional, and experimental analysis. *Clin Orthop Relat Res*. 1975;106:216.)

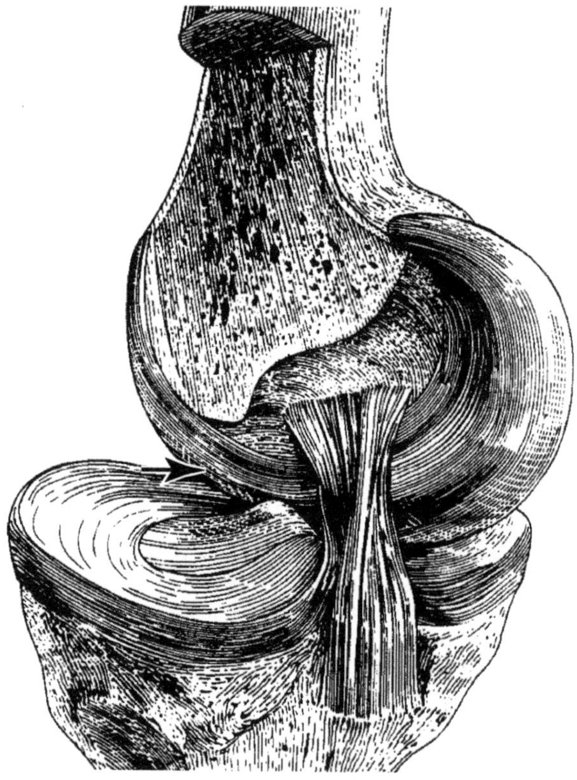

▲ **Figure 4–3. Drawing of the posterior cruciate ligament, showing the course of the ligament as it passes from the lateral aspect of the medial femoral condyle to the posterior surface of the tibia.** (Reprinted with permission, from Girgis FG, Marshall JL, Monajem A. The cruciate ligaments of the knee joint: anatomical, functional, and experimental analysis. *Clin Orthop Relat Res*. 1975;106:216.)

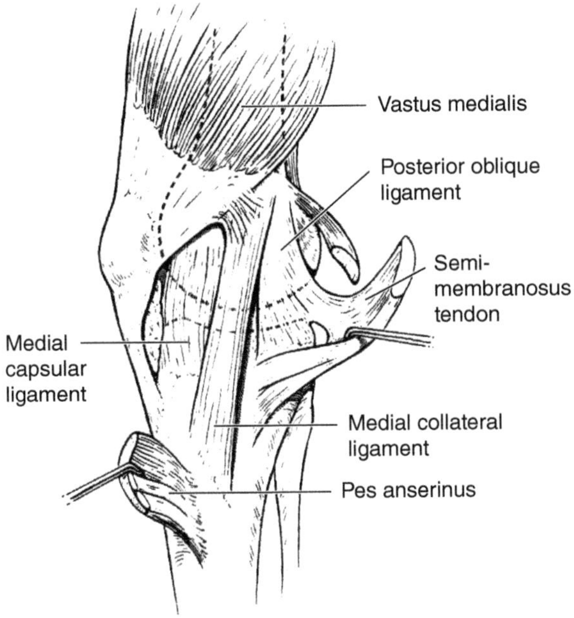

▲ **Figure 4–4.** Medial capsuloligamentous complex. (Reprinted with permission, from Feagin JA Jr. *The Crucial Ligaments*: diagnosis and treatment of ligamentous injuries about the knee. New York: Churchill Livingstone; 1988.)

knee in flexion and extension. It is important to also assess the remainder of the leg. For example, assessing hip range of motion and irritability is useful, especially in children, as referred pain from the hip to the knee area is common.

B. Collateral Ligament Evaluation

Most ligament injuries are graded as follows: grade 1, pain and no detectable instability likely from stretching or a very minor tear; grade 2, pain with mild to moderate instability from further stretching or an incomplete tear with the fibers in continuity; and grade 3, pain and severe instability from complete disruption of the ligament.

Table 4–1. History of a knee injury.

Did an injury occur?	Yes: possible ligament tear or meniscus tear. No: overuse problem or degenerative condition.
Was it a noncontact injury?	Yes: often the ACL is the only ligament torn.
Was it a contact injury?	Yes: possible multiple ligament injuries, including ACL and MCL, ACL and LCL, ACL, PCL, and a collateral ligament.
Did the patient hear or feel a pop?	Yes: a pop often occurs with ACL tears.
How long did it take to swell up?	Within hours: often an ACL tear. Overnight: often a meniscus tear.
Does the knee lock?	Yes: often a meniscus tear flipping into and out of the joint.
Does it buckle (trick knee)?	Yes: not specific; may arise from quadriceps weakness, trapped meniscus, ligament instability, or patella dislocating.
Is climbing or descending stairs difficult?	Often patellofemoral problems.
Are cutting maneuvers difficult?	ACL tear.
Is squatting (deep knee bends) difficult?	Meniscus tear.
Is jumping difficult?	Patellar tendinitis.
Where does it hurt?	Medial joint line: medial meniscus tear or medial compartment arthritis. MCL: MCL sprain. Lateral joint line: lateral meniscus tear, injury, iliotibial band tendinitis, popliteus tendinitis.

ACL, anterior cruciate ligament; LCL, lateral collateral ligament; MCL, medial collateral ligament; PCL, posterior cruciate ligament.

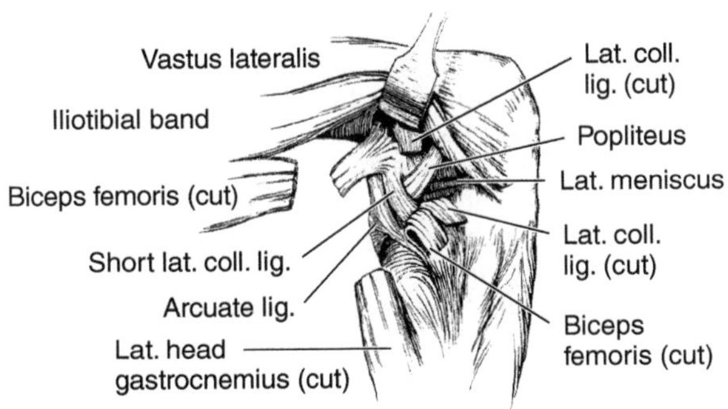

▲ **Figure 4–5. The lateral supporting structures of the knee.** (Reprinted with permission, from Rockwood CA Jr, Green DP, Bucholz RW, et al. *Fractures in Adults*, 2nd ed. New York: Lippincott; 1984.)

The collateral ligaments are evaluated with varus and valgus stability of the knee. The patient's foot can be held between the examiner's elbow and hip, leaving both hands free to palpate the joint (Figure 4–6). Stability should be determined at both full extension and 30 degrees of knee flexion. Pain but no varus or valgus instability indicates a mild ligament injury. Instability in full extension is an ominous sign that indicates disruption of key ligamentous structures. If significant valgus instability is present in full extension, the posteromedial capsule and medial collateral ligament are torn. With varus instability in full extension, the posterolateral capsular complex is torn, in addition to the lateral collateral ligament. With either varus or valgus

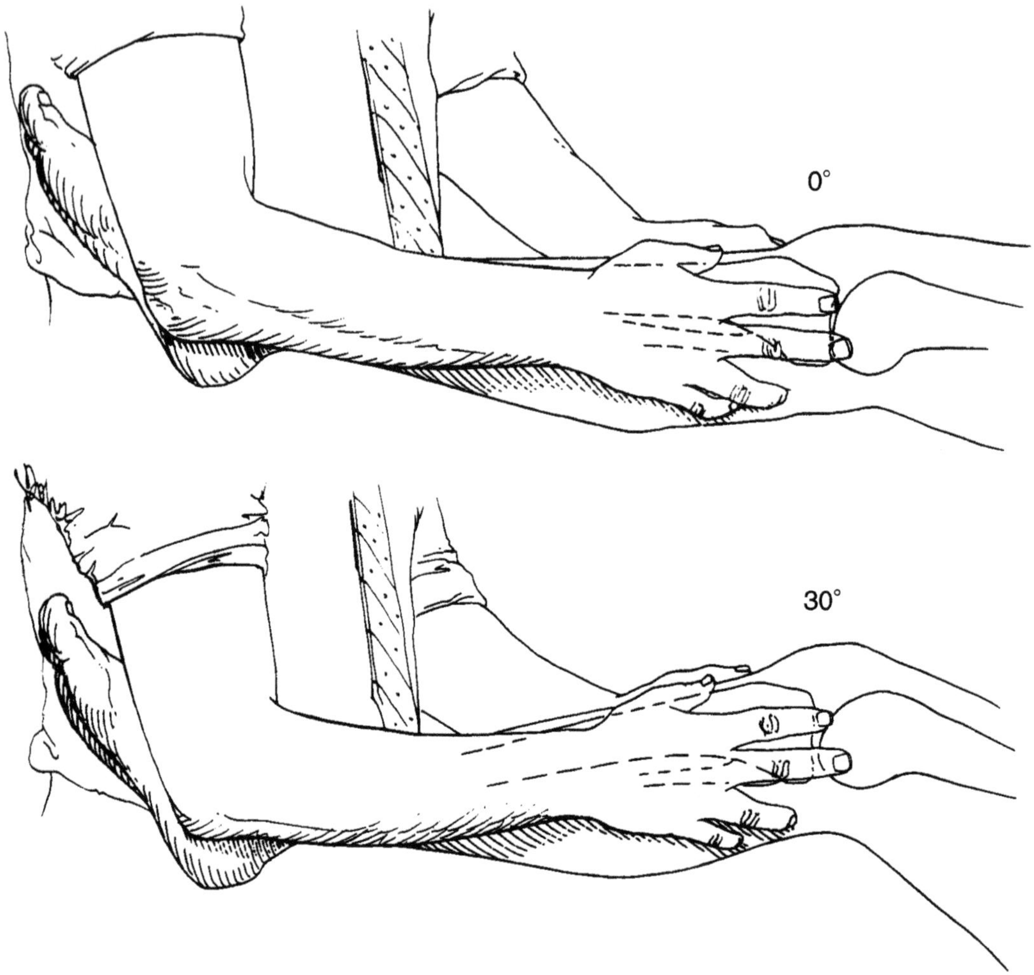

▲ **Figure 4–6. The collateral ligaments being tested in extension and 30 degrees of flexion with the foot held between the examiner's elbow and hip.** (Reprinted with permission, from Feagin JA Jr. *The Crucial Ligaments*: diagnosis and treatment of ligamentous injuries about the knee. New York: Churchill Livingstone; 1988.)

instability in full extension, cruciate ligament tears are also likely. At 30 degrees of flexion, the posterior capsule and cruciate ligaments are relaxed and the medial and lateral collateral ligaments are isolated, so varus or valgus instability will be present with collateral ligament injury.

C. Lachman Test

The Lachman test is the most sensitive test for ACL tears. It is done with the knee flexed 20 to 30 degrees, stabilizing the distal femur with one hand and pulling forward on the proximal tibia with the other hand (Figure 4–7). Cruciate ligament injuries can also be graded based on the amount of anterior translation compared to the uninjured knee and the character of an end point. With an intact ligament, minimal translation of the tibia occurs and there is a firm end point. Grade 1 is 1 to 5 mm of increased translation. Grade 2 is 6 to 10 mm of increased translation. Grade 3 is more than 10 mm of translation as compared to the uninjured knee. The character of the end point can be firm, designated as A, or soft, designated as B. The hamstring muscles must be relaxed during this maneuver to prevent false-negative findings. Comparison of the injured and uninjured knees is essential.

D. Anterior Drawer Test

The anterior drawer test is done with the knee at 90 degrees of flexion and is not as sensitive as the Lachman test but serves as an adjunct in the evaluation of ACL instability (Figure 4–8). With the patient supine and the knee

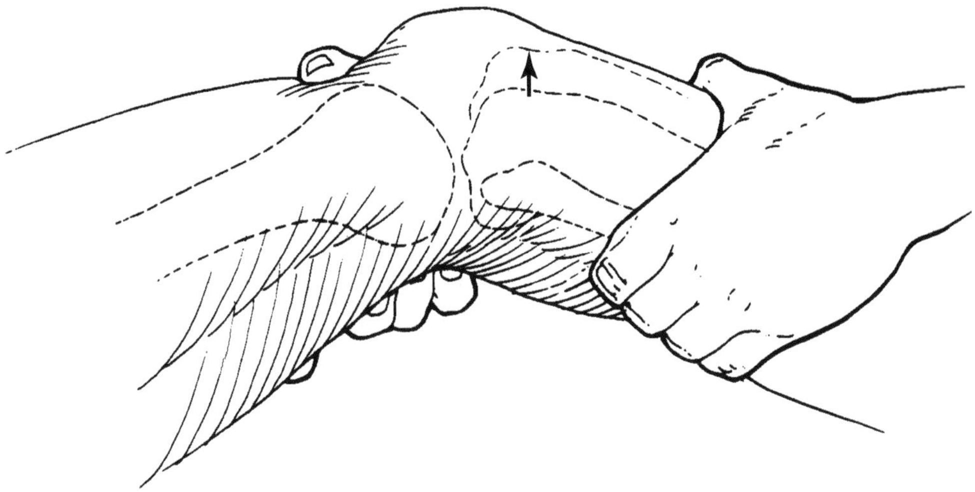

▲ **Figure 4–7. Lachman test.** (Reprinted with permission, from Feagin JA Jr. *The Crucial Ligaments*: diagnosis and treatment of ligamentous injuries about the knee. New York: Churchill Livingstone; 1988.)

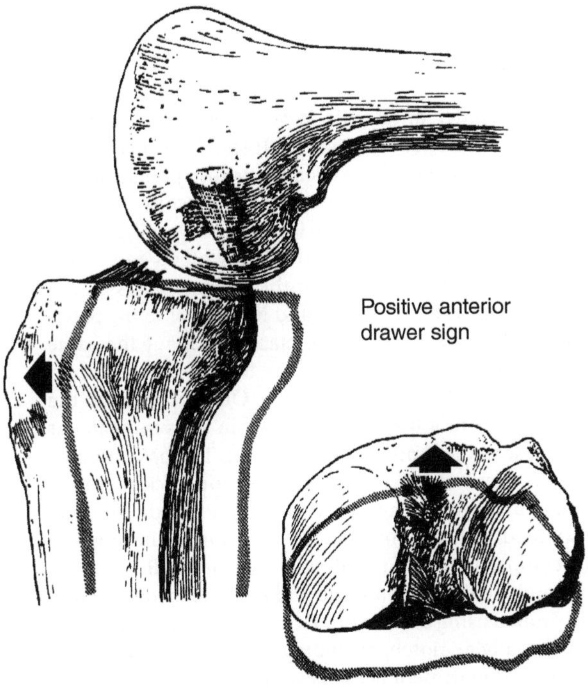

▲ **Figure 4–8. A positive anterior drawer test signifying a tear of the anterior cruciate ligament.** (Reprinted with permission, from Insall JN. *Surgery of the Knee*. New York: Churchill Livingstone; 1984.)

flexed to 90 degrees (hip flexed to about 45 degrees), the foot is restrained by sitting on it and the examiner's hands are placed around the proximal tibia. Then, while the hamstrings are felt to relax and the tibia is pulled forward, the displacement and the end point are evaluated.

E. Losee Test

The pivot shift phenomenon demonstrates the instability associated with an ACL tear. Once demonstrated, it is often difficult to repeat because the patient may find this maneuver uncomfortable and will guard against having it done again. As described by Losee, a valgus and internal rotation force is applied to the tibia (Figure 4–9). Starting at 45 degrees of flexion, the lateral tibial plateau is reduced. Extending the knee causes the lateral plateau to subluxate anteriorly with

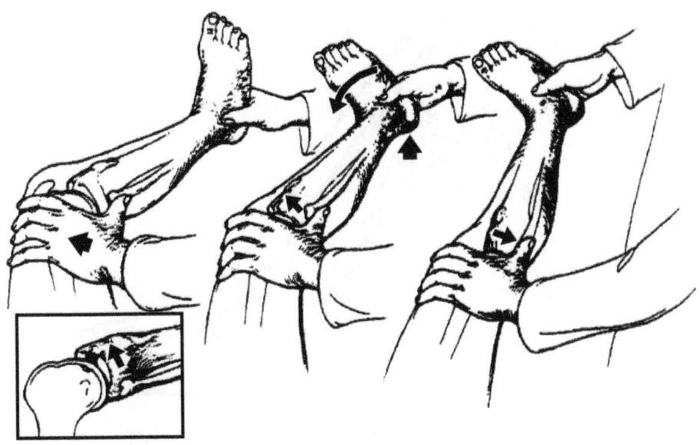

▲ **Figure 4–9. The Losee pivot shift test.** (Reprinted with permission, from Scott WN. *Ligament and Extensor Mechanism Injuries of the Knee: Diagnosis and Treatment*. New York: Mosby-Year Book; 1991.)

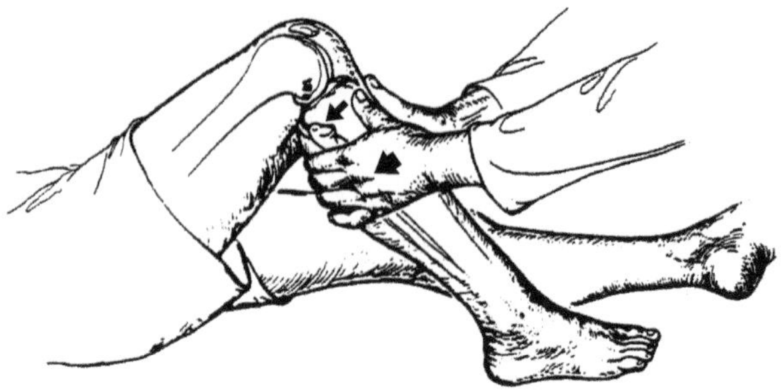

▲ **Figure 4–10. The posterior drawer test is done in the same fashion as the anterior drawer test, except that the examiner exerts a posterior force.** (Reprinted with permission, from Scott WN. *Ligament and Extensor Mechanism Injuries of the Knee: Diagnosis and Treatment.* New York: Mosby-Year Book; 1991.)

a thud at about 20 degrees of flexion. It reduces quietly at full extension. Many other ways of doing this test have been described, but the phenomenon and significance of the different tests are similar.

F. Posterior Drawer Test

The posterior drawer test evaluates the integrity of the PCL. It is performed with posterior pressure on the proximal tibia with the knee flexed at 90 degrees (Figure 4–10). Normally, the tibial plateau is anterior to the femoral condyles, and a "step-off" to the tibia is palpated when the thumb is slid down the femoral condyles. With a PCL injury, sagging of the tibial plateau may be appreciated, and no step-off is palpated (Figure 4–11).

G. McMurray Test

With the McMurray test, forced flexion and rotation of the knee will elicit a clunk along the joint line if there is a meniscus injury (Figure 4–12). Found in less than 10% of patients with a meniscus injury, joint line pain with the McMurray test is much more common.

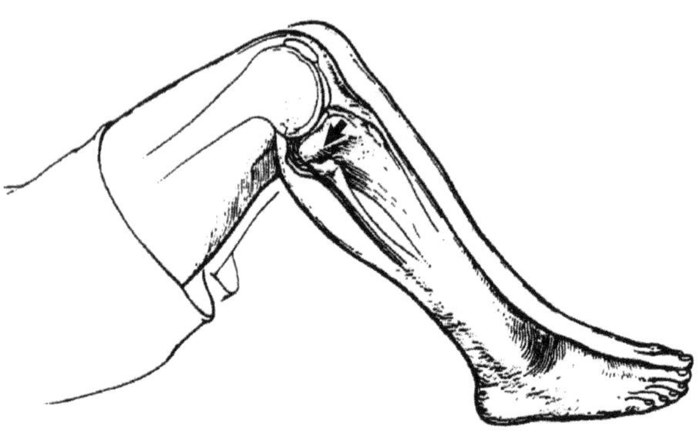

▲ **Figure 4–11. The posterior sag seen in posterior cruciate disruption.** (Reprinted with permission, from Scott WN. *Ligament and Extensor Mechanism Injuries of the Knee: Diagnosis and Treatment.* New York: Mosby-Year Book; 1991.)

Arthroscopic Examination

A. Indications for Knee Injuries

Indications for arthroscopic examination of the knee include the following:

1. Meniscus injuries
2. Loose bodies
3. Knee instability including patella instability
4. Select tibial plateau fractures
5. Chronic synovitis
6. Recurrent effusions
7. Chondral and osteochondral fractures
8. Acute knee joint infections

A specific diagnosis of the type of knee injury can usually be made with a history, physical examination, and appropriate imaging studies. With an examination under anesthesia and arthroscopic evaluation, a specific diagnosis can be confirmed, expanded, or revised, and treatment can be rendered as needed.

B. Technique

Examination under anesthesia is very helpful in diagnosing ligament injuries and instability. It should be performed before the beginning of the procedure, before preparing and draping the extremity. For diagnostic arthroscopy, the knee joint is distended with irrigating fluid (usually saline or lactated Ringer solution), which washes away blood and debris from the joint. A lateral portal for the arthroscope is placed at the level of the inferior patella and just lateral to the patellar tendon. The medial portal is placed at about the same level, but just medial to the patellar tendon for introducing arthroscopic tools such as a probe. One approach to the general inspection of the joint is to start in the suprapatellar pouch. Loose bodies and plicas are sought. The patellofemoral joint is then inspected and observed for tracking problems and cartilage damage. The lateral and medial gutters are examined with flexion of the knee, prior to entering the medial compartment. With valgus stress, the medial femoral condyle and medial tibial plateau and then the medial meniscus are probed using a nerve hook through the medial portal. The intercondylar notch, including the ACL, is inspected. The lateral compartment is then examined in a similar manner with varus stress. The posterior knee can be visualized, if needed, by placing the arthroscope through the intercondylar notch and with additional posteromedial and posterolateral portals. Documentation of findings and procedures

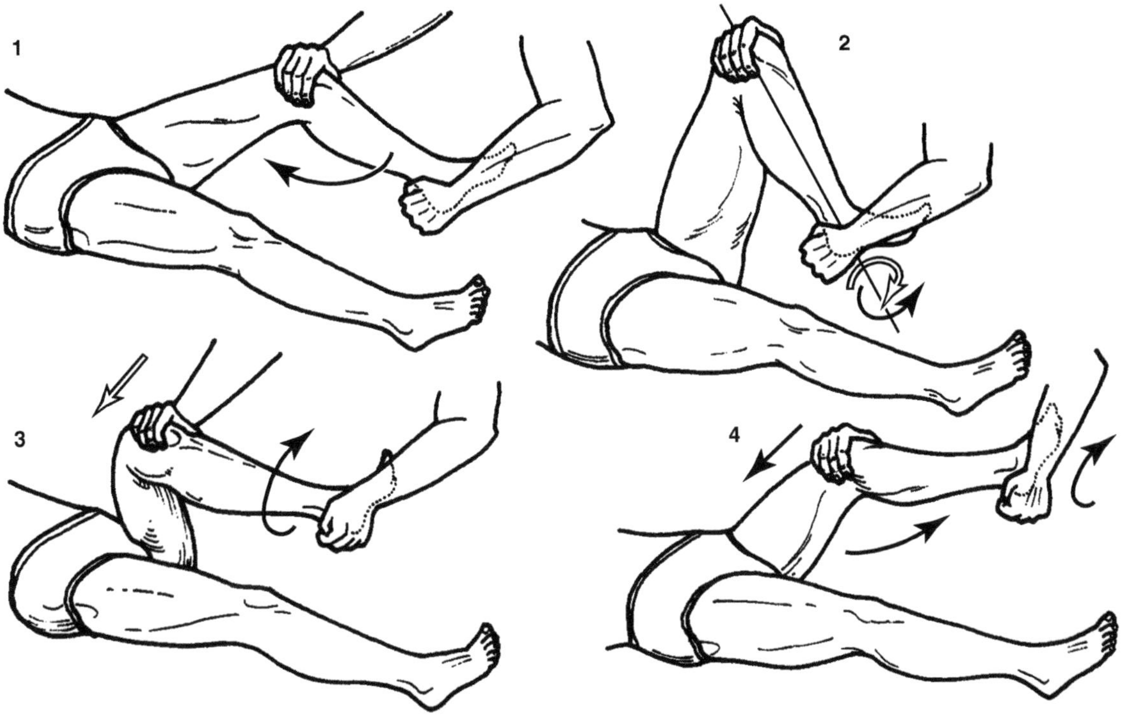

▲ **Figure 4–12. The McMurray test to produce click.** (Reproduced, with permission, from American Academy of Orthopaedic Surgeons. *Athletic Training and Sports Medicine*, 2nd ed. Burlington, MA: Jones and Bartlett; 1991.)

performed is important. With assessment of the pathologic changes, treatment can be initiated, such as debridement and repair of meniscus tears, removal of loose bodies, or ACL reconstruction.

Imaging and Other Studies

A. Magnetic Resonance Imaging

Magnetic resonance imaging (MRI) is a powerful technique for evaluation of the knee joint. While the diagnosis is usually evident from the history and physical examination, MRI can be used to confirm the suspected injury. Other times, when a physical examination is not possible because of pain or the diagnosis remains elusive, MRI can aid in a proper diagnosis. The specificity, sensitivity, and accuracy of MRI are greater than 90% for the medial and lateral menisci and the ACL and PCL. Therefore, MRI is often appropriate for ruling out the need for diagnostic arthroscopic examination. It is less helpful for the diagnosis of problems in knees with previous surgery.

B. Imaging Studies

X-rays of the knee is indicated in the evaluation of traumatic injury. In cases of minimal trauma, radiographs may not be needed if the injury proves to be self-limited. Arthrographic examination can be helpful in patients who are unable to undergo MRI because of claustrophobia, metal in the body that may be dislodged, electronic devices such as cardiac pacemakers and defibrillators that may be damaged, or other contraindications.

C. Laboratory Tests

Laboratory tests may be helpful in ruling out nonmechanical disorders such as inflammatory arthritis, as described in Chapter 7.

Lau BC, Vashon T, Janghala A, Pandya NK. The sensitivity and specificity of preoperative history, physical examination, and magnetic resonance imaging to predict articular cartilage injuries in symptomatic discoid lateral meniscus. *J Pediatr Orthop*. 2018;38(9):e501-e506. [PMID: 30036288]

Saygili A, Albayrak S. Knee meniscus segmentation and tear detection from MRI: a review. *Curr Med Imaging Rev*. 2020;16(1):2-15. [PMID: 31989889]

Suchman KI, Behery OA, Mai DH, Anil U, Bosco JA. The demographic and geographic trends of meniscal procedures in New York State: an analysis of 649,470 patients over 13 years. *J Bone Joint Surg Am*. 2018;100(18):1581-1588. [PMID: 30234622]

MENISCUS INJURY

Essentials of Diagnosis

- *Acute tears most commonly occur with axial loading combined with rotation.*
- *Sensation of clicking or catching of the knee with motion.*
- *Positive joint line tenderness and presence of effusion are important physical exam findings. There may also be a positive McMurray test.*
- *MRI can help classify location and morphology.*

Meniscal injuries are the most common reason for arthroscopy of the knee. The medial meniscus is more frequently torn than the lateral meniscus because the medial meniscus is securely attached around the entire periphery of the joint capsule, whereas the lateral meniscus has a mobile area where it is not attached. Meniscus injury is rare in childhood, occurs in the late teens, and peaks in the third and fourth decades. After the age of 50, meniscus tears are more often the result of arthritis than trauma.

Clinical Findings

Acute traumatic tears of the menisci are often caused by axial loading combined with rotation. Patients typically report pain and swelling. Patients may also have a sensation of clicking or catching in the knee. Patients with larger tears in the meniscus may complain of locking of the knee as the meniscus displaces into the joint and/or femoral notch. Loss of knee motion with a block to extension may result from a large bucket handle tear. In acute tears involving an associated ACL injury, the swelling may be more significant and acute. Acute ACL injuries often involve a meniscus tear.

Conversely, chronic or degenerative tears of the menisci often present in older patients (>50 years old) with a history of an insidious onset of pain and swelling with or without an acute increase superimposed. Often, no identifiable history of trauma is obtained, or the inciting event may be quite minor such as a bending or squatting motion.

The most important physical examination findings in the knee with a meniscus tear are joint line tenderness and an effusion. Other specialized tests include the McMurray, flexion McMurray, and Apley grind tests. The McMurray test is performed with the patient lying supine with the hip and knee flexed to about 90 degrees. While one hand holds the foot and twists it from external to internal rotation, the other hand holds the knee and applies compression (Figure 4–12). A positive test is one that elicits a pop or click that can be felt by the examiner when the torn meniscus is trapped between the femoral condyle and tibial plateau. A variation of this test is the flexion McMurray, in which the knee is held as for the McMurray test. To test the medial meniscus, the foot is externally rotated and the knee maximally flexed. A positive test occurs when the patient experiences pain over the posteromedial joint line as the knee is gradually extended. To test the lateral meniscus, the foot is internally rotated, and the knee is taken through the same range of motion. The Apley grind test requires placing the patient prone with the knee flexed to 90 degrees. The examiner applies downward pressure to the sole of the foot while twisting the lower leg in external and internal rotation. A positive test results in pain at either joint line.

Tear Classification

Meniscal tears can be classified either by etiology or by their arthroscopic and MRI appearance. Etiologic classification divides tears into either acute tears (excessive force applied to an otherwise normal meniscus) or degenerative tears (normal force applied to a degenerative structure).

Classification should describe the tear location and its associated vascularity, morphology, and stability. Tear location is described by its location in the anteroposterior plane (anterior, middle, or posterior) and its circumferential location with respect to its vascularity. The common vascular zones are named with regard to the vascularity on either side of the tear. For instance, the most peripheral zone near the meniscocapsular junction is referred to as the red-red zone due to good vascularity on either side of the tear. The intermediate red-white zone has decreased vascularity on the side farthest from the capsule, while the most central white-white zone has no vascularity on either side of the tear. As tears occur more centrally, the healing rate is lower because of a decreased blood supply. Tears can also occur at the meniscal root, which is the attachment of the meniscus to the tibia. These tears should be repaired when possible, as the circumferential fibers of the meniscus become incompetent in the setting of a root tear leading to ineffective load-dispersing abilities of the meniscus.

Tear morphology describes the orientation of the tear within the meniscus and includes vertical longitudinal tears that are perpendicular to the tibial surface and parallel to the meniscus, vertical radial tears that are perpendicular to both the tibial surface and the meniscus, horizontal tears (ie, cleavage), oblique tears (ie, flap tears that are a combination of horizontal and longitudinal), root tears, and complex tears, which are combinations of the prior and include degenerative tears (Figure 4–13). Oblique, bucket handle, and parrot beak tears can displace significantly. Vertical longitudinal tears can be complete or incomplete and usually start in the posterior horn and continue anteriorly a variable distance. When large, they have been coined bucket handle tears. Large tears can cause significant mobility of the torn meniscal fragment, allowing it to displace into the femoral notch and cause a locked knee (Figure 4–14). This more commonly occurs in the medial meniscus, possibly owing to its decreased mobility. Oblique tears commonly occur at the junction of the middle and posterior thirds. Complex or degenerative tears occur in multiple planes and are often

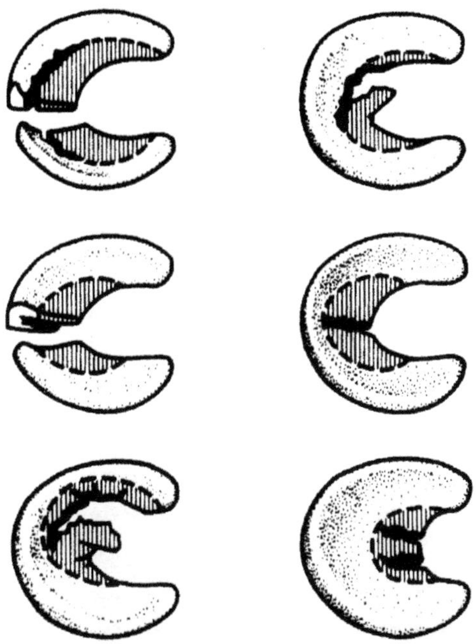

▲ **Figure 4–13. Patterns of meniscal tears: bucket handle, flap, horizontal cleavage, radial, degenerative, and double radial tear of a discoid meniscus.** (Reproduced, with permission, from Scott WN. *Arthroscopy of the Knee.* New York: WB Saunders; 1990.)

located in or near the posterior horns. Horizontal longitudinal tears are often associated with meniscal cysts. These tears usually start at the inner margin of the meniscus and extend toward the meniscocapsular junction. They are thought to result from shear stresses and, when associated with meniscal cysts, occur in the medial meniscus and cause localized swelling at the joint line. Most acute tears in younger patients are vertical or oblique tears, whereas complex and degenerative tears occur more commonly in older patients.

Treatment and Prognosis

Before the importance of the meniscus was understood and arthroscopy became available, the meniscus was often removed, even when normal. We now attempt to repair the meniscus or remove only the torn portion of the meniscus.

During arthroscopy, the meniscus can be visualized and palpated with a probe. The inner two-thirds of the adult meniscus are avascular and often require resection when torn, and the remaining meniscus is smoothed and contoured to prevent further tearing. Return to full function may be expected in 6 to 8 weeks.

Tears in the peripheral third of the meniscus, if small (<15 mm), may heal spontaneously and become asymptomatic because there is a blood supply in this portion of the adult meniscus. For larger tears of this region at a young age, every effort should be made to repair the meniscus because those who undergo meniscectomy are at risk of early osteoarthritis. Incomplete tears are likely to heal and do not need to be repaired unless the tear results in persistent pain or catching.

A. Partial Meniscal Resection

Partial meniscectomy has a 90% rate of good or excellent results in patients without knee instability or osteoarthritis. A major advantage over meniscus repair is a short recovery period. However, results diminish over time, and osteoarthritis often occurs with over 10 years of follow-up. Medial meniscus tears generally do better than lateral tears after partial resection, and an intact meniscal rim and those with normal articular cartilage and normal knee stability are associated with a better prognosis.

B. Meniscus Repair

Most surgeons will attempt a meniscus repair rather than a partial meniscectomy in young, active individuals. Other commonly accepted criteria for meniscus repair include a complete vertical longitudinal tear greater than 15 mm in length, a tear within the peripheral third of the meniscus, a peripheral tear that can be significantly displaced with a probe, the absence of secondary meniscus degeneration, absence of osteoarthritis, and a tear in a patient undergoing concurrent ligament or articular cartilage repair.

Multiple factors affect the success of meniscus repair. Although no absolute age limit exists, patients younger than 40 years are thought to have a better chance for healing. Knees with associated ligamentous instability, particularly persistent instability after ACL rupture, have inferior rates of meniscus healing. The location of the tear and the time lapsed from injury to treatment are also important. Acute tears located in the peripheral red-red or red-white zone have better healing than chronic tears located in the red-white or white-white zones. Tears 5 mm or more from the periphery are considered avascular (white zone), whereas those between 3 and 5 mm are variable in vascularity (red-white), and tears in the peripheral 3 mm are considered vascular (red). In areas with marginal vascularization, abrasion of the meniscocapsular junction or use of a fibrin clot may be performed. Finally, the stability of the meniscus repair is a factor, with vertical mattress sutures generally considered best for meniscus repair. The superiority of vertical mattress over horizontal mattress sutures may be from the vertical mattress sutures capturing the strong peripheral, circumferential fibers of the meniscus.

While persistent ACL instability decreases meniscal healing, meniscus repair is more successful when done with ACL reconstruction. Successful meniscal repair approaches up to 90% when combined with ACL reconstruction, compared to lower success rates for meniscal repairs in patients with intact ACLs. Many of the meniscus tears that occur with an

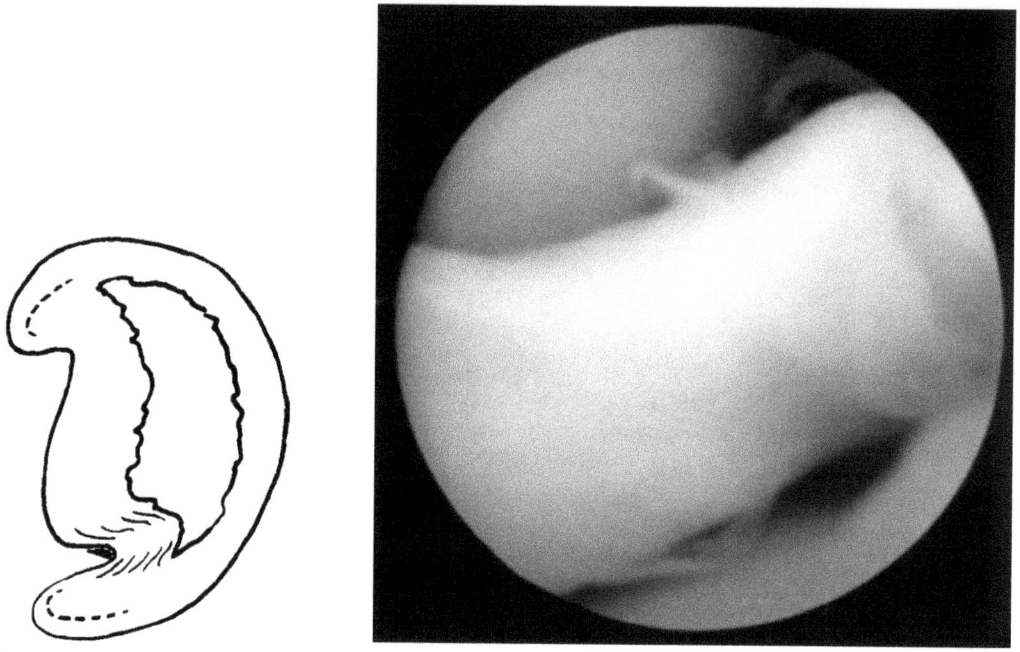

A B

▲ **Figure 4–14. A:** Diagram of a typical bucket handle tear of the medial meniscus. **B:** Arthroscopic view of a bucket-handle fragment displaced into the intercondylar notch. (Reproduced, with permission, from McGinty JB. *Operative Arthroscopy*. Baltimore: Raven Press; 1991.)

acute ACL tear are amenable to repair. Stabilizing the knee with ACL reconstruction protects the repaired meniscus from abnormal knee motion and is more successful than when the knee is unstable.

Types of repairs include the traditional open repair and arthroscopic repairs that can be done with inside-out, outside-in, or all-inside techniques. Inside-out and outside-in repairs are usually done with sutures and require a mini-incision and securing of the meniscus to the capsule with sutures. There are many options for all-inside repair, including sutures and various polymer devices. Regardless of the type of repair chosen, adequate preparation of the tear site is required. The tear edges should be debrided or abraded with a shaver or rasp to stimulate bleeding. Restoration of biomechanical function is encouraged by anatomic apposition of the tear edges to ensure good healing potential.

1. Open meniscal repair—Open repair of meniscus tears has been shown to have successful long-term results. The technique involves making a small incision through the subcutaneous tissue, capsule, and synovium to directly visualize the tear. Open repair is most useful in peripheral or meniscocapsular tears, often occurring in conjunction with open repair of a collateral ligament injury or a tibial plateau fracture. Follow-up studies of 10 years or longer have shown survival rates of 80% to 90% of repaired menisci", in part influenced by the peripheral nature of the tear and the associated hemarthrosis present in ligament tears or fracture repair cases.

2. Arthroscopic meniscal repair

A. INSIDE-OUT MENISCAL REPAIR—Arthroscopic inside-out meniscus repairs are performed using cannula systems to introduce long, flexible needles with attached sutures that are passed across the tear from inside the knee to a protected area outside the joint capsule. Sutures can be placed in various configurations for repair of common tears, but there is risk of neurovascular injury from the needles, sutures, and retraction of the soft tissues. This technique requires a posteromedial or posterolateral incision to protect the neurovascular structures and safely retrieve the exiting needles. Because surgeons are able to place vertical mattress sutures, the best biomechanical construct for meniscus repair, this technique remains the gold standard for many surgeons. Root repairs can be done with inside-out techniques. Healing of the inside-out meniscus repairs have consistently shown rates of 70% to 90% in isolated repairs, and greater than 90% when done in conjunction with an ACL reconstruction. This technique is ideal for posterior and mid-posterior horn tears. There is difficulty in passing needles in mid to anterior horn meniscus tears.

B. OUTSIDE-IN MENISCAL REPAIR—The arthroscopic outside-in repair was developed in part to decrease the neurovascular risk associated with the inside-out technique. The outside-in technique involves passing a needle from outside the joint, across the tear, and into the joint. Two options then exist for repair of the meniscus tear. One option is then to retrieve the suture through an anterior portal, tie a knot outside the knee joint, and then bring the knot back in through the anterior portal placing the knot against the reduced meniscus body fragment. A second option is to use parallel needles and retrieve the suture through the second needle. This can be done using a suture relay. A knot is then tied outside the joint over the capsule. This method is useful for tears in the anterior horn or body of the menisci but does not work for tears in or near the posterior horn. Results of the outside-in technique using MRI, arthrography, or second-look arthroscopy to assess healing have shown complete or partial healing; between 74% and 87% of meniscus repairs have been successful. As expected, repairs of the posterior horn nearer the posterior root that are technically difficult and tears in unstable knees did worse.

C. ALL-INSIDE MENISCAL REPAIR—All-inside repairs do not require accessory incisions, thereby saving operative time, and they avoid more technical arthroscopic techniques required in other types of repairs. However, repairs with some devices have been less successful compared with traditional techniques. Success rates may be comparable to inside-out techniques. Some concerns with the all-inside repairs arise from the potential complications, including devices that have migrated from their original position, broken fragments, foreign-body reactions, inflammation, chronic effusions, and articular cartilage injuries.

Recent biomechanical studies have found repair with some of these devices to have properties equivalent to vertical mattress sutures, although there is considerable variation with the type of device. What remains to be known, however, is the meniscus repair strength needed for optimal meniscus healing.

C. Meniscal Transplantation

An alternative to leaving the patient with a meniscus-deficient knee, and almost certain early osteoarthrosis, is meniscus transplantation. This technique yields satisfactory results in about two-thirds of patients, although patient selection is of the utmost importance. Appropriate patients are ligamentously stable, without significant malalignment, and free of any cartilage damage. Both medial and lateral menisci can be transplanted, although the techniques vary according to the location. Donor menisci are sized via three-dimensional imaging to match the appropriate candidates. In the future, biologic scaffolds may enable menisci to be regenerated after meniscectomy.

Bezuglov EN, Lyubushkina AV, Khaitin VY, et al. Prevalence of asymptomatic intra-articular changes of the knee in adult professional soccer players. *Orthop J Sports Med.* 2019;7(11):2325967119885370. [PMID: 32010730]

Everhart JS, Magnussen RA, Cavendish PA, et al. Subjective knee function and risk of failure are equivalent for men and women at 5 years after meniscus repair. *Arthroscopy.* 2020;36(3):816-822. [PMID: 31919022]

Krych AJ, Bernard CD, Kennedy NI, et al. Medial vs. lateral meniscus root tears: is there a difference in injury presentation, treatment decisions, and surgical repair outcomes? *Arthroscopy.* 2020;36(4):1135-1141. [PMID: 31973989]

Spang RC 3rd, Getgood A, Strickland SM, Amendola AN, Gomoll AH. Optimizing anterior cruciate ligament (ACL) outcomes: what else needs fixing besides the ACL? *Instr Course Lect.* 2020;69:653-660. [PMID: 32017758]

Thaunat M, Fournier G, O'Loughlin P, et al. Clinical outcome and failure analysis of medial meniscus bucket-handle tear repair: a series of 96 patients with a minimum 2 year follow-up. *Arch Orthop Trauma Surg.* 2020;140(11):1649-1654. [PMID: 31993744]

KNEE OSTEOCHONDRAL LESIONS

Articular cartilage injuries of the knee are infrequent, and there must be a high index of suspicion to detect them. MRI and arthroscopy are very helpful with these injuries, especially small, isolated articular cartilage injuries, where radiographs will be normal.

Essentials of Diagnosis

- *Patients usually present with vague, poorly localized complaints of knee pain.*
- *Classic location is the posterolateral aspect of the medial femoral condyle.*
- *Involvement is bilateral in up to 25% of cases, so examine both knees.*
- *Effusion, crepitus, and an antalgic gait are possible findings on exam.*
- *Radiographs and MRI can be helpful in determining the location and size of the lesion.*

Osteochondral Fracture (ie, Osteochondritis Dissecans)

The term *osteochondral injuries* is used to describe injuries ranging from acute osteochondral fractures to pure chondral injuries. Osteochondral lesions, also termed *osteochondritis dissecans* (OCD), start as potentially reversible lesions of subchondral bone resulting in delamination or fragmentation, with or without destruction of the overlying articular cartilage. OCD is subdivided into juvenile and adult forms depending on the presence of an open distal femoral physis, and there is a male predominance of 2:1. A combination of etiologies is now thought to be responsible for OCD.

Although seemingly idiopathic, a stress fracture may develop in the subchondral bone of the distal femoral condyle. Such an injury may provoke further vascular compromise, which results in injury to the subchondral bone that was initially covered with normal articular cartilage. Loss of support from the subchondral bone may result in damage to the overlying articular cartilage. The vast majority of adult OCDs are thought to have arisen from a persistent juvenile OCD lesion, although new lesions in adults are possible as well.

Both adult and juvenile OCDs that do not heal have the potential for further sequelae, including loose bodies and degenerative osteoarthritis. Juvenile OCDs, defined as knees with an open physes, generally have a better prognosis than adult lesions. The classic location of OCD is the posterolateral aspect of the medial femoral condyle, which accounts for 70% to 80%. Lateral condyle OCD is seen in 15% to 20% of patients, and patellar involvement ranges from 5% to 10%.

Clinical Findings

A common presentation of a patient with OCD is aching and activity-related knee pain that is poorly localized. Pain may worsen with stair climbing or running. Patients may also report mechanical symptoms if articular cartilage damage is present, resulting in an unstable or loose OCD lesion. Patients may present with an antalgic gait, and knee effusion or crepitus may be present upon examination. Pain with range of motion or specific tenderness with palpation of the femoral condyle may be observed with varying degrees of knee flexion. Loss of range of motion or quadriceps atrophy may be noted in more long-standing cases.

It is important to identify patients with unstable lesions. Involvement is bilateral in up to 25% of cases, so both knees should be evaluated regardless of symptoms. Initial evaluation should include anteroposterior, lateral, and tunnel (notch) views of both knees. The goal of plain radiographs is to evaluate for arthritis and loose bodies, exclude any other bony pathology, evaluate the physes, and localize the lesion. Lesion location and an estimation of size can also be assessed. An MRI is frequently helpful to localize the lesion and give an estimation of its size, the condition of the overlying cartilage, condition of underlying subchondral bone, extent of bone edema, and presence of any loose bodies and to provide clues of OCD stability. A high signal line is the most common sign in patients found to have unstable lesions that are most likely to fail nonoperative treatment. Arthroscopy remains the gold standard in evaluation of these lesions.

Treatment and Prognosis

Prognosis is good for an immature child. Predictors of poor prognosis include closed physes, larger lesion size, lesions in the lateral femoral condyle or patella, sclerosis on plain radiographs, and fluid present behind the lesion on MRI. Nonoperative management should be pursued in those with a stable OCD lesion and open physes. The goal of nonoperative treatment is for the lesion to heal before physis closure so as to prevent early-onset osteoarthritis. Even if patients are within 6 to 12 months of physeal closure, a trial of nonoperative treatment is warranted.

Because failure of the subchondral bone precedes failure of the overlying articular cartilage, most orthopedists recommend some sort of activity modification. Debate exists on whether activity modification should include the use of cast or brace immobilization. The tenet of nonoperative treatment is to reduce the activity level until the patient can perform activities of daily living without pain. However, there is no optimal immobilization protocol known.

Patients should be non–weight bearing or partial weight bearing with crutches for 3 to 6 weeks or until they are pain-free. Repeat radiographs are obtained at approximately 6-week intervals. Physical therapy with full weight bearing may be initiated once patients are pain-free. Physical therapy should focus on low-impact quadriceps and hamstring strengthening. If patients remain asymptomatic up to at least 3 months after the diagnosis was made, activity may be slowly advanced to higher-impact activities such as running or jumping. Any recurrence of symptoms or any progression of the OCD on plain radiographs should prompt a return to non–weight bearing and possible immobilization for a longer period. Patient frustration and lack of compliance (especially in adolescents) is common, and a full discussion of the risks and benefits of nonoperative and operative treatment is required.

Operative treatment should be considered in the following instances: (1) loose bodies, (2) an unstable OCD lesion, (3) persistence of symptoms despite nonoperative treatment in a compliant patient, (4) worsening appearance on imaging studies, and (5) near or complete epiphyseal closure. Goals of operative treatment should include achievement of a stable OCD lesion that maintains joint congruity and allows early range of motion.

For stable lesions with an intact articular surface, arthroscopic procedures can create channels for potential revascularization through the subchondral bone. Options include transarticular and transepiphyseal stimulation. Postoperative radiographic healing and relief of symptoms can be expected in 80% to 90% of patients with open physes. This decreases to 50% to 75% in those with closed physes.

Patients with partially unstable flap lesions should be managed by the status of the subchondral bone. Fibrous tissue between the lesion and subchondral bone should be debrided if present. If significant subchondral bone loss has occurred, it can be filled with bone graft prior to fixation of the lesion. If the OCD has sufficient bone such that an anatomic fit into its donor site is possible, fixation should be attempted. Various fixation methods have been described including screws, headless compression screws, and bioabsorbable screws or pins. Complications with these treatments include migration of devices from their original position, broken fragments, foreign-body reactions, inflammation, chronic effusions, and articular cartilage injuries.

Simple excision of the larger fragments has shown poor results with more rapid progression of osteoarthritis. For lesions greater than 2 cm^2, drilling or microfracture methods that lead to filling of the defect with fibrocartilage have yielded poor results with worsening osteoarthritis over time. For these larger lesions, there has been success with cartilage repair procedures such as osteochondral cartilage replacement and autologous chondrocyte transplantation. Disadvantages of autologous chondrocyte transplantation, also known as mosaicplasty, include donor site morbidity and incongruent articular fit. Advantages include good, immediate fixation of the patient's own articular cartilage. Autologous chondrocyte implantation, which involves harvesting of the patient's chondrocytes, proliferating them over time, and then reimplanting the chondrocytes also uses the patient's own tissue and has lessened donor site morbidity. A major disadvantage is that it requires two surgeries. Longer-term results in young adult patients show successful clinical results in up to 90% for both procedures.

Chahla J, Stone J, Mandelbaum BR. How to manage cartilage injuries? *Arthroscopy.* 2019;35(10):2771-2773. [PMID: 31604490]

Perelli S, Molina Romoli AR, Costa-Paz M, Erquicia JI, Gelber PE, Monllau JC. Internal fixation of osteochondritis dissecans of the knee leads to good long-term outcomes and high degree of healing without differences between fixation devices. *J Clin Med.* 2019;8(11):1934. [PMID: 31717628]

Tírico LEP, McCauley JC, Pulido PA, Bugbee WD. Lesion size does not predict outcomes in fresh osteochondral allograft transplantation. *Am J Sports Med.* 2018;46(4):900-907. [PMID: 29360386]

Wang D, Lin KM, Burge AJ, Balazs GC, Williams RJ 3rd. Bone marrow aspirate concentrate does not improve osseous integration of osteochondral allografts for the treatment of chondral defects in the knee at 6 and 12 months: a comparative magnetic resonance imaging analysis. *Am J Sports Med.* 2019;47(2): 339-346. [PMID: 30543757]

Wang K, Waterman B, Dean R, et al. The influence of physeal status on rate of reoperation after arthroscopic screw fixation for symptomatic osteochondritis dissecans of the knee. *Arthroscopy.* 2020;36(3):785-794. [PMID: 31870748]

KNEE LIGAMENT INJURY

Knee injuries occur during both contact and noncontact athletic activities. Advances in the diagnosis and treatment of ligament injuries have allowed athletes at all levels of ability to return to sports at their preinjury level of activity. The ligaments and menisci of the knee work in concert with one another, and frequently, more than one structure is damaged when an acute injury occurs.

Anatomy

Knee stability requires proper functioning of four ligaments. These ligaments include the ACL, the PCL, the medial collateral ligament (MCL), and the lateral collateral ligament (LCL). There are also several accessory or secondary stabilizers of the knee. Secondary stabilizers of the knee include the menisci, iliotibial band, and biceps femoris. These secondary stabilizers become more important when a primary stabilizer is injured.

The MCL is the primary static stabilizer against valgus stress at the knee. The MCL originates from the central sulcus of the medial epicondyle. The sulcus of the C-shaped medial epicondyle is located anterior and distal to the adductor tubercle. The MCL is made up of three main static medial stabilizers of the knee. These include the superficial MCL, the posterior oblique ligament, and the deep capsular ligament.

The LCL is the primary static stabilizer against varus stress at the knee. The LCL originates from the lateral epicondyle. This is the most prominent point of the lateral femoral condyle. The LCL insertion is on the styloid process of the fibular head, which projects superiorly from the posterolateral fibular head. The LCL joins with the arcuate ligament, the popliteus muscle, and the lateral head of the gastrocnemius to form a lateral arcuate complex to control statically and dynamically varus angulation and external tibial torsion. The iliotibial band and biceps femoris also contribute to stability on the lateral aspect of the knee.

The ACL is the primary static stabilizer of the knee against rotation and anterior translation of the tibia on the femur. The ACL originates anterior to the "over the top" position from the posteromedial surface of the lateral femoral condyle in the intercondylar notch. The ACL inserts on the tibial plateau anterolateral to the medial tibial spine and posterior to the intermeniscal ligament. This is just medial to the anterior horn of the lateral meniscus and about 15 mm posterior to the anterior edge of the tibial articular surface. The ACL is composed of two bands: the anteromedial band that is tight in flexion and the posterolateral band that is tight in extension. The blood supply to the ACL and PCL is the middle geniculate artery. Both the ACL and PCL are covered by a layer of synovium, making these ligaments intraarticular and extrasynovial. The PCL is the primary static stabilizer of the knee against posterior translation of the tibia on the femur. The PCL originates from the anterolateral medial femoral condyle in the intercondylar notch. The PCL inserts on the posterior aspect of the tibial plateau in a central depression just posterior and below the articular surface. The insertion extends distally along the posterior aspect of the tibia for up to 1 cm in length. The PCL is a complex structure consisting of two major bands: the anterolateral and posteromedial bands. The anterolateral band is tight in flexion and the posteromedial band is tight in extension. The cross-sectional area of the anterolateral band is twice as large as the posteromedial band. The meniscofemoral ligaments, the ligaments of Humphrey and Wrisberg, are anterior and posterior to the PCL, respectively, and run from the posterior horn of the lateral meniscus to the posteromedial femoral condyle.

Differential Diagnosis of Knee Instability

The differential diagnosis of acute or chronic knee instability can involve any of the knee ligaments and/or the structures of the posterolateral corner. There are often combinations of ligament injuries in addition to injuries of secondary stabilizing structures such as the menisci. The history and mechanism of injury are valuable. Similarly, the location of pain can help to narrow the diagnosis. A thorough physical examination helps to distinguish which ligaments have been injured. Additionally, imaging studies are often obtained to confirm clinical suspicions and to evaluate for occult injuries.

Ekås GR, Ardern CL, Grindem H, Engebretsen L. Evidence too weak to guide surgical treatment decisions for anterior cruciate ligament injury: a systematic review of the risk of new meniscal tears after anterior cruciate ligament injury. *Br J Sports Med.* 2020;54(9):520-527. [PMID: 31959673]

Verhulst FV, MacDonald P. Diagnosing PCL injuries: history, physical examination, imaging studies, arthroscopic evaluation. *Sports Med Arthrosc Rev.* 2020;28(1):2-7. [PMID: 31895325]

1. Medial Collateral Ligament Injuries

Essential of Diagnosis

- *Occurs after a valgus stress to the knee or noncontact rotational injury.*
- *Medial knee pain and instability to valgus stress at 30 degrees of flexion; consider ACL or PCL injury in addition if there is instability to valgus stress in full extension.*
- *Chronic injuries may have calcification at the insertion of the MCL on the medial femoral condyle (Pellegrini-Stieda lesion).*
- *MRI can be helpful in confirming diagnosis and helping to rule out meniscal injury.*

Symptoms (History)

Mechanism of injury and the duration of symptoms can significantly aid in diagnosis. Lower-grade MCL injuries typically occur in a noncontact external rotational injury, whereas higher-grade injuries generally involve lateral contact to the thigh or upper leg. Other important pieces of the history include the location and presence of pain, instability, timing of swelling, and sensation of a "pop" or tear. Surprisingly, grade 1 and 2 injuries are often more painful than complete MCL rupture. Immediate swelling or joint effusion should make one suspicious for an associated cruciate ligament injury, fracture, and/or patellar dislocation.

A prior history of knee injuries or instability should always be sought when evaluating a new knee injury. MCL injuries are similar in female and male athletes.

Signs (Physical Examination)

A complete knee examination is important in evaluating MCL injuries. For example, additional ACL injury, PCL injury, or patellofemoral instability may change treatment. Tenderness of the MCL is typical at the location of the tear. Pain and instability to valgus stress are assessed at 30 degrees of knee flexion where the MCL is the primary restraint. In full extension, the posterior capsule and PCL will stabilize the knee to valgus stress. Grade 1 and 2 injuries typically have a firm end point, whereas a grade 3 injury tends to have a soft end point to valgus stress.

Imaging Studies

A. Radiographs

Knee radiographs should be obtained in any patient with a suspected significant knee injury. Radiographs should be inspected for acute fracture, lateral capsular avulsion (Segond fracture; see section on ACL imaging), loose bodies, Pellegrini-Stieda lesion (MCL calcification at the medial femoral condyle), and evidence of patellar dislocation. Stress radiographs should be obtained in patients prior to skeletal maturity to rule out an epiphyseal fracture.

B. MRI

MRI is useful for confirming MCL injury and identifying the site of injury. It is also useful to detect the presence of meniscal and other injuries to the knee. Relative indications for an MRI include an uncertain cruciate injury, the patient guarding during examination and evaluation of a suspected meniscal tear, or preoperative evaluation for a planned MCL reconstruction or repair.

C. Special Tests

An examination under anesthesia can be valuable when physical examination is unreliable because of the patient guarding the knee. Diagnostic arthroscopy can also be used to evaluate for coexistent pathology. However, both of these diagnostic methods have largely been replaced by MRI.

Treatment (Nonsurgical and Surgical)

Treatment of an isolated MCL injury is generally nonoperative with protection against valgus stress and early motion. Grade 1 and grade 2 injuries can be placed in a brace and bear weight as tolerated. Generally, knee motion is started within the first week or two, and full recovery is usually achieved more rapidly with early knee range of motion.

Grade 3 injuries are a bit more controversial. Comparison of isolated grade 3 MCL tears treated with nonsurgical reconstruction and surgical management showed that the nonsurgical treatment group enjoyed better results in both subjective scoring and earlier return to activity. But there may be increased instability in grade 3 tears treated nonsurgically, although most of the studies evaluating this did not exclude knees with multiligamentous injuries. There is also controversy in regard to MCL injuries in the multiligament injured knee. Some recommend early reconstruction of the cruciate ligament injury and nonoperative treatment of the MCL injury. Others delay cruciate reconstruction until the MCL has healed. And still others reconstruct the cruciate ligament injury and attempt repair of the MCL.

Operative treatment is indicated in the setting of chronic valgus instability, bony avulsions, and entrapment of the ligament over the pes anserinus tendons. MCL surgical treatment in the acute setting can include a primary repair, with shortening if needed, of the torn ligament. Similarly, avulsion fragments, although rare, are treated with reduction and fixation in the acute setting. Primary repairs can be reinforced with autograft or allograft tissues if the remaining MCL is insufficient. Chronic reconstructions also often include autograft or allograft tissue reconstruction.

Early motion and strengthening of the knee can occur at an early stage while the ligament is protected from valgus stress. As knee motion improves, strengthening exercises are introduced. As the strength of the extremity improves, the intensity of functional rehabilitation increases accordingly.

Complications

With nonsurgical treatment becoming the standard of care, complications associated with an MCL injury have decreased. The main complication of nonsurgical therapy is residual valgus instability or medial knee pain. After healing, radiographs may show calcification of the MCL at the medial femoral condyle (Pellegrini-Stieda lesion). Potential surgical complications also include stiffness, infection, and damage to the saphenous nerve or vein.

Results/Return to Play

In general, good outcomes can be achieved with nonsurgical treatment and rehabilitation of isolated MCL injuries. Return to professional football after nonsurgical treatment of isolated MCL injuries is 98%.

Kramer DE, Miller PE, Berrahou IK, Yen YM, Heyworth BE. Collateral ligament knee injuries in pediatric and adolescent athletes. *J Pediatr Orthop*. 2020;40(2):71-77. [PMID: 31923166]

Motamedi AR, Gowd AK, Nazemi AK, Gardner ST, Behrend CJ. Incidence, positional distribution, severity, and time missed in medial collateral ligament injuries of the knee in NCAA Division I football athletes. *J Am Acad Orthop Surg Glob Res Rev*. 2017;1(5):e019. [PMID: 30211356]

Stanley LE, Kerr ZY, Dompier TP, Padua DA. Sex differences in the incidence of anterior cruciate ligament, medial collateral ligament, and meniscal injuries in collegiate and high school sports: 2009-2010 through 2013-2014. *Am J Sports Med*. 2016;44(6):1565-1572. [PMID: 26940226]

2. Lateral Collateral Ligament Injuries

Essentials of Diagnosis

- *Patients may complain of lateral knee pain and a varus thrust gait.*
- *Lateral knee pain and instability to varus stress at 30 degrees of flexion; consider ACL or PCL injury in addition if there is instability to varus stress in full extension.*
- *Frequently part of a multiligamentous injury to the knee.*
- *There is a high incidence of peroneal nerve injury; document neurovascular status to the involved leg.*
- *MRI should be obtained as a useful adjunct to help diagnose associated posterolateral corner injuries.*

Symptoms (History)

The most consistent symptom of an acute LCL injury is lateral knee pain. However, the symptoms of lateral and posterolateral instability are quite variable and depend on the severity of injury, patient activity level, overall limb alignment, and other associated knee injuries. For example, a sedentary individual with minimal laxity and overall valgus alignment will have few, if any, symptoms. However, if LCL laxity is combined with overall varus alignment, hyperextension, and high activity level, symptoms will be quite pronounced. These patients may complain of lateral joint line pain and a varus thrust of their leg with everyday activities. This is often described as the knee buckling into hyperextension with normal gait.

Signs (Physical Examination)

Patients with an LCL and/or posterolateral corner injury may also have cruciate ligament injuries or a knee dislocation. Therefore, a thorough knee examination should be performed to evaluate for other knee pathology. Additionally, a careful neurovascular examination should be performed as the incidence of neurovascular injury, particularly peroneal nerve injury, has been reported in 12% to 29% of posterolateral knee injuries.

The LCL is assessed with a varus stress of the knee in full extension and 30 degrees of flexion. Exam findings with an isolated LCL injury are varus instability at 30 degrees of knee flexion and none in full extension due to the stabilizing effect of the intact cruciate ligaments. Because laxity at 30 degrees of knee flexion is variable, it should be compared to the uninjured leg. The average baseline for varus laxity is 7 degrees.

It is important to note that a significant posterolateral knee injury can be present without significant varus laxity. The most useful test to evaluate for posterolateral instability is the dial test. This is done by externally rotating the tibia and noting the angle subtended between the thigh and the foot. The dial test is performed at both 30 and 90 degrees of knee flexion, with a significant difference being an angle 10 degrees or greater than the uninjured leg. Injury to the posterolateral corner alone is confirmed with greater external rotation at 30 degrees only, while an isolated PCL injury is confirmed with greater rotation at 90 degrees. Injury to both structures presents with greater external rotation of the foot at both 30 and 90 degrees compared to the uninjured leg.

Imaging Studies

A. Radiographs

A series of knee radiographs should be obtained in any patient with a suspected knee injury. Radiographs should be inspected for acute fractures, lateral capsular avulsion (Segond fracture; see section on ACL imaging), loose bodies, fibular head avulsions, and evidence of patellar dislocation. With chronic posterolateral instability, degenerative changes of the lateral compartment are often noted by lateral joint space narrowing with osteophytes and subchondral sclerosis. Stress radiographs can help to better quantify the amount of varus angulation present.

B. MRI

MRI is often a useful adjunct for diagnosing posterolateral corner and LCL injuries in the severely injured knee. As mentioned earlier, posterolateral corner injuries can go unnoticed during an initial evaluation as pain and guarding can obscure the full extent of the injury. MRI can be extremely helpful as findings can refocus the examination on the posterolateral corner.

C. Special Tests/Examinations

1. Reverse pivot shift test—This test involves starting with the knee flexed to 90 degrees. While the knee is extended, the leg is loaded axially with a valgus stress applied to the knee, and the foot is held in external rotation. A palpable shift is noted as the tibia reduces from its posteriorly subluxed position as the knee is extended, indicating a posterolateral corner injury.

2. External rotation recurvatum test—This test is performed with the patient supine and the hip and knee fully extended. The leg is lifted off the bed by the toes. Hyperextension, varus instability, and external rotation of the tibial tubercle occur with adequate quadriceps relaxation in a patient with posterolateral corner instability.

3. Posterolateral drawer test—A standard posterior drawer test (see section on PCL physical examination) can be performed with the tibia in internal rotation, neutral, and externally rotated positions. With posterolateral corner injuries, the magnitude of the posterior drawer displacement will be greatest with external tibial rotation.

4. Examination under anesthesia—An examination while the patient is relaxed under general anesthetic is extremely useful, particularly in the acute setting. If a patient with a multiligamentous knee injury is taken to the operating room, this is an excellent opportunity to examine the knee without guarding to improve the accuracy of the examination.

Treatment

A. Nonsurgical

Isolated LCL ligament injuries, as noted earlier, are rare injuries. However, in the case of an isolated grade 1 or 2 LCL ligament injury, a period of immobilization from 2 to 4 weeks followed by a quadriceps strengthening program will usually yield good results. Grade 3 injuries often have better results with surgical treatment. The combination of delayed diagnosis along with an uncertain natural history of posterolateral instability makes the treatment of these injuries a challenge.

B. Surgical

LCL and posterolateral corner injuries, as discussed earlier, rarely occur in isolation. Therefore, other injuries must also be considered in the treatment plan of the multiligamentous knee injury. Ideally, the posterolateral corner and LCL injuries are diagnosed in the acute setting. This allows the preferred surgical treatment of a primary repair of the injured structures with augmentation as needed. Primary repair is generally only feasible in the first few weeks following the knee injury.

The knee with chronic posterolateral instability will often require ligament. The key biomechanical concept of any lateral ligamentous reconstruction is that the LCL is isometric between the fibular head and the lateral epicondyle. Therefore, regardless of the graft material used to reconstruct the lateral ligamentous complex, a portion of the graft must pass between the lateral femoral epicondyle and the fibular head.

To improve the success rate of reconstruction of chronic lateral knee ligamentous instability, a proximal tibial valgus osteotomy may be performed to decrease the stress on the lateral structures of the knee.

Rehabilitation

The rehabilitation of the knee after posterolateral corner reconstructions or repairs is largely guided by associated injuries to the ACL or PCL. It is generally necessary to limit weight bearing for at least 6 weeks and protect the lateral structures with a brace for at least 3 months.

Complications

The peroneal nerve runs along the posterolateral knee, following the medial border of the biceps femoris and then wrapping around the fibular head. It is important to isolate the peroneal nerve prior to any lateral knee exposure to minimize the complication of nerve injury.

Results

If injuries to the posterolateral corner of the knee are diagnosed and repaired acutely, the results are good for restoration of varus stability and return to sports. Chronic posterolateral corner injury reconstructions also perform well when an isometric or anatomic lateral reconstruction is achieved, but chances of return to sports remain uncertain.

Pfeiffer TR, Herbst E, Kanakamedala AC, Naendrup JH, Debski RE, Musahl V. The use of fluoroscopy leads to improved identification of the femoral lateral collateral ligament origin site when compared with traditional tactile techniques. *Arthroscopy*. 2018;34(8):2487-2493.e1. [PMID: 29859771]

3. Anterior Cruciate Ligament Injuries

Essentials of Diagnosis

- *Mechanism is either noncontact deceleration/rotation injury of a slightly flexed knee or contact injury with valgus force to an extended knee.*
- *Patients often hear a "pop." Patients may have feelings of instability and the knee giving out with twisting activities.*
- *Substantial knee effusion is present within first 12 hours after injury.*
- *There is a high incidence of associated injuries, including meniscus tears.*
- *Lachman is most sensitive test for diagnosis; pivot shift or Losee test helps evaluate rotational instability.*
- *Segond sign (avulsion of the anterolateral capsule of the tibia) may be seen on plain radiographs.*
- *MRI is helpful to confirm diagnosis and evaluate for other knee injuries.*

Symptoms (History)

The mechanism of injury can guide evaluation of other injured structures. ACL injury can occur in a variety of ways; however, a few mechanisms predominate. The most common noncontact ACL injury mechanism involves a deceleration and rotational injury of the slightly flexed knee during running, cutting, or jumping activities. The most common contact injury involves either hyperextension and/or valgus forces to the knee by a direct blow.

ACL injury is often associated with a "pop" heard by the patient at the time of injury, although this is not specific. Upon return to sports, the patient will often notice instability of the knee or describe the knee "giving out" with twisting activities. Substantial knee swelling secondary to a hemarthrosis typically occurs within the first 4 to 12 hours after injury. ACL injuries are more common in female than male athletes.

Signs (Physical Examination)

With the aforementioned history obtained and a proper physical examination, an ACL tear can usually be diagnosed without any additional tests. A complete examination of the knee should be performed to evaluate for any associated injuries. The uninjured knee is examined first to familiarize the patient with the knee examination.

The Lachman test is the most useful test for anterior instability of the knee. The Lachman test is performed with the knee in 20 to 30 degrees of flexion as an anterior force is applied to the tibia while the other hand stabilizes the distal femur.

The anterior drawer test is another test to evaluate anterior tibial translation. This is performed with the knee in 90 degrees of flexion as an anterior force is applied to the tibia. This test is less sensitive than the Lachman test. The examiner should also ensure that the patient's tibia is starting in a normal resting position, which means the anterior tibial plateau is about a centimeter anterior to the medial femoral condyle in 90 degrees of flexion. A PCL incompetent knee can appear to have significant anterior translation on anterior drawer testing when in truth the tibia is starting posteriorly subluxed due to posterior instability.

After acute ACL tear, physical examination is best before knee swelling and hemarthrosis result in guarding. Aspiration of the hemarthrosis can help to decrease pain and improve the physical examination when it has already occurred.

The pivot shift test (Losee test) is performed to test the rotational instability associated with an ACL tear. The test is based on the lateral tibial plateau subluxing anteriorly with extension and reduction of the lateral compartment with flexion. The most effective method of achieving this result is by flexing the knee with an axial load from full extension with valgus stress at the knee and internal rotation of the tibia. The reduction of the subluxation should occur at approximately 30 degrees of flexion. MCL injury and some meniscal tears may produce a false-negative test.

The pivot shift test is considered the most functional test to evaluate knee stability after ACL injury, but it is usually uncomfortable. An examination under anesthesia is then useful in obtaining a more accurate pivot shift test. This can be useful in a patient with an unclear history of instability and an equivocal examination in the office.

Imaging Studies

Plain radiographs of the knee should be obtained to rule out fractures about the knee. The Segond fracture is an avulsion of the anterolateral capsule of the tibia. Most common before skeletal maturity, avulsion fractures of the tibial insertion of the ACL can also be seen radiographically. MRI is useful for evaluation of associated injuries. Although generally not needed, MRI can diagnose an ACL tear with 95% or better accuracy. Bone bruises of the lateral femoral condyle and lateral tibial plateau are noted in up to 80% of ACL injuries.

Treatment

A. Nonsurgical

Rehabilitation following an isolated ACL injury should include an effort to regain knee motion and strengthen the muscles about the knee. Returning to activities that produce episodes of instability is discouraged. Once motion and strength have been restored, a gradual return to activities can be attempted to determine the functional level that can be attained without instability.

The decision for ACL reconstruction is individualized and based on the patient's other knee injuries, desire to return to activity, age, presence of prior osteoarthritis, and objective and subjective knee instability. For example, a young, active patient with continued desire to compete in cutting and jumping sports with severe objective instability and subjective instability may be best treated with surgical reconstruction. On the other hand, an older patient with osteoarthritis and minimal desire for continued competitive athletics and mild objective instability and no subjective instability would be much more suited to nonsurgical care.

Significant episodes of instability resulting in pain, swelling, and disability follow nonoperative treatment of an ACL rupture in about 80% of individuals participating in twisting activities such as tennis, football, and soccer. These episodes of instability put the menisci and articular cartilage of the knee at increased risk of injury (Figure 4–15).

B. Surgical

The goal of ACL reconstruction is to reproduce the strength, function, and location of the intact ACL. The anterolateral ligament can be injured with the ACL, and some advocate its repair, but its role in knee instability remains controversial.

1. ACL repair—Early in the history of ACL surgery, primary repairs had poor results because the ACL did not heal. Recently, several new techniques of ACL repair have been developed in an effort to improve healing. These may allow

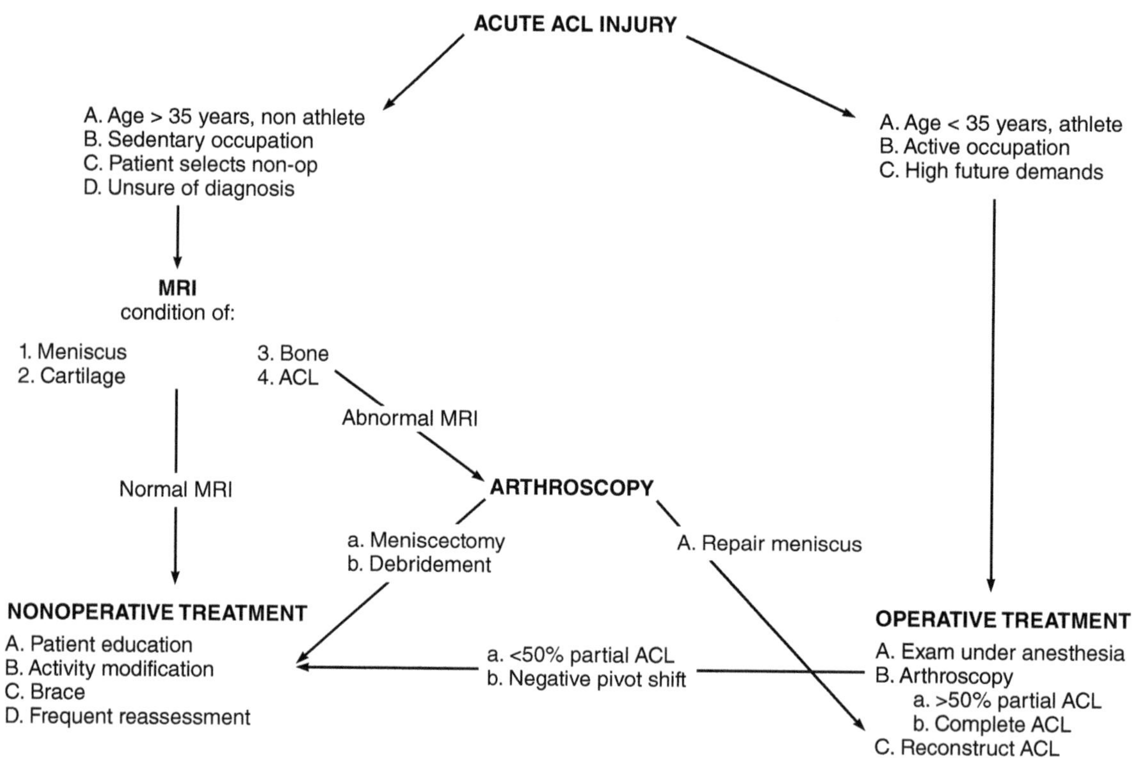

▲ **Figure 4–15.** Flow chart that summarizes the current management of acute anterior cruciate ligament (ACL) injuries. MRI, magnetic resonance imaging. (Reproduced, with permission, from Marzo JM, Warren RF. Results of nonoperative treatment of anterior cruciate ligament injury: changing perspectives. *Adv Orthop Surg*. 1991;15:59.)

repair of insertion site ruptures, use a scaffold soaked in autologous blood products, or use sutures or other devices to augment and aid in repair of the torn ACL. One potential advantage of repair is that it may maintain proprioception of the ACL. Studies reporting outcome of ACL repair have small numbers and short follow-up.

2. ACL reconstruction—ACL reconstruction is currently the standard, and grafts ranging from synthetics to autograft and allograft tissues have been used. Bone-patellar tendon-bone, semitendinosus/gracilis hamstring, and bone-quadriceps tendon autografts and allografts are most commonly used.

Single-bundle ACL reconstruction is most common, but recurrent instability occurs in up to 30% of patients, and only 60% to 70% return to their preinjury level of sports. In an effort to improve outcomes, double-bundle ACL reconstruction was developed. With this technique, both the anteromedial and posterolateral bundles of the ACL are reconstructed. The anteromedial bundle is thought to provide anteroposterior stability, and the posterolateral bundle rotational control. The double-bundle ACL reconstruction may resist rotatory loads and mimic normal knee kinematics more closely than the single-bundle ACL reconstruction. But there is probably not a significant clinical difference between the two with regard to outcome scores, graft failure, or radiographic changes of osteoarthritis. Regardless of whether single-bundle or double-bundle ACL reconstruction is used, it is important to put the tunnels in the tibia and femur (Figures 4–16 and 4–17) at the insertion sites of the ACL and fix the graft securely. Not doing so significantly increases the chances of graft failure.

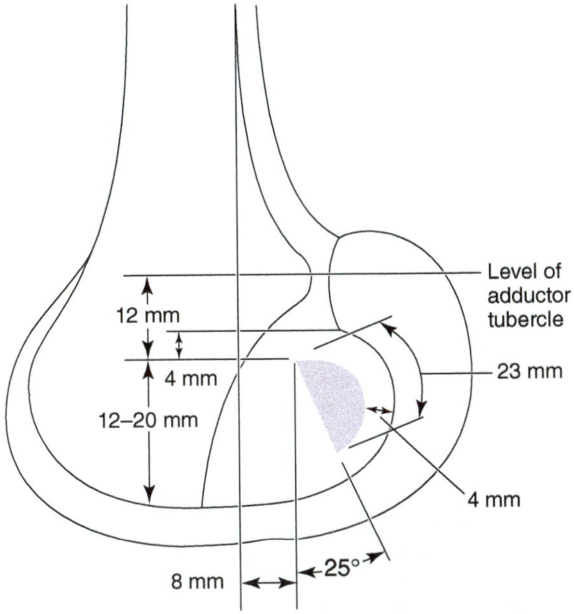

▲ **Figure 4–16. Drawing of the medial surface of the right lateral femoral condyle showing the average measurements and body relations of the femoral attachment of the anterior cruciate ligament.** (Reprinted with permission, from Arnoczky SP. Anatomy of the anterior cruciate ligament. *Clin Orthop Relat Res*. 1983;172:19.)

Complications

Although ACL reconstruction often results in a successful outcome, there are several complications that can occur. The more common complications are recurrent instability from graft failure and loss of knee motion. This can be minimized with good surgical technique, by avoiding postoperative graft injury, and by obtaining and maintaining full knee extension as soon as possible following surgery. Knee flexion exercises are begun as soon as possible also with a goal of 90 degrees by 1 week after surgery. Additionally, patellar mobilization is performed in an attempt to minimize patellofemoral scarring. Persistent knee pain, and particularly anterior knee pain, has an etiology that is often unclear. It is thought that harvesting the patellar tendon autograft may increase the incidence of patellofemoral pain. Less common complications (<1%) include patellar fracture, patellar tendon rupture, and quadriceps tendon rupture depending on the graft harvest site.

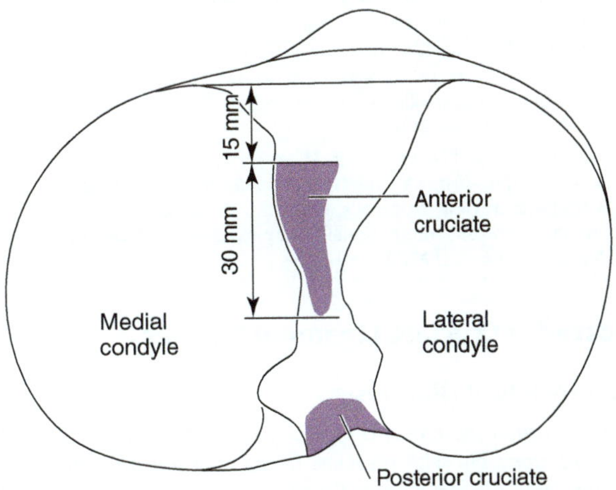

▲ **Figure 4–17. The upper surface of the tibial plateau to show average measurements and relations of the tibial attachments of the anterior cruciate ligament.** (Reprinted with permission, from Girgis FC, Marshall JL, Monajem A. The cruciate ligaments of the knee joint: anatomical, functional, and experimental analysis. *Clin Orthop Relat Res*. 1975;106:216.)

Results/Return to Play

The goal of rehabilitation after ACL reconstruction is to return the patient to their full desired level of activity in as short amount of time as possible while avoiding any complications or setbacks. With improved surgical techniques and accelerated rehabilitation protocols, there was hope of better return to play and higher patient satisfaction. But return to sport is about 80%, and only 65% return to their preinjury level of sport. Patients generally are able to return between 4 and 6 months postoperatively, with some professional athletes returning successfully to competition in 3 months. Specific criteria for return to sports vary, with a combination of functional testing, subjective reporting, and clinical examination contributing to the decision. In general, the criteria for return to sports include full range of motion, anterior tibial translation within 2 to 3 mm of the uninjured knee, 85% or greater quadriceps strength and full hamstring strength, and overall functional strength testing within 85% of the uninjured leg.

Belk JW, Kraeutler MJ, Houck DA, McCarty EC. Knee osteoarthritis after single-bundle versus double-bundle anterior cruciate ligament reconstruction: a systematic review of randomized controlled trials. *Arthroscopy.* 2019;35:996-1003. [PMID: 30733027]

Bell KM, Rahnemai-Azar AA, Irarrazaval S, et al. In situ force in the anterior cruciate ligament, the lateral collateral ligament, and the anterolateral capsule complex during a simulated pivot shift test. *J Orthop Res.* 2018;36(3):847-853. [PMID: 28782837]

Chen H, Chen B, Tie K, Fu Z, Chen L. Single-bundle versus double-bundle autologous anterior cruciate ligament reconstruction: a meta-analysis of randomized controlled trials at 5 year minimum follow up. *J Orthop Surg Res.* 2018;13:50. [PMID: 29523208]

Farraro KF, Sasaki N, Woo SL, et al. Magnesium ring device to restore function of a transected anterior cruciate ligament in the goat stifle joint. *J Orthop Res.* 2016;34(11):2001-2008. [PMID: 26916011]

Hoogeslag RA, Brouwer RW, Boer BC, et al. Acute anterior cruciate ligament rupture: repair or reconstruction? Two-year results of a randomized controlled trial. *Am J Sports Med.* 2019;47(3): 567-577. [PMID: 30822124]

Kandhari V, Vieira TD, Ouanezar H, et al. Clinical outcomes of arthroscopic primary anterior cruciate ligament repair: a systematic review from the Scientific Anterior Cruciate Ligament Network International Study Group. *Arthroscopy.* 2020;36(2):594-612. [PMID: 32014188]

4. Posterior Cruciate Ligament Injuries

Essentials of Diagnosis

- *Most common mechanisms of injury are a direct blow to the anterior tibia with the knee flexed or a fall onto the ground with the foot plantar flexed.*
- *Patients complain of knee pain, swelling, and stiffness.*
- *Physical examination may show positive posterior drawer, Godfrey, and reverse pivot shift tests.*
- *Must perform thorough knee exam because other knee injuries are common with PCL injury, particularly the posterolateral corner and the menisci.*
- Imaging studies should include plain radiographs as well as confirmatory MRI. Radiographs are helpful in chronic PCL injuries to assess patellofemoral and medial compartment arthritis.

Symptoms (History)

When evaluating a patient for a PCL injury, it is important to obtain the mechanism of injury. One of the most common mechanisms of PCL injury is the "dashboard" injury when the anterior tibia strikes the car dashboard with the knee in 90 degrees of flexion during a motor vehicle collision resulting in a posterior-directed force. Sports injuries to the PCL most commonly result from a blow, in contrast to the typical deceleration twisting mechanism of an ACL injury. Another common mechanism of a sports PCL injury is from a fall onto a flexed knee with the foot in plantar flexion. Additionally, significant multiligamentous knee injuries with PCL tears can result from a varus or valgus blow to the extended knee.

In contrast to an ACL tear, it is rare for patients with isolated acute PCL injuries to report hearing a "pop" or feelings of instability. More commonly, patients will complain of knee pain, swelling, and stiffness. However, patients with combined injuries involving the posterolateral corner of the knee will often complain of feelings of instability and giving way. A patient with a subacute or chronically injured PCL may be asymptomatic.

Signs (Physical Examination)

As with other ligamentous injuries, a thorough knee examination is necessary. Specific cues to injury to the PCL on initial inspection include abrasions or ecchymosis of the proximal anterior tibia and ecchymosis in the popliteal fossa. Assessment for associated ligamentous injury and meniscal damage should be performed. Evaluation of ACL instability in the presence of an acute PCL injury is challenging due to the lack of a stable reference point to perform a Lachman or anterior drawer test as the tibia will be resting in a posterior subluxed position.

Examination of the PCL in the acutely injured knee can be challenging. Despite increased awareness of the injury, many PCL injuries go undiagnosed in the acute setting. The most accurate clinical test of PCL integrity is the posterior drawer test. The knee is flexed to 90 degrees with the patient supine, and a posteriorly directed force is applied to the proximal tibia. The amount of posterior translation and the presence and character of the end point are noted. Translation is assessed as the change in the distance of the step-off between the anteromedial tibial plateau and the medial femoral condyle. Normally the tibial plateau is approximately 1 cm anterior to the medial femoral condyle. The uninjured knee must be examined to establish a baseline. Grade 2 instability is when the tibial plateau translates to about the medial femoral condyle and grade 3 when the tibial plateau translates posterior to it.

Another test for examination of the PCL is the posterior sag or Godfrey test. For this test, the patient is positioned supine and both the hip and knee are flexed with the foot resting on the examination table. The amount of tibial "sag" is then noted as posterior subluxation of the proximal tibia on the femoral condyles resulting from gravity. One can also watch for reduction of this subluxation with active quadriceps contraction, known as the quadriceps activation or active drawer test. With the patient supine, the foot is held in place on the examination table. The patient is then asked to slide their foot anteriorly to induce quadriceps activation. A positive test is when the posterior subluxed proximal tibia reduces to its normal position anterior to the femoral condyles.

It is very important to evaluate the posterolateral corner structures when there is a suspected PCL injury. Please see the section on LCL physical examination for descriptions of the dial test, reverse pivot shift, external rotation recurvatum test, and posterolateral drawer test.

Imaging Studies

A. Radiographs

Given the magnitude of the forces required to injure the PCL, plain radiographs of the knee are essential to evaluate for bony injuries, dislocation, or evidence of other associated injuries. Subtle posterior subluxation on the lateral radiograph may indicate PCL injury. Stress posterior drawer radiographs and comparison to the uninjured knee may also increase the sensitivity for detecting PCL injuries with plain radiographs. In the chronic setting of PCL injury, radiographs are useful to assess for patellofemoral and medial compartment osteoarthritis that can occur over time.

B. MRI

Although plain films are necessary and useful in the evaluations of these injuries, MRI has become the diagnostic study of choice for the knee with a presumed PCL injury. MRI is reported to be 96% to 100% sensitive at diagnosing PCL tears. Equally or more importantly, MRI is extremely valuable in its ability to detect associated injuries. This is particularly important in diagnosing associated posterolateral corner injuries because these can often be missed on the initial clinical examination. In multiligamentous knee injuries, MRI can also be of use in assessing the ACL because clinical examination of the ACL is challenging in the setting of a complete PCL tear.

C. Special Studies

With chronic, isolated PCL tear, pain in the medial and patellofemoral compartments is generally evaluated with radiographs. If these are normal, some surgeons will proceed with a bone scan to evaluate for increased uptake in these areas because increased uptake can occur before there is osteoarthritis on radiographs. These patients may benefit from a PCL reconstruction to decrease the stress and delay osteoarthritis.

Treatment

The decision for PCL reconstruction is individualized and based on the other injuries of the knee, the patient's desire to return to activity, age, presence of prior osteoarthritis, and objective and subjective knee instability. Since patients complain less of instability after isolated PCL injuries, there is more controversy as to which patients should have surgery than with isolated ACL injuries.

A. Nonsurgical

Most patients do well with nonsurgical treatment of a PCL tear. Rehabilitation of the PCL-injured knee is often largely dependent on other knee injuries, particularly with posterolateral corner injuries. Regaining motion and strength are two key objectives of a rehabilitation program. Obtaining full quadriceps strength is essential for achieving the optimal result with nonsurgical treatment. The initial treatment is aimed at reducing abnormal joint motions and minimizing stress on the injured PCL. Bracing is generally ineffective in controlling PCL instability. With grade 1 and 2 injuries, the prognosis is quite good, and rehabilitation of early motion, weight bearing as tolerated, and strengthening are usual. For grade 3 injuries, the knee can be immobilized in extension to protect the posterolateral structures. Early strengthening exercises focus on quadriceps strength with quadriceps sets, straight leg raises, and partial weight bearing in extension. Resisted hamstring strengthening should be avoided in the early phases of rehabilitation.

Despite objective instability on examination, most patients are subjectively satisfied with the function of their knee. But nonoperative care of these injuries is not without consequences. Although subjective results in these patients are good in the short term, a PCL-deficient knee places significantly increased stresses on the patellofemoral and medial compartments of the knee, and many develop osteoarthritis of these compartments at long-term follow-up. It is common for those with PCL-deficient knees at an average of 15 years after injury to have persistent pain, and about half have chronic effusions.

B. Surgical

In those with grade 3 PCL injures, subjective instability, and multiligamentous injury, surgical reconstruction of the PCL is a reasonable choice. Surgical management is also indicated for avulsion fractures, and although rare, if significantly displaced, they are best treated with open reduction and internal fixation. If nondisplaced, an avulsion fracture will usually heal.

Current PCL reconstruction methods involve either autograft or allograft tendons secured at the insertion sites of the PCL. Classically, PCL reconstruction was done with a single-bundle technique and, in some cases, may have reconstructed only the anterolateral bundle. Double-bundle techniques were developed to reconstruct both the anterolateral and posteromedial bundles of the PCL and may be superior.

Severe instability multiligamentous knee injuries involving the PCL make the argument for ligament reconstruction more compelling. Acute treatment of these complex knee injuries can be repair, and subjective results are generally good, but residual excessive, objective instability is common. PCL reconstructions with allograft or autograft are the most common methods of treatment after this challenging knee injury.

Complications

A more common complication following PCL reconstruction is the return of objective posterior instability on physical examination. This does not usually result in symptomatic instability, and patient satisfaction is usually high. Decreased range of motion, especially after acute PCL reconstruction with surgery for multiligamentous knee injury that can result in arthrofibrosis with extensive scarring, is also a common complication.

Results/Return to Play

Even with nonsurgical management of a PCL injury, the prognosis for a functional recovery and return to competition is very good. A strong quadriceps muscle and extensor mechanism can significantly compensate for PCL instability. Athletes should spend a minimum of 3 months in rehabilitation before attempting a return to competition. However, some patients experience significant instability with a grade 3 PCL injury that does not allow a return to competition, and they may benefit from PCL reconstruction.

The prognosis for a PCL tear associated with a multiligamentous knee injury is guarded with respect to return to play. Although prompt recognition of a multiligamentous injury and appropriately timed treatment, reconstruction, and rehabilitation are essential for optimal recovery, these injuries are such that a significant percentage of patients will not be able to return to full competition.

LaPrade RF, Chahla J, DePhillipo NN, et al. Single-stage multiple-ligament knee reconstructions for sports-related injuries: outcomes in 194 patients. *Am J Sports Med.* 2019;47(11):2563-2571. [PMID: 31381372]

LaPrade RF, Cinque ME, Dornan GJ, et al. Double-bundle posterior cruciate ligament reconstruction in 100 patients at a mean 3 years' follow-up: outcomes were comparable to anterior cruciate ligament reconstructions. *Am J Sports Med.* 2018;46(8):1809-1818. [PMID: 29953296]

Lee DY, Kim DH, Kim HJ, Ahn HS, Lee TH, Hwang SC. Posterior cruciate ligament reconstruction with transtibial or tibial inlay techniques: a meta-analysis of biomechanical and clinical outcomes. *Am J Sports Med.* 2018;46(11):2789-2797. [PMID: 29328888]

Lee DY, Kim DH, Kim HJ, Nam DC, Park JS, Hwang SC. Biomechanical comparison of single-bundle and double-bundle posterior cruciate ligament reconstruction: a systematic review and meta-analysis. *JBJS Rev.* 2017;5(10):e6. [PMID: 29040171]

Wright JO, Skelley NW, Schur RP, Castile RM, Lake SP, Brophy RH. Microstructural and mechanical properties of the posterior cruciate ligament: a comparison of the anterolateral and posteromedial bundles. *J Bone Joint Surg Am.* 2016;98(19):1656-1664. [PMID: 27707852]

5. Patella Dislocation

Essentials of Diagnosis

- *Almost always a lateral dislocation.*
- *Pain, swelling, and tenderness over the medial border of the patella and apprehension when the patella is pushed laterally with the knee slightly flexed.*
- *An osteochondral fragment may be found on radiographs.*

Dislocation of the patella is a potential cause of acute hemarthrosis and must be considered when evaluating a patient with an acute knee injury. The injury occurs when valgus force and external rotation of the tibia are applied to a flexed leg. It most commonly occurs in the second and third decades of life and is about the same in males and females.

Clinical Findings

The patella almost always dislocates laterally. The patient may notice the patella sitting laterally or might say that the rest of the knee has shifted medially. It is unusual for a patient to present with the patella dislocated; rather, the reduction occurs when the knee is extended and the patient presents with a reduced patella.

Examination will demonstrate tenderness over the medial retinaculum and adductor tubercle, as the origin of the medial patellofemoral ligament is between the medial epicondyle and the adductor tubercle. The patient will also have pain and apprehension when the patella is pushed laterally with the knee slightly flexed. Rather than apprehension, some patients will rapidly contract the quadriceps muscle when the patella is pushed laterally with the knee slightly flexed. Radiographs, including axial superior-to-inferior views known as Merchant or sunrise views, should be obtained to evaluate for osteochondral fractures. A displaced osteochondral fracture will require excision or internal fixation. A small fleck of bone on the medial aspect of the patella may be avulsed with the retinaculum. It is not intraarticular and does not require removal. Examination of the uninjured knee as well as the injured knee is recommended to aid in determining whether there are predisposing factors for dislocation, such as patella alta, patellofemoral dysplasia such as hypoplasia of the trochlear groove, increased femoral anteversion, increased knee valgus, tibial tubercle to trochlear groove (TT to TG) distance, and hypermobility, specifically genu recurvatum. The patellofemoral joint constraint increases as knee flexion increases. A high-riding patella necessitates more knee flexion before the patella is constrained in the trochlear groove. There are multiple radiographic methods to assess for patella alta, or high-riding patella. The Insall-Salvati ratio is calculated by measuring the length of the patellar tendon and dividing by the length of the patella. The upper limit of normal is 1.2, with greater values indicating patella alta. The Q angle is the formed by the intersection of a line along the patellar tendon and a line from the anterior superior iliac spine to the center of the patella. A normal Q angle is less than about 15 degrees in males and a few degrees more in females. Using cross-sectional imaging, a TT to TG distance can be measured, with greater than 20 mm often defined as abnormal. Because it is quantitative, TT to TG distance is replacing the Q angle, which is qualitative. Patients with generalized hypermobility have increased extension of the knee, or genu recurvatum, which in effect gives them patella alta. They also often have abnormal static stabilizers such as the retinaculum and the medial patellofemoral ligament, giving them significant patella hypermobility in that there is excessive medial and/or lateral motion.

Treatment and Prognosis

Treatment of the first patella dislocation is usually strengthening exercises and a patella stabilization brace as long as there are no osteochondral fragments. Little is lost by this functional treatment, similar to the treatment of isolated MCL sprains, and it is often successful. Treatment may be altered by predisposing factors, and then tibial tubercle realignment, for example, may be warranted. If patella dislocation recurs, patellofemoral ligament reconstruction may be performed. Medial patellofemoral ligament reconstruction decreases recurrent dislocation rates after first-time traumatic dislocation but may have no effect on subjective or objective outcome scores compared to knee brace treatment. Degenerative changes in the patellofemoral ligament after nonanatomic patellofemoral stabilizing procedures may occur more often compared to those treated nonoperatively, although this may be skewed by there being more osteochondral injuries in operative patients.

Askenberger M, Mostrom B, Ekström W, et al. Operative repair of medial patellofemoral ligament injury versus knee brace in children with an acute first-time traumatic patellar dislocation. *Am J Sports Med.* 2018;46:2328-2340. [PMID: 29847145]

KNEE TENDON INJURY

Ruptures of the quadriceps and patellar tendons usually result from a tremendous eccentric contraction of the quadriceps muscle, as may occur when an athlete stumbles and tries not to fall. Both types of ruptures are more common in patients with underlying disorders of the tendon.

1. Rupture of the Quadriceps Tendon

Essentials of Diagnosis

- *Occur in patients older than 40 years.*
- *Patient will be unable to actively extend the knee.*
- *Radiographs will reveal patella baja.*
- *The quadriceps will retract proximally if left untreated.*

Quadriceps tendon ruptures occur most frequently in patients over 40 years old. Biopsies of fresh rupture sites show local degenerative changes already present, consistent with the theory that normal tendons do not rupture. Rarely the injury occurs bilaterally and is often associated with gout, diabetes, or steroid use. When it does occur bilaterally with only a small amount of trauma, the diagnosis may be difficult to make because of the small amount of swelling or symptoms of injury.

The cardinal symptom is inability to actively extend the knee. The patella is slightly lower than the contralateral side. A defect is palpable above the patella, and the anterior border of the femoral condyles may be palpated. When extension is attempted, a gap develops in the suprapatellar region.

Acute complete quadriceps tendon ruptures should be repaired surgically. If left untreated, proximal migration and scarring of the quadriceps muscle will occur. Direct-end repair of the quadriceps to the patella along with repair of the medial and lateral retinaculum produces excellent results. Immobilization in extension is recommended initially, followed by increases in range of motion over the next 2 months and strengthening after about 3 months. Repair of ruptures more than a few weeks old may be difficult and may require quadriceps lengthening, muscle or tendon transfers, or a combination of these procedures.

Serino J, Mohamadi A, Orman S, et al. Comparison of adverse events and postoperative mobilization following knee extensor mechanism rupture repair: a systematic review and network meta-analysis. *Injury.* 2017;48(12):2793-2799. [PMID: 29050687]

2. Rupture of the Patellar Tendon

Essentials of Diagnosis

- *Typically occurs in patients younger than 40.*
- *Patient will be unable to actively extend the knee.*
- *Radiographs will reveal patella alta.*

Rupture of the patellar tendon occurs more frequently in patients younger than 40 years old. The patient cannot actively extend the knee, the patella is high-riding, and a defect is palpable beneath the patella. Surgical repair is the treatment of choice. The tendon, along with the medial and lateral retinaculum, should be sewn end to end. A stress-relieving retention suture may be placed around the patella and through the tibial tubercle. Chronic patellar tendon ruptures are very hard to treat. The quadriceps must be freed up from the femur and the patella pulled down to the proper location. The gracilis and semitendinosus tendons can be used as autografts for treatment of chronic patellar tendon rupture.

The extensor mechanism may also be disrupted at the inferior pole of the patella where the patellar tendon originates. This usually occurs in children aged between 8 and 12 years old. The distal pole of the patella along with a large sleeve of articular cartilage is pulled off (Figure 4–18). This may be easily misdiagnosed if the fragment of bone is small. Reestablishment of an intact extensor mechanism is necessary. With displaced fractures, open reduction and internal fixation with tension band wiring is recommended.

Hantes ME, Mathews R, Raoulis V, Varitimidis S, Karachalios T, Malizos KN. Better knee function after surgical repair of acute quadriceps tendon rupture in comparison to acute patellar tendon rupture. *Orthop Traumatol Surg Res.* 2019;105(1):119-123. [PMID: 30455100]

KNEE PAIN

Pain in the knee region is a very common complaint of athletes. If there is no history of an acute injury, then overuse is commonly the cause. The patient is often able to point to the area of pain. The history of activity must be obtained as well as overall evaluation of the extremities.

1. Anterior Knee Pain

Patellofemoral Disorders

A. Essentials of Diagnosis

- *Pain with activity involving stairs or hills.*
- *Commonly involves young females.*
- *Check Q angle, femoral anteversion, patellar mobility, and quadriceps strength and tone.*
- *On radiographs, look for valgus alignment of knee, OCD, and patella alta.*

B. Clinical Findings

1. Symptoms and signs—This is a common complaint and is frequently bilateral. It is most common in females during the second decade of life. The patellofemoral joint is often the source of pain. Entities such as chondromalacia patella (softening of the patellar cartilage), patellofemoral arthralgia, lateral patellofemoral compression syndrome, and patella instability are diagnostic considerations.

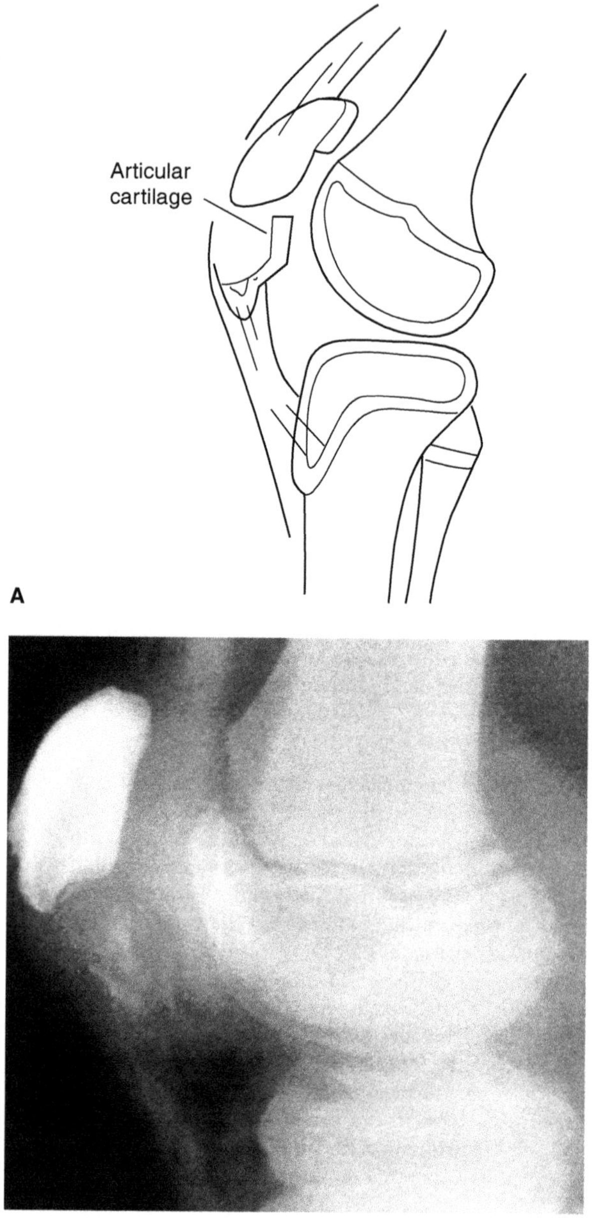

▲ **Figure 4–18.** Sleeve fracture of the patella. **A:** A small segment of the distal pole of the patella is avulsed with a relatively large portion of the articular surface. **B:** Lateral radiograph of the knee with a displaced sleeve fracture of the patella. Note that the small osseous portion of the displaced fragment is visible, but the cartilaginous portion is not seen. (Reproduced, with permission, from Rockwood CA Jr, ed. *Fractures in Children*, 3rd ed. Philadelphia: Lippincott; 1991.)

Patellar pain is often felt when going up or down hills or stairs, and there may be complaints of instability during walking, running, or other sports activities. These activities may create a joint reaction force of several times the body weight on the patella with each step. Swelling is seldom a complaint. If the pain is in one knee only, the patient may alter the way of climbing and descending stairs so that the affected leg is kept straight and each step leads with the same foot. This strategy significantly decreases the joint reaction force on the patellofemoral joint.

Many of these problems arise because of a problem with patellofemoral constraint. The degree of constraint is dependent on a number of factors, including variations in the trochlear groove, position of the patella such as patella alta, and variations in ligamentous laxity. In addition, femoral anteversion and increased Q angle (Figure 4–19) predispose the patella to subluxation or dislocation. The degree of congruity is variable and may lead to high-contact stresses caused by the anatomic configuration and static and dynamic constraints on the patella. Increased pressure may cause pain and patellofemoral osteoarthritis.

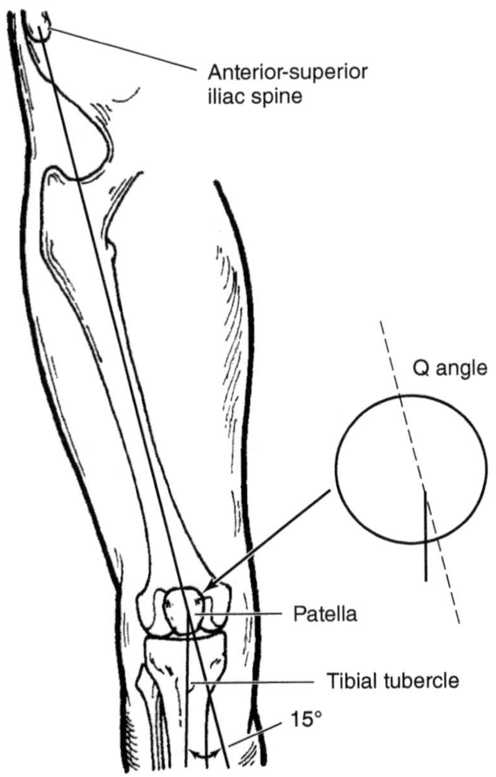

▲ **Figure 4–19.** Q angle and valgus angulation. (Reproduced, with permission, from American Academy of Orthopaedic Surgeons. *Athletic Training and Sports Medicine*, 2nd ed. Burlington, MA: Jones and Bartlett; 1991.)

On physical examination of the patient with patellofemoral subluxation, minimal findings in relation to complaints may be present. Occasionally, crepitus, a crackling or clicking sound, is found with flexion and extension. Quadriceps strength, tone, and bulk are usually reduced. Pain may be elicited at a particular angle of flexion by putting the knee through its range of motion with resistance. Subluxation may often be diagnosed with pain and apprehension or rapid contraction of the quadriceps when the patella is pushed laterally with the knee slightly flexed.

2. Imaging studies—X-rays may show a valgus angulation of the knee on anteroposterior views. Occasionally, patella alta may be identified on the lateral view, and tangential views of the patella at various knee flexion angles will reveal a lack of contact of the medial facet of the patella with the medial facet of the trochlear groove of the femur. Lateral subluxation of the patellofemoral joint may also be observed.

This syndrome with normal x-rays is frequently called chondromalacia patella, or with subluxation is referred to as patellofemoral subluxation. A more accurate term would be patellofemoral arthralgia, because patellofemoral subluxation was probably present prior to the onset of pain and because chondromalacia patella is an arthroscopic or pathologic diagnosis. Patellofemoral arthralgia is a clinical diagnosis.

C. Treatment

1. Chondromalacia patella/patellofemoral arthralgia—Initially, treatment is conservative, with the intent of improving quadriceps strength and stamina to stabilize the patellofemoral joint. Weight loss is prescribed to decrease the stress on the patellofemoral joint; reduction in loading the knee in the flexed position also accomplishes pressure reduction. Knee orthotics may be beneficial. When subluxation and fear of dislocation are major concerns, an orthotic that limits extension of the knee may be beneficial because the patella becomes inherently more stable with knee flexion. Nonsteroidal anti-inflammatory drug may be beneficial. Only when conservative treatment has been exhausted is surgical treatment considered. Alteration in the alignment of the patellofemoral joint may be beneficial, and distal realignment may be necessary to achieve appropriate alignment and reduction in pain in those cases with an abnormality such as valgus knee, increased Q angle, or increased femoral anteversion. Cartilage repair procedures, such as transplanting cartilage cells or osteochondral grafts into defects when rarely indicated, may be helpful.

2. Lateral patellofemoral compression syndrome—With lateral patellofemoral compression syndrome, there is tenderness along the lateral facet of the patella or along the femoral condyle. Without cartilage damage, an effusion is rarely present. Treatment includes decreasing the activity level, including avoiding hills or step aerobics. Ice massage, quadriceps and hamstring stretching, and short-arc quadriceps exercises against resistance are recommended to strengthen the vastus medialis obliquus muscle without aggravating the pain. Patellar supports or neoprene sleeves may also be helpful. Most patients will respond to this regimen and gradually resume their activities. The role of lateral retinaculum release is controversial.

3. Patellar tendinitis—Patellar tendinitis, or jumper's knee, is seen in basketball and volleyball players. There is tenderness along the tendon, most notably at the inferior pole of the patella. Treatment with ice and avoiding jumping usually suffice. In refractory cases, debridement of mucinous degenerative material from the tendon may be successful.

D. Prognosis

The prognosis of anterior knee pain is extremely varied, because the term encompasses so many disparate diagnoses. Patellofemoral arthralgia and lateral patellofemoral compression syndrome can last several years. The prognosis for jumper's knee is quite good because the condition, while often persistent, is self-limiting. The patient can usually alleviate symptoms by avoiding the activities that cause the problem.

Stephen J, Ephgrave C, Ball S, Church S. Current concepts in the management of patellofemoral pain: the role of alignment. *Knee*. 2020;27(2):280-286. [PMID: 32014409]

2. Lateral Knee Pain

Iliotibial Band Friction Syndrome

A. Essentials of Diagnosis

- *Lateral knee pain.*
- *Commonly affects runners and cyclists.*
- *Tenderness over lateral epicondyle and positive Ober test.*

Lateral knee pain that is not located on the joint line may result from iliotibial band friction syndrome. This is a form of bursitis caused by rubbing of the iliotibial band against the lateral epicondyle. Tenderness over the lateral epicondyle at about 30 degrees of flexion when the knee is being extended is indicative of this diagnosis. The Ober test is used to detect tightness of the iliotibial band in a lateral decubitus position. Reproduction of pain or tightness that occurs when the hip is brought from a flexed and abducted position into extension and adduction is considered a positive finding. There is occasionally crepitus at the lateral femoral condyle. Runners and cyclists are commonly afflicted. Crossover gait or running on banked terrain is thought to be a causative factor.

Treatment involves decreasing the athlete's activities, ice massage, and stretching of the iliotibial band. Running on flat terrain and changing the gait pattern may be helpful. In cyclists, lowering the seat height so the full extension of the knee is not reached and adjusting the pedals so that the toes are not internally rotated should help. Steroid injections are infrequently needed, and release of the inflamed portion of the iliotibial band is seldom necessary. As for other overuse syndromes of the knee, the prognosis is good.

Baker RL, Fredericson M. Iliotibial band syndrome in runners: biomechanical implications and exercise interventions. *Phys Med Rehabil Clin N Am*. 2016;27(1):53-77. [PMID: 26616177]

Everhart JS, Kirven JC, Higgins J, Hair A, Chaudhari AAMW, Flanigan DC. The relationship between lateral epicondyle morphology and iliotibial band friction syndrome: a matched case-control study. *Knee*. 2019;26(6):1198-1203. [PMID: 31439366]

ANKLE OR FOOT PAIN

Evaluation of foot and ankle injuries is described in Chapter 10. Keep in mind that foot and ankle pain is very common in those over 55 years of age. Injury specific to athletics includes chronic Achilles tendinopathy, heel pain, plantar fasciitis, and posterior tibial syndrome.

Clinical Findings

Achilles tendinopathy is a frequent complaint in runners. This may result from a contracted gastrocnemius and soleus or hyperpronation that may cause overpulling of the medial insertion. Additionally, there may be a bony prominence on the superior-posterior aspect of the calcaneus, causing retrocalcaneal bursitis.

Heel pain is a common problem in runners and is difficult to treat because of the uncertainty as to cause. Theories include painful heel spurs, bursitis, fat-pad atrophy, stress fracture, plantar fasciitis, or entrapment of the terminal branches of the posterior tibial nerve.

Many patients have pain localized in the posteromedial surface of the foot just distal to the attachment of the plantar fascia to the calcaneus. When plantar fasciitis is the cause, the pain is often worse on initially getting up in the morning and decreases as the day goes on.

Posterior tibial syndrome occurs in runners with hyperpronation. As the longitudinal arch flattens out, the posterior tibial musculotendinous unit that normally elevates the arch has abnormal strain placed upon it.

Treatment

Treatment depends on the cause of the injury but includes decreasing running activities, using a heel lift, and performing stretching exercises. If hyperpronation is thought to be the cause, an arch support orthotic may be used. Steroid injections are not recommended as they could lead to weakening and subsequent rupture of the tendon.

Surgical intervention for chronic Achilles tendinopathy or retrocalcaneal bursitis is rarely necessary. This would be done to remove areas of fibrosis or calcium within the tendon and possibly some bone from the posterior process of the calcaneus. The treatment for plantar fasciitis includes rest, ice massage, and possibly anti-inflammatory medications, insoles, heel cups, and splints at night to avoid plantar flexion. A steroid injection may be given in recalcitrant cases. Acute rupture of the plantar fascia may occur. The pain is usually quite sharp and may cause significant disability for 6 to 12 weeks.

Hyperpronation may also cause fibular stress fractures. A semirigid orthosis may be recommended for this to decrease the amount and angular velocity of pronation. Using an orthosis while running actually increases the work of running, but if it decreases abnormal stresses in those who hyperpronate, it may be quite helpful.

Keenan AM, Drake C, Conaghan PG, Tennant A. The prevalence and impact of self-reported foot and ankle pain in the over 55 age group: a secondary data analysis from a large community sample. *J Foot Ankle Res.* 2019;12:53. [PMID: 31788030]

Maffulli N, Longo UG, Kadakia A, Spiezia F. Achilles tendinopathy. *Foot Ankle Surg.* 2020;26(3):240-249. [PMID: 31031150]

Schuitema D, Greve C, Postema K, Dekker R, Hijmans JM. Effectiveness of mechanical treatment for plantar fasciitis: a systematic review. *J Sport Rehabil.* 2019:1-18. [PMID: 31629333]

OTHER INJURIES OF THE LOWER BODY

The differential diagnosis of some injuries in athletes must be carefully made to rule out severe injuries and those that require surgery. Once done, a period of rest followed by gradual return to activities is often the best treatment. During convalescence, application of ice packs, stretching exercises, and gradual strengthening of the injured limb will facilitate return to sports activities.

OVERUSE SYNDROMES OF THE LOWER EXTREMITIES

Athletes such as runners, cyclists, aerobics enthusiasts, volleyball players, and basketball players can develop painful disorders of the lower extremities without an acute injury. History taking is very important, and the examiner should ask specific questions about the circumstances in which the discomfort occurs. In a runner, for example, the examiner should ask whether there was an increase in the distance run or a change in the running surface, when the pain was felt, and what home remedies have been tried before the runner sought advice from a physician.

The physical examination should include not only the affected area but also evaluation of the back, pelvis, leg lengths, genu varum or valgum, femoral and tibial torsion, and cavus or flatfoot deformities. The presence of hamstring and heel cord contracture should be determined, and the gait pattern should be observed. Running shoes should be inspected for wear patterns, which may be quite helpful.

1. Muscle Strains

Essentials of Diagnosis

- *Classically involves muscles that span two joints (ie, gastrocnemius).*
- *Patient will feel muscle "grab" and localized pain in the involved area.*
- *Eccentric forces thought to be causative factors.*

Muscle strains of the lower extremity are frequent and disabling muscle injuries, with strain of the distal muscle tendon junction being most common. Muscles may stretch to about 125% of their resting length before tearing. Strains are graded as mild, moderate, and severe, based on the degree of pain, spasm, and disability that the strain causes. A severe strain would be complete disruption of the muscle, with a palpable defect and balling up of the muscle proximally.

Despite the frequency of muscle strains and the disability they produce, there is little scientific information on their pathologic basis. Muscles susceptible to more stretching are more susceptible to strains. In the lower extremity, the muscles most frequently injured are the hamstring, quadriceps, and gastrocnemius muscles. Each of these muscles crosses two joints, and they may be unable to resist full stretching across both joints. The most powerful muscles are more likely to be strained, and strains are more common in "explosive"-type athletics. Eccentric contraction (muscle contraction while the muscle is lengthening) is often thought to be causative.

Clinical Findings

The diagnosis is relatively easy. Often the athlete will feel the muscle "grab" with injury. There is localized tenderness over the muscle and pain on stretching of the muscle. Because the two joint muscles are most frequently involved, the muscles should be stretched over both of the joints during examination.

Treatment and Prognosis

The treatment of muscle strains should begin with ice immediately after the injury. Flexibility and strength should be regained prior to return to activity. This may take many months, and if the patient returns to activity too early, there may be a setback.

Strengthening of the muscles might make them less susceptible to being torn. It is commonly believed that flexibility will help prevent muscle strains, but there are conflicting reports regarding this.

Mehta N, Alter T, Beck EC, et al. Endoscopic repair of proximal hamstring tear with double-row suture bridge construct. *Athrosc Tech.* 2019;8(7):e675-e678. [PMID: 31467836]

Orchard JW, Chaker Jomaa M, Orcahrd JJ, et al. Fifteen-week window for recurrent muscle strains in football: a prospective cohort of 3600 muscle strains over 23 years in professional Australian rules football. *Br J Sports Med.* 2020;54(18): 1103-1107. [PMID: 32024646]

2. Shin Pain

Essentials of Diagnosis

- *Pain over the anterior tibia.*
- *Associated with increase in training or activity level.*
- *Radiographs will be negative for fracture.*

Clinical Findings

A. Shin Splints

The term *shin splints* is widely used for shin pain, but it is not a diagnostic term. A more specific diagnosis should be made if possible. Shin splints usually occur in the beginning of training after a relatively inactive period. The pain and tenderness are located over the anterior compartment and disappear in 1 to 2 weeks as the athlete becomes conditioned to the exercise. Care must be taken to differentiate shin splints from stress fractures of the tibia, which cause more localized pain and have many more potential complications if not cared for properly.

B. Medial Tibial Stress Syndrome

Medial tibial stress syndrome is also seen in runners, occurring along the medial border of the distal tibia. After 3 to 4 weeks, some hypertrophy of the cortical bone and periosteal new bone formation may be seen on radiograph. It is thought to be either a periostitis or possibly an incomplete stress fracture. The pull of the tibialis posterior muscle from its origin on the tibia and posterior tibial tendinitis are also thought to be causes.

Treatment

Treatment for shin splints and medial tibial syndrome is rest and resumption of athletic activities in a graduated fashion.

3. Stress Fractures

Essentials of Diagnosis

- *Localized pain after an increase in training or activity.*
- *Plain radiographs often normal initially; MRI and bone scan are better diagnostic tests.*

Stress fractures may occur in the pelvis, femoral neck, tibia, navicular, and metatarsals. They are usually the result of a significant increase in training and activity. In the female athlete, a triad of eating disorders, amenorrhea, and osteoporosis is associated with a higher prevalence of stress fractures.

The history is important in differentiating stress fractures from infection or neoplasm, particularly when there is a finding on radiographs. Plain radiographs are normal at first, so MRI and technetium bone scans are better diagnostic tests. If symptoms persist for over a month, radiographs may become positive.

Treatment of stress fractures involves rest and avoidance of high-impact activities until healing has occurred. This includes resolution of the tenderness with radiographic evidence of fracture healing on plain films. Continuous activity with stress fractures may lead to complete fractures. Patients must be made aware of this and all the complications that may develop with a complete fracture.

Abbott A, Bird M, Brown SM, Wild E, Stewart G, Mulcahey MK. Part I: epidemiology and risk factors for stress factors in female athletes *Phys Sportsmed.* 2019;11:1-8. [PMID: 31213104]

Abbott A, Bird M, Brown SM, Wild E, Stewart G, Mulcahey MK. Part II: presentation, diagnosis, classification, treatment and prevention of stress factors in female athletes. *Phys Sportsmed.* 2019;11:1-8. [PMID: 31295036]

4. Exertional Compartment Syndromes

Essentials of Diagnosis

- *Recurrent claudication/pain during exertional activity and relieved by rest.*
- *Measure compartment pressures while exercising on treadmill (pressures >30 mm Hg 1 minute after exercise or >20 mm Hg 5 minutes after exercise or absolute values >15 mm Hg while resting are consistent with this diagnosis).*

Exertional compartment syndromes may result from muscle hypertrophy within the confining osseofascial compartment. As the muscles hypertrophy and the amount of edema within the compartment increases, the blood supply to the nerves and muscles within the involved compartment is diminished, and the pressure continues to increase.

The syndrome presents as recurrent claudication during exertional activity and is relieved by rest. After exercise, the findings of localized pain, pain on passive motion, and hypesthesia are indicative. Diagnosis involves measuring the pressures of the concerning compartments before and then 1 minute and 5 minutes after exercising on a treadmill. The aforementioned diagnostic values will provide the diagnosis.

Treatment consists of activity modification including gradual resumption of training. If nonoperative treatment is ineffective, surgical fasciotomies can be performed in the appropriate compartments.

Scully WF, Benevides JM. Surgical tips for performing open fasciotomies for chronic exertional compartment syndrome of the leg. *Foot Ankle Int.* 2019;40(7):859-865. [PMID: 30966780]

Waterman BR, Laughlin M, Kilcoyne K, Cameron KL, Owens BD. Surgical treatment of chronic exertional compartment syndrome of the leg: failure rates and postoperative disability in an active patient population. *J Bone Joint Surg.* 2013;95(7A):592-596. [PMID: 23553293]

CONTUSIONS AND AVULSIONS OF THE LOWER BODY

1. Contusion to the Quadriceps Muscle

Essentials of Diagnosis

- *History of direct trauma.*
- *Peripheral calcification on radiographs (as opposed to parosteal osteosarcoma, which has central calcification).*

Clinical Findings

A severe contusion to the quadriceps muscle (charley horse) is disabling, results in prolonged inactivity, and frequently occurs in football players. With significant bleeding into the muscle, there is inhibition of movement. Rarely, a compartment syndrome will occur.

Myositis ossificans may occur after these injuries and is apparent 2 to 4 weeks after the injury as peripheral calcification. Radiographically and histologically, myositis ossificans may be similar to parosteal osteosarcoma; therefore, the history of contusion is very important. Radiographs should be obtained after such a contusion to minimize myositis ossificans being confused with cancer.

Treatment and Prognosis

Quadriceps contusions should be treated with compression, elevation of the leg, and the knee flexed to tolerance to minimize bleeding. If it can be tolerated, the knee can be immobilized in 120 degrees of flexion for 24 hours. After this, the knee can be moved with continuous passive motion or "drop-and-dangle," gravity-assisted exercises. For the latter, the patient is seated on a table high enough to keep the feet off the floor. The patient then hooks the uninjured foot behind the ankle of the injured leg. The uninjured leg extends the knee of the injured leg, and gravity flexes the injured knee. The average length of disability for mild contusions is 2 weeks, and for severe contusions is 3 to 6 weeks.

If heterotopic ossification is present, no specific treatment is recommended other than treatment for the contusion. Normal function may be obtained, but the recovery period is longer. Because early surgery may cause exacerbation of the heterotopic ossification, it should be avoided.

Rossettini G, Ristori D, Testa M. Myositis ossificans: delayed complication of severe muscle contusion. *J Orthop Sports Phys Ther.* 2018;48(5):420. [PMID: 29712545]

Ueblacker P, Müller-Wohlfahrt HW, Ekstrand J. Epidemiological and clinical outcome comparison of indirect ('strain') versus direct ('contusion') anterior and posterior thigh muscle injuries in male elite football players: UEFA Elite League study of 2287 thigh injuries (2001-2013). *Br J Sports Med.* 2015;49(22):1461-1465. [PMID: 25755277]

CONTUSIONS ABOUT THE HIP AND PELVIS

Clinical Findings

Contusions about the pelvis and hip region may be very painful and disabling. Because of the subcutaneous location of the iliac crests and the greater trochanters, these regions are at risk in contact sports.

A contusion over the greater trochanter may cause persistent bursitis, tenderness directly over the greater trochanter, and increased pain with adduction of the leg. Females are more prone to trochanteric bursitis because of their broader pelvis.

A hip pointer is a very painful contusion over the iliac crest that can occur during a variety of contact sports. It must be differentiated from an avulsion fracture in a child and a tear of the muscle aponeurosis in an adult. Profuse bleeding may occur and can be very painful.

Treatment and Prognosis

For a contusion over the greater trochanter, treatment consists of ice and decreased activities. Padding may be helpful to prevent recurrent injuries. The prognosis is good. For hip pointer injuries, initial treatment with ice is helpful. Protective pads are useful in preventing these injuries and returning the athlete to activities sooner.

AVULSION OF THE TIBIAL TUBERCLE

Essentials of Diagnosis

- *Occurs in adolescent athletes between 14 and 16 years of age.*
- *Result of a forceful contraction by the quadriceps against a fixed tibia.*
- *Significant swelling and tenderness over the tubercle; palpable defect with substantial displacement.*
- *Patient will not be able to actively extend the knee.*
- *Radiographs will be helpful to determine amount of displacement and guide treatment course.*

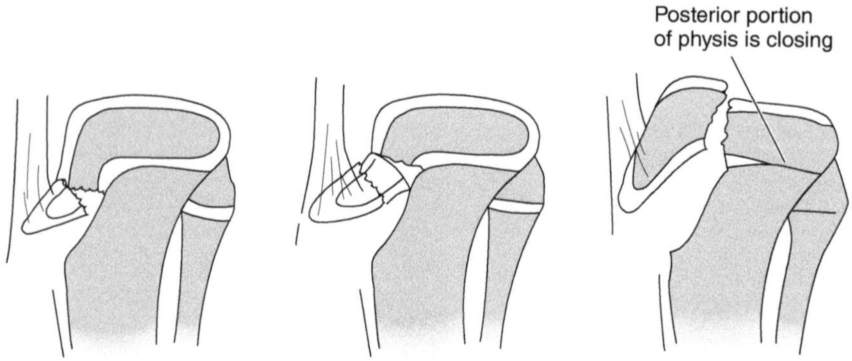

▲ **Figure 4–20.** Classification of avulsion fractures of the tibial tubercle. Type 1 fracture (**left**) across the secondary ossification center at level with the posterior border of the inserting patellar ligament. Type 2 fracture (**center**) at the junction of the primary and secondary ossification centers of the proximal tibial epiphysis. Type 3 fracture (**right**) propagates upward across the primary ossification center of the proximal tibial epiphysis into the knee joint. This fracture is a variant of the Salter-Harris III separation and is analogous to the fracture of Tillaux at the ankle because the posterior portion of the physis of the proximal tibia is closing. (Reprinted with permission, from Odgen JA, Tross RB, Murphy MJ. Fractures of the tibial tuberosity in adolescents. *J Bone Joint Surg Am.* 1980;62:205.)

Clinical Findings

Tibial tubercle avulsions occur in adolescent athletes, most often in males aged between 14 and 16 years. They result from a powerful contraction of the quadriceps muscle against a fixed tibia. This can occur by forced flexion of the knee against a powerful quadriceps contraction, as in an awkward landing at the end of a jump or fall. In addition to this lengthening mechanism, avulsion of the tubercle may occur with a sudden shortening of the quadriceps. The patellar tendon must be pulled hard enough to overcome the strength of the growth plate, the surrounding perichondrium, and the adjacent periosteum.

Swelling and tenderness are located over the proximal anterior tibia. A tense hemarthrosis may be present. A palpable defect in the anterior tibia is associated with a displaced avulsion fracture. Proximal migration of the patella occurs, and the patella may seem to float off the anterior aspect of the femur. The knee is held flexed, and the patient is unable to actively extend the knee.

Originally there were three types (Figure 4–20): type 1, in which there is a fracture across the secondary ossification center at the level of the posterior border of the patellar ligament; type 2, in which the fracture propagates between the primary and secondary ossification centers; and type 3, in which the fracture propagates upward through the main portion of the proximal tibial epiphysis. Two others were added later: type 4, with fracture through the entire proximal physis, and type 5, when the periosteal sleeve is avulsed with the extensor mechanism from the secondary ossification center. The degree of displacement depends on the severity of injury to the surrounding soft-tissue moorings. A lateral radiograph with the tibia slightly internally rotated is the best view to see the fracture and the degree of displacement.

Treatment

Full function of the extensor mechanism is necessary, and therefore, treatment of tibial tubercle avulsion fractures is aimed at this goal. If the fracture is minimally displaced and the patient is able to fully extend the knee against gravity, nonoperative treatment is acceptable. A cylinder cast should be applied with the knee extended and worn for 4 weeks. Active range of motion and strengthening exercises should then commence. At 6 weeks, quadriceps exercises against resistance are initiated. For displaced fractures, open reduction and internal fixation are recommended, with screws if the segment is large enough. If rigid fixation of large fragments is obtained, early active flexion and passive extension may be initiated. If a tenuous repair is obtained, protection in a cast is advisable.

Prognosis

Because the injury occurs in children who are close to skeletal maturity, meaningful growth abnormalities at the proximal tibial physis do not occur. Return to activities is allowed after the athlete develops quadriceps mass and strength equal to the uninjured side.

Young EY, Shlykov MA, Hosseinzadeh P, Abzug JM, Baldwin KD, Milbrandt TA. Fractures around the knee in children. *Instr Course Lect.* 2019;68:463-472. [PMID: 32032063]

OSGOOD-SCHLATTER DISEASE

Osgood-Schlatter disease, or osteochondrosis of the tibial tuberosity, usually occurs between 10 and 15 years of age in athletes and should not be confused with an acute avulsion

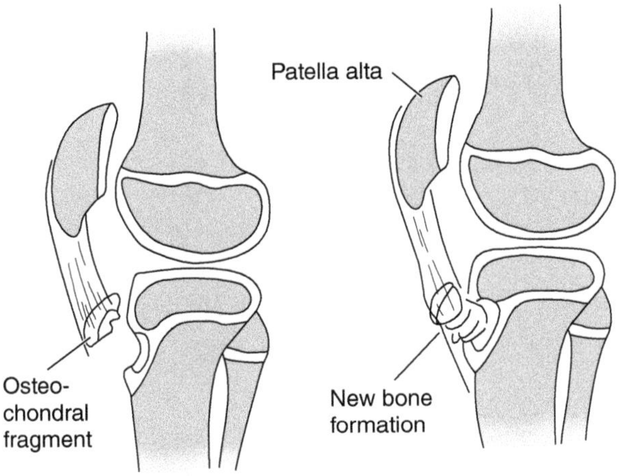

▲ **Figure 4–21.** Development of Osgood-Schlatter lesion. (**Left**) Avulsion of osteochondral fragment that includes surface cartilage and a portion of the secondary ossification center of the tibial tubercle. (**Right**) New bone fills in the gap between the avulsed osteochondral fragment and the tibial tubercle. (Reproduced, with permission, from Rockwood CA Jr, ed. *Fractures in Children*, 3rd ed. Philadelphia: Lippincott; 1991.)

fracture of the tibial tubercle. It occurs younger in females than males and is bilateral in about one-quarter of patients. Pain is located at the tibial tubercle and is usually present intermittently over a period of several months to a few years. Walking on a flat surface is not difficult, but ascending or descending stairs causes difficulty. Physical examination reveals tenderness and prominence of the tibial tubercle. Radiograph examination shows slight separation of the tibial tubercle with new bone formation beneath it (Figure 4–21).

Treatment for Osgood-Schlatter disease initially focuses on decreasing pain. This involves activity modification, ice, and quadriceps stretching. Patella tendon straps may also help. The long-term prognosis for pain relief is excellent. Early short-term immobilization may shorten the period of discomfort. Explaining the benign nature of the problem to both the patient and the parents, reassuring them that the long-term prognosis is good, and decreasing activity usually allow continued participation in athletics. The pain will go away when the tubercle unites with the tibia. In a very small number of cases, chronic pain will be present if the ossicle fails to unite. Painful ossicles in the adult are successfully treated with simple excision.

AVULSIONS ABOUT THE PELVIS

Clinical Findings

In the skeletally immature athlete, the apophysis, or growth plate where the muscle attaches to bone, is the weak link in the bone-muscle-tendon unit. Therefore, just as the growth plate is prone to breaking in children's fractures, the bony origin of muscles may be pulled off. This most commonly occurs in athletes between 14 and 25 years of age, with the majority of patients falling in the lower aspect of this age range. Comparison radiographs may be helpful to make sure the avulsion fracture is not just a normal anatomic variant. In the pelvis, this may occur at the iliac crest (abdominal muscles), anterior superior iliac spine (sartorius origin), anterior inferior iliac spine (rectus femoris origin), ischial tuberosity (hamstring origin), and lesser trochanter of the femur (iliopsoas insertion). Injury usually occurs from a forceful contraction or lengthening of the activated muscle that puts a force on the previously mentioned tendinous origins and insertions. Patients often perceive a "crack" or "pop" followed by intense pain.

Treatment and Prognosis

Symptomatic care with a few days of rest followed by ambulation with crutches for about a month is recommended. It is usually 6 to 10 weeks before athletic activities may be resumed. Long-term athletic activity will probably not be affected. Nonoperative care of protected weight bearing, avoiding tension on the affected muscle, ice, and activity modification usually results in healing. Operative fixation for large fragments (>2 cm) displaced greater than 1.5 to 2 cm has been advocated. These operative criteria may decrease the possibility of nonunion or heterotopic ossification that may occur in the ischial tuberosity region and be the cause of chronic bursitis and pain but add the potential postoperative complications of transient or permanent numbness and implant irritation. Excision of the painful nonunion fragment and excision of the exuberant callous, when present, resolve these problems.

Calderazzi F, Nosenzo A, Galavotti C, Menozzi M, Pogliacomi F, Ceccarelli F. Apophyseal avulsion fractures of the pelvis. A review. *Acta Biomed* 2018;89(4):470-476. [PMID: 30657114]

5 Disorders, Diseases, and Injuries of the Spine

Elliott Kim, MD
Bobby K.B. Tay, MD
Brett A. Freedman, MD
Scott D. Boden, MD
John M. Rhee, MD

INFLAMMATORY DISEASES OF THE SPINE

RHEUMATOID ARTHRITIS

Essentials of Diagnosis

- *Up to 71% of patients with rheumatoid arthritis have C-spine involvement.*
- *C1-C2 instability, basilar invagination, and subaxial subluxation are common disease patterns.*
- *Inflammatory pannus causes synovial joint destruction.*
- *Eighty percent of patients are rheumatoid factor positive.*

General Considerations

Rheumatoid arthritis is the most common form of inflammatory arthritis. It affects 3% of women and 1% of men. The disease frequently affects the spine. Up to 71% of patients with rheumatoid arthritis show involvement of the cervical spine. Risk factors for cervical spine involvement include female gender, positive rheumatoid factor, long-term corticosteroid treatment, peripheral joint erosions, younger age, and markers of higher disease activity including erythrocyte sedimentation rate (ESR) and C-reactive protein (CRP). The most common patterns of involvement are C1-C2 instability, basilar invagination, and subaxial subluxation. Of these patterns, both C1-C2 instability and basilar invagination have become less frequently encountered as a result of improvements in pharmacologic therapy. Sudden death associated with rheumatoid arthritis, most probably secondary to brainstem compression or vertebrobasilar insufficiency, is reported.

Pathogenesis

The same inflammatory cells that destroy peripheral joints affect the synovium of apophyseal and uncovertebral joints of the spine, causing painful instability with or without neurologic compromise. The pannus, a combination of hypertrophic synovium and inflammatory cells, often causes facet joint and transverse ligament destruction, leading to painful instability. The hypertrophic tissue can also cause direct compression of the spinal cord and nerve roots at the affected levels.

Prevention

Prevention of rheumatoid instability centers on control of the inflammatory component of the disease. Pharmacotherapeutic strategy initially involves the use of anti-inflammatory medication and application of disease-modifying antirheumatic drugs (DMARDs). Over the past decade, biologic agents such as infliximab, etanercept, and adalimumab have been shown to be effective in helping to control disease activity and suppress joint destruction. Biologic agents work by targeting specific steps in the inflammatory process, unlike DMARDs, which target the entire immune system. Furthermore, evidence has shown that biologic agents help prevent new cervical lesions from developing in patients with rheumatoid arthritis.

Clinical Findings

A. Symptoms and Signs

From 7% to 34% of patients present with neurologic problems. Documentation of neurologic function can be difficult because loss of joint mobility leads to general muscle weakness. Although many patients complain of nonspecific neck pain, atlantoaxial subluxation is the most common cause of pain in the upper neck, occiput, and forehead in patients with rheumatoid arthritis. Symptoms are aggravated by motion. Increased compression of the spinal cord can result in severe myelopathy with gait abnormalities, weakness, paresthesia, and loss of dexterity. Findings may also include Lhermitte sign (a tingling or electrical feeling that occurs in the arms, legs, or trunk when the neck is flexed), increased muscle tone of the upper and lower extremities, and pathologic reflexes.

B. Imaging Studies

Instability of the upper cervical spine is determined on lateral flexion-extension radiographs. An atlantodens interval (ADI) that exceeds 3.5 mm is abnormal. Subluxation with an ADI of 10 to 12 mm indicates disruption of all supporting ligaments of the atlantoaxial complex (transverse and alar ligaments). The spinal cord in this position is compressed between the dens and the posterior arch of C1. Although the ADI is an important measurement for traumatic instability of the C1-C2 complex, the posterior ADI (PADI) is more prognostic to assess neurologic compromise. The PADI is a direct measure of the space available for the spinal cord at the C1-C2 level. The PADI is measured from the posterior aspect of the odontoid process to the nearest posterior structure (the foramen magnum or the posterior ring of the atlas). If the space available for the spinal cord is less than 13 mm, the likelihood that the patient will develop myelopathy is extremely high.

Cranial settling is present in 5% to 32% of patients. The odontoid process should not project more than 3 mm above the Chamberlain line, which is a line between the hard palate and the posterior rim of the foramen magnum. The tip of the dens should not project more than 4.5 mm above the McGregor line, which is a line connecting the posterior margin of the hard palate to the occiput. The Clark classification divides the axis into thirds in the sagittal plane. In severe cases of cranial settling, the anterior arch of C1 moves from station 1 (the upper third of C2) to station 3 (the lower third of C2). Neurologic compromise occurs as a result of impingement of the dens into the brainstem and the upper cervical spinal cord. The vertebral arteries can also become occluded as they course between the dens and the foramen magnum to enter the skull.

Lateral subluxation and posterior atlantoaxial instability are less frequent. From 10% to 20% of patients with rheumatoid arthritis present with subaxial subluxation. Erosion of the facet joints and narrowing of the disks leads to subtle anterior subluxations often found on several levels. This results in the characteristic so-called stepladder deformity that occurs most commonly at the C2-C3 and C3-C4 levels.

C. Laboratory Studies

Rheumatoid factor is positive in up to 80% of patients. The ESR and CRP rate are elevated and the hemoglobin is decreased in the active phase of the disease. After plain radiographs, which should include lateral flexion-extension views, magnetic resonance imaging (MRI) is the study of choice to evaluate the degree of neural compression and deformity.

Differential Diagnosis

- Osteoarthritis
- Other inflammatory arthritides

Complications

Untreated instability can lead to loss of neurologic function, paralysis, and sudden death. Medical treatment using DMARDs can cause immunosuppression and lead to a higher risk of contracting infections. Complications of surgical treatment include a higher rate of infection, poor wound healing, lower fusion rate, and potentially a higher rate of instrumentation failure due to poor bone quality.

Treatment

Indications for surgery are severe neck pain and increasing loss of neurologic function. Most commonly, a posterior arthrodesis between C1 and C2 is performed. A Gallie type or Brooks type of fusion can be done, or segmental C1 and C2 screw fixation can be used (Figure 5–1). The latter obviates the need for postoperative halo immobilization, avoids intrusion of instrumentation into the spinal canal, and is generally the preferred technique. In cases of basilar invagination (cranial settling), extension of the fusion to the occiput may be necessary. However, there is evidence that C1-C2 fusion alone can have long-term successful outcomes as long as there is no active destruction of the occipital-C1 joints (Figure 5–2). Preoperative halo traction is often required to reduce the subluxation or pull the odontoid process out of the foramen magnum. Often a suboccipital craniectomy is necessary to decompress the brainstem adequately. Good fixation can be obtained through the use of plate-screw and rod-screw constructs. Subaxial subluxation with spinal cord compression should be treated with decompression and stabilization with spinal fusion. This can be done most easily via a posterior approach with laminectomy and posterior instrumented fusion or a combined anterior and posterior decompression and fusion for patients with poor bone stock or significant sagittal plane deformity (Figure 5–3).

Kaito T, Ohshima S, Fujiwara H, Makino T, Yonenobu K, Yoshikawa H. Incidence and risk factors for cervical lesions in patients with rheumatoid arthritis under the current pharmacologic treatment paradigm. *Mod Rheumatol.* 2017;27(4):593-597. [PMID: 27830965]

Lopez-Medina C, Molto A, Dubremetz M, et al. Assessment of adherence to disease-modifying drugs in patients with chronic inflammatory rheumatic disease: results of a survey of 1594 patients. *Joint Bone Spine.* 2019;86(5):610-614. [PMID: 30738192]

Miura K, Morita O, Hirano T, et al. Prevalence and factors associated with dysfunctional low back pain in patients with rheumatoid arthritis. *Eur Spine J.* 2019;28(5):976-982. [PMID: 30850879]

Werle S, Ezzati A, ElSaghir H, Boehm H. Is inclusion of the occiput necessary in fusion for C1-2 instability in rheumatoid arthritis? *J Neurosurg Spine.* 2013;18(1):50-56. [PMID: 23157277]

Zhu S, Xu W, Luo Y, Zhao Y, Liu Y. Cervical spine involvement risk factors in rheumatoid arthritis: a meta-analysis. *Int J Rheum Dis.* 2017;20(5):541-549. [PMID: 28524646]

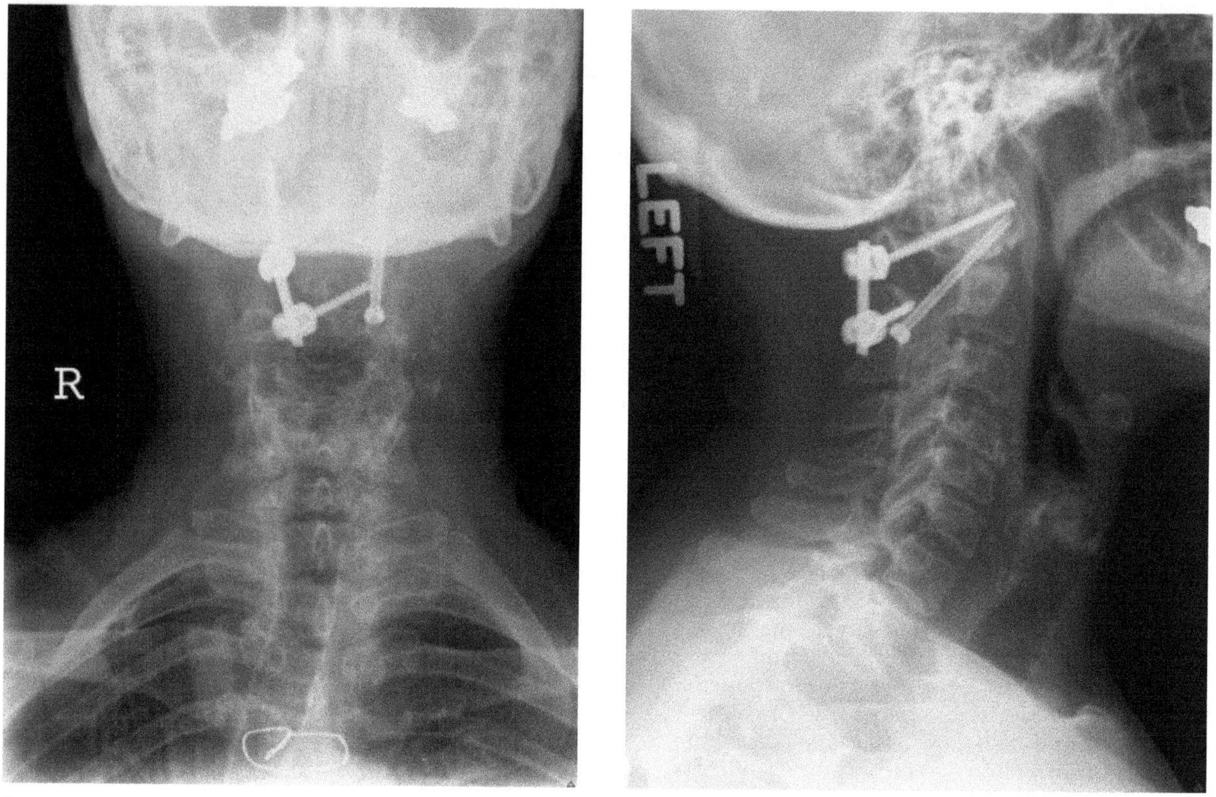

A B

▲ **Figure 5–1.** (**A and B**) Anteroposterior and lateral radiographic images of a 50-year-old woman with rheumatoid arthritis who suffered a fracture of the odontoid treated with posterior C1-C2 fusion with a transarticular screw construct on the right and a C1 lateral mass/C2 translaminar screw construct on the left.

ANKYLOSING SPONDYLITIS

Essentials of Diagnosis

- *Seronegative spondyloarthropathy.*
- *Juvenile ankylosing spondylitis has a predisposition to hip involvement.*
- *Unlike rheumatoid arthritis, males are more often affected than females.*
- *Eighty-eight percent to ninety-six percent of patients with ankylosing spondylitis are HLA-B27 positive.*

General Considerations

Ankylosing spondylitis is a chronic seronegative inflammatory disease that affects the axial skeleton, especially the sacroiliac joints, hip joints, and spine. Extraskeletal involvement is found in the aorta, lung, and uvea. The incidence of ankylosing spondylitis is 0.5 to 1 per 1000 people. Although males are affected more frequently than females, mild courses of ankylosing spondylitis are more common in the latter. The disease usually has its onset during early adulthood. However, juvenile ankylosing spondylitis affects adolescents (younger than 16 years) and has a predisposition to hip involvement.

Pathogenesis

The human leukocyte antigen (HLA)-B27 surface antigen is found in 88% to 96% of patients, and investigators postulate that an endogenic component (ie, HLA-B27) and an exogenic component (eg, *Klebsiella* or *Chlamydia*) are responsible for triggering of the disease process. The ESR is elevated in up to 80% of the cases but does not accurately reflect disease activity. The serum creatine phosphokinase (CPK), however, is a good indicator of the severity of the disease process.

Prevention

No preventive measures are available to avoid developing the disease. However, agents such as tumor necrosis factor-α (TNF-α) antagonists have been shown to slow the radiographic progression of the disease. Appropriate bracing prior

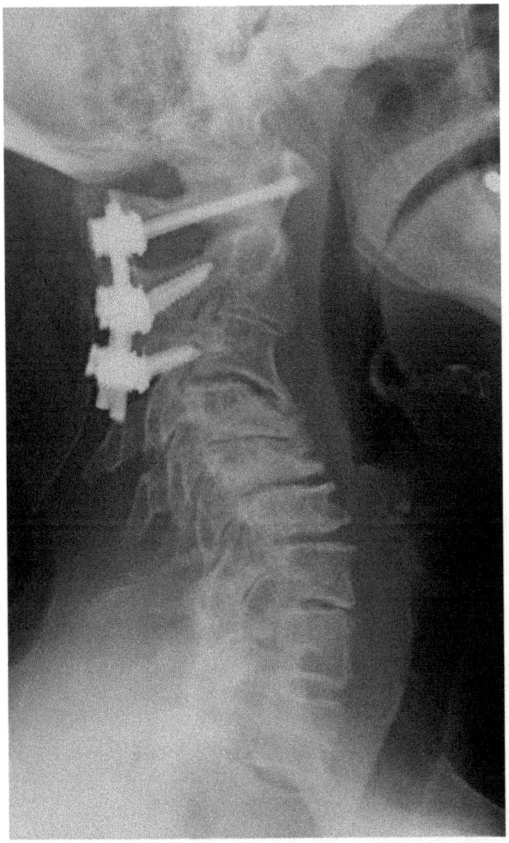

▲ **Figure 5–2.** A 72-year-old woman with rheumatoid arthritis on etanercept and C1-C2 instability. She underwent segmental screw fixation C1-C3 (C2-C3 was autofused) and posterior spinal fusion using structural iliac crest bone graft.

to the onset of spinal ankylosis can minimize or prevent the development of spinal deformity.

Clinical Findings

A. Symptoms and Signs

The onset is insidious, with early symptoms including pain in the buttocks, heels, and lower back. Patients complain typically of morning stiffness, the improvement of symptoms with activity during the day, and the return of symptoms in the evening. The earliest changes involve the sacroiliac joints and then extend upward into the spine. Spinal disease results in loss of motion and subsequent loss of lordosis in the cervical and lumbar spine. Synovitis in the early stages leads to progressive fibrosis and ankylosis of the joints during the reparative phase. Enthesitis occurs at the insertion of the annulus fibrosus on the vertebral body with eventual calcification that results in the characteristic "bamboo spine." The pain from the inflammatory process subsides after full ankylosis of the affected joints occurs. Approximately 30% of patients develop uveitis, and 30% have chest tightness. Limited chest expansion indicates thoracic involvement. Fewer than 5% of patients have involvement of the aorta, characterized by dilation and possible conduction defects. In addition, patients may suffer from renal amyloidosis and pulmonary fibrosis. Due to the severe rigidity of the spine, patients with ankylosing spondylitis are more prone to fractures after low-energy trauma and have a much higher incidence of spinal cord injuries with spine fractures. Careful evaluation is needed to avoid missing potentially devastating neurologic injuries in this patient population.

B. Imaging Studies

The earliest radiographic changes are visible in the sacroiliac joints. Symmetric bilateral widening of the joint space is followed by subchondral erosions and ankylosis. Bony changes in the spine affect the vertebral body. Changes include loss of the anterior concavity of the vertebral body, squaring of the vertebra, and marginal syndesmophyte formation, which give the spine the appearance of bamboo. Ankylosis of the apophyseal joints also develops. The disease generally starts in the lumbar spine and migrates cephalad to the cervical spine. Atlantoaxial instability is seen occasionally.

Differential Diagnosis

Early stages of the disease can appear to be similar to other inflammatory spondyloarthropathies.

Complications

The main complications of untreated cervical spinal deformity include significant loss of functionality from inability to look forward (loss of horizontal gaze). Complications of surgical treatment include infection, paralysis, spinal cord or nerve root injury, and proximal junctional kyphosis in cases of deformity correction. Because of medical treatments, these patients are at a higher risk for wound complications and postsurgical infections. TNF-α antagonists should be stopped for at least 2 weeks prior to surgical treatment to minimize the risk for infection. Prolonged use of a halo vest in the postoperative period (up to 6 months) can lead to halo-related complications, including pin site infection and intracranial perforation of the halo pins over time. The patient's osteoporotic bone (especially in the cervical spine lateral masses) increases the risk of hardware pullout.

Treatment

The natural history of ankylosing spondylitis, with its slow progression over several decades, has to be considered in planning treatment. Initially, treatment consists of exercises and nonsteroidal anti-inflammatory drugs (NSAIDs) such as

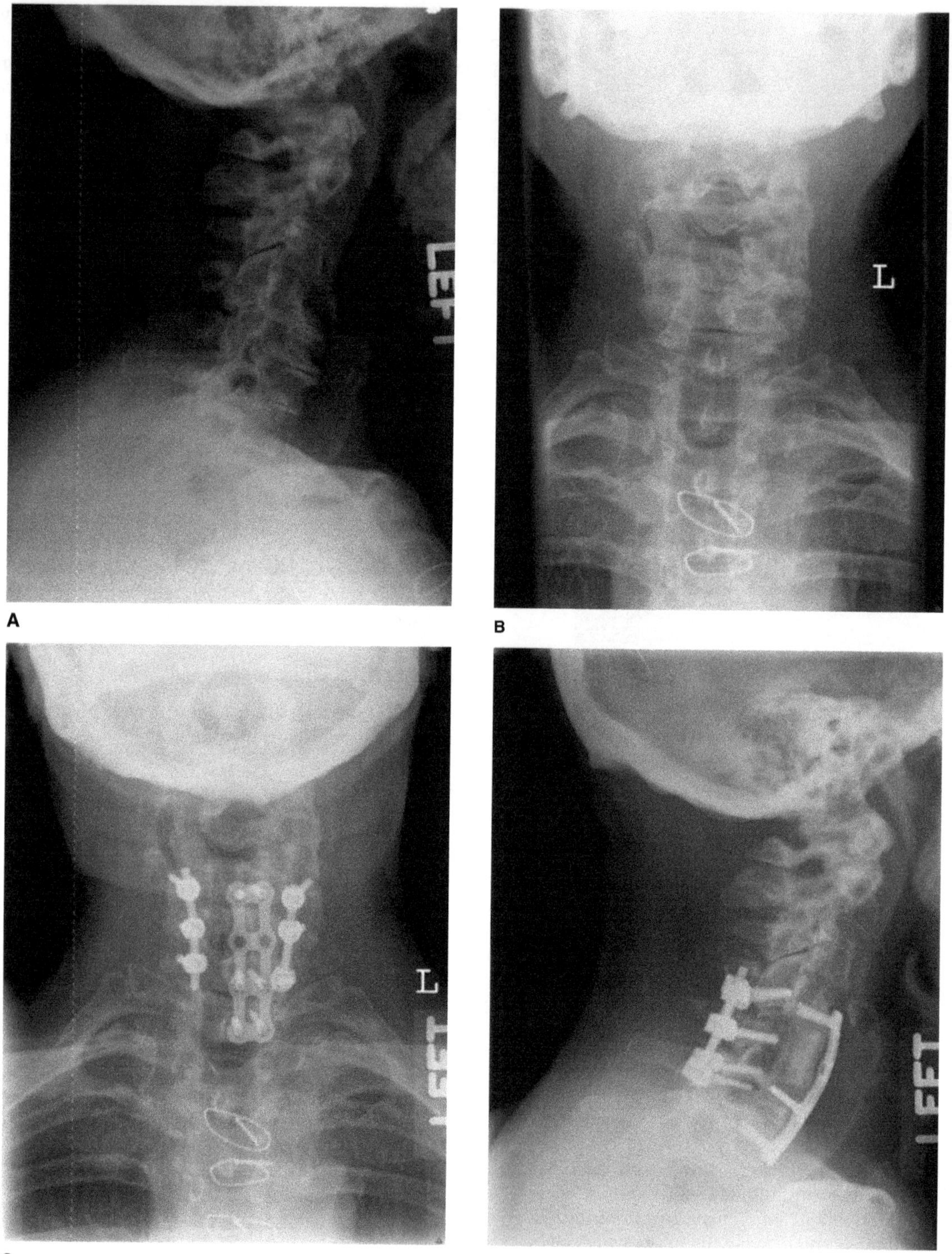

A B C D

▲ **Figure 5–3.** (**A and B**) Preoperative anteroposterior (AP) and lateral images of a 58-year-old man with inflammatory arthritis demonstrating severe joint damage and subaxial subluxation. (**C and D**) Postoperative AP and lateral radiographic images after treatment with anterior and posterior decompression and reconstruction with fusion.

naproxen and indomethacin. Approximately 10% of patients develop severe bony changes that eventually require surgical intervention. These changes characteristically include a fixed bony flexion deformity that limits their ambulatory potential. When planning surgical treatment, it is important to stop treatment with TNF-α inhibitors for at least 2 weeks prior to surgery to minimize the risk for wound infection. Furthermore, up to a third of patients with ankylosing spondylitis are concomitantly diagnosed with osteoporosis. An appropriate workup including a bone mineral density study may be needed prior to surgical intervention. Relative contraindications to surgery are poor general health and significant calcification of the major vessels, which may be injured when the spine is extended. Preoperative planning is crucial for successful outcomes in deformity correction in ankylosing spondylitis patients. The surgeon should analyze the overall sagittal alignment as well as the shape of the deformity. It is important to determine mobile segments in a stiff spine for planning purposes as well as understanding possible compensatory mechanisms through the hip and knee joints. Hip disease should be addressed before correction of spinal deformities because correction of hip flexion deformities may allow significant compensation of the spinal kyphosis to allow adequate horizontal gaze. Understanding these factors can help the surgeon determine whether the most effective correction will be in the thoracolumbar or cervical spine. Correction through the midthoracic spine is not recommended given the rigidity of the costosternal and costovertebral articulations preventing significant correction.

Loss of lumbar lordosis can be treated by multilevel V-shaped osteotomies posteriorly (the Smith-Petersen procedure), by a decancellation procedure (the Heinig procedure), or by pedicle subtraction osteotomy (Thomassen osteotomy) (Figure 5–4). The L2, L3, and L4 levels are commonly used because they correlate with the apex of the normal lumbar lordosis and allow for adequate distal fixation to hold the osteotomy in a stable configuration.

The spine is then fused in the corrected position. Utilization of pedicle screw-rod constructs allows for early mobilization of the patient. Thorough preoperative assessment of the deformity and measuring of the chin-eyebrow-to-floor angle are helpful for the exact planning of the corrective osteotomy.

The cervical osteotomy is typically performed between C7 and T1. This approach avoids injury to the vertebral artery that usually enters the transverse foramen at the C6 level. Historically, the procedure was usually performed under local anesthesia in the semisitting position with facet wiring and halo application as the only forms of fixation. However, the evolution of somatosensory and transcranial motor evoked potential monitoring of the spinal cord permits the use of general anesthesia. After removal of the posterior elements and neural decompression, the kyphotic deformity is corrected with gentle extension of the head. The ossified disk space fractures under the extension force and hinges on

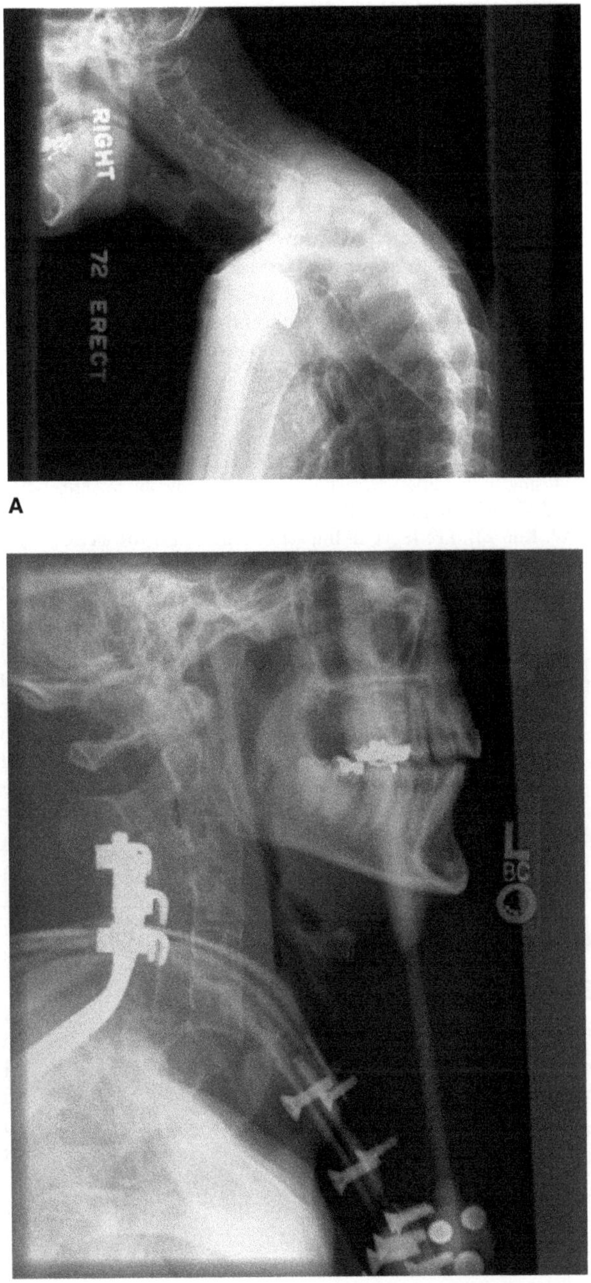

A

B

▲ **Figure 5–4.** Preoperative (**A**) and postoperative (**B**) lateral radiographs of a 38-year-old man with cervicothoracic kyphosis and loss of horizontal gaze who was treated with a posterior cervicothoracic osteotomy and instrumented fusion.

the posterior longitudinal ligament. The head is held in the corrected position using internal fixation typically with rod-screw constructs or, traditionally, with hook-rod constructs supplemented with a halo (see Figure 5–4). Long constructs with multiple levels of fixation often to C2 or C3 are necessary to obtain sufficient purchase in the ossified but osteoporotic bone to allow for adequate biomechanical stability. Other procedures, such as a decancellation wedge osteotomy of C7, have also been described. However, great care must be taken in these cases to avoid inadvertent spinal translation at the osteotomy site that can cause injury to the nerves or the spinal cord. Adoption of circumferential fusion and fixation techniques has allowed the potential to avoid halo vest immobilization.

Koller H, Koller J, Mayer M, Hempfing A, Hitzl W. Osteotomies in ankylosing spondylitis: where, how many, and how much? *Eur Spine J.* 2018;27(suppl 1):70-100. [PMID: 29290050]

Park JW, Kim MJ, Lee JS, et al. Impact of tumor necrosis factor inhibitor versus nonsteroidal antiinflammatory drug treatment on radiographic progression in early ankylosing spondylitis: its relationship to inflammation control during treatment. *Arthritis Rheumatol.* 2019;71(1):82-90. [PMID: 29984487]

Qian BP, Huang JC, Qiu Y, et al. Complications of spinal osteotomy for thoracolumbar kyphosis secondary to ankylosing spondylitis in 342 patients: incidence and risk factors. *J Neurosurg Spine.* 2018;30:91-98. [PMID: 30485225]

Teunissen FR, Verbeek BM, Cha TD, Schwab JH. Spinal cord injury after traumatic spine fracture in patients with ankylosing spinal disorders. *J Neurosurg Spine.* 2017;27(6):709-716. [PMID: 28984512]

DISEASES AND DISORDERS OF THE CERVICAL SPINE

Essentials of Diagnosis

- *Adequate imaging is essential to diagnosis.*
- *Imaging must include the entire cervical spine and the occipitocervical and cervicothoracic junctions.*
- *Lateral cervical spine view is the most important view in radiographic imaging of the cervical spine.*
- *Inadequate imaging will miss over 20% of cervical injuries.*

General Considerations

In evaluating the cervical spine, the use of appropriate imaging studies is critical to a timely and precise diagnosis. Available imaging techniques include plain radiography, tomography, myelography, computed tomography (CT), CT with myelography, three-dimensional reconstruction CT, MRI, and scintigraphy. An understanding of the advantages and disadvantages of each technique is necessary for the proper selection of imaging studies and interpretation of results.

A. Plain Radiography

In evaluating the patient with neck pain, cervical spine radiographs are important in the initial search for a possible lesion. In the trauma setting, when a head or neck injury is suspected, radiographic studies must be carried out appropriately or a life-threatening lesion may be overlooked. The trauma series includes anteroposterior (AP), right oblique, left oblique, and open-mouth (odontoid) views in addition to an initial cross-table lateral view. When all five views are taken, sensitivity is 92%. Cervical spine precautions must be implemented throughout the radiographic evaluation (see the section on injuries of the cervical spine). In the absence of a history of trauma, the oblique and odontoid views are not always required.

The lateral view reveals the majority of traumatic lesions if performed correctly. Inadequate views can miss more than 20% of cervical spine injuries, however. All seven vertebrae should be clearly visible. Gentle traction on the upper extremities may be necessary to view C7. If this is unsuccessful, a swimmer's view may be necessary. Careful scrutiny of the prevertebral soft tissue, the anterior border of the vertebral bodies, the vertebral bodies themselves, the posterior border of the bodies, the spinal canal proper, and the posterior elements must be done.

The prevertebral region may reveal swelling consistent with a hematoma, and this may serve as the only clue to a traumatic lesion. The upper limits for the prevertebral space are 10 mm at C1; 5 mm at C2; 7 mm at C3 and C4; and 20 mm at C5, C6, and C7. The contours of the cervical bony structures are regular, and subtle incongruities may indicate significant instability. Variations in normal cervical anatomy do exist, however, and a familiarity with them may prevent an overzealous workup. The ADI normally measures less than 3 mm in adults and less than 4 mm in children.

In reviewing the AP radiograph, careful assessment of the interspinous distance must be undertaken. Vertical widening at a given level greater than 1.5 times the level above and below indicates a hyperflexion injury with posterior instability or interlocking of the posterior facets. Traumatic tilting may also be noted in the AP plane while not appreciated on the lateral view.

Oblique views taken at 45 degrees allow visualization of the articulations of the facet joints. The open-mouth view permits evaluation of the odontoid process, the lateral masses, and the articulations of the lateral masses, and it also permits assessment of the distance between each lateral mass and the odontoid process. In atlantoaxial rotatory subluxation, the lateral mass of the atlas that is rotated forward is closer to the midline (medial offset); the opposite mass is farther away from the midline (lateral offset). Burst fractures of the C1 ring cause overhang of the C1 lateral masses on C2. A combined overhang exceeding 6.9 mm is highly correlated with insufficiency of the transverse ligament and C1-C2 sagittal instability.

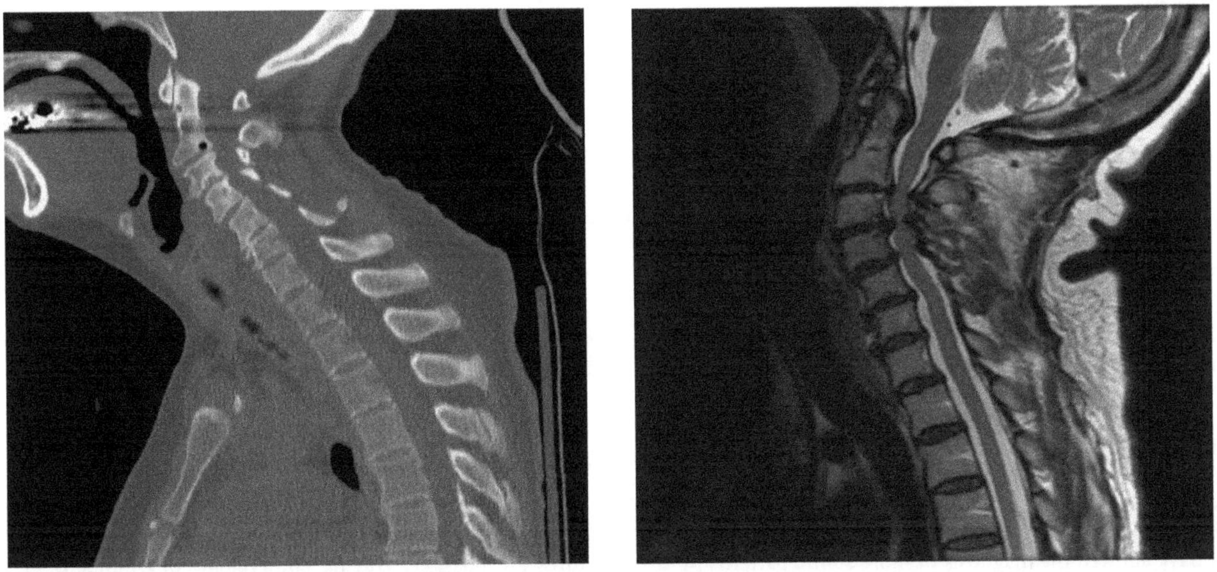

A B

▲ **Figure 5–5.** Sagittal CT (**A**) and MRI (**B**) images of a patient with cervical spondylotic myelopathy and spinal stenosis. CT demonstrates excellent bony detail, and the MRI allows assessment of the spinal cord and disks.

This radiographic series is equally important in evaluating infants and children with suspected congenital or developmental defects and adults with insidious neck pain. Arthritic changes may be subtle or readily apparent with osteophytes, disk space narrowing, and facet sclerosis. Bone quality can also be assessed on plain radiographs.

B. Computed Tomography

CT scans allow excellent visualization of the bony architecture and the paravertebral soft tissues of the cervical spine. The pedicles, laminae, spinous processes, and bony spinal canal can be examined with significantly better resolution when CT is used than when conventional radiographs are taken (Figure 5–5). CT with myelography or intrathecal contrast enhancement permits visualization of the spinal canal contents.

CT is an appropriate modality for evaluating congenital variations and malformations, including spinal canal stenosis and spina bifida. Pars defects, atlantoaxial joint diseases, inflammatory changes, primary tumors, and metastatic carcinoma are well appreciated with CT. Although cervical disk disease is detectable when thin cuts and contrast enhancement are used with CT, it is better visualized with MRI.

In the trauma patient, CT is integral in evaluating possible fractures or instability. Atrophy, deformity, and displacement of the spinal cord from acute or chronic injury are all appreciable with the use of intrathecal contrast. With the advent of MRI, however, CT is now typically reserved for the assessment of the bony architecture, which it does better than MRI. However, CT angiography may be added to help increase the detection of vertebral artery injuries (Figure 5–6).

Three-dimensional reconstruction of CT images can be rotated to evaluate the anatomy from almost any perspective.

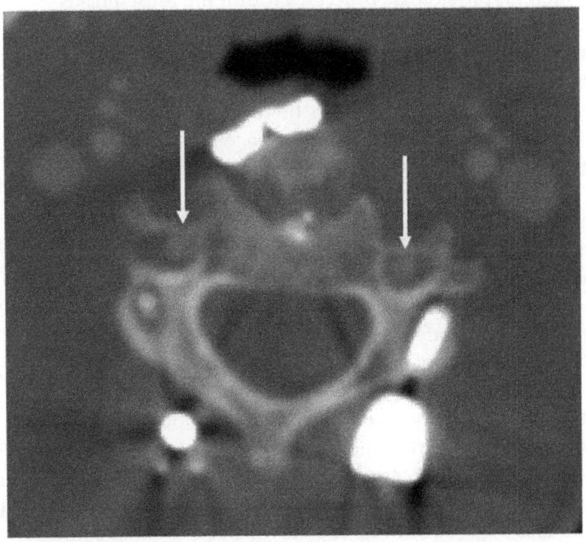

▲ **Figure 5–6.** This patient underwent anterior posterior cervical spine surgery from C1-C3 and presented with nonunion and instrumentation failure. Workup included a CT angiogram to evaluate the bony anatomy. Note the contrast material highlighting the vascular structures, including the vertebral arteries (*arrows*).

This technique is valuable in understanding atlantoaxial rotatory subluxations or complex fractures of the spinal column. Three-dimensional reconstructions can also aid in understanding complex deformities.

C. Magnetic Resonance Imaging

MRI permits axial, sagittal, coronal, or oblique plane analysis of the anatomy. It is routinely noninvasive, requiring contrast material in only selected cases.

MRI is the standard for assessing cervical spinal cord damage. Spinal cord tumors and trauma, as well as central disk herniation, can be easily visualized. In the preoperative evaluation of patients with spondylosis or disk herniation, MRI is the neuroimaging test of choice (see Figure 5–5).

Intravenous paramagnetic agent gadolinium is commonly used to differentiate tissues receiving higher blood flow. This is helpful in the diagnosis of infection, tumor, and postsurgical scar.

High-resolution dynamic (flexion/extension/upright) MRIs have allowed the diagnosis of more subtle patterns of spinal impingement that may not be apparent in a supine (nonloaded) MRI study with the neck in a neutral position. These can allow imaging to be done in a neck position that reproduces the patient's symptoms. However, in the majority of cases, a noncontrasted, supine cervical MRI is sufficient.

D. Scintigraphy

Bone scans that employ technetium-99m phosphate permit assessment of physiologic processes within the musculoskeletal system. Metabolic, metastatic, and inflammatory abnormalities can be detected. Technetium-99m phosphate is a bisphosphonate. Its chemical similarity to pyrophosphate promotes its incorporation into bone hydroxyapatite and accumulates in areas of increased osteogenesis. Early-phase imaging with technetium-99m gives blood flow information. Accordingly, subtle fractures, avascular necrosis, and osteomyelitis can be detected. Other radioisotopes used in scintigraphy include gallium-67 citrate, which labels serum proteins, and indium-111, which labels white blood cells. These labeling techniques are helpful in discerning areas of neoplasia or acute infection.

Currently, positron emission scintigraphy combined with high-resolution CT provides a more precise image of the affected areas due to the level of anatomic bony detail that CT scans can provide. Furthermore, the two modalities prove to be effective for unique cases such as diagnoses of postoperative infection where CT or MRI scan alone may create metallic artifact, making it difficult to discern which can be overcome with positron emission tomography (PET) modalities.

Tobert DG, Le HV, Blucher JA, Harris MB, Schoenfeld AJ. The clinical implications of adding CT angiography in the evaluation of cervical spine fractures: a propensity-matched analysis. *J Bone Joint Surg*. 2018;100(17):1490-1495. [PMID: 30180057]

CONGENITAL MALFORMATIONS

Essentials of Diagnosis

- *Os odontoideum is a congenital nonunion of the dens that can lead to significant C1-C2 instability.*
- *Injuries can occur after minimal trauma.*
- *Klippel-Feil syndrome exhibits a triad of clinical features: a short "web" neck, a low posterior hairline, and limited cervical neck motion.*
- *Syndromic conditions such as VATER (vertebrae, anus, trachea, esophagus, and renal abnormalities) must be ruled out in the presence of congenital failure of formation or segmentation in the cervical spine.*

General Considerations

The atlanto-occipital region is a frequent location for abnormalities. Various combinations involving bone and nervous structures are possible. During embryologic development, 42 somites are formed from the paraxial mesoderm. The somites divide into sclerotomes, which form the vertebral bodies after separation into a caudal and cephalad portion. The middle portion builds the intervertebral disk. The second, third, and fourth somites fuse and become the occiput and posterior part of the foramen magnum. The fate of the first somite is unclear. The development of the neural tube progresses simultaneously with that of the cartilaginous skeleton.

Disturbances of embryologic development can result in incomplete development or absence of a tissue or part, as found in dysraphism, aplasia of the odontoid process, incomplete closure of the atlas, or absence of the atlas facet. Lack of segmentation results in atlanto-occipital fusion, block vertebrae, and possible instability at adjacent cervical levels. A disturbance of neurologic development, alone or in combination with bony defects, can lead to basilar impression, Arnold-Chiari malformation, and syringomyelia, all of which manifest in various states of spinal cord dysfunction (myelopathy).

1. Os Odontoideum

Pathogenesis

Os odontoideum is an uncommon type of pseudarthrosis between the odontoid process and the body of the axis (Figure 5–7). It can cause significant atlantoaxial instability and myelopathy and can result in sudden death. Gross instability at the C1-C2 level can lead to spinal cord impingement or injury as it is compressed against the anterior portion of the axis or the posterior ring of the atlas. In some cases, extrinsic compression of the vertebral arteries results in ischemic insult to the brain.

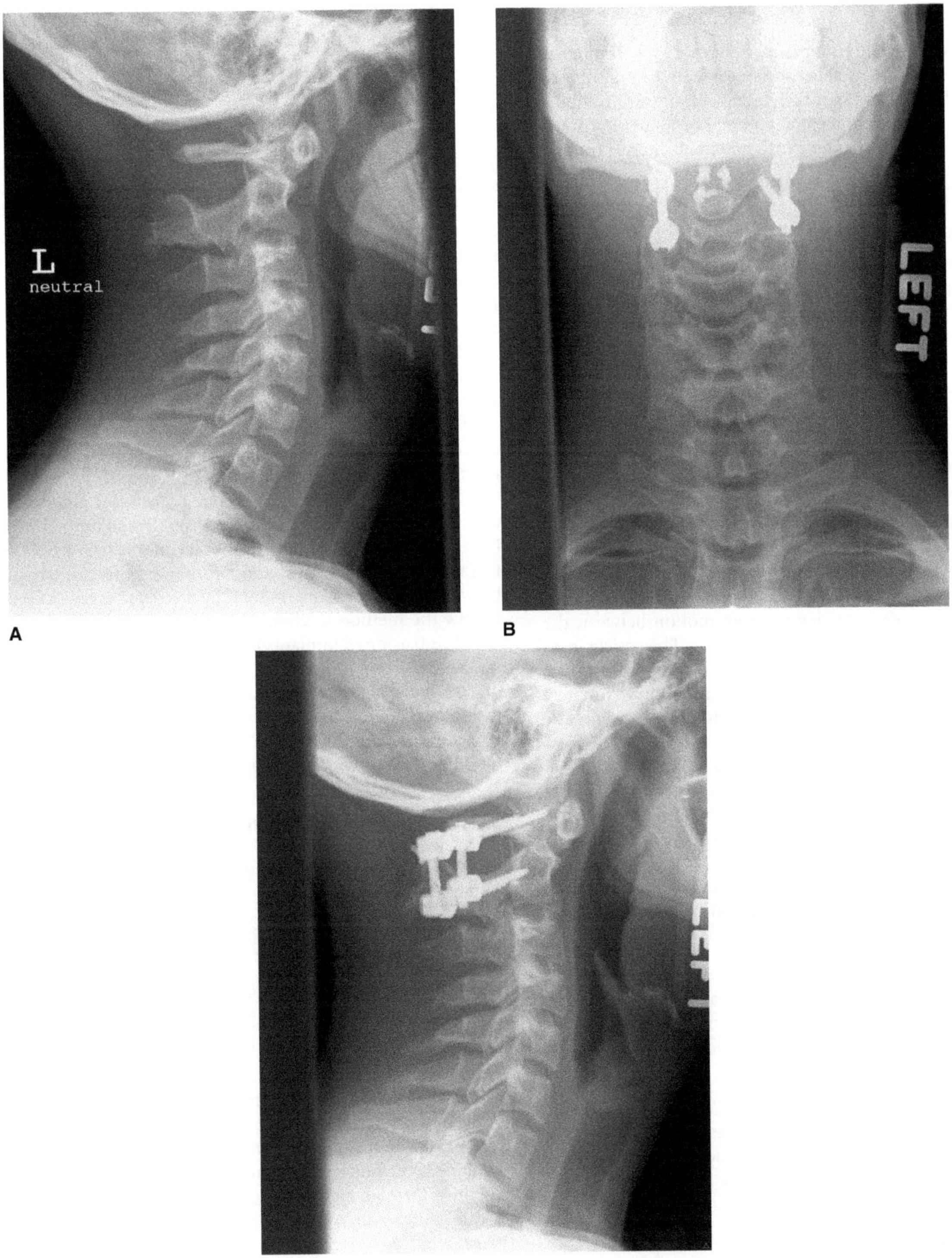

A B C

▲ **Figure 5–7.** (**A**) Lateral radiograph of a 24-year-old man with a symptomatic os odontoideum. (**B and C**) Anteroposterior and lateral radiographs after stabilization and fusion of C1-C2 to stabilize the os odontoideum.

Prevention

There is no preventive measure to avoid this congenital anomaly. However, a stable os odontoideum (no motion on flexion and extension) may be treated without surgical stabilization. In this case, the patient should be counseled about the risks of neurologic injury with potentially minor trauma.

Clinical Findings

A. Symptoms and Signs

Patients with os odontoideum may be asymptomatic or may present with symptoms and signs that relate to atlantoaxial instability, such as ill-defined neck complaints or focal or diffuse neurologic deficits. A careful history may be needed to rule out trauma, although congenital os odontoideum may come to the attention of the surgeon secondary to a reported but inconsequential neck injury.

B. Imaging Studies

The radiographic findings may be extremely subtle and difficult to distinguish. In the mature skeleton, os odontoideum appears as a radiographic lucency. In children younger than 5 years, however, an anomalous gap may be confused with a normal neural synchondrosis. Flexion-extension views must therefore be obtained to demonstrate motion between the odontoid process and the body of the axis. The ossicle in os odontoideum is either round or ovoid, with a smooth surface and uniform cortical thickness. It is usually approximately half the size of the normal odontoid process. In traumatic nonunion, the edge is irregular with a narrow gap. The fracture line may involve the body of C2 as well. An additional radiologic finding in os odontoideum is hypertrophy of the anterior ring of the atlas with a corresponding hypoplastic posterior ring. In flexion-extension views, the ossicle travels with the anterior ring of the atlas (see Figure 5–7). In cases that are difficult to diagnose, further studies include open-mouth views, tomograms, and CT reconstructions.

Differential Diagnosis

Dens fractures may appear similar to an os odontoideum. However, these fractures are often associated with more significant trauma (eg, motor vehicle accident).

Complications

Complications of nonsurgical treatment include neurologic injury, chronic neck pain, and sudden death. Complications of surgical treatment include paralysis, infection, stroke, or death from vertebral artery injury.

Treatment

Patients diagnosed with os odontoideum must be warned of the gravity of the situation because trauma to the spinal cord at this level can be fatal. Patients with cervical myelopathy can be treated with traction, immobilization, or both, but they often require subsequent posterior fusion. Direct osteosynthesis of the os odontoideum fragment is often not possible due to its small size. Sometimes symptoms are reversible with or without intervention. Management of asymptomatic patients with instability is controversial. The benefits of surgical stabilization in an attempt to avoid potentially lethal injury from trauma are counterbalanced by the possible complications of surgery. However, more recent evidence suggests that even asymptomatic patients should be strongly considered for surgical evaluation especially for those who are young, have anatomy favorable for surgical intervention, and show evidence of instability.

If fusion is indicated, usually a posterior fusion of C1-C2 is adequate. Different fusion techniques are available. Most surgeons use internal fixation of C1 lateral mass/C2 screw fixation with rods or transarticular screws. This can be combined with the Gallie or Brooks technique of structural bone grafting. The Gallie technique involves the use of a single block-shaped bone graft between the posterior ring of C1 and the spinous process of C2. A single sublaminar wire holds the graft in place. The Brooks technique uses from two to four sublaminar wires, and two bone grafts are wedged between the laminae of C1 and C2. In general, screw fixation is now the method of choice because it is more secure and avoids intrusion of implants into the spinal canal. The loss of motion between atlas and axis results in an overall decrease of 50% of cervical rotation. Use of screw-rod constructs that purchase into the lateral masses of C1 and the pedicle, pars, or lamina of C2 are rigid enough to allow the patient to mobilize with or without a soft cervical collar.

2. Klippel-Feil Syndrome

Essentials of Diagnosis

- *Syndrome associated with congenital fusion of cervical vertebrae.*
- *"Classic triad."*
- *Look for associated anomalies including scoliosis, renal disorders, deafness, and Sprengel deformity.*

Pathogenesis

Klippel-Feil syndrome refers to an array of clinical disorders associated with congenital fusion of one or more cervical vertebrae. The fusion, which may be multilevel, results from a failure of the normal division of the cervical somites during the third through eighth weeks of embryogenesis. The cause of this failure is unknown. The syndrome was first described in 1912 by M. Klippel and A. Feil as a triad of clinical features: a short "web" neck, a low posterior hairline, and limited cervical neck motion. Interestingly, only 50% of patients with the syndrome that now bears the names of Klippel and

Feil present with this classic triad. This condition is typically underreported given that many instances are found only incidentally on imaging studies.

Various conditions were subsequently seen in association with congenitally fused cervical vertebrae. These include scoliosis (seen in approximately 60% of cases), renal abnormalities (in 35%), deafness (in 30%), Sprengel deformity (in 30%), synkinesis or mirror movement (in 20%), congenital heart defects (in 14%), brainstem anomalies, congenital cervical stenosis, adrenal aplasia, ptosis, Duane contracture, lateral rectus palsy, facial nerve palsy, syndactyly, and upper extremity diffuse or focal hypoplasia.

Prevention

There is no preventive measure to avoid this congenital anomaly. Children with mild involvement can be expected to grow up to lead healthy, normal lives. Patients with more severe involvement can do comparably well if the associated conditions are successfully treated at an early age.

Clinical Findings

A. Symptoms and Signs

Decreased range of motion is the most frequent finding in patients with cervical spine involvement. Involvement of only the lower cervical spine or fusion of fewer than three vertebrae results in minimal loss of motion, however. Patients may also be able to compensate at other cervical interspaces, masking any loss of motion.

Neck shortening is difficult to detect unless extreme. Webbing of the neck (pterygium colli), facial asymmetry, or torticollis is seen in fewer than 20% of patients. Webbing of the neck can nevertheless be dramatic, with underlying muscle involvement extending from the mastoid to the acromion. Sprengel deformity, which results from a failure of either or both scapulae to descend from their embryologic origin at C4, is seen in approximately 30% of patients. Sometimes an omovertebral bone bridges the cervical spine to the scapulae and limits the neck and shoulder motion.

Cervical spine symptoms in Klippel-Feil syndrome are related to the secondary hypermobility of the unfused vertebrae. Except for atlantoaxial joint involvement, resulting in a significant decrease in occipital rotation, the fused joints at a given level are asymptomatic. Because of the increased mechanical demands placed on the uninvolved joints, secondary osteoarthritis, disk degeneration, spinal stenosis, and instability may result at these levels. Neurologic sequelae, usually confined to the head, neck, and upper extremities, result from impingement of the cervical nerve roots. Furthermore, due to the altered pattern of degenerative changes, patients with congenital cervical fusions appear to be more predisposed to cervical myelopathy compared to the general population. With progressive cervical instability, the spinal cord may become involved, leading to spasticity, weakness, hyperreflexia, and even quadriplegia or sudden death from minor trauma.

B. Imaging Studies

Radiographic findings of congenital cervical vertebral fusion are diagnostic of Klippel-Feil syndrome (Figure 5–8). This may present as synostosis of two vertebral bodies or as a multilevel fusion, as originally described in 1912. Other noteworthy findings are flattening of the involved vertebral bodies and the absence of disk spaces. Hypoplastic cervical disks in a child are often hard to appreciate radiographically. If suspected, flexion-extension views can be taken. CT scanning and MRI have can provide more detailed assessment of bony and nerve root involvement.

Spinal canal stenosis is not usually seen until adulthood. Although anterior spina bifida is infrequent, the posterior form is not. Enlargement of the foramen magnum with fixed hyperextension often accompanies the cervical spina bifida. Hemivertebrae can also occur in this syndrome.

Involvement of the upper thoracic spine may be the first sign of an undiagnosed cervical synostosis. Because of the potential for multiorgan involvement in patients with Klippel-Feil syndrome, an electrocardiogram and renal ultrasound are also recommended.

Differential Diagnosis

In the presence of associated congenital abnormalities such as hemivertebra, other syndromic conditions such as VATER should be ruled out.

Complications

Complications are directly related to the treatment of the specific symptomatic conditions. The complications of surgical treatment include nerve injury and paralysis. Nonfusion-type procedures can lead to kyphosis because the levels adjacent to the congenitally fused levels are often degenerated at the time of presentation. Anterior fusion surgery can often span more than one motion segment and can lead to loss of range of motion (from fusion) and can potentially accelerate the rate of wear of the segments adjacent to the surgical fusion. Extensile anterior approaches can be complicated by postoperative swallowing disorders or unilateral vocal cord paralysis.

Treatment

Treatment of cervical spine abnormalities is limited. Multilevel involvement leads to hypermobility at uninvolved joints, so affected patients should be cautious in their activities. Prophylactic surgical stabilization is not routinely performed in asymptomatic patients because the risk-benefit ratio has not been well defined. In some cases, however, surgical fusion is performed.

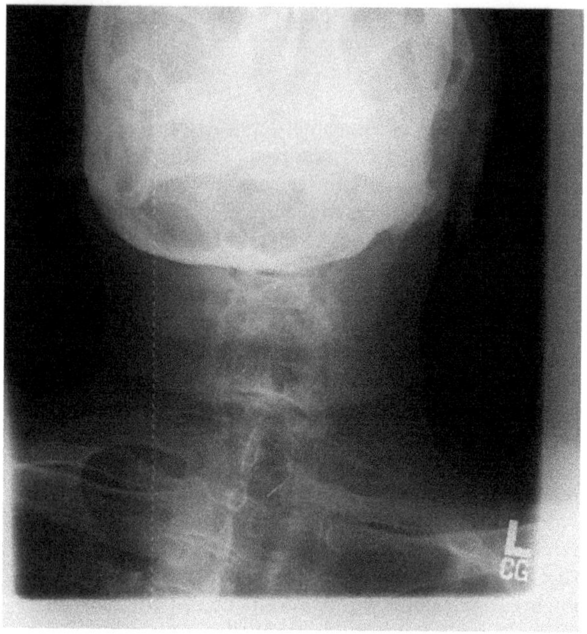

A

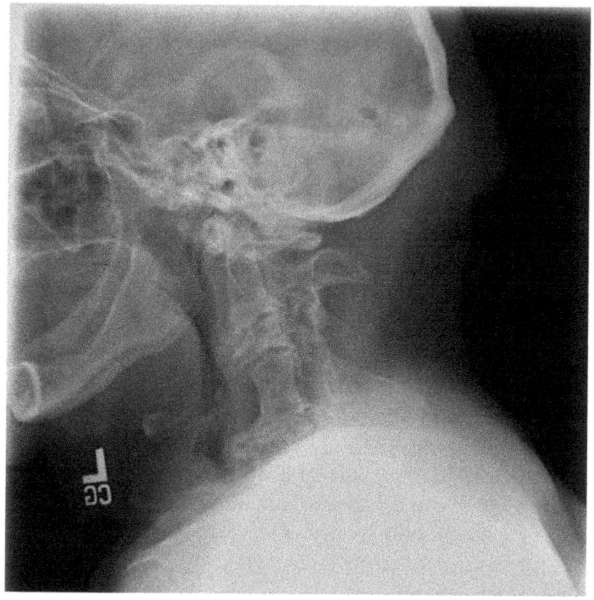

B

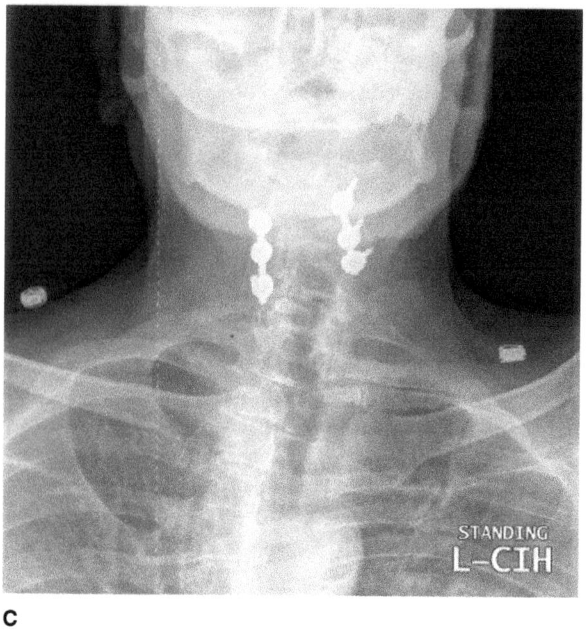

C

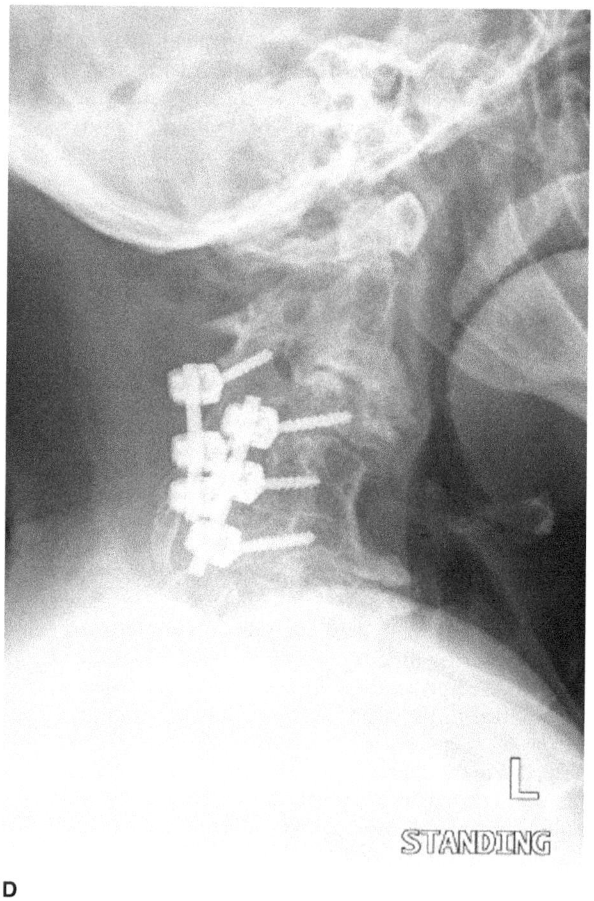

D

▲ **Figure 5–8.** (**A and B**) Anteroposterior (AP) and lateral radiographs of a 60-year-old man with Klippel-Feil demonstrating the congenitally fused cervical vertebrae that have led to deterioration of the adjacent disk segments, leading to severe spinal stenosis. (**C and D**) AP and lateral radiographs after posterior laminectomy and fusion with instrumentation.

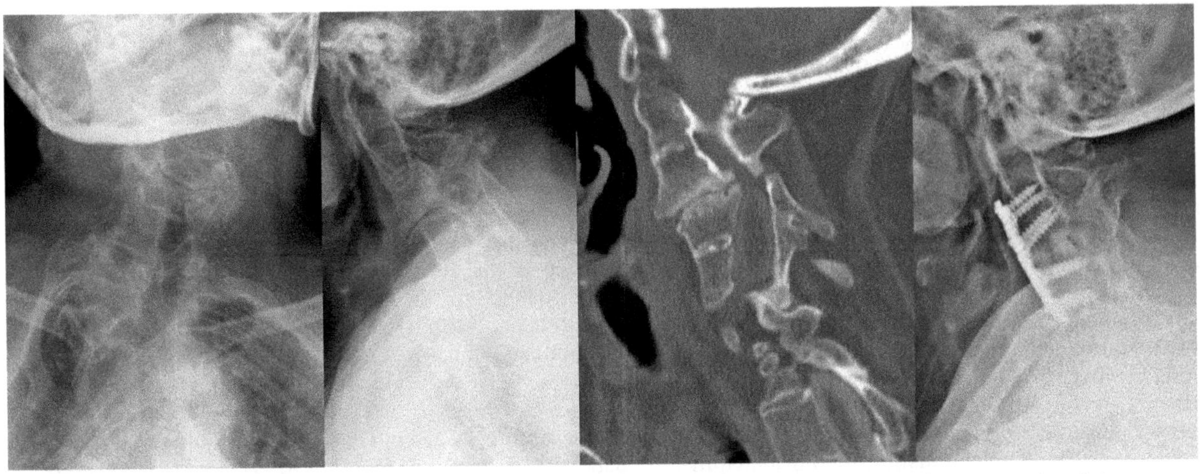

▲ **Figure 5–9.** A 55-year-old woman with multiple congenital anomalies of the spine, including cervical and thoracolumbar scoliosis, as well as congenital autofusions leaving only a single mobile segment at C3-C4 in the occipitocervical spine. She presented with progressive myelopathy at the C3-C4 level and was treated with C3-C4 anterior cervical diskectomy and fusion (ACDF). Supplemental fixation was placed into the autofused segments above and below.

Secondary osteoarthritis may be treated in the usual manner, including use of a cervical collar, traction, and anti-inflammatory agents. Nerve root impingement and canal stenosis require careful evaluation before surgical decompression because more than one level may be involved (Figure 5–9).

Surgical correction of the aesthetic deformities is only moderately successful. Carefully selected candidates may benefit from soft-tissue Z-plasty or tenotomies. This may improve the appearance of the patient but does not affect cervical motion.

Gruber J, Saleh A, Bakhsh W, Rubery PT, Mesfin A. The prevalence of Klippel-Feil syndrome: a computed tomography-based analysis of 2,917 patients. *Spine Deform.* 2018;6(4):448-453. [PMID: 29886918]

Nouri A, Martin AR, Lange SF, Kotter MRN, Mikulis DJ, Fehlings MG. Congenital cervical fusion as a risk factor for development of degenerative cervical myelopathy. *World Neurosurg.* 2017;100:531-539. [PMID: 28130167]

CERVICAL SPONDYLOSIS

Essentials of Diagnosis

- *Cervical spondylosis is directly associated with disk degeneration.*
- *The most frequently involved levels are the more mobile segments: C5-C6, C6-C7, and C4-C5.*
- *Spinal canal stenosis is present when the canal diameter becomes less than 13 mm.*
- *Extension of the cervical spine often exacerbates the symptoms of spinal cord and nerve root compression.*

General Considerations

Cervical spondylosis (International Classification of Diseases, 10th Revision [ICD-10] M47.812, M47.12) is defined as a generalized disease process affecting the entire cervical spine and related to chronic disk degeneration. In approximately 90% of men older than 50 years and 90% of women older than 60 years, degeneration of the cervical spine can be demonstrated by radiographs, but the vast majority of these are asymptomatic. Initial disk changes are followed by facet arthropathy, osteophyte formation, and ligamentous instability. Myelopathy, radiculopathy, or both may be seen secondarily. Cervical myelopathy is the most common form of spinal cord dysfunction in people older than 55 years. People older than 60 years are more likely to have multisegmental disease. The incidence of cervical myelopathy is twice as great in men as in women.

Pathogenesis

The relationship between the spinal cord and its bony arcade has been studied extensively. The first publication on the subject was written in the early 1800s and gave the first account of a "spondylotic bar," which was actually a thickened posterior longitudinal ligament protruding into the canal secondary to disk degeneration. Subsequent work revealed that disk degeneration and osteoarthritis could lead to spinal cord and nerve root impingement.

Acute traumatic disk herniation was distinguished from the chronic spondylotic process in the mid-1950s. Concurrently, anterior spinal artery impingement by the disk or osteophyte was proposed as part of the pathogenesis. As indicated in these studies, disk degeneration starts with tears in the posterolateral region of the annulus. The subsequent loss of water content and proteoglycans in the nucleus then leads to a decrease of disk height. The longitudinal ligaments degenerate and form bony spurs at their insertion into the vertebral body. These so-called hard disks have to be distinguished from soft disks, which represent acute herniation of disk material into the spinal canal or into the neural foramen. The most frequently involved levels are the more mobile segments: C5-C6, C6-C7, and C4-C5. The converging of the cervical disk space may result in buckling of the ligamentum flavum, with further narrowing of the spinal canal. Segmental instability results in hypertrophic formation of osteophytes by the uncovertebral joint of Luschka and by the facet joints. These prominent spurs result in compression of both the exiting nerve roots and the spinal cord.

Further work revealed that the sagittal cervical canal diameter was appreciably smaller (3 mm on average) in the myelopathic spondylotic spine than in the normal spine. The anterior-posterior dimensions of the cervical spinal canal measure between 17 and 18 mm in normal individuals. Spinal canal stenosis is present when the canal diameter becomes less than 13 mm. With extension of the neck, both the spinal canal diameter and the neuroforaminal diameter decrease.

Prevention

Cervical spondylosis is generally progressive with aging. However, it is critical to understand that radiologic degenerative changes do not necessarily correlate with symptoms and that the overwhelming majority of degenerative changes in the cervical spine are asymptomatic and, in and of themselves, do not constitute indications for treatment (Figure 5–10). It is not possible, on the basis of imaging findings alone, to determine whether spondylosis is symptomatic or not. Even neurologic impingement, in the absence of symptoms or clinical findings, does not necessarily warrant treatment. Over a long period of time, many patients have decreased pain, but those with the most severe involvement do not usually improve. Maintaining overall aerobic conditioning and fitness and awareness, early diagnosis, and appropriate treatment of spinal cord compression can reduce or prevent functional losses.

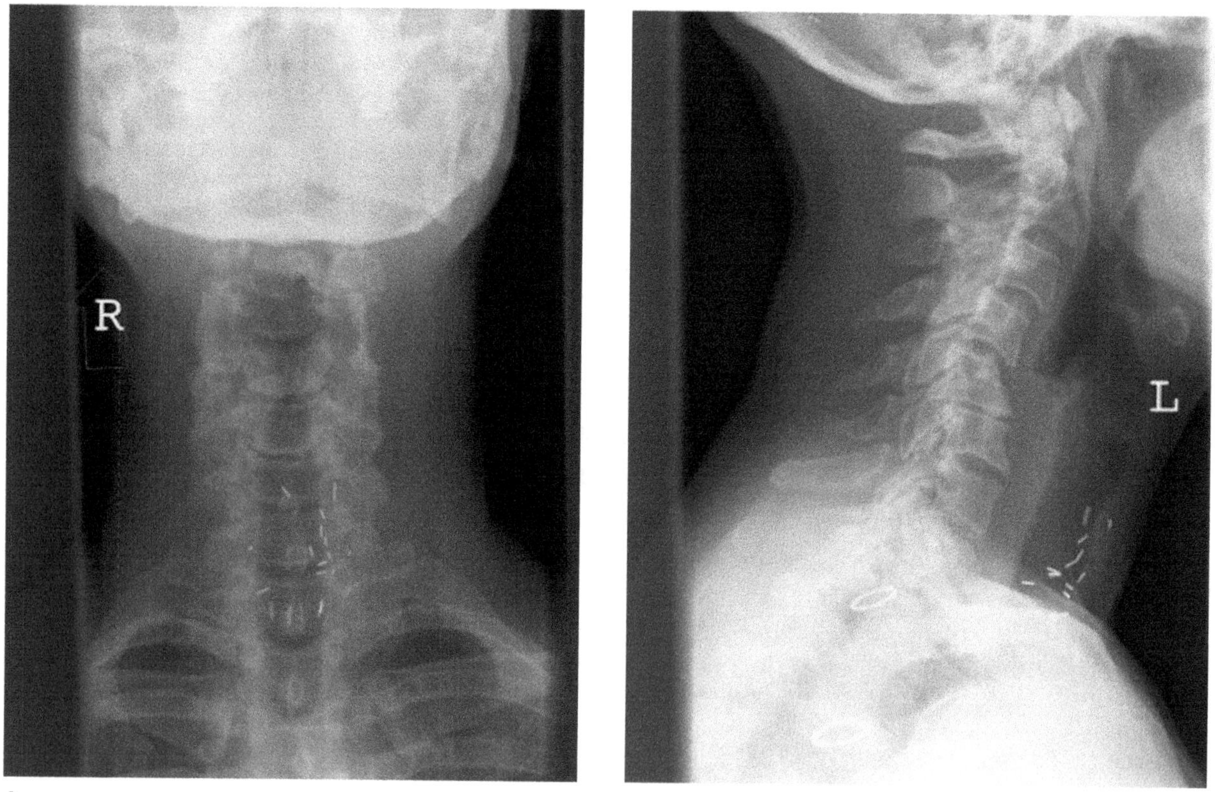

A B

▲ **Figure 5–10.** (**A and B**) Anteroposterior and lateral radiographs of a 53-year-old woman with multilevel cervical spondylosis.

Clinical Findings

A. Symptoms and Signs

Headache may be the presenting symptom of cervical spondylosis. Usually, the headache is worse in the morning and improves throughout the day. It is commonly located in the occipital region and radiates toward the frontal area. Infrequently, patients complain of a painful, stiff neck. Signs include decreased range of motion, crepitus, or both. With more advanced cases, radicular or myelopathic symptoms may be present.

1. Cervical spondylotic radiculopathy—Cervical radiculopathy in spondylosis can be quite complex, with nerve root involvement seen at one or more levels and occurring either unilaterally or bilaterally. The onset may be acute, subacute, or chronic, and impingement on the nerve roots may be from either osteophytes or disk herniation. With radiculopathy, sensory involvement in the form of paresthesias or hyperesthesia is more common than motor or reflex changes. Several dermatomal levels may be involved, with radiation into the anterior chest and back. The chief complaint is radiation of pain into the interscapular area and into the arm. Typically, patients have proximal arm pain and distal paresthesias. However, "classic" symptoms that neatly follow a dermatomal pattern are often not present, and thus meticulous detective work is often necessary on the part of the practitioner to make an accurate diagnosis, particularly with respect to the spinal level(s) involved. Extension of the neck with rotation toward the side of neural impingement (Spurling sign) can reproduce the patient's pain pattern.

2. Cervical spondylotic myelopathy—Cervical myelopathy has a variable clinical presentation, given the complex pathogenic mechanisms involved. These include static or dynamic canal impingement, facet arthropathy, vascular ischemia, and the presence of spondylotic transverse bars. In addition, given its neuronal topography, the cord may be affected in dramatically different ways by relatively minor differences in anatomic regions of compression. The clinical course of myelopathy is usually progressive, leading to worsening disability over a period of months to years with stepwise deteriorations in function.

Patients often present with paresthesias, dyskinesias, or weakness of the hand, the entire upper extremity, or the lower extremity. Deep aching pain of the extremity, broad-based gait, loss of balance, loss of hand dexterity, and general muscle wasting are found in patients with advanced myelopathy. Impotence is not uncommon in these patients but can be difficult to attribute to myelopathy versus other etiologies. Patients with severe myelopathy may exhibit a positive Lhermitte sign. In this situation, dropping the head rapidly into flexion elicits a "lightning/electrical" sensation that radiates into the arms and down the thoracic spine. Lhermitte sign is also positive in patients suffering from multiple sclerosis. Appropriate imaging studies, including a brain MRI, are necessary to rule this diagnosis out.

Hyperextension injuries of the spondylotic cervical spine can precipitate a central cord syndrome in which motor and sensory involvement is typically greater in the upper extremities than the lower extremities. Recovery from this injury is usually incomplete. Complete quadriplegia can also occur if the preexisting stenosis is severe. In this setting, the 1-year mortality approaches 80%.

Deep tendon reflexes can be either hyporeflexic or hyperreflexic, with the former seen in anterior horn cell (upper extremity) involvement and the latter seen in corticospinal tract (lower extremity) involvement. Hyporeflexia is found at the level of compression; hyperreflexia occurs on the level below. Long-tract signs, such as the presence of the Hoffmann reflex or Babinski reflex, indicate an upper motor neuron lesion. Clonus is often present although asymmetric. Physical signs, however, are not always present in myelopathy and can be present in nonmyelopathic (even neurologically normal) patients; thus, their absence or presence neither rules out nor rules in the diagnosis. Upper extremity involvement may be unilateral, whereas lower extremities are affected bilaterally. Multiple compressions of the spinal cord cause more severe deterioration functionally and electrophysiologically than does a single-level compression.

B. Imaging Studies

Although spondylosis results from cervical spine degeneration, not every patient with radiographic evidence of cervical disk degeneration has symptoms. Furthermore, patients with all the radiographic stigmas of cervical spondylosis may be asymptomatic, and others with clinical evidence of myelopathy may show only modest radiographic changes. This paradox is explainable by canal size differences, with the smaller-diameter canal having less space to buffer the degenerative lesion.

The average AP diameter of the spinal canal measures 17 mm from C3 to C7. The space required by the spinal cord averages 10 mm. The dural diameter increases by 2 to 3 mm in extension. The smallest sagittal AP diameter is measured between an osteophyte on the inferior aspect of the vertebral body to the base of the spinous process of the next vertebra below. An absolute spinal canal stenosis exists with a sagittal diameter of less than 10 mm. The stenosis is relative if the diameter measures 10 to 13 mm.

Plain film findings also vary according to the stage of spondylosis at which they were taken. Radiographs may appear normal in early disk disease. Alternatively, they may show single-level or multilevel disk space narrowing with or without osteophytes. C5-C6 and C6-C7 are the two most commonly involved segments. Vertebral body sclerosis at the adjacent base plates may also be seen. Cortical erosion is uncommon and indicates an inflammatory process such as rheumatoid arthritis.

Oblique views permit evaluation of the facet joints and detection of osteophytosis and sclerosis. The superior facets undergo degeneration more frequently than their inferior counterparts. The superior joints may then subluxate posteriorly and erode into the lamina below. Inferior osteophytes, however, may prevent significant slippage. If instability seen on flexion-extension views is significant (>3.5 mm when measured at the posteroinferior corner of the vertebral body), foraminal stenosis may result.

MRI permits visualization of the entire cervical canal and spinal cord by showing the spinal cord and nerve roots in two planes (Figure 5–11). MRI can provide valuable information about degree of spinal cord or foraminal stenosis as well as possible damage to the cord based on T1- and T2-weighted signal changes. The use of a CT scan may be required in elderly patients with advanced degenerative bony changes of the cervical spine. CT scan may reveal facet arthrosis, spondylotic bars, disk-osteophyte complexes, and ossification of the posterior longitudinal ligament (OPLL) lesions, all of which are important to recognize in the process of disease treatment. CT scans are also helpful in surgical planning to identify fixation points and identify changes in bony anatomy that may not be appreciable on MRI and plain x-ray. Accurate identification of the location and extent of pathologic changes is necessary to determine the optimal approach for decompression. Selective nerve root blocks and electromyography may be useful to identify the level of involvement.

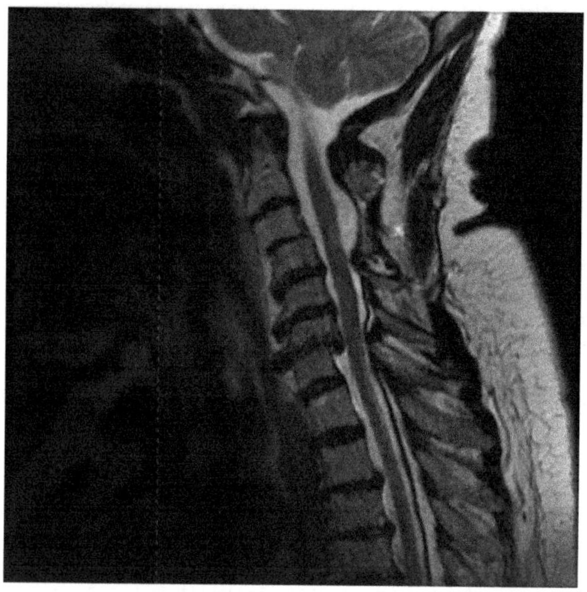

▲ **Figure 5–11.** Sagittal T2-weighted MRI image of a patient with cervical spondylotic myelopathy demonstrating severe multisegmental spinal stenosis.

Differential Diagnosis

Inflammatory, neoplastic, and infectious conditions can mimic cervical spondylotic radiculopathy and myelopathy.

The cervical spine is affected in most rheumatoid arthritis patients. Atlantoaxial subluxation or subaxial instability can cause symptoms similar to those seen in degenerative cervical myelopathy. A primary tumor or metastatic disease can present with unremitting neck pain, often more intense at night. MRI can distinguish neoplastic conditions from degenerative disorders. Infections of the cervical spine occur in children and in elderly (>60 years) or immunocompromised individuals. Multiple sclerosis should be considered in the differential diagnosis. It occurs in younger patients but can present with similar motor signs. Pancoast tumors may invade the brachial plexus, resulting in upper extremity symptoms. Syringomyelia presents with tingling sensations plus motor weakness. A low protein concentration in the cerebrospinal fluid and characteristic changes on MRI are found. Disorders of the shoulder, especially rotator cuff tendinitis, can imitate cervical radiculopathy. Compressive peripheral neuropathies, such as thoracic outlet syndrome, also have to be ruled out. Parsonage-Turner syndrome can also mimic cervical cord or root compression.

Treatment

Patients should be divided into three groups, according to the predominance of their symptoms: neck pain alone, radiculopathy, and myelopathy. The duration and progression of symptoms need to be considered in the planning of treatment. Several studies suggest that patients with cervical myelopathy may have better long-term results from surgery if symptoms are of short duration.

Prevention

Initial management of patients with cervical spondylosis may involve a soft collar, anti-inflammatory agents, and physical therapy consisting of mild traction and the use of isometric strengthening and range-of-motion exercises. The soft cervical collar should be worn only briefly, until the acute symptoms subside. Analgesics are important in the acute phase, and muscle relaxants are helpful in breaking the cycle of muscle spasm and pain. Diazepam should be avoided because of its side effects as a clinical depressant. Epidural corticosteroid injections may be efficacious in patients with radicular pain. Trigger point injections are an empirical form of therapy that seem to work well in patients with chronic neck pain.

The value of cervical traction remains unclear. It is contraindicated in patients with cord compression, rheumatoid arthritis, infection, or osteoporosis. A careful screening of roentgenograms before treatment is mandatory. No evidence indicates that home traction is more effective than manual traction. Isometric strengthening exercises of the paravertebral musculature should be started after the acute symptoms resolve. The patient should be instructed to start a home exercise program early to avoid long-term dependency on passive therapy modalities. Although ice, moist heat, ultrasound, transcutaneous electrical nerve stimulation (TENS), and interferential stimulation are safe to use, there is no scientific proof of their efficacy.

Complications

Complications of surgical treatment include nerve injury, paralysis, and infection. If anterior approaches are employed, dysphagia and vocal cord paralysis can occur. Postsurgical kyphotic deformity can develop after multilevel laminectomy, which is not a procedure that is recommended. If fusions are performed, failure of fusion (nonunions) that will require surgical augmentation/repair can occur.

Surgical Treatment

Surgical intervention should be considered if the patient does not respond to a conservative treatment protocol or shows evidence of deteriorating myelopathy or radiculopathy. The spinal cord can be effectively decompressed by anterior, posterior, or combined approaches. The choice of approach will depend on a number of factors.

The anterior approach allows for multilevel diskectomy, vertebrectomy, foraminotomy, preparation of the interspaces, and fusion with structural autograft taken from the iliac crest bone, structural allografts, or synthetic fusion cages supplemented with autograft, allograft, or synthetic matrices (Figure 5–12). Cervical plating improves fusion rate, decreases the potential for bone graft dislodgement, and helps to maintain cervical alignment during the healing process. However, supplemental posterior fixation and fusion should be considered after two-level vertebrectomy

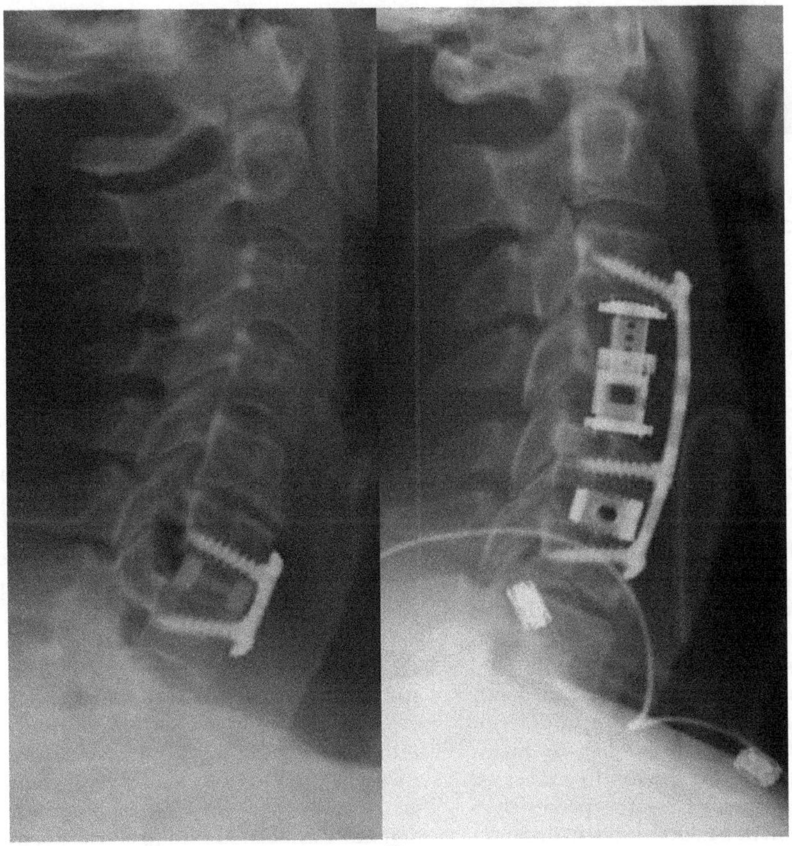

A B

▲ **Figure 5–12.** (**A**) Anterior cervical diskectomy and fusion (ACDF) at C6-C7 to decompress the spinal cord. Two allograft bone spacers were used to fill the entire disk space. (**B**) In this patient with multilevel cord compression, a corpectomy was performed at C4 for retrovertebral spinal cord decompression, combined with ACDF at C6-C7 for disk space decompression. Titanium cages were used for reconstruction in this case.

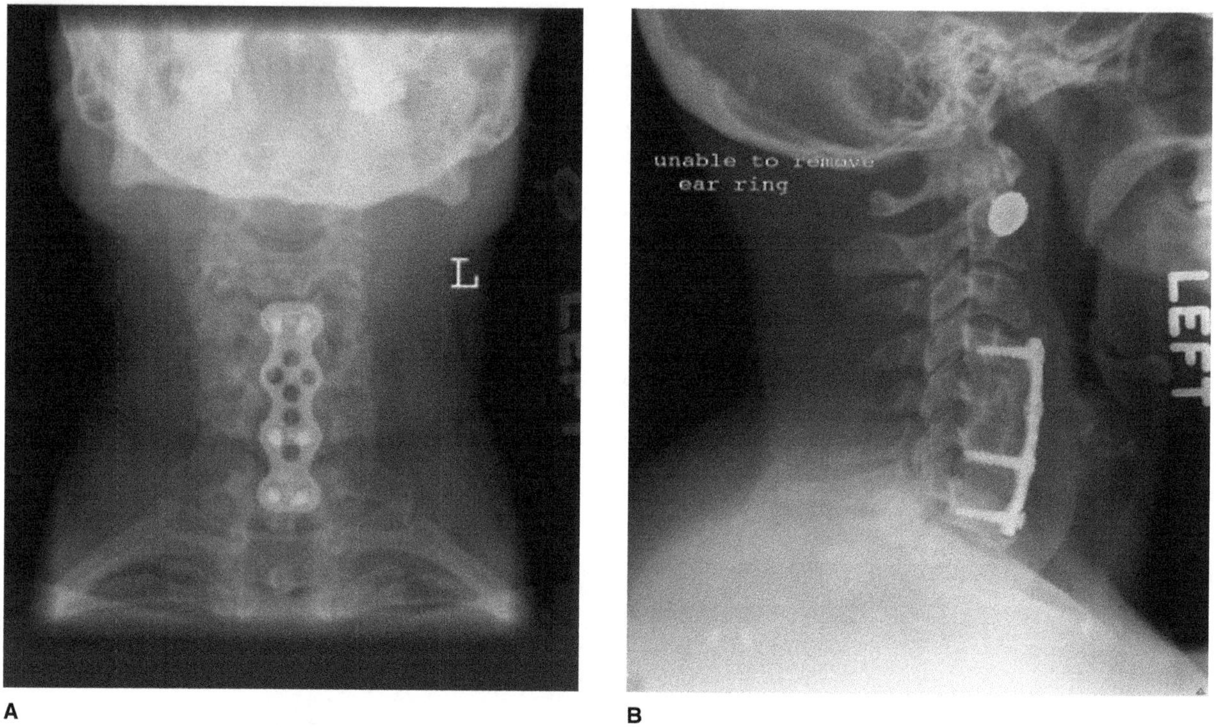

▲ **Figure 5–13.** (**A and B**) Anteroposterior and lateral radiographs of a patient treated with an anterior decompression and fusion with a corpectomy of C5 and diskectomy of C6-C7 and anterior plating.

and should be definitely performed after a three-level corpectomy. Posterior fixation minimizes the risk of anterior dislodgement of the graft even in the presence of solid anterior fixation. Alternatively, short (one-level) corpectomy combined with diskectomy for long fusions (three or more levels) improves fixation and thus decreases the potential for graft dislodgement (Figure 5–13). Anterior interbody fusion after decompression for a herniated cervical disk has a high success rate. However, fusion does lead to increased biomechanical stresses and intradiskal pressures at the adjacent unfused disk spaces. This may lead to premature degeneration of those adjacent levels.

Cervical disk replacement prostheses were also developed to provide a motion-sparing alternative to anterior cervical diskectomy and fusion (Figure 5–14). By maintaining existing motion or restoring motion to a diseased motion segment, these prostheses have the potential to decrease the rate of symptomatic adjacent segment degeneration. Currently, 10-year data from clinical trials approved by the US Food and Drug Administration (FDA) provide evidence that the disk prosthesis for one-level cervical disk disease achieves neurologic and neck pain relief comparable to anterior cervical diskectomy and fusion while maintaining motion at the treated level. Furthermore, other studies have also demonstrated long-term satisfactory outcomes with cervical disk replacement for two-level disease as well. Cervical arthroplasty, however, is not indicated in all cases. Potential contraindications include OPLL, severe spondylosis, significant facet arthropathy, kyphosis, and instability.

The number of involved levels is one important factor in deciding which of the surgical approaches to use. Patients with cervical myelopathy and involvement of more than three vertebral body levels may be best managed by a posterior approach. Multilevel laminectomy and fusion or laminoplasty shows excellent results. Postkyphotic deformities after laminectomy can be avoided with simultaneous posterior fusion using lateral mass fixation (Figure 5–15). Laminoplasty is advantageous in that the cervical spinal cord can be decompressed without the morbidity associated with fusion and some cervical motion can be preserved (Figure 5–16). The ideal indication for laminoplasty is in the patient with multilevel cord compression (three or more motion segments), with preserved lordotic alignment, and minimal axial neck pain arising from spondylosis.

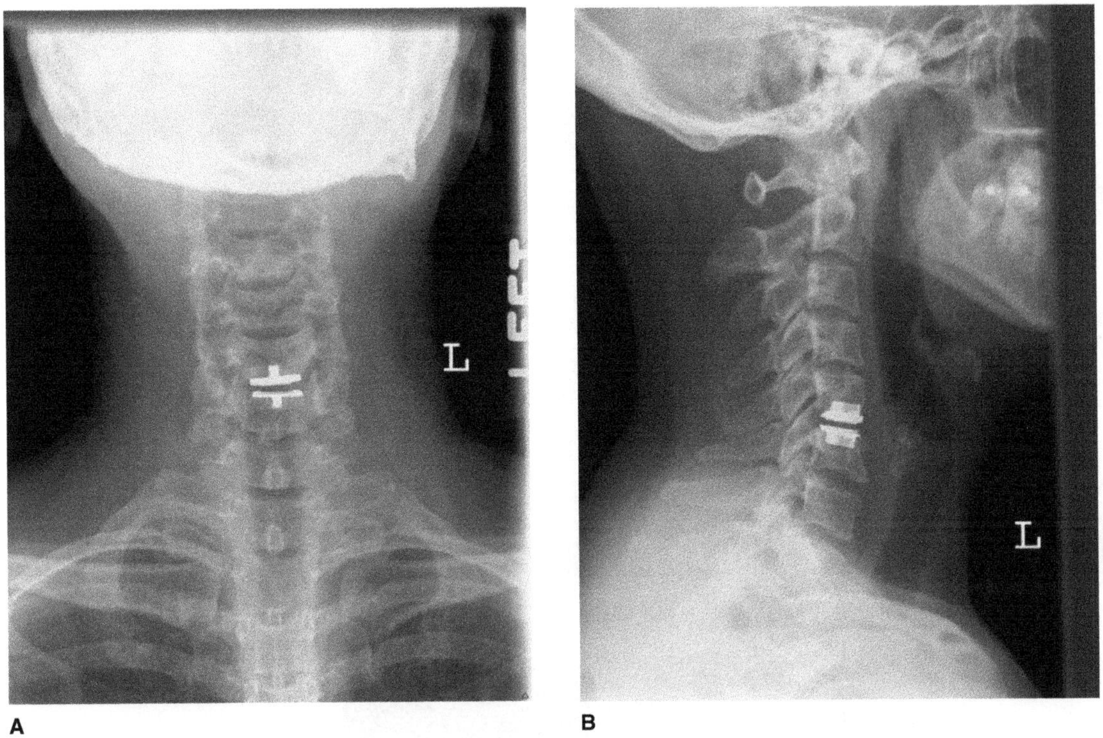

▲ **Figure 5–14.** (**A and B**) Anteroposterior and lateral radiographs of a 45-year-old woman with a C5-C6 herniated disk treated with a diskectomy and reconstruction with a cervical disk replacement.

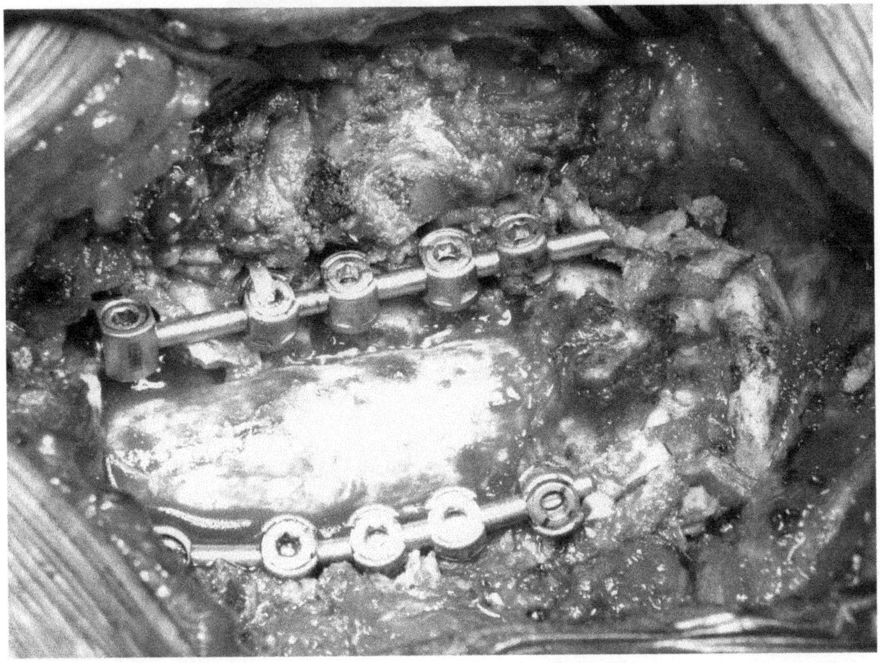

▲ **Figure 5–15.** Intraoperative image of the decompressed dura and stabilized spine after a posterior C3 to C7 laminectomy and fusion with instrumentation.

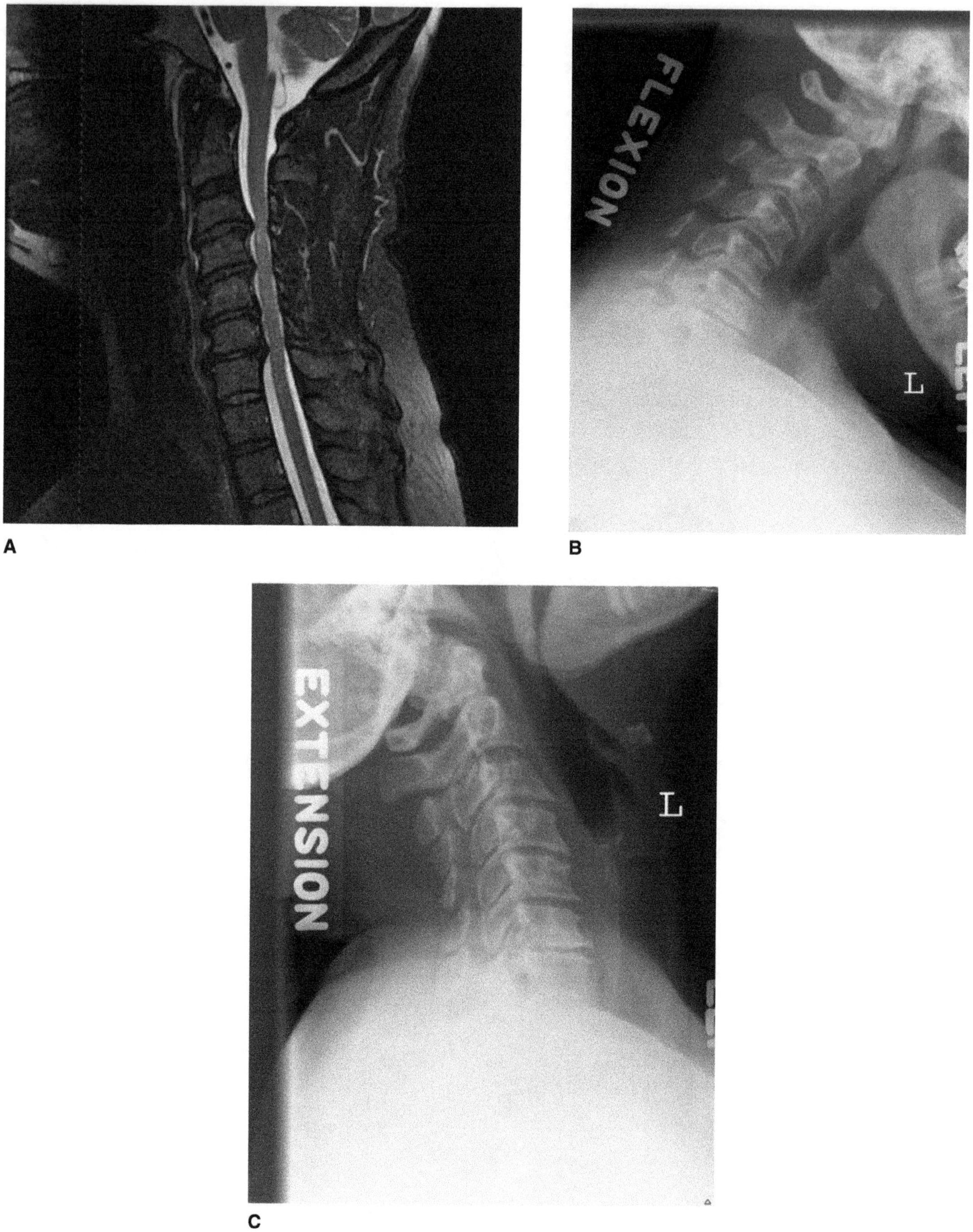

▲ **Figure 5–16.** (**A**) Preoperative sagittal T2-weighted MRI image of a patient with multilevel cervical spinal stenosis and myelopathy. (**B and C**) Lateral flexion and extension radiographs after decompression with a posterior C3 to C7 laminoplasty demonstrating excellent cervical motion.

Operative treatment in cases of cervical spondylotic radiculopathy and myelopathy must be individualized for every patient.

Fehlings MG, Santaguida C, Tetreault L, et al. Laminectomy and fusion versus laminoplasty for the treatment of degenerative cervical myelopathy: results from the AOSpine North America and International prospective multicenter studies. *Spine J.* 2017;17(1):102-108. [PMID: 27597512]

Kato S, Nouri A, Wu D, Nori S, Tetreault L, Fehlings MG. Comparison of anterior and posterior surgery for degenerative cervical myelopathy: an MRI-based propensity-score-matched analysis using data from the prospective multicenter AOSpine CSM North America and international studies. *J Bone Joint Surg.* 2017;99(12):1013-1021. [PMID: 28632590]

Lanman TH, Burkus JK, Dryer RG, Gornet MF, McConnell J, Hodges SD. Long-term clinical and radiographic outcomes of the Prestige LP artificial cervical disc replacement at 2 levels: results from a prospective randomized controlled clinical trial. *J Neurosurg Spine.* 2017;27(1):7-19. [PMID: 28387616]

Lavelle WF, Riew KD, Levi A, Florman JE. Ten-year outcomes of cervical disc replacement with the BRYAN(R) cervical disc: results from a prospective, randomized, controlled clinical trial. *Spine.* 2019;44(9):601-608. [PMID: 30325888]

Lebl DR, Bono CM. Update on the diagnosis and management of cervical spondylotic myelopathy. *J Am Acad Orthop Surg.* 2015;23(11):648-660. [PMID: 26498584]

McAnany SJ, Rhee JM, Baird EO, et al. Observed patterns of cervical radiculopathy: how often do they differ from a standard, "Netter diagram" distribution? *Spine J.* 2019;19(7):1137-1142. [PMID: 30121324]

OSSIFICATION OF THE POSTERIOR LONGITUDINAL LIGAMENT

Essentials of Diagnosis

- *Common cause of myelopathy in Asian population.*
- *Peak age of onset in the sixth decade of life.*
- *Disorder associated with other rheumatologic conditions.*
- *Males are more affected than females.*

General Considerations

OPLL is a relatively common cause of spinal canal stenosis and myelopathy in the Asian population (Figure 5–17). Its overall incidence is 2% to 3% in Japan, compared with 0.6% in Hawaii and 1.7% in Italy. Males are affected more often than females, and the peak age at onset of symptoms is the sixth decade.

Pathogenesis

Although the cause of the disorder is unknown, it may be controlled by autosomal dominant inheritance because it is found in 26% of the parents and 29% of the siblings of affected patients. The disorder is associated with several rheumatic conditions, including diffuse idiopathic skeletal hyperostosis, spondylosis, and ankylosing spondylitis.

Prevention

Currently, there are no preventive measures that affect the development of OPLL. Once symptomatic, fusion of the affected area can slow the growth of the ossification.

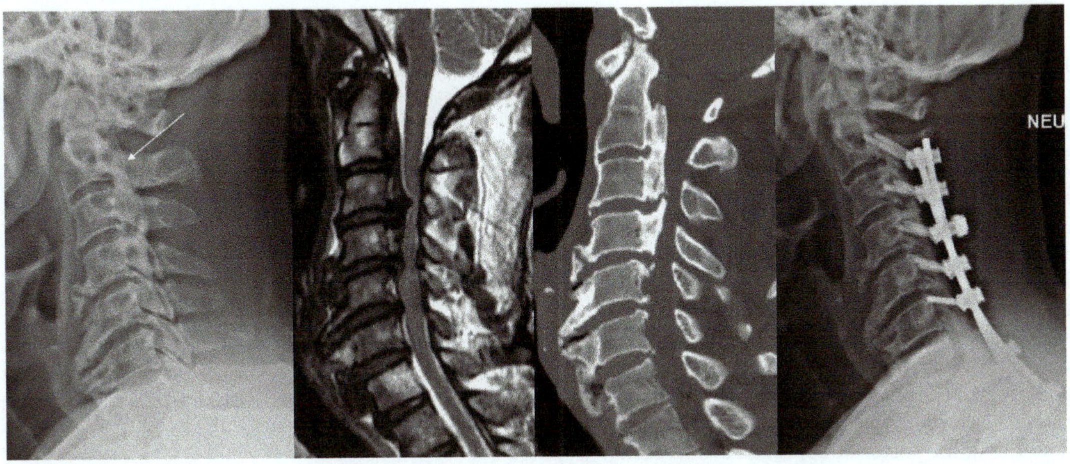

▲ **Figure 5–17.** A 51-year-old man with progressive cervical myelopathy due to ossification of the posterior longitudinal ligament (OPLL). Note the OPLL can be seen on the lateral x-ray (*arrow*). Severe spinal cord compression is noted on the MRI. CT scan shows extensive mixed segmental-continuous ossification. He was treated with posterior laminectomy with fusion and improvement in myelopathic symptoms.

Clinical Findings

Almost all patients have only mild subjective complaints at the onset, although 10% to 15% of them complain of clumsiness and spastic gait. Nevertheless, minor trauma can lead to acute deterioration of symptoms and can result in quadriplegia. Spastic quadriparesis is the most common neurologic presentation.

OPLL can easily be diagnosed on plain lateral radiographs. The levels most frequently involved are C4, C5, and C6. A segmental type of disorder is distinguished from the continuous, local, and mixed type based on the distribution of lesions behind the vertebral bodies. CT scanning is helpful in assessing the thickness, lateral extension, and AP diameter of the ossified ligament. More than 95% of the ossification is localized in the cervical spine, although extension into the thoracic spine is reported to be a cause of persistent myelopathy following cervical decompression.

Endochondral ossification is mainly responsible for the formation of the ossified mass, which connects to the upper and lower margins of the vertebral bodies. In many cases, the ossified material is closely adherent to the underlying dura and makes excision potentially hazardous. Compression of the spinal cord results in atrophy and necrosis in the gray matter and demyelination of the white substance.

Differential Diagnosis

OPLL must be considered in every case of cervical spondylotic myelopathy. OPLL must also be distinguished from idiopathic disk space calcification.

Complications

Complications of surgical treatment include nerve injury (especially C5 root neurapraxia), paralysis, and infection. Removal of the ossification through an anterior approach has a high incidence of durotomy and subsequent spinal fluid leakage.

Treatment

Neurologic outcomes are comparable to surgical treatment seen in other forms of degenerative cervical myelopathy. Patients with severe myelopathy require neural decompression by an anterior, posterior, or combined approach. Most cases of severe OPLL are treated by a posterior laminectomy with fusion. No attempt is made to remove the OPLL; instead, the decompression is indirect by allowing the cord to drift posteriorly away from the anterior compression. Fusion decreases the growth of OPLL and maintains sagittal alignment. In addition, the posterior approach avoids complications related to direct removal of OPLL, such as large dural deficiencies and cerebrospinal fluid fistula. Nonfusion approaches, such as laminoplasty, can be considered but may allow for continued growth of OPLL and can be associated with recurrent ventral cord compression from the OPLL if sagittal alignment worsens. Anterior surgery is considered if the OPLL is less severe or if the indirect decompression of a posterior approach will not allow for adequate spinal cord decompression.

Nakashima H, Tetreault L, Nagoshi N, et al. Comparison of outcomes of surgical treatment for ossification of the posterior longitudinal ligament versus other forms of degenerative cervical myelopathy: results from the prospective, multicenter AOSpine CSM-international study of 479 patients. *J Bone Joint Surg.* 2016;98(5):370-378. [PMID: 26935459]

DISEASES AND DISORDERS OF THE LUMBAR SPINE

OVERVIEW

Symptomatic degenerative conditions of the lumbar spine are among the most common reasons for referral to a spine surgeon. The differential diagnosis of back and radiating lower extremity pain is extensive (Table 5–1). Five of the most common forms of symptomatic degenerative lumbar spinal conditions, as well as spinal infections, tumors, and scoliosis, will be addressed.

DISK HERNIATION

General Considerations

A disk herniation occurs when a piece of the nucleus pulposus (central gelatinous portion of the disk) pushes through a tear in the tougher annulus fibrosis, a dense collagenous ring

Table 5–1. Differential diagnoses for degenerative lumbar spinal conditions.

- Myofascial pain, "lumbar strain"; myofascial low back pain (second most common pain generator after disk) tends to respond more to muscle relaxers; possible role for Botox (botulinum toxin)
- Medical neuropathy (eg, vitamin B_{12} deficiency, thyroid disease)
- Central nervous system disease (eg, cerebrovascular accident, multiple sclerosis)
- Referred pain (eg, chronic pancreatitis, splenomegaly)
- Spondylodiskitis, epidural abscess, infected facet cyst
- Malignancy (metastatic disease most common neoplasm; night pain, atypical, nonpostural/mechanical, constitutional symptoms)
- Peripheral vascular disease, vascular claudication (VC); riding a bike makes VC worse and not neurogenic claudication (NC), standing makes NC worse and not VC; VC is typically associated with a specific distance tolerance and weak pulses
- Diabetes mellitus
- Degenerative joint disease of the hip
- Piriformis syndrome; about 20% of the time the sciatic nerve goes through the piriformis; with contraction of this muscle, sciatica occurs; steroids for inflammation and Botox have been used

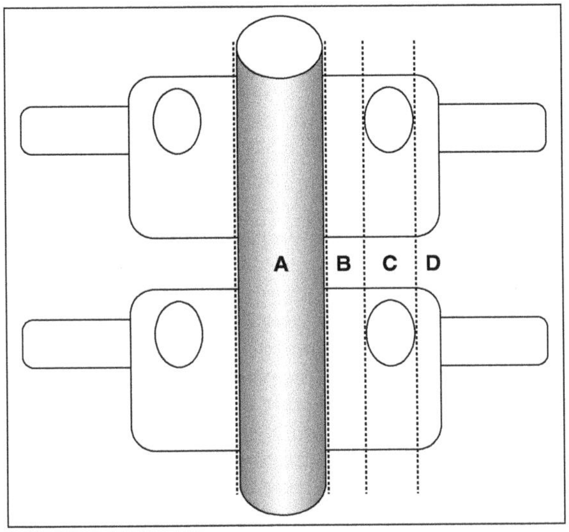

▲ **Figure 5–18.** Diagram depicting the four locations/zones for a disk herniation.

encircling the nucleus pulposus. This can occur in the central (Figure 5–18A), posterolateral (Figure 5–18B), foraminal (Figure 5–18C), and extraforaminal zones (Figure 5–18D). The more central the herniation, the more likely it is to compress the traversing nerve root (ie, S1 at the L5/S1 disk), whereas the more lateral the herniation, the more likely it is to compress the exiting nerve root (ie, L5 at L5/S1 disk). Thus, a disk herniation at one spinal level can have different clinical presentations.

Herniated nucleus pulposus (HNP) can cause nerve root symptoms by two mechanisms. First, the herniation can cause a mechanical deformation of the nerve root. Second, the release of various inflammatory mediators by the herniated disk elicits a robust inflammatory response and irritates the nerve root. It is thought that most cases of symptomatic radiculopathy from disk herniations have both a mechanical and inflammatory basis, which helps to explain in part why the size of the herniation does not necessarily correlate with the severity of symptoms.

Annually, about 5 to 20 per 1000 adults sustain disk herniations, resulting in a 13% to 40% lifetime incidence, occurring most commonly in the fifth decade. The L4/5 and L5/S1 levels are most commonly affected (80%); however, with age, proximal levels (eg, L2/3 and L3/4) become increasingly involved. Genetic inheritance has been identified as one of the most important risk factors for developing lumbar disk herniations. Recently, newer studies have shown an association between low-grade infections with organisms such as *Propionibacterium acnes* and degenerative disk disease, possibly suggesting another etiology for disk herniations. Occupational and recreational exposures, obesity, and smoking are also important potentially modifiable risk factors.

Table 5–2. Lumbar spine physical exam.

- Inspection: skin, signs of previous surgery, palpation, spasm
- Posture: alignment (scoliosis), sagittal balance, coronal balance, stance
- Range of motion: amount and motion that elicits pain
- Motor strength (5-point manual muscle testing scale; 0 = flaccid, 5 = normal)
- Sensation: by dermatome (L1-S1) + low sacral (anal sensation)
- Tension signs
  - Supine and sitting straight leg raise test (L5-S1 radiculopathy)
  - Femoral stretch test (L2-L4 radiculopathy)
- Sacroiliac joint testing: palpation, lateral compression, FABER (flexion, abduction, external rotation)
- Gait: heel walk, toe walk, in-line walk, standing squat, balance
- Mental status (mood/affect, orientation) and Waddell sign
- Targeted extremity exam: pulses, hip/knee range of motion

Clinical Findings

A. Signs and Symptoms

Disk herniations classically present with prodromal low back pain that acutely changes to a radiating leg pain. When this occurs, the low back pain may resolve or remain, but the leg symptoms most commonly predominate. More than 50% of the time, there is no inciting event noted. Along with pain, the patient can have numbness and/or weakness in the pattern of the compressed nerve. Diskogenic problems typically are worse in forward flexion and better in extension. Because sitting increases intradiskal pressure, many with symptomatic disk herniations feel more pain sitting than in other positions, such as lying down or even standing. Additionally, positions that put tension on the nerve root (ie, fully extending the knee) tend to reproduce or exacerbate the radiating pain.

All patients presenting with painful lumbar degenerative conditions need a thorough neurologic and physical examination (Tables 5–2 to 5–4). Representative dermatomes of the L1-S1 nerve roots should be assessed for light touch and pinprick sensation and should be compared to the contralateral side. The patient should be asked to stand and ambulate. Gait should be assessed for independence, stability, and antalgia. Frequently, patients will not bear full weight on the

Table 5–3. Motor strength grades.

0–No motion, no twitch, complete paralysis
1–Muscle twitch/contraction or fasciculation, no motion
2–Full AROM[a] with gravity eliminated
3–Full AROM against gravity, but not against resistance
4–Able to overcome gravity and some degree of resistance
5–Normal muscle strength (ie, symmetric to contralateral side)

[a]AROM, active range of motion. "+" and "–" can be added to provided further degrees of description; this is helpful in more subtle degrees of motor loss (the more common clinical scenario), since the motor grading scale is skewed toward more profound deficit.

Table 5–4. Major motor groups and their innervation.

Nerve Root	Muscle	Action
L1, 2	Iliopsoas	Hip flexion
L3, 4	Quadriceps Adductors	Knee extension Hip adduction
L4, 5	Tibialis anterior	Ankle dorsiflexion
L5	Extensor hallucis longus	Great toe extension
L5, S1	Peroneal longus/brevis	Ankle eversion
S1	Gastrosoleus	Ankle plantarflexion

leg ipsilateral to a large disk herniation and may list to the contralateral side. To further test motor strength and coordination, patients should be asked to walk on their heels and toes. If possible, spine range of motion should be assessed, specifically seeking out whether spinal flexion or extension is more provocative. Last, tension signs should be assessed. In the supine position, each lower extremity should be elevated between 20 and 70 degrees. Reproduction of pain down the leg below the knee constitutes a positive straight leg raise (SLR) test. A crossed SLR occurs when elevation of the contralateral extremity reproduces pain in the symptomatic extremity. Prone SLR (femoral stretch test) can be performed to test for tension in the upper lumbar roots (L2, L3, and L4), indicated by anterior thigh pain. The SLR can be repeated in the sitting position, during motor strength testing of the quadriceps as the patient fully extends the knee.

B. Imaging

MRI is the gold standard for detecting and defining lumbar disk herniations but can be overly sensitive, because high proportions of asymptomatic volunteers may have abnormal-appearing disks on MRI. Thus, it is paramount to correlate MRI findings with clinical signs and symptoms when diagnosing and treating HNPs. In instances where MRI may be not be available or contraindicated (ie, pacemakers or cochlear implants), CT myelography can be used as an alternative to confirm the diagnosis of disk herniations. Disk herniations typically have three distinct morphologies on MRI—protrusion (often called a "disk bulge"), extrusion, and sequestration. A protrusion is a general bulge of the posterior disk that is seen both in conjunction with disk degeneration and the normal aging process. It is the most common form of HNP, seen in 20% to 30% of asymptomatic adults under the age of 40, 60% between age 40 and 60, and 80% to 100% over the age of 60. Protrusions have the most variable outcomes following diskectomy, with a 7% to 13% reherniation rate and up to 38% with persistent sciatica complaints. Protrusions are a relatively poor prognosticator for either operative or nonoperative outcomes with treatment since a protrusion tends to indicate global disk failure, which is less likely to respond to focal interventions like injections or microdiskectomy. Disk extrusion is an HNP in which nuclear material pushes through and beyond the annulus, yielding a mushroom-like appearance with a cap and a stalk. Extrusions represent the HNP morphology most commonly treated with diskectomy (approximately two-thirds of cases) (Figure 5–19). Sequestration is a progression of extrusion, in which the herniated nuclear fragment is no longer in

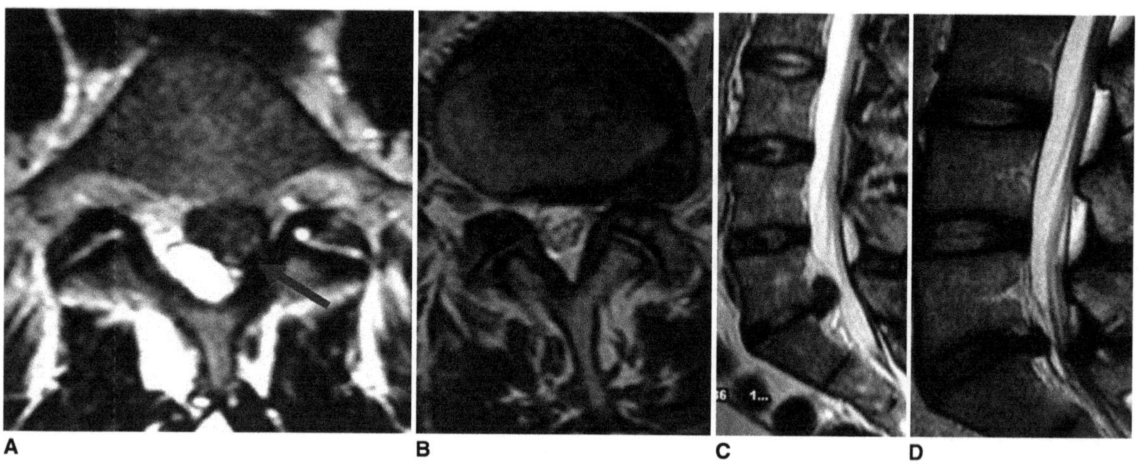

▲ **Figure 5–19.** Different types of disk herniations. (**A**) Axial T2 MRI of a large, extruded, posterolateral disk herniation at L5-S1 compressing the S1 root (*purple arrow*). (**B**) Axial T2 MRI of an extraforaminal disk herniation at L4-L5 (*purple arrow*). This herniation compresses the exiting L4 root. (**C**) Sagittal MRI demonstrates disk herniation (extrusion type) that has migrated cephalad from the disk space of origin (L5-S1). (**D**) Sagittal MRI demonstrates disk herniation that has stayed at the level of the disk space (L5-S1).

continuity with the disk of origin. Extrusions and sequestrations typically have better outcomes than protrusion. Unlike protrusions or bulges, extrusions and sequestrations are seen in fewer than 1% to 10% of asymptomatic volunteers. Thus, the clinical relevance of extrusion and sequestration is generally more certain than that of a protrusion or disk bulge.

Treatment

The first-line treatment for most degenerative, symptomatic conditions of the lumbar spine is nonoperative. Nonoperative treatment is initially attempted because of the overall favorable natural history of the disorder. Symptoms in 60% to 90% of HNPs will resolve spontaneously in the first 6 to 12 weeks. Table 5–5 lists some of the more common nonoperative treatment options. Treatments are added in a stepwise fashion, beginning with medications such as NSAIDs. A short course of oral steroids often provides significant symptom relief as well. Muscle relaxants may help diminish spasms and pain. Narcotics should generally be used sparingly and only for a short period of time due to their addictive potential. Physical therapy may be helpful in those whose symptom level allows them to participate. Insufficient evidence exists to determine whether spinal manipulation or manual/mechanical traction may provide any benefit. Epidural steroid injections (ESIs) are a common nonoperative treatment option. These are best performed under fluoroscopic guidance, with the medication placed transforaminally at the level and side of the herniation to provide the maximal dose at the needed area. The results of clinical studies on ESIs have been variable, but there is level 1 evidence indicating that they may be superior to placebo at least in the acute phase. It is unclear, however, whether ESIs change the natural history of disk herniations. Regardless, the immediate response to these injections can be diagnostic and prognostic. Patients with good to excellent initial response, regardless of whether it diminishes with time, have better outcomes following diskectomy than those with little to no response at any point following injection.

Table 5–5. Nonoperative treatment options.

Physical therapy/exercise
Counseling/education
Activity modification
NSAIDs/celecoxib
Narcotics pain medications
Muscle relaxers
Nerve-modulating agents (ie, gabapentin)
Oral steroids
Epidural or nerve root injection of steroids
Chiropractor/manipulation/traction
Massage/heat/cold/transcutaneous electrical nerve stimulation/ acupuncture
Psychology/biofeedback/psychiatry

NSAIDs, nonsteroidal anti-inflammatory drugs.

Indications for operative treatment include (1) persistent symptoms despite a reasonable course of nonoperative treatment, (2) profound or progressive motor deficit, (3) cauda equina syndrome, (4) intractable pain, and (5) patient preference. Level 1 studies have consistently shown that surgical decompression of the nerve root by removal of the offending disk fragment is associated with greater improvements than nonoperative care. These advantages exist for all outcomes commonly assessed, including pain reduction, functional improvement, and even improvement in mental health. Without question, the single most consistent finding is that the time to achieve maximal clinical outcome is substantially reduced with surgery compared with nonoperative care. The most impactful of these studies is the Spine Patient Outcomes Research Trial (SPORT), a National Institutes of Health–funded, 13-site multicenter study with observational and randomized clinical trial arms that evaluated the outcomes of surgical treatment versus conservative care for three of the most common degenerative spinal conditions—disk herniation, spinal stenosis, and spondylolisthesis. The ample data collected from this landmark 5-year prospective study have been subanalyzed to evaluate the impact of multiple factors, including cost and complications. The more proximal the herniated level (ie, L3/4 or L4/5 and above), the more likely surgical decompression is superior to nonoperative care. Eight-year outcomes data have demonstrated that patients undergoing surgery for lumbar disk herniation achieve greater improvement than those pursuing nonoperative care.

For all comers, the major advantage of surgery over nonoperative care is quicker time to resolution of symptoms, especially radicular pain. This faster symptom resolution leads to a cost-benefit advantage over nonoperative care. Most patients who undergo microdiskectomy notice substantial improvement in radicular leg pain in the immediate postoperative period. Not infrequently, preoperative weakness and less commonly numbness may also improve quickly, although usually not as quickly or as completely as pain does, particularly if the numbness and weakness were long-standing and constant rather than intermittent. Diabetic patients may also have less recovery of nerve root function.

Conversely, nonoperatively treated patients have an overall slower time to improvement, with maximal outcomes not achieved until 1 to 2 years following symptom onset; however, at the 1- to 2-year mark, some studies have shown that the significant clinical advantage of surgery over nonoperative care may lessen or no longer exist. On the other hand, the results of the SPORT study show that patients who presented for both surgical and nonsurgical treatment after 6 or more months of symptom duration had significantly less improvement than those who received treatment more acutely, which is consistent with prior prospective studies. Thus, there appears to be an optimal time window for maximal benefit from surgery that is somewhere between 6 weeks and 6 months. In the end, it is patient preference that should most direct treatment following symptomatic HNPs that do not resolve spontaneously or fail to respond to initial attempts at nonoperative care. Those with the most significant symptoms tend to select surgery, and those with more mild or intermittent symptoms may be best treated in a nonoperative fashion. There is little evidence that the method of surgery (eg, microdiskectomy, minimally invasive diskectomy, traditional "open" diskectomy) has a significant effect on outcomes as long as the nerve root is appropriately decompressed.

While the decision to treat an HNP with surgery or nonoperative therapy is largely one of patient and surgeon preference, there are rare exceptions in which acute operative treatment is absolutely indicated. The most agreed upon urgent surgical indication following HNP is cauda equina syndrome. Patients with cauda equina syndrome may demonstrate acute, profound bilateral lower extremity neurologic deficits, with saddle anesthesia and bowel/bladder incontinence (usually bowel incontinence and urinary retention). Cauda equina syndrome represents one of the true emergent/urgent conditions of the lumbar spine. Thus, all patients with suspected cauda equina syndrome should be immediately referred to a spine surgeon and undergo emergent MRI. Neurologic outcomes are traditionally thought to be best when decompression occurs within the first 48 hours, although recently, it has been shown that the severity (regardless of duration) of incontinence is the most important preoperative predictor of bowel/bladder functional recovery. Even when treated quickly, about 25% to 50% of patients will have continued bowel/bladder dysfunction. In addition to cauda equina syndrome, patients with any form of progressive neurologic deficit or those in whom pain is not well controlled in an outpatient setting are also candidates for early surgery.

Careful patient selection is mandatory when considering surgery. In addition to the disk pathology, psychosocial factors weigh heavily on outcomes. The presence of three or more of the five Waddell signs is associated with poor outcomes following surgical treatment due to underlying psychosocial issues. These signs include (1) a discrepancy between the seated and the supine SLR; (2) superficial and widespread tenderness that is nonanatomic; (3) pain with axial loading of the head or twisting the pelvis; (4) nondermatomal sensory deficits ("my whole leg is numb"); and (5) overreaction on exam. Expectations with treatment also play a significant additional role in outcomes. In a more recent subgroup analysis of SPORT data, patients who had low expectations of outcomes with surgery were predicted to have poorer outcomes regardless of their treatment, whereas those who had higher expectations of nonoperative management were predicted to have better outcomes with nonoperative care.

Complications

The most common complications of lumbar diskectomy include infection (1%-3%), dural tears (3%-10%), nerve root injury (<1%), and recurrent herniations (4%-27%). Persistent low back pain is a not uncommon complaint despite excellent relief of radicular pain. It must be understood by the patient preoperatively that the primary goal of surgery is to relieve radicular nerve root pain and that midline axial low back pain may or may not improve even with an otherwise successful surgery.

Benzakour T, Igoumenou V, Mavrogenis AF, Benzakour A. Current concepts for lumbar disc herniation. *Int Orthop.* 2019;43(4):841-851. [PMID: 30506088]

Lurie JD, Henderson ER, McDonough CM, et al. Effect of expectations on treatment outcome for lumbar intervertebral disc herniation. *Spine.* 2016;41(9):803-809. [PMID: 26641853]

SPINAL STENOSIS

Essentials of Diagnosis

- *Often due to degenerative conditions of the spine but can also occur from congenitally narrowed spinal canal or inflammatory and traumatic conditions.*
- *Symptoms are exacerbated by extension of the spine and improved by flexion of the spine.*
- *Need to assess for vascular insufficiency and osteoarthritis of the hips and knees.*

General Considerations

Spinal stenosis refers to a narrowing of the spinal canal, most commonly due to the accumulation of space-occupying, degenerative material such as hypertrophic ligamentum flavum, osteophytes, and disk herniations or bulges (Figure 5–20). In rare instances, accumulation of epidural fat can also lead to spinal stenosis. Stenosis can occur in the central portion of the canal, the lateral recess (ie, the area underneath the facet joints), or the foramen. In most cases, stenosis occurs at the level of the facet joints. It is at that level that pathologic changes in the disk, facets, and ligamentum flavum hypertrophy converge to produce the greatest amount of narrowing. In contrast, stenosis is relatively uncommon at the level of the pedicles, and when it occurs at this level, it often indicates an underlying congenital or developmental stenosis of the bony canal.

Spinal stenosis is often seen in patients with a developmentally narrow spinal canal. Such patients may have had sufficient room for their nerve roots in youth, but possess little reserve capacity for the accumulation of degenerative lesions, which occur in all humans with age. Concomitant spinal instability (lateral listhesis or spondylolisthesis) and/or deformity (eg, scoliosis) may accentuate spinal stenosis: as one vertebra translates on the other, the portion of the spinal canal in between the two segments becomes narrowed in a manner similar to the closing of a cigar cutter. When foraminal stenosis occurs, it is usually due to the hypertrophy and/or proximal migration of the superior articular facet from

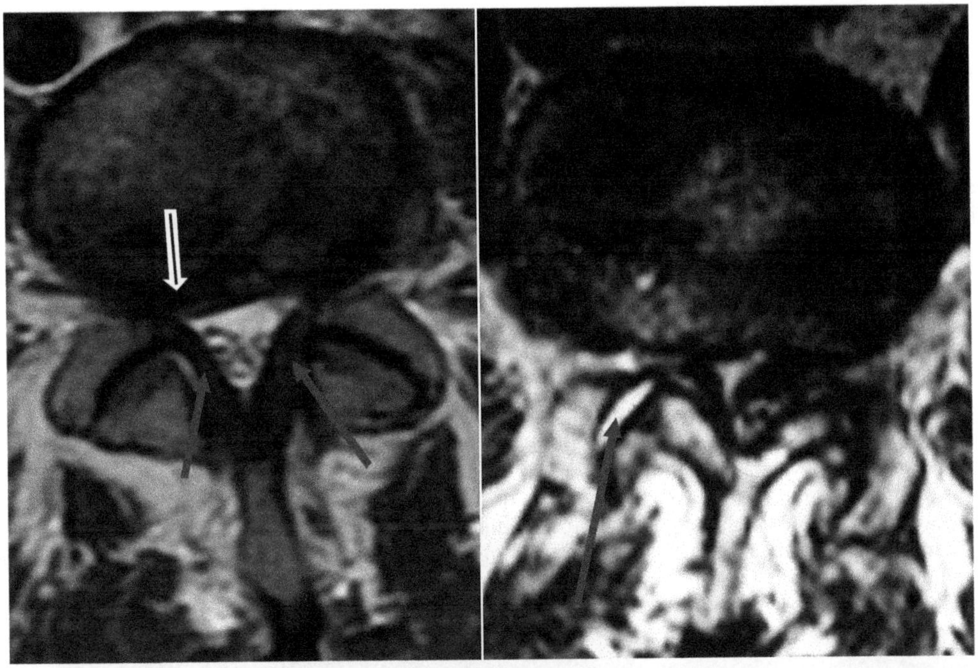

▲ **Figure 5–20.** (**A**) Axial MRI demonstrating lateral recess (subarticular) stenosis due to thickening of the ligamentum flavum (*purple arrows*). There is also an associated right posterolateral disk bulge (*white arrow*). (**B**) Severe central stenosis causing a pinhole-size spinal canal. Note associated facet joint synovitis and arthropathy (*purple arrow*).

the level below (ie, the S1 superior facet in L5-S1 foraminal stenosis), along with associated encroachment of the ligamentum flavum into the foramen. A decrease in disk height or disk herniation or annular bulging into the foramen can also lead to foraminal stenosis. The L4/5 level is the most commonly involved segment in spinal stenosis. Symptomatic patients can present at any adult age, with congenitally stenotic patients presenting as early as their late teen years, but most degenerative stenosis patients present in their 50s and beyond.

Clinical Findings

A. Signs and Symptoms

Classically, patients complain of the insidious onset of radiating buttock and leg pain that is worse as the compromised spinal canal is further narrowed in extension (eg, standing upright or walking [downhill especially]) and improved as the canal is relatively enlarged in flexion (eg, sitting, lying down in a "fetal" position, or walking while bent over a shopping cart). Associated numbness, weakness, or a feeling of "heaviness" or easy fatigue in the legs with walking may be present. Patients may also complain of concomitant low back pain. Not all patients, however, present with these classic symptoms. Many will have significant radicular leg pain even at rest. Not infrequently, the leg symptoms may not radiate all the way down the leg but rather localize only to the buttock or posterior thigh area.

A thorough physical examination is necessary but is commonly nonfocal. Severe motor and sensory deficits are relatively uncommon. The hips and knee joints of all patients should be assessed, as osteoarthritis of those joints may often mimic spinal stenosis symptoms. Greater trochanteric bursitis can also masquerade as radiating leg pain. Sacroiliac joint pain, which can be very difficult to definitively diagnose, can also mimic stenotic pain localized only to the buttocks. In addition, a vascular examination should be performed in all patients to rule out vascular claudication.

B. Imaging

A noncontrast MRI scan is the most useful diagnostic tool for identifying spinal stenosis. AP and cross-sectional diameter should be assessed on both sagittal and axial images. The presence of a "sedimentation sign," the absence of sedimentation of the lumbar nerve roots along the dorsal part of the dural sac on supine MRI, shows significant reliability in diagnosing lumbar spinal stenosis. In those who cannot have MRI scans (eg, those with pacemakers), a CT myelogram is the next best imaging study. There is little role for a plain CT scan in evaluating spinal stenosis, although it may be useful in identifying associated bony abnormalities or for surgical planning. Standing plain AP, lateral, and flexion-extension x-rays should be taken to rule out associated spinal instability or deformity. Electromyography is not routinely used in the diagnosis of lumbar spinal stenosis but may be beneficial when the diagnosis is unclear and when attempting to differentiate from other diseases with similar clinical presentations, such as peripheral neuropathy.

Treatment

Nonoperative treatment modalities include the same ones used to treat lumbar disk herniations. Because stenosis rarely leads to progressive neurologic injury, nonoperative modalities are generally attempted first. However, whereas disk herniations may spontaneously resolve over time with resorption of fragments, spinal stenosis due to bony or ligamentous hypertrophy does not spontaneously regress with either time or nonoperative treatment. Similar to lumbar disk herniations, nonoperative treatment in lumbar spinal stenosis is purely symptomatic, meaning that it may help to improve pain symptoms but does not modify the underlying stenosis or make it "go away." As such, it is debatable whether nonoperative therapies alter the natural history of spinal stenosis, and the literature shows little evidence of such. Evidence in support of various nonoperative treatments is low grade at best. ESIs are a common nonoperative treatment; however, unlike for disk herniation, there does not appear to be a clinical advantage between intralaminar and transforaminal techniques. In milder cases of lumbar spinal stenosis, nonoperative treatment may lead to long-term improvement in symptoms. More commonly, however, especially in those with severe stenosis, the symptoms tend to recur and progress with time.

In those with persistent symptoms or progressive neurologic deficits, surgical treatment affords excellent outcomes. In the majority of cases of central and lateral recess stenosis, the procedure of choice is a decompressive laminectomy of the stenotic areas (Figure 5–21). A fusion is not generally indicated for spinal stenosis in the absence of instability. In those with symptomatic foraminal stenosis, a foraminotomy is additionally performed. If there is symptomatic foraminal

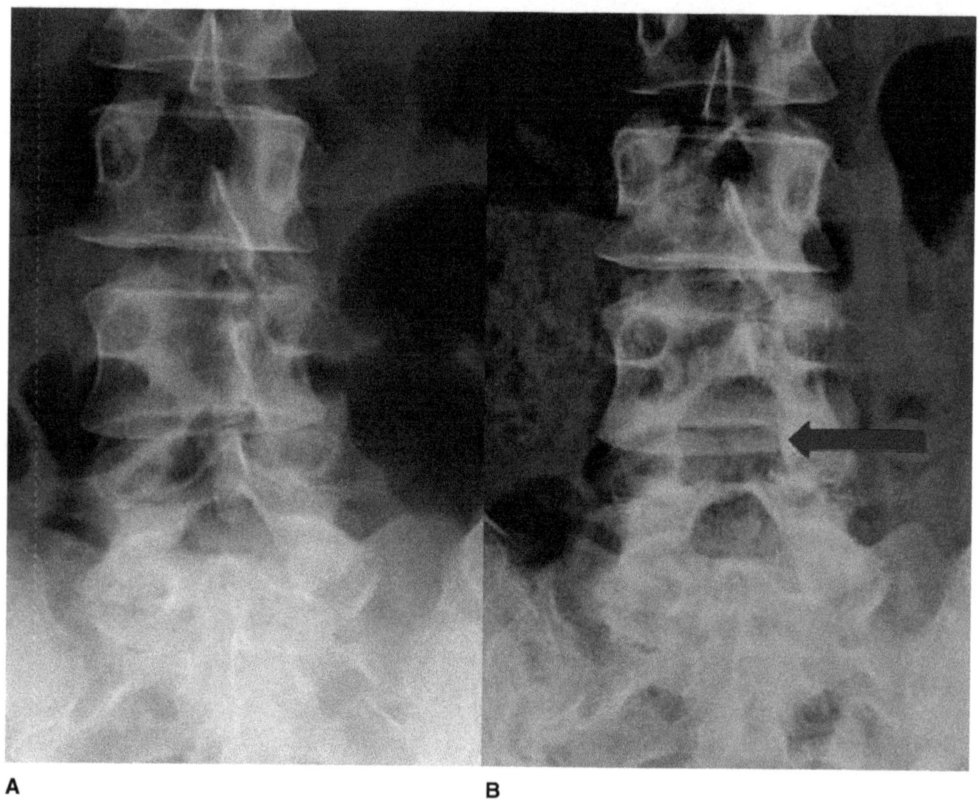

▲ **Figure 5–21.** Anteroposterior radiographs before (**A**) and after (**B**) L4-L5 laminectomy for spinal stenosis. In most cases, central and lateral recess stenoses occur at the level of the disk space, where the facets, ligamentum flavum, and disk can converge to compress the neural elements. Thus, adequate decompression is generally achieved when the area spanning the rostral to the caudal portion of the facet joints has been relieved of neurologic compression (*purple arrow*).

stenosis with height loss causing vertical stenosis, then a fusion may be necessary to keep the foraminal height sufficient to relieve root compression postoperatively, even if a foraminotomy has been performed.

Multiple studies have attempted to compare outcomes between operative and nonoperative management in patients with spinal stenosis, but the conclusions are heterogeneous and difficult to interpret due to low-quality evidence and issues with study bias such as high crossover rates. However, in the properly chosen patient, laminectomy provides excellent improvement in spinal stenosis symptoms. Reduction or elimination of radicular/claudicatory pain and improvement in physical function can be expected in 70% to 90% of cases. Again, patients should be counseled that the primary goal of treatment is relief of neurogenic rather than axial back pain, although a reduction in the latter may occur in up to 75% of cases. Multiple factors have been associated with poorer outcomes in patients undergoing operative management including depression, cardiovascular comorbidity, disorders that affect walking ability, scoliosis, and smoking. These should be taken into consideration when deciding the appropriate treatment regimen.

Lurie J, Tomkins-Lane C. Management of lumbar spinal stenosis. *Br Med J*. 2016;352:h6234. [PMID: 26727925]

DEGENERATIVE DISK DISEASE

Essentials of Diagnosis

- *Aging of the disk leads to dehydration and internal disk disruption.*
- *Most degenerative disks are asymptomatic.*
- *It is not possible to diagnose a painful disk by imaging studies alone.*

General Considerations

Aging of the intervertebral disk leads to a loss of water content, decrease in height, and an alteration in its normal mechanical properties. As a result, motion segment hypermobility, along with tears in the annulus, may occur. Although this degenerative cascade occurs ubiquitously in all spines with aging, it becomes symptomatic in only a small minority. It is currently unclear why some degenerative disks cause pain, whereas the vast majority do not, and there are no MRI or other imaging criteria that reliably differentiate symptomatic from nonsymptomatic degenerative disks. Thus, it is not possible to diagnose a painful degenerative disk on the basis of imaging studies alone.

We differentiate the term "degenerative disk," which is a radiographic and anatomic description, from "degenerative disk disease" (DDD), which refers to the clinical syndrome of pain in the presence of a degenerative disk (Figure 5–22). Because the diagnosis of DDD is difficult to make, surgically treating diskogenic low back pain has relatively low success rates compared to other types of spinal surgery. Thus, surgical treatment of DDD is reserved for patients with severe symptoms who fail to respond to extensive nonoperative measures and in whom a clear disk pain generator has been identified (see Table 5–5). Heritability and genetics have been shown to be important risk factors for developing DDD. Potentially modifiable risk factors include smoking, obesity, and occupational exposures.

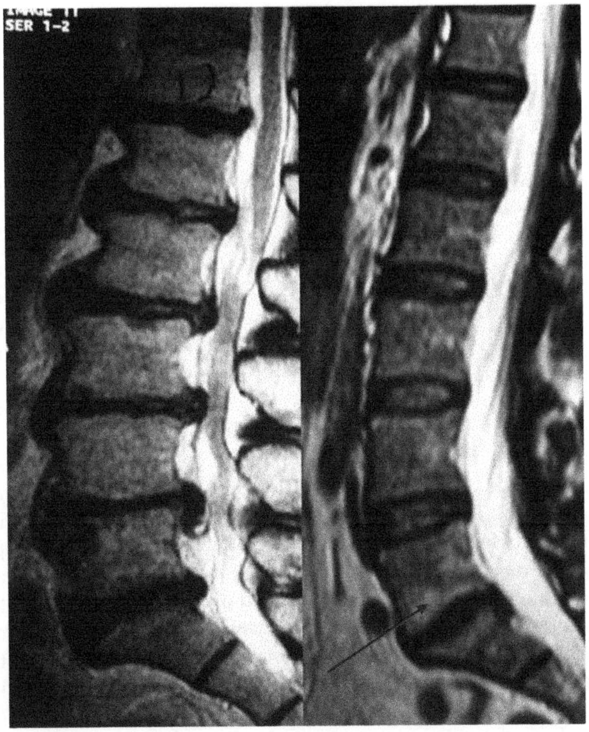

A B

▲ **Figure 5–22.** (**A**) A 75-year-old man with symptoms of spinal stenosis and multilevel disk degeneration, but no low back pain. For reasons that are unclear, the majority of degenerative disks do not cause axial low back pain. Thus, one must not presume that degenerative changes found on imaging studies are necessarily responsible for symptoms, although they certainly can be. (**B**) A 37-year-old woman with single-level symptomatic degenerative disk disease at L5-S1. Note the relative loss of hydration (the central portion of the disk is darker, essentially black, compared to the more proximal disks) and disk height, along with Modic endplate changes (*purple arrow*).

Clinical Findings

A. Signs and Symptoms

Diskogenic low back pain classically is worse in flexion and better in extension. As with disk herniations, sitting is often the most aggravating position because it leads to the highest intradiskal pressures. Axial back pain may radiate to the buttock, thigh, or groin, but usually not past the knee in the absence of neurologic compression. Radiation past the knee in a dermatomal distribution typically indicates concomitant nerve root compression/irritation. It is important to determine the degree of relief afforded by rest. Pain that never improves, even at rest, suggests that mechanically based procedures such as spinal fusion may be unlikely to improve the pain.

B. Imaging

Radiographs typically show disk space narrowing, vertebral body osteophytes, or endplate and facet sclerosis. Radiographs should be taken upright to evaluate for potential deformities or instabilities that may not be apparent in the recumbent position. Flexion-extension films may rule out spondylolisthesis and instability. CT scans may rule out occult spondylolysis or tumors. MRI without contrast is the study of choice and demonstrates decrease in disk height and water content (dark on T2 imaging) with disk degeneration. High-intensity zones (HIZs) are focal areas of increased signal on T2-weighted images in the normally dark posterior/outer annulus indicative of annular tears or fissures. Associated endplate changes ("Modic" changes) indicative of endplate edema, fatty degeneration, or sclerosis may occur with disk degeneration as well. Patients with HIZs and Modic changes who undergo surgery for DDD tend to have better outcomes than those without such MRI findings. However, the presence of these findings is not diagnostic of symptomatic DDD.

Diskography is a useful but imperfect diagnostic modality. Because it is impossible to determine whether a disk is painful simply by its radiographic appearance, the concept behind provocative diskography is to identify the symptomatic disk by injecting it with contrast material under pressure. If the injection reproduces the patient's typical low back pain (ie, demonstrates "concordant" pain), then that disk may be symptomatic. The limited information to be gained from this test must be balanced against the risk of the procedure. A matched cohort study of patients who underwent diskography demonstrated significantly more disk degeneration and herniation at the side and levels of disks that had undergone diskography. This finding was consistent with those of previous animal studies.

Treatment

DDD is a challenging problem to manage, and there are no excellent treatment options. In general, because the outcomes are overall not favorable, we recommend avoiding surgery for discogenic low back pain in the absence of neurologic compression or neurologic symptoms. Because surgery is appropriate for only a select few, treatment always starts in a nonoperative fashion. Nonoperative options include those listed in Table 5–5. Lifestyle modifications, behavioral therapies, and management of associated psychosocial stressors may help DDD patients better cope with and manage their pain. Level 1 evidence demonstrates that patients with symptomatic DDD that is refractory to at least 6 months of nonoperative therapy may benefit from surgical treatment.

The most common surgical treatment of symptomatic DDD is spinal fusion. Surgery can be performed either anteriorly or posteriorly. Anterior surgery has the benefits of high fusion rates and avoiding the morbidity related to disruption of lumbar extensor muscles, but carries risks intrinsic to the anterior approach, such as vascular injury, retrograde ejaculation in men, and injury to the abdominal contents (Figure 5–23). Posterior fusion (either posterolateral and/or posterior interbody) generally involves pedicle screw instrumentation and provides rigid fixation, but it requires posterior muscle dissection, which may exacerbate low back pain in some patients. Overall, only about 60% of patients obtain significant improvement in axial lumbar pain after spinal fusion surgery for DDD. It should be noted that these results are substantially inferior, in general, to the outcomes of treating lumbar stenosis and radiculopathy. In contrast to surgery for DDD, low back pain relief is much more likely and reliable after surgery that treats spinal deformity (eg, scoliosis, kyphosis), nonunions of prior surgery, and instability (eg, spondylolisthesis).

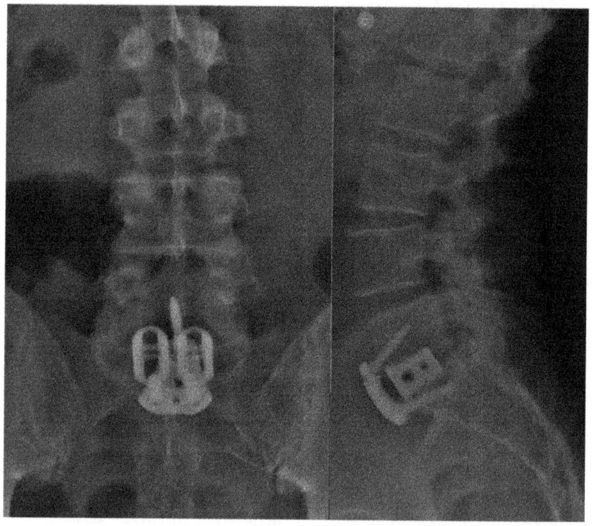

▲ **Figure 5–23.** Anteroposterior and lateral radiographs of a 43-year-old man status post-anterior lumbar interbody fusion with cage and plate construct. Although this particular threaded, lumbar-tapered interbody cage can be used quite successfully (>95% fusion rate) as a stand-alone device, when the vascular anatomy permits and cage fixation is suboptimal, a plate can be added to further secure the construct. Excellent relief of symptoms was obtained.

Nonfusion approaches such as anterior lumbar disk arthroplasty are an alternative to fusion procedures. In some studies, arthroplasty demonstrates equivalent or superior clinical outcomes over fusion. However, the long-term functionality and survival characteristics for lumbar arthroplasties are unknown. Catastrophic implant failures, including potentially life-threatening expulsion of implants into the iliac vessels, have been reported, tempering enthusiasm for this approach. For a variety of reasons, lumbar arthroplasty has been less frequently used over time since the initial enthusiasm during its introduction, and we do not recommended it.

Complications

Complications of instrumented posterior fusions include infection, nonunions, and implant-related issues such as malposition, loosening of screws, or backout of cages. Anterior complications include vascular injury (up to 3%), retrograde ejaculation due to hypogastric plexus injury (up to 5%), and cage migration. Fusion rates of anterior lumbar interbody fusions using rhBMP-2 approach 100%. However, the rate of retrograde ejaculation may be higher when rhBMP-2 is used versus autograft. Fusion rates for posterior one- and two-level arthrodesis are 80% to 95%. The most common issue associated with surgery for axial lumbar pain due to DDD is failure to significantly improve low back pain.

Prognosis

DDD displays relatively poor outcomes compared to other lumbar spinal diagnoses regardless of either surgical or nonoperative management. About one-third of patients fail to respond to all forms of treatment. Careful patient selection is the key to successful surgical outcomes. Patients with refractory low back pain and untreated underlying psychosocial conditions that exacerbate pain perception consistently have poorer surgical outcomes. Other poor prognostic factors include worker's compensation status, pending litigation, obesity, and smoking. Proper counseling as to realistic expectations for pain reduction following surgery is paramount.

Saifi C, Cazzulino A, Park C, et al. National trends for primary and revision lumbar disc arthroplasty throughout the United States. *Global Spine J.* 2018;8(2):172-177. [PMID: 29662748]

Sandhu F, Blumenthal S, Grunch B, Kimball B, Ferko N, Hollmann S. Barriers to and budget impact of lumbar total disc replacement utilization. *Spine.* 2017;42(suppl 24):S112-S114. [PMID: 29176487]

Zigler J, Gornet MF, Ferko N, Cameron C, Schranck FW, Patel L. Comparison of lumbar total disc replacement with surgical spinal fusion for the treatment of single-level degenerative disc disease: a meta-analysis of 5-year outcomes from randomized controlled trials. *Global Spine J.* 2018;8(4):413-423. [PMID: 29977727]

FACET SYNDROME

General Considerations

Facet arthropathy and facet syndrome are relatively common but often underappreciated pain generators in patients with degenerative lumbar conditions. Unlike disk degeneration, which is ubiquitous in symptomatic and asymptomatic people, 15% to 90% of patients with chronic low back pain have obvious arthritic changes to their lumbar facet joints, whereas fewer than 15% of asymptomatic volunteers have arthritic changes on advanced imaging. Upward of 10% of patients following diskectomy may develop clinically symptomatic lumbar facet joint syndrome, which can be responsive to facet blocks. Revision or radical diskectomies significantly increase this risk.

Facet joints appear to be an independent generator of back pain. Although facet arthrosis may follow disk degeneration, facet syndrome and diskogenic back pain syndrome usually do not occur concurrently, as facet anesthetic blocks and diskogram are positive at the same level in fewer than 3% to 10% of cases. L5/S1 is the most commonly involved level, followed by L4/5 and L3/4. Facet degeneration is characterized by changes similar to those seen at other synovial joints—osteophytes, subchondral cysts, cartilage wear, joint space narrowing, and deformation (Figure 5–24).

The facet capsule is richly innervated by the medial branch of the posterior ramus. Each posterior ramus divides to innervate two to three facet joints, including

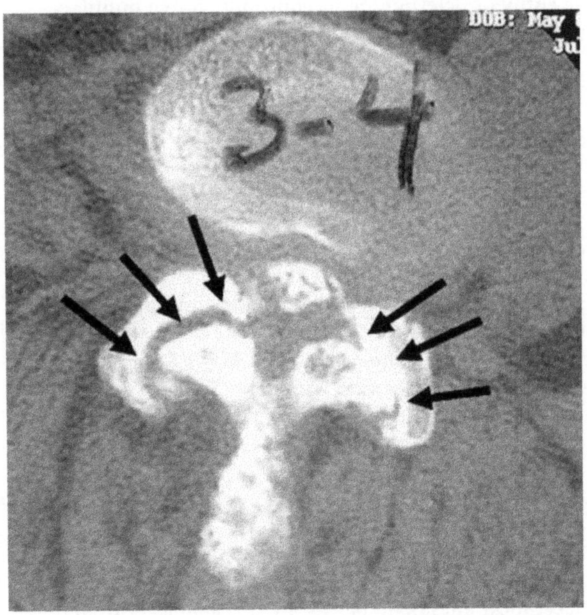

▲ **Figure 5–24.** CT myelogram demonstrates severe spinal stenosis at L3-L4 along with bilateral facet arthropathy (*black arrows*).

the joints associated with its neuroforamen and the ones above and below.

Clinical Findings

A. Signs and Symptoms

One of the challenges with diagnosing facet syndrome (the cluster of chronic low back pain worse in extension, in the setting of facet arthritic changes that respond to facet local anesthetic blocks) is that it has no reliable signs or symptoms. Often there is referred pain that radiates into the buttock and posterior thigh (not below the knee) and sometimes into the groin as well. Lumbar extension, especially with the addition of truncal rotation, is often limited and painful. Controlled, comparative local anesthetic blocks are the diagnostic modality of choice. Diagnostic blocks may include a local anesthetic with or without steroids. Debate exists as to the appropriate diagnostic criteria when using blocks to determine whether facet arthropathy is a primary pain generator. Some authors have argued for repeat blocks in multiple sessions given the high false-positive rate (30%-45%) that can be seen with a single block session. Some also recommend a block at two contiguous levels given the dual nerve supply of the facet joint from the same level and level above. Unfortunately, multiple studies have demonstrated poor or no correlation between response to facet injections and response to nonoperative treatment or subsequent spinal fusion. Thus, while many spine surgeons believe facet degeneration is a pain generator in chronic low back pain, defining it as a unique entity or determining its contribution to a multifactorial etiology for low back pain remains unclear.

B. Imaging

It is thought in most instances that disk degeneration and height loss precede facet arthrosis. Facet orientation, which is best measured on CT scan, tends to become progressively more sagittal as arthrosis progresses. Patients with more sagittally oriented facet joints are more prone to develop spondylolisthesis. MRI and CT scans often demonstrate lateral recess and foraminal stenosis from hypertrophy of the superior articulating process in advanced facet arthropathy. Like other synovial joints, arthrosis can lead to the formation of synovial cysts. Facet cysts most commonly form on the posterior aspect of the joint, but those on the ventral or medial surface can compress nerve roots, causing radiculopathy.

Treatment

Facet syndrome is primarily treated nonoperatively with the modalities listed in Table 5–5. After clinical examination, facet local anesthetic blocks are a potential next step for the diagnosis and treatment of facet syndrome. Patients who have a positive response to facet blocks (>50%-80% pain reduction) are candidates for intraarticular steroid injections or radiofrequency ablations (RFAs). Steroid injections provide long-term back pain relief in 16% to 63% of patients. Currently, there is no consensus as to whether an intraarticular block is more effective than medial branch blocks for pain relief. RFA involves placing a radiofrequency probe under radiographic guidance and thermocoagulating the medial branch of the posterior ramus as it enters the facet capsule. Using strict selection criteria (positive controlled comparative blocks), it is thought that RFA provides up to 1 year of 80% to 90% pain relief in 60% of patients, with 87% of patients getting at least 60% pain relief. Randomized controlled trials have shown that RFA is superior to placebo. Other studies have found no significant treatment effect following facet steroid injections or RFA compared to saline placebo. RFA and intraarticular steroid injections, like many nonoperative interventions, tend to produce diminishing returns with repeated application. Last, posterior fusion may be a final treatment option for facet syndrome, with limited and contradictory evidential support. In general, facet syndrome should not be viewed as a surgical disease; further, favorable results from facet injections may not predict good outcomes from fusion surgery.

Perolat R, Kastler A, Nicot B, et al. Facet joint syndrome: from diagnosis to interventional management. *Insights Imaging.* 2018;9(5):773-789. [PMID: 30090998]

SPONDYLOLISTHESIS

Essentials of Diagnosis

- *There are six distinct types of spondylolisthesis.*
- *Signs and symptoms are dependent on type but often include a combination of low back pain and leg pain.*
- *Degree of slippage and slip angle and overall sagittal balance are important considerations in choosing the optimal treatment.*

General Considerations

Spondylolisthesis is derived from the Greek *spondylo* (meaning spine) and *olisthesis* (meaning slip) and refers to an abnormal slippage of one vertebra over the next. There are six types of spondylolisthesis (Table 5–6). The overall lifetime incidence of spondylolisthesis is 9% to 10%, with isthmic and degenerative being the most common types.

Clinical Findings

A. Signs and Symptoms

1. Degenerative spondylolisthesis—Patients are typically older (50 years and up) and complain of varying amounts of low back and/or leg pain. The radicular leg symptoms are similar to those of spinal stenosis, as central and lateral recess stenosis is exacerbated by the slip. Foraminal stenosis

Table 5–6. Wiltse classification of spondylolisthesis.

I	**Dysplastic/congenital:** marked by dome-shaped sacrum, abnormal L5/S1 facet joints, elongated, thin L5 pars with a trapezoidal shape of the L5 vertebral body; prone to high-grade slip (ie, >50%).
II	**Isthmic** (most common in adolescents/adults): due to a defect or acute fracture in the bilateral L5 pars interarticularis; allows L5 to slip forward up to 50%. Spondylolysis typically occurs spontaneously by age 5-6. It occurs in about 5%-6% of Caucasians (higher rate in other races), but only about one-third go on to develop listhesis. There is a familial predilection. If the lysis occurs from a traumatic cause, it can be treated nonoperative with a good outcome. Lytic spondylolisthesis does not predict low back pain; therefore, when a low-grade slip is incidentally found, it does not require spine surgical consultation. When low back pain and/or radiating lower extremity symptoms are present and fail to respond to nonoperative measures, spinal fusion with or without decompression and reduction provides favorable results for most.
III	**Degenerative** (most common in older adults): the final outcome of progressive disk degeneration, height loss, instability, and facet arthropathy, most commonly at L4/5 level (>85% of cases) and often associated with neurogenic claudication. Strong female predilection (4-6:1). Decompression and fusion are indicated following failure of nonoperative treatment for symptomatic patients, typically in their 50s to 60s, with good to excellent outcomes in >75%.
IV	**Traumatic:** spondylolisthesis following a destabilizing fracture of the lumbar spine other than a pars fracture. This injury requires spinal stabilization surgery.
V	**Pathologic:** spondylolisthesis occurring secondary to primary or metastatic lesions weakening the supportive structures of the spinal unit. This condition requires spinal stabilization surgery with or without tumor resection and adjuvant therapies. This is a rare condition.
VI	**Iatrogenic:** typically used to describe spondylolisthesis that occurs following lumbar decompression surgery without fusion, where the pars is thinned too much, resulting in acute or insufficiency pars fracture. Fusion is indicated in these cases.

can also occur. Thus, the radicular symptoms may be associated with both the exiting and traversing roots at the level of stenosis. The L4/5 level is by far the most common level affected by degenerative spondylolisthesis, although it can occur at other lumbar levels. Associated axial low back pain from instability should typically be better with rest and worse with standing or walking.

2. Isthmic spondylolisthesis—Patients may present in their preteen to teen years or be relatively asymptomatic until their adulthood (30s to 50s). L5-S1 is by far the most common level involved, although isthmic defects can be seen at other levels (Figure 5–25). Central stenosis is relatively uncommon with isthmic defects, as the pars defect actually enlarges the spinal canal with slippage of the associated vertebrae. Instead, foraminal narrowing and the resulting exiting root compression are typical, with the L5 root being most commonly involved with an L5-S1 isthmic slip. Low back pain, when present, tends to be mechanical (worse with activity) and may be acutely associated with a "clunking" sensation in flexion and extension.

B. Imaging

The degree of spondylolisthesis is commonly classified according to the Meyerding grade (Table 5–7). Degenerative slips tend to be low grade, with the majority being grade I or, less frequently, grade II or III. Standing lateral x-rays are paramount to diagnosis, as the slip may not be visible on recumbent films such as supine x-rays or CT/MRI scans. Flexion-extension films may demonstrate dynamic worsening of instability (>2-4 mm motion). Lateral listhesis (slippage in the coronal plane) can also occur alone or in combination with spondylolisthesis. MRI scans are obtained

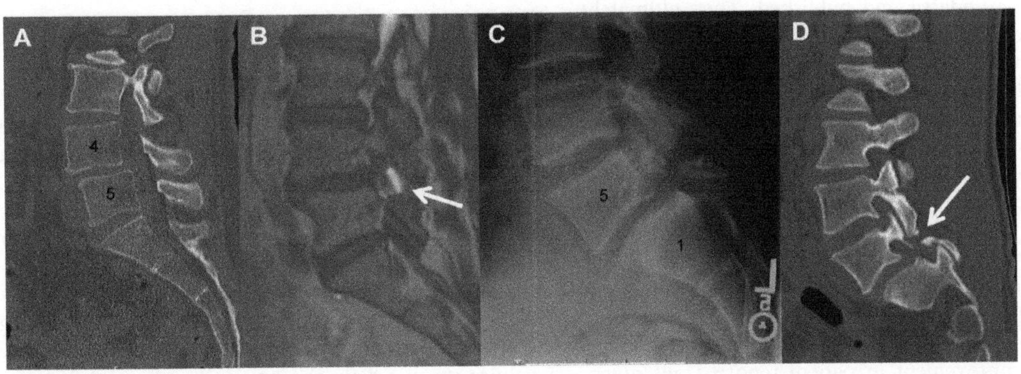

▲ **Figure 5–25.** (**A**) Degenerative spondylolisthesis at L4-L5, the most common level at which they occur. (**B**) MRI of same patient showing fluid (*white arrow*) in the severely degenerative L4/5 facet. (**C**) Isthmic spondylolisthesis at L5-S1 (grade 1) (0%-25% slippage). Although isthmic defects occur most commonly at L5-S1, they can occur elsewhere. (**D**) Note the pars defect (*white arrow*).

Table 5–7. Meyerding slippage grade.

Percent slippage is measured as the distance from the inferior posterior corner of L5 to the superior posterior corner of S1, divided by the length of the S1 superior endplate. Spondylolisthesis is often classified as low grade (0%-50%) versus high grade (>50%) because this distinction impacts surgical treatment.	
I	0%-25%
II	26%-50%
III	51%-75%
IV	76%-100%
V	Spondyloptosis: the condition in which the L5 (and the entire spinal column above) has slipped completely anterior to the S1 vertebra

to evaluate associated neural impingement. Facet fluid seen on MRI may also be indicative of spondylolisthesis and possibly even instability. CT scans with sagittal reformatting can be helpful in identifying pars defects that may not be evident on x-ray or MRI. Bone scans are occasionally useful in identifying occult pars defects.

Treatment

Slips in adults with isthmic or degenerative spondylolisthesis rarely progress. However, growing children with isthmic defects may progress. In addition, children with dysplastic slips and adults with iatrogenic slips (typically resulting from a pars insufficiency fracture after previous diskectomy/decompression procedure) are much more likely to progress and thus should be fused or at least followed carefully. The standard nonoperative treatment options (see Table 5–5) apply to the initial treatment of spondylolisthesis. Decompression alone is rarely appropriate for patients with any form of spondylolisthesis as it can further destabilize the segment or leave persistent symptoms (back and/or leg pain) related to instability. In 2016, the North American Spine Society's (NASS) Evidence-Based Clinical Guideline for the Diagnosis and Treatment of Degenerative Lumbar Spondylolisthesis was updated and published. They ultimately concluded that there was fair evidence that surgical decompression with fusion would better improve clinical outcomes compared with decompression alone. Furthermore, they stated there was poor-quality evidence that direct surgical decompression alone may be considered for the treatment of patients with symptomatic spinal stenosis associated with low-grade degenerative lumbar spondylolisthesis. The most common treatment for either degenerative or isthmic spondylolisthesis is a posterior lumbar decompression and fusion. Interbody fusions are routinely becoming performed more often, especially in the setting of instability; however, the literature continues to be inconclusive as to whether this provides any improvement in patient-reported outcomes. Randomized controlled trials have shown that surgery in the form of one- to two-level posterior decompression and fusion for degenerative spondylolisthesis with stenosis reliably and significantly outperforms nonoperative care at all times points out to 5 years. Fusion for degenerative and isthmic spondylolisthesis tends to be a very successful operation, with 75% or more of patients reporting major improvement in their condition that lasts 2 to 4 years or longer. To put this in generic terms, the improvement in overall measures of general health and well-being (eg, Short Form-36) following fusion for spondylolisthesis is equivalent to that for hip/knee arthroplasty.

Challier V, Boissiere L, Obeid I, et al. One-level lumbar degenerative spondylolisthesis and posterior approach: is transforaminal lateral interbody fusion mandatory? A randomized controlled trial with 2-year follow-up. *Spine.* 2017;42(8):531-539. [PMID: 27548582]

Matz PG, Meagher RJ, Lamer T, et al. Guideline summary review: an evidence-based clinical guideline for the diagnosis and treatment of degenerative lumbar spondylolisthesis. *Spine J.* 2016;16(3):439-448. [PMID: 26681351]

Spiker WR, Goz V, Brodke DS. Lumbar interbody fusions for degenerative spondylolisthesis: review of techniques, indications, and outcomes. *Global Spine J.* 2019;9(1):77-84. [PMID: 30775212]

SPINAL INFECTIONS

Essentials of Diagnosis

- *Most common forms of spinal infections include diskitis, osteomyelitis, epidural abscess, and postoperative infections.*
- *Lumbar spine is most commonly involved followed by the thoracic spine in bacterial infections.*
- *Thoracic spine most commonly involved in fungal infections.*
- *Pathophysiology of infection differs between children and adults.*
- *Back pain is the most common symptom and is severe and unremitting.*

General Considerations

Spinal infections represent fewer than 5% of orthopedic infections. The lumbar spine is the most common region involved (50%), followed by the thoracic spine (35%). The most common forms of spinal infection include (1) diskitis, (2) osteomyelitis, (3) epidural abscess, and (4) postoperative (infection complicates 0%-5% of spinal surgeries). *Staphylococcus aureus* is the most common (40%-60%) organism for all types of spinal infection, followed by coagulase-negative *Staphylococcus* and gram-negative enteric organisms, and a culture-specific diagnosis remains paramount to treatment. *P acnes* and *Staphylococcus epidermidis* are common pathogens in late-onset spinal infections following instrumented spinal fusion. Newer evidence suggests that *P acnes* may even be associated with DDD. These low-virulence pathogens are cultured from the skin in over 80% of subjects prior to skin preparation for surgery.

The pathoanatomy of pyogenic diskitis and osteomyelitis is different in children versus adults. In children, the disk can become primarily infected via blood vessels that cross the endplate and connect the vertebrae to the nucleus. In adults, the disk is avascular and becomes secondarily infected from a primary focus of infection in the vertebral body (ie, osteomyelitis). Hematogenous osteomyelitis typically starts in the anterior-inferior corner of the vertebral body. In this portion of the vertebral body, the end-arterioles loop and create sluggish blood flow. Additionally, the venous drainage of the vertebral body is valveless (Batson plexus) and communicates with the pelvic venous system. These two anatomic features may facilitate bacterial sludging and extravasation. As the infection progresses, the endplates erode, allowing spread of infection into the adjacent avascular disk (Figure 5–26). It is the involvement of adjacent

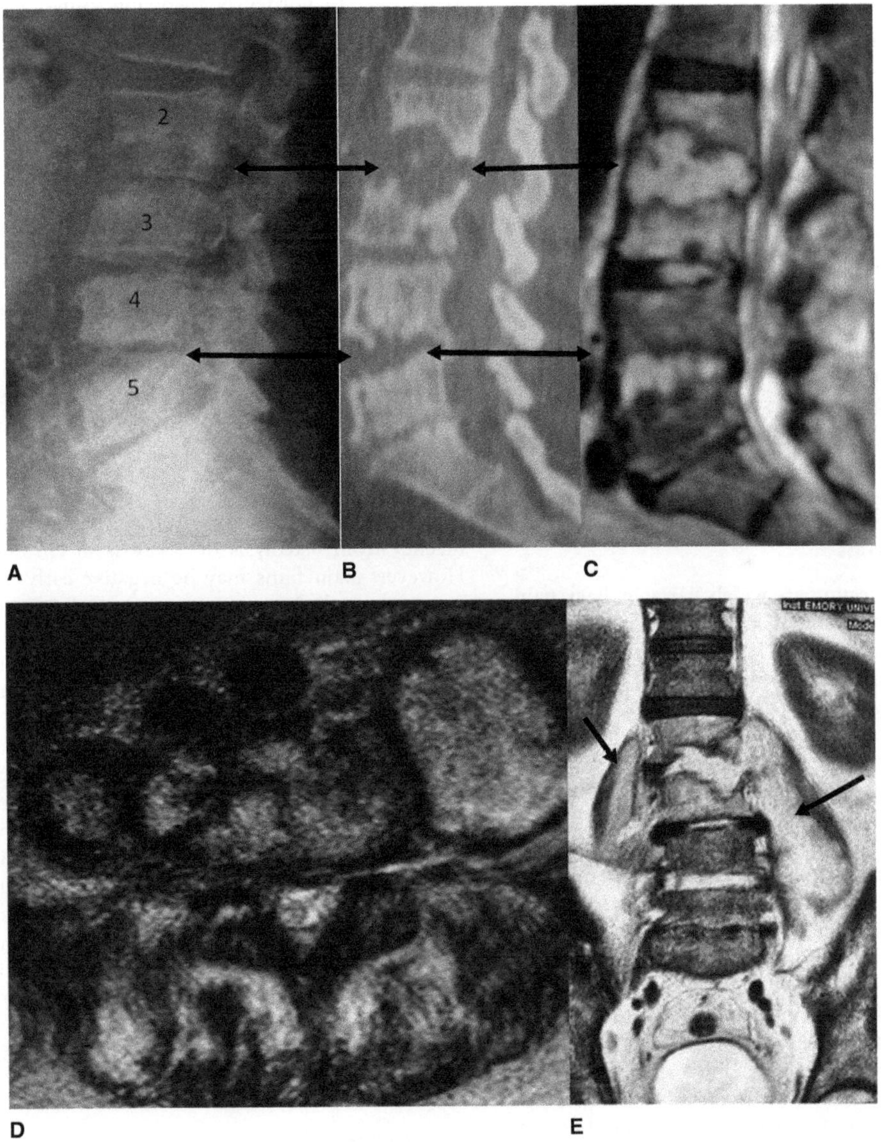

▲ **Figure 5–26.** (**A**) Lateral radiograph of a morbidly obese brittle diabetic man with osteomyelitis-diskitis involving L2-L3 and L4-L5. (**B**) CT reconstruction demonstrates erosion of the endplates at the bottom of L2, top of L3, bottom of L4, and top of L5 due to infection. (**C, D, and E**) Sagittal, axial, and coronal MRIs show extensive infection at L2-L3 and L4-L5 with bilateral psoas abscesses (*black arrows*).

vertebral levels and the intervening disk that most reliably differentiates pyogenic diskitis from neoplasm, as tumors rarely cross the disk space. From the disk space, infection can spread to adjacent vertebral bodies and/or paravertebral structures. In some advanced cases (5%-18%), infection can spread posteriorly into the spinal canal as an epidural abscess. Epidural abscess can also form hematogenously into the posterior epidural space without associated diskitis/osteomyelitis. An epidural abscess is the most urgent of spinal infections due to the potential for progressive neurologic deficit.

Nonbacterial infections are less common. Fungal infections are often indolent but can lead to multilevel involvement and significant deformity. Tuberculous spinal infection (Pott disease) is also an indolent infection, which has a predilection for the thoracic spine, but only affects about 1%-5% of patients with tuberculosis (TB). With fungal infections, kyphotic deformity is often the most clinically significant adverse effect. TB may mimic tumor because it tends to spare the disk space, presumably because TB is an obligate aerobic organism and the oxygen tension in the disk space is low. A purified protein derivative test will be positive in more than 95% of immune-competent patients, but may be anergic in immunocompromised patients. Traditional TB cultures took 21 days or longer for results, but recently, polymerase chain reaction has become the test of choice to confirm TB infection.

Clinical Findings

A. Signs and Symptoms

Symptoms of spinal infection are widely variable. Back pain localized to the area of infection is the most common symptom. Back pain associated with infections is classically more severe and unremitting (often worse at night) compared to that seen with degenerative disorders, although many patients do have mechanical symptoms that modulate with level of activity. Constitutional symptoms such as fever are not sensitive and may be present in only about 33% to 50% of spinal infections. Furthermore, fever is a common (>40%, >75% following major fusion surgery) phenomenon in the immediate postoperative period for uncomplicated spinal surgeries. Neurologic symptoms, such as radiating pain, numbness, or weakness, may occur and are associated with epidural extension of infection or pathologic fracture of infected vertebrae causing kyphosis and compression of the neural elements. Risk factors for infection include advanced patient age, diabetes, HIV, chronic steroids, substance abuse, and obesity. One of the most influenceable risk factors affecting spinal infection is spine surgery itself.

Hemodynamically unstable septic shock is rare but can occur with spinal infections. The physical exam may be normal or demonstrate limited range of motion of the affected spine. Neurologic deficits are relatively uncommon at presentation (10%-17%).

B. Laboratory Studies

Baseline laboratories for patients presenting with suspected spinal infection include complete blood count (CBC) with differential, CRP, ESR, and blood cultures from two separate sites. Leukocytosis and a left shift will be present in less than 50%, but CRP and ESR will be elevated in more than 90% at presentation. The CRP starts to elevate within 24 to 48 hours of infection onset, whereas ESR can take up to 1 week to elevate. In addition to being first to elevate, CRP is the first to normalize following initiation of successful treatment. As such, it is an important tool in monitoring treatment response. Blood cultures are positive in only 30% to 50% of patients. Procalcitonin is potentially a promising marker to distinguish between bacterial and nonbacterial infection, but unfortunately has lower sensitivity than CRP in patients with infection. Antibiotics should be withheld until blood cultures and preferably tissue cultures can be obtained. CT-guided needle biopsy of the most accessible site of presumed infection is the culture method of choice and yields positive results in 50% to 80% of patients, but it is imperative to obtain large enough samples to culture. If an organism cannot be identified or in patients with obvious infections requiring surgical debridement and reconstruction, open biopsy is performed with 80% to 90% positive yield in patients without recent antibiotic exposure.

C. Imaging

Plain radiographs in osteomyelitis may demonstrate radiolucency from osteolysis or sclerosis in chronic infections. However, plain films may be negative early in the disease process, as radiolucency is not seen until 30% to 50% of the trabeculae have been lost, which may take up to 3 to 4 weeks to develop. Disk space narrowing is an early radiographic finding of diskitis. As the infection progresses, spinal deformities such as focal kyphosis may be seen.

MRI with gadolinium contrast is the study of choice for diagnosing all forms of spinal infections. Its sensitivity and specificity are more than 95%. MRI changes occur within 24 to 48 hours of infection onset. MRI additionally allows for evaluation of neurologic compression (Figure 5–27). However, the true extent of bony destruction is better evaluated on CT scans but may take up to 3 to 6 weeks to become apparent. Typically, both an MRI and CT scan are needed to fully evaluate spinal infections. Nuclear medicine studies (technetium-99 or gallium studies) reliably (90% accuracy) show uptake in areas of infection within 3 to 7 days of onset but are less commonly used now that MRI is widely available and provides better anatomic detail.

Treatment

The goals of treating pyogenic infections are four-fold: (1) to eradicate the infection; (2) relieve pain; (3) preserve or improve neurologic function; and (4) maintain or restore

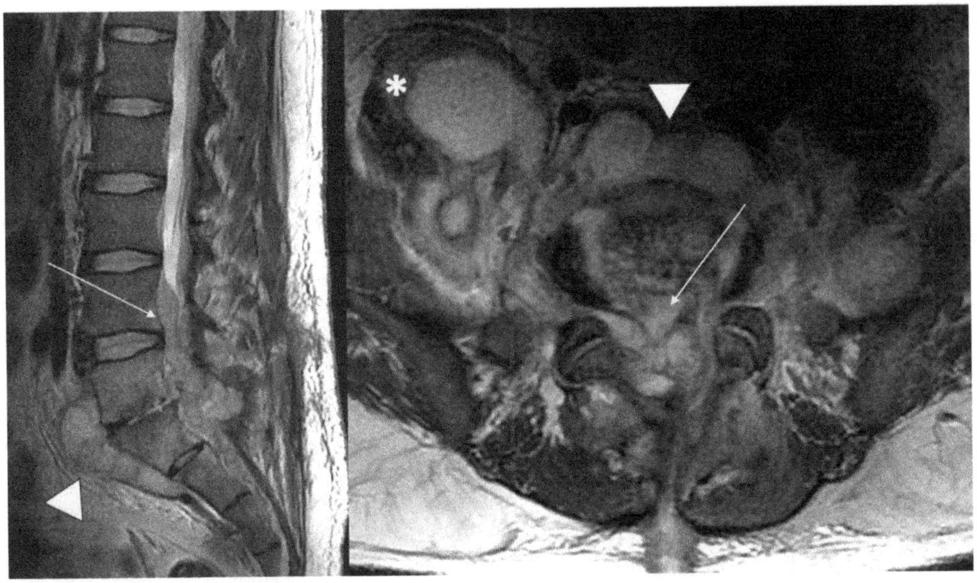

▲ **Figure 5–27.** A 35-year-old man with spinal infection secondary to brucellosis. Extensive epidural abscess (*arrow*) and prevertebral (*triangle*) and psoas abscess (*asterisk*) are present.

spinal alignment and stability. Indications for surgical treatment include the following: (1) to obtain a microbiologic diagnosis; (2) presence of abscess (intradiskal, bony, soft tissue, or epidural); (3) presence of neurologic deficit; (4) spinal instability; (5) progressive or severe spinal deformity; and (6) failure of nonoperative treatment, including refractory pain. The major goal of surgery is thorough debridement of all infected, nonviable tissue. Spinal reconstruction with instrumentation is often used to stabilize the spine after debridement. Although somewhat counterintuitive, the use of spinal implants, particularly those made of titanium, to fuse and stabilize the infected spine helps to successfully eradicate the infection, provided there has been adequate debridement and institution of culture-specific antibiotics. In the absence of the aforementioned indications, a term of nonoperative treatment may be considered. Failure of nonoperative treatment is indicated by lack of improvement in pain, fever, and/or laboratory parameters despite 6 weeks of appropriate antibiotic coverage.

In most cases, an anterior approach is necessary to radically debride the infection. Supplemental posterior instrumentation and fusion are usually needed to provide additional stability in the majority of cases, as the spine is rendered unstable either by the infection or the debridement needed to remove the infection. Anterior bone quality is generally poor in patients with infection and should not routinely be relied upon alone for fixation. Epidural abscesses are most commonly drained through a dorsal approach and are most common in the thoracolumbar spine. Classically, autograft has been used to graft anterior column deficits. More recently, allograft and titanium mesh cages combined with rhBMP-2 have been used with success to avoid the morbidity of autograft harvest. A prolonged course of postoperative antibiotics, typically parenteral for a minimum of 6 weeks, is needed. Nutritional supplementation plays a crucial role in healing of these patients, who are or become malnourished by the chronic infection.

Prognosis

Spinal infection is a serious disease, which historically was fatal in 50% to 70% of cases and even today has an overall mortality rate of 5% to 20%. Debridement and instrumented fusion can be successfully performed in a single stage with 90% to 100% initial response and less than 10% recurrence. When postoperative infections are identified and adequately treated in the acute phase (<4-6 weeks after surgery), originally placed implants can generally be left.

Berbari EF, Kanj SS, Kowalski TJ, et al. Executive summary: 2015 Infectious Diseases Society of America (IDSA) clinical practice guidelines for the diagnosis and treatment of native vertebral osteomyelitis in adults. *Clin Infect Dis.* 2015;61(6):859-863. [PMID: 26316526]

Khalil JG, Gandhi SD, Park DK, Fischgrund JS. *Cutibacterium acnes* in spine pathology: pathophysiology, diagnosis, and management. *J Am Acad Orthop Surg.* 2019;27(14):e633-e640. [PMID: 30520801]

Lener S, Hartmann S, Barbagallo GMV, Certo F, Thome C, Tschugg A. Management of spinal infection: a review of the literature. *Acta Neurochir.* 2018;160(3):487-496. [PMID: 29356895]

SPINAL TUMORS

Essentials of Diagnosis

- *Metastatic tumors are the most common tumors of the spine.*
- *Eighty percent of metastases to the spine come from cancer of the prostate, breast, or lung.*
- *Most common benign primary tumor of the spine is hemangioma.*
- *Back pain is the most common presenting symptom.*

General Considerations

Metastases represent the most common tumors of the spine. The spine is the most common location for skeletal metastasis, with the thoracic spine being the most commonly involved region. Typical spinal metastases include tumors of the prostate, breast, lung, thyroid, and kidney. Not unexpectedly, since they are the most prevalent cancers, 80% of spinal metastases originate from prostate, breast, or lung primary malignancies. In contrast, primary malignant bone tumors are comparatively rare and include chondrosarcoma, osteosarcoma, and chordoma. Lymphomas, solitary plasmacytomas, and multiple myelomas are also seen in the spine. Most (70%) malignant tumors arise in patients older than 21 years and typically occur in the anterior spine (vertebral body and pedicles). Chondrosarcoma is a notable exception that typically arises from the posterior elements.

The most common benign tumor of the spine is hemangioma, present in 10% to 12% of people. Most patients present with asymptomatic, incidental findings on MRI scans for other reasons (eg, back pain or sciatica), but in rare cases, hemangiomas can become large and symptomatic. Other than hemangiomas, which are frequently seen in older patients, benign bone tumors are much more common in younger patients. Osteoid osteomas and osteoblastomas are benign primary bone tumors that tend to involve the posterior elements. They are classically associated with nonmechanical back pain that tends to be worse at night and that improves with NSAIDs. Other benign bone tumors of the spine include aneurysmal bone cyst, fibrous dysplasia, and giant cell tumors. Giant cell tumors, although histologically benign, may be locally aggressive and even metastasize.

Another tumorlike finding that is a relatively common incidental finding on routine MRI for evaluation of back pain or sciatica is syrinx (a fluid-filled space within the spinal cord) or persistence of the central canal of the spinal cord. When seen, pathologic reasons, such as intramedullary tumor, Chiari malformation, spinal canal anomaly, tethered cord, or severe spinal stenosis, can be excluded with a screening MRI of the whole spine, preferably with contrast. However, about 90% of syrinxes are stable incidental findings not correlated with the clinical symptoms that elicited the MRI. In such cases, in the absence of progressive neurologic deficits or planned surgical intervention, expectant observation is a reasonable option as well.

Clinical Findings

A. Signs and Symptoms

The presentation of spinal tumors is often similar to that of spinal infections. Axial back pain is the most common complaint, present in about 90% of cases. Associated neurologic symptoms may be present if the tumor impinges neural elements or is associated with pathologic fracture and neural compression (ie, metastatic spinal cord compression). The presence of constitutional symptoms such as fevers, night sweats, or weight loss should be elicited. Back pain is often constant and unremitting, classically worse at night time, but may also have a component made worse by mechanical loading. Patients with new-onset back pain and a history of cancer need to be ruled out for metastatic disease to the spine. Physical findings include local tenderness over the tumor, limited range of motion, and, in advanced cases, deformity from vertebral body collapse and kyphosis.

B. Imaging and Laboratory Data

The radiologic workup of spinal tumors is similar to that of spinal infections. MRI remains the mainstay of diagnosis, with CT scans also obtained to assess the degree of bony destruction, the pattern of bone response to the lesion, and the presence of matrix and weight-bearing plain films to assess overall alignment and deformity. Plain films are poorly sensitive for tumors: approximately 40% trabecular bone loss must be present before being detectable on plain film as a lucent area. Thus, advanced imaging is critical to making a prompt diagnosis. Because of its ability to provide fine bony detail, CT scans are helpful in determining the aggressiveness of lytic lesions. Slow-growing benign tumors usually display a sharp transition zone with reactive, sclerotic bone surrounding the tumor as the bone has had time to respond. Aggressive, fast-growing tumors usually demonstrate a moth-eaten appearance with little reactive bone and a wide transition zone. Biopsy should be considered for spinal tumors that cannot be diagnosed based on imaging alone. Most commonly, needle biopsy under CT guidance is sufficient, but several large-bore specimens should be obtained to ensure a tissue diagnosis. In the case of widely metastatic disease, biopsy of a more superficial tumor may be considered if it is easier to access. If a needle biopsy is inconclusive, then open biopsy may be needed. In cases in which a curative resection is contemplated, the biopsy must be planned appropriately to allow for excision of the biopsy tract during the definitive operation.

A metastatic workup should be considered in all patients with spinal tumors, which includes a CT scan of the chest, abdomen, and pelvis. Whole-body bone scan can also be helpful in detecting malignant or metastatic foci. Unfortunately, only about 50% of multiple myelomas display increased uptake on bone scans. Bone scans detect tumors based on increased regional blood flow to the tumor and by radiolabeling (with technetium-99) phosphates, which are deposited in areas of active bone formation. However, uptake is nonspecific and can also be seen in trauma, infection, and arthropathy. [^{18}F]-Fluorodeoxyglucose PET/CT can also play a valuable role in staging and monitoring by providing not only information on anatomy but also metabolic activity. Its utility depends on the type of tumor involved given its substantially higher sensitivity in lytic lesions over blastic lesions. Routine laboratory data include CBC with differential, calcium, magnesium, Po_4, and liver function tests. Serum and urine electrophoresis can be helpful in diagnosing multiple myeloma.

Preoperative embolization of tumors may be helpful in decreasing intraoperative bleeding, making surgery safer, easier, and more effective. Likewise, selective embolization is a treatment option for large, symptomatic hemangiomas. In addition, with tumors involving the lower thoracic spine, angiography may be helpful in identifying the major feeding vessel to the spinal cord (the artery of Adamkiewicz) so that it can be spared surgically and avoid potential vascular infarction of the spinal cord.

Treatment

Treatment is dictated by a number of factors, including age (<65 or >65 years), tumor type and stage, symptom severity, overall physical condition, presence of neurologic compression or neurologic symptoms (most importantly, ambulatory status), expected life span (<3 or >3 months), and mechanical stability. Over the past decade, multiple algorithms such as NOMS (neurologic, oncologic, mechanical, and systemic decision framework) and LMNOP (location of disease in the spine [L]; mechanical instability [M]; neurology [N]; oncology [O]; patient fitness, prognosis, and response to prior therapy [P]) have been created to help create a common language by which a multidisciplinary oncologic team can devise the best treatment plan. Most benign asymptomatic lesions require no treatment, but depending on the certainty of the diagnosis, periodic follow-up with CT scans is prudent. Timely repeat imaging is also indicated if symptoms worsen during clinical observation. Indications for surgery include absence of viable nonsurgical treatment modalities, intractable pain despite nonsurgical treatment, mechanical instability, neurologic preservation or need for decompression, and, rarely, in certain primary tumors of the spine, curative resection. Percutaneous cement augmentation is a minimally invasive intervention with an expanding role in the treatment of painful spinal neoplastic lesions. The treatment of hemangiomas was the initial indication for this technique, which is now most commonly used to treat osteoporotic vertebral compression fractures.

Steroids are often used in the setting of tumors causing myelopathy from spinal cord compression. Bisphosphonates are also commonly used by oncologists to manage bone loss associated with neoplastic disease of the spine. They have been shown to significantly reduce the incidence of skeletally related (adverse) events (pathologic fracture, need for radiation or surgery to bone, or spinal cord compression) in patients with multiple myeloma and osteolytic metastases.

A. Metastatic Tumors

Most metastatic tumors without neurologic compression are treated nonsurgically with radiation and/or chemotherapy, depending on the tumor type and its responsiveness to those modalities. Over the past couple of decades, radical advancements have been made from more traditional en bloc resections combined with conventional external beam radiotherapy (cEBRT) to newer, more effective, and less invasive techniques including stereotactic body radiotherapy (SBRT) and spine stereotactic radiosurgery (SRS). cEBRT uses near full-dose radiation across the entire width of the patient, which is why doses must be kept low due to surrounding sensitive structures such as the spinal cord. In contrast, SBRT/SRS allows for multiple beams to focus on the tumor with millimetric precision and a steep dose fall-off allowing for higher, more effective doses. However, there are limits to this newer therapy, which is primarily limited to treating one- to two-level disease, with the involvement of three or more contiguous vertebral bodies being a general contraindication.

However, in the presence of symptomatic spinal cord compression, level 1 evidence that has been corroborated in other studies concludes that surgery prior to radiation therapy is superior to radiation therapy alone or radiation prior to surgery in terms of neurologic outcomes. An exception arises if neurologic compression is due solely to a highly radiosensitive tumor with no significant spinal instability or bony compressive component, in which case radiation may be considered first. Unless the tumor is highly radiosensitive or the patient is a poor surgical candidate, we generally advocate performing surgery first in patients with symptomatic neurologic compression in order to avoid progressive neurologic deterioration and complications associated with surgery through a previously irradiated field.

Surgery may also be considered in those without actual but impending neurologic compromise due to spinal instability. In general, those with more than 50% vertebral body involvement or destruction of the facet joints, pars, and pedicles are at risk for instability and resultant neurologic compromise. Unfortunately, in clinical practice, the assessment of spinal stability is often not straightforward, typically requiring a nuanced interpretation of biomechanical criteria based on the "personality" or pattern of tumor involvement seen on a combination of plain film, CT, and MRI.

The choice of surgical approach depends on a number of factors. In the vast majority of metastatic cases, the goal is palliation of pain and prevention or reversal of neurologic impairment. Thus, the operation should be designed to achieve those goals while minimizing morbidity. Depending on the location and pattern of compression, the decompression and reconstruction can be performed anteriorly, posteriorly, or combined. Given the increased precision and effectiveness of SRS/SBRT, there has been a large paradigm shift over the past couple of decades to less invasive and morbid surgical procedures and more focus toward "separation surgery." The surgical intent is to decompress the spinal cord and create enough separation between the neural matter and the tumor to allow for SRS/SBRT postoperatively in contrast to a gross radical resection of the tumor.

The choice of spinal reconstruction will depend on the patient's overall prognosis. Those with a reasonable life expectancy beyond 1 to 2 years may benefit from achieving solid bony union, but this must be balanced against the potentially higher bleeding and infection risks associated with bone grafting and fusion. Those with poor prognoses for survival may be best managed with decompression and instrumentation only. In these circumstances, cement can be used to augment vertebral corpectomies and provide immediate mechanical stability of vertebral body defects. Pain related to impending or actual pathologic fractures may be managed in certain instances with percutaneous cement procedures, such as vertebroplasty or kyphoplasty, which have the advantage of being less invasive.

B. Benign Primary Bone Tumors

Osteoid osteomas are typically seen in the posterior elements of teenagers (10-20 years old) and may be associated with acute scoliosis. CT scans demonstrate a central (lucent) nidus of tumor (sometimes with a small focus of bone at its center) surrounded by a sclerotic rim of reactive bone. Spontaneous regression can occur. If the symptoms are severe or persist despite time and NSAIDs, thorough curettage of the lesion yields good outcomes. If the nidus is removed, recurrence is relatively unlikely. Good results have also been reported with RFA. Most cases of osteoid osteoma or osteoblastoma-related scoliosis are not structural and spontaneously improve after tumor resection.

Osteoblastomas represent osteoid osteomas that are larger than 2 cm. They typically occur in patients younger than 30 years and can also be associated with scoliosis. When they occur in the spine, they tend to be in the posterior arch. Marginal excision provides excellent outcomes with relatively low recurrence rates. Depending on the extent of the excision, a fusion may be necessary.

Aneurysmal bone cysts cause hyperemic lytic lesions, most commonly in the posterior elements but not infrequently extending into the anterior column of the lumbar spine as well (Figure 5–28). As with most benign primary bone tumors, patients tend to be younger, typically younger

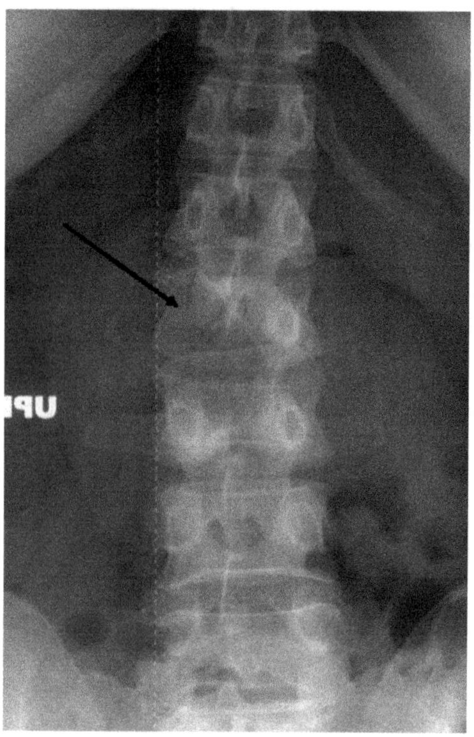

A

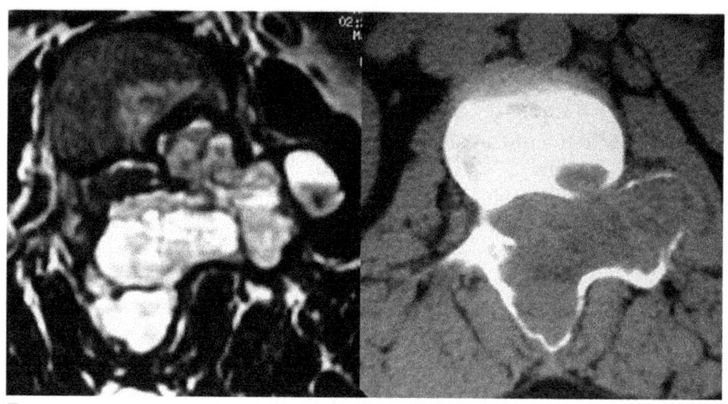

B C

▲ **Figure 5–28.** Aneurysmal bone cyst of the spine in a 27-year-old woman with severe low back pain and leg weakness. (**A**) Anteroposterior radiograph demonstrates destruction of the L2 pedicle along with lytic changes in the L2 vertebra (*black arrow*). (**B**) Axial MRI shows an expansile, cystic lesion with fluid-fluid level causing compression of the spinal canal. (**C**) CT scan shows expansile cortical margin with lytic erosion.

than 20 years. Expansion may cause neural compression and radiculopathy or myelopathy. MRI demonstrates characteristic fluid-fluid levels due to the layering of blood within the lesion. Curettage and resection of aneurysmal bone cysts with bone grafting is the treatment of choice. Again, fusion may be needed depending on the extent of the lesion. Preoperative embolization should strongly be considered to limit intraoperative bleeding.

Giant cell tumors are seen in slightly older individuals (20s to 40s) and arise most commonly in the anterior spine. Curettage and bone grafting may be performed but have a high recurrence rate of up to 45%. Thus, en bloc resection should be considered when feasible to prevent long-term recurrences. Radiation treatment may be associated with sarcomatous transformation in up to 15% of patients and thus is not routinely recommended.

C. Malignant Primary Bone Tumors

Multiple myeloma is the most common primary malignant bone tumor of the spine and is usually seen in patients in their 50s to 60s. It and its unifocal counterpart, solitary plasmacytoma, are B-cell lymphoproliferative cancers. In the absence of instability, myeloma can be treated with radiation, chemotherapy, and stem-cell transplants. However, surgery may be the option of choice in the face of neurologic compression associated with spinal instability, pathologic fractures, or impending fractures. Typically, patients will receive an antiresorptive medicine (eg, bisphosphonates) to reduce the incidence of skeletally related adverse events.

Chordomas are tumors arising from notochordal cells within the vertebral body, typically during the fifth and sixth decades and beyond. The sacrum accounts for over half of cases involving the spine, with the occipitocervical region accounting for another third. Because the local recurrence rate of chordoma is extremely high, care must be taken to obtain wide margins and avoid tumor contamination into the surgical field. Adjuvant radiation therapy may be helpful, particularly if complete resection is not possible or tumor contamination occurs during resection. Most patients with chordoma eventually die from complications related to local recurrence.

Chondrosarcomas are cartilaginous tumors typically arising in the posterior elements of the spine in patients in their 40s to 60s. Radiographs and CT scans demonstrate calcification within the tumor. Because they are radio-resistant, wide surgical excision is the mainstay of treatment. It is important to try to obtain clean surgical margins in order to avoid local recurrences, because local recurrence and progression are the most common causes of death from chondrosarcoma.

Prognosis

The prognosis will vary widely depending on the tumor. In the case of acute myelopathy associated with metastatic disease, it has been shown in a randomized controlled trial that immediate surgical decompression followed by radiation therapy is superior to radiation therapy alone. In general, surgical counseling must include specific discussion of quality of remaining life weighed against the degree of pain and/or actual versus impending neurologic deficit. Patients with less than 3 months of expected survival are typically provided nonoperative care. Surgery becomes a more reasonable option in those with better prognoses, and it should at least be considered in all patients with actual or impending neurologic deficits, especially spinal cord level compression. Even in those with relatively poor prognoses, surgery may provide substantial benefit in terms of neurologic preservation and pain relief during a patient's remaining life.

Gibbs WN, Nael K, Doshi AH, Tanenbaum LN. Spine oncology: imaging and intervention. *Radiol Clin North Am.* 2019;57(2):377-395. [PMID: 30709476]

DEFORMITIES OF THE SPINE

SCOLIOSIS

Essentials of Diagnosis

- *Scoliosis is deviation of the spine from the vertical axis greater than 10 degrees.*
- *Ninety percent of cases do not progress.*
- *Curve magnitude greater than 45 degrees is likely to progress into adulthood.*
- *Most cases in young people are asymptomatic; adults are more likely to have symptoms of back pain and sciatica.*

General Considerations

Scoliosis as defined by the Scoliosis Research Society is any lateral deviation of the spine from the normal vertical line of 10 degrees or greater. Minor "wiggles" less than 10 degrees are termed spinal asymmetry and do not require follow-up. Using the 10-degree standard, about 2% to 4% of the US population has scoliosis with an equal distribution between the sexes. At this low threshold for diagnosis, over 90% of cases will not progress to the point of warranting further intervention. Thus, referral to a spine surgeon is typically reserved for curves that are more than 15 to 20 degrees, for curves that demonstrate progression on serial assessment by the primary care provider, or for patients with worrisome history or physical exam findings. When coronal curvature is greater than 20 to 30 degrees, a strong female predominance (8-10:1) is noted. Idiopathic scoliosis is a disease that is driven by skeletal growth until a significant magnitude of curvature is obtained (>30-50 degrees). As such, there are essentially three stages of treatment for scoliosis—observation alone (the most common), bracing (only appropriate in the skeletally immature), and surgical correction.

If by skeletal maturity the coronal curve has not exceeded 30 degrees, then this mild spinal deformity is not likely to progress in adulthood, and it is unlikely to have future clinical impact on the patient. On the other hand, when the magnitude of curvature exceeds 45 to 50 degrees, progression in adulthood is predicted, typically at a pace of 1 degree per year. With continued progression, clinical manifestations are likely, which include back pain and radiculopathy/sciatica (especially when the major curve involves the lumbar spine), and in the most severe cases (>75-90 degrees), pulmonary and gastrointestinal (GI) compromise can occur. As such, surgery, in the form of instrumented spinal fusion, is typically indicated when coronal curvature exceeds 45 to 50 degrees. The goals of surgical correction are to arrest curve progression and provide sufficient curve correction to produce a stable, well-balanced spine centered over the pelvis by fusing as few segments as possible. In addition to this primary structural goal, additional benefits may include improved cosmesis and reduced back pain and neurologic dysfunction. Traditionally, scoliosis clinical research has focused on the primary goal, which has been deformity correction. Recent clinical studies have focused on the overall well-being of scoliosis patients as assessed by validated outcome tools.

Scoliosis is most commonly divided into subsets, based on the age at diagnosis. When scoliosis is present at birth, it is termed congenital scoliosis, which occurs by one of two structural anomalies. Either there is a failure of formation of part of the spine (eg, a hemivertebra, which is the most common anomaly producing congenital scoliosis), or there is failure of segmentation (ie, a block vertebra). The crucial period for formation and segmentation of the spine occurs in the fourth to sixth week of gestation, which is also a critical time for spinal cord, renal, and cardiac development. As a result, when congenital scoliosis is diagnosed, the health of these additional structures should be screened as well. When scoliosis presents within the first 3 years of life, it is termed infantile scoliosis. Infantile scoliosis is a rare (<1% of all cases) form of scoliosis that has strong genetic associations, and it too requires further screening (ie, screening MRI of the spine). It commonly produces a left thoracic curve, and the vast majority of cases (~90%) resolve spontaneously. When it presents between 3 and 10 years of age, it is called juvenile scoliosis. This type behaves and is treated like adolescent scoliosis, although the greater growth potential predisposes to a greater risk of progression to the point of surgical indication. Adolescent idiopathic scoliosis, the most common type of scoliosis, is diagnosed when scoliosis presents after 10 years of age and prior to skeletal maturity (typically 2 years after menarche in females). Adult scoliosis refers to scoliosis detected after skeletal maturity. It typically has two primary distinctions—de novo (meaning it developed in adulthood, often as an advanced form of spinal degeneration, typified by low-degree lumbar curves with significant rotatory subluxation[s]) and progressive (meaning it was the progression of a curve that started earlier in life). Aside from congenital and infantile forms of scoliosis, which have unique anatomic considerations, the distinctions between juvenile, adolescent, and adult are not as significant.

Last, the aforementioned classifications describe idiopathic scoliosis, which is the etiology of 85% of cases; however, scoliosis can be associated with skeletal syndromes (eg, Marfan syndrome or neurofibromatosis), termed syndromic scoliosis, or neuromuscular conditions (cerebral palsy being most common). These two rarer causes of scoliosis tend to produce more significant degrees of curvature and more commonly require surgical intervention. Neuromuscular scoliosis is often treated with fusion of the entire thoracic and lumbar spine to the pelvis. An important consideration for these two rare forms of scoliosis is that they are part of a syndrome. When diagnosed, comprehensive evaluation for other known associated manifestations (eg, aortic dilation in Marfan syndrome) of the syndrome should be undertaken.

Clinical Findings

A. Signs and Symptoms

Scoliosis is most commonly detected incidentally on screening examinations or during routine pediatric appointments in the preteen years. Uneven ribs, shoulders, or pelvis may be noted by the patient or parents and should be assessed on examination. While the vast majority of patients are asymptomatic at presentation, about one-third of patients will complain of back pain, which is often in the interscapular area. When it is in the low lumbar area, radiographs should be inspected for evidence of spondylolisthesis, which can coexist in scoliotic patients. Since reports of back pain can be elicited in a similar percentage of young adults with straight spines, the clinical significance of this complaint and the direct association with the underlying spinal deformity may not be clear. That being said, reports of severe back pain may prompt further evaluation, to include screening whole-spine MRI to ensure that no intraspinal anomalies (eg, syrinx, tumor, or diastematomyelia) are present. The yield from these additional studies is exceedingly low and likely does not offset the cost and difficulty (eg, some level of sedation is often needed to obtain the MRI). Since indications for MRI in the setting of scoliosis are not universally accepted, this determination is probably best left to the consultant. When patients present with positive findings on neurologic examination (eg, weakness, sensory deficits, altered gait, bowel or bladder problems), then screening MRI should be ordered.

The Adams forward bend test is the classic screening assessment for scoliosis. It is carried out in most states on an annual basis in school for adolescent females (and commonly males as well). This test requires the examiner to stand posterior to the patient, while the child bends over at the waist until their trunk is level with the ground. Scoliosis is not simply a lateral deviation, but a rotation of the spine. The rotation at the thoracic level causes the ribs to rise up on the side of the curve apex, which is most commonly the right side (90% of cases). It is so common for the main thoracic curve to be apexed to the right that many experts feel screening MRI is indicated whenever the main thoracic curve points to the left. This truncal rotation can simply be viewed or palpated, but a scoliometer is a device that looks like a carpenter's level and is used to directly measure the degree of rotation in the chest cavity. Screening thresholds for radiograph and/or spine surgical consultation vary between 5- and 7-degree tilt, as measured by the scoliometer. The lower threshold is more sensitive (minimal to no false negatives), whereas the upper limit is more specific (less false positives).

B. Imaging

The gold standard for diagnosing scoliosis is an upright posterior-anterior long cassette (36") frontal and lateral radiograph of the entire thoracic and lumbar spine. This is often called a scoliosis survey. This should be obtained at a radiology suite that is versed in the proper protocol for obtaining high-quality scoliosis films. The radiologist or spine surgeon then views the spine and looks for the three common curves that occur in scoliosis—proximal thoracic, main thoracic, and lumbar. The magnitude of the curvature is measured using the Cobb method, which subtends the angle between lines drawn at the upper endplate of the upper vertebra in the measured curve (termed the upper end vertebrae) to the lower endplate of the lower vertebrae (lower end vertebra). The apex is the direction that the convex side of the curve points (often reported using the Latin prefixes *dextro*, meaning right, or *levo*, meaning left); specifically, it is the lateral-most deviated point in the curve, which can be a vertebral body or disk space. The largest of the curves is called the major curve. Any additional curves are called minor curves. The major curve, in addition to having the greatest degree of coronal curvature, also has the greatest degree of rotation. Rotation is graded based on the degree to which the apical vertebral pedicles are rotated from their normal owl's eyes appearance. Minor curves are frequently compensatory. Compensatory curves typically do not have a rotatory component, as they are simple lateral deviations in the spine that naturally occur to compensate for the major curve, thereby keeping the head centered over the pelvis.

The most common method in current use for classifying adolescent idiopathic scoliosis curves is the Lenke classification system. It replaces the King classification system, because it is more reliable, better predicts surgical plan, and takes into account the three-dimensional nature of scoliosis. In addition to standing scoliosis films, supine bending films are also needed to assess the flexibility and structural nature of each curve. The Lenke classification system has three components. First, there are six curve types. Then there is a lumbar modifier, which demonstrates the degree to which the lumbar curve deviates from the vertical midline. Last, there is a sagittal modifier, which assesses the degree of thoracic (T5-T12) kyphosis.

Many patients with main thoracic scoliosis (Lenke type 1, most common type) have flat (hypokyphotic) thoracic spines, as the normal thoracic kyphosis has rotated into the coronal plane. Kyphosis (abnormal forward curvature of the spine; normal = 10-50 degrees) can occur in the setting of scoliosis or as an independent deformity. When global thoracic kyphosis of more than 50 degrees occurs in the setting of three or more consecutive thoracic vertebral bodies having a wedging of 5 degrees or more, typically with Schmorl nodes present, it is termed Scheuermann kyphosis. Most cases of Scheuermann kyphosis require no specific treatment, although bracing can be attempted during growth. Corrective surgical fusion may be considered in severe cases (>75-90 degrees).

Treatment

As stated earlier, there are three stages of treatment for scoliosis. The first and commonly the only stage needed is serial observation. Because scoliosis is a disease of progression, it takes at least two points in time to fully assess the significance of the deformity, unless the deformity is severe at presentation. Three factors most affect the likelihood of progression: (1) female gender, (2) growth remaining, and (3) current curve magnitude. To minimize repeated radiation exposure, serial follow-up typically occurs at 4-month intervals during periods of peak growth and 6-month intervals during periods of less expected growth, especially in lower magnitude curves (<20 degrees). Curves that are less than 30 degrees in adulthood do not require routine follow-up. While there is some variation, a consensus of the reported methods for predicting progression to more than 40 to 45 degrees shows that major curves that are less than 20 to 30 degrees at or in the year prior to menarche or the start of the skeletal growth spurt in males have less than 5% to 20% risk of progression to the point of requiring surgical intervention. Asymptomatic curves of less than 30 degrees detected as incidental findings in females more than 2 years out from menarche and skeletally mature males do not require spine surgical consultation solely for evaluation of scoliosis. Since curve progression in adulthood occurs at a much slower pace than in adolescence, serial images, when indicated, should be separated by 1 to 3+ years in adults. The measurement error for coronal curve measurement on scoliosis films is 3 to 5 degrees. Thus, with an expected progression of 1 degree per year in adulthood, it would take at least 3 years to demonstrate a real progression exceeding measurement error. Indications for scoliosis surgery in adults are largely based on clinical complaints, as opposed to curve magnitude and deformity.

If the major curve progresses to 20 to 25 degrees (up to 35 degrees) in a skeletally immature patient, then bracing is the next stage of treatment offered. There are several types of braces, with two major subsets—thoracolumbar orthoses and nighttime braces. Thoracolumbar orthoses (eg, Boston brace) are the most common type of brace and are intended to be worn 20 to 22 hours a day. They are typically made of thin plastic, so they can be worn under clothes to reduce the stigma of wearing a brace. Compliance significantly affects the ability of braces to prevent progression, which is the goal of bracing. Bracing is not intended to permanently correct scoliosis, but rather to arrest curve progression at a magnitude below which it is unlikely to produce lifelong impact (ie, <30 degrees). With compliant wear, bracing can arrest or slow scoliosis progression and prevent need for surgical intervention in up to 75% of those treated. Bracing is a challenging treatment for image-conscious adolescents to tolerate, because when it is started, it must be maintained through the remainder of skeletal growth and then some time after (often 2-3 years of total wear time). To avoid brace wear during school, nighttime braces were introduced, which hold the spine in an overcorrected position during nighttime only. This technique is more painful and may be less effective. Physical therapy and activity modification do not influence the natural history of scoliosis. There is no reason to restrict activity in patients diagnosed with scoliosis. That being said, reducing the weight of book bags, encouraging the wear of both shoulder straps (versus using just one shoulder), and best yet, rolling book bags with two sets of books (one for school and one for home) can help reduce back pain complaints and do demonstrate short-term measurable differences in curvature.

Last, when the degree of curvature exceeds 45 to 50 degrees, surgical intervention in the form of instrumented spinal fusion is indicated. This can occur via posterior, anterior, or combined posterior-anterior spinal fusion. Clear clinical superiority between the approaches is uncertain. Each has its own specific risk-benefit profile. Multiple techniques exist for correcting the curvature seen in scoliosis. All methods include rigid fixation of the spine, some degree of destabilization of the instrumented spinal segment (ie, facetectomies and ligament releases), correction of the deformity via forces applied through the implants, and securing the correction by locking the screws (or fixation devices) to rods and then placement of bone graft to encourage solid fusion across the instrumented segment. The most common means for instrumenting the spine is a pedicle screw and rod construct. Pedicle screws provide strong three-column fixation capable of delivering three-dimensional corrective forces to the spine. In the setting of early-onset or congenital scoliosis where significant growth remains, growing rods have been shown to be safe and effective in select patients in an attempt to control the deformity and delay fusion.

Outside the scope of this chapter is the complex decision process that goes into level selection and whether to fuse all curves or only the major curve, expecting the minor/compensatory curves to spontaneously correct. Current surgical techniques, especially in young healthy patients, produce solid fusions with excellent correction in the vast majority of patients with very low rates of complications. The most dreaded complication is spinal cord injury (<1%). This can occur through implant malposition, but more commonly is related to the acute correction of the deformity, especially in the setting of significant kyphosis. Intraoperative neuromonitoring allows for real-time or near real-time assessment of spinal cord function during scoliosis surgery to reduce the risk of this severe complication. Comorbidities, such as osteoporosis, obesity, cardiac disease, and diabetes, increase the rate of complication associated with adult scoliosis surgery. Further, younger patients have significantly more flexible curves, which can be more effectively corrected with simpler techniques, than the rigid curves seen in adult scoliosis. When the primary presenting symptom is pain or neurologic deficit, deformity correction in the setting of low-magnitude curves (30-50 degrees) in patients with neutral sagittal balance (ie, the spine is maintained in a rather vertical stature, without fixed forward tipping of the spine) is not always a goal of surgery in adult scoliosis. When sagittal imbalance is present through scoliosis or kyphoscoliosis, long-segment thoracolumbar fusions are often indicated to secure the spine and restore the sagittal balance in adults. This is crucial, because sagittal balance is the structural parameter most predictive of successful clinical outcome following adult scoliosis surgery. More recently, it has been shown that in addition to achieving these technical goals, scoliosis surgery significantly improves cosmesis, pain, and overall well-being (Figure 5–29).

Helenius L, Diarbakeli E, Grauers A, et al. Back pain and quality of life after surgical treatment of adolescent idiopathic scoliosis at 5-year follow up: comparison with healthy controls and patients with untreated idiopathic scoliosis. *J Bone Joint Surg*. 2019;101(16):1460-1466. [PMID: 3146653]

Howard A, Wright JG, Hedden D. A comparative study of TLSO, Charleston, and Milwaukee braces for idiopathic scoliosis. *Spine (Phila Pa 1976)*. 1998;23(22):2404-2411. [PMID: 9836354]

Louer C Jr, Yaszay B, Cross M, et al. Ten-year outcomes of selective fusions for adolescent idiopathic scoliosis. *J Bone Joint Surg*. 2019;101(9):761-770. [PMID: 31045663]

Ramirez N, Johnston CE, Browne RH. The prevalence of back pain in children who have idiopathic scoliosis. *J Bone Joint Surg Am*. 1997;79:364-368. [PMID: 9070524]

Thompson RM, Hubbard EW, Jo CH, Virostek D, Karol LA. Brace success is related to curve type in patients with adolescent idiopathic scoliosis. *J Bone Joint Surg*. 2017;99(11):923-928. [PMID: 28590377]

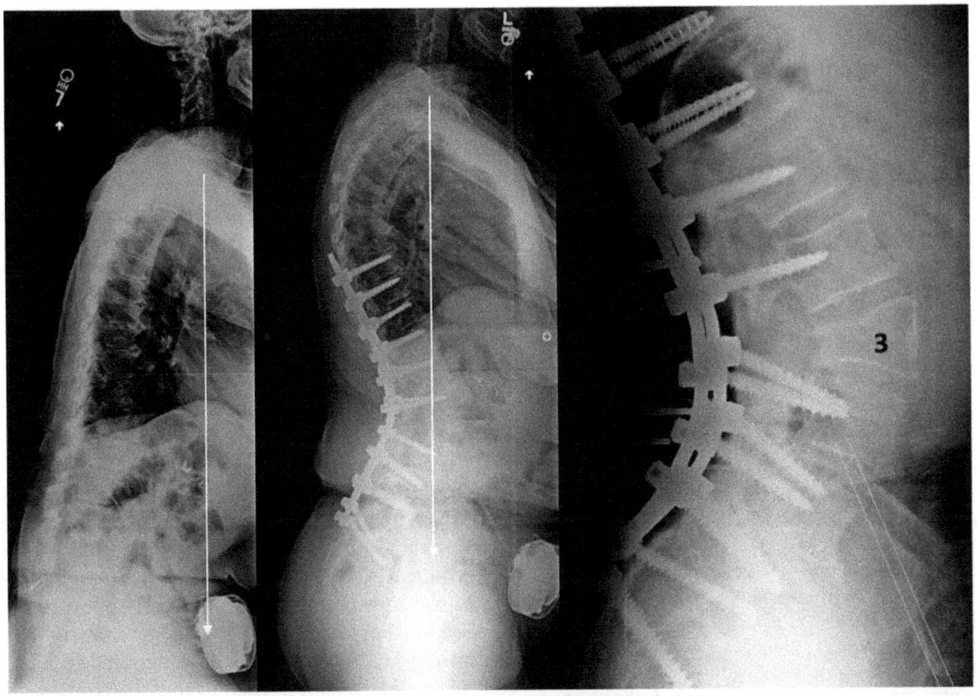

A B C

▲ **Figure 5–29.** (**A**) A 59-year-old woman with severe sagittal plane imbalance after multiple prior lumbar surgeries that left her fused in 10 degrees of lumbar kyphosis. Sagittal vertical axis (SVA) is markedly positive (*arrow*) at +15 cm. (**B**) Postoperative after L3 pedicle subtraction osteotomy (PSO) and multiple level posterior column osteotomies to realign the sagittal plane. Note significant improvement in SVA (*arrow*) to +5 cm with lumbar lordosis now 53 degrees. Normal sagittal spinal contours have been obtained. (**C**) Intraoperative image showing a close up view of the wedge-shaped PSO at L3.

NEUROFIBROMATOSIS

Spinal deformity associated with neurofibromatosis poses some special considerations. Curvatures seen in affected patients may be of the idiopathic type or the dysplastic type. Curvatures of the first type exhibit the same curve patterns as seen in patients with idiopathic scoliosis and are most commonly right thoracic curves and may be managed in a similar manner. Curvatures of the second type can be much more malignant in behavior.

Dysplastic curves can be identified by evidence of dysplastic bone: penciling of the ribs or transverse processes, enlargement of the foramina, erosion of the vertebrae, and evidence of a shorter, more abrupt curve than that seen in idiopathic scoliosis. Dysplastic curves usually are associated with kyphosis, which also exists through a fairly short sharp segment. They may occur in the thoracic, thoracolumbar, or lumbar spine.

Dysplastic curves in patients with neurofibromatosis can progress rapidly and lead to severe deformity. Bony erosion can occur secondary to neurofibromas or dural ectasia (expansions of the dural sac, which can account for enlargement of the foramina or erosion of the vertebrae). The short kyphotic curves and erosion of bone can, in severe cases, result in neurologic impairment, including paraplegia.

Historically, a combined anterior and posterior approach was typically used due to increased success rates of fusion with a combined approach especially in dysplastic curves, which have a higher incidence of pseudoarthrosis. However, over the past two decades, the rate of combined approaches has been decreasing, while the rate of the posterior-only approach has significantly increased almost three-fold. Recent studies have demonstrated successful outcomes via satisfactory curve correction with a low complication risk in the setting of posterior-only instrumentation for both dysplastic and nondysplastic scoliosis. Because of the dysplastic bone stock, it may be necessary to use a combination of sublaminar wires, hooks, and screws. Growing rods are also a potential option to treat early-onset scoliosis associated with neurofibromatosis with the ability to help control curve progression. However, some studies have shown higher complication rates compared to fusion including hardware failure, proximal junctional kyphosis, and continued curve progression. Preoperative MRI may be useful in assessing the extent of dural ectasia. Fusion levels are selected according to the end vertebra of the curvature. The end fusion level must lie centered over the middle of the sacrum (the Harrington stable zone), much like the selection for idiopathic scoliosis. Clearly, however, the fusion should not end above or below a dysplastic vertebra, although it would be rare for such a level not to be within the curve.

Carbone M, Vittoria F, Del Sal A. Treatment of early-onset scoliosis with growing rods in patients with neurofibromatosis-1. *J Pediatr Orthop B.* 2019;28(3):278-287. [PMID: 30855545]

Deng A, Zhang HQ, Tang MX, Liu SH, Wang YX, Gao QL. Posterior-only surgical correction of dystrophic scoliosis in 31 patients with neurofibromatosis type 1 using the multiple anchor point method. *J Neurosurg Pediatr.* 2017;19(1):96-101. [PMID: 27739946]

Jain VV, Berry CA, Crawford AH, Emans JB, Sponseller PD. Growing rods are an effective fusionless method of controlling early-onset scoliosis associated with neurofibromatosis type 1 (NF1): a multicenter retrospective case series. *J Pediatr Orthop.* 2017;37(8):e612-e618. [PMID: 28234734]

Kurucan E, Bernstein DN, Thirukumaran C, et al. National trends in spinal fusion surgery for neurofibromatosis. *Spine Deform.* 2018;6(6):712-718. [PMID: 30348349]

Lyu Q, Zhou C, Song Y, Liu L, Wang L, Zhou Z. Does spinal deformity correction of non-dystrophic scoliosis in neurofibromatosis type I with one-stage posterior pedicle screw technique produce outcomes similar to adolescent idiopathic scoliosis? *Spine J.* 2017;17(12):1850-1858. [PMID: 28645674]

Yao Z, Guo D, Li H, et al. Surgical treatment of dystrophic scoliosis in neurofibromatosis type 1: outcomes and complications. *Clin Spine Surg.* 2019;32(1):e50-e55. [PMID: 30273186]

CONGENITAL SCOLIOSIS

Congenital scoliosis is caused by one of the two types of structural bony abnormality (Figure 5–30). Type I is a failure of formation, such as that seen with hemivertebrae. Type II is a failure of segmentation, such as that seen with block vertebrae and that seen with unsegmented bars, where there is a tether to growth on one side of the spine. Mixed abnormalities are also found in patients with congenital scoliosis. Unilateral unsegmented bars with contralateral hemivertebrae have the greatest tendency for rapid progression and should be surgically fused as soon as the bony abnormality is evident. Unilateral unsegmented bars also tend to progress.

With respect to progression, hemivertebrae have a variable prognosis, depending on whether a contralateral hemivertebra is present that results in overall balance of the spine, whether multiple hemivertebrae are on one side of the spine, and how much growth potential is predicted for each endplate of the hemivertebra. Hemivertebrae at the cervicothoracic junction and the lumbosacral junction have a relatively poor prognosis because the spine above or below the abnormality cannot compensate. Hemivertebrae should be observed so as to delineate their growth potential and progression.

In patients with congenital scoliosis, the incidence of cardiac abnormalities is increased, as is the incidence of renal abnormalities (20%-30%) and intracanal abnormalities (10%-50%). Abdominal ultrasound or other imaging tests should be used to rule out absent or abnormal kidneys. Intracanal abnormalities may include a syrinx (cyst within the cord), diastematomyelia or diplomyelia (division or reduplication of the cord, respectively), and tethered cord (presence of a tight filum terminale that does not permit the conus medullaris to migrate upward normally with growth).

Bracing is ineffective in treating congenital scoliosis because the curves are inflexible. Bracing is sometimes used to prevent progression of the compensatory curve, however. More recently, serial derotational casting has been used as a "time-buying" strategy to delay surgery for up to 2 years.

If surgical intervention in patients with congenital scoliosis is indicated, several options are available. "Growth-friendly" surgical management is preferred in early-onset scoliosis so that the curve can be controlled while the spine and thorax continue to grow. Multiple studies have shown that vertical expandable prosthetic titanium rib (VEPTR) allows for continued growth while still allowing for curve correction. Furthermore, VEPTR in congenital scoliosis has also compared favorably to outcomes seen in adolescent idiopathic scoliosis when evaluating Scoliosis Research Society 22-Item (SRS-22) outcome scores. Fusion in situ is the simplest procedure. For very young (<10 years) patients, however, a posterior fusion alone results in tethering of the posterior elements while the anterior elements continue to grow. This situation may lead to the crankshaft phenomenon, whereby the anterior growth in the spine results in a twisting deformity around the fused posterior elements. For this reason, combined anterior and posterior fusion is usually recommended for very young patients, halting growth circumferentially about the spine. However, newer studies evaluating patients treated for congenital scoliosis under the age of 10 years with posterior hemivertebrae excision and posterior fusion alone have not demonstrated crankshaft phenomenon. (The crankshaft phenomenon can also occur in very young patients with noncongenital forms of scoliosis who were treated by posterior fusion. Age younger than 10 years, Risser stage 0 or 1, and the presence of an open triradiate cartilage are indicators of skeletal maturity at risk for development of crankshaft.)

In some cases of hemivertebra, hemiepiphysiodesis may be performed, arresting growth on the curve convexity but permitting continued growth on the curve concavity, with resultant gradual curve correction. This procedure has good results in selected patients but can be unpredictable with respect to the amount of actual correction that can be achieved.

In cases in which a hemivertebra is accompanied by significant coronal decompensation and compensatory growth would not be adequate to result in spinal balance, consideration can be given to hemivertebra excision via a combined

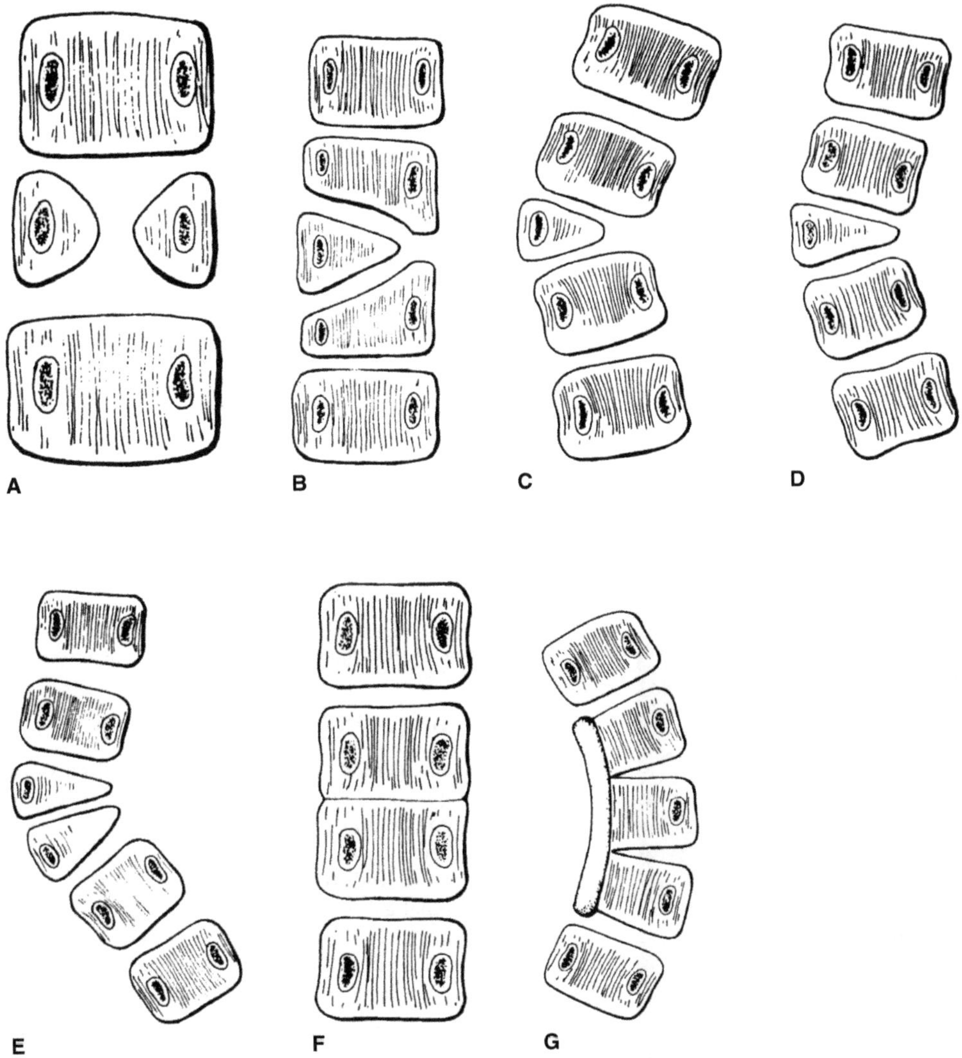

▲ **Figure 5–30.** The major types of congenital scoliosis are failure of formation, as shown in diagrams **A** through **E**, and failure of segmentation, as shown in diagrams **F** and **G.** (Reprinted, with permission, from Hall JE. Congenital scoliosis. In Bradford DS, Hensinger RN, eds. *The Pediatric Spine*. New York: Thieme; 1985.)

anterior and posterior approach. Although this procedure is technically more demanding and has greater potential risks, it allows for better overall curve correction and improvement of coronal balance. Newer studies have demonstrated satisfactory outcomes with hemivertebra excision and posterior-only fusion without risk of crankshaft phenomena. Hemivertebra excision may be the preferred option in the lumbar spine or lumbosacral junction, where the neurologic risk is to the cauda equina rather than the spinal cord and where oblique takeoff of the vertebra above the hemivertebra can result in significant truncal decompensation.

Chang DG, Kim JH, Ha KY, Lee JS, Jang JS, Suk SI. Posterior hemivertebra resection and short segment fusion with pedicle screw fixation for congenital scoliosis in children younger than 10 years: greater than 7-year follow-up. *Spine.* 2015;40(8):E484-E491. [PMID: 25835484]

Chang DG, Suk SI, Kim JH, Ha KY, Na KH, Lee JH. Surgical outcomes by age at the time of surgery in the treatment of congenital scoliosis in children under age 10 years. *Spine J.* 2015;15(8):1783-1795. [PMID: 25862509]

Demirkiran HG, Bekmez S, Celilov R, Ayvaz M, Dede O, Yazici M. Serial derotational casting in congenital scoliosis as a time-buying strategy. *J Pediatr Orthop.* 2015;35(1):43-49. [PMID: 24887080]

Pahys JM, Guille JT. What's new in congenital scoliosis? *J Pediatr Orthop.* 2018;38(3):e172-e179. [PMID: 28009797]

Sullivan BT, Abousamra O, Puvanessarajah V, et al. Deep infections after pediatric spinal arthrodesis: differences exit with idiopathic, neuromuscular or genetic and syndromic causes of deformity. *J Bone Joint Surg.* 2019;101(24):2219-2225. [PMID: 31609894]

KYPHOSIS

The normal sagittal contour of the spine includes cervical lordosis, thoracic kyphosis, and lumbar lordosis (Figure 5–31). Increases or decreases in any of these can be seen. If they are severe enough, they can cause disability, as in the cases of congenital kyphosis and Scheuermann kyphosis.

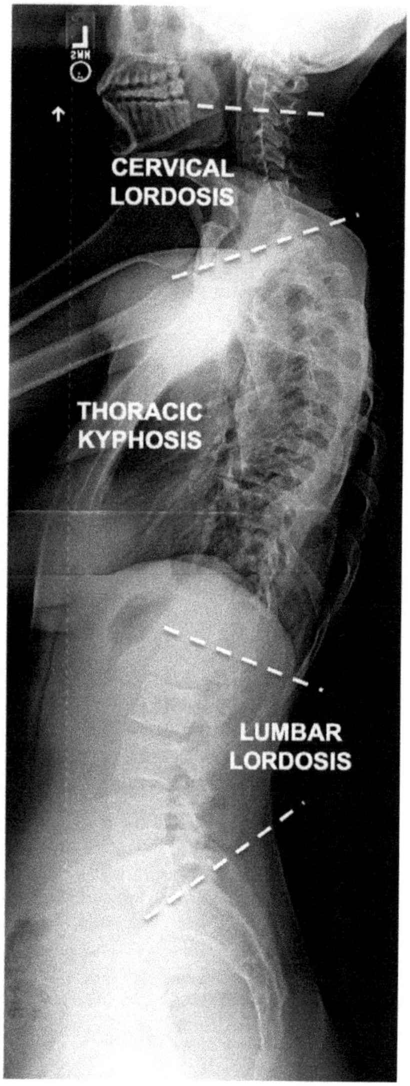

▲ **Figure 5–31.** Contours of the spine: cervical lordosis, thoracic kyphosis, lumbar lordosis.)

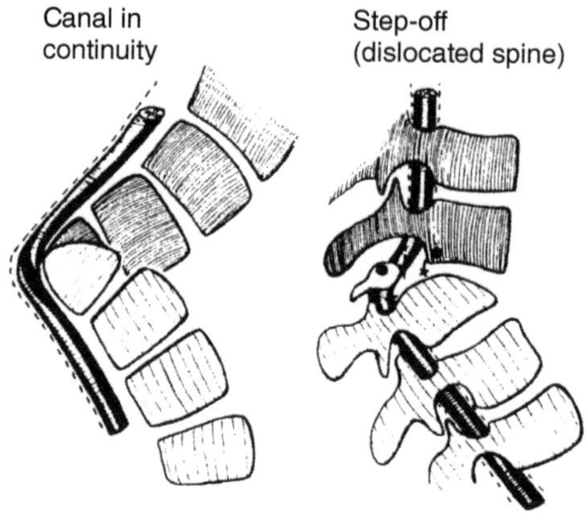

▲ **Figure 5–32. Congenital kyphosis and congenital "dislocation" of the spinal column.** (Reproduced, with permission, from Dubousset J. Congenital kyphosis. In Bradford DS, Hensinger RN, eds. *The Pediatric Spine.* New York: Thieme; 1985.)

1. Congenital Kyphosis

As in congenital scoliosis (see previous discussion), congenital kyphosis can result from a failure of formation or a failure of segmentation. In congenital kyphosis, however, failures of formation have a much more dangerous clinical prognosis. These can lead to congenital or progressive "dislocation" of the spinal column (Figure 5–32) and paralysis if not treated appropriately. If performed early enough, posterior fusion may be sufficient to prevent neurologic problems. Severe deficiencies, however, may require anterior and posterior fusion to achieve stability.

2. Scheuermann Kyphosis

Normal thoracic kyphosis ranges from 25 to 45 degrees. Postural kyphosis can increase this curvature, but if no abnormalities are present, the curve is flexible and the posture can be easily corrected by the child. If endplate abnormalities are present and three or more vertebral bodies are wedged as seen on the lateral radiograph, the diagnosis of Scheuermann kyphosis can be made. Schmorl nodules, characterized by herniation of the disk material at the vertebral endplates, and increased thoracic kyphosis are also seen. Clinically, patients with this type of kyphosis have a curvature that is more abrupt than that observed in people with postural roundback, and this type is only partly correctable by forced extension. It can be demonstrated either by having the patient hyperextend or by taking a lateral radiograph with the patient lying over a bolster at the apex of the kyphosis so the Cobb angle can be measured. Deformity is usually the most common complaint and the reason younger patients will seek medical evaluation. Thoracic curves may cause pain and discomfort, although some report that pain is more commonly seen in thoracolumbar curves.

For mild deformities, exercises and physical therapy focused on hyperextension have shown to have some benefit. Bracing can be instituted if the kyphosis measures more than 45 or 55 degrees in a skeletally immature patient, particularly if the curvature is progressive or accompanied by pain. If lesser degrees of deformity are symptomatic, they can be treated with physical therapy exercises and observed for progression. Brace treatment requires the use of the Milwaukee brace, with two paraspinal pads placed over the apical ribs posteriorly. Radiographs should be taken with the patient in the brace to confirm that adequate correction is being effected. The brace can be removed for sports and bathing but should otherwise be worn 23 hours a day. Repeat lateral radiographs should be taken at intervals of 4 to 6 months. If bracing is successful at controlling the curve, it should be continued until the patient nears skeletal maturity. Weaning should be performed slowly, so as to maintain correction. Although some correction may be lost, proper use of the Milwaukee brace can result in long-lasting improvement in many patients with kyphosis (which is not the case with brace treatment of adolescent idiopathic scoliosis).

Surgical treatment of kyphosis may be indicated if the curve magnitude increases despite bracing, if the patient has significant associated symptoms, or if the patient who is nearing skeletal maturity has a severe curvature (>80 degrees). Posterior spinal fusion with multilevel posterior Smith-Peterson osteotomies is the treatment of choice in these cases. Segmental instrumentation using pedicle screws with a compression-type construct is used to correct the deformity and hold the correction until fusion occurs. If the curve flexibility does not permit adequate correction as demonstrated on a hyperextension lateral radiograph, an anterior release and fusion prior to the posterior spinal fusion is indicated. Care should be taken to extend the fusion to the upper thoracic spine, sometimes to T1, to minimize the risk of developing junctional problems at the cervicothoracic junction.

Reports describe the natural history of Scheuermann kyphosis, suggesting some functional limitations but little actual interference with lifestyle. The deformity can worsen over time. It appears clear, however, that many patients have their symptoms of back pain and deformity improved by surgery. Proper patient education and selection are essential for appropriate treatment of these patients.

Polly DW Jr, Ledonio CGT, Diamond B, et al. What are the indications for spinal fusion surgery in Scheuermann kyphosis? *J Pediatr Orthop*. 2019;39(5):217-221. [PMID: 30969249]

MYELODYSPLASIA

Neural tube defects can result in complex spinal deformities secondary both to the neuromuscular collapsing nature of the spine and to the vertebral anomalies that can give rise to congenital kyphosis or congenital scoliosis. Myelomeningocele or meningocele is present at birth in a patient whose neural tube failed to close in utero. Sac closure is usually performed shortly after birth. In many cases, the affected infant also requires placement of a ventriculoperitoneal shunt because of hydrocephalus. The level of neurologic function usually corresponds to the level of the defect. For example, a low thoracic myelomeningocele patient has no lumbar nerve roots functioning and therefore no lower extremity function. An L4 myelomeningocele patient has a functioning tibialis anterior but no extensor hallucis and no gastrocnemius and usually no voluntary bowel and bladder control.

Neurologic function in patients with myelodysplasia is static and should not deteriorate with growth. Neurologic changes, especially during growth spurts, require evaluation for tethered cord, a common occurrence in affected children, which results in traction on the spinal cord.

Orthopedic management includes maximizing the function of patients through the use of braces, ambulatory aids, wheelchairs, or surgery. The degree of spinal deformity is related to the neurologic level, with spinal collapse more likely in those with a higher neurologic level of involvement than in those with a lower level. The presence of bony abnormalities can affect this prognosis, of course.

As with many neuromuscular spinal deformities, curvatures may present early in life. If the clinician elects to treat a patient with bracing, it is important to remember that bracing in the presence of insensate skin can result in pressure sores if the brace is not adequately padded and the parents are not instructed regarding skin care.

In many cases, the curvature eventually requires surgical stabilization. Because of the magnitude and stiffness of the curvature as well as the absence of posterior elements, the preferred treatment is anterior and posterior fusion. Anterior instrumentation may improve rigidity of the surgical construct as well as fusion rates. In patients with myelodysplasia, fusion to the sacrum is invariably required because of pelvic obliquity or lack of sitting balance. Instrumentation from the pelvis (iliac fixation) to the proximal thoracic spine is preferred, as with many neuromuscular deformities.

The lack of posterior elements in the myelodysplastic spine can lead to congenital kyphosis. Although kyphosis in these patients does not compromise neurologic function, it can lead to pressure sores over the prominent area. The treatment of choice for this problem is posterior kyphectomy and fusion. The neural elements can be cut and tied off at the site of the kyphotic deformity since the patient usually has no neurologic function below the kyphus.

Ramirez N, Valentin P, Mayer OH, et al. The spinal structure and lung function relationship in an untreated nonambulatory myeloleningocele group of patients. *J Am Acad Orthop Surg.* 2019;27(9):327-334. [PMID: 30252790]

THORACIC DISK DISEASE

Disk herniation is found much less commonly in the thoracic spine than in the cervical and lumbar spine, presumably because of the decreased mobility seen in this region with the rib cage and sternum. Herniated thoracic disks account for 1% to 2% of operative disks, although the reported incidence in autopsy series is 7% to 15%.

Patients with thoracic disk disease may present with radicular symptoms at the level of involvement and complain of back or lower extremity pain, extremity weakness, numbness corresponding to the level of the disk herniation or below, and bowel or bladder dysfunction. They may demonstrate a spastic gait, with long-tract signs, if the disk is more central. Diagnosis is made by MRI or CT myelogram for those with contraindications to MRI.

In the absence of long-tract signs and paraparesis, conservative measures may include rest, anti-inflammatory medications, and physical therapy, with a 70% to 80% success rate.

Surgical treatment is recommended for patients with signs of myelopathy, including paraparesis or hyperreflexia. A variety of approaches have been described, with anterior or anterolateral thoracoscopy or thoracotomy approaches being safest for central disk herniations, while posterolateral approaches can be suitable for those disk herniations that are paracentral or lateral and do not cross the midline. A bilateral posterolateral approach may potentially be used for central disk herniations in the setting of bilateral facetectomies. Anterolateral retropleural approaches have begun to gain popularity due to their ability to leave the pleura intact and provide a more direct route to the thoracic spine. Furthermore, recent studies are beginning to demonstrate that more minimally invasive approaches using either mini-open approaches or endoscopy may provide favorable outcomes compared to more traditional methods. Ossified or calcified thoracic disk herniations associated with severe cord compression can be very challenging to safely remove, much more so than soft disk herniations that are not ossified.

Bouthors C, Benzakour A, Court C. Surgical treatment of thoracic disc herniation: an overview. *Int Orthop.* 2019;43(4):807-816. [PMID: 30406842]

OSTEOPOROSIS AND VERTEBRAL COMPRESSION FRACTURES

Osteoporosis is characterized by a decline in overall bone mass in the axial and appendicular skeleton. The disease affects between 15 and 20 million people in the United States. Peak bone mass, attained between 16 and 25 years of age, slowly declines with age as the rate of bone resorption exceeds that of bone formation. This phenomenon occurs in both men and women and is known as senile osteoporosis. Women are also susceptible to postmenopausal osteoporosis that occurs during the 15 to 20 years after the onset of menopause and is directly linked to estrogen deficiency. Environmental factors also play a role in accelerating the rate of skeletal bone loss. These include chronic calcium deficiency, smoking, excessive alcohol intake, hyperparathyroidism, and inactivity. Genetic influences may also play a role.

Vertebral compression fractures are one of the most frequent manifestations of osteoporosis in the elderly (>60 years). Over 700,000 vertebral compression fractures occur each year. Given that the US population age greater than 50 years is expected to increase by 60% by 2025, this number is only expected to increase. Fortunately, the overwhelming majority of patients are asymptomatic or become asymptomatic after a period of conservative care.

Clinical Findings

Patients with symptomatic vertebral compression fractures typically complain of axial pain localized to the fractured level. Occasionally, the patient's family notices that the patient's back is becoming increasingly rounded, and significant loss of height has occurred. This spinal deformity is known as the "dowager's hump." In general, there is no neurologic dysfunction and no radiation of the pain in any dermatomal distribution. There is often no history of significant trauma or an inciting event.

Imaging

Plain radiographs and densitometric scans are the major imaging modalities in the assessment of osteoporotic bone and their pathologic counterpart, insufficiency fractures. Dual-energy x-ray absorptiometry (DXA or DEXA) is the most useful of the densitometric imaging techniques because it carries a high degree of precision (0.5%-2%) and subjects the patient to minimal amounts of radiation. It is also quite accurate for assessment of osteoporosis in both the axial and appendicular skeleton. It is important to note, however, that hypertrophic osteophytes in the spine that are radiodense can cause an inaccurate reading on the DXA and should not be used as the sole site of assessment for osteoporosis. Other imaging modalities include single-energy x-ray absorptiometry (SXA), quantitative CT (QCT), and radiographic absorptiometry.

Posterior/anterior and lateral radiographs of the affected area of the spine are likely to reveal the location and severity of the osteoporotic fracture(s). In the thoracic spine, wedge compression fractures are most commonly encountered. In the lumbar spine, both compression and burst fractures can occur. Other imaging modalities include technetium bone scans and MRI scans. These studies should be reserved for the evaluation of fractures that remain symptomatic or progress after a course of conservative treatment. MRI is extremely useful in differentiating nonunited fractures from those that have healed and in differentiating osteoporotic fractures from those caused by malignancy.

Bone biopsy is indicated if a metabolic bone disease or a malignancy is suspected as the cause of the osteoporosis. The sample, typically retrieved from the anterior iliac crest or from the vertebral body at the time of vertebral augmentation, is examined using bone histomorphometry.

Treatment

Prevention still remains the best treatment for osteoporosis. Maximizing bone mineral density prior to the onset of bone loss and minimizing the bone loss that occurs is the optimal regimen to prevent the painful sequelae of the disease. Nutritional health focusing on supplementation of vitamin D and calcium has played an increasing role during the past couple of decades. For patients greater than the age of 70, the Institute of Medicine recommends 800 IU of vitamin D and 1200 mg of calcium daily. In women, estrogen replacement therapy can be initiated if there is no history of breast cancer, thromboembolic disease, or endometrial disease. Routine gynecologic examination is necessary once therapy is initiated. Calcitonin therapy can be used if estrogen therapy is contraindicated. Teriparatide (recombinant parathyroid hormone) is an anabolic bone agent used to treat severe osteoporosis and is the drug of choice for fragility fractures.

The bisphosphonates etidronate and alendronate prevent osteoclastic resorption of bone. They are the only FDA-approved compounds in widespread use that increase bone mineral density. However, the increase is relatively small. The use of chronic continuous bisphosphonate therapy has been linked to insufficiency fractures of the proximal femur.

The initial treatment of symptomatic vertebral compression fractures involves a trial of analgesic therapy and bracing for comfort. Evaluation and treatment for osteoporosis can be initiated if not done already. Conservative therapy should be attempted for at least 6 to 12 weeks or longer if the patient is improving.

Surgical Treatment

Patients who have fractures that cause neurologic deficits or significant spinal cord compression should be treated with anterior decompression and fusion followed by posterior segmental instrumentation and fusion. The poor bone quality makes correction of deformity and maintenance of posterior only constructs a challenging task (Figure 5–33).

Patients who have recalcitrant back pain from a nonunited vertebral compression fracture and have failed a course of conservative management can obtain excellent symptomatic relief from fracture stabilization through injection of polymethylmethacrylate (PMMA) bone cement into the fracture through a percutaneous technique. The two most popular procedures are vertebroplasty and kyphoplasty. In both techniques, a cannula is inserted intrapedicularly or extrapedicularly (lateral to the pedicle) into the anterior portion of the affected vertebral body, and acrylic cement is instilled into the fractured bone under fluoroscopic control. Once the cement cures, the fracture is immediately stabilized. In the kyphoplasty technique, a balloon is inflated in the vertebral body in an attempt to compress the existing bone, create a void for instillation of more viscous cement under lower pressure, and correct the wedge deformity. This technique has the theoretical advantage of allowing some deformity correction and preventing high-pressure-related extrusion of PMMA into the spinal canal. In 2010, the American Academy of Orthopaedic Surgeons evidence-based guidelines strongly recommended against the use of vertebroplasty but stated that kyphoplasty was a viable option for treatment of painful compression fractures. However, since that time, multiple studies have been published including randomized control trials as well as meta-analyses that demonstrate no clinical differences between vertebroplasty and kyphoplasty. While kyphoplasty demonstrated superior radiographic outcomes, it is also known to be more costly. This newer data suggest that vertebroplasty still has a role in treatment of compression fractures refractory to nonoperative care.

The mechanism of pain relief achieved through vertebroplasty and kyphoplasty is unclear. Multiple mechanisms may play a role, including fracture stabilization, denervation of pain fibers by the heat generated during the cement curing process, and neurotoxicity of the PMMA monomer. In addition, longer follow-up has raised concerns over predisposing the adjacent segment to fracture by overstiffening the affected level. These concerns are currently under active investigation.

Choma TJ, Rechtine GR, McGuire RA Jr, Brodke DS. Treating the aging spine. *J Am Acad Orthop Surg*. 2015;23(12):e91-e100. [PMID: 26510625]

Dang DT, Zetumer S, Zhang AL. Recurrent fragility fractures: a cross-sectional analysis. *J Am Acad Orthop Surg*. 2019;27(2): e85-e91. [PMID: 30169444]

Karlsson MK, Kherad M, Hasserius R, et al. Characteristics of prevalent vertebral fractures predict new fracture in elderly men. *J Bone Joint Surg*. 2016;98(5):379-385. [PMID: 26935460]

INJURIES OF THE CERVICAL SPINE

The cervical spine is the most mobile area of the spine, and as such, it is prone to the greatest number of injuries. Injuries to the cervical spine and spinal cord are also potentially the most devastating and life altering of all injuries compatible with life. In the United States, approximately 10,000 spinal cord injuries occur each year (about 39 per million). An estimated 80% of the victims are younger than 40 years, with the

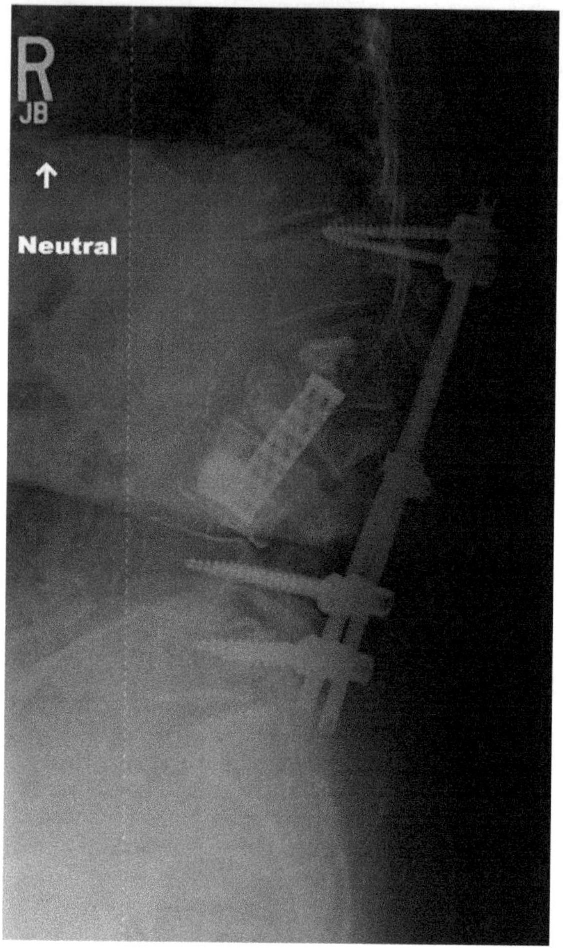

A

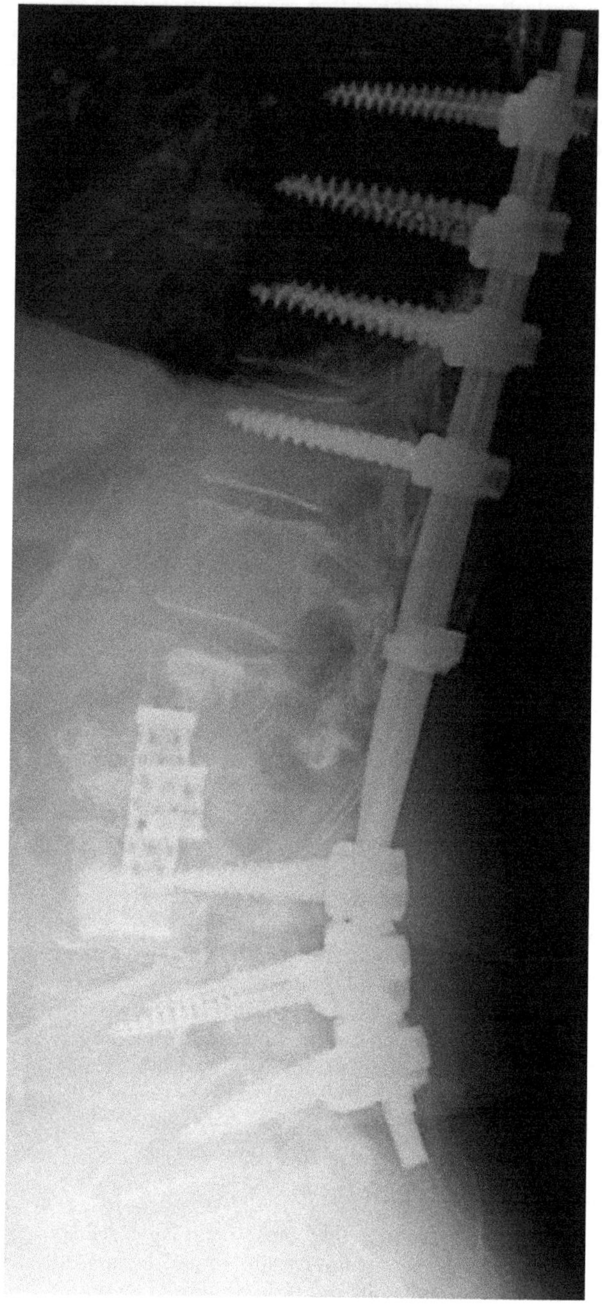

B

▲ **Figure 5–33.** Complex revision osteotomy surgery. A 65-year-old woman with incapacitating back and leg pain after two failed prior operations done at an outside hospital for an osteoporotic burst fracture. (**A**) Preoperative lateral x-ray demonstrates pullout of the screw construct, multiple nonunions, sagittal imbalance, and inability to walk due to pain. She underwent third-time revision decompression, complete removal of the L2 vertebral body (vertebral column resection [VCR]), and revision instrumentation and fusion, all done through a posterior approach. This procedure allows for shortening of the spinal column and correction of kyphotic deformity. (**B**) Postoperative lateral x-ray demonstrates markedly improved alignment. Patient was able to walk with minimal pain.

highest proportion of injuries reported in those between 15 and 35 years of age. Approximately 80% of all people who suffer from spinal column injuries are male. Falls account for 60% of injuries to the vertebral column in patients older than 75 years. In younger patients, 45% of injuries result from motor vehicle accidents, 20% from falls, 15% from sports injuries, 15% from acts of violence, and the remainder from other causes.

With the use of seat belts and air bags in motor vehicles and the advent of trauma centers and improved emergency service awareness of potential cervical injuries, fewer patients with cervical spine injuries are dying secondary to respiratory complications. The approach in treating these patients is early recognition of cervical spine injuries with rapid immobilization to prevent neurologic deterioration while the evaluation and treatment of associated injuries are carried out. After the patient is stabilized, the goals are restoration and maintenance of spinal alignment to provide stable weight bearing and facilitate rehabilitation.

Identification and Stabilization of Life-Threatening Injuries

Eighty-five percent of all neck injuries requiring medical evaluation are a result of a motor vehicle accident. Many of the affected patients are multiple-trauma victims and therefore may have more urgent life-threatening conditions. The ABCs of trauma are followed in order of priority, with *a*irway, *b*reathing (ventilation), and *c*irculation secured before further evaluation proceeds. Throughout the evaluation of other body systems, the cervical spine should be presumed injured and thus immobilized. Approximately 20% of patients with cervical trauma are hypotensive upon presentation. The hypotension is neurogenic in origin in approximately 70% of cases and related to hypovolemia in 30%. Concomitant bradycardia is suggestive of a neurogenic component. Another finding suggestive of cervical spine injury is an altered sensorium secondary to head trauma or lacerations and facial fractures. Appropriate diagnosis and fluid management are critical in the early hours of postinjury management. After all life-threatening injuries are identified and stabilized, the secondary evaluation, including an extremity examination and neurologic examination, can be safely carried out.

History and General Physical Examination

Details of the history of the injury should be obtained. If the patient is conscious, much of the information can be obtained directly. If not, family members or witnesses of the injury should be questioned. In the case of a motor vehicle accident, for example, pertinent questions include the following: Which part of the patient's body was the point of impact? Was the patient thrown from the car? Was there head trauma or a loss of consciousness? Were there any transient signs of paresis? Was the patient able to move any of his or her extremities at any time following the accident and before loss of function? What were the speeds of the involved motor vehicles? Was the patient restrained with a seat belt? Did an air bag deploy?

The history taken from the patient or family members should also include information about preexisting conditions such as epilepsy or seizures and about preexisting injuries. If the patient had any previous radiographic examinations, the radiographs might be useful for comparison.

It is helpful to question patients about what they are experiencing at the time of the examination. Are there areas of numbness, paresthesia, or pain? Can they move their extremities? The examiner should then proceed with the physical evaluation, beginning by observing the face and head of the patient for any areas of potential injury and attempting to determine the potential mechanism of injury. For instance, any lacerations or contusions to the forehead might indicate a hyperextension-type injury because as the head hits the windshield and stops, the body continues to move forward from the momentum of the impact. Observation should next include watching the extremities for any signs of motion. A genital examination should be performed because a sustained penile erection may be indicative of severe spinal cord injury. Then without moving the patient, palpation can be performed. Although palpation (the sense of touch is carried through the posterior columns) can be helpful in identifying potential levels of injury of the spine, it should not be used as the sole screening examination because false-negative results are possible.

Neurologic Evaluation

A meticulous neurologic examination should be performed following the history and general physical examination.

A. Neurologic Tests

The neurologic evaluation should start with documentation of the function of the cranial nerves, working proximally to distally. Observation is particularly important in the unconscious patient. Spontaneous motion in an extremity may be a sole source of information regarding spinal cord function. Respiratory efforts made with intrathoracic musculature versus abdominal musculature are also significant. In the conscious patient who is able to follow commands, a motor examination should be fairly straightforward. Rectal and perianal sensations should be documented because these may be the sole signs of intact distal spinal cord function.

An extensive sensory examination should also be performed with careful attention to dermatomal innervation. In the acute setting, it is useful to document sharp and dull sensations as well as proprioception. Sharp and dull sensations are carried via the lateral spinothalamic tract, whereas proprioception is carried through the posterior columns. Sharp and dull sensations are effectively tested with the sharp

Table 5–8. Evaluation of reflexes in patients with injuries of the cervical spine.

Reflex	Root	Positive Response	Significance
Babinski	Upper motor neurons	Extension and spread of toes	Upper motor neuron lesion is present
Bulbocavernosus	S3 and S4	Contraction of anal sphincter	Spinal shock is over
Cremasteric	T12 and L1	Retraction of scrotal sac	Spinal shock is over
Anal wink	S2, S3, and S4	Contraction of anal sphincter	Spinal shock is over

and blunt ends of a pen, and proprioception is tested by having the patient verify the position of the large toe and other joints as the examiner places them in dorsiflexion and plantarflexion. It is helpful to make ink markings directly on the patient's skin to show the level of the dermatomal deficit, which decreases the chance for intraobserver or interobserver error over sequential examinations.

Reflexes should be checked bilaterally. In the upper extremity, the biceps reflex at the flexor side of the elbow evaluates the C5 nerve root, and the brachioradialis stretch reflex at the radial aspect of the forearm just proximal to the wrist checks the C6 nerve root. The triceps reflex is innervated by C7. In the lower extremity, the knee jerk reflex is innervated by L4, and the ankle jerk is innervated by S1.

The presence or absence of the four reflexes listed in Table 5–8 should be checked. The Babinski reflex (plantar reflex) is evaluated by firmly stroking the lateral plantar aspect of the foot distally and then medially over the metatarsal heads and then observing the toes. If the toes flex, the response is considered negative (normal). If the toes extend and spread, the response is considered positive (abnormal) and indicative of an upper motor neuron lesion. The bulbocavernosus reflex has its root in the S3 and S4 nerves and is evaluated by squeezing on the glans in a male patient or applying pressure to the clitoris in a female patient. This action should elicit a contraction of the anal sphincter. If a Foley catheter is in place, simply pulling on the Foley catheter can stimulate the anal sphincter contraction. The cremasteric reflex is evaluated by stroking the inner thigh and observing the scrotal sac, which should retract upward secondary to contraction of the cremasteric muscle. This function is innervated by T12 and L1. Finally, the anal wink, innervated by S2, S3, and S4, is elicited by stimulating the skin about the anal sphincter and eliciting a contraction.

The presence of spinal shock causes the absence of all reflexes below the level of injury and typically lasts up to 24 hours after the injury. The bulbocavernosus reflex is the reflex that returns first (see Table 5–8), thus marking the end of spinal shock. This point has prognostic importance because recovery from a complete neurologic deficit that is still present at the end of spinal shock is extremely unlikely. A complete neurologic examination should be repeated over time as the patient is manipulated and treated.

B. Anatomic Considerations

The ability to interpret the results of a patient's neurologic examination appropriately depends on a thorough knowledge of the anatomy of the spinal cord and peripheral nerves.

Peripheral nerves are a combination of afferent fibers, which carry information from the periphery to the central nervous system, and efferent fibers, which carry information away from the central nervous system. As the peripheral nerve approaches the spinal cord, it becomes known as the spinal nerve. Prior to entering the spinal cord, the fiber splits, with the afferent fibers becoming the dorsal root or sensory root and the efferent fibers becoming the ventral root. The afferent fibers are often regrouped in various plexuses that are located between the spinal cord and the periphery. This regrouping takes place before the fibers enter the dorsal root, therefore leading to significant overlap between the dorsal root and the respective dermatomes. The implications of this anatomic fact should be kept in mind by the clinician when performing a sensory examination. For example, a sectioned peripheral nerve is demonstrated by a highly specific sensory loss in that particular area served by that nerve, whereas the clinical findings are more variable for a sectioned dorsal root.

The spinal cord is a caudal continuation of the brain, extending in an organized fashion from the foramen magnum at the base of the skull down to the proximal lumbar spine. The spinal cord has three primary functions: it provides a relay point for sensory information; it serves as a conduit for ascending sensory information and descending motor information; and it mediates body and limb movements because it contains both interneurons and motor neurons. Headed from caudal to cephalad, the spinal cord is highly organized with a central butterfly-shaped area of gray matter and surrounding white matter.

The overall diameter of the spinal cord varies as a relative percentage of the spinal canal. The cord fills approximately 35% of the canal at the level of the atlas but increases to approximately 50% of the canal in the lower cervical spine. This variation results from the relative increasing and decreasing size of the spinal gray matter and spinal white matter. As the spinal roots become larger, as occurs at the base of the cervical spine, the size of the gray matter increases relative to the white matter, whereas the size of the white matter decreases linearly from cephalad to caudal.

The gray matter, so called because it appears gray on unstained cross sections, is divided into three zones: the dorsal horn, the intermediate zone, and the ventral horn. Made up predominantly of lower motor neurons, it is prominent in the cervical swellings and lumbar swellings, where axons concentrate before exiting to innervate the upper extremities and lower extremities, respectively.

The white matter derives its name from the fact that the axons in this area are myelinated, casting a white hue on unstained sections. White matter is functionally and anatomically divided into three bilaterally paired columns: the anterior columns, the lateral columns, and the posterior columns.

The two major ascending systems that relay somatic sensory information are the posterior columns and the anterolateral system. The ascending axon has its cell body located in the dorsal root ganglion before proceeding without synapsing through the dorsal horn at that level and then ascending in the posterior column before synapsing at the approximate level of the medulla and crossing over to the contralateral side before proceeding to the cerebral cortex. The topography of the posterior column is such that the sacrum and lower extremities are medial, with the trunk and cervical region being lateral. The anterolateral system carries pain and temperature sensorium. The afferent fibers have a cell body in the dorsal root ganglion and then synapse at that given level in the dorsal horn before crossing directly to the contralateral side and traveling up the anterolateral column.

Motor pathways originate in the cerebral cortex and travel distally to the contralateral side approximately at the level of the medulla and travel down the lateral corticospinal tract before synapsing with the lower motor neuron in the ventral horn of the gray matter. The topography of the corticospinal tract is such that the sacrum and legs lie lateral to the trunk and cervical axons. Thus, at the level of the cervical spine, the spinal cord contains both lower motor neurons traversing to the upper extremities and upper motor neurons being transmitted to the lower extremities. Therefore, injury in this area can give both upper and lower motor findings.

The anatomy of the reflex arc and especially its relationship to spinal shock should be kept in mind. The basic reflex circuitry is an afferent nerve coming from a stretch receptor through the dorsal horn of gray matter before synapsing with the lower motor neuron in the ventral horn of the gray matter, which sends a positive signal to the same muscle via an alpha motor neuron. This simple arc, however, is modulated by input from higher centers. If all descending influence is interrupted, such as would occur in a traumatic transection of the spinal cord, all reflexes are lost. This is also seen during spinal shock. If the local circuitry of the reflex arc is not disturbed, reflexes return at the end of spinal shock. The earliest reflex to return is the bulbocavernosus reflex, which typically returns within 24 hours of injury. Peripheral reflexes may take several months before they return.

C. Risk of Neurologic Damage

As mentioned earlier, the spinal cord varies in its diameter from cephalad to caudad. In the upper cervical spine, it occupies approximately a third of the spinal canal. In the lower cervical spine, it occupies approximately half of the canal. As inferred from this anatomy, the risk of neurologic damage from injury is greater in the lower cervical spine.

Cord compromise extends from two causes: mechanical destruction resulting directly from the trauma and vascular insufficiency. With vascular insufficiency, hypoxia and edema follow and result in further tissue damage. By approximately 6 hours after the trauma, axonal transport ends, and by 24 hours, cord necrosis begins.

D. Classification of Neurologic Status

1. Intact—Approximately 60% of injuries to the cervical spine result in no neurologic sequelae. In most of these cases, the injuries are in the upper cervical spine, where the ratio of the spinal cord to the spinal canal is smaller. It is obviously critical to identify unstable injuries of the cervical spine in the intact patient because the evolution of neurologic deficits is both potentially catastrophic and preventable.

2. Nerve root injuries—Eight cervical nerve roots correspond to the seven cervical vertebral bodies. Each of the first seven nerve roots exits above its respective body (the C1 nerve exiting above the C1 vertebral body, the C2 nerve exiting above the C2 body, and so forth), whereas the C8 nerve root exits through the foramen between the C7 and T1 vertebral bodies. Nerve root injuries can happen either in isolation or in conjunction with more severe spinal cord injuries. Injury to the nerve root alone may result from a compression or fracture of the lateral bone mass and thus impingement on the neural foramen. The clinical findings of a root injury would be those of a lower motor neuron lesion. If the nerve root is still intact and the ongoing pressure to the root is removed, the prognosis for recovery of nerve root function is good.

3. Incomplete versus complete neurologic injury—In the acute setting, any evidence of neurologic function distal to the level of injury is significant and defines the lesion as being incomplete rather than complete. As Lucas and Ducker reported in a prospective study published in 1979, "The less the injury, the greater the recovery," and "partial lesions partially recover, whereas complete lesions do not."

The motor and sensory examination outlined by the American Spinal Injury Association (ASIA) is the most widely accepted and used system to assess the impact of spinal cord injury on the patient. It involves the use of a grading system to evaluate the remaining sensory and motor function. The system allows the patients to be assessed through scales of impairment and functional independence.

The sensory level is determined by the patient's ability to perceive pinprick (using a disposable needle or safety pin) and light touch (using a cotton ball). Testing of a key point in each of the 28 dermatomes on the right and the left sides of the body and evaluation of perianal sensation are required. The variability in sensation for each individual stimulus is graded on a three-point scale:

0 = absent

1 = impaired

2 = normal

NT = not testable

In the cervical spine, the C3 and C4 nerve roots supply sensation to the entire upper neck and chest in a cape-like distribution from the tip of the acromion to just above the nipple line. The next adjacent sensory level is the T2 dermatome. The brachial plexus, C5-T1, supplies the upper extremities.

ASIA also recommends testing of pain and deep pressure sensation in the same dermatomes as well as an evaluation of proprioception by testing the position sense of the index fingers and great toes on each side.

The motor level is determined by manual testing of a key muscle in the 10 paired myotomes from cephalad to caudal. The strength of each muscle is graded on a six-point scale:

0 = total paralysis

1 = palpable or visible contraction

2 = full range of motion of the joint powered by the muscle with gravity eliminated

3 = full range of motion of the joint powered by the muscle against gravity

4 = active movement with full range of motion against moderate resistance

5 = normal strength

NT = not testable

For myotomes that are not clinically testable by manual muscle evaluation, the motor level is presumed to be the same as the sensory level (C1-C4, T2-L1, S2-S5).

ASIA also recommends evaluation of diaphragmatic function (via fluoroscopy, C4 level) and the abdominal musculature (via the Beevor sign, which is the upward migration of the umbilicus from upper abdominal contraction in the absence of lower abdominal contraction due to paralysis at the T10 level). Evaluation of medial hamstring and hip adductor strength is also recommended but not required.

E. Clinical Features of Spinal Cord Syndromes

Combining the findings on examination with knowledge of the cross-sectional anatomy of the spinal cord allows the examiner to identify specific injury patterns (Figure 5–34).

1. Central cord syndrome—The most common of the incomplete cord syndromes is the central cord syndrome, which occurs most frequently in elderly (>65 years) people with underlying degenerative spondylosis but can also be found in younger people who have had a severe hyperextension injury with or without evidence of a fracture, known as spinal cord injury without radiographic abnormality (SCIWORA). Central cord syndrome is defined by ASIA as a clinical presentation characterized by "dissociation in degree of motor weakness with lower limbs stronger than upper limbs and sacral sensory sparing." The syndrome typically occurs following a hyperextension injury and is thought to be caused by an expanding hematoma or edema forming in the central aspect of the spinal cord. Central cord syndrome can be quite variable in presentation and in recovery. A mild presentation may consist of a slight burning sensation in the upper extremities, whereas a severe central cord syndrome includes motor impairment in both the upper and lower extremities, bladder dysfunction, and a variable sensory deficit below the level of injury. The pattern of clinical presentation is directly related to the cross-sectional anatomy of the spinal cord. Because the lower extremity and sacral tracts of the spinothalamic and corticospinal tracts are lateral, these areas are often spared in central cord syndrome. In cases in which they are involved, they are the areas whose function returns first. The upper extremity deficit is caused by a lesion in the gray matter, and the damage here is largely irreversible.

From 50% to 75% of patients with central cord lesions show some neurologic improvement, but the amount of improvement varies considerably among patients. The usual order in which motor function recovery occurs is as follows: return of lower extremity strength, return of bladder function, return of upper extremity strength, and return of intrinsic function of the hand.

2. Anterior cord syndrome—The patient with an anterior cord syndrome typically presents with immediate paralysis and loss of pain and temperature sensation. Both the spinothalamic and corticospinal tracts are located in the anterior aspect of the spinal cord and are therefore involved. With the posterior columns preserved, the patient still has intact proprioception and vibratory sense as well as intact sensation to deep pressure. This clinical presentation is the most common in the younger (<35 years) trauma victim. The mechanism of injury is typically a flexion injury to the cervical spine. It is usually associated with an identifiable lesion of the cervical spine, most commonly a vertebral body burst fracture or a herniated disk. Return of useful motor function is reported in only 10% to 16% of patients with anterior cord syndrome. The prognosis is slightly improved, however, if evidence of spinothalamic tract function is present early.

3. Brown-Séquard syndrome—Patients with this syndrome have a motor weakness on the ipsilateral side of the lesion and a sensory deficit on the contralateral side caused by a functional hemisection of the spinal cord. For example, a cervical lesion on the right side of the spinal cord disrupts the ipsilateral corticospinal tract, which is the tract that carries

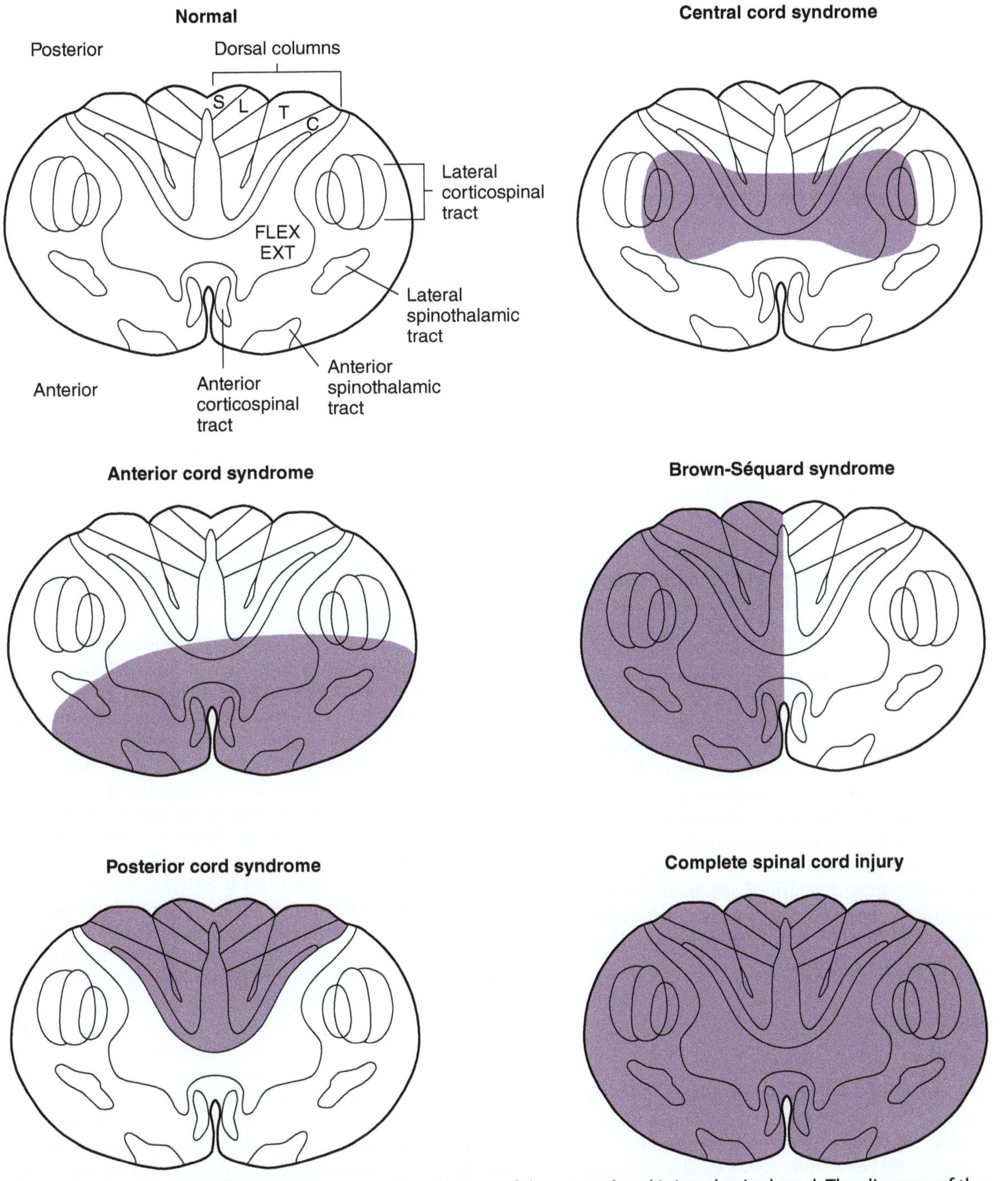

▲ **Figure 5–34.** Diagrams illustrating cross-sectional views of the normal and injured spinal cord. The diagram of the normal spinal column shows the segmental arrangement (C, cervical; L, lumbar; S, sacral; T, thoracic) and the area of flexors and extensors (FLEX and EXT). Central cord syndrome, anterior cord syndrome, Brown-Séquard syndrome, and posterior cord syndrome are incomplete injuries, with affected areas shaded. In complete spinal cord injury, all areas are affected.

motor function to the right side of the body distal to the level of the lesion. The right spinothalamic tract is also disrupted. This tract carries pain and temperature fibers from the contralateral side of the body distal to the level of injury. Position sense and vibratory sense, which are carried in the posterior column, have not yet crossed the midline; therefore, these sensory functions are disrupted on the ipsilateral side of the injury.

Brown-Séquard syndrome may result from a closed rotational injury such as a fracture-dislocation or may result from a penetrating trauma such as a stab wound or from iatrogenic injury while placing surgical instruments within the spinal canal. The prognosis in cases resulting from a closed injury is quite favorable, with 90% of patients regaining function of the bowel and bladder as well as the ability to walk.

4. Posterior cord syndrome—The posterior cord syndrome is the least common of the incomplete syndromes and typically a result of an extension-type injury. Its clinical presentation is one of loss of position and vibratory sense below the level of injury secondary to disruption of the posterior columns. With these deficits as isolated findings, the prognosis for recovery of ambulation and function of the bowel and bladder is excellent.

5. Complete spinal cord injury—A complete neurologic deficit is characterized by a total absence of sensation and voluntary motor function caudal to the level of spinal cord injury in the absence of spinal shock. Initial evaluation must rule out any evidence of sacral sparing and the presence of a bulbocavernosus reflex. In the absence of sacral sparing and with the return of the bulbocavernosus reflex, which typically occurs within 24 hours, the spinal cord injury is termed complete and there is virtually no likelihood of functional spinal cord recovery. Affected patients may gain some root function about the level of the injury—a phenomenon called root escape because this damage to nerve roots is a peripheral nerve injury. Although the presence of root escape should not be taken as a potential return of spinal cord function, it can significantly improve the patient's rehabilitation efforts because vital function of the upper extremities may be regained.

Imaging Studies

A. Radiography

1. Screening radiograph—A lateral radiograph of the cervical spine may be the only screening tool obtained upon initial radiographic evaluation of the multiple-trauma patient. This radiograph must be carefully reviewed. Should a patient present with a complete neurologic injury or a densely affected incomplete neurologic injury indicating a traumatically malaligned cervical spine, closed reduction of the cervical spine should be urgently attempted with axial traction through Gardner-Wells tongs. Once the patient is fully evaluated and life-threatening injuries are stabilized, secondary diagnostic studies can then be undertaken. If the patient is fully alert, has full pain-free rotational range of motion, no palpable tenderness, and no other injuries, the cervical spine can be cleared on clinical grounds.

2. Subsequent plain radiographs—Full radiographic evaluation of the cervical spine with plain radiographs includes lateral, AP, open-mouth (odontoid), right oblique, and left oblique views. The lateral radiograph, if adequate, visualizes approximately 85% of significant cervical spine injuries. It must display the base of the skull with all seven cervical vertebrae, as well as the proximal half of the T1 vertebral body. If the C7-T1 junction is not visualized, a repeat radiograph should be done with axial traction on the upper extremities caudally to attempt to visualize the C7-T1 junction. If this is unsuccessful, a swimmer's view, which is a transthoracic lateral with the patient's arm fully abducted, should be taken. If this plain radiograph is not satisfactory and if suspicion of injury is still high, a CT scan must be obtained.

When evaluating a lateral cervical spine radiograph, the clinician should first evaluate the bony anatomy. Four lines or curves should be kept in mind (Figure 5–35). The anterior spinal line and the posterior spinal line are imaginary lines drawn from the anterior cortex and posterior cortex, respectively, of the cervical vertebral body from C2 all the way down to T1. The spinal laminar curve is an imaginary line drawn from the posterior aspect of the foramen magnum connecting the anterior cortex of each successive spinous process. These three lines (labeled A, B, and C in Figure 5–35) should have a gentle, continuous lordotic curve with no areas of acute angulation. The fourth line (labeled D in Figure 5–35) is known as the basilar line of Wackenheim, and it is drawn along the posterior surface of the clivus and should thus be tangent to the posterior cortex of the tip of the odontoid process. After the clinician examines the radiograph in terms of these four lines or curves, he or she should look at the individual vertebral bodies to see if there is loss of height of any of them or if a rotational deformity is present with alterations in the alignment of the facets.

The evaluation of soft tissues can also prove valuable diagnostically. Prevertebral soft tissues have an upper limit of normal width beyond which a prevertebral hematoma indicative of vertebral injury can be suspected. The upper limits of normal are 11 mm at C1, 6 mm at C2, 7 mm at C3, and 8 mm at C4. The measurements below C4 become more variable and therefore less reliable clinically.

The AP view of the cervical spine is at first a confusing projection to those who are unfamiliar with cervical anatomy, yet careful attention to bony detail in the AP view can be of significant diagnostic aid in picking up subtle injuries. The bony and soft-tissue anatomy seen on the AP projection should be symmetric. The spinous processes should be equally spaced because a single level of increased intraspinous process distance suggests posterior instability. Abrupt

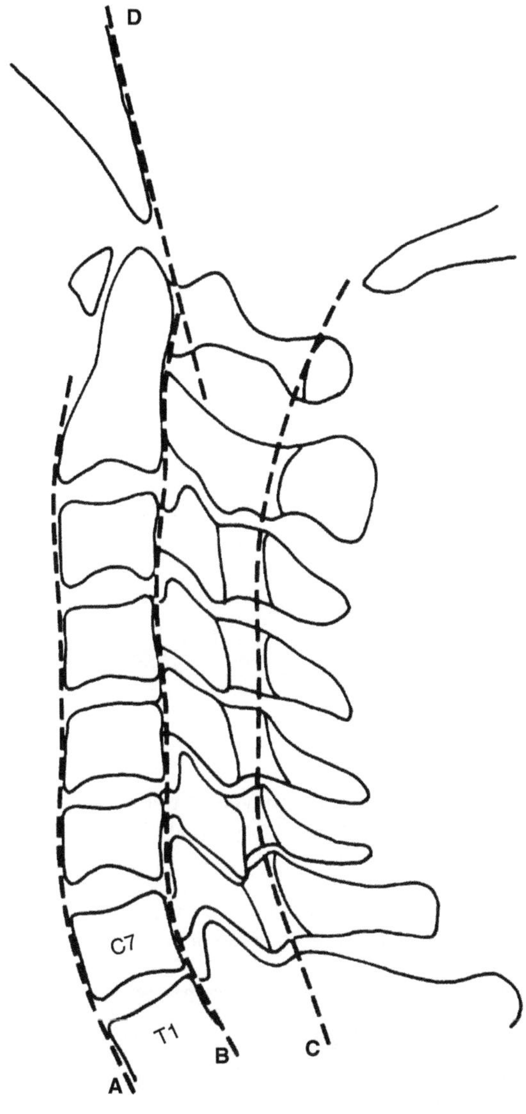

▲ **Figure 5–35.** **Diagram illustrating normal lines and curves in the bony anatomy of the cervical spine. The anterior spinal line (line A), the posterior spinal line (line B), and the spinal laminar curve (line C) should have a gentle, continuous lordotic curve. The basilar line of Wackenheim (line D) is drawn along the posterior surface of the clivus and should thus be tangent to the posterior cortex of the tip of the odontoid process.** (Reprinted with permission, from El-Khoury GY, Kathol MH. Radiographic evaluation of cervical spine trauma. *Semin Spine Surg.* 1991;3:3.)

malalignment of the spinous processes suggests a rotatory injury such as a unilateral facet dislocation. After checking for these problems, the clinician should inspect the lateral masses. The facet joints are typically angled away from the vertical and therefore not clearly seen on the AP projection. If, however, the facet joint can be seen at a particular level, this is indicative of a fracture through the lateral masses and a rotational malalignment of the facet.

The open-mouth (odontoid) view is the projection most useful for looking at C1-C2 anatomy. It permits visualization of both the dens in the AP plane and the lateral masses of C1 on C2.

The right and left oblique views of the cervical spine can be taken with the patient in the supine position. These views are useful as confirmatory studies in ruling in or out lateral mass injuries.

3. Stress radiographs—Two techniques are used in obtaining cervical stress radiographs. The first is to apply axial distraction to the cervical spine through a halo or traction device and obtain a lateral radiograph. This technique should be carefully performed in the presence of a physician and only after gross instabilities of the cervical spine are ruled out. Serial lateral radiographs are taken as weight is sequentially added, reaching an amount equivalent to approximately a third of body weight or 30 kg, depending on the level of suspected injury. Occult instability can be inferred by noting an interspace angulation of at least 11 degrees or an interspace separation of at least 1.7 mm (Figure 5–36).

The second technique, which should only be performed in a fully alert and cooperative patient, is used to obtain flexion-extension lateral radiographs that are helpful in the diagnosis of late instability. The technique is to have the patient flex the head forward as far as possible while a lateral radiograph is taken and then to have the patient put the head in full extension while another radiograph is taken. Findings presumptive of instability are facet subluxation, forward subluxation of 3.5 cm of one vertebral body on the next, and interbody angulation of greater than 11 degrees.

B. Computed Tomography

CT scanning is the most useful means for definitive delineation of bony fracture anatomy. Its advantages are its ready availability and its ability to be performed with a minimal amount of patient manipulation. CT scans provide excellent axial detail, and if thin enough sections are taken, the computer can reconstruct images in sagittal, coronal, or oblique planes. CT scans can be reformatted into a three-dimensional construct for excellent visualization of the bony anatomy.

C. Magnetic Resonance Imaging

MRI is the most effective way to evaluate the soft-tissue component of cervical trauma. The major advantage of MRI is that it can visualize occult disk herniation, hematoma, or

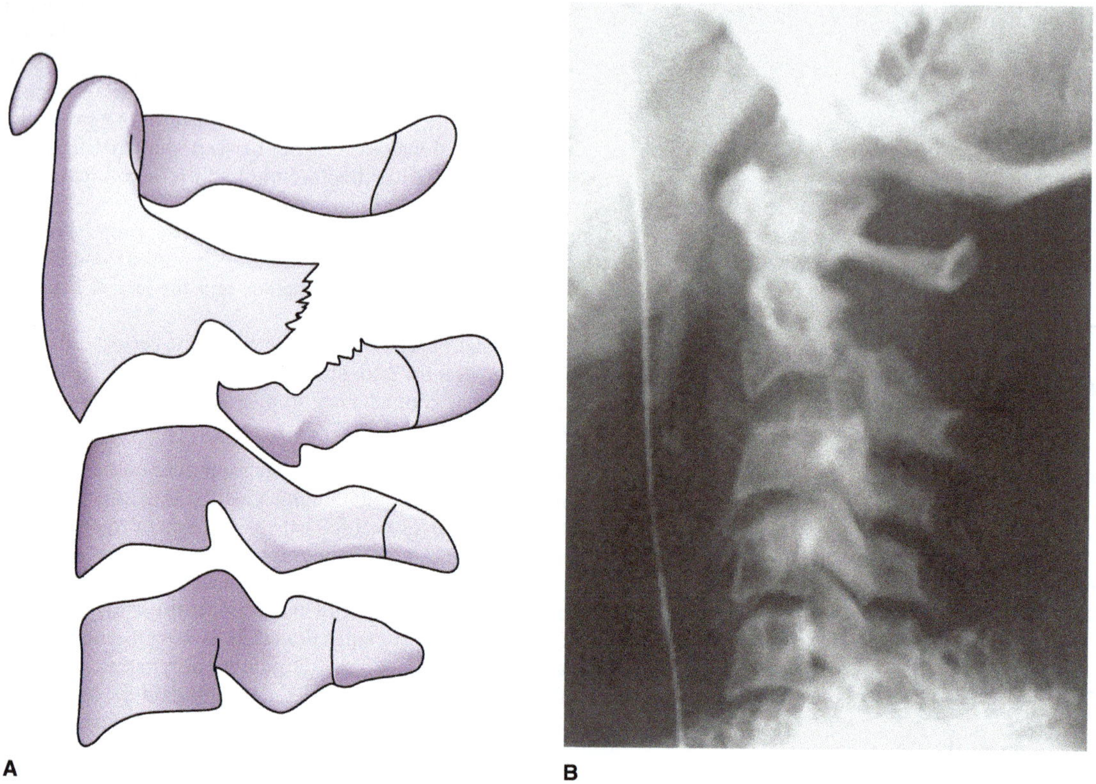

▲ **Figure 5–36.** (**A**) Diagram illustrating an increase of the C2-C3 interdisk space in a patient with type IIA traumatic spondylolisthesis. (**B**) Radiograph demonstrating an increased space. (Reprinted with permission, from Levine AM, Rhyne AL. Traumatic spondylolisthesis of the axis. *Semin Spine Surg*. 1991;3:47.)

edema about the spinal cord, as well as ligamentous injury. Current disadvantages are that MRI is disrupted by metallic objects, so these should be removed from the area of examination, and it also requires a prolonged amount of time to perform, therefore making close monitoring of the acutely ill patient difficult.

Diagnostic Checklist of Spinal Instability

The concept of spinal stability is central to the understanding and treatment of cervical spine injuries. In a broad sense, patients with injuries that are deemed unstable require surgical intervention, whereas those deemed to have stable injury patterns can be treated nonoperatively. Spinal injuries, however, are not readily divided into unstable and stable injuries, and in actuality, they fall along a spectrum of spinal instability.

White and Panjabi's diagnostic checklist of spinal instability (Table 5–9) has nine categories, each of which is assigned a point value. If a total of 5 points is present in a given patient, the injury is deemed unstable.

Table 5–9. White and Panjabi's diagnostic checklist of spinal instability.

Checklist Category	Description	Point Value[a]
1	Disruption of the anterior elements, with >25% loss of height	2
2	Disruption of the posterior elements	2
3	Sagittal plane translation of >3.5 mm or >20% of the anteroposterior diameter of the vertebral body	2
4	Intervertebral sagittal rotation of >11 degrees	2
5	Intervertebral distance of >1.7 mm on a stretch test	2
6	Evidence of cord damage	2
7	Evidence of root damage	1
8	Acute intervertebral disk space narrowing	1
9	Anticipated abnormally large stress	1

[a]If a total of 5 points is present in a given patient, the injury is deemed unstable.

Reprinted and adapted, with permission, from White AA III, Panjabi MM. Update on the evaluation of instability of the lower cervical spine. *Instr Course Lect*. 1987;36:513.

Denis's three-column theory, proposed for application to the thoracolumbar spine, is also applied to the cervical spine in an attempt to better predict stability in the neck. This theory divides the spine into the anterior column (anterior longitudinal ligament, anterior two-thirds of the body and annulus), middle column (posterior longitudinal ligament, posterior one-third of the body and annulus), and posterior column (pedicles, lamina, facets, spinous processes, posterior ligamentous complex) in order to characterize injury patterns. The Spine Trauma Study Group created the Subaxial Injury Classification (SLIC) system composed of three main categories (injury morphology, diskoligamentous complex injury, and neurologic status) and has been shown to have inter- and intrarater reliability.

General Principles of Managing Acute Injuries of the Cervical Spine

Management of acute cervical spine injury is predicated on two principles: protection of the uninjured spinal cord and prevention of further damage to the injured spinal cord. This is accomplished by following spine precaution principles from the very onset of medical care, starting at the accident scene. The cervical spine should be considered injured until proven otherwise and securely immobilized before the patient is transported to a medical center. The equipment for initial immobilization should not be removed until the definitive means of immobilization can be put in place or the cervical spine is cleared of injury. Use of a spinal board, with the patient's head taped to the board and held between two sandbags, is the most secure form of immobilization readily available in the field. This technique can be supplemented by a Philadelphia collar. When the medical center is reached, if a definitive cervical spine injury is identified and deemed unstable, skeletal traction for immobilization, reduction, or both may be applied. Gardner-Wells traction is easily applied and adequate for axial traction. Halo traction affords the added advantage of four-point fixation and thus controlled traction in three planes. Prior to application of traction, it is important to make sure that the patient does not have an occipitocervical dislocation. In these cases, application of traction can lead to worsening of the dislocation and neurologic injury. These specific cases should be treated with immediate application of a halo vest. Halo traction can also be easily converted at a later time to halo-vest immobilization.

Among the various agents that show potential benefits in laboratory studies of models of spinal cord injury are corticosteroids, opiate receptor antagonists (eg, naloxone or thyrotropin-releasing hormone), and diuretics (eg, mannitol). The National Acute Spinal Cord Injury Studies (NASCIS) II and III reported neurologic improvement with steroid treatment given within 8 hours of injury. However, the conclusions drawn from these analyses have come under scrutiny given the incomplete reporting of primary outcome data as well as post hoc analysis. Correlating with these criticisms, the percentage of spine surgeons using corticosteroids for acute spinal cord injury has significantly declined from almost 90% in 2006 to just 50% in 2014.

Denis F. The three-column spine and its significance in the classification of acute thoracolumbar spinal injuries. *Spine (Phila Pa 1976)*. 1983;8:817-831. [PMID: 6670016]

Haller J, Bice M, Lawrence B. Mediating the secondary effects of spinal cord injury through optimization of key physiologic parameters. *J Am Acad Orthop Surg*. 2016;24(3):160-171. [PMID: 26855116]

Kwon BK, Banaszek D, Kirshblum S. Advances in rehabilitation of the spinal cord-injured patient: the orthopedic surgeons' perspective. *J Am Acad Orthop Surg*. 2019;27(21):e945-e953. [PMID: 31045690]

Schoenfeld AJ, Beck AW, Harris MB, Anderson PA. Evaluating the cervical spine in the blunt trauma patient. *J Am Acad Orthop Surg*. 2019;27(17):633-641. [PMID: 31135560]

INJURIES OF THE UPPER CERVICAL SPINE

With the exception of occipitoatlantal dissociation, traumatic injuries to the upper cervical spine are less frequently associated with significant neurologic injury than are traumatic injuries to the lower cervical spine. This is secondary to the fact that the spinal cord occupies only a third of the upper spinal canal versus a half of the lower spinal canal.

Occipitoatlantal Dissociation

Occipitoatlantal dissociation is a disruption of the cranial vertebral junction, and it implies a subluxation or complete dislocation of the occipitoatlantal facets. This injury is typically fatal, yet the clinician must be aware of it because unrecognized occipitoatlantal dissociation may have catastrophic results. The mechanism of dissociation is poorly understood, but it most likely results from either a severe flexion or distraction type of injury. Anterior translation of the skull on the vertebral column is a common presentation and most likely a hyperflexion injury. Bucholz, however, presented the pathologic anatomic findings of fatal occipitoatlantal dissociation and proposed a mechanism of hyperextension with resultant distractive force applied across the craniovertebral junction.

When the dissociation is a frank dislocation, the findings are clear on a lateral radiograph. When the dissociation is a subluxation, however, findings may be more subtle. In normal individuals, the distance between the tip of the dens and the basion (the anterior aspect of the foramen magnum) should be no greater than 1.0 cm, and the previously described Wackenheim line should run from the base of the basion tangentially to the tip of the dens. If the dens penetrates this line, anterior translation of the cranium is implied. Calculation of the Powers ratio can also be helpful in securing

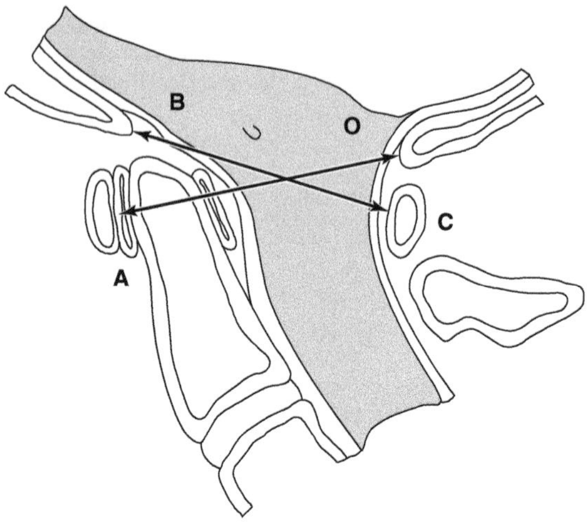

▲ **Figure 5–37.** Diagram showing lines used in the calculation of the Powers ratio, which is helpful in diagnosing occipitoatlantal dissociation. The distance between the basion (point B) and the posterior arch (point C) is divided by the distance between the anterior arch of C1 (point A) and the opisthion (point O). The normal ratio of BC to AO is 1:1. A ratio of greater than 1 suggests the head is dislocated anteriorly on the spine.

the diagnosis. Powers and his colleagues described a ratio of two lines (Figure 5–37), the first of which runs from the tip of the basion to the midpoint of the posterior lamina of the atlas (line BC) and the second of which runs from the anterior arch of C1 to the opisthion (line AO). When the ratio of BC to AO is greater than 1:1, anterior occipitoatlantal dissociation is present. Other radiographic signs include marked soft-tissue swelling and the presence of avulsion fractures at the occipitovertebral junction. CT scan–based measurements assessing condyle-C1 intervals have shown high sensitivity in diagnosing occipitoatlantal dissociation injuries when compared to traditional radiographic measurements. MRI may provide more detail to a potential injury at the occipitoatlantal joint when radiographs and CT are normal but suspicion for injury remains high.

Early recognition and surgical stabilization via occipitocervical fusion are the mainstays of treatment in cases of occipitoatlantal dissociation.

Fractures of Vertebra C1 (Atlas Fractures)

The mechanism of injury in the fracture of the atlas is most typically axial compression with or without extension force, and the anatomic findings of the fracture are indicative of the specifics of the force and the position of the head at the time of impact. In 1920, Jefferson presented his classic description of the four-part fracture of the atlas following an axial injury. This fracture is a burst type that occurs secondary to the occipital condyles being driven into the interior portions of the ring of the atlas and driving the lateral masses outward, resulting in a two-part fracture of the anterior ring of the atlas as well as a two-part fracture of the posterior ring. More common than the classic four-part atlas fracture, however, are the two-part and three-part fractures. Isolated anterior arch fractures are the least common, and they are typically associated with fractures of the dens, whereas the more common posterior arch fracture is typically the result of a hyperextension injury.

A fracture of the atlas is typically diagnosed on plain radiographs. Findings may be subtle on the lateral cervical spine radiograph. The open-mouth (odontoid) view may show asymmetry of the lateral masses of C1 on C2 with overhang (Figure 5–38). A bilateral overhang totaling more than 6.9 mm is presumptive evidence of a disruption to the transverse ligament and suggests potential late instability. Presumptive evidence for transverse ligament disruption can also be seen on the lateral radiograph if the ADI is greater than 4 mm. MRI may potentially show direct visualization of transverse ligament disruption, whereas CT scan can reveal ligament avulsion injuries or further assessment of lateral mass overhang and ADI.

The treatment for fractures of the atlas as isolated injuries is typically nonoperative with rigid collars (Figure 5–39). If there are signs of transverse ligament disruption, halo-vest application may be attempted; however, surgical stabilization is typically favored with C1-C2 fusion. At completion of bony union, flexion-extension views should be obtained to rule out any evidence of late instability. If late instability is present and the bony elements were allowed to heal, a limited C1-C2 fusion can address the instability. If a nonunion is present or if the posterior arch remains disrupted, an occiput to C2 fusion is necessary to control the late instability.

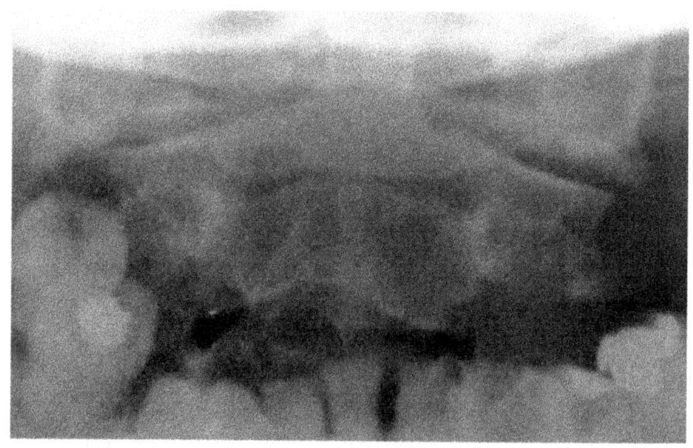

▲ **Figure 5–38.** **Open-mouth (odontoid) radiographic view demonstrating asymmetry of the lateral masses of C1 on C2 with overhang in a patient with a Jefferson fracture.** (Reprinted with permission, from El-Khoury GY, Kathol MH. Radiographic evaluation of cervical spine trauma. *Semin Spine Surg.* 1991;3:3.)

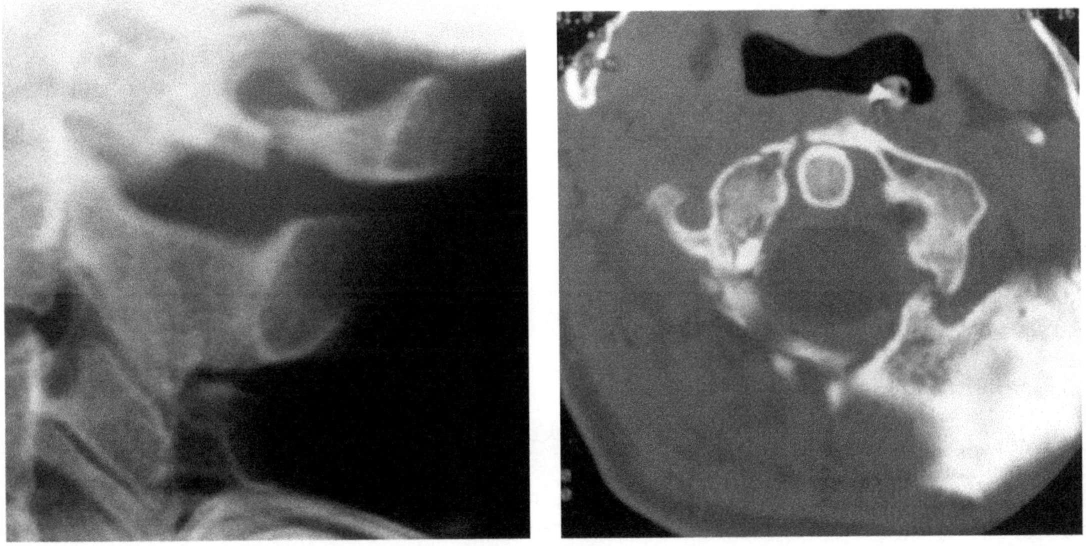

A B

▲ **Figure 5–39.** Imaging studies in a patient who was in a motor vehicle accident and sustained a distractive extension injury to his cervical spine and a three-part fracture of his atlas (a Jefferson fracture). (**A**) Lateral radiographic view showing a fracture of the posterior arch. (**B**) Axial section of a CT scan further delineating the fracture anatomy. This injury was deemed stable and treated nonoperatively in a halo vest.

Dislocations and Subluxations of Vertebrae C1 and C2

A. Atlantoaxial Rotatory Subluxation

Atlantoaxial rotatory subluxation is most common in children and may be associated with minimal trauma or even occur spontaneously. Although some patients are asymptomatic, others present with neck pain or torticollis (a position in which the head is tilted toward one side and rotated toward the other). Inasmuch as the mechanism of injury is often unclear, the propensity for the C1-C2 location is based on anatomic factors. In approximately 50% of cases, cervical spine rotation occurs at the C1-C2 junction, where the facet joints are more horizontal and less inherently stable in rotation.

The diagnosis of atlantoaxial rotatory subluxation is typically suspected on the basis of radiographs taken in several views. The odontoid view may show displacement of the lateral masses with respect to the dens; a lateral view may show an increased ADI; and the AP view may show a lateral shift of the spinous process of C1 on C2. CT scanning can be used to confirm the diagnosis, and a dynamic CT scan with full attempted right and left rotation can demonstrate a fixed deformity.

There are four types of atlantoaxial rotatory subluxations. In type I, the ADI is less than 3 mm, which suggests the transverse ligament is still intact. In type II, the interval is 3 to 5 mm, which suggests the transverse ligament is not structurally intact. In type III, the interval exceeds 5 mm, which is indicative of disruption of the transverse ligament as well as secondary stabilization of the alar ligament. In type IV, there is a complete posterior dislocation of the atlas on the axis, a finding typically associated with a hypoplastic odontoid process such as that seen in several forms of mucopolysaccharidosis (eg, Morquio syndrome).

Treatment of atlantoaxial subluxation is typically conservative, consisting of traction followed by immobilization. Approximately 90% of patients respond to this treatment regimen. There is a high incidence of recurrence, however. For patients who do not respond to conservative measures and for patients with recurrent problems or instability, C1-C2 arthrodesis may be required to control the deformity.

B. Disruption of the Transverse Ligament

The transverse ligament and secondarily the alar ligament are the main constraints to anterior displacement of C1 on C2. It was previously presumed that because anterior subluxation of C1 on C2 typically involves a fracture through the dens, the transverse ligament is in fact stronger than the bony elements of the dens. Fielding and his colleagues, however, showed that experimentally this was not the case, yet clinically the higher association of anterior dislocation of dens fractures still holds true.

The mechanism of disruption is typically a flexion injury, and the diagnosis is made on lateral radiographs. The ADI should not exceed 3 mm in the adult. If the interval is 4 mm or larger and the dens is intact, a rupture of the transverse ligament is presumed.

High-resolution CT scan can be used to categorize this injury into two types. Type 1 is a disruption in the substance of the transverse ligament, whereas type 2 involves an avulsion fracture of the insertion of the transverse ligament on the lateral mass of C1. Type 1 injuries predictably fail conservative treatment and should be managed with a C1-C2 arthrodesis. A trial of nonoperative care in type 2 injuries using a rigid cervical orthosis or halo immobilization may be a reasonable alternative. A 74% success rate can be anticipated, with surgery reserved for patients who fail nonoperative care, showing persistent instability after 12 weeks in mobilization.

C. Fracture of the Odontoid Process

Fracture of the odontoid process is typically associated with high-velocity trauma, and the mechanism of injury is flexion in most cases. Depending on the fracture pattern, extension may be the predominant force in a smaller subset of cases. Associated injuries, particularly fractures of the ring of the atlas, should be ruled out. Neurologic involvement is relatively rare with odontoid fractures. In a study of 60 patients with acute fractures of the odontoid process, Anderson and D'Alonzo reported that 15 had some neurologic deficit on presentation, but only 5 of the 15 had major neurologic involvement, and only 2 of this group of 5 remained quadriparetic at follow-up.

Odontoid fractures may be suspected on the basis of clinical presentation and confirmed on plain radiographs, although spasm and overlying shadows can obscure the diagnosis. CT scan with sagittal and coronal reconstruction is the most sensitive study to diagnose these injuries. CT scan with axial sectioning alone may miss the horizontal fracture line typical of these injuries; thus, the reconstructions are necessary.

Both the risk of nonunion with delayed instability and the method of treating odontoid fracture depend on the

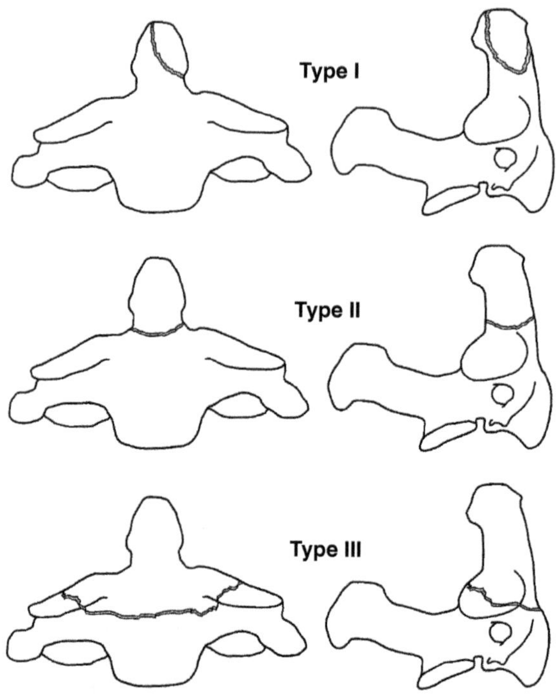

▲ **Figure 5–40.** Diagram showing the three types of fractures of the odontoid process.

classification of the fracture. Reported rates of nonunion range from 20% to 63%. According to the classification system proposed in 1974 by Anderson and D'Alonzo, there are three types of fracture of the odontoid process (Figure 5–40).

Type I is a fracture through the tip of the odontoid process. In this configuration, the blood supply is maintained through the base of the odontoid process and through the attachment of the alar transverse ligaments. The mechanical stability of this fracture pattern is left intact. Symptomatic care and immobilization are the treatment of choice.

Type II, the most common type, is a fracture through the base of the odontoid process at its junction with the body of the axis. In this configuration, soft-tissue attachments to the fracture fragment cause distraction at the fracture site. Because the amount of cancellous bone available for opposition is limited, a high nonunion rate is expected, particularly if displacement is significant or the patient is older (>60 years). In this case, primary surgical treatment may be indicated. Anterior screw fixation of the odontoid process is now the treatment of choice for most type II odontoid fractures when the fracture pattern is amenable. Although it is technically demanding, it does allow for the maintenance of motion at C1-C2 (Figure 5–41). For patients treated conservatively who go on to have nonunion, C1-C2 posterior

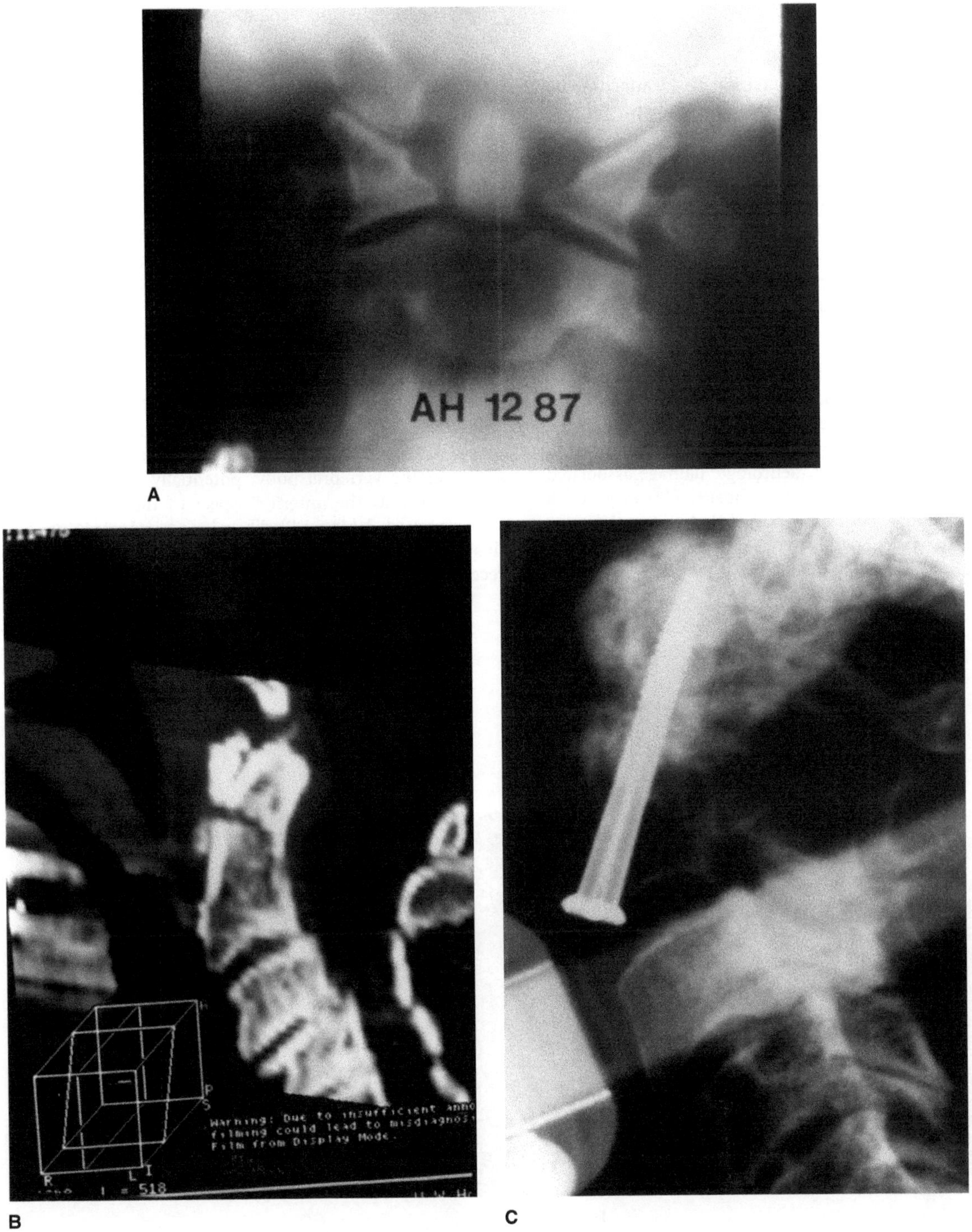

▲ **Figure 5–41.** Imaging studies in a patient with a type II odontoid fracture nonunion. (**A**) Open-mouth radiographic view showing the fracture line at the base of the odontoid process. (**B**) Sagittal reconstruction using CT scanning to better delineate the fracture anatomy. (**C**) Radiograph taken after the patient underwent anterior placement of two odontoid screws under fluoroscopic control using a cannulated screw system.

instrumentation and arthrodesis have proven to be a reliable treatment even in the elderly.

Type III is a fracture through the body of the axis. The blood supply is maintained through soft-tissue attachments, and abundant cancellous bone opposition at the fracture site facilitates a high rate of union. The treatment, therefore, is conservative, consisting of immobilization via rigid cervical collar until bony union occurs. Although the rate of union is acceptable, there is a relatively high rate of malunion that may limit the patient's cervical rotation.

D. Hangman's Fracture (Traumatic Spondylolisthesis of Vertebra C2)

Hangman's fracture occurs when a fracture line passes through the neural arch of the axis. The anatomy of the axis is such that the superior facets are anterior and the inferior facets are posterior, thus concentrating stress through the neural arch. Because of the high ratio of spinal canal size to spinal cord size at this level, neurologic damage associated with hangman's fracture should be unusual. However, in his postmortem studies, Bucholz reported that traumatic spondylolisthesis was second only to occipitoatlantal dislocations in cervical injuries leading to fatalities.

According to the scheme proposed by Levine and Rhyne, hangman's fractures can be classified on the basis of anatomic factors and the presumed mechanism of injury. Treatment depends on the type of fracture. Imaging studies in a patient with hangman's fracture are shown in Figure 5–42.

Type I is typically caused by hyperextension with or without additional axial load. There is no angulation of the deformity, and the fracture fragments are separated by less than 3 mm. Treatment should consist of immobilization in a cervical collar or halo vest until union occurs, which is typically 12 weeks.

Type II is thought to be caused by hyperextension and axial load with a secondary flexion component leading to displacement of the fracture. Reduction of the anterior angulation in this type of fracture is necessary and typically obtained by traction therapy and then followed by placement of a halo vest until union occurs. An atypical type II hangman's fracture is described. This fracture occurs through the posterior aspect of the vertebral body, potentially resulting in cord compromise as the anterior aspect of the vertebral body flexes forward. A higher likelihood of neurologic injury with this atypical pattern is seen, and halo-vest immobilization is recommended.

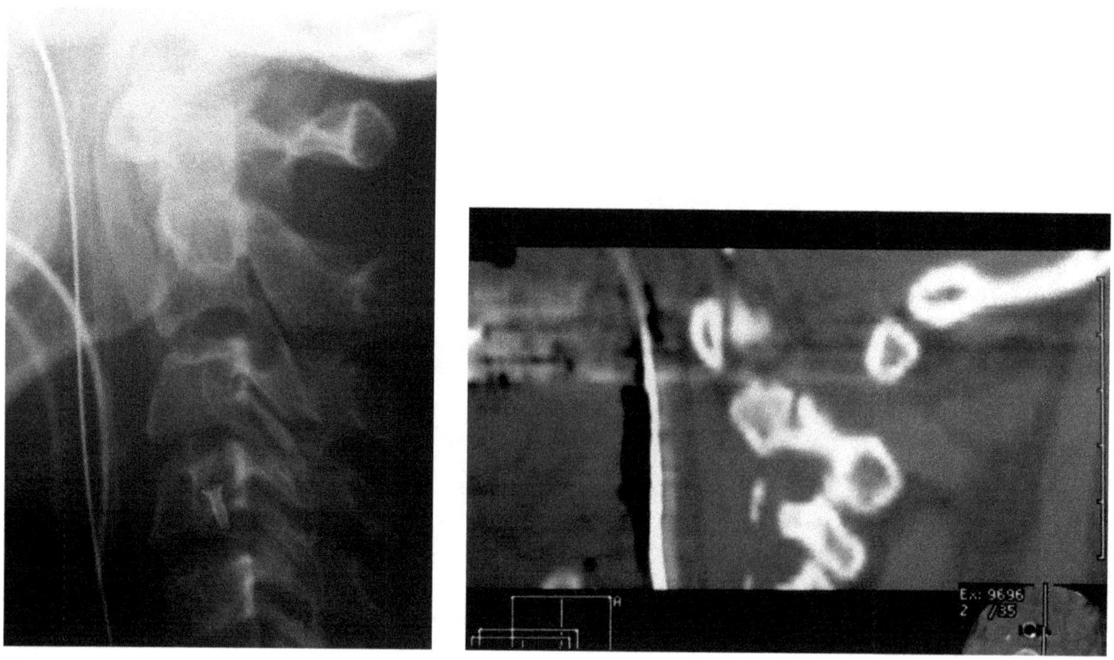

A B

▲ Figure 5–42. Imaging studies in a patient who was in a motor vehicle accident and sustained a hangman's fracture, or traumatic spondylolisthesis of C2. (**A**) Lateral radiographic view, which is largely unremarkable. (**B**) Sagittal reconstruction using CT scanning to better delineate the fracture site at the base of the posterior elements. The patient was treated nonoperatively.

Type IIA has the same fracture pattern as type II but with a component of distraction that also occurred at the time of injury and led to disruption of the C2-C3 disk space, rendering this injury inherently unstable. Traction should be avoided in cases of type IIA fracture because it exacerbates the injury. Treatment should consist of C2-C3 anterior or posterior fusion.

Type III includes a fracture through the neural arch, a facet dislocation, and a disruption of the C2-C3 disk space that renders the injury highly unstable. Treatment generally consists of open posterior reduction and stabilization with fusion.

Joestl J, Lang NW, Tiefenboeck TM, Hajdu S, Platzer P. Management and outcome of dens fracture nonunions in geriatric patients. *J Bone Joint Surg Am.* 2016;98(3):193-198. [PMID: 26842409]

Pearson AM, Martin BI, Lindsey M, Mizra SK. C2 fractures in the Medicare population: incidence, outcomes, and costs. *J Bone Joint Surg.* 2016;98(6):449-456. [PMID: 26984912]

Uei H, Tokuhashi Y, Maseda M. Radiographic and clinical outcomes of C1-C2 intra-articular screw fixation in patients with atlantoaxial subluxation. *J Orthop Surg Res.* 2018;13(1):273. [PMID: 30373599]

INJURIES OF THE LOWER CERVICAL SPINE

As stated earlier, fractures and dislocations of the lower cervical spine have a greater frequency of catastrophic neurologic involvement because of the decreased ratio of spinal canal to spinal cord in the lower levels. Treatment of affected patients again relies on early recognition of the injury, recognition of inherent stability or instability of the injury pattern, and institution of appropriate definitive care.

In 1982, Allen and colleagues developed a classification system for closed indirect fractures and dislocations of the lower cervical spine. After reviewing numerous cases previously described by other authors as well as 165 of their own cases, they grouped the injuries into six categories, based on the position of the cervical spine at the time of impact and on the dominant mode of failure. The six categories were compressive flexion, vertical compression, distractive flexion, compressive extension, distractive extension, and lateral flexion. Of these, the distractive flexion injuries were the most common, followed by the compressive extension injuries and the compressive flexion injuries. Some of the categories were further divided into stages, as described next.

Compressive Flexion Injury

There are five stages of compressive flexion injuries, which are labeled compression flexion stage (CFS) I through V (Figure 5–43). CFS I shows a slight blunting and rounding to the anterior superior vertebral margin, without any evidence of posterior ligamentous damage. CFS II shows some additional loss of height of the anterior vertebral body, again sparing the posterior elements. CFS III has an additional fracture line passing from the anterior surface of the vertebral body through to the inferior subchondral plate, with minimal displacement. CFS IV has less than 3 mm of displacement of the inferior posterior vertebral fragment into the neural canal. CFS V has severe displacement of the inferior posterior fragment into the canal, with widening of the spinous processes posteriorly, indicative of three-column disruption.

Within the compressive flexion category are two types of fractures, more commonly referred to as the **compression fracture** and the **teardrop fracture.** Most compression fractures without disruption of the posterior elements are thought to be stable, so no surgical intervention is required. The more severe compression fracture injuries, however, can result in displacement of bone into the spinal canal, and if a neurologic injury is present, these require anterior decompression and stabilization. All patients should be carefully checked with flexion-extension views at the completion of their treatment to rule out any evidence of late instability.

Vertical Compression Injury

Vertical compression spinal (VCS) injuries occur secondary to axial loading and are divided into three stages. VCS I consists of an endplate central fracture with no evidence of ligamentous failure. VCS II is a fracture of both vertebral endplates, again with only minimal displacement. VCS III is the more commonly termed **burst fracture** with a spectrum of fragmentation of the vertebral body, with or without posterior element disruption.

The treatment for VCS injuries is typically nonoperative. Traction is applied to obtain and maintain alignment, and bony union is generally complete after 3 months of immobilization. In the setting of a burst fracture and posterior element disruption, surgical stabilization should be considered. Flexion-extension views should be obtained at the completion of healing because a posterior ligamentous injury can result in late instability.

Distractive Flexion Injury

The category of distractive flexion spinal (DFS) injury was the most common injury category reported by Allen and colleagues, and it includes both unilateral and bilateral facet subluxation and dislocation. There are four stages of DFS injury. DFS I, termed a **flexion sprain,** is characterized by subluxation of the facet joint, with possible interspinous process widening. This injury has subtle radiographic findings and may easily be missed during initial evaluation and therefore result in late symptomatic instability (Figure 5–44). DFS II is a unilateral facet dislocation, the diagnosis of which can be confirmed on plain radiographs. The lateral radiograph would reveal an anterior subluxation of one vertebra of approximately 25% of vertebral body width at the affected

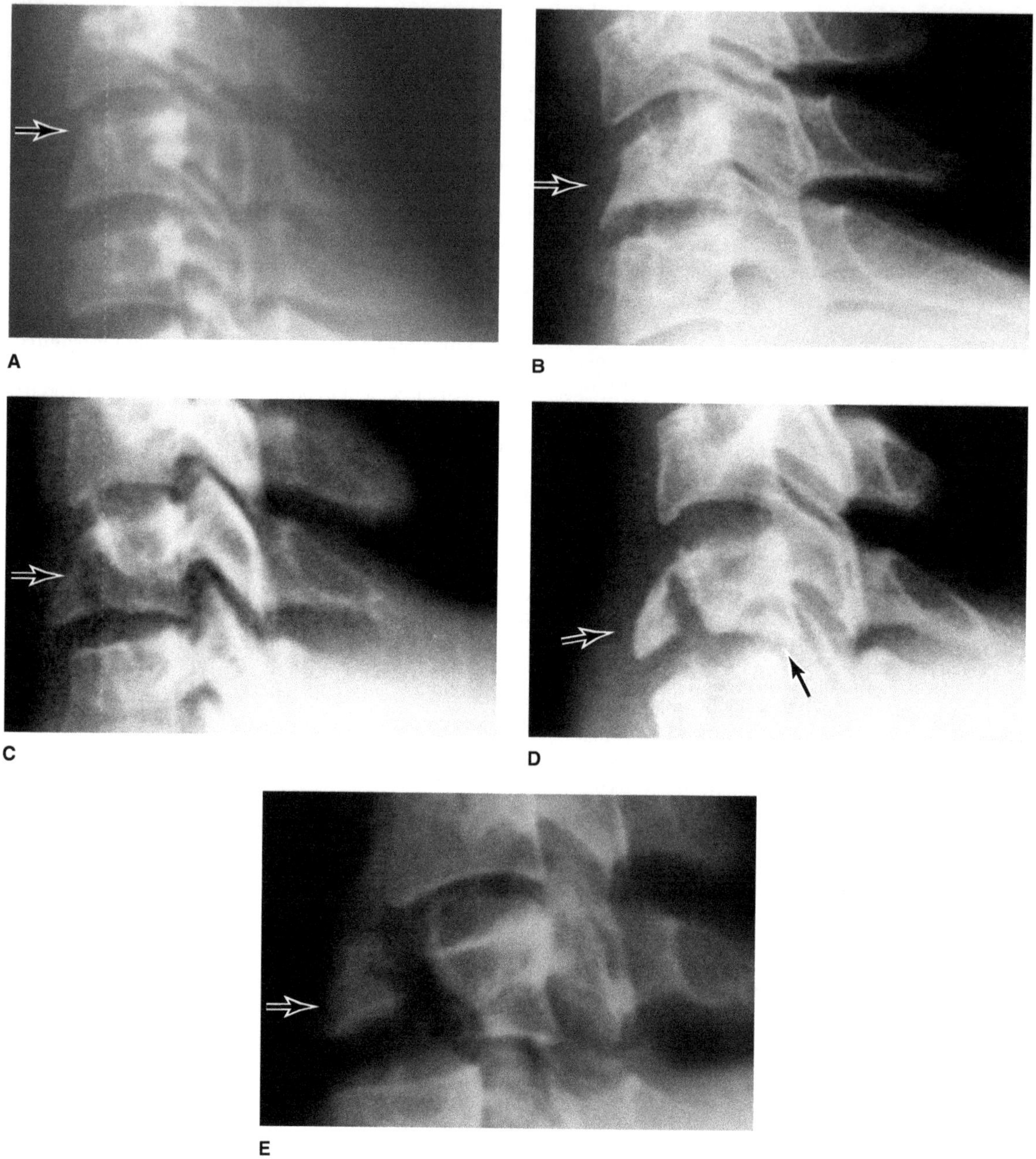

▲ **Figure 5–43.** Radiographs showing the five stages of compressive flexion injury. **A** shows compression flexion stage (CFS) I. **B** shows CFS II. **C** shows CFS III. **D** shows CFS IV. **E** shows CFS V. (Reprinted with permission, from Allen BL, Ferguson RL, Lehmann TR, et al. A mechanistic classification of closed, indirect fractures and dislocations of the lower cervical spine. *Spine (Phila Pa 1976)*. 1982;7:1.)

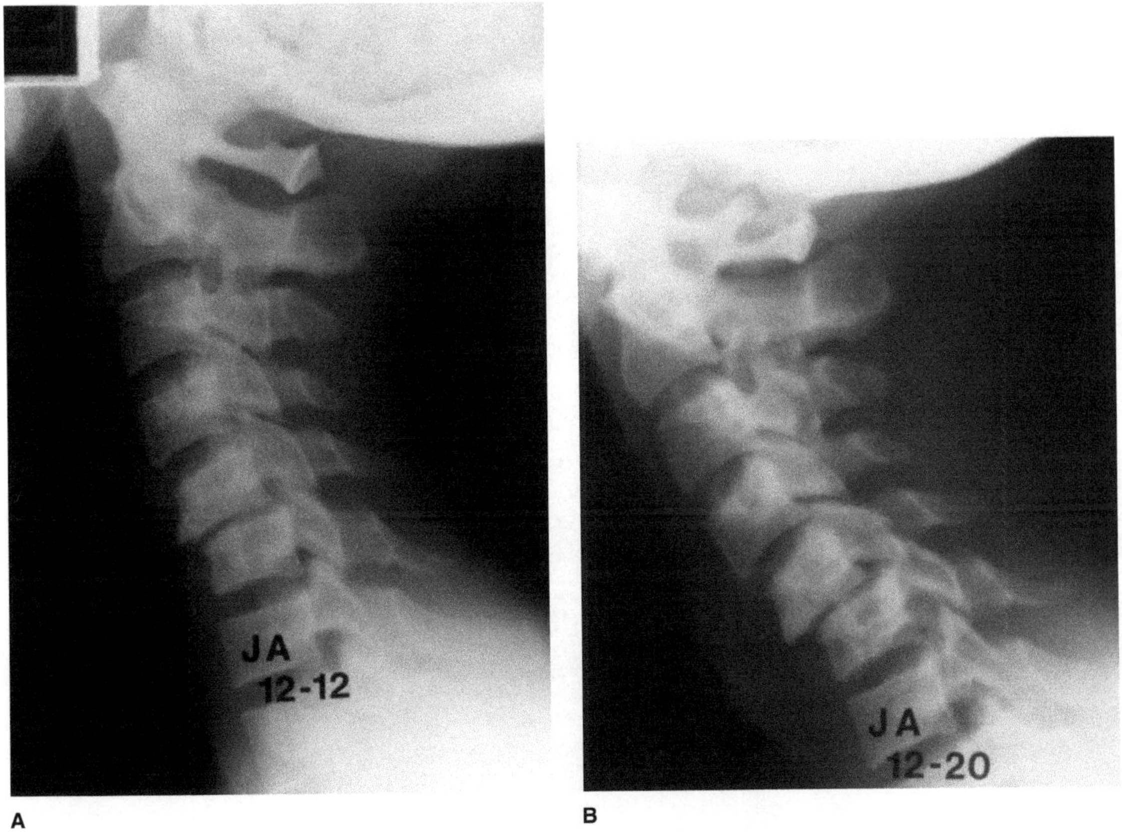

▲ **Figure 5–44.** Imaging studies in a patient with a distractive flexion injury of the cervical spine. (**A**) This lateral radiographic view demonstrates anterior subluxation of C5 on C6. (**B**) The follow-up radiograph shows progression of the subluxation. The patient was treated with a posterior spinal fusion of C5-C6.

level. The facet itself may be perched or fully dislocated. DFS III is a bilateral facet dislocation with approximately 50% anterior dislocation at the affected level. DFS IV, which is also termed a **floating vertebra,** is a bilateral facet dislocation with displacement of a full vertebral width.

Treatment of DFS injuries depends on the severity of the injury. Achievement of anatomic alignment and spinal stability yields the best results. Patients with unilateral facet dislocation should be treated with closed reduction in the acute phase, followed by immobilization. If closed reduction is not possible, open reduction and fusion are indicated (Figure 5–45). Bilateral facet dislocations are associated with a higher incidence of both neurologic injury and instability. Treatment consisting of closed reduction and immobilization is feasible, but because it results in a high percentage of late instability, which eventually requires fusion, the use of early anterior or posterior fusion is indicated.

Another fracture pattern that should be included in the discussion on flexion injuries is the clay shoveler's fracture, which is a fracture of the spinous process, typically at level C6, C7, or T1. This is an avulsion injury that generally occurs in flexion by the counteractive forces of the muscular attachments. As an isolated injury, it is considered stable and usually treated nonoperatively.

Compressive Extension Injury

The category of compressive extension (CES) injury was the second most common injury category reported by Allen and colleagues. It is divided into five stages. CES I is a fracture of the vertebral arch unilaterally, with or without displacement, and CES II is a bilateral fracture. CES III and CES IV were not encountered in the series reported by Allen and colleagues but are theoretic interpolations between CES II and CES V. CES III is a bilateral fracture of the vertebral arch articular processes, lamina, or pedicle without vertebral displacement, whereas CES IV is the same fracture pattern but with moderate vertebral body displacement. Three patients in the Allen series had CES V injuries, which were bilateral vertebral arch fractures with 100% anterior displacement.

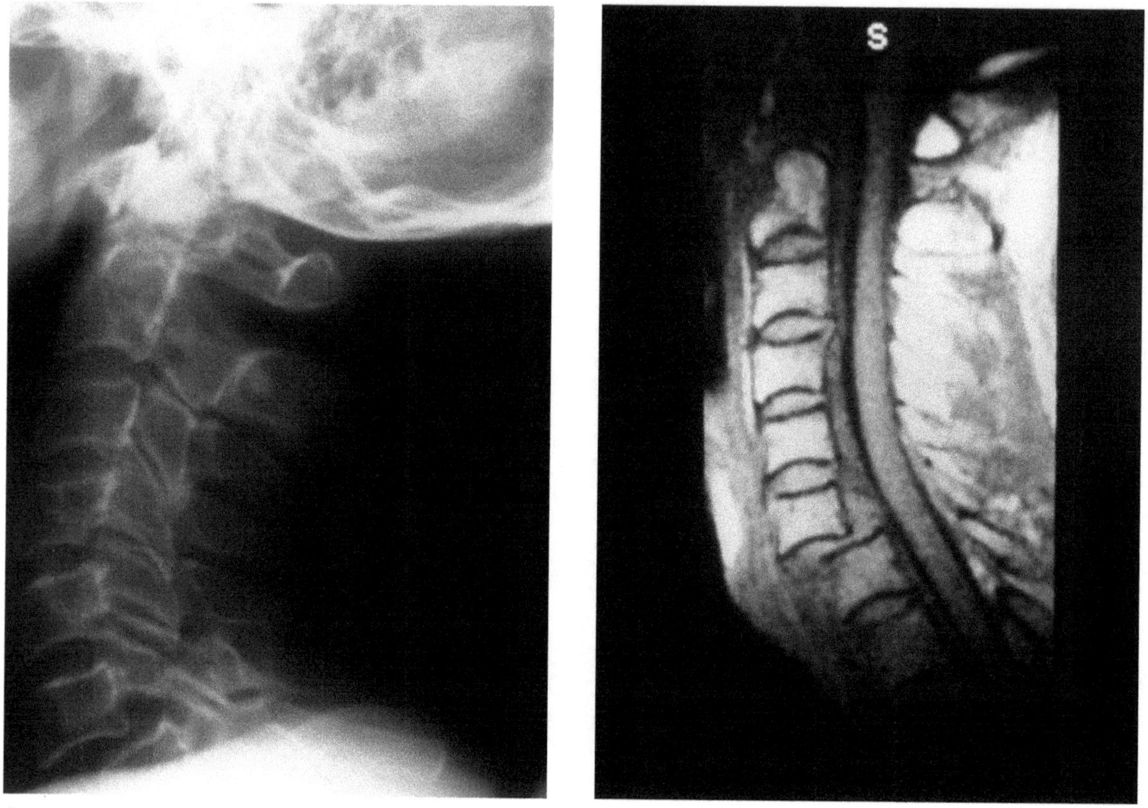

A B

▲ **Figure 5–45.** Imaging studies in a man who fell from a height and suffered a C6-C7 fracture-dislocation with a perched facet but remained neurologically intact. (**A**) Lateral radiographic view demonstrating the fracture-dislocation at C6-C7. (**B**) MRI demonstrating the anterior subluxation of C6 on C7, with the intervertebral disk retropulsed behind the C6 vertebral body. The patient was treated with an anterior diskectomy, reduction, and fusion.

Treatment of CES injuries is related to the three-column theory. Stabilization with a posterior, anterior, or combined approach is indicated if there is significant disruption of the middle column or of two of the three columns.

Distractive Extension Injury

Distractive extension (DES) injuries are typically soft-tissue lesions and divided into two stages. DES I is a disruption of the anterior ligamentous complex or, rarely, a nondisplaced fracture of the vertebral body. Radiographs may appear entirely normal. One clue to the diagnosis is widening of the disk space, which is sometimes present. DES II is a disruption of the posterior soft-tissue complex, which can allow posterior displacement of the upper vertebral body into the spinal canal. This lesion is often reduced at the time of lateral radiographs and may show only subtle or no changes on routine radiographs. When neurologic involvement is present, it is most commonly a central cord syndrome, and provided that no coexisting compression lesions are present, some neurologic recovery is expected.

The DES injury is usually stable and does not require surgical intervention for the fracture itself. Lateral flexion-extension views, however, are indicated to rule out any evidence of late instability.

Lateral Flexion Injury

Allen and colleagues included the injuries of five patients in the category of lateral flexion (LFS) injury. This category is further divided into two stages. LFS I is an asymmetric compression fracture of the vertebral body and ipsilateral posterior arch, with no displacement in the coronal plane. LFS II has a similar fracture pattern but with displacement in the coronal plane, which suggests ligamentous disruption on the tension side of the injury. This mechanism can lead to brachial plexus injuries of varying degrees on the distracted side.

Because of the rarity of LFS injuries, treatment protocols are not well established. Surgical stabilization should be considered if late instability is expected or if there is a neurologic deficit.

Treatment Decisions

Ultimately, the treating physician must decide on a treatment plan. The Allen classification, although quite useful to describe an injury, is a mechanistic system that is challenging to apply to the individual patient to assess operative indications. The decision whether to operate is based on a spectrum of spinal stability and neurologic compromise. A patient with a three-column injury, continued neurologic compression, and neurologic symptoms has a clear operative indication either through an anterior, posterior, or combined approach. A fully neurologically intact patient with a one-column injury generally does fine in a brace. The SLIC system, which takes into account three main clinical characteristics (injury morphology, diskoligamentous complex injury, and neurologic status), compared very well to the Allen classification system and can potentially be used to help guide decision-making.

CERVICAL STRAINS AND SPRAINS (WHIPLASH INJURY)

Cervical strains and sprains, which are commonly referred to as a whiplash injury when associated with motor vehicle accidents, can produce a protracted and confusing clinical picture. Pain is typically the one unifying feature, yet there may be numerous other complaints, including local tenderness, decreased range of motion, headaches that are typically occipital, blurred or double vision, dysphagia, hoarseness, jaw pain, difficulty with balance, and even vertigo. It is often difficult for the physician to correlate radiographic findings, diagnostic test results, and other objective findings with the subjective complaints of the patient. The constellation of symptoms is fairly uniform, however, and should certainly not be discounted, and many investigators propose an anatomic basis for the clinical complaints. McNabb proposed that paresthesias in the ulnar distribution may be secondary to spasm of the scalenus muscle, and certainly symptoms such as hoarseness and dysphagia can be related to retropharyngeal hematoma. The cervical zygapophysial joint and facet capsule are implicated as a source for chronic pain after whiplash injury.

Radiographs should be taken because the amount of neck trauma that the patient has sustained may be significant. Radiographic findings, however, may be subtle or entirely negative. Cervical lordosis may be reversed, indicating spasm. Subtle signs of instability may also be present, and these can be further delineated on flexion-extension views if symptoms persist. The prevertebral soft-tissue window should be within normal limits to rule out any prevertebral hematoma. MRI is not helpful in the acute setting to definitively diagnose whiplash injury.

Once the stability of the spine is ensured, the care of the cervical sprain or whiplash injury should be symptomatic. Initial rest, bed rest if necessary, and soft collar immobilization are indicated, along with the use of anti-inflammatory medications. Early mobilization with progressive range of motion and weaning from external supports should be encouraged, however. Frequent reassurance is often necessary because the symptoms may be long lasting. Some patients with chronic unrelenting symptoms, despite maximal conservative management, may benefit from facet injections and rhizotomies.

Approximately 42% of patients have persistent symptoms beyond 1 year, with approximately a third having persistent symptoms beyond 2 years. Most patients who do improve do so within the first 2 months. Factors associated with a poor prognosis include the presence of occipital headaches, interscapular pain, or reversal of cervical lordosis. Women have a worse prognosis than men, and hyperextension injuries are thought to have a worse prognosis than hyperflexion injuries.

Onoue K, Farris C, Burley H, et al. Role of cervical spine MRI in the setting of negative cervical spine CT in blunt trauma: critical additional information in the setting of clinical findings suggestive of occult injury. *J Neuroradiol.* 2019;May 24. [Epub ahead of print] [PMID: 31132384]

Schliecher P, Kobbe P, Kandziora F, et al. Treatment of injuries to the subaxial cervical spine: recommendations of the spine section of the German Society for Orthopedics and Trauma (DGOU). *Global Spine J.* 2018;8(2 suppl):25S-33S. [PMID: 30210958]

6 Musculoskeletal Oncology

Nicholas M. Bernthal, MD
Zachary D.C. Burke, MD
Gideon W. Blumstein, MD
Danielle Greig, MD
Akash Shah, MD

Musculoskeletal oncology is a field of medicine that involves the diagnosis and management of neoplastic conditions affecting the musculoskeletal system. This not only entails neoplasia of mesenchymal origin (derived from embryonic mesoderm), but also metastatic carcinoma and a variety of pseudotumorous conditions. Mesenchymal tumors are an extremely heterogeneous group of neoplasms including over 200 benign conditions and 90 types of sarcoma. The majority of this chapter is dedicated to these conditions. The relative incidence of benign to malignant disease is 200:1. These tumors are classified histomorphologically based on features of differentiation, but there is considerable overlap. It is reasonable to consider these separate conditions as points on a continuum, rather than entirely distinct entities. Classification, nevertheless, is important because it may yield insight to the behavior, treatment response, and overall prognosis. Benign disease, by definition, exhibits little tendency to locally recur or metastasize, and is generally not aggressive in terms of local tissue destruction. However, some benign lesions are more likely to exhibit aggressive growth than others, and several lesions traditionally described as benign have relatively high rates of local recurrence and the potential to metastasize. Sarcomas (malignant tumors of mesenchymal origin) are often rapidly destructive, have metastatic potential, and have a tendency to locally recur.

Neoplastic processes arise in tissues of mesenchymal origin far less frequently than those of ectodermal or endodermal origin. According to the National Cancer Institute's Surveillance, Epidemiology, and End Results (SEER) program, approximately 12,300 new soft-tissue sarcomas and 3300 new bone sarcomas developed in the United States in 2016, with over 4900 sarcoma-related deaths. When compared with the overall cancer mortality of 595,000 cases in 2016, sarcomas are a small fraction of the problem. While they are a relatively uncommon form of cancer, these tumors behave in an aggressive fashion, with currently reported mortality rates that may be greater than 50%. The associated morbidity is much higher. These tumors inflict a tremendous emotional and financial toll on individuals and society alike. Furthermore, sarcomas preferentially affect older patients, with only 15% occurring in patients younger than 15 years and 40% in patients older than 55 years. Accordingly, as the population ages, the incidence of these conditions will increase.

ETIOLOGY OF MUSCULOSKELETAL TUMORS

Tumorigenesis is a multifactorial process, which, despite considerable fiscal and intellectual interest, is still poorly understood. Generally, genetic mutations that cause cells to replicate in an unregulated fashion are the driving force behind tumorigenesis. Many such mutations have been identified, each often associated with multiple neoplastic processes. The development of a colony of abnormally proliferating cells out of normal tissue is referred to as transformation. This process involves acquired mutations in oncogenes, tumor suppressor genes, and other genes that directly or indirectly control proliferation, cell motility, and properties of invasiveness. Such a process may progress beyond the state of benign disease to an aggressive, dedifferentiated state with considerable genomic instability.

To appreciate how bone or soft-tissue tumors develop, one must have a basic understanding of the cell cycle and the regulation thereof. The cell cycle is divided into four distinct phases: G1 (gap 1), S (DNA synthesis), G2 (gap 2), and M (mitosis). After a copy of the entire cellular genome has been synthesized, duplicate chromosomes are separated, and the cell divides during mitosis. The majority of cell growth occurs during G1. The mature state for mesenchymal cells is normally in a resting, nonproliferative phase designated G0.

Control of the cell cycle is a function of numerous regulatory proteins and checkpoints. These checkpoints allow for the monitoring and repair of the genetic sequence. These proteins are encoded by two basic gene types: oncogenes (stimulatory) and tumor suppressor genes (inhibitory).

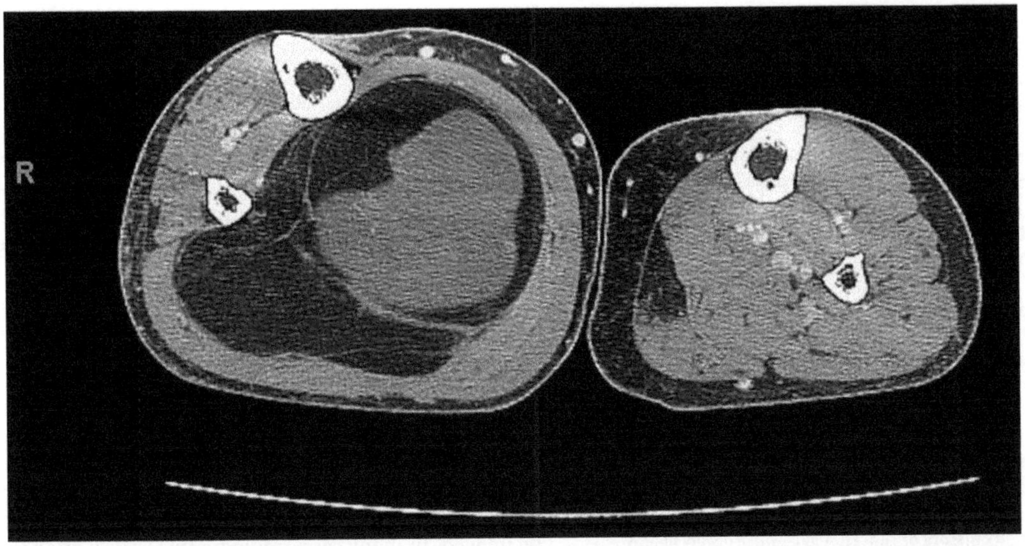

▲ **Figure 6–1.** CT scan of a myxoid liposarcoma within the substance of a long-standing intramuscular lipoma.

Oncogenes are genes encoding proteins, which have the inherent ability to transform the host cell to a neoplastic phenotype. Protooncogenes (eg, *RAS*, *WNT*, *MYC*) are wild-type genes that can become oncogenes upon mutation or dysregulation of expression. Tumor suppressor genes (eg, *p53*, *Rb*, *p21*) typically require loss-of-function mutations or mutations in other regulatory genes to impart the neoplastic phenotype. These genes are primarily involved with cell-cycle checkpoints.

Inherited mutations in these genes result in neoplastic predisposition syndromes. In syndromes such as hereditary retinoblastoma and Li-Fraumeni syndrome, one mutated copy of a tumor suppressor gene (*Rb* and *p53*, respectively) is inherited. Through a variety of causes including deletion, translocation, point mutation, promoter silencing, or other means of loss of heterozygosity, the remaining function of that gene product is lost, and from that cell, a tumor is born. Once checkpoint machinery has been disrupted, additional mutations may be accumulated at an increasing rate, allowing genomic instability to spiral out of control. At the extreme, as seen commonly in osteosarcoma, cells contain up to four times the normal number of chromosomes with multiple chromosomal aberrations.

In addition to hereditary factors that predispose one to the development of neoplasia, many well-described environmental factors exist, such as radiation exposure, chemical carcinogens, and certain oncogenic viral infections. More of these factors may surface as meticulous investigation continues in the field of cancer research.

The neoplastic process may arrest in the so-called benign state, with further genomic instability curtailed, or it may progress to a sarcomatous state. For example, if a cell type of origin is a lipoblast, then a lipoma or a liposarcoma may develop. Furthermore, a liposarcoma may progress in its differentiation such that its phenotype, as a high-grade lesion, minimally reflects its lipoblastic origin. This principle is illustrated in Figure 6–1, which shows a myxoid liposarcoma within the substance of a typical intramuscular lipoma. This possibility does not imply, however, that all benign lesions are necessarily at risk for malignant degeneration. It is not a surgical indication to resect a lipoma because of concern for secondary liposarcoma.

Although a plethora of molecular pathways are being studied, understanding of the details of genomic instability and subsequent tumor formation is lacking. There is no single pathway by which all neoplasms arise; instead, multiple genetic targets are altered in a variety of sequences and combinations with the common result of cellular proliferation that is tumorigenesis.

EVALUATION AND STAGING OF TUMORS

History and Physical Examination

When evaluating a new patient with a possible tumor, the workup should begin with a thorough history and physical examination. Prior to ordering any diagnostic studies, certain questions must be answered, and the physical characteristics of the mass in question must be assessed. This procedure prevents unnecessary tests and better enables the physician to determine which tests will be most helpful in diagnosing the condition as well as facilitating therapeutic interventions if needed.

Table 6–1. Questions that must be asked in the workup of a possible tumor.

1. **The patient's age.** Certain tumors are relatively specific to particular age groups.
2. **Duration of complaint.** Benign lesions generally have been present for an extended period (years). Malignant tumors usually have been noticed for only weeks to months.
3. **Rate of growth.** A rapidly growing mass, as in weeks to months, is more likely to be malignant. Growth may be difficult to assess by the patient if it is deep seated, as can be the case with bone. Deep lesions may be much larger than the patient thought ("tip-of-the-iceberg" phenomenon).
4. **Pain associated with the mass.** Benign processes are usually asymptomatic. Osteochondromas (see text) may cause secondary symptoms because of encroachment on surrounding structures. Malignant lesions may cause pain.
5. **History of trauma.** With a history of penetrating trauma, one must rule out osteomyelitis. With a history of blunt trauma, healing fracture must be entertained.
6. **Personal or family history of cancer.** Adults with a history of prostate, renal, lung, breast, or thyroid tumors are at risk for developing metastatic bone disease. Children with neuroblastoma are prone to bony metastases. Patients with retinoblastoma are at an increased risk for osteosarcoma. Secondary osteosarcomas and other malignancies can result from treatment of other childhood cancers. Family history of conditions such as Li-Fraumeni syndrome must raise suspicion of any bone lesion. Furthermore, certain benign bone tumors can run in families (eg, hereditary multiple exostoses; see text).
7. **Systemic signs or symptoms.** Generally, there should be no significant findings on the review of systems with benign tumors. Fevers, chills, night sweats, malaise, change in appetite, weight loss, and so on should alert the physician that an infectious or neoplastic process may be involved.

The clinical history is of paramount importance (Table 6–1). The age of the patient allows the clinician to develop a list of potential diagnoses (Table 6–2). When combined with the history, physical examination, and a few additional studies, this information is often sufficient to make a diagnosis. The duration and timing of symptoms, rate of growth, presence of pain, and a history of trauma can help elucidate the diagnosis. Specifically, pain or other symptoms occurring at rest or that awaken a patient from sleep are particularly concerning for a neoplastic process. Additionally, a careful past medical history, family history, and review of systems must not be overlooked.

A thorough physical examination is also critical (Table 6–3). The clinician must assess the location and size of the mass, the quality of the overlying skin, the presence of warmth, any associated swelling, the presence of tenderness, and the firmness of the lesion. For superficial lesions, transillumination and auscultation may also be beneficial. Range of motion of all joints in proximity to the tumor must be recorded, and a complete neurovascular exam must be performed. An assessment of the related lymph node chains and an examination for an enlarged liver or spleen should also be performed.

The clinician must also consider pseudotumors in addition to true neoplastic conditions. A history of trauma suggests possible stress fracture or myositis ossificans as a diagnosis. The association of symptoms with physical activity and variations of symptoms with the passage of time are important considerations in establishing a differential diagnosis.

Imaging Studies

A. Radiography

Initial evaluation should begin with plain radiography. In every patient with a suspected tumor, orthogonal anteroposterior (AP) and lateral views of the affected area should be obtained. This includes soft-tissue masses as well. Furthermore, in the case of a bone lesion, the entire bone should be imaged. In many cases, radiographic examination is diagnostic, although in the case of a more aggressive process, further evaluation with advanced studies is usually indicated to determine the extent of disease involvement, relation to essential anatomic structures, and the degree of systemic involvement (staging).

The initial radiographic images must be scrutinized. For bone lesions, the location within the bone (eg, diaphyseal, metaphyseal, or epiphyseal; eccentric or central; medullary or surface) facilitates the diagnosis. Epiphyseal tumors have a narrow differential diagnosis and are usually benign. Primary sarcomas of bone are usually metaphyseal where growth is occurring most rapidly; however, round cell tumors, such as Ewing sarcoma, multiple myeloma, and lymphoma, are usually medullary diaphyseal lesions. A tumor arising from the surface of a bone may be benign, such as an osteochondroma, or may be malignant, such as a parosteal osteosarcoma.

Terms such as *geographic*, *well-circumscribed*, and *permeative* are useful in describing radiographic abnormalities. Geographic or well-circumscribed implies that the lesion has a distinct, sharply marginated boundary, and suggests a benign lesion (Figure 6–2). Lesions with this feature may exhibit sclerotic borders if the bone itself has reacted to contain the process. A poorly defined, infiltrative process is described as permeative or moth-eaten and reflects a more aggressive process such as malignancy (Figure 6–3), although more aggressive benign processes can exhibit this radiographic feature as well (Figure 6–4). An exception to this rule is multiple myeloma, which frequently demonstrates a punched-out, well-demarcated appearance but in multiple locations.

Matrix quality is another radiographic feature that aids in diagnosis. Lesions may be entirely radiolucent, sparsely mineralized, or predominantly mineralized, and mineralization may be spiculated, stippled, or composed of rings and arcs. Most osteosarcomas, for example, have a spiculated pattern

Table 6–2. Distribution of bone tumors by age (years).

Type of Tumor	0	10	20	30	40	50	60	70	80
Benign bone tumors									
Osteoid osteoma									
Osteoblastoma									
Osteofibrous dysplasia									
Enchondroma									
Periosteal chondroma									
Osteochondroma									
Chondroblastoma									
Chondromyxoid fibroma									
Fibrous cortical defect									
Nonossifying fibroma									
Fibrous dysplasia									
Solitary bone cyst									
Aneurysmal bone cyst									
Epidermoid cyst									
Giant cell tumor									
Hemangioma									
Malignant bone tumors									
Classic osteosarcoma									
Hemorrhagic osteosarcoma									
Parosteal osteosarcoma									
Periosteal osteosarcoma									
Secondary osteosarcoma									
Low-grade intramedullary osteosarcoma									
Irradiation-induced osteosarcoma									
Multicentric osteosarcoma									
Primary chondrosarcoma									
Secondary chondrosarcoma									
Clear cell chondrosarcoma									
Dedifferentiated chondrosarcoma									
Mesenchymal chondrosarcoma									
Ewing sarcoma									
Lymphoma									
Multiple myeloma									
Solitary plasmacytoma									
Fibrosarcoma									
Malignant fibrous histiocytoma									
Adamantinoma									
Vascular sarcoma									
Chordoma									
Metastatic carcinoma									

Table 6–3. Aspects of physical examination that should be documented when evaluating a patient with a mass.

1. **Skin color**
2. **Warmth**
3. **Location**
4. **Swelling.** Swelling, in addition to the primary mass effect, may reflect a more aggressive process.
5. **Neurovascular exam.** Changes may reflect a more aggressive process.
6. **Joint range of motion** of all joints in proximity to the region in question, above and below.
7. **Size.** A mass greater than 5 cm should raise the suspicion of malignancy.
8. **Tenderness.** Tenderness may reflect a more rapidly growing process.
9. **Firmness.** Malignant tumors tend to be firmer on examination than benign processes. This applies more to soft-tissue tumors than osseous ones.
10. **Lymph nodes.** Certain sarcomas (eg, rhabdomyosarcoma, synovial sarcoma, epithelioid, and clear cell sarcomas) all have increased rates of lymph node involvement.

of mineralization expanding out from the host bone in a sunburst appearance. In contrast, chondroid matrix characteristically forms rings and arcs of mineralization. In soft-tissue lesions, matrix mineralization can be very helpful in diagnosis, as in hemangiomas showing smooth, round mineralized phleboliths, as opposed to synovial sarcoma frequently showing irregular mineralization.

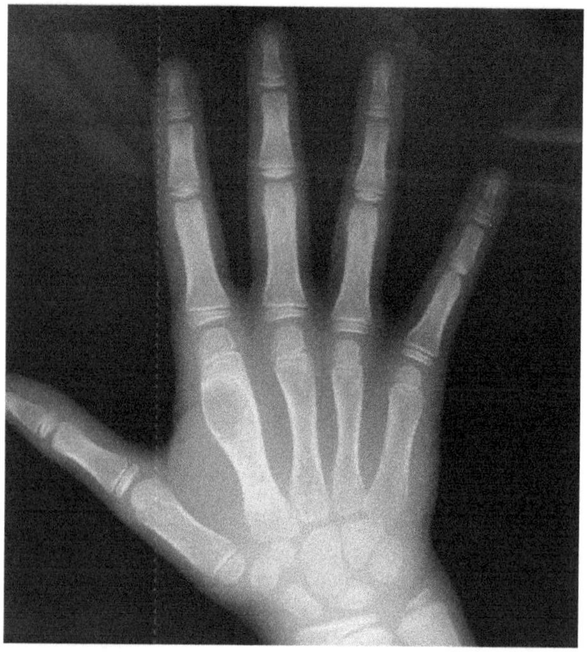

▲ **Figure 6–2.** Radiograph of an enchondroma of the second metacarpal. Notice its geographic appearance.

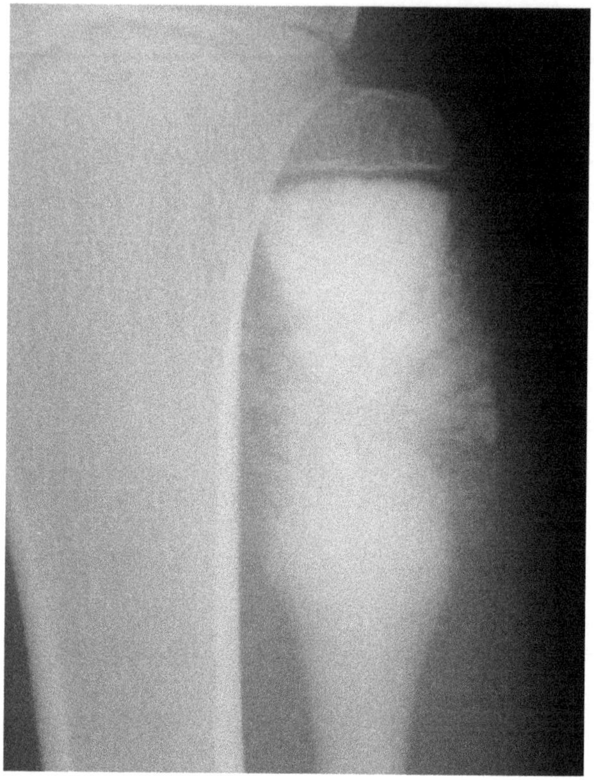

▲ **Figure 6–3.** Radiograph of a proximal fibular osteosarcoma demonstrating the destructive, permeative nature of malignant bone tumors.

With a careful history, physical examination, and appropriate radiographs, the physician can usually reach a working diagnosis of the lesion. Although some benign and malignant tumors mimic each other, many diagnoses can be ruled out based on information gained without advanced imaging. Factors such as patient age and tumor location as well as radiographic features such as boundary, matrix quality, and reaction of the bone to the lesion can be used to narrow the differential diagnosis. It should be noted that infection can have an extremely variable radiographic appearance and frequently remains on the differential until ruled out by laboratory studies or biopsy. Tables 6–1 through 6–6 can be used in a step-wise fashion to illustrate the process of focusing the differential diagnosis prior to any advanced imaging and can assist in obtaining the most appropriate studies.

B. Isotope Bone Scanning

Technetium-99 radioisotope scans are used to assess the degree of osteoblastic activity (and indirectly the degree of new bone formation) of a given lesion (Figure 6–5). In general, they are quite sensitive for active lesions of bone, with a

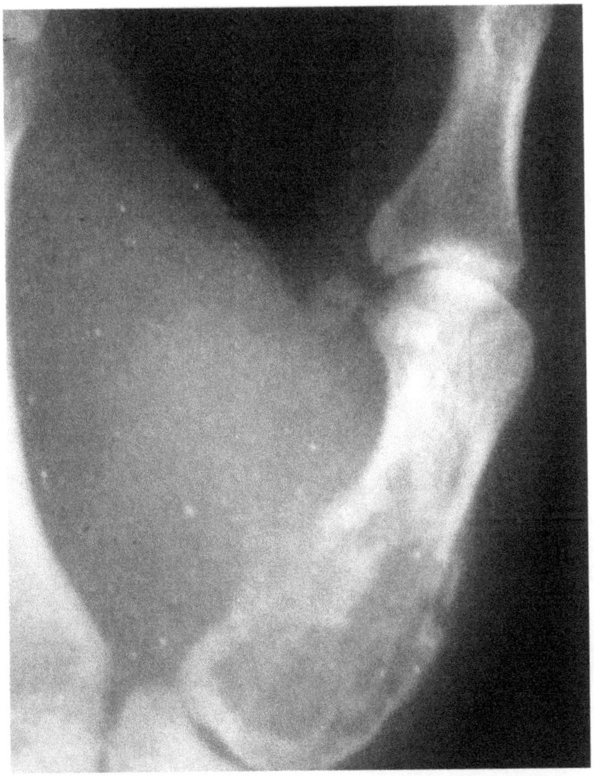

▲ **Figure 6–4.** Radiograph of a giant cell tumor of the thumb. This is a typical moth-eaten appearance.

few exceptions. Accordingly, technetium-99 scans are excellent screening studies for remote lesions (staging). The best indication for a bone scan is suspected multiple bony lesions, such as in metastatic carcinomas and lymphomas of bone. Isotope bone scanning is far simpler to perform, less expensive, and requires less total-body irradiation than skeletal surveys. It is common practice to use serial isotope scans to follow patients with suspected metastatic disease and, at the same time, evaluate the effectiveness of their systemic therapy.

Isotope scanning is also used in the staging process of a primary sarcoma of bone such as osteosarcoma to rule out an asymptomatic remote skeletal lesion. Technetium-99 scans are also useful in distinguishing blastic lesions of bone. Given that the study reflects osseous metabolic activity, dormant lesions such as enostoses (bone islands) would not demonstrate significantly increased tracer uptake compared with a blastic prostate metastasis. Inflammatory and traumatic lesions also demonstrate increased activity. It is important to note, however, that multiple myeloma and some metastatic carcinomas (eg, renal cell carcinoma) may not demonstrate increased uptake (ie, false-negative result). Skeletal surveys are preferable for screening for distant involvement in such cases.

C. Computed Tomography, Magnetic Resonance Imaging, and Positron Emission Tomography

Computed tomography (CT) remains a standard imaging procedure for use in well-selected clinical situations. Perhaps the best indication for CT is for smaller lesions that involve cortical structures of bone or spine (Figure 6–6). In such cases, CT is superior to magnetic resonance imaging (MRI) because the resolution of cortical bone using MRI is inferior. Sarcomas in general have a predilection for metastasis to the lungs, making chest CT an essential component of staging. When a skeletal metastasis is identified and the primary tumor remains unknown after initial workup, CT scans of the chest and abdomen/pelvis identify the primary lesion in the majority of patients. For tumors involving the pelvis and sacrum, CT can help elucidate the extent of bone involvement (Figure 6–7).

MRI of the entire involved bone is often performed after plain radiographs when a sarcoma is suspected. This allows for evaluation of intramedullary involvement and assesses for noncontiguous lesions within the involved bone (ie, skip lesions). MRI with and without contrast is generally considered the gold standard for evaluating soft-tissue sarcomas. The two most common sequences are the T1-weighted and T2-weighted spin echo (Figure 6–8). Short tau inversion recovery (STIR) sequences have been shown to further delineate tumors and bone marrow edema against a nonpathologic background. MRI can also demonstrate the normal anatomy of soft structures, including nerves and vessels, thereby eliminating the need for arteriography and myelograms. Dynamic-enhanced MRI, with its ability to estimate tumor blood flow by examining the rate of contrast uptake and clearance, may serve as a predictor of clinical outcome or tumor response to chemotherapy.

Positron emission tomography (PET), most often combined with CT (PET-CT), is increasingly used in the diagnosis and staging of high-grade sarcomas. The use of PET-CT is limited in low- and intermediate-grade sarcomas given their relatively low avidity for isotope uptake. Recent evidence suggests that PET-CT may be superior to bone scan for the detection of metastatic disease. However, PET-CT has been shown to be inferior to conventional chest CT for the evaluation of pulmonary metastases.

▶ Laboratory Studies

A. Biopsy

The biopsy is usually the last staging procedure. It is preferred to obtain advanced imaging prior to biopsy to avoid postsurgical artifact on these studies, which may aid in determining a definitive diagnosis. There are three types of biopsy for musculoskeletal neoplasia: excisional, incisional, and needle biopsies. Excisional biopsy is discouraged unless the lesion is particularly small (2-3 cm) or in a location where a cuff of healthy tissue can be resected as a margin without significantly increased morbidity.

Table 6–4. Skeletal distribution of bone tumors, ranked from most common (1) to least common (5) sites.

Type of Tumor	Femur	Tibia	Foot or Ankle	Humerus	Radius	Ulna	Hand or Wrist	Scapula	Clavicle	Rib	Vertebra	Sacrum	Pelvis	Skull	Face
Benign bone tumors															
Osteoid osteoma	1	2		4			5				3				
Osteoblastoma	3	4		5							1				2
Osteofibrous dysplasia		1													
Chondroma	2		4	3		5	1								
Osteochondroma	1	3		2				5					4		
Chondroblastoma	1	3		2				5					4		
Chondromyxoid fibroma	3	1	2		5								4		
Fibrous cortical defect	2	1		3	4				5						
Nonossifying fibroma	2	1		3	4				5						
Solitary bone cyst	2	3		1		5							4		
Aneurysmal bone cyst	1	2		4							3		5		
Giant cell tumor	1	2		5	3							4			
Hemangioma	3	4		5							2			1	
Malignant bone tumors															
Classic osteosarcoma	1	2		3									4		
Hemorrhagic osteosarcoma	1	2		3							5		4		
Parosteal osteosarcoma	1	2		3		4									
Periosteal osteosarcoma	1	2	5	3		4									
Secondary osteosarcoma	2	5		3									1	4	
Low-grade intramedullary osteosarcoma	1	2													
Irradiation-induced osteosarcoma	1			2							3	5			4
Primary chondrosarcoma	1			4						3	5		2		

Secondary chondrosarcoma	2			3				4			5		1		
Dedifferentiated chondrosarcoma	1			3				4		5			2		
Mesenchymal chondrosarcoma	5									3	2		1		4
Ewing sarcoma	1			3				5		4			2		
Lymphoma	1			4						5	3		2		
Myeloma	4			5						2	1		3		
Fibrosarcoma	1	2		4									3		5
Malignant fibrous histiocytoma	1	3		5									2	4	
Adamantinoma	3	1			4	2									
Vascular sarcoma		4		3						5	1		2		
Chordoma											3	1		2	
Metastatic carcinoma	2			5						4	1		3		

Table 6–5. Bone tumors: imaging characteristics, location in a long bone, and beneficial studies, ranked from most common or most beneficial (1) to least common or least beneficial (3).

	Imaging Characteristics			Location in a Long Bone					Beneficial Studies				
Type of Tumor	Geographic	Moth Eaten	Permeative	Epiphyseal	Metaphyseal	Metadiaphyseal	Diaphyseal	Surface	Plain Radiograph	CT Scan	MRI	Isotope Bone Scan	Blood Studies
Benign bone tumors													
Osteoid osteoma	1				1	2	3		1	2		3	
Osteoblastoma	2	1			2	1	3		1	2		3	
Osteofibrous dysplasia		1				2	1		1	2		3	
Chondroma	1				3	1	2		1	2		3	
Osteochondroma	1				2			1	1	2			
Chondroblastoma	1	2		1	2				1	2			
Chondromyxoid fibroma	1	2			1	2			1	2		3	
Fibrous cortical defect	1				1	2			1				
Nonossifying fibroma	1	2			1	2			1	2			
Solitary bone cyst	1				1	2	3		1				
Aneurysmal bone cyst	3	2	1		1	2		3	1	2	3		
Giant cell tumor	3	1	2	1	2				1	2			3
Hemangioma	2	1			3	1	2		1	2			
Malignant bone tumors													
Classic osteosarcoma	3	1	2		1	2	3		1		2	3	
Hemorrhagic osteosarcoma		1	2		1	2			1		2		3
Parosteal osteosarcoma	2	1			2	3		1	2	1			
Periosteal osteosarcoma	2	1			3	2		1	2	1			
Secondary osteosarcoma		1	2		1	2	3		2	1	3		
Low-grade intramedullary osteosarcoma		1			1	2			1	2		3	
Irradiation-induced osteosarcoma		1	2		1	2	3		1		2	3	

Primary chondrosarcoma	2	1		3	1	2			2	1	3		
Secondary chondrosarcoma	2	1			2	3		1	2	1			
Dedifferentiated chondrosarcoma		1	2		1	2	3		2	3	1		
Mesenchymal chondrosarcoma		1	2		1	2			2	3	1		
Ewing sarcoma		2	1		1	2	3		2		1	3	
Lymphoma		2	1		3	1	2		3		1	2	
Myeloma	1	2			1	3	2		1			3	2
Fibrosarcoma		1	2		1	2	3		2		1		
Malignant fibrous histiocytoma		1	2		1	2	3		2		1		
Adamantinoma	2	1			3	2	1		1	2	3		
Vascular sarcoma	2	1	3		1	2	3		1		2	3	
Chordoma	2	1				1	2		3	2	1		
Metastatic carcinoma	3	1	2		1	2	3		2	3		1	

Table 6–6. Distribution of soft-tissue tumors by age.

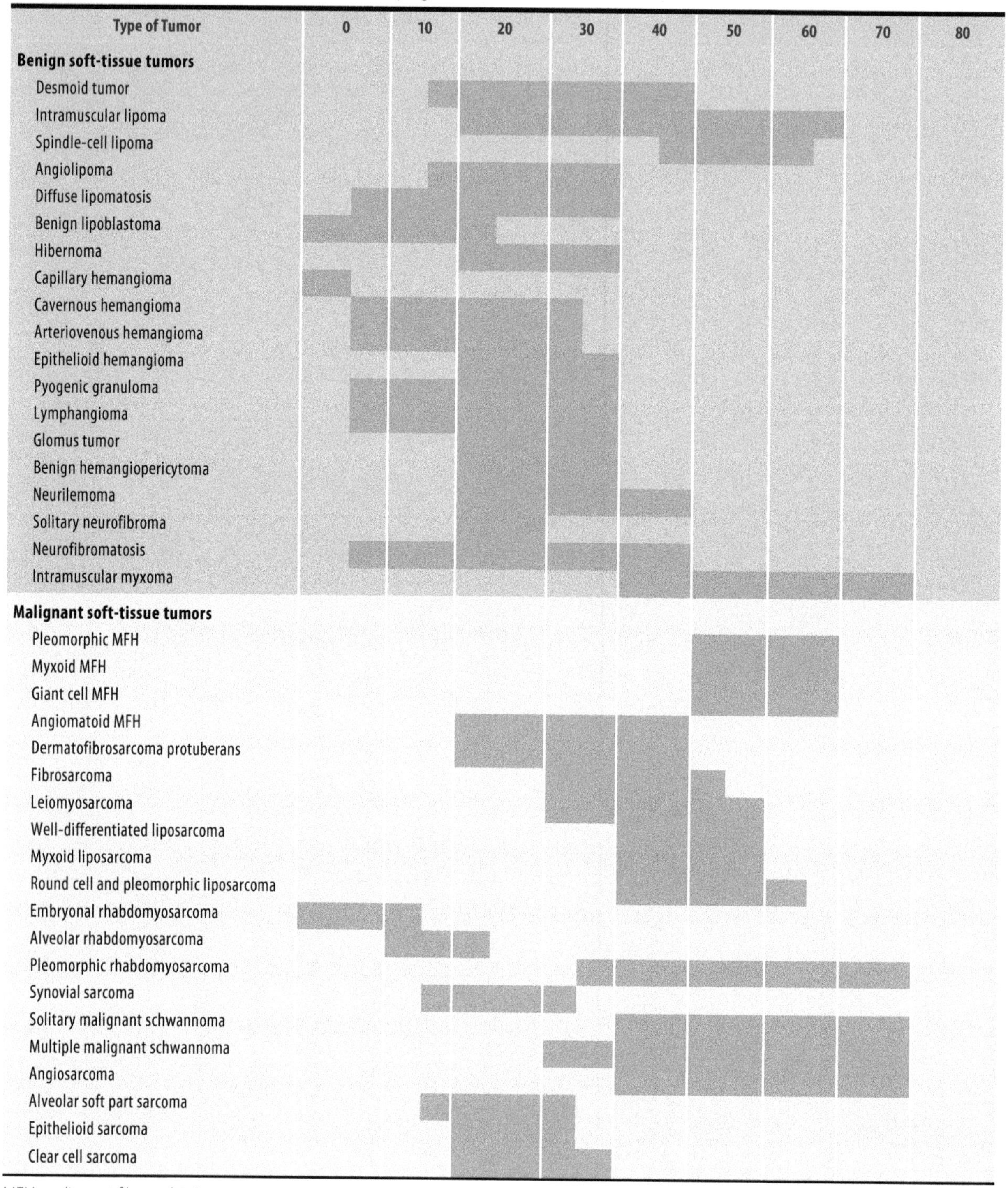

MFH, malignant fibrous histiocytoma.

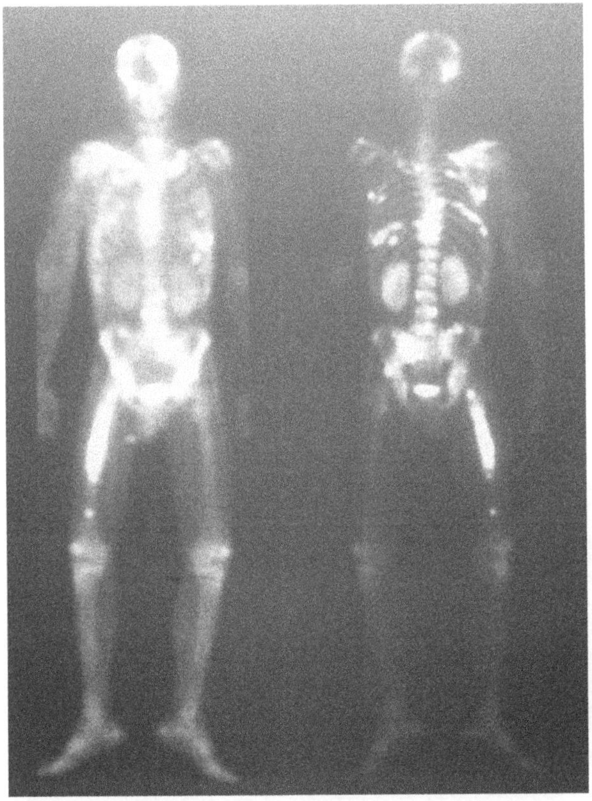

▲ **Figure 6–5.** Technetium-99 scan demonstrating extensive osteoblastic activity in a patient with metastatic adenocarcinoma.

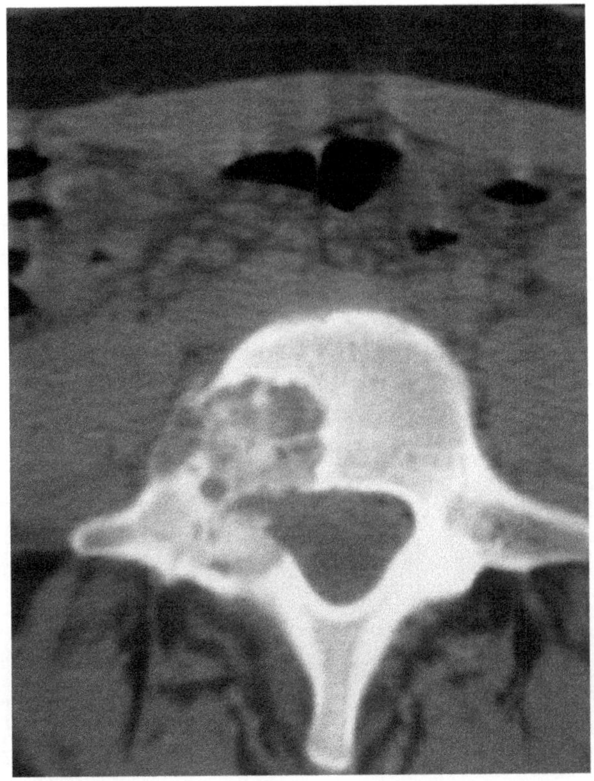

▲ **Figure 6–6.** CT scan of an osteoblastoma arising from the right pedicle of a lumbar vertebra.

Complications relating to biopsy are very common. Accordingly, careful preoperative planning is imperative. Imaging studies aid the surgeon in planning biopsy approach and technique. The highest-quality diagnostic tissue is usually found at the periphery of the lesion, where it interfaces with the normal surrounding tissue. In the case of extracompartmental primary bone lesions, the periphery of the soft-tissue extension can be sampled without further compromising the structural integrity of the bone. In the case of intramedullary lesions, a round or ovular window should be developed to decrease the risk of fracture, and the defect should be filled with bone wax or cement to avoid unnecessary contamination of the uninvolved soft tissue. There is also evidence that biopsies performed by the treating oncologic surgeon have a lower complication rate than those performed by inexperienced practitioners prior to referral.

The placement of the biopsy site is a major consideration, since resection of the biopsy tract is necessary for many malignant diagnoses. To facilitate resection, the biopsy tract should be placed in the plane of the planned resection whenever possible. Given this, it is strongly recommended that the biopsy be performed or coordinated by an oncologic surgeon who plans to carry out any subsequent sarcoma resection. Serious contamination of vital structures such as the popliteal artery or sciatic nerve may result in amputation rather than limb-sparing surgery. Furthermore, transverse

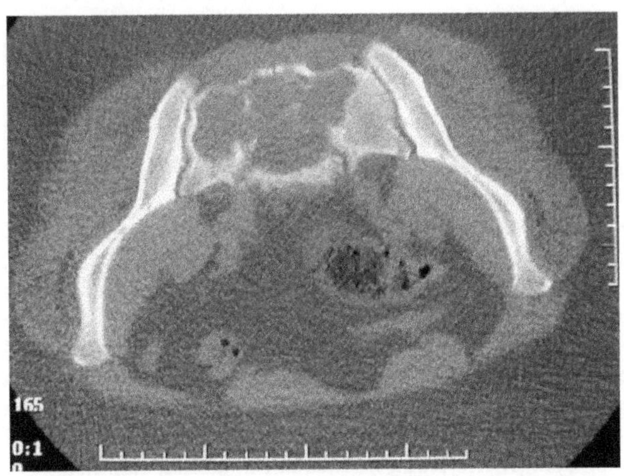

▲ **Figure 6–7.** Pelvic CT demonstrating the bony destruction of the sacrum caused by a giant cell tumor.

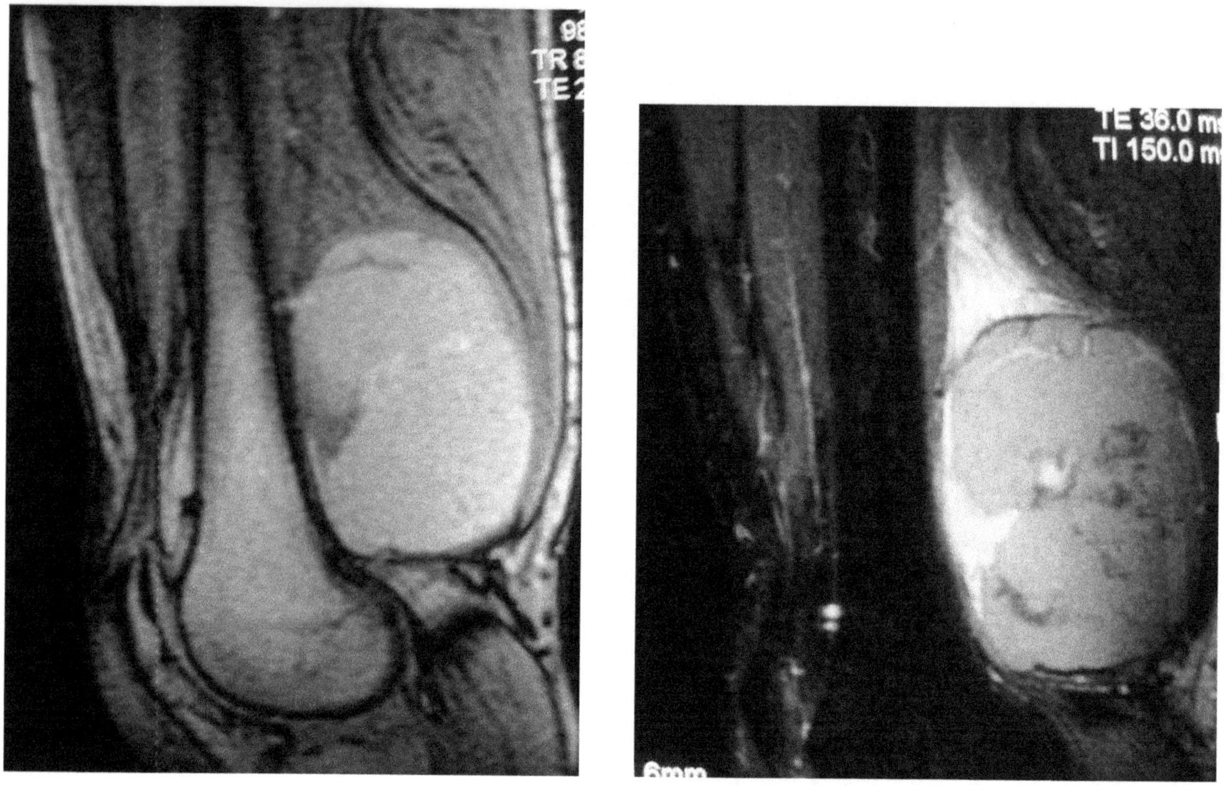

A B

▲ **Figure 6–8.** Synovial sarcoma involving the popliteal fossa. (**A**) T1-weighted. (**B**) T2-weighted.

incisions should be avoided as they often involve multiple anatomic compartments (rather than a single compartment with a longitudinal incision) that would be at risk for contamination in the case of sarcoma diagnosis. When multiple compartments are contaminated, the use of free or rotational flap coverage or amputation may be necessary. Meticulous hemostasis is also mandatory to avoid the formation of a contaminating hematoma. In rare instances, a drain may be helpful, but should exit the skin in line with the biopsy incision.

Obtaining an adequate specimen is critical. A frozen section determines whether viable, diagnostic tissue has been obtained. Definitive diagnosis is rarely possible based on frozen section. In most circumstances, definitive resection should be delayed until final histopathologic diagnosis has been rendered. For the diagnosis of some histologies, special studies may be required such as immunohistochemistry, flow cytometry, fluorescence in situ hybridization, or other cytogenetic studies. Adequate material, handled appropriately, is required for the completion of many of these studies.

Needle biopsies, either core or fine needle, are increasingly being used at experienced tumor centers where multidisciplinary teams of surgeons, medical oncologists, and pathologists work together to interpret results from smaller histologic samples. Image-guided needle biopsy offers the advantages of reduced morbidity and precise tissue sampling. Furthermore, recent data suggest that needle biopsy tracts are at significantly reduced risk for tumor contamination compared to open biopsy. For spine or deep pelvic lesions, image-guided needle biopsy is ideal because it avoids excessive multicompartmental contamination. Because the subtype of tumor frequently determines treatment, architecture of the tumor is generally needed, which requires core-needle rather than fine-needle biopsy. Highly lytic or highly sclerotic lesions may be difficult to sample using core-needle biopsy, and open biopsy may be preferred. In the case of heterogenous tumors, image-guided biopsy allows for targeting of high-yield tumor regions (eg, the periphery). Needle biopsy may be reasonable for presumed lesions that are easily diagnosed histologically, such as round cell tumors or metastatic carcinoma. Fine-needle biopsy should be reserved for use in consultation with an experienced cytopathologist. Most current studies show a diagnostic accuracy of 75% to 85% for needle biopsy compared with more than 95% accuracy for incisional biopsy.

B. Cultures and Special Studies

The damage of biopsy specimens after retrieval can make it impossible to perform special studies such as immunohistochemistry, cytogenetics, flow cytometry, and electron microscopy. For this reason, the surgeon should consult with the pathologist prior to biopsy. For example, formalin preservation of the specimen will preclude many of the aforementioned studies. Not only is it important for the operating room personnel to be aware of this, but it is also important for the pathologist to be aware of the clinical history and differential diagnoses, so that the specimen is handled appropriately. It is also wise to culture for bacteria, fungus, and acid-fast bacilli when clinical suspicion warrants.

Molecular diagnostics continue to revolutionize sarcoma diagnostics. Specific genomic rearrangements and mutations have been identified in a variety of tumors (Table 6–7). This is not only improving diagnostics, but also treatment. Gastrointestinal stromal tumor (GIST), a malignant mesenchymal neoplasm of the gastrointestinal tract, omentum, and mesentery, expresses a mutant form of *c-kit*. The *KIT* gene encodes a tyrosine kinase receptor for which targeted therapy has been developed and has shown significant efficacy. Targeted therapy has also been developed for some subtypes of lymphoma based on the expression pattern of cell surface markers. The status of these cell surface proteins is most often established using flow cytometry.

Staging Systems

Staging refers to a critical assessment of the grade and size of a tumor and the extent to which the disease has spread. There are two dominant staging systems for both soft-tissue sarcoma and primary bone sarcoma, which are described in the following sections. The goals of cancer staging include treatment guidance, prognostic stratification, and investigation continuity.

Table 6–7. Common translocations seen in sarcomas.

Ewing/primitive neuroectodermal tumor: t(11;22) (q24;q12), (t21;22) (q22;q12), (t7;22) (p22;q12)
Myxoid chondrosarcoma: t(9;22) (q22;q12)
Myxoid and round cell liposarcoma: t(12;16) (q12;p11)
Synovial sarcoma: t(X;18) (p11;q11)
Alveolar rhabdomyosarcoma: t(2;13) (q35;q14), t(1;13) (p36;q14)
Alveolar soft parts sarcoma: t(X;17) (p11.2;q25)
Desmoplastic small round cell tumor: t(11;22) (p13;q12)
Congenital fibrosarcoma: t(12;15)

A. System of the American Joint Committee on Cancer

The American Joint Committee on Cancer (AJCC) system (8th edition) is used by most surgical oncologists. This is the four-stage tumor, node, metastasis (TNM) classification system that provides staging criteria for both soft-tissue sarcoma and primary bone sarcoma, as well as all other major malignancies. The distinct staging systems for both soft-tissue sarcoma and primary bone sarcoma entail the size and grade of the primary tumor as well as presence of nodal or distant metastases. The AJCC system is updated regularly based on recent evidence. Notable recent changes include adoption of a three-tier staging system, rather than a four-tier system, and elimination of tumor depth as a factor in staging soft-tissue sarcomas.

For soft-tissue sarcoma, stage I represents any histologic grade 1 (out of 3) tumor without nodal or distant metastases. This is further subdivided by size, with stage IA including tumors of less than 5 cm in largest dimension and stage IB including tumors of 5 cm or greater diameter. Stage II and III tumors are grade 2 or 3 tumors without metastases. The distinction is in size, where stage II is any tumor less than 5 cm, stage IIIA is tumors measuring 5 to 10 cm, and stage IIIB is any tumor larger than 10 cm. Stage IV is any grade or size tumor with nodal or distant metastases.

For primary bone sarcoma, stage I represents any grade 1 (out of 3) tumor without metastatic disease. This is further subdivided by size, with stage IA including tumors of less than 8 cm in largest dimension and stage IB including tumors of 8 cm or greater or noncontiguous boney disease ("skip lesions"). Stage II represents any grade 2 or 3 tumor without noncontiguous or metastatic disease. This group also is divided into stage IIA and IIB based on 8-cm size. Stage III is any grade or size tumor with noncontiguous disease in the same bone and no distant metastases. Stage IV is any grade or size tumor with distant metastatic disease and is divided into stage IVA and IVB based on isolated pulmonary metastases versus extrapulmonary disease including lymph nodes, respectively.

B. Musculoskeletal Tumor Society System (Surgical Staging System or Enneking System)

Many orthopedic oncologists prefer the Enneking system, which addresses both primary bone and soft-tissue sarcoma, and specifically addresses unique problems associated with sarcoma affecting the extremities. It is a three-stage system with stage I representing low-grade tumors without metastases. Stage II represents high-grade tumors without metastases. The first two groupings are further subdivided into types A and B based on intra- or extracompartmental designation, respectively. Stage III is any tumor with metastatic disease. Although compartmentalization is an important surgical concept, to date, it has not been shown to be a statistically significant prognostic factor.

C. Future Directions of Sarcoma Staging

Data gathered from biopsy and surgical resection of sarcomas have been increasingly used to facilitate accurate staging. As the cellular and molecular understanding of sarcomas increases, specific genetic information collected from biopsy and surgical samples has shown promise in predicting clinical outcomes. When preoperative (neoadjuvant) chemotherapy is used, as is often the case in osteosarcoma, the percent necrosis of the resected or biopsied tumor sample has been shown to be highly correlated with clinical course.

Essentials of Diagnosis

- *Meticulous history and physical examination are critical in the diagnosis of bone and soft-tissue tumors.*
- *Plain radiography should be the initial imaging modality in the evaluation of bone and soft-tissue tumors. Frequently, it is diagnostic, obviating the need for advanced imaging and, at times, biopsy.*
- *When biopsy is necessary, it should be performed with careful planning by the surgeon prepared to definitively treat all possible diagnoses.*

Baheti AD, O'Malley RB, Kim S, et al. Soft-tissue sarcomas: an update for radiologists based on the revised 2013 World Health Organization classification. *Am J Roentgenol.* 2016;206(5):924-932. [PMID: 26998884]

Barrientos-Ruiz I, Ortiz-Cruz EJ, Serrano-Montilla J, et al. Are biopsy tracts a concern for seeding and local recurrence in sarcomas? *Clin Orthop Relat Res.* 2017;475(2):511-518. [PMID: 27655183]

Jaffe CC. Response assessment in clinical trials: implications for sarcoma clinical trial design. *Oncologist.* 2008;13:14. [PMID: 18434633]

Jeys LM, Thorne CJ, Parry M, et al. A novel system for the surgical staging of primary high-grade osteosarcoma: the Birmingham classification. *Clin Orthop Relat Res.* 2017;475(3):842-850. [PMID: 27138473]

Li Y, Du Y, Luo TY, et al. Factors influencing diagnostic yield of CT-guided percutaneous core needle biopsy for bone lesions. *Clin Radiol.* 2014;69(1):e43-e47. [PMID: 24268511]

Ordonez JL, Martins AS, Osuna D, et al. Targeting sarcomas: therapeutic targets and their rational. *Semin Diagn Pathol.* 2008;25:304-316. [PMID: 19013896]

Shimada H, Setoguchi T, Yokouchi M, et al. Metastatic bone tumors: analysis of factors affecting prognosis and efficacy of CT and 18F-FDG PET-CT in identifying primary lesions. *Mol Clin Oncol.* 2014;2(5):875-881. [PMID: 25054061]

Steffner RJ, Jang ES. Staging of bone and soft-tissue sarcomas. *J Am Acad Orthop Surg.* 2018;26(13):e269-e278. [PMID: 29781819]

Surveillance, Epidemiology, and End Results (SEER) Program. Research Data (1975-2016), National Cancer Institute, DCCPS, Surveillance Research Program, released April 2019. Accessed November 8, 2020. www.seer.cancer.gov.

DIAGNOSIS AND TREATMENT OF TUMORS

BENIGN BONE TUMORS

Benign bone tumors have certain characteristics that favor their diagnosis over malignant conditions. Benign lesions are frequently asymptomatic and, many times, are detected incidentally during workup of an unrelated condition such as minor trauma. The diagnosis can often be made with plain radiography alone. Benign bone tumors are usually well circumscribed, and there is evidence of the host bone successfully reacting to contain the lesion, characterized radiographically by sclerotic margins or a dense osteoblastic reactive zone. In contrast, if the condition is malignant, the patient usually complains of pain, and the radiograph commonly shows a more permeative lesion with lytic destruction and poorly defined margins that suggest rapid progression. Further studies such as MRI or bone scintigraphy are unnecessary for typical benign lesions, such as fibrous dysplasia, enchondroma, or nonossifying fibroma. There is far less cytogenetic information available for benign bone tumors, likely because there is less implication in the treatment. A system of staging exists for benign bone tumors. Stage 1 lesions are considered latent. They are generally asymptomatic, but not always. Although they can progress, they usually resolve. Initially, these lesions should be observed. Stage 2 lesions are considered active. They tend not to resolve spontaneously and are less well demarcated than stage 1 lesions. They frequently require surgical intervention with meticulous attention to complete extirpation because of their propensity for recurrence. Stage 3, or aggressive, lesions demonstrate extensive destruction. Treatment often requires wide en bloc resection.

The more common types of benign bone tumors are discussed in this section.

Benign Osteoid-Forming Tumors

A. Osteoid Osteoma

The most common benign osteoid-forming tumor is the osteoid osteoma, accounting for 10% of all benign bone tumors. It is more common in males than in females with a peak incidence in the second decade of life. Although it may be present in almost any bone, the proximal femur is the most common location. Dull, aching, nocturnal pain is characteristic, and it is commonly relieved entirely by nonsteroidal anti-inflammatory drugs (NSAIDs) secondary to a high concentration of prostaglandins in the nidus. Osteoid osteoma may have a unique pathogenic nerve supply as well, a unique finding among the bone tumors.

The characteristic radiographic feature of the osteoid osteoma is a central, lytic nidus usually 1 cm or less in diameter. The more common cortically based lesion (Figure 6–9) exhibits extensive reactive sclerosis, creating a fusiform bulge on the bone surface. However, if the nidus is more centrally

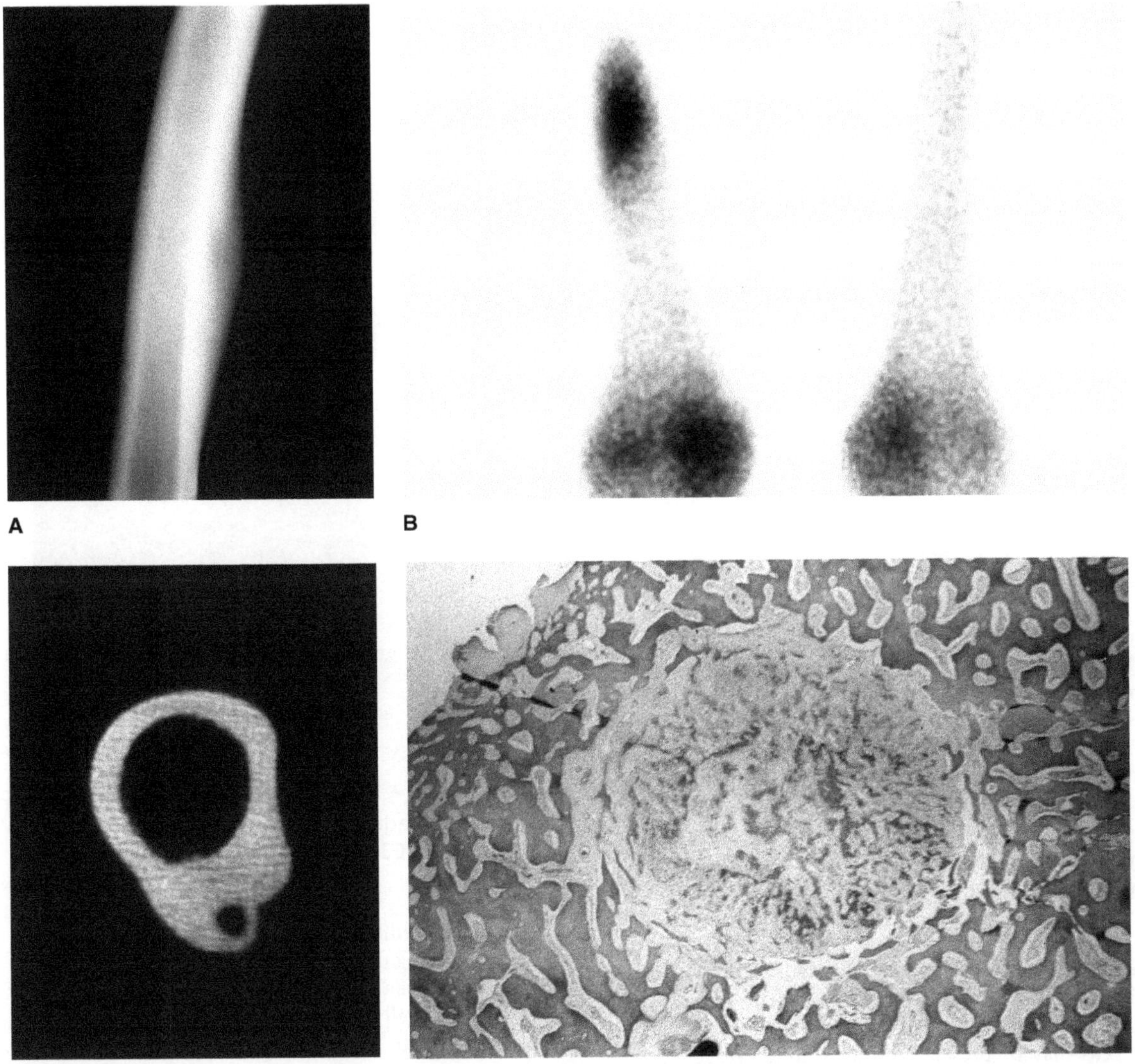

A B C D

▲ **Figure 6–9.** Radiograph (**A**), isotope bone scan (**B**), CT scan (**C**), and photomicrograph (**D**) of an osteoid osteoma in the femur of a 19-year-old man.

located in metaphyseal bone, less sclerosis is seen and the radiographic appearance is less diagnostic. If the nidus is close to, or actually in, a joint, as in a femoral neck lesion, the resulting reactive synovitis may mimic a pyarthrosis or rheumatoid arthritis. Technetium bone scans are invariably positive. A CT scan is recommended to better anatomically locate the nidus and confirm the diagnosis.

In the spine, the typical location for an osteoid osteoma is in the posterior elements. The lumbar spine is most commonly involved, followed by the thoracic spine. A secondary scoliosis is usually associated with this presentation with the lesion located at the apex of the concavity. Furthermore, if the nidus is in proximity to a nerve root, radicular pain may develop, which may obscure timely diagnosis.

Histologically, the nidus is seldom larger than 1 cm, and for lesions greater than 2 cm, the term *osteoblastoma* is reserved, suggesting somewhat more aggressive proliferative features. The nidus is composed of loose, vascular connective tissue and immature, lacy osteoid lined by plump osteoblasts. At the periphery of the nidus, there is bone organized into a tiny trabecular network with centripetally increasing maturity. There is a paucity of cytogenetic data for this entity, which is unlikely to increase rapidly, secondary to diagnostic tissue being rarely procured for diagnosis or treatment.

Many cases of osteoid osteoma are stage 1 lesions and can be treated symptomatically with aspirin or NSAIDs until they spontaneously resolve. If the patient fails such treatment, intervention is warranted. CT-guided radiofrequency ablation has emerged as the preferred treatment modality in many cases. This method employs probes with high-frequency alternating current to induce ionic agitation and frictional heat to induce tumor necrosis. Radiofrequency ablation is used extensively as a less invasive treatment modality with similar success rate as surgical excision.

If open surgical excision is undertaken, the entire nidus must be eradicated. Resection of surrounding sclerotic bone should not be excessive, because it can severely compromise the structural integrity of the host bone. The so-called burr-down technique is preferred over en bloc resection. The nidus is recognized by the hyperemic, pink hue and is removed by curettage. The burr is then used to advance the margin another 2 to 3 mm.

B. Osteoblastoma

Osteoblastoma is closely related to osteoid osteoma and demonstrates a propensity for the posterior elements of the spine. Like osteoid osteomas, osteoblastomas are found more commonly in males than in females with peak incidence in the second decade of life. Osteoblastomas are less common than osteoid osteomas, accounting for 1% of all benign bone tumors. They can occur in the metaphyses of long bones, raising concern of osteosarcoma, and may rarely be seen in the ankle and wrist. These are usually stage 1 to 2 lesions.

Radiographically, the osteoblastoma has a more lytic and destructive appearance than the osteoid osteoma. Its nidus, which is greater than 2 cm, has a less sclerotic boundary and may take on the appearance of an aneurismal bone cyst. Histologically, however, the nidus is identical to that of an osteoid osteoma. There is rich vascularity in a bed of disorganized, immature osteoid and microtrabeculae lined with a single layer of plump osteoblasts. Multinucleated, osteoclast-like giant cells may be present. Although little cytogenetic data are available, preliminary evidence suggests moderately increased genetic instability over that of osteoid osteoma.

In the spine, the effects of osteoblastoma are similar to osteoid osteoma, although at times more pronounced, including radiating pain and other effects of nerve root or spinal cord impingement (Figure 6–10).

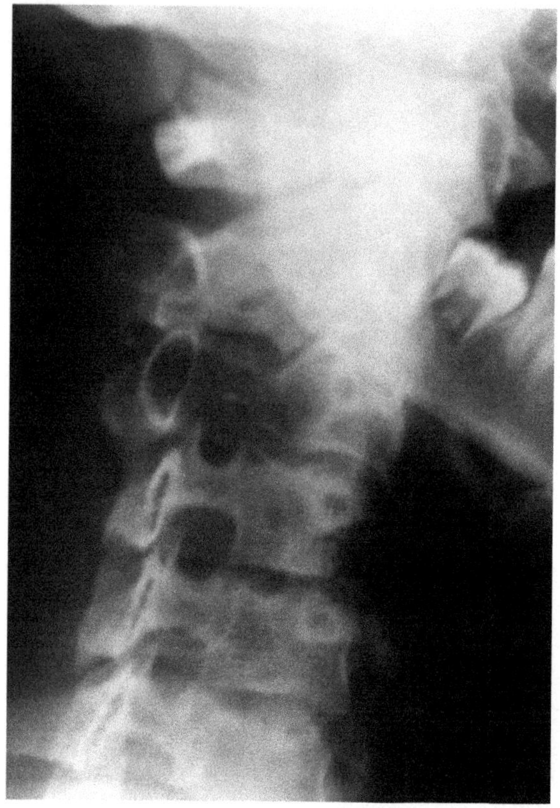

▲ **Figure 6–10.** Radiograph of an osteoblastoma in the pedicle area of the C3 vertebra of a 14-year-old boy.

In patients with osteoblastoma, treatment usually consists of vigorous curettage of the lesion, which may require structural bone grafting if instability results. Radiofrequency ablation may also prove useful in the management of this lesion in certain circumstances.

C. Osteofibrous Dysplasia

Osteofibrous dysplasia is a rare condition, usually presenting as a stage 1 or 2 lesion, that is seen almost exclusively in the tibia of children during the first two decades of life. There is a strong male predilection. It commonly affects the anterior cortex, resulting in an anterior tibial bow. Osteofibrous dysplasia can be seen in the fibula and, even more rarely, can be seen bilaterally. It is most likely a hamartomatous process and tends to involute spontaneously with skeletal maturity.

In osteofibrous dysplasia (Figure 6–11), lytic changes are seen in the anterior tibial cortex surrounded by sclerotic margins creating a soap-bubble appearance similar to the radiographic picture of fibrous dysplasia and adamantinoma. Histologically, the lytic lesion shows a benign trabecular alphabet soup pattern in a fibrous stroma. Notably, there is prominent osteoblastic rimming of the trabeculae, in contrast with fibrous dysplasia.

As previously eluded to, there is a significant diagnostic dilemma in distinguishing between osteofibrous dysplasia and the potentially malignant adamantinoma. There is significant debate as to whether these lesions represent a continuum of the same process or are discrete entities. If progression is documented or there are other alarming features, diagnostic biopsy is warranted. Osteofibrous dysplasia is vimentin positive but keratin negative, whereas

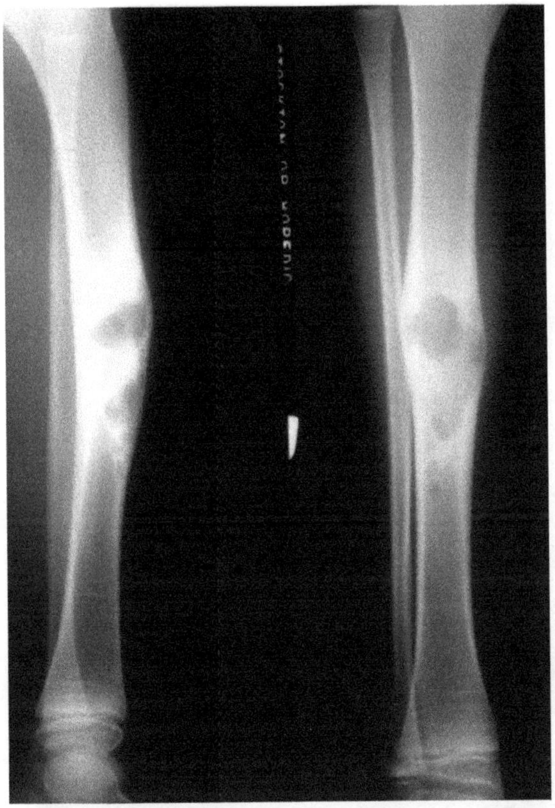

▲ **Figure 6–11.** Radiograph of osteofibrous dysplasia in the tibia of an 8-year-old boy.

adamantinoma exhibits prominent nests of keratin-positive epithelial cells. When a few scattered keratin-positive cells are seen, it is termed osteofibrous dysplasia–like adamantinoma.

Treatment consists of observation, often until skeletal maturity when the disease spontaneously arrests before proceeding with curettage and grafting if indicated.

Essentials of Diagnosis

- *Benign osteoid-forming lesions of bone are typically painful and, especially in the case of osteoid osteoma, may be relieved by aspirin or NSAIDs.*
- *Osteoblastoma is very similar to osteoid osteoma, but larger, and both show a predilection to the posterior elements of the spine. If there is an associated painful scoliosis, the convexity will point away from the side of the lesion.*
- *Osteofibrous dysplasia is characterized histologically by the presence of osteoblastic rimming of the immature trabeculae, in contrast to fibrous dysplasia, which has absent osteoblastic rimming.*

Benign Chondroid-Forming Tumors

A. Enchondroma and the Multiple Enchondromatoses

Enchondroma refers to a centrally located chondroma of bone. These tumors are relatively common, accounting for greater than 10% of benign bone tumors. In 50% of cases, the tumor is found in the small tubular bones of the hands and feet. It arises in growing bones as a hamartomatous process but is frequently asymptomatic and may avoid detection until the patient reaches adulthood, at which time it may be discovered in association with a pathologic fracture or as an incidental finding.

Radiographs of enchondromas show geographic lysis with sharp margination and central calcification (Figure 6–12). In the case of an enchondroma of the hand, the cortex is frequently thinned out with slight expansion. In contrast, with involvement of the large long bones, the lesion is centrally located with minimal cortical erosion. Enchondromas are either stage 1 or 2 lesions.

Multiple enchondromatosis, or Ollier disease (Figure 6–13), is a rare nonfamilial dysplasia typically seen on half of the body and appears similar to fibrous dysplasia. This condition can be quite extensive with significant involvement of the metaphyses resulting in bowing and shortening of the long bones. Such dramatic changes are not seen in solitary enchondroma. In patients with Maffucci syndrome, multiple enchondromatosis is seen in association with multiple soft-tissue hemangiomas.

A large solitary enchondroma converts to low-grade chondrosarcoma in fewer than 5% of cases, and the conversion takes place during adulthood. A solitary enchondroma in the hand rarely converts to chondrosarcoma, although histologically, these appear more biologically active. A

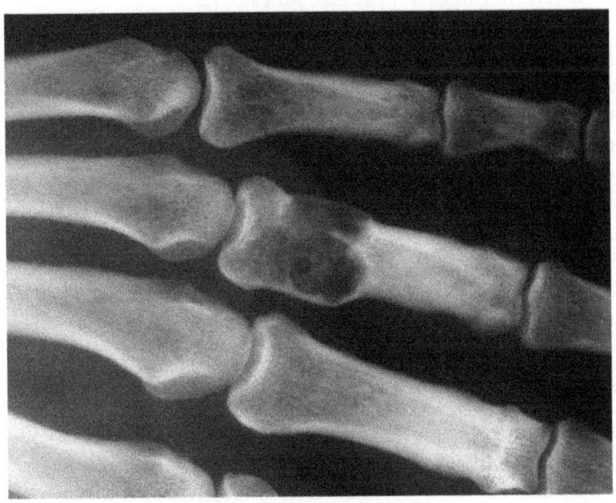

▲ **Figure 6–12.** Radiograph of an enchondroma of the proximal phalanx of the ring finger.

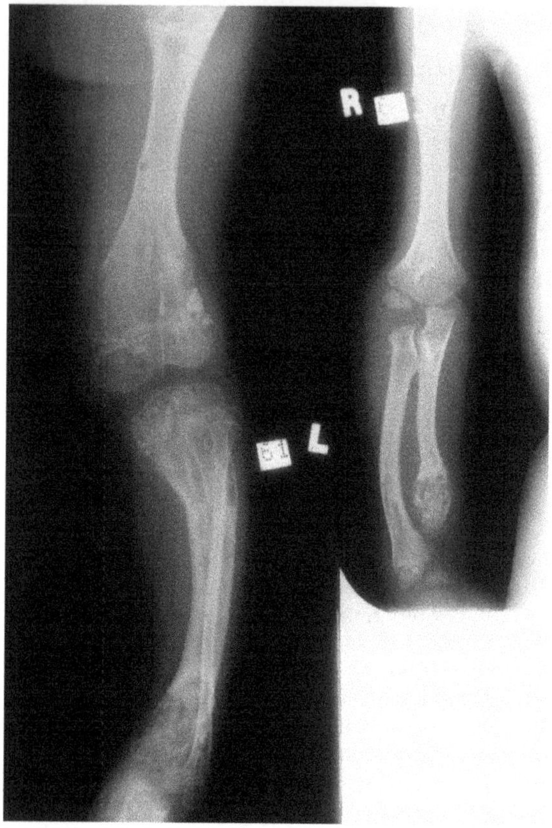

▲ **Figure 6–13.** Radiograph of Ollier disease of the upper and lower extremities.

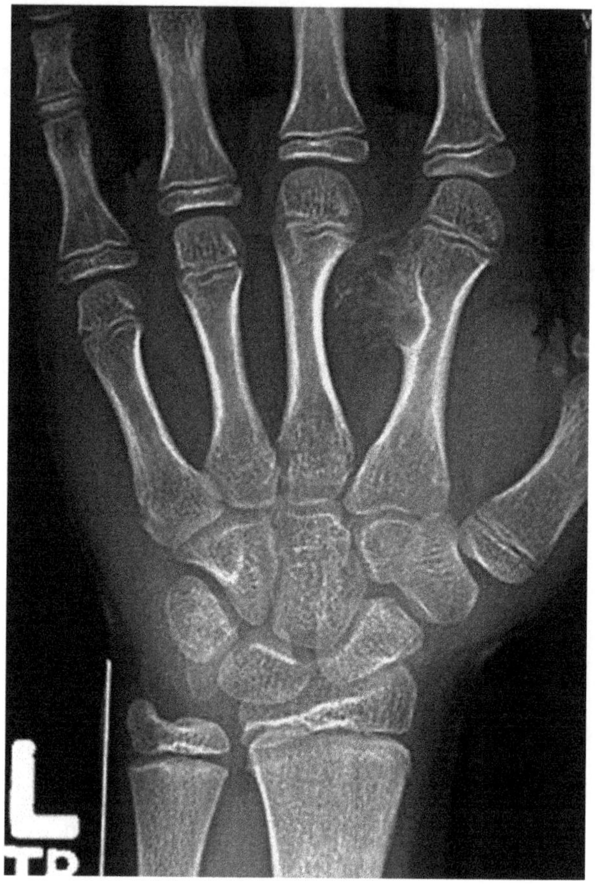

▲ **Figure 6–14.** Radiograph of a periosteal chondroma on the index metacarpal of a 12-year-old boy. Notice the buttress of bone proximally and the characteristic matrix mineralization.

secondary chondrosarcoma can occur in enchondromatosis up to 20% of the time and may be related to acquired inactivation of certain tumor suppressor genes.

There is no need to treat an asymptomatic patient with a solitary enchondroma, but the patient should be followed radiographically for changes suggesting dedifferentiation. In cases of impending fracture or persistently symptomatic lesions, curettage with margin extension and bone grafting may be performed with a low risk of recurrence. Patients with multiple enchondromatosis must be followed closely because of the increased risk of secondary chondrosarcoma. Patients with Maffucci syndrome are at additional risk for the development of other mesenchymal neoplasia, including hemangiosarcoma and lymphangiosarcoma.

B. Periosteal Chondroma

A benign chondroma seen on the surface of a bone is called a periosteal chondroma. Patients frequently have more than one lesion, and the most common location is on the proximal humeral metaphysis. Radiographically, the lesions appear to saucerize the underlying cortex (Figure 6–14). These stage 1 or 2 lesions may grow to a sizable mass, but those larger than 4 cm suggest peripheral chondrosarcoma. Management usually consists of serial imaging to ensure it does not continue growing into adulthood. In concerning cases, simple excision results in low recurrence rates.

C. Osteochondroma

The nonossifying fibroma is the most common benign bone tumor, and the osteochondroma is the second most common. Like the enchondroma, the osteochondroma is a developmental, or hamartomatous, process that arises from a defect in the outer edge of the metaphyseal side of a growth plate, resulting in an exostosis that points away from the joint and moves away from the physis with growth.

Macroscopically, there is a bony base, sharing a medullary communication with the host bone, and a cartilaginous

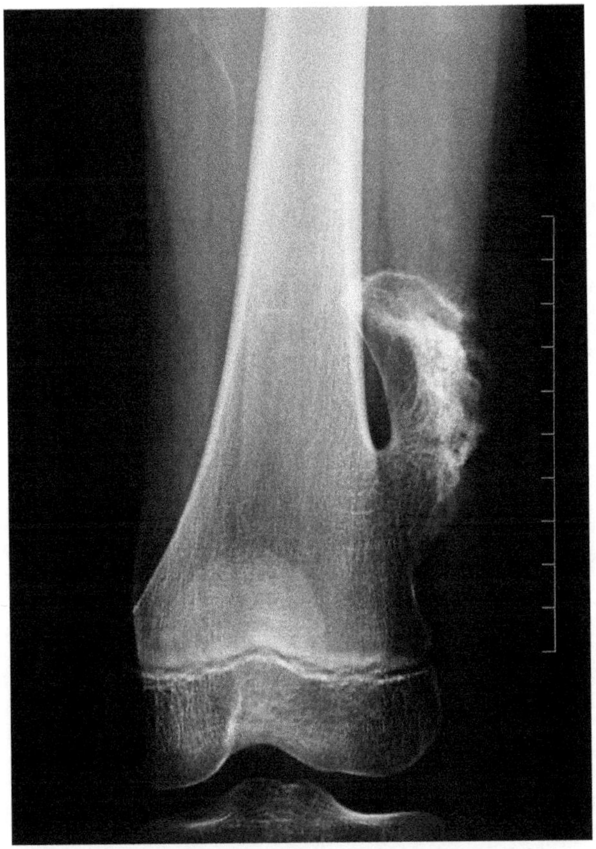

▲ **Figure 6–15.** Radiograph of a solitary osteochondroma on the distal femur of a skeletally immature individual.

cap (Figures 6–15 and 6–16). They may be pedunculated or sessile. The cartilage cap has a similar columnar organization as a growth plate and synchronously stops growth at skeletal maturity.

A familial form of osteochondromata, called multiple hereditary exostosis (MHE), is an autosomal dominant disorder that is one-tenth as common as solitary osteochondroma. Three genetic loci are associated with MHE involving the tumor suppressor *EXT* genes (*EXT1, EXT2,* and *EXT3*). This condition exhibits variable penetrance, with the severest forms resulting in severe angular deformities and limb shortening from hundreds of osteochondromata. Forearm involvement can be quite deforming. The metaphyseal portions of the long bones are deformed and widened (Figures 6–17 and 6–18). The histologic findings in the lesions of MHE are similar to those in solitary osteochondroma.

Conversion to chondrosarcoma is exceedingly rare in solitary osteochondroma (<1%) and occurs in adulthood. The lifetime risk of malignant transformation across all lesions in patients with MHE is higher, although the exact transformation rate is a topic of debate. It is often reported to be approximately 5%, with rates in the literature ranging from 1% to 25%. When transformation does occur, it is in the cartilaginous cap, usually in the larger proximal lesions.

Osteochondromas are stage 1 lesions. Most children with a solitary osteochondroma are asymptomatic and therefore do not require surgical treatment. In some cases, the lesion may be palpable and irritating. Surgical resection is appropriate in these cases to address the symptoms only and not as a prophylaxis for chondrosarcomatous degeneration. In MHE, symptomatic lesions are addressed surgically as needed. Corrective osteotomy is occasionally required for angular deformity. If a previously quiescent lesion begins to enlarge in an adult, it should be removed. The surgical margin should be wide enough to include the entire cartilaginous cap.

D. Chondroblastoma

The chondroblastoma is a benign cartilage-forming tumor that occurs in the epiphyses or apophyses. When it is diagnosed near or at skeletal maturity, it may expand across the physis or physeal scar. The peak incidence is during the second decade of life with a slight male predominance. The long bones are most often affected, but the patella, talus, and calcaneus are also commonly reported locations. There may be joint involvement presenting with an effusion.

Radiographically, there is sharp demarcation of a radiolucent lesion in the epiphysis with stippled or flocculent calcification. There may be erosion of the subchondral bone with collapse or pathologic fracture (Figure 6–19). There may also be a recognizable aneurysmal component. Histologically, there is a background of uniform polyhedral cells with grooved nuclei producing sparse, amorphous chondroid. The cells may be separated by a fine lace of mineralization producing a "chicken wire" appearance. Osteoclast-like giant cells and macrophages are present, especially near areas of hemorrhage or aneurismal conversion.

Although chondroblastoma presents in a younger age group than giant cell tumor, the two are comparable. Similarities include the location, radiographic appearance, and strikingly similar histologic features. They both typically present as stage 2 or 3 lesions. Also in common is the rare incidence of pulmonary metastasis. When pulmonary metastasis develops, the histology is the same, and they respond well to resection, carrying an excellent prognosis.

Treatment of chondroblastoma usually consists of intralesional curettage with margin extension and bone grafting or structural supplementation with polymethyl methacrylate. Adjuvant treatments such as phenol, liquid nitrogen, or high-speed burr may also be used. The recurrence rate is less than 10% with this form of treatment. When the subchondral bone has been destroyed or the lesion is otherwise more locally aggressive, wide resection with osteoarticular allograft reconstruction has been used with success. Transformation

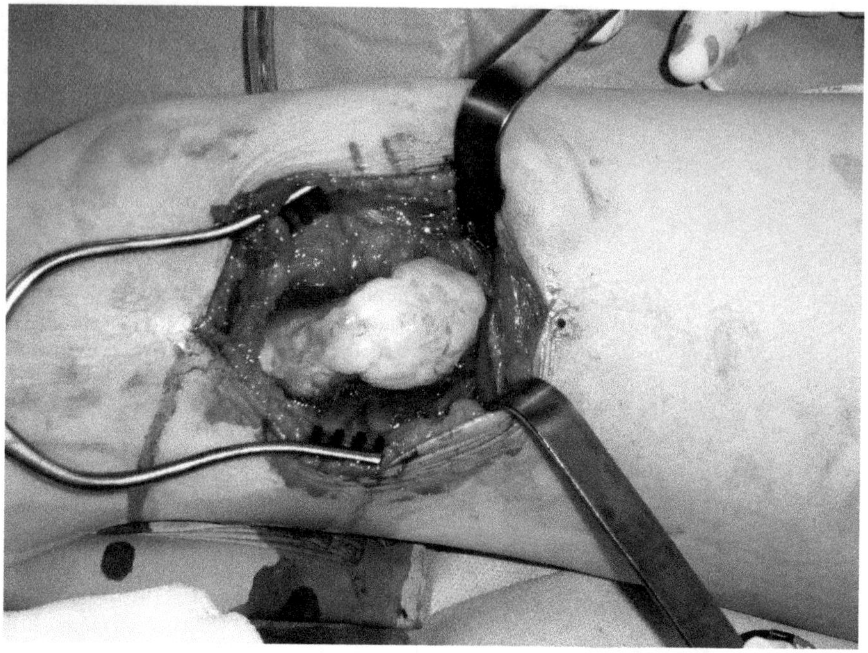

▲ **Figure 6–16.** Typical glistening white appearance of the cartilage cap seen on the same osteochondroma in Figure 6–15.

to secondary chondrosarcoma is extremely rare but occurs with increased frequency following radiation therapy.

E. Chondromyxoid Fibroma

The chondromyxoid fibroma, a very rare tumor, generally affects males in the second or third decade of life. The most common location is the proximal tibial metaphysis, followed by the distal femur and the metatarsals. The tumor is slow growing and accompanied by mild pain and symptoms.

Radiographs of chondromyxoid fibroma show a lytic tumor with sharp sclerotic margins and a pseudoloculated pattern resembling that of a bone cyst. They are eccentric in metaphyseal bone with thinning of the involved cortex (Figure 6–20). Histologic findings include a strange but specific mixture of fibrous, myxomatous, and chondroid tissues, which could mistakenly suggest the diagnosis of chondrosarcoma. There are also frequent osteoclast-like giant cells. The expression pattern of collagens seems to be unique to this entity with predominantly type II, but also types I, III, and VI.

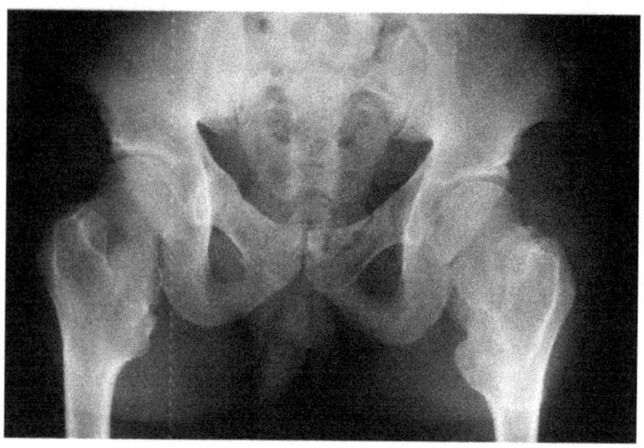

▲ **Figure 6–17.** Radiograph of multiple exostoses involving both hips.

Chondromyxoid fibroma usually presents as a stage 2 lesion and has a markedly high propensity for local recurrence. With recurrence rates approaching 25% following simple curettage and bone grafting, aggressive margin extension should be performed. The conversion of chondromyxoid fibroma to secondary chondrosarcoma is extremely rare.

Essentials of Diagnosis

- *The matrix of chondroid tumors is characterized by stippled calcification or the presence of rings and arcs of calcification.*
- *The hallmark of osteochondroma is continuity of the medullary portion of the lesion with the host bone in contrast to the periosteal chondroma, where the host cortex separates the medullary canal of the host bone from the lesion itself.*
- *Chondromyxoid fibroma is a rare lesion but may be aggressive and have a very high rate of local recurrence.*

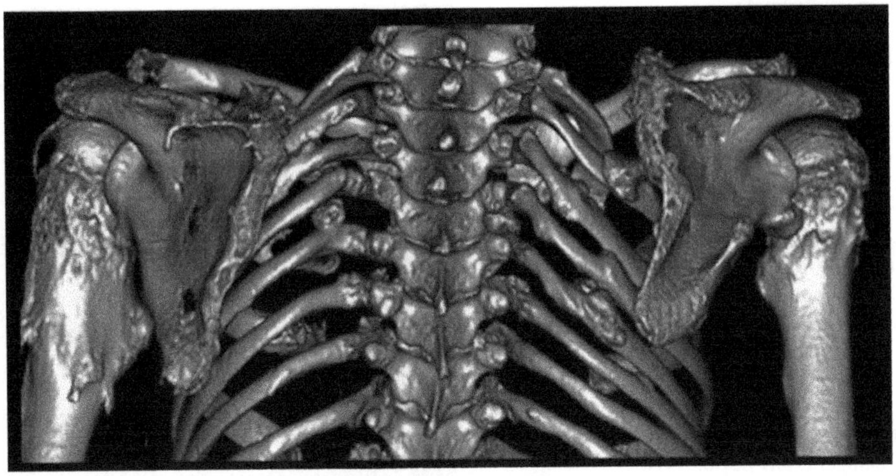

▲ **Figure 6–18.** Three-dimensional reconstructed CT scan of the bilateral shoulders and upper thorax of a skeletally immature female with hereditary multiple exostoses.

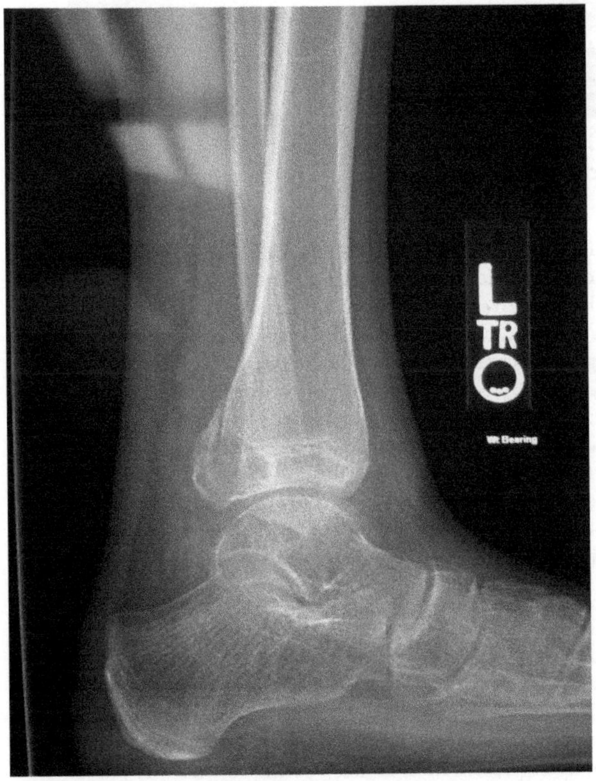

▲ **Figure 6–19.** Radiograph of a chondroblastoma in the distal tibia of a 15-year-old boy.

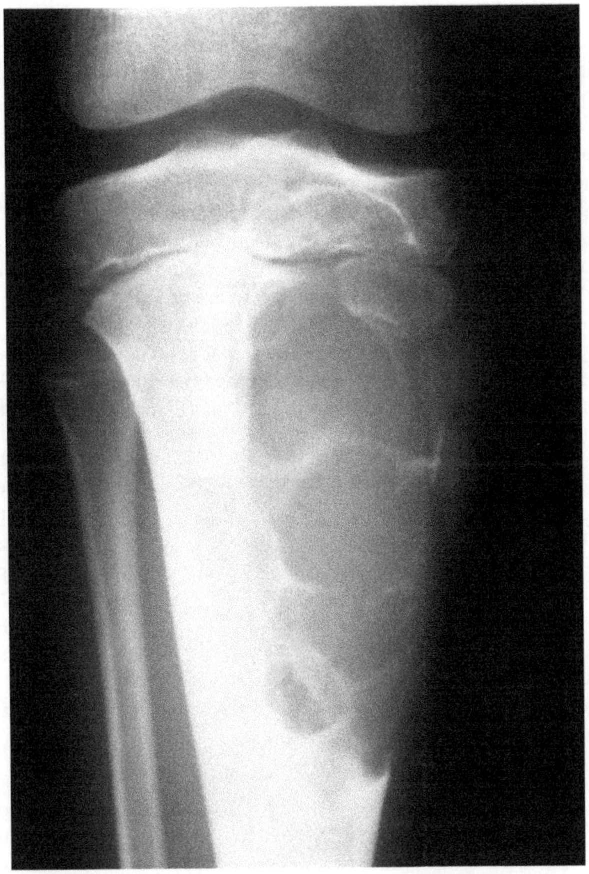

▲ **Figure 6–20.** Radiograph of a chondromyxoid fibroma in the proximal tibia of an 11-year-old boy.

Benign Fibrous Tumors of Bone

A. Fibrous Cortical Defect

Fibrous cortical defects, or cortical desmoids, are small, hamartomatous fibromas seen almost exclusively in the metaphyseal areas of the lower extremities of growing children. They can be multiple, and as many as 25% of normal children demonstrate these asymptomatic lesions at 5 years of age. The lesions tend to disappear as a result of bone remodeling before skeletal maturity. They may show increased uptake on isotope bone scans.

In the case of fibrous cortical defects, microscopic studies show benign-appearing fibroblasts in a whorled pattern with occasional histiocytes, foam cells, and benign giant cells. The radiographic appearance is so characteristic of this entity (Figure 6–21) that a biopsy is usually not necessary. These are stage 1 lesions and can generally be observed.

B. Nonossifying Fibroma

Just as the osteoblastoma is considered a larger or more extensive form of osteoid osteoma, the nonossifying fibroma is considered a larger form of the fibrous cortical defect. It is typically seen in the lower extremity of children. Because of its size, it may not entirely resolve by skeletal maturity and can persist into adult life. If the lesion is quite large, approaching 50% of the diameter of the bone, pathologic fracture may ensue. The fracture healing process may facilitate resolution of the lesion. Careful consideration to fracture prophylaxis should be reserved for large lesions in children older than 10 years. Nonossifying fibromas are stage 1 lesions, and neither they nor fibrous cortical defects require biopsy because their radiographic appearance is so characteristic.

With nonossifying fibroma, multiple lesions may take on the appearance of fibrous dysplasia and can be associated with café-au-lait skin defects. Large defects in the tibia can assume the appearance of chondromyxoid fibroma (Figure 6–22).

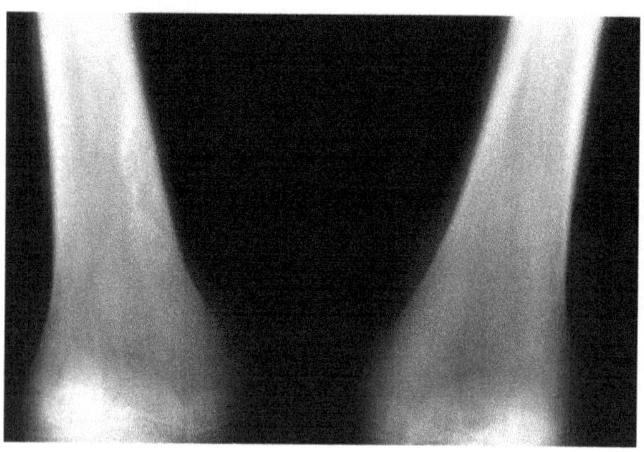

▲ **Figure 6–21.** Radiograph of a metaphyseal fibrous cortical defect in a 15-year-old boy.

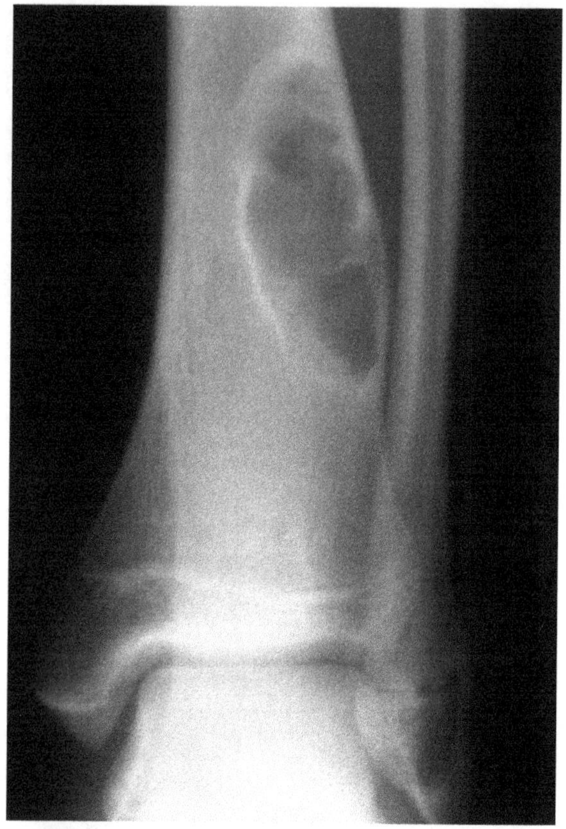

▲ **Figure 6–22.** Radiograph of a nonossifying fibroma of the distal tibia.

The lesions have a well-defined sclerotic margin with a pseudoloculated lytic center that gives them a soap-bubble radiographic appearance. Histologically, they appear identical to fibrous cortical defects and are characterized by abundant benign fibrous tissue speckled with areas of histiocytes, foam cells, and giant cells. As the lesion involutes in adulthood and the number of giant cells and histiocytes diminishes, large areas of cholesterol deposits become evident, which may suggest the diagnosis of xanthofibroma or xanthoma of bone. Nonossifying fibromas are clearly separated from fibrous dysplasia by the absence of metaplastic osteoid formation in the fibrous stroma.

C. Fibrous Dysplasia

Fibrous dysplasia can present in a variety of ways: monostotic, polyostotic, and with or without associated syndromes (Figure 6–23). Most cases are diagnosed in the first three decades and have a distinct female predilection. The monostotic presentation is more common than the polyostotic. This condition is a dysplastic anomaly of bone forming mesenchymal tissue with an inability to produce mature

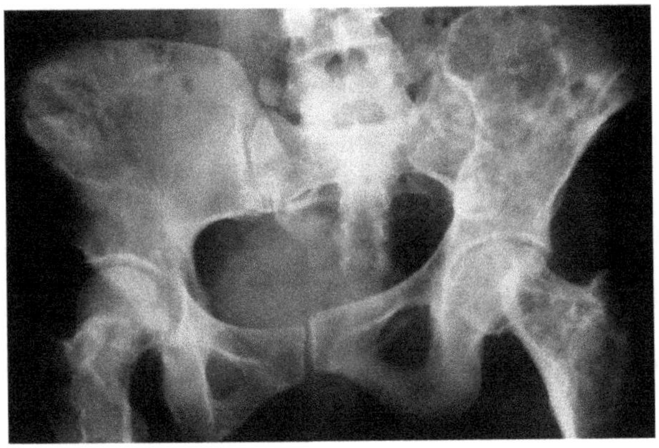

▲ **Figure 6–23.** Radiograph of polyostotic fibrous dysplasia of the pelvis.

lamellar bone. Accordingly, the bone is arrested in an immature woven state with a resultant proliferation of spindled fibroblasts. In the polyostotic form, it tends to be unilateral rather than bilateral. Nevertheless, it can involve any bone in the body. The most common location is the proximal femur where it results in the so-called shepherd's crook deformity. Other areas frequently involved include the tibia, pelvis, humerus, radius, and ribs.

In addition to bony involvement, patients can demonstrate café-au-lait skin pigmentation. These patches usually have a rough border, in contrast to the smooth border of those seen in neurofibromatosis. Patients with fibrous dysplasia may have associated endocrine problems. For example, 5% of patients with the polyostotic form of fibrous dysplasia also exhibit precocious puberty (McCune-Albright syndrome). Other associated endocrine abnormalities include hyperthyroidism, acromegaly, Cushing disease, and hypophosphatemic osteomalacia. Polyostotic fibrous dysplasia with soft-tissue myxomas is known as Mazabraud syndrome. Fibrous dysplasia can also involve the skull and jaw bones, mimicking ossifying fibroma of jaw bone.

Radiographically, fibrous dysplasia has a ground-glass appearance due to the fine mineralization pattern of the immature woven trabeculae. There is surrounding remodeling of the host bone, which is often expansile. In fibrous dysplasia, microscopic findings include an alphabet soup pattern of metaplastic woven bone scattered through a benign fibrous tissue stroma. The woven trabeculae have a characteristic absence of osteoblastic rimming. Foam cells, giant cells, and cholesterol deposits can be seen. Large cystic areas and even areas of cartilage formation are commonly present.

The molecular basis for fibrous dysplasia is associated with mutations affecting the alpha subunit of G protein. Cells of the osteoblastic lineage are affected, resulting in decreased differentiation and increased proliferation. These mutations cause constitutive elevation of cyclic adenosine monophosphate (cAMP) in fibrous dysplasia and thus alter cAMP target genes such as *c-fos*, *c-jun*, *IL-6*, and *IL-11*.

Fibrous dysplasia tends to be active during the growing years and then burns out in adult life. Less than 1% of lesions convert to osteosarcoma, fibrosarcoma, or even chondrosarcoma. If conversion does occur, it almost always happens during adulthood. Generally, this disease is either stage 1 or 2.

In pediatric patients with active disease, curettage and grafting should be avoided because of high recurrence rates. The goals in treating pediatric patients should be the prevention and treatment of deformity, especially in the lower extremity. Most cases should become quiescent with skeletal maturity. If not, the best surgical treatment in adults consists of rigid fixation with an intramedullary implant with strut grafting as needed. Medical management with bisphosphonates is of benefit in some cases. Irradiation is contraindicated because it may lead to irradiation-induced sarcoma at a later date.

Essentials of Diagnosis

- *Nonossifying fibromas/fibrous cortical defects may be present in up to one-third of the population and are usually detected incidentally.*
- *If fibrous dysplasia is suspected, a careful examination of the skin should be performed for café-au-lait spots, which are seen in McCune-Albright syndrome.*

Cystic Lesions of Bone

A. Simple Bone Cyst

Simple bone cysts are a common pseudotumor of bone and the most frequent cause of pathologic fractures in children. Bone cysts usually affect patients between 5 and 15 years of age and occur more often in boys than in girls (2:1) with an incidence of 1 per 10,000 children per year. They are found in the proximal humerus in 50% of cases and in the upper femur in 25%. The calcaneus and pelvis are also uniquely common locations. Patients are asymptomatic until a pathologic fracture occurs. The cystic process continues to grow away from the physis. When it remains in contact with the physis, it is termed "active." When it separates, it is termed "inactive."

Radiographs typically show a solitary cyst that is centrally located in the metaphyseal area and has marked thinning of the adjacent cortical bone and a pseudoloculated appearance (Figure 6–24). The bone cyst is filled with a clear serous fluid, and there is increased pressure during the active phase. The fact that this pressure gradually decreases as the cyst becomes inactive suggests a hydrodynamic mechanism. If there is associated fracture, radiographs may show the characteristic "fallen leaf" sign (Figure 6–25).

The cyst cavity, lined with a fibrinous membrane that contains giant cells, foam cells, and a slight osteoid formation, is similar to the fibrous tissues seen in other fibrous

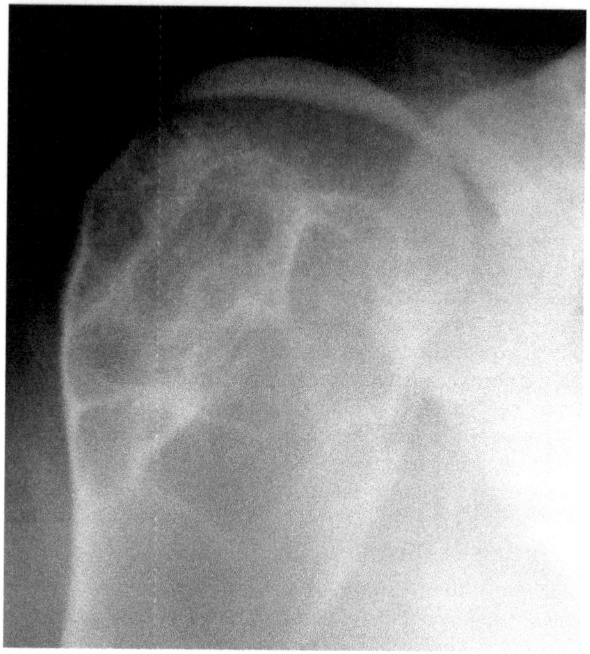

▲ **Figure 6–24.** Radiograph of a solitary bone cyst on the proximal humerus of a 13-year-old boy.

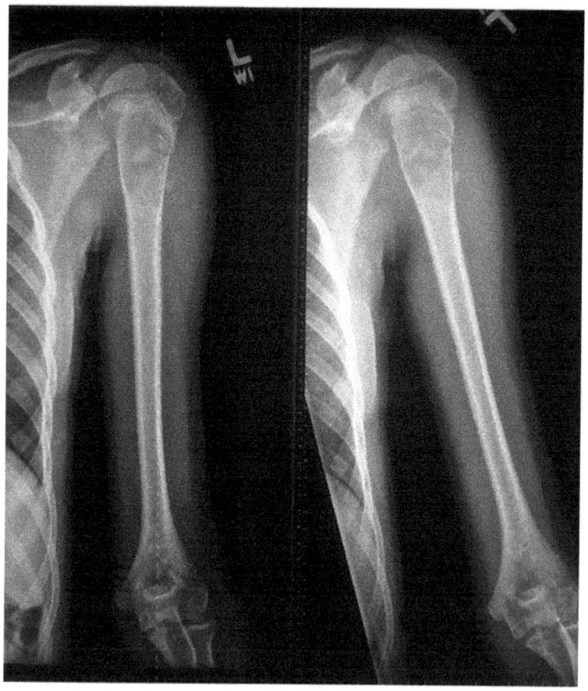

▲ **Figure 6–25.** Radiographs of a solitary bone cyst with associated pathologic fracture and a "fallen leaf" sign in a 12-year-old girl.

bone lesions, including fibrous dysplasia. The periosteal covering in the area of a cyst is normal, and thus, the pathologic fractures heal normally and in most cases do not require surgery. Unfortunately, the cyst usually persists after fracture union and requires further treatment. Bone-resorbing factors, such as matrix metalloproteinases, prostaglandins, interleukin (IL)-1, IL-6, tumor necrosis factor-alpha (TNF-α), and oxygen-free radicals, are demonstrated in the cyst fluid. Nitrate and nitrite levels are also noted to be higher than in serum.

Before the mid-1970s, the standard treatment for a solitary bone cyst was aggressive curettage or even resection followed by bone grafting. In patients with active disease, the recurrence rate was 30% to 50%, and repeated grafting was frequently necessary. In patients with inactive disease, particularly those older than 15 years, the surgical results were much better and the recurrence rate was lower. Unicameral bone cysts are generally considered stage 1 lesions, but occasionally, they may be stage 2. Currently, treatment is a function of location. In weight-bearing bones, such as the proximal femur, lesions should be treated aggressively. Initial management usually involves aspiration/injection with either bone marrow or corticosteroid. The injections are carried out with bone biopsy needles and are repeated three to five times at intervals of 2 to 3 months, depending on the radiographic response. The best results are when the patient is between 5 and 15 years of age, at which time the disease is active and macrophage activity is greatest in the cyst lining. Curettage and bone grafting may also be an effective modality. Demineralized bone matrix injected in combination with autogenous bone marrow shows encouraging results, with a relatively low recurrence rate and low morbidity.

Physicians should note that sarcomas can take on the radiographic appearance of a solitary bone cyst. For this reason, if needle aspiration does not reveal cystic fluid or if it is impossible to inject contrast material and obtain radiologic confirmation of the diagnosis, an open biopsy is indicated to rule out a sarcoma.

B. Aneurysmal Bone Cyst

Aneurysmal bone cyst is a hemorrhagic lesion with many characteristics of a giant cell tumor but occurs only half as frequently. Although 75% of the cases of aneurysmal bone cyst occur in patients aged 10 to 20 years old, giant cell tumor is rare in patients younger than 20 years of age. Both aneurysmal bone cyst and giant cell tumor are more common in females than in males. The femur is the most frequently affected site, followed by the tibia, pelvis, and spine. In the spine, two-thirds of aneurysmal bone cysts arise from the posterior elements, and one-third arise from the vertebral body.

Initially, the aneurysmal bone cyst appears on radiograph as an aggressive osteolytic lesion with extensive permeative cortical destruction that gives the impression of a malignant process such as Ewing sarcoma or telangiectatic osteosarcoma. Next, a large aneurysmal bulge occurs outside the bone, with a thin reactive shell of bone forming at the outer

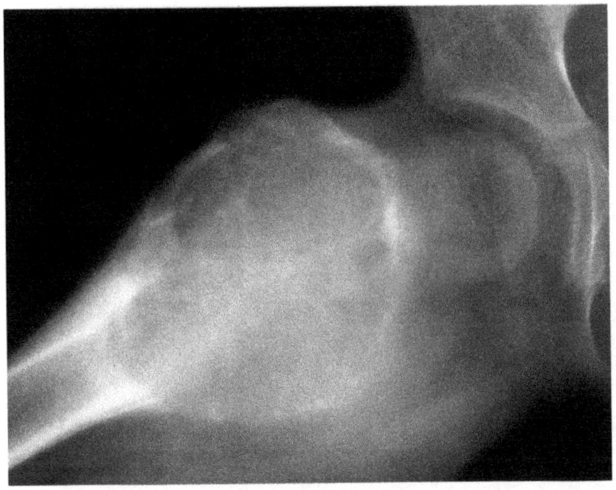

▲ **Figure 6–26.** Radiograph of an aneurysmal bone cyst on the proximal femur of a 5-year-old boy.

edge. Less soap-bubbly pseudoseptation is seen in an aneurysmal bone cyst than in a solitary bone cyst (Figure 6–26). MRI demonstrates multiple fluid-fluid levels representing the separation of blood components and often shows a soft-tissue component to the lesion.

At the time of biopsy, the aneurysmal bone lesion demonstrates large hemorrhagic cysts, but bleeding is modest. The hemorrhagic cysts are broken up by thick spongy fibrous septae that histologically contain great numbers of large giant cells and have thin osteoid seams. Even if a few mitotic figures are seen, the diagnosis of a benign lesion can remain. A carefully placed biopsy with multiple samples is needed to rule out other well-known skeletal tumors that may demonstrate an aneurysmal component. These include giant cell tumor, chondromyxoid fibroma, and telangiectatic osteosarcoma. Some believe there is no such entity as the aneurysmal bone cyst and that it is merely a morphologic variant of some other underlying neoplastic process. Like the solitary bone cyst, this cyst may have a hydraulic pressure origin that is secondary to hemorrhage and could be traumatically induced. However, abnormal cytogenetic findings were noted in aneurysmal bone cysts, which may suggest a distinct cellular pathogenetic etiology. Specifically, a t(16;17) translocation resulting in a *CDH11-USP6* fusion gene product is frequently observed in aneurismal bone cyst. Aneurysmal bone cyst is either a stage 2 or 3 lesion and frequently symptomatic.

If an aneurysmal bone cyst is left untreated, it may involute spontaneously, during which time it develops a heavy shell of reactive bone at the periphery. Surgical treatment is often required and entails aggressive curettage with local adjuvants such as phenol, high-speed burr, argon beam, or liquid nitrogen, followed by reconstruction with bone graft of polymethyl methacrylate. En bloc resection may be required in some cases. Radiation is no longer recommended. Another option for treating extremely large lesions is repeated embolization to reduce the rate of hemorrhagic expansion. Less invasive treatment such as systemic bisphosphonate or denosumab therapy and percutaneous doxycycline injection are under investigation.

C. Epidermoid Cyst

The least common bone cyst is the epidermoid bone cyst. This lesion is found either in the distal phalanx or in the skull. No other bone is affected. In the case of the phalanx, the cyst is usually the result of nail bed epithelium being driven into the distal phalanx by a crushing blow. The ectopic squamous epithelium produces a keratinized cavity that is filled with clear fluid and creates surface erosion with a sclerotic reactive base (Figure 6–27). The bulbous cyst seen at the fingertip transilluminates with flashlight examination. Other conditions that might have a similar appearance are the glomus tumor and the enchondroma. The epidermoid cyst is treated with a simple curettage and, in some cases, a bone graft.

Essentials of Diagnosis

- *In the treatment of solitary bone cysts, there is a significant rate of recurrence, but the cysts will usually resolve with skeletal maturity.*
- *If an aneurysmal bone cyst is suspected in the differential diagnosis prior to biopsy, then a telangiectatic osteosarcoma should also be considered.*

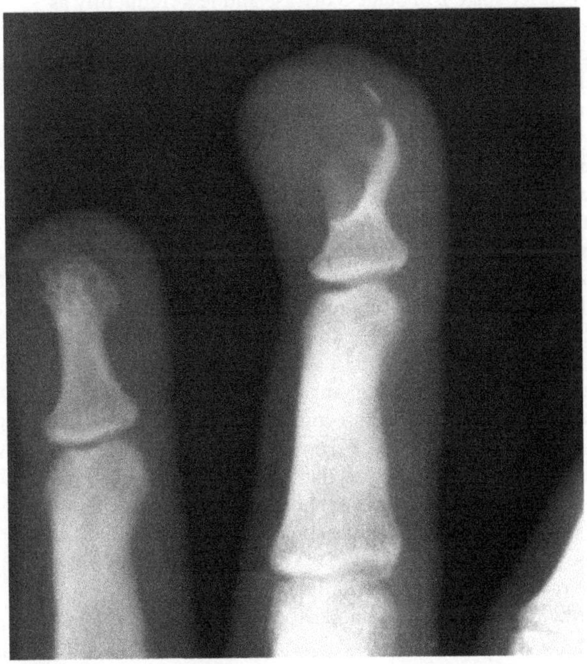

▲ **Figure 6–27.** Radiograph of an epidermoid cyst in the distal phalanx.

Giant Cell Tumor of Bone

Numerous types of tumors contain giant cells but are not true benign giant cell tumors of bone. Most of the variants are seen in children and include aneurysmal bone cyst, chondroblastoma, simple bone cyst, osteoid osteoma, and osteoblastoma. The giant cell–rich osteosarcoma is the most malignant of the variants, and it is sometimes difficult to distinguish from an aggressive benign giant cell tumor. The giant cell reparative granuloma is a benign variant seen in jaw bones or hand bones and has more spindle cells than a classic giant cell tumor. Only after all of the variant conditions are excluded can the diagnosis of benign giant cell tumor be made. Giant cell tumor of bone is associated with an imbalance in the receptor activator of nuclear factor kappa B/ receptor activator of nuclear factor kappa B ligand (RANK/ RANKL) system, which is normally associated with osteoclastogenesis. Specific gene mutations in the *H3F3A* histone gene have been identified and may assist with differentiating giant cell tumor of bone from its many variants.

Between 5% and 10% of all benign bone tumors are true giant cell tumors, occurring most frequently in the third decade of life. They are more frequently found in females than in males. In approximately half of the cases, the tumor is found about the knee. The next most common locations are the distal radius and the sacrum. The tumor is usually painful for several months prior to diagnosis and can cause a pathologic fracture. It can also cause a painful effusion because of its juxtaposition to a major joint. Giant cell tumors may present as either stage 2 or stage 3 disease and less frequently as stage 1. On radiograph, the lesion appears lytic in nature and is located in the epiphyseal-metaphyseal end of a long bone (Figure 6–28). The lesion grows toward the joint surface and frequently comes into contact with articular cartilage but rarely breaks into the joint.

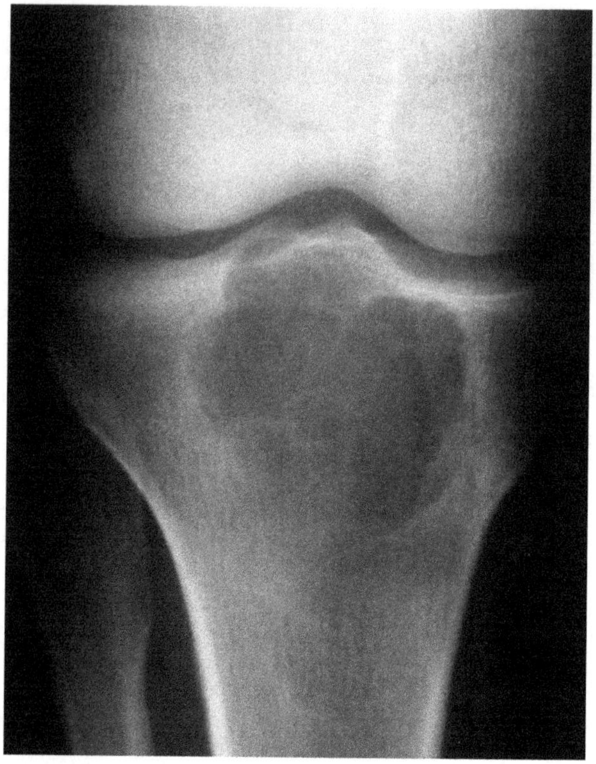

▲ **Figure 6–28.** Radiograph of a giant cell tumor on the proximal tibia of a 22-year-old woman.

Like the chondroblastoma, the benign giant cell tumor has a 1% to 2% chance of metastasizing to the lung, and recurrent tumors have up to a 10% chance. Accordingly, pulmonary staging is an important component in the initial evaluation and follow-up of giant cell tumor of bone. The prognosis for survival with this complication is favorable, and the tumors may resolve spontaneously. The benign giant cell tumor can later convert to a malignant condition such as an osteosarcoma or malignant fibrous histiocytoma. It is generally believed that this is secondary to treatment. A conversion rate of 15% to 20% is reported in patients who were treated previously with more than 3000 cGy of radiation, with conversion occurring 3 or more years after treatment. The conversion rate in patients who do not receive radiation is less than 5%. This finding has come into question with newer radiation therapy modalities.

Until recent years, the standard treatment for giant cell tumor was curettage and bone grafting. The recurrence rate with this treatment was reported to be up to more than 50%. Follow-up treatment consisted of an aggressive resection of the lesion and reconstruction with a large osteoarticular allograft, endoprosthesis, or an excisional arthrodesis. Currently, most surgeons elect for an aggressive curettage, followed by high-speed burring and adjuvant phenol, hydrogen peroxide, or liquid nitrogen and by subsequent packing of the defect with bone cement. With this new approach, the recurrence rate is between 10% and 25%. When giant cell tumor infrequently involves an expendable bone, such as the fibula or ilium, it should be primarily resected. En bloc resection continues to be used to treat multiple recurrent tumors, intensive soft-tissue involvement, or massively destructive cases. Embolization may also prove palliative or curative in unresectable cases. Systemic denosumab therapy for giant cell is under investigation but remains controversial. Close follow-up for locally recurrent disease and pulmonary involvement is critical. Surveillance should include a plain chest radiograph every 6 to 12 months for the first 2 to 3 years at least.

Hemangioma

Hemangioma of bone is a hamartomatous process that occurs more frequently in females than in males. It is most commonly found in vertebral bodies. It is found only rarely in the diaphysis of a long bone (Figure 6–29). Hemangiomas

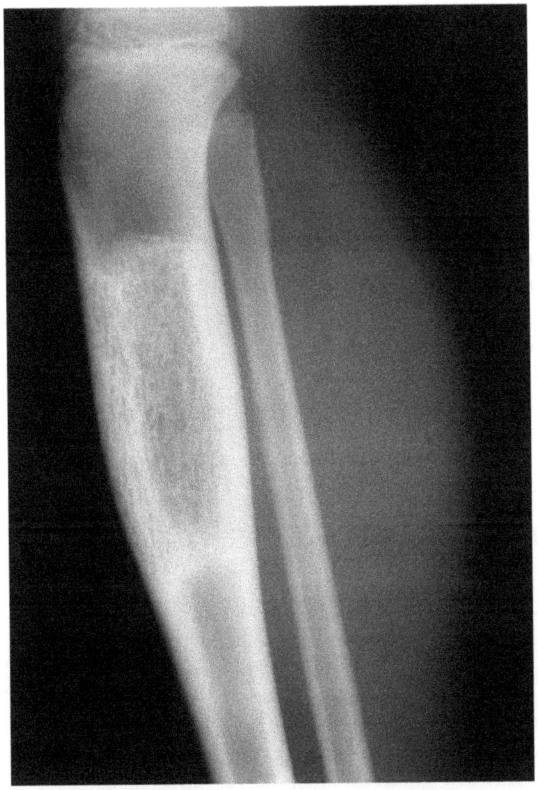

▲ **Figure 6–29.** Radiograph of a hemangioma of the tibia in a 14-year-old boy.

of bone can be associated with hemangiomas of soft tissue. The spinal lesion is usually discovered as an incidental radiographic finding and demonstrates a characteristic vertically oriented honeycombed or moth-eaten appearance. On rare occasions, a lesion can cause cord compression that may require surgical resection. In such cases, preoperative angiography is critical in evaluating the blood supply to the spinal cord. Alternatively, an attempt at arterial embolization may prove successful and is less aggressive.

Gorham disease, characterized by massive osteolysis in children or young adults, is usually associated with the presence of benign cavernous hemangiomas or lymphangiomas of bone. This strange condition usually affects a particular area (such as the spine or the hip) but can involve multiple bones of the area and tends to resolve spontaneously (Figure 6–30).

Essentials of Diagnosis

- *Plain radiography is usually diagnostic, and advanced imaging is usually not required except for preoperative planning in benign bone lesions.*
- *Surgical treatment of most benign bone tumors is reserved for symptomatic lesions unresponsive to conservative measures, those at significant risk of fracture, or for documented enlargement over time.*
- *Giant cell tumor of bone and chondroblastoma both have an incidence of pulmonary seeding, and chest imaging should be included in the workup and surveillance of these entities.*

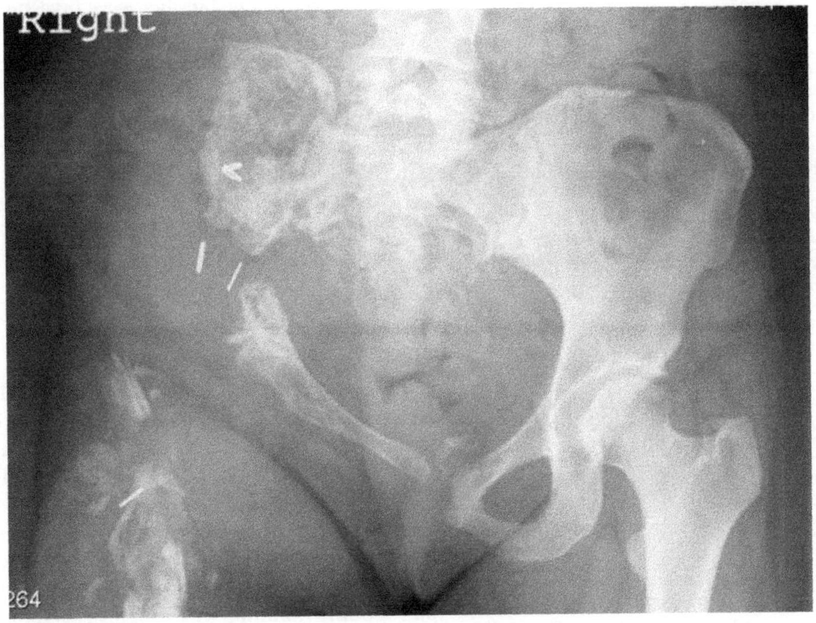

▲ **Figure 6–30.** Radiograph of a pelvis affected with Gorham disease in a 48-year-old woman.

Agyeman K, Pretell-Mazzini J, Subhawong R, et al. Gorham disease. *Am J Orthop.* 2017;46(6):E458-E462. [PMID: 29309464]

Atesok KI, Alman BA, Schemitsch EH, et al. Osteoid osteoma and osteoblastoma. *J Am Acad Orthop Surg.* 2011;11:678-689. [PMID: 22052644]

Behjati S, Tarpey PS, Presneau N, et al. Distinct H3F3A and H3F3B driver mutations define chondroblastoma and giant cell tumor of bone. *Nat Genet.* 2013;45(12):1479. [PMID: 24162739]

Bousson V, Rey-Jouvin C, Laredo JD, et al. Fibrous dysplasia and McCune–Albright syndrome: imaging for positive and differential diagnoses, prognosis, and follow-up guidelines. *Eur J Radiol.* 2014;83(10):1828-1842. [PMID: 25043984]

Czajka CM, DiCaprio MR. What is the proportion of patients with multiple hereditary exostoses who undergo malignant degeneration? *Clin Orthop Relat Res.* 2015;473(7):2355-2361. [PMID: 25582066]

Montgomery C, Couch C, Emory CL, Nicholas R. Giant cell tumor of bone: review of current literature, evaluation, and treatment options. *J Knee Surg.* 2019;32(4):331-336. [PMID: 30449024]

Muthusamy S, Conway SA, Temple HT. Five polyostotic conditions that general orthopedic surgeons should recognize (or should not miss). *Orthop Clin North Am.* 2014;45(3):417-429. [PMID: 24975767]

Noordin S, Allana S, Umer M, et al, Unicameral bone cysts: current concepts. *Ann Med Surg.* 2018;34:43-49. [PMID: 30224948]

Park HY, Yang SK, Sheppard WL, et al. Current management of aneurysmal bone cysts. *Curr Rev Muscoloskelt Med.* 2016;9(4):435-444. [PMID: 27778155]

Puri A, Gulia A, Hegde P, et al. Neoadjuvant denosumab: its role and results in operable cases of giant cell tumour of bone. *Bone Joint J.* 2019;101(2):170-177. [PMID: 30700112]

Riddle ND, Bui MM. Fibrous dysplasia. *Arch Pathol Lab Med.* 2013;137(1):134-138. [PMID: 23276185]

Romeo S, Hogendoorn PC, Dei Tos AP. Benign cartilaginous tumors of bone: from morphology to somatic and germline genetics. *Adv Anat Path.* 2009;16(5):307-315. [PMID: 19700940]

Sampath Kumar V, Tyrrell PN, Singh J, et al. Surveillance of intramedullary cartilage tumours in long bones. *Bone Joint J.* 2016;98(11):1542-1547. [PMID: 27803232]

Scholfield DW, Sadozai Z, Ghali C, et al. Does osteofibrous dysplasia progress to adamantinoma and how should they be treated? *Bone Joint J.* 2017;99(3):409-416. [PMID: 28249983]

Shields DW, Sohrabi S, Crane EO, et al. Radiofrequency ablation for osteoid osteoma: recurrence rates and predictive factors. *Surgeon.* 2018;16(3):156-162. [PMID: 28807571]

Wang B, Han SB, Jiang L, et al. Percutaneous radiofrequency ablation for spinal osteoid osteoma and osteoblastoma. *Eur Spine J.* 2017;26(7):1884-1892. [PMID: 28391383]

Traub F, Eberhardt O, Fernandez FF, Wirth T. Solitary bone cyst: a comparison of treatment options with special reference to their long-term outcome. *BMC Musculoskelet Disord.* 2016;17(1):162. [PMID: 27075249]

Xu H, Nugent D, Monforte HL, et al. Chondroblastoma of bone in the extremities: a multicenter retrospective study. *J Bone Joint Surg Am.* 2015;97(11):925-931. [PMID: 26041854]

MALIGNANT BONE TUMORS

Malignant bone tumors are primarily treated with wide resection followed by limb salvage surgery in current treatment regimens. Depending on the histology, this is augmented with the use of adjuvant chemotherapy or radiation therapy or both. Limb salvage surgery has been advanced significantly in the past two decades with improvements in megaprostheses and techniques associated with the use of allografts. Recent series report survival of megaprostheses about the knee of 80% to 90% and 60% to 80% at 5 and 10 years, respectively. Newer methods of fixation of megaprostheses are showing promising results for long-term survival and ease of revision surgery.

Allograft reconstruction continues to be useful but is used less frequently in the reconstruction of a major weight-bearing joint and is now primarily used in metadiaphyseal reconstructions.

Osteoid-Forming Sarcomas

Aside from multiple myeloma, osteosarcoma of bone is the most common primary malignant tumor of bone, constituting 20% of all primary malignancies of bone. In the United States, between 500 and 1000 new cases are diagnosed each year. The global incidence is felt to be between 1 and 3 per million people annually. There are currently many subtypes of osteoid-forming sarcomas, ranging from the extremely low-grade variants, such as parosteal osteosarcoma, to the extremely high-grade variants, such as osteosarcoma secondary to Paget disease.

The molecular pathobiology is a subject of intense investigation. Several gene families were investigated as potential biomarkers of disease progression. Among these are genes involved with angiogenesis (eg, vascular endothelial growth factor [VEGF]), growth factors and their receptors (eg, transforming growth factor beta, Wnt receptor LRP5, *HER2*), cytoskeletal protein (eg, ezrin), and cellular senescent protein (ie, telomerase).

This discussion begins with the more common, central form of sarcoma that is seen in children and known as classic osteosarcoma.

A. Classic Osteosarcoma

The classic form of osteosarcoma is typically seen in patients in their second or third decade, with a peak in the adolescent growth spurt. It occurs more frequently in males than in females and is found in the metaphyseal areas of long bones, with 50% of lesions about the knee joint (Figures 6–31 and 6–32). The distal femur is the most common site, followed by the proximal tibia and then the proximal humerus. It is rare to see osteosarcoma in the small bones of the feet and hands or in the spine. When seen in the foot, it occurs in the larger bones of the hindfoot. The prognosis is more favorable for a tumor in a small bone than for one in a large bone.

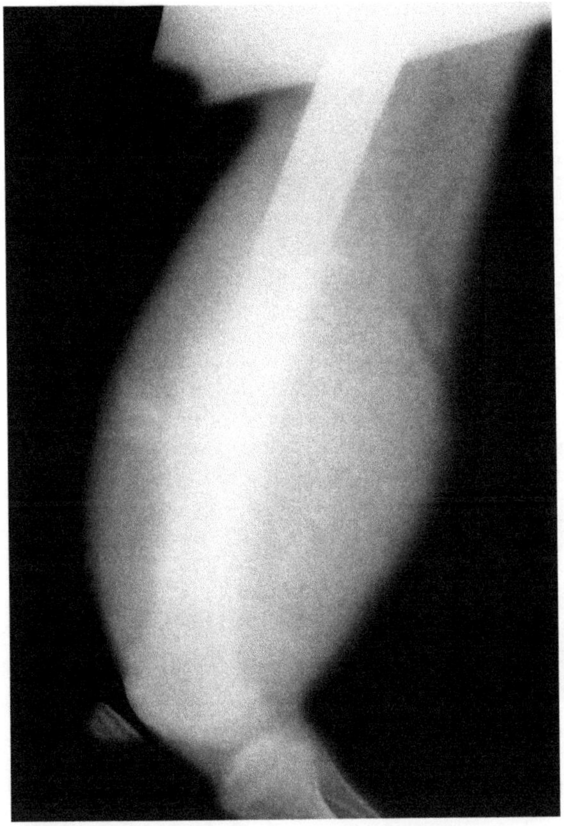

▲ **Figure 6–31.** Osteosarcoma of the distal femur of a 15-year-old female patient. Notice the sunburst appearance.

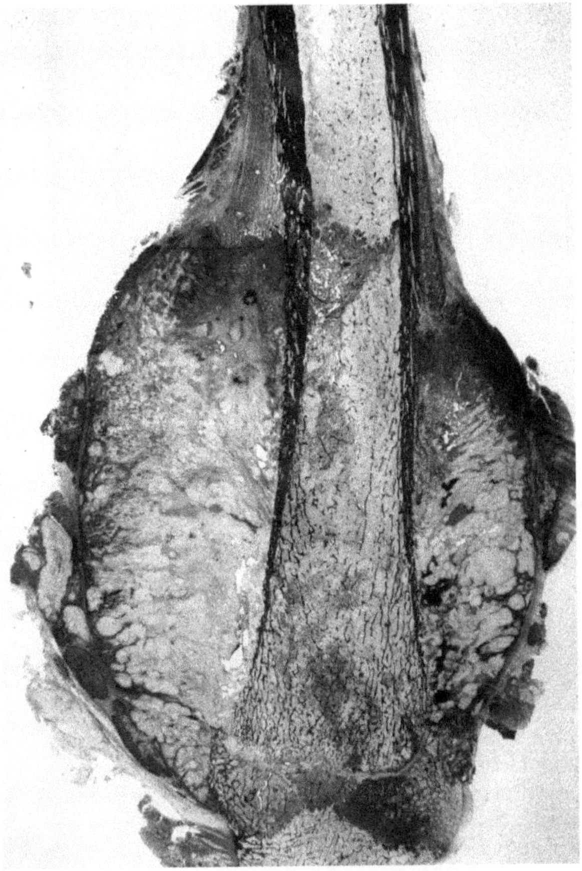

▲ **Figure 6–32.** Gross surgical specimen from Figure 6–31. Notice the sharp upper medullary margin located about the same level as the extracortical mass. The tumor has not invaded the growth plate.

Most patients with classic osteosarcoma have symptoms of pain before a tumor is noticeable. A mass near a major joint may exist for several weeks or even months before a diagnosis is made. Dilated veins may be seen in the overlying skin. The radiographic findings include permeated lytic destruction of metaphyseal bone, with eventual cortical breakthrough into the subperiosteal space and subsequent formation of a Codman triangle at the diaphyseal end of the tumor (Figure 6–33). As the tumor continues to push its way into the extracortical soft tissue, a typical sunburst pattern of neoplastic bone may be seen outside the involved bone.

In approximately 2% to 25% of cases, an additional lesion may be found at a higher level in the femur. These skip lesions may portend a worse probability of survival and should be considered a true metastatic focus. Approximately 50% of osteosarcomas are of the more typical osteoblastic type, followed by chondroblastic, with a small percentage of them fibroblastic. Whether the subtype portends a better or worse prognosis is controversial. Confounding variables such as multidrug resistance (P-glycoprotein expression) may be differentially expressed in different subtypes. P-glycoprotein overexpression itself bears a substantial relationship to clinical outcome. More recently, higher serum VEGF levels as a presumed surrogate marker for higher levels of tumor VEGF production have been associated with increased risk of developing osteosarcoma as well as poorer survival.

Staging of osteosarcoma must include an MRI of the entire involved bone (Figure 6–34). This technique offers excellent visualization of the extracortical portion of the tumor as well as excellent intramedullary contrast of the high-signal tumor next to a low-signal fatty marrow. The periphery of the tumor can be readily appreciated and represents the most anaplastic and rapidly growing region. This region represents the best target for a biopsy because it is easy to reach, soft enough for a diagnostic frozen section, and representative of the most aggressive portion of the tumor. Furthermore, MRI provides the necessary anatomic data to determine the level of transection through the host bone for

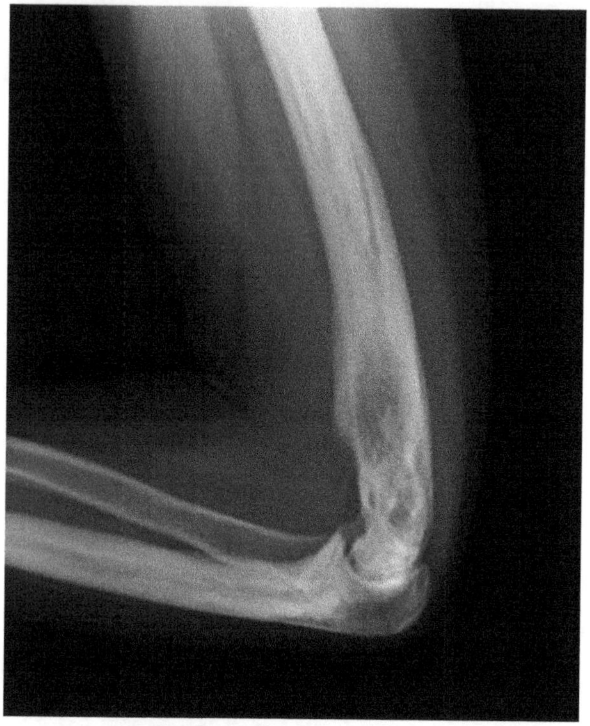

▲ **Figure 6–33.** Radiograph of the elbow of a 16-year-old patient who carries diagnoses of hereditary retinoblastoma and melorheostosis. Increasing elbow pain and the anterior diaphyseal Codman triangle were the presentation of an underlying osteosarcoma.

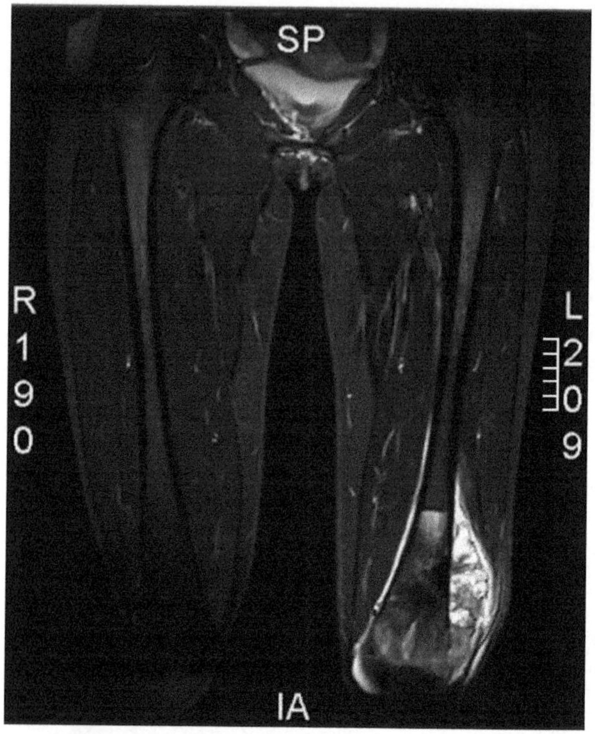

▲ **Figure 6–34.** Short tau inversion recovery sequence MRI of osteosarcoma of the femur of a 19-year-old woman.

a safe margin and to determine whether a limb-sparing procedure is feasible.

Before the advent of adjuvant multidrug chemotherapy, the treatment of osteosarcoma was radical amputation. Eighty percent of these patients proceeded to die from disseminated pulmonary disease. Today, with the combination of chemotherapy and surgical treatment, the prognosis for 5-year survival is 70% to 80%.

The drugs commonly used today include high-dose methotrexate, doxorubicin, cisplatin, and ifosfamide. The use of interferon in high-grade osteosarcoma is an area of active investigation. Neoadjuvant chemotherapy is administered intravenously in cyclic intervals of 3 to 4 weeks for approximately 11 to 15 weeks prior to surgery. Surveillance imaging studies are performed during this period to assess possible reduction in tumor volume. Tumor necrosis secondary to neoadjuvant chemotherapy, determined at the time of tumor resection, is an important prognostic factor. In a recent study, tumor necrosis of 90% or greater with margins greater than 2 mm was associated with 98% 5-year survival, whereas necrosis of less than 90% with margins of 2 mm or less was associated with 76% survival. Furthermore, the postoperative drug regimen can be adjusted based on evaluation of percent necrosis.

In osteosarcoma of the extremities, limb-sparing surgery with wide resection of the tumor is the standard approach. Amputation is reserved for the exceptional or recurrent case. In fewer than 10% of cases, amputation is performed at a level approximately 5 cm above the upper pole of the tumor. Limb salvage techniques include reconstruction options using large prostheses, structural allografts, and composite reconstructions. Endoprosthetics are composed of modular components in various lengths, linked together with taper fittings (Figures 6–35 and 6–36). The intramedullary stems are of various diameters and lengths and are usually cemented. Endoprosthesis failure rate varies according to anatomic location, with recent data demonstrating 16% failure for proximal femoral replacements to 43% for combined distal femoral-proximal tibial replacement. Soft-tissue failure, aseptic loosening, and structural failure compose mechanical modes of failure, whereas nonmechanical modes include infection and tumor progression. Infection is the most common cause of failure in tumor endoprostheses. Newer methods of fixation of megaendoprosthetics are showing promising results. Another limb-sparing procedure consists of the use of an osteoarticular allograft alone or in combination with a

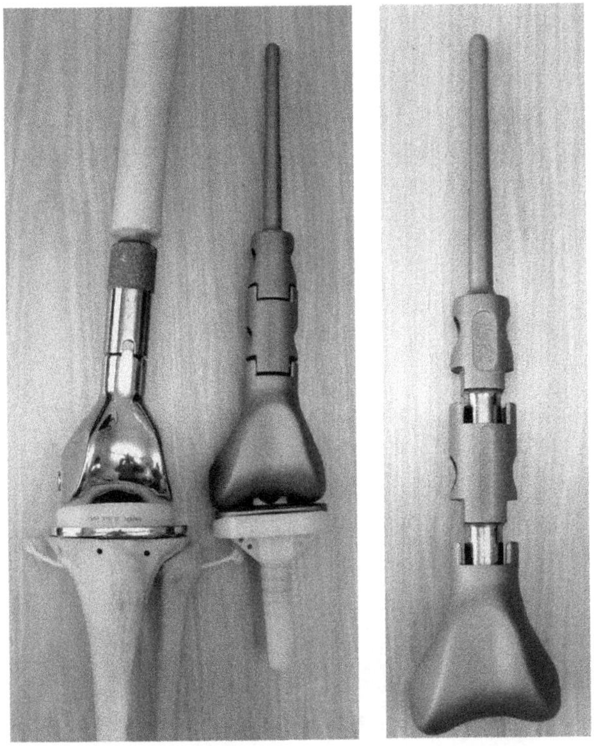

A B

▲ **Figure 6–35.** (**A**) Two examples of distal femoral replacement systems. (**B**) Modularity of system allows different-size intercalary body segments.

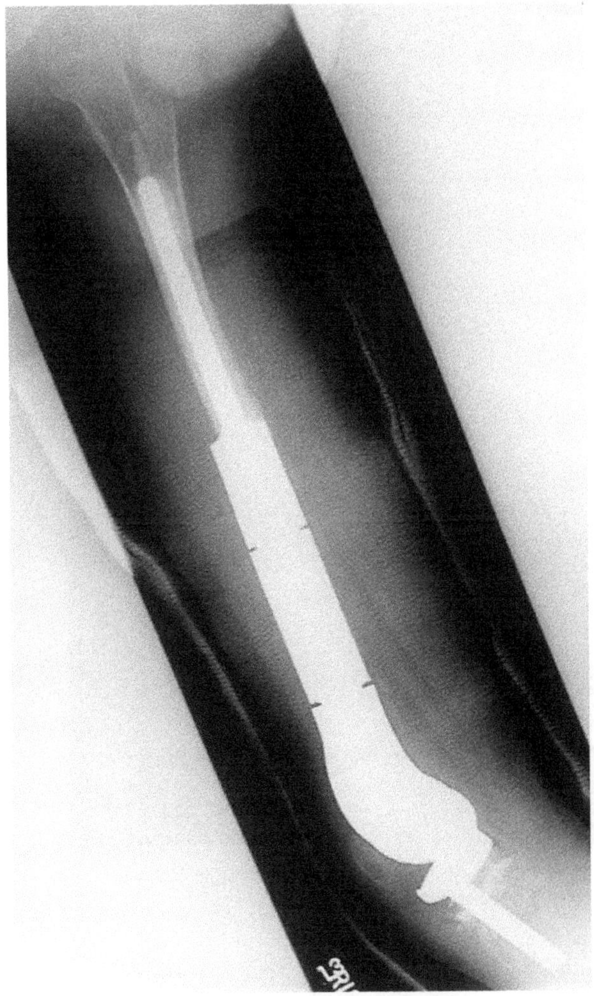

▲ **Figure 6–36.** Lateral radiograph of distal femoral replacement system in a skeletally immature patient. Expansion with larger intercalary body segment is possible.

prosthesis. The major drawback with large bone allografts is a 10% to 15% chance of infection, nonunion, or stress fracture, especially in the immunosuppressed patient receiving chemotherapy. Recent data comparing the failure of osteoarticular allografts and endoprostheses suggest that infection rates may be higher in allografts than endoprostheses. The use of an excisional arthrodesis was more popular in the past but is rarely employed today because patients have better function with a mobile joint.

Prior to the introduction of chemotherapy, the finding of pulmonary metastasis portended a poor prognosis. Today, however, in larger tumor centers where aggressive surgical approaches with multiple thoracotomies and continued chemotherapy are used, the 5-year survival rate is approximately 30%. Patients with skeletal metastases, or so-called metachronous osteosarcoma, have a significantly worse prognosis. The exception to this is a solitary, resectable metastasis.

Molecular oncologic evaluation of osteosarcoma specimens is beginning to elucidate factors involved in its pathogenesis. The *p53* suppressor genes have an increased mutation rate in osteosarcoma. Osteosarcomas with a mutation in the *p53* gene have a significantly higher rate of genomic instability, including multiple duplicate chromosomes and frequent hyperdiploid state. However, wild-type *TP53* and *MDM2* in and of themselves are not of prognostic value. Loss of heterozygosity of the *Rb* gene is a predictive feature of osteosarcoma. The *F33* isoform also demonstrates a strong correlation with osteosarcoma disease progression. *ErbB-2* (*HER2/neu*), a protooncogene, and transforming growth factor-beta, isoform 3 expression is also correlated with a worse prognosis in osteosarcoma patients. Controversy surrounds the significance of cytoplasmic versus membranous staining in *HER2/neu* expression as it relates to prognosis in osteosarcoma.

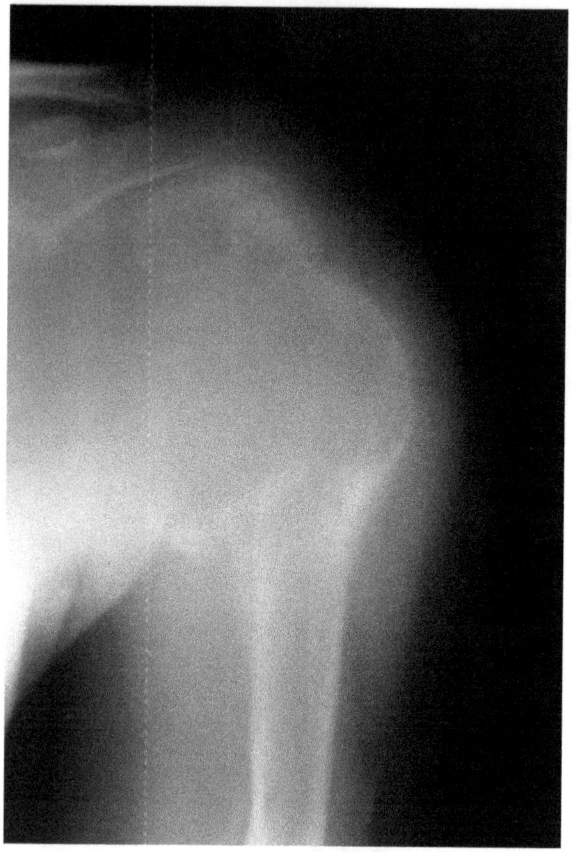

▲ **Figure 6–37.** Radiograph of hemorrhagic osteosarcoma in a 6-year-old girl.

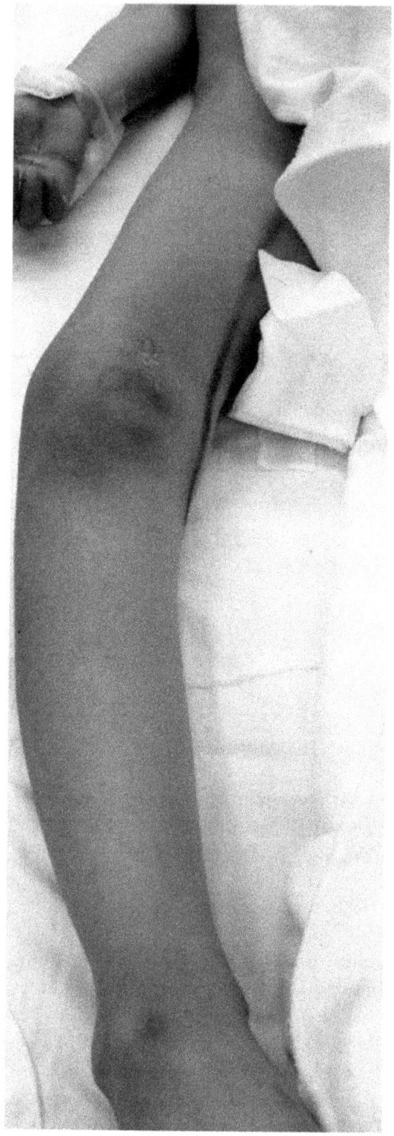

▲ **Figure 6–38.** Clinical photograph of patient who sustained pathologic fracture through a distal femoral osteosarcoma contaminating the neurovascular structures precluding limb salvage.

B. Hemorrhagic or Telangiectatic Osteosarcoma

Telangiectatic osteosarcoma, an extremely lytic and destructive variant of classic osteosarcoma, is seen in the same age group and location. Its radiographic appearance is similar to that of an aneurysmal bone cyst, thereby making the diagnosis difficult (Figure 6–37). The pathologic specimen is hemorrhagic, with microscopic evaluation demonstrating the presence of malignant-appearing stromal cells with giant cells.

Because hemorrhagic osteosarcoma is a high-grade, purely lytic tumor, the incidence of pathologic fracture in the early course of the disease is high. If significant contamination of the adjacent neurovascular structures results, a pathologic fracture may necessitate amputation rather than limb salvage (Figure 6–38). This situation must be carefully evaluated with a preoperative MRI. Accordingly, in cases with significant risk for fracture during the preoperative treatment regimen, it may be appropriate to immobilize the involved extremity or proceed with limb-sparing surgery earlier than usual. Prior to the advent of aggressive multidrug chemotherapy, the prognosis for patients with hemorrhagic osteosarcoma was extremely poor. At present, however, it is the same as the prognosis for patients who have classic osteosarcoma and is treated with similar protocols.

C. Parosteal Osteosarcoma

Parosteal osteosarcoma is a low-grade variant arising in an exophytic pattern from the cortical surface of bone. There is no medullary involvement. It is low grade, with a 5-year survival rate in excess of 90% and a 10-year survival rate over 80%. It accounts for 3% to 4% of all osteosarcomas.

The tumor is composed of a spindle cell fibroblastic component with well-developed bone trabeculae. There also may be areas of cartilage present. Osteoblasts are well differentiated, and few mitotic figures are present.

Parosteal osteosarcoma is more common in females than in males and affects a slightly older age group than classic osteosarcoma (see Table 6–2). It is a slow-growing tumor with minimal symptoms initially. It is metaphyseal in origin, with the vast majority of cases involving the posterior aspect of the distal femur (Figure 6–39).

Because the parosteal osteosarcoma is low grade, it does not respond well to either chemotherapy or radiation therapy. Therefore, the only treatment is wide surgical resection. This usually requires distal femur resection. In select cases, limited resection of the posterior cortex and tumor may be feasible, sparing the knee joint. Nevertheless, achieving negative tumor margins is imperative. Otherwise, recurrence is likely. Recurrence may occur as late as 5 to 10 years because of the tumor's slow growth.

On occasion, low-grade parosteal osteosarcoma can dedifferentiate into a high-grade sarcoma. Such a lesion carries a similar prognosis to classic osteosarcoma.

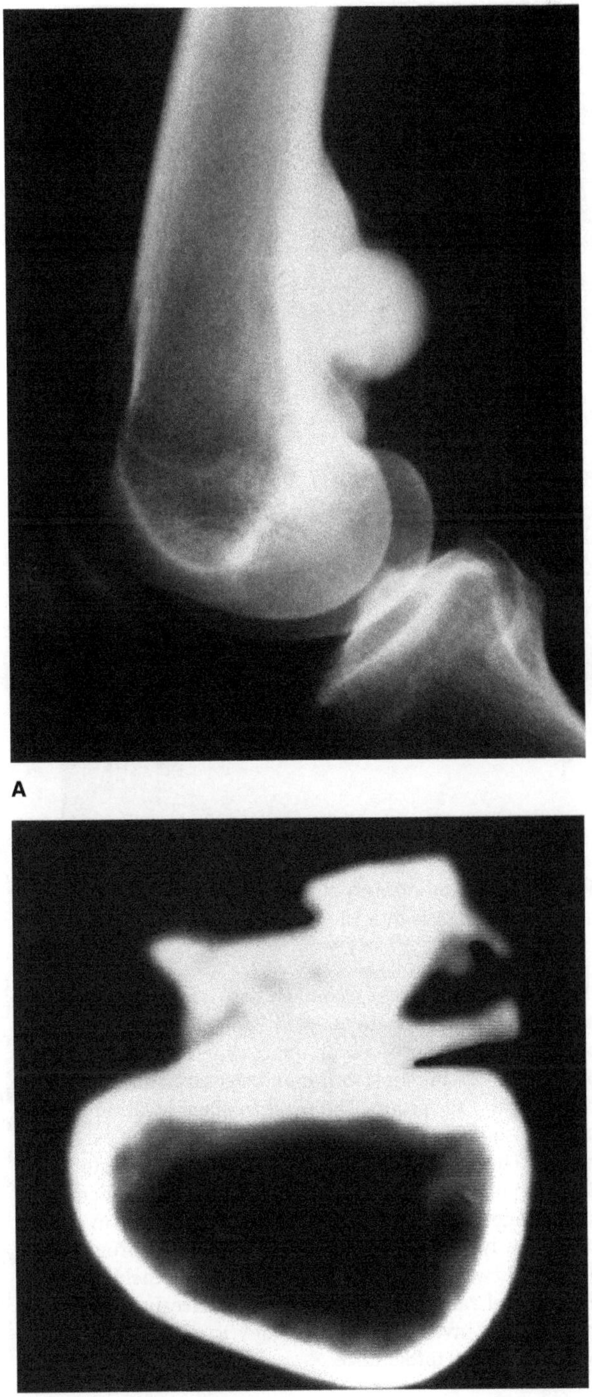

A

B

▲ **Figure 6–39.** Radiograph (**A**) and CT scan (**B**) of a parosteal osteosarcoma of the distal femur in a 21-year-old woman.

D. Periosteal Osteosarcoma

Periosteal osteosarcoma is another surface osteosarcoma of low to intermediate grade. This lesion represents less than 2% of all osteosarcomas. It arises beneath the periosteum, elevating it and inducing vigorous neo-osteogenesis with a predominant chondroblastic differentiation. It is slightly more common in females, with a peak incidence in the second decade of life. It almost exclusively arises in the long bones. The lesion can mimic an aneurysmal bone cyst or periosteal chondroma radiographically (Figure 6–40).

Because of its low to intermediate grade, periosteal osteosarcoma is not generally treated with chemotherapy, although it may be indicated in more advanced cases. Wide surgical resection is the modality of choice. It also carries a better prognosis than classic osteosarcoma. Approximately 25% of patients succumb to metastatic disease within 2 to 3 years. The surgical treatment is usually a limb-sparing procedure, and because the tumor is more diaphyseal in location, the adjacent joints may often be spared.

E. Secondary Osteosarcoma

Osteosarcoma can arise from benign disease through a process that may involve a second mutation and usually occurs at a later age (see Table 6–2). Among the benign conditions that can result in secondary osteosarcoma are Paget disease, osteoblastoma, fibrous dysplasia, benign giant cell tumor, bone infarction, and chronic osteomyelitis.

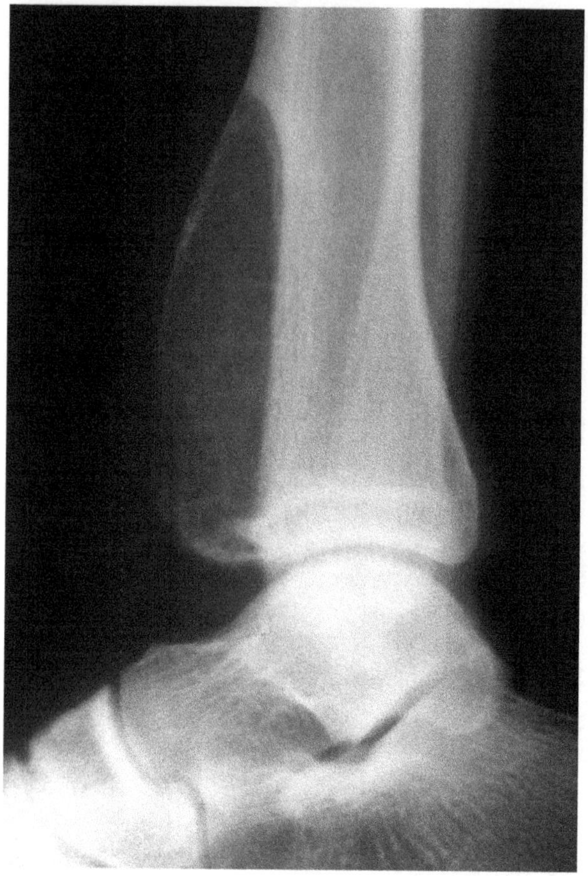

▲ **Figure 6–40.** Radiograph of a periosteal osteosarcoma of the distal tibia in a 15-year-old boy.

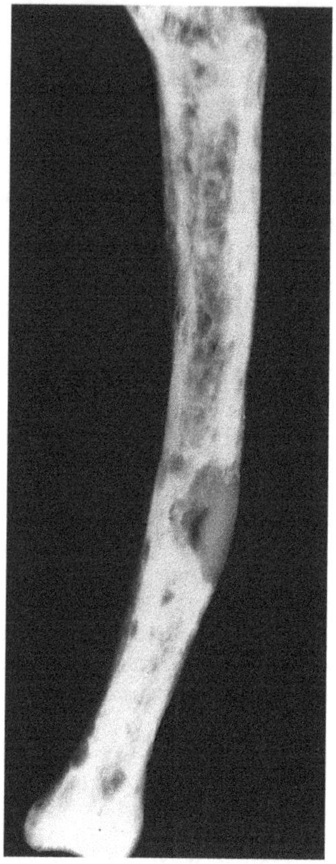

▲ **Figure 6–41.** Radiograph of a pagetic osteosarcoma of the tibia.

The classic example of a secondary osteosarcoma is seen in a small percentage of patients with Paget disease. Pagetic osteosarcomas, which represent approximately 3% of all osteosarcomas, are the most common osteosarcomas in the older (>65 years) age group. The most frequent location for pagetic osteosarcoma is the humerus, followed by the pelvis and femur. The typical presentation involves a long history (15-25 years) of dull, aching pain associated with the inflammation of Paget disease before a new acute pain arises in an area of recent lytic destruction (Figure 6–41). The prognosis for patients with pagetic osteosarcoma is extremely poor (5-year survival rate of approximately 8%). Because of the older age group involved, chemotherapy is usually not an option secondary to intolerance.

F. Low-Grade Intramedullary Osteosarcoma

Another rare and low-grade osseofibrous variant of osteosarcoma is the central or intramedullary form. Although this variant has a microscopic appearance similar to that of parosteal osteosarcoma, it is usually located in metaphyseal bone about the knee joint in adults between 15 and 65 years of age. Males and females are equally affected. Radiographically, intramedullary osteosarcoma creates a sclerotic density in metaphyseal bone (Figure 6–42). Like parosteal osteosarcoma, low-grade intramedullary osteosarcoma carries an excellent prognosis and can be treated with local surgery alone.

G. Radiation-Induced Osteosarcoma

Radiation-induced osteosarcoma may arise after any form of significant radiation exposure (in excess of 30 Gy) (Figure 6–43). Onset is usually delayed an average of 15 years (range, 3-55 years). Other radiation-induced sarcomas, besides the osteosarcoma type, include fibrosarcoma and malignant fibrous histiocytoma. These secondary sarcomas tend to be high grade and carry a poor prognosis for survival, with a very high rate of metastasis.

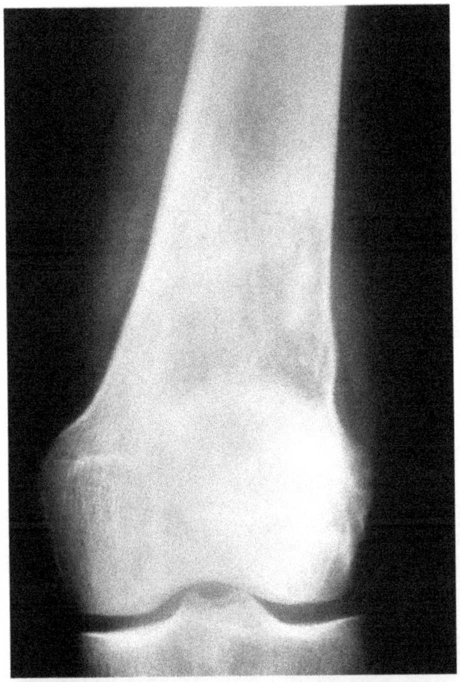

A

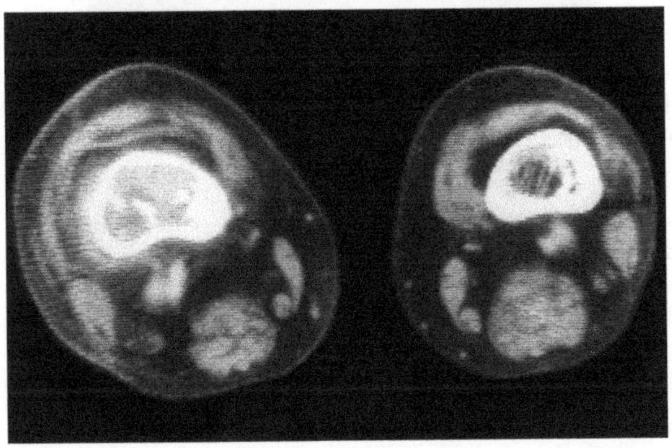

B

▲ **Figure 6–42.** Radiograph (**A**) and CT scan (**B**) of a low-grade intramedullary osteosarcoma in the distal femur of a 65-year-old man.

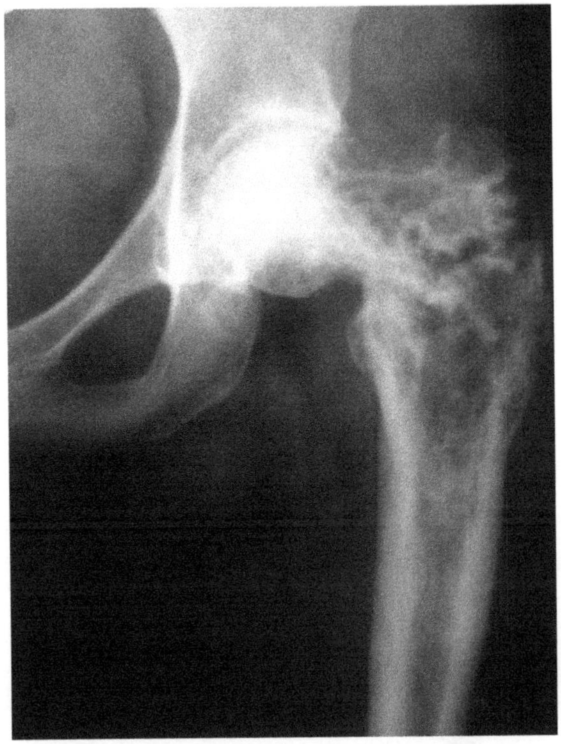

▲ **Figure 6–43.** Radiograph of irradiation-induced osteosarcoma of the peritrochanteric area in a 35-year-old woman.

H. Multicentric Osteosarcoma

Multicentric osteosarcoma has two clinical presentations: (1) synchronous, occurring in childhood and adolescence, and (2) metachronous, occurring in adults. In the synchronous type, multiple skeletal lesions occur simultaneously. In the metachronous form, the lesions occur sequentially (Figure 6-44). Multicentric osteosarcoma is rare, representing approximately 1.5% of all osteosarcoma, and has a poor prognosis. Patients with synchronous lesions have lower survival than those with metachronous lesions; it has been hypothesized that many of the lesions in the synchronous type are skeletal metastases from a primary lesion.

I. Soft-Tissue Osteosarcoma

Osteosarcoma can occur in muscle tissue outside bone and accounts for approximately 4% of all osteosarcomas (Figure 6–45). Soft-tissue osteosarcoma is rarely seen in patients younger than 40 years. The number of cases is equal in females and males, and the tumor is usually seen in large muscle groups of the pelvis and thigh areas.

Soft-tissue osteosarcoma must be differentiated from the more common myositis ossificans. An important distinction is that soft-tissue osteosarcoma has heavy mineralization in the central area (see Figure 6–45), while myositis ossificans has a zonal pattern of ossification, with the mature, dense ossification at the periphery of the lesion.

The treatment of soft-tissue osteosarcoma is the same as for the high-grade osseous form and includes a wide

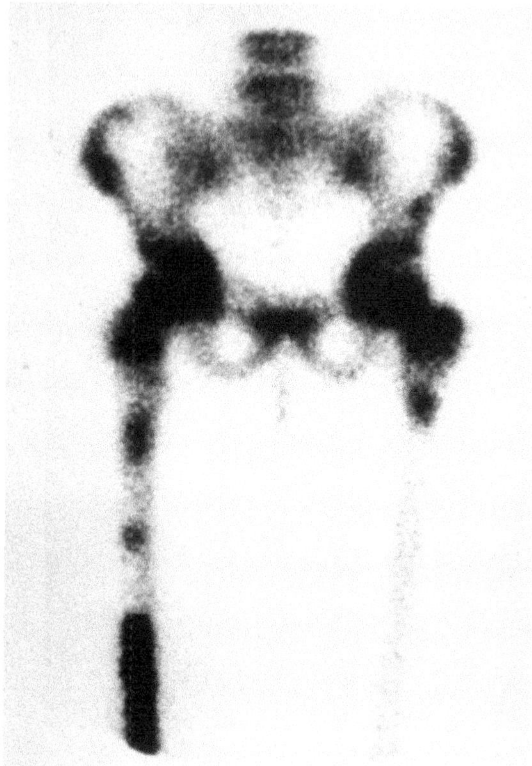

▲ **Figure 6–44.** Isotope bone scan of multicentric osteosarcoma in an 8-year-old girl.

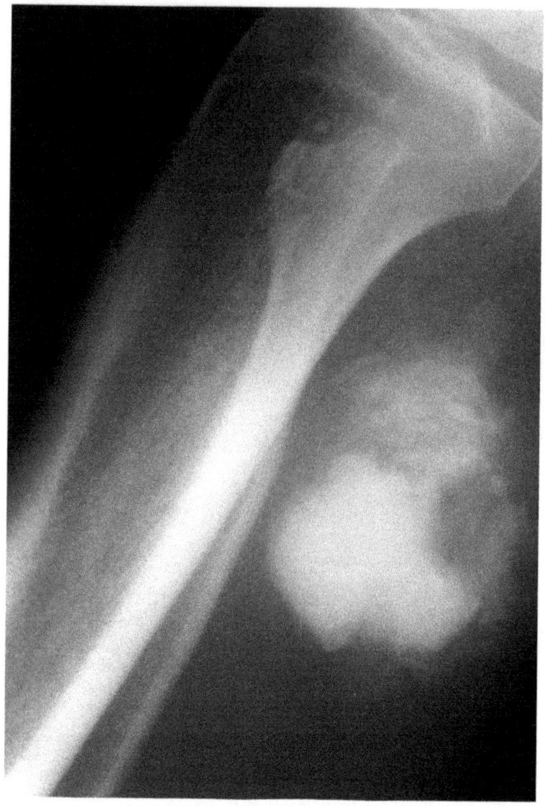

▲ **Figure 6–45.** Radiograph of a soft-tissue osteosarcoma in the calf area of a 67-year-old woman.

resection and adjuvant chemotherapy. The prognosis is worse with the soft-tissue form of osteosarcoma, with a high rate of chemotherapy resistance.

Essentials of Diagnosis

- *Osteosarcoma is best confirmed by biopsy of the leading edge of the soft-tissue component if possible.*
- *Parosteal osteosarcoma usually occurs on the posterior aspect of the distal femur, exhibiting a "stuck-on" appearance.*

Chondroid-Forming Sarcomas

Chondroid-forming sarcomas are a heterogeneous group of neoplasms consisting of a cartilage-based histology. A cornerstone to the diagnosis of chondrosarcoma is the absence of osteoid formation. If any osteoid is present with a malignant stroma, the tumor is considered an osteosarcoma with chondroblastic features. It is important to make the distinction because chondrosarcomas behave differently from osteosarcomas. However, this can be a difficult task. The surgeon must consider the age of the patient and carefully assess the radiographic and histologic features to confirm the diagnosis.

A. Primary or Central Conventional Chondrosarcoma

The typical primary chondrosarcoma is a low-grade tumor seen in adults between 30 and 60 years of age. The tumor is found more frequently in men than in women. Minimal symptoms of pain may occur over a period of several years before a radiograph is obtained. The pelvis and femur are the most common locations, followed by the rib cage, proximal humerus, scapula, and upper tibia. Primary chondrosarcoma is extremely rare in small bones, including the hand and foot. The metaphysis is the most common location in a long bone; however, a diaphyseal location is not unusual.

Approximately 85% of central chondrosarcomas are low-grade lesions with atypical matrix calcification that can be described as flocculated with multiple rings and arcs. Radiographic rather than histologic criteria are more useful in distinguishing between enchondroma and low-grade chondrosarcoma. Frequently cited radiographic criteria suggestive of more aggressive biologic potential include endosteal scalloping greater than 50% of the cortical width, change

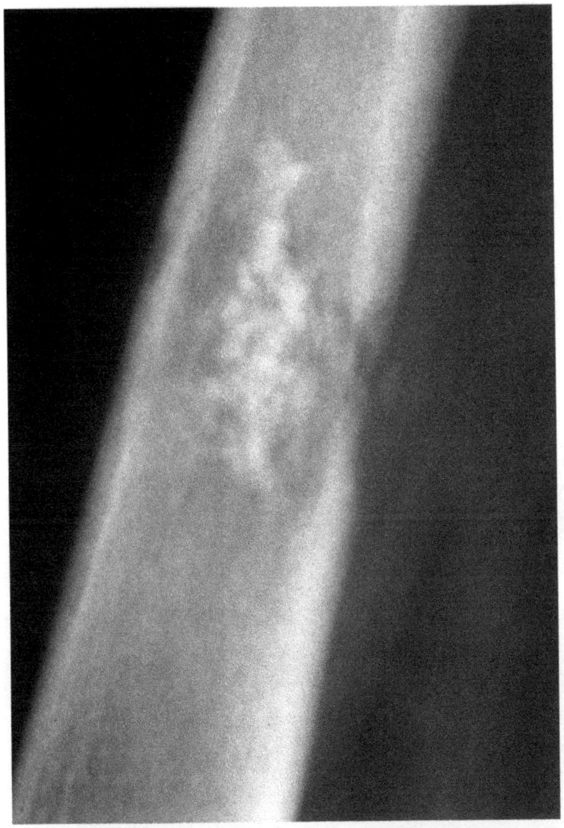

▲ **Figure 6–46.** Radiograph of a low-grade primary chondrosarcoma in the distal femur of an 83-year-old man.

over time, and adjacent radiolucency near an area of typical chondroid matrix calcification (Figure 6–46). High-grade lesions are rare. Radiographically, they lose their typical lobulated and calcific pattern and take on the appearance of a more permeative high-grade tumor, such as malignant fibrous histiocytoma. High-grade chondrosarcomas do not have a chondroid matrix pattern, and instead are a more aggressive spindle cell tumor.

Because of the weakened cortex in chondrosarcoma, the patient usually complains of local pain not typically experienced with enchondroma. Because most chondrosarcomas are low grade, they do not respond well to adjuvant irradiation or chemotherapy. Therefore, aggressive surgical management is imperative. The optimal surgical management is controversial. Although wide en bloc resection is ideal from the standpoint of achieving negative margins, it is associated with considerable morbidity. On the contrary, aggressive intralesional resection (curettage) and margin expansion with adjuvant therapy (eg, phenol or liquid nitrogen) can reduce morbidity and may provide equal local control. In fact, some authors found that for grade 1 chondrosarcoma, the margin of resection is not significant in terms of local recurrence or disease progression.

In general, the prognosis for low-grade central chondrosarcoma is very good, with a low rate of pulmonary metastasis if the primary lesion is widely resected. Nevertheless, recurrences can occur late, even over 15 years later. For any intermediate- or high-grade chondrosarcomas, wide en bloc resection is mandatory (Figure 6–47).

B. Secondary Chondrosarcoma

The vast majority of secondary chondrosarcomas arise from osteochondromas in patients afflicted with MHE. Transformation occurs at the cartilaginous cap. Patients with solitary osteochondromas do not generally form secondary chondrosarcomas in their lesions, making resection unnecessary unless the solitary lesion is otherwise symptomatic. Reported lifetime rates of malignant transformation across all lesions in patients with MHE range from 1% to 25%. Patients with secondary chondrosarcoma tend to be younger than those with primary chondrosarcomas (see Table 6–2). The lesions tend to be slow growing with minimal to mild symptoms. The most common site is the pelvis, followed by the proximal femur, proximal humerus, and ribs. Plain radiographs demonstrate a flocculated calcific pattern (Figure 6–48). An osteochondroma with a cartilage cap thicker than 1 to 2 cm should raise suspicion of a secondary chondrosarcoma. The overall prognosis for patients with secondary or peripheral chondrosarcoma is better than that for patients with primary or central chondrosarcoma. Surgical removal, without violation of the cartilage cap, is the only effective treatment modality.

C. Dedifferentiated Chondrosarcoma

Dedifferentiated chondrosarcoma is the most malignant variant of chondrosarcoma, accounting for between 5% and 10% of all chondrosarcomas. It is heralded by the transformation of areas of conventional chondrosarcoma into malignant fibrous histiocytoma or osteosarcoma. Histologically, it is characterized by two distinct but neighboring areas of low- to intermediate-grade malignant chondroid tumor and heterogeneous high-grade sarcoma. Dedifferentiated chondrosarcoma occurs in older patients, usually between 50 and 70 years of age. It is found in the same areas affected by central primary chondrosarcomas, including the pelvis, femur, and proximal humerus (Figure 6–49). Radiographs show areas of rarefaction within the tumor with cortical attenuation. Pathologic fracture is not uncommon.

The prognosis for dedifferentiated chondrosarcoma is bleak, with the majority of patients developing and dying from metastatic disease within 1 year. Chemotherapy and radiation therapy are less effective than in malignant fibrous histiocytoma or osteosarcoma that arose de novo. Surgical resection remains the mainstay of treatment, with adjuvant modalities employed in younger patients.

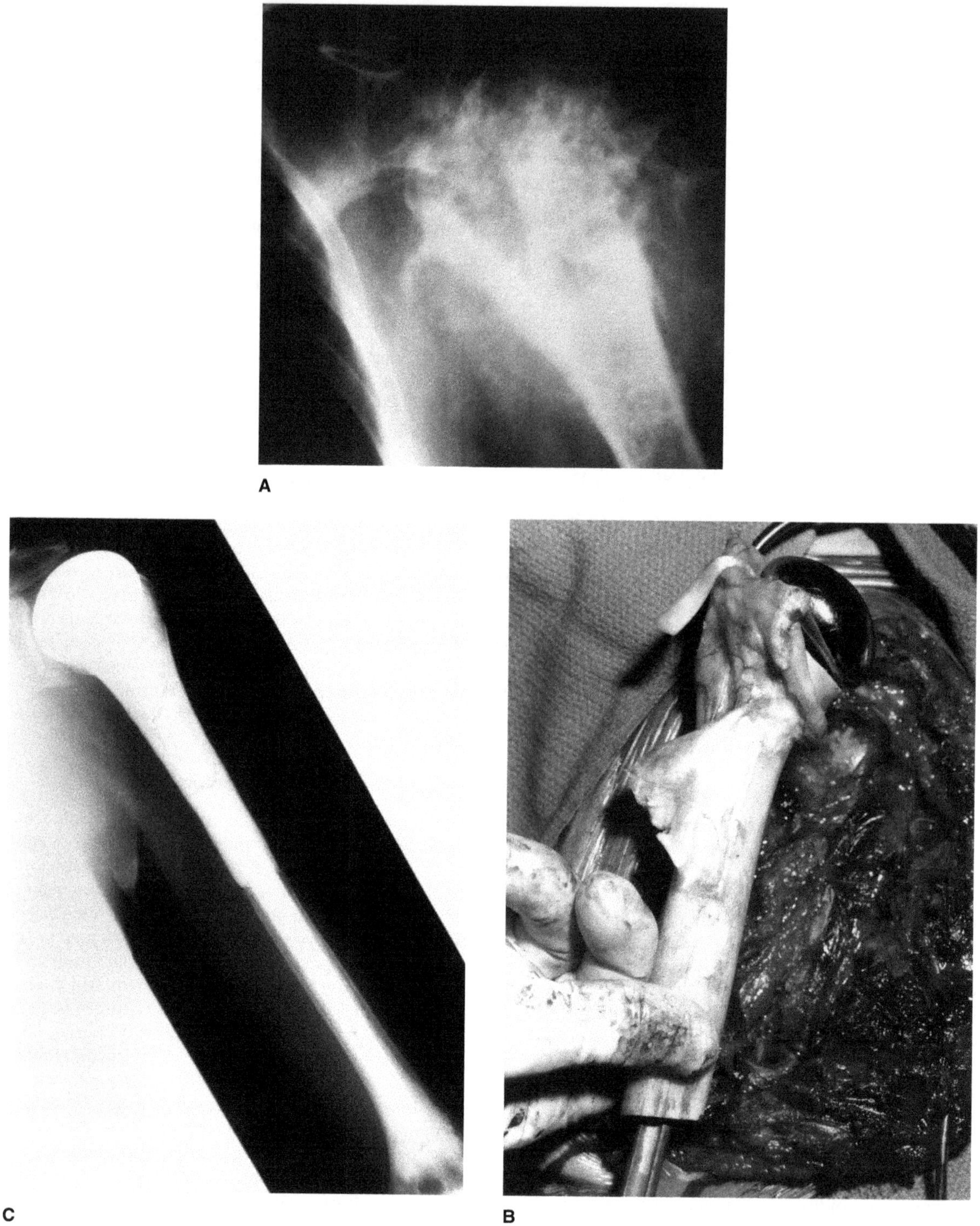

▲ **Figure 6–47.** Preoperative radiograph of a large central chondrosarcoma in the proximal humerus of a 52-year-old woman (**A**), placement of a Neer prosthesis (**B**), and postoperative radiograph (**C**).

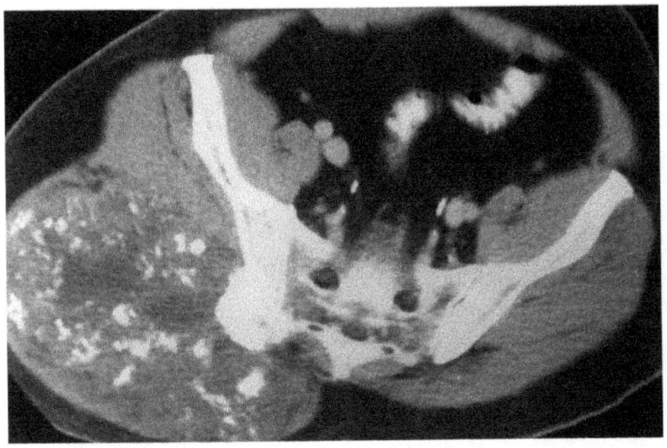

▲ **Figure 6–48.** CT scan of a secondary peripheral chondrosarcoma in the ilium of a 56-year-old man with hereditary multiple exostoses.

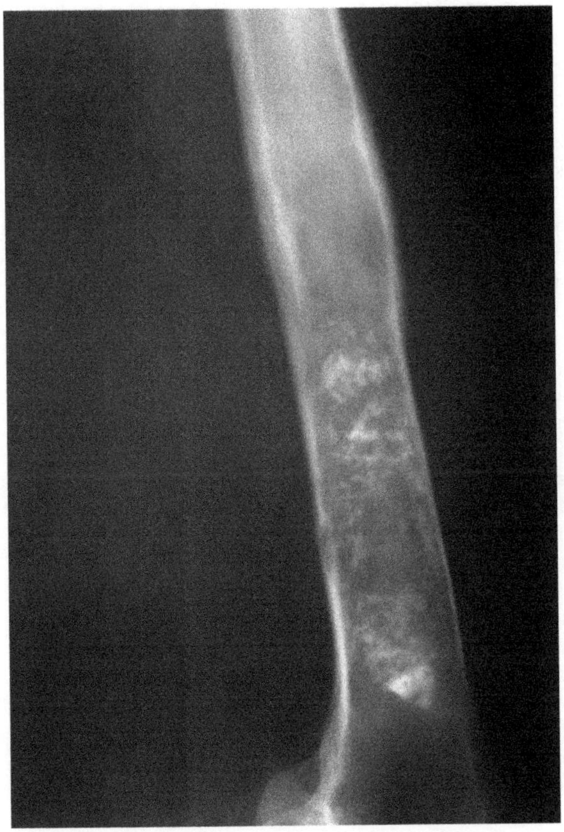

▲ **Figure 6–49.** Radiograph of dedifferentiated chondrosarcoma in the distal femur of a 73-year-old woman.

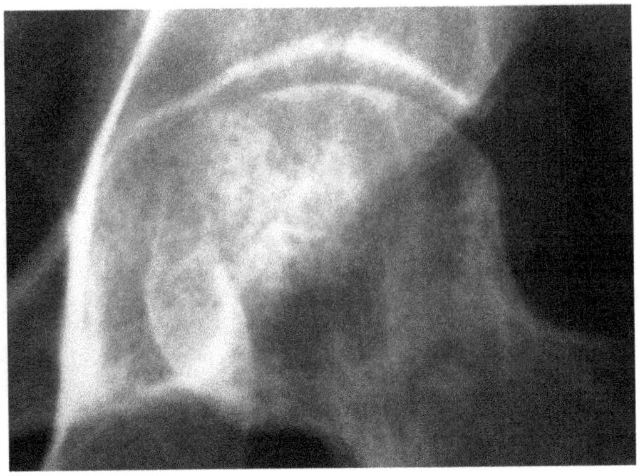

▲ **Figure 6–50.** Radiograph of clear cell chondrosarcoma of the femoral head in a 25-year-old man.

D. Clear Cell Chondrosarcoma

Clear cell chondrosarcoma is a rare low-grade variant of chondrosarcoma. Clear cell lesions occur more often in males than in females and are usually seen in patients between 20 and 50 years of age. These lesions often occur in the epiphysis, one of only a few lesions that commonly occur in this area. The vast majority of lesions are found in the femoral head (Figure 6–50). The radiographic appearance is one of a lytic tumor with sharp margination and a central matrix calcification, creating the appearance of a chondroblastoma. Although microscopic examination reveals the presence of some giant cells, as seen in chondroblastoma, areas of low-grade chondrosarcoma are also evident in which no giant cells are seen. Even on gross examination, clear cell chondrosarcoma does not look like a chondrosarcoma; indeed, it is frequently mistaken for chondroblastoma in younger adult patients. Abundant glycogen in the tumor cells results in the characteristic clear cell phenotype. Although no significant genetic alteration has been identified in clear cell chondrosarcoma, it has been found that alkaline phosphatase activity may correlate with prognosis.

The treatment for clear cell chondrosarcoma is a wide excision and reconstruction. The prognosis with this type of treatment is good. In contrast, when lesions are mistaken for chondroblastomas and treatment consists of simple curettage and bone grafting, the prognosis is poor and the recurrence rate is high.

E. Mesenchymal Chondrosarcoma

Another rare variant of chondrosarcoma is the mesenchymal chondrosarcoma. It is a highly cellular tumor composed of primitive mesenchymal cells with foci of cartilage differentiation. This tumor involves the soft tissue in a third of cases, occurs more frequently in females than in males, and is seen in young adults (see Table 6–2). The jaw is the most common location, followed by the spine and ribs, with few cases noted in long bones.

Mesenchymal chondrosarcoma is a high-grade tumor with histologic features of low-grade chondrosarcoma. Heavily calcified areas, mixed with areas of malignant round cells, may give it the appearance of Ewing sarcoma or solitary fibrous tumor.

Treatment consists of resection, with a wide margin if possible, and adjuvant chemotherapy and radiation therapy. Despite aggressive treatment, the prognosis is very poor with a high incidence of pulmonary metastasis.

Essentials of Diagnosis

- *Typical chondroid-forming sarcomas are not sensitive to radiation therapy or chemotherapy and are treated with surgery alone.*
- *Pain, endosteal scalloping greater than 50% of the cortical width, or radiolucency adjacent to an otherwise typical-appearing enchondroma should alert the practitioner to the possibility of chondrosarcoma.*

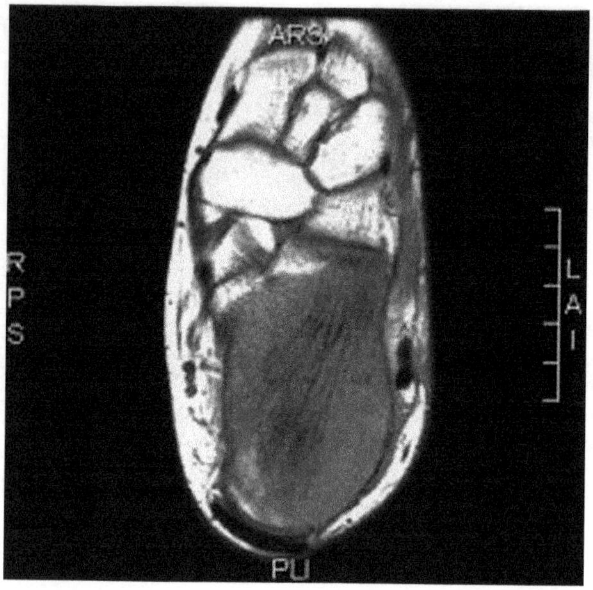

▲ **Figure 6–51.** MRI of the hindfoot of a 9-year-old girl with calcaneal Ewing sarcoma.

Round Cell Tumors

This so-called group of tumors is composed of distinct tumors that—other than their similar microscopic appearance using hematoxylin-eosin stain—are quite heterogeneous. They behave and are treated in a variety of ways, given that each arises from a different cell type.

A. The Ewing Sarcoma Family of Tumors

1. Ewing sarcoma—Ewing sarcoma is a well-known clinical entity originally described by James Ewing as a diffuse endothelioma of bone. Since the time of his description, many theories have evolved regarding the tumor's true histogenesis. Based on electron microscopy and immunohistochemistry findings, it is thought that the tumor represents an undifferentiated member of the family of neural tumors distinct from neuroblastoma. The Ewing sarcoma family of tumors (ESFT) also includes the less common primitive neuroectodermal tumor (PNET) and Askin tumors. ESFTs have been shown to express chimeric transcription factors that result from reciprocal translocations involving chromosome 22, containing the Ewing sarcoma gene (*EWS*). Ninety percent of the time, t(11;22) is seen, resulting in a *EWS/FLI-1* chimera. Less frequently, t(21;22) and t(7;22) are seen. The resulting transcription factors are put under the control of the *EWS* promoter. Recently, investigations have elucidated a handful of downstream targets including VEGF (encoding vascular endothelial growth factor) and CAV1 (encoding caveolin-1), which are thought to be necessary for tumorigenesis. Furthermore, they are being investigated as possible targets for directed therapy.

In 90% of cases, Ewing sarcoma is found in patients between 5 and 25 years of age. If the patient is younger than 5 years, the most likely diagnosis is metastatic neuroblastoma. Males are affected more frequently than females and carry a worse prognosis. The pelvis is the most common location, followed by the femur, tibia, humerus, and scapula. As a myelogenous tumor, Ewing sarcoma may be found in any bone of the body (Figure 6–51).

Ewing sarcoma appears radiographically as a central lytic tumor of the diaphyseal-metaphyseal bone. There is often a large associated soft-tissue component. It creates extensive permeative destruction of cortical bone, and as it breaks through under the periosteum, it takes on a typical onionskin, multilaminated appearance. Another radiographic feature is the reactive hair-on-end appearance created by bone forming along the periosteal vessels that run perpendicularly between the cortex and the elevated periosteum (Figure 6–52).

Ewing sarcoma can frequently masquerade as osteomyelitis because it is a high-grade lesion with resultant areas of necrosis; liquefaction may occur that may be mistaken for pus. Furthermore, patients frequently present with systemic symptoms of low-grade intermittent fever and elevated white cell count and erythrocyte sedimentation rate (ESR). Microscopically, small roundlike cells predominate in densely packed sheets. Formation of pseudorosettes may also be seen (in <20%). The rosette-like patterns are more frequently seen in PNET.

Ewing sarcoma is an aggressive malignancy with high local recurrence and metastatic rates. Patients with locally resectable disease treated with multidrug chemotherapy have a 5-year survival rate of approximately 70% (Figure 6–53).

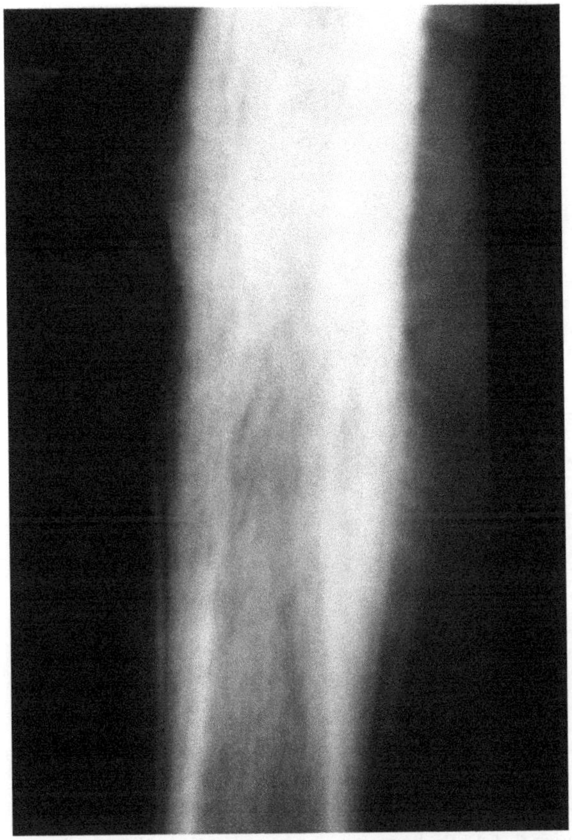

▲ **Figure 6–52.** Radiograph of periosteal response in Ewing sarcoma of the femur in a 15-year-old boy.

Currently, most chemotherapy is driven by large cooperative trials including induction and adjuvant multidrug chemotherapy with drugs such as vincristine, doxorubicin, cyclophosphamide, dactinomycin, and ifosfamide. Unfortunately, 15% to 25% of patients present with nonlocalized disease. For the patient who presents with advanced metastatic disease, the 5-year survival rate is 30%. Resection of lung metastasis, if possible, does improve survival.

Ewing sarcoma is a radiosensitive tumor. Historically, 45 to 50 Gy over 5 weeks was employed to treat local disease. Because of the risk of secondary sarcomas, surgery has since become the primary modality for local control. In the event of positive margins, local irradiation must still be used postoperatively. Adjuvant radiotherapy is also generally accepted after complete resection of a tumor showing a poor response to neoadjuvant chemotherapy, with improved local control rates having been illustrated. Neoadjuvant radiotherapy, although not generally used, may have a role in lesions that are on the border of resectability.

2. Primitive neuroectodermal tumor—PNET is the less common relative of Ewing sarcoma. Like Ewing sarcoma, this tumor demonstrates expression of neural markers by immunocytochemistry. PNET also exhibits the t(11;22) translocation with the resulting EWS/FLI-1 fusion protein. Due to their similarities, it has been suggested that PNET and Ewing sarcoma may represent two ends of a spectrum of disease.

By strict criteria, PNET is a rare tumor, representing approximately 10% of Ewing-like tumors. The patient demographics are similar to those of Ewing-like tumors. Treatment of PNET is similar to that of Ewing sarcoma; however, the survival rate is slightly less. Accordingly, some authors feel it should be distinguished from Ewing sarcoma.

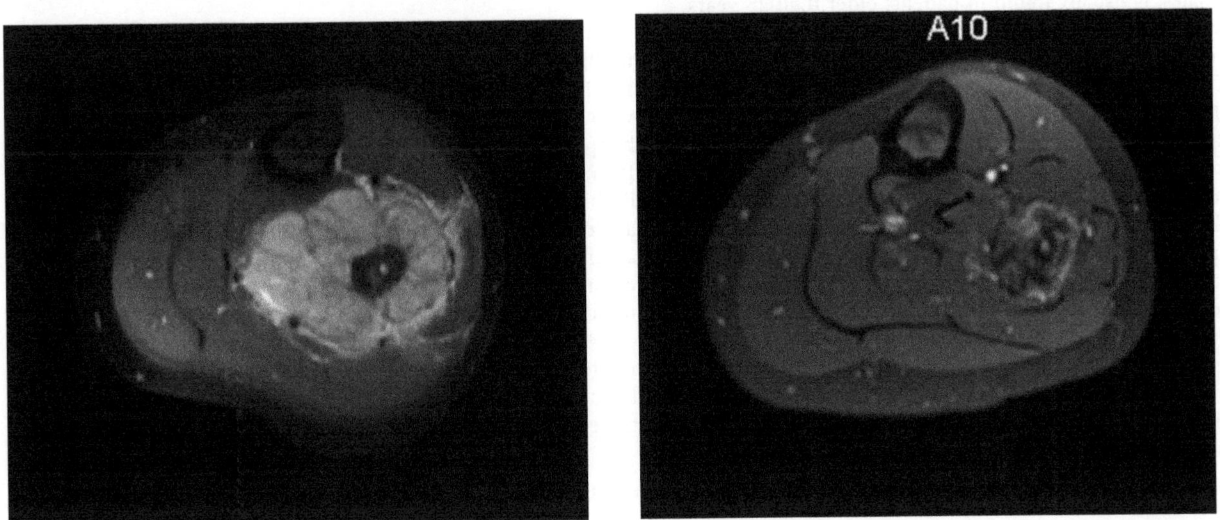

A B

▲ **Figure 6–53.** Pretreatment MRI (**A**) and MRI following 10 weeks of neoadjuvant chemotherapy (**B**) of Ewing sarcoma of the fibula in a 14-year-old boy.

B. Lymphoma

Lymphoblastic tumors are considered systemic neoplasms of the lymphatic organs, including the bone marrow, and they account for 7% of all malignant bone tumors. They can be roughly divided into Hodgkin lymphomas and non-Hodgkin lymphomas, both of which can affect bone. Of the two groups, the lymphomas associated with Hodgkin disease carry a much better prognosis. When they are found in bone, they tend to be localized and have a considerable blastic response, especially when involving the vertebra.

There are two main types of non-Hodgkin lymphomas. The type emphasized in this section is primary lymphoma of bone, in which a localized lytic destruction occurs in a single bone and the staging studies (including an isotope bone scan, a CT scan of the chest and abdomen, and marrow aspiration) rule out other areas of involvement. The second type is the more generalized or systemic form of lymphoma, in which many lymphoid organs are involved including the lymph nodes, liver, spleen, and bone. The prognosis is better for an isolated primary lymphoma of bone, although this may progress to generalized or systemic and carry a worse prognosis. This is similar to the case with plasma cell tumors, in which the findings in a patient can progress from that of a solitary plasmacytoma with an excellent prognosis to that of the multiple myeloma form of the disease with a poor prognosis.

Primary lymphoma of bone, formerly known as reticulum cell sarcoma of bone, accounts for approximately half of all lymphomas. To meet the criteria of being a primary bone lymphoma, there must be a 4- to 6-month interval from the onset of skeletal manifestations to the development of systemic disease. It occurs more frequently in males than in females, is usually found in patients older than 25 years, and affects the spine or pelvis in more than 50% of the cases. In the extremities, the femur is the most commonly involved area, followed next by the humerus and the tibia. Polyostotic involvement occurs in 10% to 40% of cases.

Radiographic findings in primary lymphoma include extensive lytic permeation of cortical bone, with minimal sclerotic response in diaphyseal, metaphyseal, and epiphyseal locations (Figure 6–54). MRI studies demonstrate that the actual marrow involvement is frequently more extensive than the cortical disruption seen on simple radiographs suggests.

The most common histologic types of lymphoma of bone are the large cell or mixed small and large cell types. The cells tend to demonstrate little cytoplasmic structure. However, the nuclear pattern shows indented and folded nuclear patterns and a prominent pink-staining nucleolus, which may help to distinguish it histologically from Ewing sarcoma. Immunohistochemical staining is often necessary to differentiate Ewing sarcoma from the B-cell and T-cell subtypes of lymphoma. In the case of lymphomas, the glycogen stain is usually negative, but the reticulum stain is often positive.

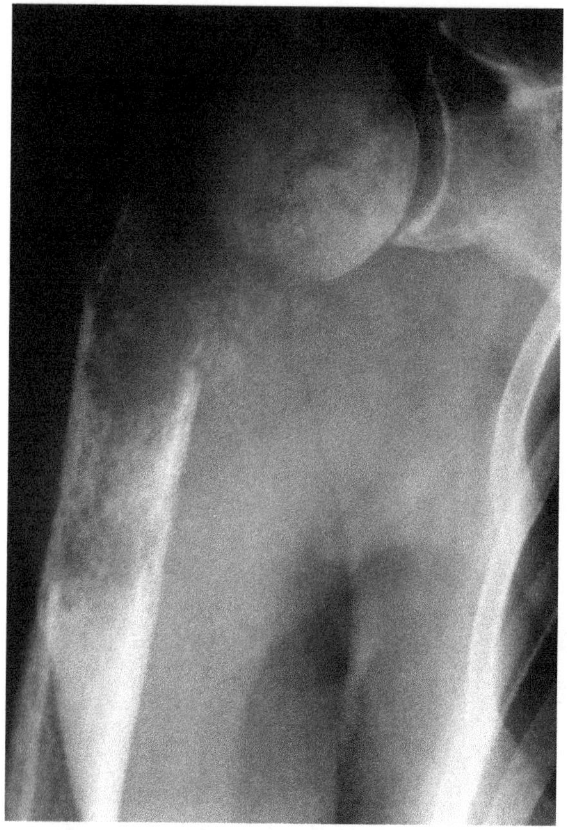

▲ **Figure 6–54.** Radiograph of a lymphoma in the proximal humerus of a 64-year-old woman.

In primary lymphoma of bone, as in Ewing sarcoma, multidrug chemotherapy has greatly improved the 5-year survival rate, which now is approximately 70% for patients with either of these tumors. Like Ewing sarcoma, primary lymphoma of bone is highly sensitive to local irradiation. If the primary lymphoma is localized, a wide resection and limb-salvage reconstruction may be carried out, thereby avoiding the need for local irradiation, and possibly effect a cure. However, if the involvement is more extensive, as is commonly the case, it is necessary to use intralesional techniques such as cemented intramedullary nails or a long-stem prosthesis and subsequently use whole bone irradiation, similar to the management of metastatic carcinoma with pathologic fractures. In cases of extensive systemic involvement, bone marrow transplantation can be used.

C. Plasma Cell Tumor

A bone tumor composed of malignant monoclonal plasma cells is referred to as a myeloma or plasmacytoma. It is rare for a patient to have a solitary myeloma or plasmacytoma.

Tumors are almost always found on multiple bony sites, in which case the term *multiple myeloma* is used.

1. Myeloma—Multiple myeloma, which is the most common primary tumor of bone, accounts for 45% of all malignant bone tumors. It is the second most common hematopoietic malignancy. An estimated 90% of cases are in patients older than 40 years. It accounts for 1% of all malignancies in Caucasians and 2% in African Americans.

The disease is characterized by a triad of osteolytic punched-out lesions (multifocal) (Figure 6–55), neoplastic proliferation of atypical plasma cells, and a monoclonal gammopathy. Diagnostic criteria are established for myeloma. Major criteria include plasmacytosis on biopsy of a lesion, marrow plasmacytosis, and an abnormal serum protein electrophoresis and light (Bence Jones) proteinuria. It causes bony destruction similar to that caused by lymphomas, with most lesions occurring in the trunk, hip, and shoulder areas. Knowledge of the biology of multiple myeloma continues to increase at an astounding rate, and investigation toward targeted therapy grows proportionally. Targeted therapy trials have included inhibitors of cell surface receptors such as VEGF-R and IGF-1R, inhibitors of cell signaling pathways such as the MAPK pathway and the MTOR pathway, Janus kinase inhibitors, proteasome inhibitors, and histone deacetylase inhibitors.

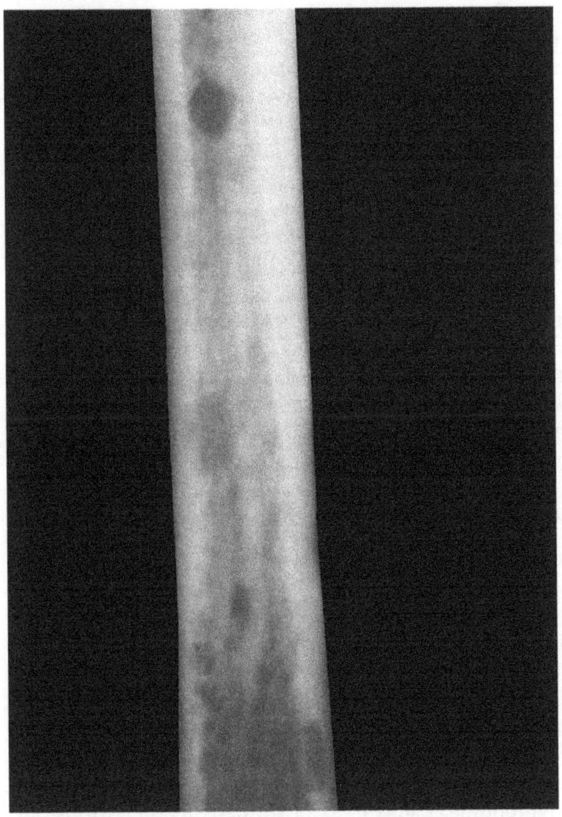

▲ **Figure 6–55.** Radiograph of multiple myeloma in the femoral shaft of a 72-year-old man.

Lesions are rarely found distal to the knee or elbow. Approximately 3% of patients with myeloma have a sclerotic form of the disease, which appears to carry a better prognosis and is associated with peripheral neuropathy. The serum protein electrophoresis shows an elevated monoclonal immunoglobulin on either the *a* or *y* spike. Bence Jones proteinuria is secondary to light-chain immunoglobulin spillover. Occasionally, electrophoresis of a urine sample yields positive results, whereas that of a serum sample yields negative results. In aggressive forms of myeloma, the extensive bone breakdown causes hypercalcemia, which can lead to a semicomatose state and, over a long period, results in nephrocalcinosis. Renal damage also results from protein plugging of the renal tubules, and renal failure may ensue.

A marrow aspirate usually demonstrates the abnormal plasma cells. These cells show an eccentrically placed nucleus in a well-structured eosinophilic cytoplasm. Although normal B-cell–derived plasma cells produce antibodies, the abnormal B-cell–derived plasma cells produce immunoglobulin that is ineffective, which helps explain the increased infection rate in patients with myelomas. Patients may also demonstrate extraosseous infiltrates, with the majority seen in the upper airway and oral cavity. Amyloidosis may be seen concurrently in 10% to 15% of cases. A quarter of these have extensive cardiac involvement. In such cases, the median survival is 4 months.

Plain radiographs show myeloma lesions to be sharply demarcated lytic lesions with minimal periostitis. Pathologic fixation is frequent. Bone scans have a high false-negative rate thought to be caused by almost exclusive osteoclast activity. For this reason, a skeletal survey instead of a bone scan is important in the staging of this disease.

Fewer than 2% of myeloma cases demonstrate the POEMS syndrome (*p*olyneuropathy, *o*rganomegaly, *e*ndocrinopathy, *M*-component spike, *s*kin changes, *s*cleroses of bone).

Although treatment and prognosis have improved, myeloma remains a fatal disease, with more than 90% of patients dying within 2 to 3 years. Chemotherapy such as melphalan and cortisone may induce a transient remission in 50% to 70% of cases. Bisphosphonates have been introduced to the treatment algorithm with results showing reduced skeletal-related events, pain, and increased time to progression.

Surgical management of multiple myeloma is largely a palliative procedure. The decision to operate is dependent on the overall clinical status of the patient. The employed surgical procedure ranges from biopsy and kyphoplasty to instrumented spinal fusion and cephalomedullary nail fixation for fractures of the spine or femur, respectively. The amount of bleeding at the surgical site is often extensive, similar to that encountered with surgery for metastatic renal cell carcinoma and certain thyroid metastases.

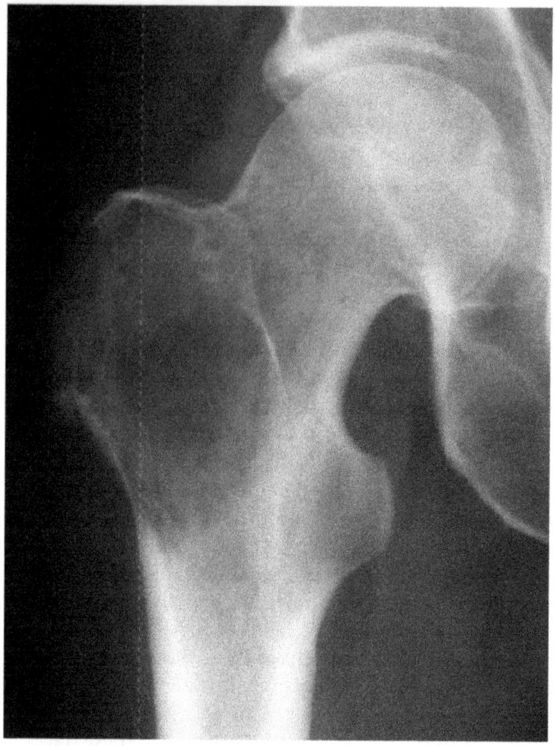

▲ **Figure 6–56.** Radiograph of a solitary plasmacytoma in the proximal femur of a 46-year-old man.

2. Solitary myeloma—Solitary lesions are rare (Figure 6–56). By definition, there must be no marrow involvement. Seventy-five percent of these cases have an entirely normal serum protein electrophoresis (SPEP) and urine protein electrophoresis (UPEP). The remaining 25% may have mild abnormalities. Vertebral involvement is the most common site. Patients also tend to be younger (<50 years old). Unfortunately, 70% of these solitary cases develop multiple myeloma within 3 years. Until progression to myeloma, the treatment is only local, with wide resection if possible or intralesional debridement and reconstruction followed by radiation therapy.

Essentials of Diagnosis

- *Ewing sarcoma is characterized by a chimeric transcription factor that is a product, most often, of the t(11;22), resulting in an altered expression pattern in the neoplastic lineage.*
- *Because of the high level of sensitivity of lymphoma to chemotherapy and radiation therapy, wide resection is infrequently performed.*
- *Because of the propensity for myeloma to remain cold on isotope bone scanning, a skeletal survey is the study of choice for skeletal staging.*

Fibrous Sarcomas of Bone

Malignant fibrous tumors of bone are clinically similar to osteosarcoma, but they affect an older (<20 years) age group of patients and show a complete absence of tumor osteoid formation. The two major tumors in this category are fibrosarcoma and malignant fibrous histiocytoma.

A. Fibrosarcoma of Bone

Fibrosarcoma of bone is a malignant spindle cell tumor seen in an older patient population with a peak incidence in the fourth decade. It is 10 times less frequent than osteosarcoma but tends to involve similar locations. The most common site of fibrosarcoma is the distal femur, followed next in order by the proximal tibia, pelvis, proximal femur, and proximal humerus. It is rarely seen in the spine, hand, or foot.

On radiograph, fibrosarcomas appear to be almost purely osteolytic and permeative, similar to lymphomas. For this reason, they are painful and can lead to a pathologic fracture. Microscopically, myofibroblastic differentiation with osteoid formation or histiocytes permits distinction from fibroblastic osteosarcoma and malignant fibrous histiocytoma (MFH) of bone. The low-grade form is characterized by malignant-appearing fibroblasts that form a large amount of collagen fiber, giving the appearance of an aggressive desmoplastic fibroma. The high-grade form is characterized by a more anaplastic fibroblast with a higher index of mitotic activity and less collagen fiber formation. It is common to see a basket-woven or storiform pattern in the microscopic picture.

The prognosis and treatment are directly related to the histologic grade of the tumor. Low-grade fibrosarcoma has a better prognosis than osteosarcoma does, but it must be treated aggressively with wide resection to avoid local recurrence. Because the low-grade form has a low mitotic index, adjuvant chemotherapy and radiation therapy are of little help. High-grade fibrosarcoma has a prognosis and a rate of metastasis that are similar to those of osteosarcoma, and it is usually treated in a similar manner with a combination of surgery and, if the patient is young enough to tolerate the systemic toxicity, adjuvant chemotherapy.

B. Malignant Fibrous Histiocytoma of Bone

Prior to 1970, MFH was rarely diagnosed in bone but was commonly found in soft tissue. Now MFH is more common in bone than fibrosarcoma, but the two types of tumor run a similar clinical course. MFH of bone is seen in middle-age and older adults (see Table 6–2), is more common in males than in females, and affects the same bony sites as fibrosarcoma and osteosarcoma.

MFH is a purely lytic tumor that shows aggressive permeation of metaphyseal-diaphyseal bone, similar to the findings in lymphoma (Figure 6–57). Lytic destruction is diffuse, with no evidence of a periosteal response of blastic repair.

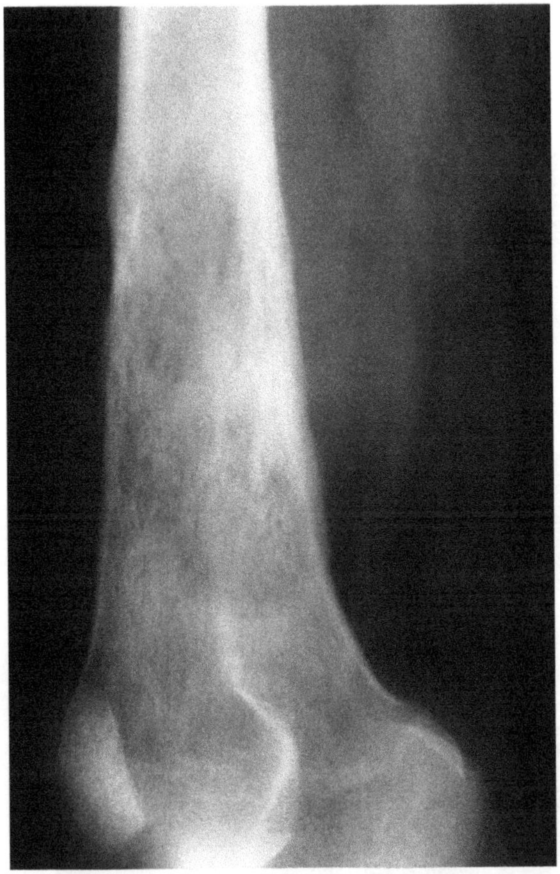

A

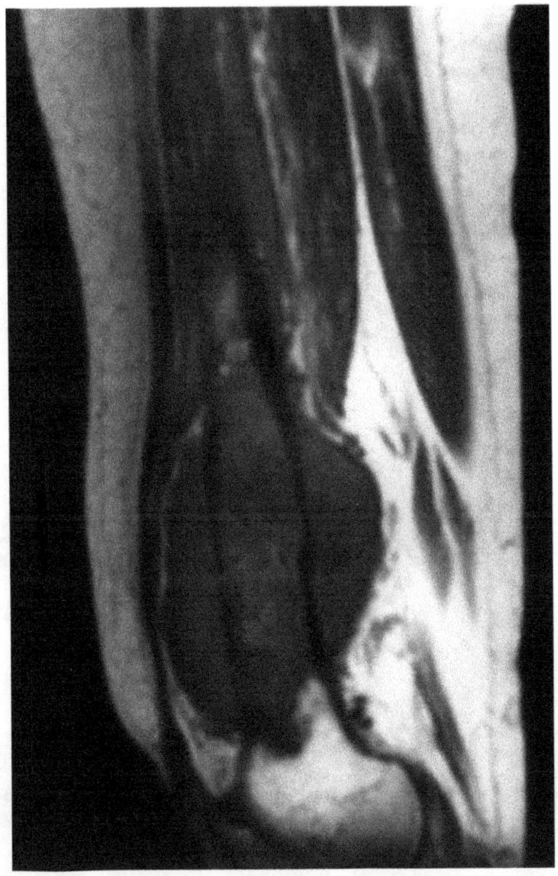

B

▲ **Figure 6–57.** Radiograph (**A**) and T1-weighted MRI (**B**) of malignant fibrous histiocytoma in the distal femur of a 50-year-old woman.

Histologic analysis of MFH typically shows the tumor to be high grade and have highly anaplastic fibroblasts mixed with malignant histiocytes and a few giant cells in a typical storiform pattern.

Because MFH is closely related to the high-grade fibrosarcoma, it carries a poor prognosis with high rates of local recurrence and metastasis. The treatment regimen is therefore similar to that for high-grade fibrosarcoma and osteosarcoma, and it includes an aggressive wide resection and the use of adjuvant chemotherapy.

Adamantinoma of Bone

Adamantinomas account for only 0.33% of all malignant bone tumors; occur with equal frequency in males and females, usually during the second and third decades of life; are found in the tibia in 90% of cases; and are usually diaphyseal in location, frequently starting in the anterior cortex. The cause of adamantinoma remains unknown, although angioblastic synovial cells and epithelial cells were considered in the past. Newer investigations, including immunohistochemistry and electron microscopic studies, lend support to the hypothesis of an epithelial origin, which goes along with the histologic appearance of a basal cell carcinoma and might explain the common site of origin subcutaneously in the anterior tibial cortex.

In patients with adamantinoma, the radiograph shows a benign tumor with a lytic central core that is surrounded by reactive sclerotic bone that typically bulges the anterior cortex and thus takes on the appearance of either fibrous dysplasia or osteofibrous dysplasia (Figure 6–58). One consideration in the differential diagnosis is that osteofibrous dysplasia is painless, whereas pain is a frequent symptom in adamantinoma. Another is that benign fibrous lesions of bone stop growing at bone maturity, whereas the adamantinoma continues on into adult life, at which point a biopsy

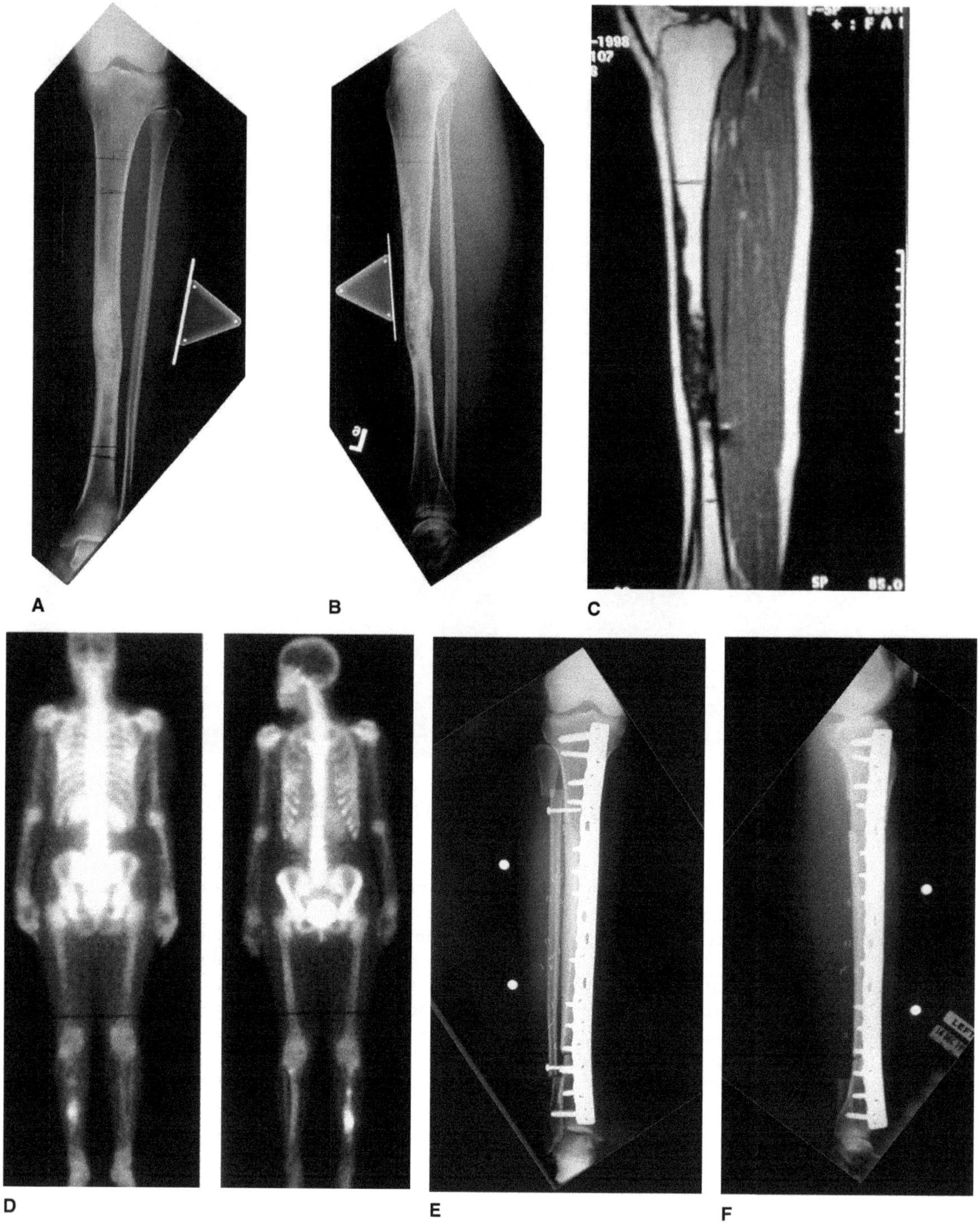

▲ **Figure 6–58.** Adamantinoma of the tibia. Initial anteroposterior radiograph (**A**), lateral radiograph (**B**), bone scan (**C**), and MRI (**D**). Immediate postoperative radiographs after resection with intercalary allograft reconstruction and vascularized fibula transport are shown in **E** and **F**. Anteroposterior and lateral radiographs from 3 years postoperatively are shown in **G** and **H**. Clinical photographs from 3 years postoperatively are shown in **I–K**.

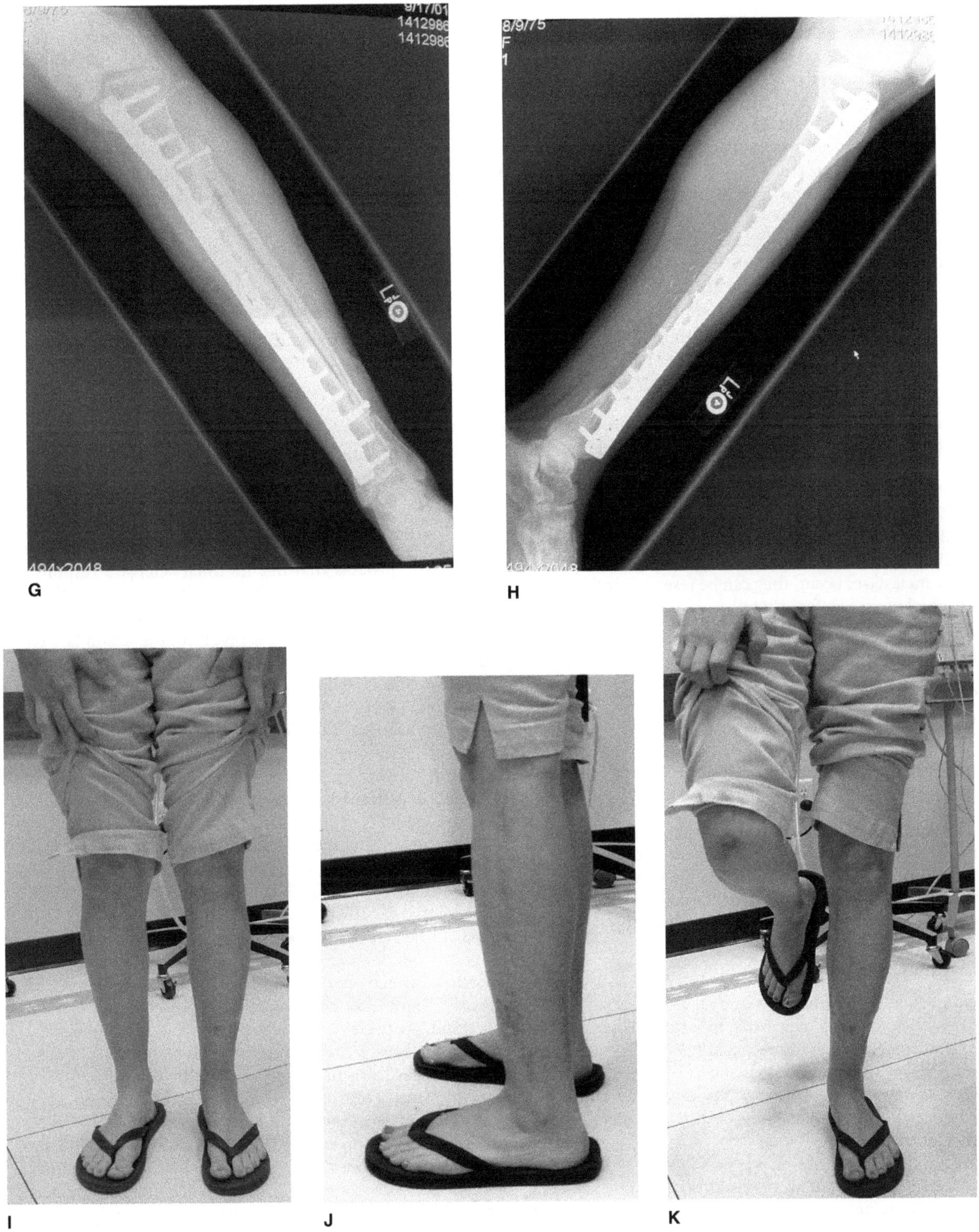

▲ **Figure 6–58.** (*Continued*)

of the progressive lytic portion of the disease should be performed. There have been cases of osteofibrous dysplasia combined with small areas of adamantinoma scattered in the benign osseofibrous tissue. In fact, more recently, one variant has been termed osteofibrous dysplasia–like adamantinoma and appears to have less overall biologic potential. Adamantinoma is also occasionally found in both the tibia and fibula, so the physician should look for multiple sites. It is an area of ongoing investigation whether osteofibrous dysplasia and adamantinoma represent distinct entities or if osteofibrous dysplasia is a precursor lesion to adamantinoma.

Microscopic findings include nests or cords of epithelial or angioid tissue growing in a fibrous tissue stroma, which can give adamantinoma the appearance of a low-grade angiosarcoma or a metastatic carcinoma. Cytologically, chromosomal abnormalities are frequent, especially gains of chromosomes 7, 8, 12, and 19.

Adamantinoma grows extremely slowly, over many years, but on occasion metastasizes to regional lymph nodes and the lung. For this reason, it should be treated by a wide resection, which in most cases is a segmental diaphyseal resection followed by an allograft reconstruction over an intramedullary nail. Because of the low-grade nature of this tumor, adjuvant irradiation or chemotherapy is rarely indicated. Even if pulmonary metastases occur, they can be resected, and there is a fairly good prognosis for survival.

Essentials of Diagnosis

- *Adamantinoma and osteofibrous dysplasia should be distinguished by increasing pain and radiographic progression.*

Vascular Sarcomas of Bone

Vascular sarcomas are relatively rare. They include hemangioendothelioma, angiosarcoma, and hemangiopericytoma of bone. The terms *hemangioendothelioma* and *angiosarcoma* are frequently used synonymously; however, the first term refers to a low-grade tumor, and the second term usually suggests a higher-grade lesion with a poorer prognosis.

A. Hemangioendothelioma

The hemangioendothelioma, also known as angiosarcoma, which is more common in males than in females, is seen in a wide range of ages between the second and seventh decades. The femur, pelvis, spine, and ribs are the usual sites of origin, and the diaphyses and metaphyses of the long bones are also involved. One-third of cases are multicentric, usually in the same bone or limb.

Radiographically, the lesion appears purely lytic. The more anaplastic the disease process is, the less reactive bone is. The clinical picture varies widely, depending on the histologic grade of the tumor. The low-grade lesions look like benign hemangiomas, are slow growing, and carry an excellent prognosis. The high-grade lesions are fast-growing lytic lesions with a poor prognosis.

Treatment depends on the histologic grade. The low-grade lesions do well with simple curettage and bone graft, but the high-grade lesions require a more aggressive wide resection and reconstruction. Adjuvant chemotherapy and radiation therapy can be considered for high-grade lesions, especially in patients with multifocal disease.

Chordomas

Chordoma of bone is rare and accounts for 4% of malignant bone tumors. It takes its origin from the primitive notochord and has the clinical appearance of a chondrosarcoma. Chordomas affect males more frequently than females and are seen in patients between 30 and 80 years of age. Although 50% of the tumors are sacrococcygeal in origin, 37% arise in the sphenoccipital area, and the remainder of tumors arise from vertebral bodies of the cervical, thoracic, or lumbar spine. The cranial lesions are seen in a younger age group and carry a poor prognosis because of proximity to the brain, where surgical removal is difficult.

On radiograph, the chordoma appears as a centrally located lytic process that has minimal sclerotic response at the periphery and may show slight matrix calcification, as in a chondrosarcoma. By definition, chordoma is a midline lesion. If the sacrum is involved, the lesion is seen usually in the lower three sacral segments and presents as an extracortical lobulated mass both in front and behind the sacrum. Because of the slow tumor growth, pain may not occur early, but constipation can be an early symptom that results from pressure on the rectum. Because the true anatomic borders are not readily defined by routine radiography, it is best to image this tumor with CT or MRI (Figure 6–59).

Microscopically, nests or cords of cells, sprinkled in a sea of mucinous tissue, give an appearance similar to low-grade chondrosarcoma. Classically, chordomas are found to have large vacuolated cells with small round nuclei that appear like a signet ring, referred to as physaliferous cells.

Treatment for the sacral lesions is an aggressive wide resection, which can be difficult because of excessive bleeding. Significant neurogenic bowel and bladder deficits can result. At present, it is common to use high-dose neoadjuvant radiation therapy. Adjuvant radiation is not currently standard practice, especially in the case of negative margins. Local recurrence is unfortunately common after surgical resection of chordomas, with reported rates between 19% and 54%. Recurrence as late as 10 to 15 years following surgery is not uncommon. Because of the low-grade characteristics of the chordoma, it is rare to encounter pulmonary metastasis, even after a local recurrence following an inadequate local surgical resection.

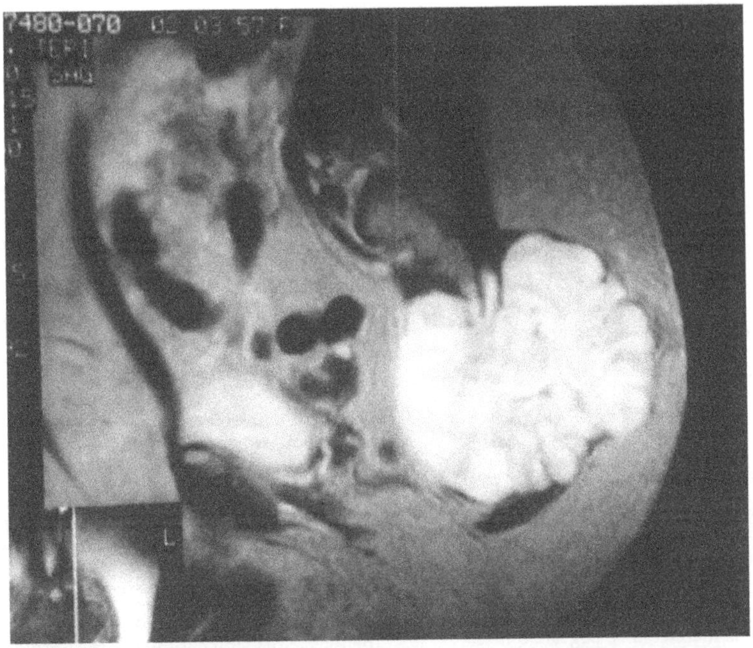

A

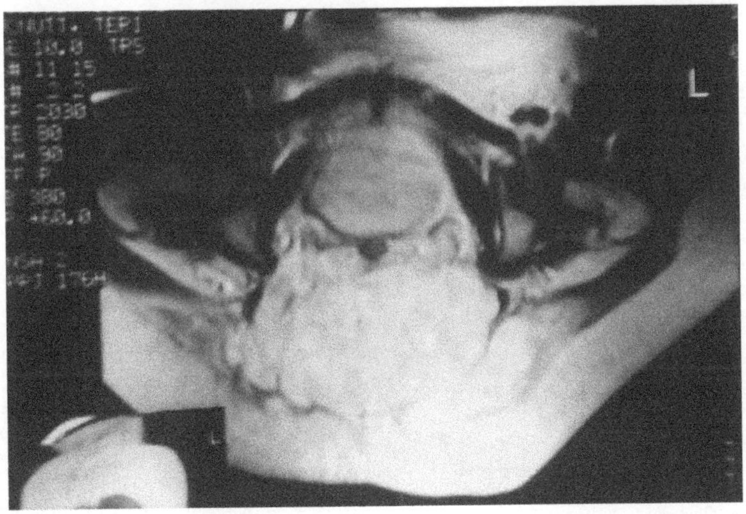

B

▲ **Figure 6–59.** Sacral chordoma in middle-aged woman: T2 sagittal image (**A**) and T2 transverse image (**B**).

Essentials of Diagnosis

- *Information provided in the history and physical examination is critical in determining malignant versus benign characteristics of bone tumors.*
- *Survival in Ewing sarcoma and osteosarcoma has been dramatically improved with refined neoadjuvant chemotherapy, and the timing and duration of that treatment modality can affect outcome.*
- *Biopsy of bone lesions with suspected malignant potential should include a portion of the periphery of the lesion, particularly when there is an associated soft-tissue component, as this is where the most diagnostic tissue is found.*

Ailon T, Torabi R, Fisher CG, et al. Management of locally recurrent chordoma of the mobile spine and sacrum. *Spine (Phila Pa 1976).* 2016;41(suppl 20):S193-S198. [PMID: 27753782]

Albergo JI, Gaston CL, Aponte-Tinao LA, et al. Proximal tibia reconstruction after bone tumor resection: are survivorship and outcomes of endoprosthetic replacement and osteoarticular allograft similar? *Clin Orthop Relat Res.* 2017;475(3): 676-682. [PMID: 27103142]

Anwer F, Gee KM, Iftikhar A, et al. Future of personalized therapy targeting aberrant signaling pathways in multiple myeloma. *Clin Lymphoma Myeloma Leuk.* 2019;19(7):397-405. [PMID: 31036508]

Avnet S, Longhi A, Salerno M, et al. Increased osteoclast activity is associated with aggressiveness of osteosarcoma. *Int J Oncol.* 2008;33:1231-1238. [PMID: 19020756]

Bacci G, Balladelli A, Palmerini E, et al. Neoadjuvant chemotherapy for osteosarcoma of the extremities in preadolescent patients: the Rizzoli Institute experience. *J Pediatr Hematol Oncol.* 2008;30:908-912. [PMID: 19131777]

Bacci G, Forni C, Longhi A, et al. Local recurrence and local control of non-metastatic osteosarcoma of the extremities: a 27-year experience in a single institution. *J Surg Oncol.* 2007;96:118-123. [PMID: 17577221]

Bielack SS, Smeland SS, Whelan JS, et al. Methotrexate, doxorubicin, and cisplatin (MAP) plus maintenance pegylated interferon alfa-2b versus MAP alone in patients with resectable osteosarcoma and good histologic response to preoperative MAP: first results of the EURAMOS-1 good response randomized controlled trial. *J Clin Oncol.* 2015;33(20):2279-2287. [PMID: 26033801]

Chen X, Yu LJ, Peng HM, et al. Is intralesional resection suitable for central grade 1 chondrosarcoma: a systematic review and updated meta-analysis. *Eur J Surg Oncol.* 2017;43(9): 1718-1726. [PMID: 28666625]

Corradi D, Wenger DE, Bertoni F, et al. Multicentric osteosarcoma: clinicopathologic and radiographic study of 56 cases. *Am J Clin Pathol.* 2011;136(5):799-807. [PMID: 22031320]

Czajka CM, DiCaprio MR. What is the proportion of patients with multiple hereditary exostoses who undergo malignant degeneration? *Clin Orthop Relat Res.* 2015;473(7):2355-2361. [PMID: 25582066]

Dea N, Fisher CG, Reynolds JJ, et al. Current treatment strategy for newly diagnosed chordoma of the mobile spine and sacrum: results of an international survey. *J Neurosurg Spine.* 2018;30(1):119-125. [PMID: 30497218]

Dierselhuis EF, Goulding KA, Stevens M, et al. Intralesional treatment versus wide resection for central low-grade chondrosarcoma of the long bones. *Cochrane Database Syst Rev.* 2019;3:CD010778. [PMID: 30845364]

El Beaino M, Roszik J, Livingston JA, et al. Mesenchymal chondrosarcoma: a review with emphasis on its fusion-driven biology. *Curr Oncol Rep.* 2018;20(5):37. [PMID: 29582189]

Ferrari S, Meazza C, Palmerini E, et al. Nonmetastatic osteosarcoma of the extremity. Neoadjuvant chemotherapy with methotrexate, cisplatin, doxorubicin and ifosfamide. An Italian Sarcoma Group study (ISG/OS-Oss). *Tumori.* 2014;100(6):612-619. [PMID: 25688494]

Gandolfi S, Laubach JP, Hideshima T, et al. The proteasome and proteasome inhibitors in multiple myeloma. *Cancer Metastasis Rev.* 2017;36(4):561-584. [PMID: 29196868]

Gelderblom H, Hogendoorn PC, Dijkstra SD, et al. The clinical approach towards chondrosarcoma. *Oncologist.* 2008;13: 320-329. [PMID: 18378543]

Hang JF, Chen PC. Parosteal osteosarcoma. *Arch Pathol Lab Med.* 2014;138(5):694-699. [PMID: 24786129]

Harrison DJ, Schwartz CL. Osteogenic sarcoma: systemic chemotherapy options for localized disease. *Curr Treat Options Oncol.* 2017;18(4):24. [PMID: 28391422]

Huang R, Sun Z, Zheng H, et al. Identifying the prognosis factors and predicting the survival probability in patients with non-metastatic chondrosarcoma from the SEER database. *Orthop Surg.* 2019;11(5):801-810. [PMID: 31663279]

Jeys LM, Thorne CJ, Parry M, et al. A novel system for the surgical staging of primary high-grade osteosarcoma: the Birmingham classification. *Clin Orthop Relat Res.* 2017;475(3):842-850. [PMID: 27138473]

Lagares-Tena L, Garcia-Monclus S, Lopez-Alemany R, et al. Caveolin-1 promotes Ewing sarcoma metastasis regulating MMP-9 expression through MAPK/EK pathway. *Oncotarget.* 2016;7(35):56889-56903. [PMID: 27487136]

Laitinen M, Parry M, Albergo JI, et al. The prognostic and therapeutic factors which influence the oncological outcome of parosteal osteosarcoma. *Bone Joint J.* 2015;97-B(12):1698-1703. [PMID: 26637687]

Liu JQ, Bai X, Duan DC, et al. Role of five small nucleotide polymorphisms in the VEGF gene on the susceptibility to osteosarcoma and overall survival of patients. *Oncol Lett.* 2015;10(3):1481-1486. [PMID: 26622695]

Lozano Calderon SA, Kuechle J, Raskin KA, et al. Lower extremity megaprostheses in orthopaedic oncology. *J Am Acad Orthop Surg.* 2018;26(12):e249-e257. [PMID: 29781818]

Nagano A, Ohno T, Shimizu K, et al. EWS/Fli-1 chimeric fusion gene upregulates vascular endothelial growth factor-A. *Int J Cancer.* 2010;126(12):2790-2798. [PMID: 19642105]

Parrondo RD, Sher T. Prevention of skeletal related events in multiple myeloma: focus on the RANK-L pathway in the treatment of multiple myeloma. *Onco Targets Ther.* 2019;12:8467-8478. [PMID: 31686861]

Rotondo RL, Folkert W, Liebsch NJ, et al. High-dose proton-based radiation therapy in the management of spine chordomas: outcomes and clinicopathological prognostic factors. *J Neurosurg Spine.* 2015;23(6):788-797. [PMID: 26340383]

Scholfield DW, Sadozai Z, Ghali C, et al. Does osteofibrous dysplasia progress to adamantinoma and how should they be treated? *Bone Joint J.* 2017;99-B(3):409-416. [PMID: 28249983]

Smeland S, Bielack SS, Whelan J, et al. Survival and prognosis with osteosarcoma: outcomes in more than 2000 patients in the EURAMOS-1 (European and American Osteosarcoma Study) cohort. *Eur J Cancer.* 2019;109:36-50. [PMID: 30685685]

Surgeon's Committee of the Chinese Myeloma Working Group of the International Myeloma Foundation. Consensus on surgical management of myeloma bone disease. *Orthop Surg.* 2016;8(3):263-269. [PMID: 27627707]

BENIGN SOFT-TISSUE TUMORS

Soft tissue can be defined as nonepithelial, extraskeletal mesenchymal tissue exclusive of the reticuloendothelial system and glia. This definition would include fat, fibrous tissue, muscle, and the relating neurovascular structures.

Benign soft-tissue tumors, by definition, represent a differentiated neoplastic process with a limited capacity for autonomous growth. They generally demonstrate a marginal capacity to invade locally with infrequent local recurrence. Because of the extensive numbers of benign soft-tissue tumors, discussion is limited here to the more common entities.

Lipomas

The lipoma is by far the most common soft-tissue tumor, accounting for approximately 50% of all soft-tissue tumors. Lipomas occur in about 2% of the population and typically present between the ages of 40 and 60 years. Lipomas are rarely seen in childhood, with multiple lesions highly suggestive of hamartomatous polyposis syndromes. Lipoma outnumbers liposarcoma by a ratio of 100:1. Cytogenetic abnormalities have been reported in 50% to 80% of lipomas. There are a large number of variants including the superficial subcutaneous lipoma; the intramuscular lipoma; the spindle cell lipoma; the angiolipoma; the benign lipoblastoma; and the lipomas of tendon sheaths, nerves, synovium, periosteum, and lumbosacral area.

A. Superficial Subcutaneous Lipoma

The most frequently seen type of lipoma is the superficial subcutaneous type, which can be solitary or multiple. Subcutaneous lipomas occur with equal frequency in men and women and seem to arise spontaneously during the fifth and sixth decade of life. The most common locations are the back, shoulder, and neck.

On palpation, this tumor is soft and ballotable. Although it is found more commonly in obese patients, the size of the lipoma does not correlate with the weight of the patient. Lipomas do not reduce in volume with weight loss. They generally grow to a limited size of about 1 to 3 cm, although occasional giant lipomas are 10 to 20 cm, and sarcomatous transformation does not occur. Surgical treatment is usually cosmetic in nature, and the recurrence rate is less than 5%.

B. Intramuscular Lipoma

The deep intramuscular lipoma is seen in adults between 30 and 60 years of age, affects men more frequently than women, and is commonly found in the large muscles of the extremities. The lesions are slow growing and painless. The intramuscular lipoma has a characteristic radiolucency that contrasts with the surrounding muscle (Figure 6–60). On MRI, this tumor demonstrates a uniform high-signal image on the T1-weighted spin-echo sequence. On gross examination, the tumor can appear quite infiltrative in surrounding muscle and has a faint yellow color on sectioning. Histologic studies show that the intramuscular lipoma, like the subcutaneous lipoma, is composed of benign lipocytes with small pyknotic nuclei that are difficult to see on the surface of the large fat-laden cell. When samples are taken for biopsy purposes, the pathologist must take care to rule out a low-grade, well-differentiated liposarcoma that can coexist with a benign lipoma. On rare occasions, a lipoma can have chondroid or osseous hamartomatous elements that have caused it to be classified as a mesenchymoma in the past. In other cases, evidence of hemorrhage or necrosis can be found in a lipoma and creates low-signal changes on the MRI that are similar to the changes seen in liposarcoma.

A marginal surgical excision is indicated for treatment of intramuscular lipoma. Local recurrence rates of 15% to 60% are reported.

C. Spindle Cell Lipoma

The spindle cell lipoma is seen typically in the posterior neck and shoulder area in men between 45 and 64 years of age. On gross examination, the spindle cell lipoma has the appearance of an ordinary lipoma but with areas of gray-white gelatinous foci streaking through it. Microscopic examination of these areas reveals the presence of benign fibroblasts. Thus, with imaging studies, dense areas are scattered throughout the normal radiolucent areas of a lipoma. On MRI, findings generally consist of a low-signal streaking through the typical high-signal pattern of a benign lipoma. The treatment for this lesion is a simple marginal resection. The chance for local recurrence is minimal.

D. Angiolipoma

The angiolipoma (Figure 6–61) is a subcutaneous lesion seen in young adults (see Table 6–6), usually on the forearm. Multiple lesions are frequently present and usually painful because of their vascularity. Grossly, the lobular lipoma demonstrates vascular channels. Treatment of angiolipoma consists of marginal excision.

E. Diffuse Lipomatosis

An extremely rare variant of the lipoma is diffuse lipomatosis, characterized by the presence of multiple superficial and deep lipomas that involve one entire extremity or the trunk and usually have their onset during the first 2 years of life. Histologically, an individual lesion in a patient with diffuse lipomatosis looks no different from a typical solitary lipoma. When lipomatosis of a nerve occurs, the involved limb or digit may become massive in size, sometimes making it impossible to remove the fatty tumors surgically. If this is the case, amputation may be indicated.

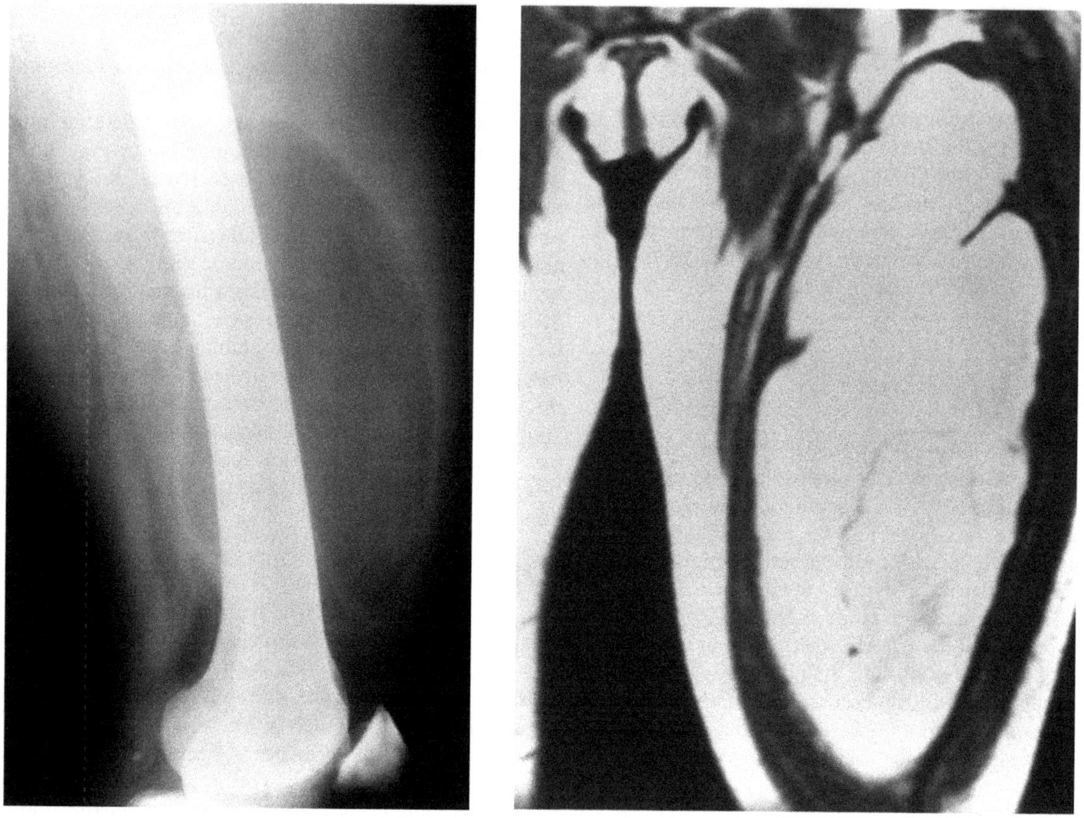

A B

▲ **Figure 6–60.** Radiograph (**A**) and coronal view T1-weighted MRI (**B**) of an intramuscular lipoma in the quadriceps muscle of a 72-year-old man.

F. Lumbosacral Lipoma

The lumbosacral lipoma occurs in the lumbosacral area posterior to a spina bifida defect. It is frequently associated with both intradural and extradural lipomas and thus can result in neurologic deficits. Although lumbosacral lipoma is generally considered a pediatric tumor, it can be seen in adults (Figure 6–62).

Surgical treatment consists of a marginal resection of the entire lipoma, including the portion arising from the vertebral canal and lumbosacral roots.

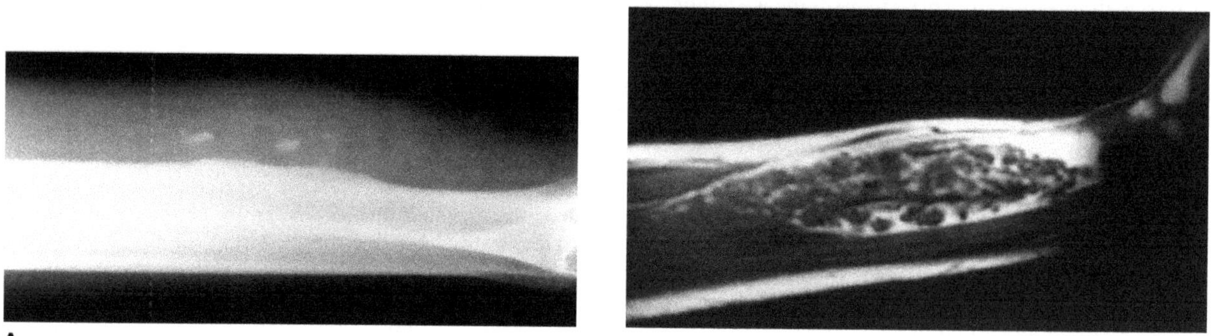

A B

▲ **Figure 6–61.** Radiograph (**A**) and T1-weighted MRI (**B**) of a soft-tissue angiolipoma in the volar aspect of the forearm of a 27-year-old woman.

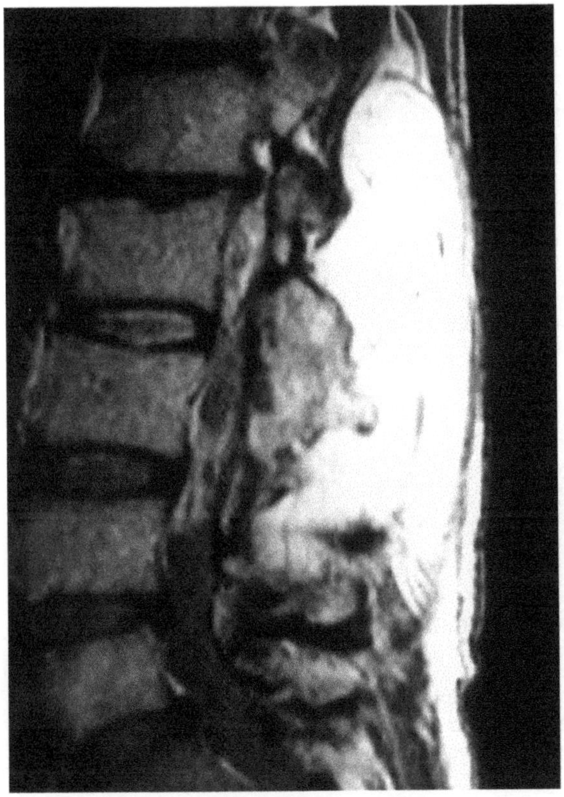

▲ **Figure 6–62.** T1-weighted MRI of a lumbosacral lipoma.

G. Benign Lipoblastoma and Diffuse Lipoblastomatosis

The benign and diffuse types of lipoblastoma arise from embryonic white fat and are typically seen in the extremities or trunk of infants before the age of 3 years. The lesions, solitary or multiple, can be superficial or deep in muscle tissue. They demonstrate cellular immaturity, with lipoblasts similar to the myxoid form of liposarcoma. Even with the cellular aggressiveness of the lesions, the prognosis is excellent following simple surgical resection.

H. Hibernoma

Hibernoma, a rare lipoma usually seen in young adults (see Table 6–6), commonly occurs in the scapular and interscapular regions, is painless and slow growing, and ranges between 10 and 15 cm in diameter. The hibernoma is composed of finely granular or vacuolated cells characteristic of brown fat and contains a considerable amount of glycogen. The treatment is marginal surgical resection with a low potential for recurrence.

Essentials of Diagnosis

- *In the histologic characterization of lipomatous lesions, biopsy is subject to considerable sampling error. Therefore, if incisional biopsy is indicated, the most suspicious portion of the lesion should be obtained.*
- *The differential diagnosis of macrodactyly should include lipomatosis of nerve.*
- *MRI findings of a lesion that shares the same signal intensity as subcutaneous fat on all sequences are diagnostic of a benign to low-grade lipomatous lesion.*

Benign Vascular Tumors

Benign vascular proliferative tumors are the second most common benign tumor after lipomas. Three types of vascular tumors are discussed here: hemangiomas, lymphangiomas, and glomus tumors.

Like lipomas, angiomas occur in a wide variety of clinical conditions seen more often in females than in males. The most common type of angioma is the hemangioma, which can be a superficial cutaneous lesion or a deep, intramuscular one. The lymphatic counterpart of the hemangioma is known as the lymphangioma or hygroma. In most cases, the lesion is solitary or localized. If it is extensive and involves an entire limb, the term *angiomatosis* is used. Because most hemangiomas and lymphangiomas are congenital, the term *hamartomatous* or *arteriovenous malformation* is applied in their classification. Hemangiomas and lymphangiomas arise from developmental dysplasias of the endothelial tube, whereas glomus tumors arise from pericytes, which are cells that lie outside the endothelial tube. Most vascular anomalies arise sporadically, but some familial, autosomal dominant inheritance patterns are also described. Genetic analysis of these families identified specific gene mutations supporting the genomic role in the regulation of angiogenesis.

A. Hemangioma

Hemangiomas are the most frequently seen tumors of childhood and account for 7% of all benign tumors.

1. Capillary hemangioma—The most common type of hemangioma is the solitary capillary type, also referred to as the port-wine stain, which appears as an elevated red to purple cutaneous lesion on the head or neck. The lesion occurs during the first few weeks after birth, grows rapidly over a period of several months, and regresses over a 7-year period in 75% to 90% of cases.

Because of the spontaneous regression, no treatment is needed in most cases. In the past, treatment consisted of cryosurgery, sclerotherapy, or irradiation, but frequently, this treatment was worse than the disease itself. Today, when treatment is required, the treatment of choice involves the use of selective laser coagulation.

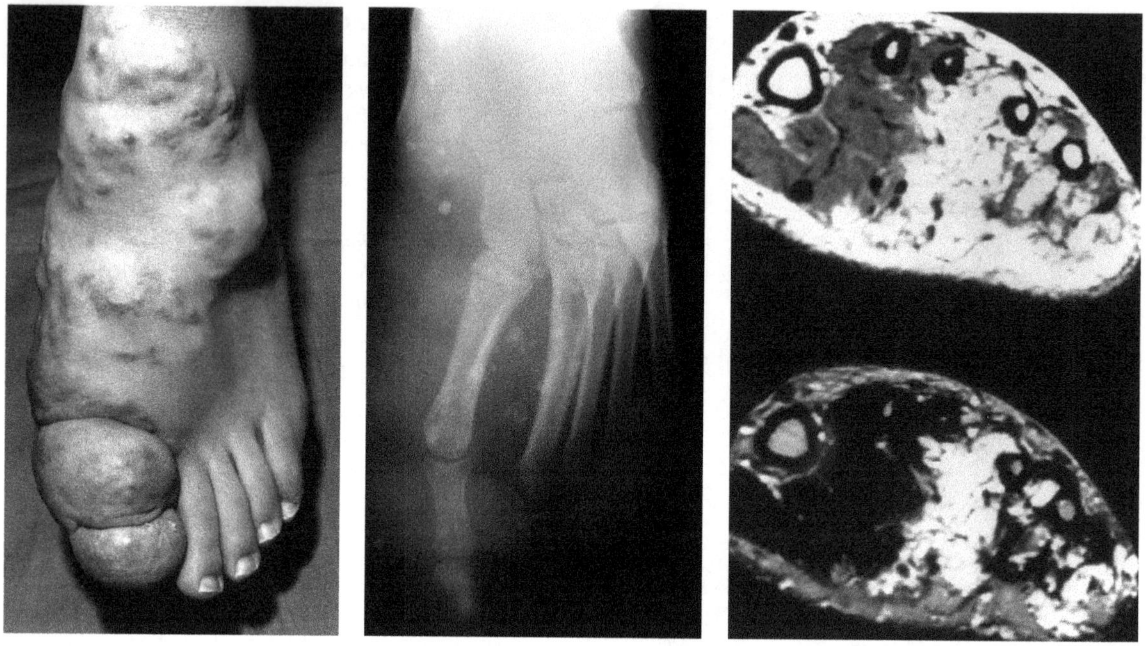

A B C

▲ **Figure 6–63.** Clinical appearance (**A**) and radiographic appearance (**B**) of a cavernous hemangioma in the foot of one patient, and T1-weighted and T2-weighted MRIs (**C**) of a cavernous hemangioma of another patient.

2. Cavernous hemangioma—The cavernous hemangioma is larger and less common than the capillary hemangioma. The enlarged vascular spaces of the cavernous lesion give it the appearance of a cluster of purple grapes. It lies deep in the extremity, with common involvement of muscles and even the synovial membrane of the joints (synovial hemangioma).

Imaging may be characteristic (Figure 6–63). In some patients with deep intramuscular forms of hemangioma, the skin shows no abnormalities and no phleboliths are apparent on radiograph. With MRI, deep intramuscular hemangiomas can be easily detected by the characteristic mixed-signal serpiginous pattern seen in the T1-weighted image.

The muscle lesions are usually asymptomatic until intralesional hemorrhage occurs either spontaneously or after a minor injury. The pain symptoms are usually short lived but recur infrequently. In some patients, the pain is more severe and associated with muscle contracture and joint deformity. These patients may require surgical resection of the scarred-down lesion to allow for better joint function and to reduce the pain. In rare cases of multiple hemangiomas involving the entire limb, amputation may be indicated. Vascular embolization of the feeder vessels can be attempted but may lead to a significant compartment syndrome, with severe contractures or with loss of muscle strength and limitation of joint movement.

3. Arteriovenous hemangioma—The arteriovenous hemangioma is seen in young patients (see Table 6–6), usually in the head, neck, or lower extremity. It is associated with significant arteriovenous shunting in the tumor, which creates increased perfusion. This results in increased local temperature, pain, and continuous thrill or bruit over the mass. In the extremity, it also results in an overgrowth of the limb (Klippel-Trenaunay syndrome).

If shunting is excessive, surgical removal of the hemangioma may be necessary to prevent consumptive coagulopathy and high-output cardiac failure (Kasabach-Merritt syndrome). Arteriograms are helpful in determining the degree of shunting prior to treatment. Embolization or surgical ligation of feeder vessels is frequently not a successful form of treatment.

4. Epithelioid hemangioma (Kimura disease)—This cutaneous hemangioma is found on the head or neck in women between 20 and 40 years old. It is associated with inflammatory changes and eosinophilia, and it sometime ulcerates. Its name is derived from the epithelial appearance of the endothelia-lined capillary structures.

5. Pyogenic granuloma—The pyogenic granuloma is a polypoid capillary hemangioma that affects the skin or mucosal surfaces of males and females in all age groups. It may be associated with trauma and is found about the mouth, gingivae, or fingers. The lesions have a purple-red color, bleed easily, and ulcerate.

B. Lymphangioma

The lymphangioma is nothing more than an angioma composed of lymphatic endothelial tubes filled with lymphatic fluid, rather than being filled with blood, as the hemangioma is. Lymphangiomas can be localized, which occurs with the cystic hygroma, and they are usually seen about the head, neck, or axilla of young boys and girls (see Table 6–6). As with hemangiomas, the larger lymphomas are cavernous lesions seen in older patients with deeper involvement. In both lymphangioma and hemangioma, because of increased regional perfusion, bony overgrowth can occur (Figure 6–64).

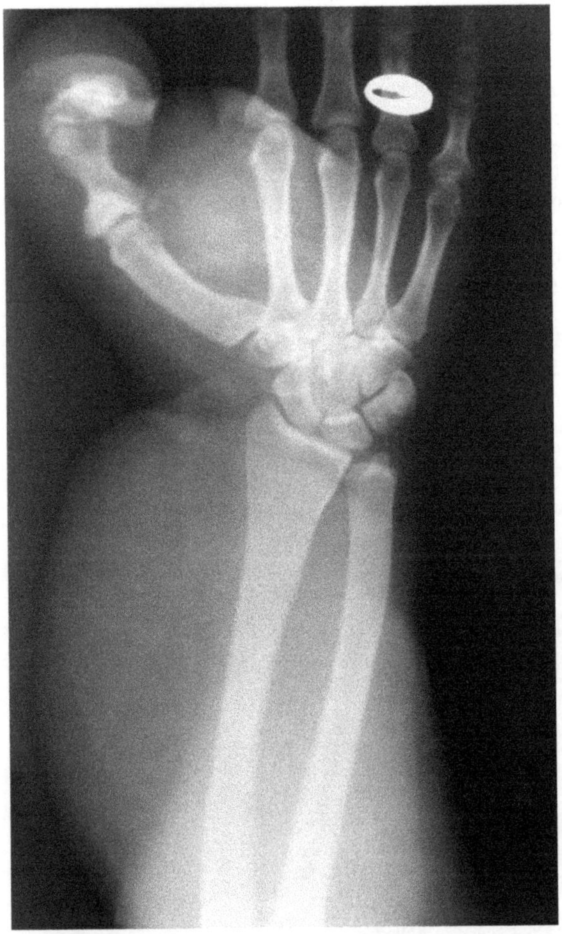

▲ **Figure 6–64.** Radiograph of a lymphangioma in the forearm and hand of a 23-year-old woman.

C. Glomus Tumor

The glomus tumor arises from the hemangiopericyte, which is a cell seen at the periphery of the capillary vascular network and normally involved with the regulation of blood flow through the capillary system. Microscopic examination of the tumor reveals large vascular spaces surrounded by a homogeneous field of round epithelioid hemangiopericytes, with no evidence of mitotic activity.

The glomus tumor is a pink lesion that usually measures less than 1 cm in diameter. It represents 1.6% of all soft-tissue tumors and occurs with equal frequency in men and women, usually between 20 and 40 years of age. Although the tumor is found most commonly in the subungual area of a digit, where it is readily visible, it also occurs subcutaneously on the hand, wrist, forearm, or foot, where it may be invisible and thus difficult to diagnose until localized lancinating pain leads to a surgical exploration. Glomus tumors have sporadically been reported in deep soft tissues, viscera, and intraosseous locations as well. After the lesion is surgically removed, the pain subsides and recurrence occurs in fewer than 10% of cases.

Essentials of Diagnosis

- *Radiographic findings of phleboliths are diagnostic of hemangioma.*
- *Glomus tumors are usually diagnosed at a very small size due to characteristic location in the fingertip and extreme cold sensitivity.*

Extraabdominal Desmoid Tumors (Aggressive Fibromatosis)

In comparison with the infantile fibrous lesions mentioned earlier, the desmoid tumor is seen in older children and young adults up through 40 years of age. Whereas abdominal desmoids are seen in the abdominal wall of women following pregnancy, the extraabdominal desmoids usually occur in men and are more common in proximal areas about the shoulder and buttock, followed next by the posterior thigh, popliteal area, arm, and forearm. In most cases, it presents as a solitary tumor. Multicentric involvement is seen at times, however, and can be associated with Gardner syndrome, which is characterized by polyposis of the large bowel and by craniofacial osteomas. In patients with familial adenomatous polyposis (FAP), an inherited disease caused by mutations in the *APC* gene, desmoids are a significant source of morbidity and mortality. The *APC* gene, located on chromosome 5, encodes for a 300-kDa protein, in which a germline mutation is an early event in tumor formation.

Desmoids are deep-seated tumors that arise from muscle fascial planes and infiltrate extensively into adjacent muscle tissue, tendons, joint capsules, and even bone. Compared with malignant fibrosarcomas, desmoids are poorly marginated and thus difficult to resect surgically. Desmoids can engulf surrounding vessels and nerves, whereas fibrosarcomas usually push these structures aside. A desmoid may cause local pain and grow quite rapidly, suggesting a malignant tumor. The desmoid tends to grow more longitudinally along muscle planes to a considerable size, frequently resulting in restricted joint motion about the shoulder, hip, or knee. Because the local aggressiveness of desmoids is so similar to that of malignant fibrosarcomas or MFHs, some experts believe the desmoid may be a low-grade fibrosarcoma that has lost its potential to metastasize; however, molecular analyses may suggest otherwise.

On gross examination, a desmoid tumor is firm and heavily collagenized. Microscopically, it has a low mitotic index, similar to that of a plantar or palmar fibromatosis. Radiographically, a desmoid is noncalcified and appears dense in comparison with normal muscle. It is easily seen in soft window CT scanning. More exact presurgical imaging can be obtained with MRI (Figure 6–65). As with an abdominal desmoid, an extraabdominal desmoid physical injury may play a role in the activation of a preexisting oncogene located in the damaged fibroblast.

Desmoids are usually treated surgically with an aggressive wide resection similar to that used in treating a primary sarcoma. Even following a margin-negative resection of the desmoid, the recurrence rate may approach 50%. For this reason, it is common to administer 50 Gy of radiation to the surgical site starting 2 weeks postoperatively. With radiation therapy, the recurrence rate decreases to 15%. In rare cases, an amputation may be necessary after multiple recurrences. A few cases of spontaneous involution of desmoid tumors are reported after 40 years of age.

Based on clinical and experimental evidence, estrogen may play a role in the development of desmoid tumors. Accordingly, agents such as tamoxifen are being used in some centers because of their antiestrogen effects. NSAIDs were also implemented in attempts to treat aggressive cases. Cytotoxic chemotherapy has also been instituted in selected unresectable cases, especially associated with familial adenomatous polyposis, with some success.

Essentials of Diagnosis

- *Desmoids are benign but may be extremely locally aggressive, with up to 50% recurring locally after margin-negative resection alone.*

Benign Tumors of Peripheral Nerves

Benign tumors of peripheral nerve sheaths are common and take their origin from Schwann cells, which normally produce myelin and collagen fiber.

A. Neurilemmoma

The neurilemmoma (neurinoma or benign schwannoma) is the least common of the benign tumors of peripheral nerve sheaths. It usually affects individuals between 20 and 50 years of age and occurs with equal frequency in men and women. It has a predilection for spinal roots and for superficial nerves on the flexor surfaces of both upper and lower extremities. In most cases, the lesion is solitary, but multiple lesions are occasionally seen in neurofibromatosis type 1 (von Recklinghausen disease). The neurilemmoma is slow growing and rarely causes pain or a neurologic deficit.

Unlike the neurofibroma, which has a fusiform appearance, the neurilemmoma is round (Figure 6–66). Microscopic studies reveal the presence of a characteristic Verocay body, which consists of palisading Schwann cells and is found in the fibrotic Antoni A substance of the tumor. Other areas reveal a more mucinous Antoni B substance. Neurilemmomas may occur in an axial fashion involving spinal roots, often presenting as a dumbbell-shaped extradural defect (Figure 6–67). In comparison with the less restricted peripheral lesions, the nerve root lesions are more apt to

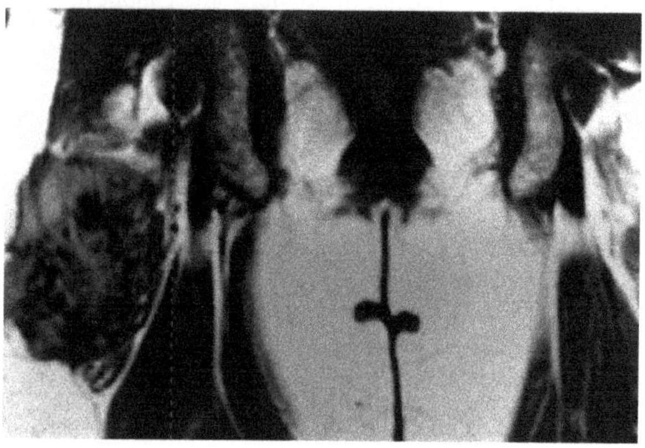

▲ **Figure 6–65.** T1-weighted MRI of a desmoid tumor in the gluteal area of a 45-year-old woman.

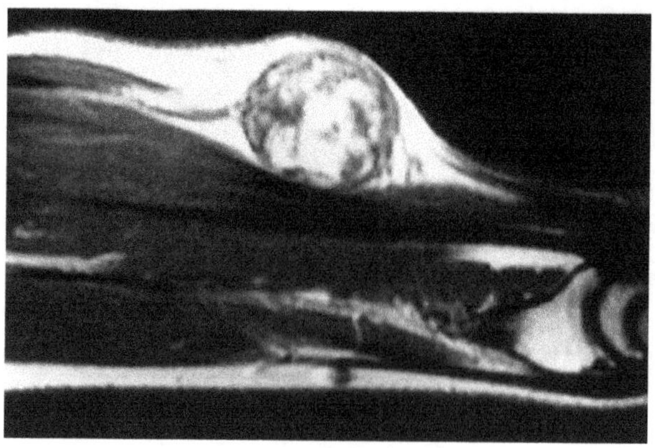

▲ **Figure 6–66.** T1-weighted MRI of a neurilemoma of the ulnar nerve in a 69-year-old man.

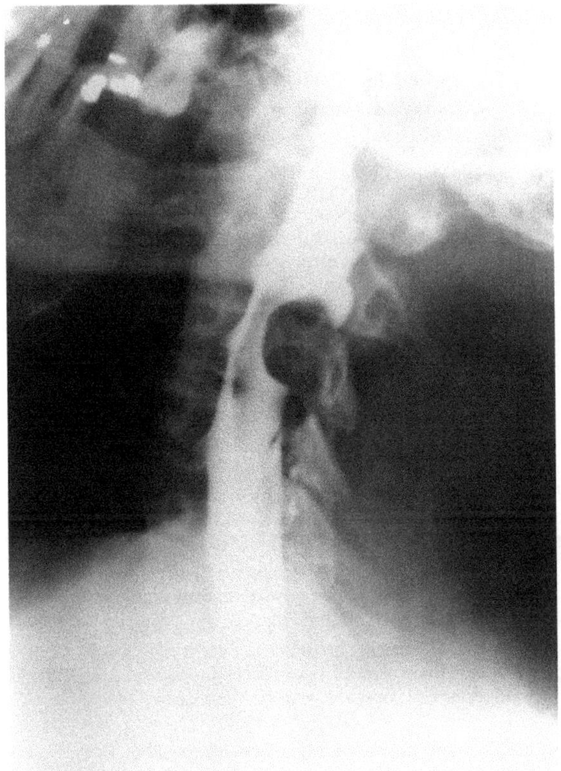

▲ **Figure 6–67.** Myelogram of a neurilemoma in the cervical spine.

cause pain associated with neurologic deficiency because of their bony constriction.

In some cases, simple excision of the neurilemmoma is clinically indicated, which often can be performed without serious damage to the nerve. If the patient is asymptomatic, observation is appropriate because there is little chance for malignant degeneration.

B. Solitary Neurofibroma

The solitary neurofibroma is a fusiform fibrotic tumor arising centrally from a smaller peripheral nerve (Figure 6–68). The tumor is seen with equal frequency in men and women, usually between 20 and 30 years of age. It is 10 times more common than the multiple form seen in von Recklinghausen disease (neurofibromatosis type 1), is usually smaller, and carries less chance of malignant degeneration. Microscopic examination of the solitary neurofibroma shows interlacing bundles of elongated spindle cells with benign-appearing nuclei and occasionally with areas resembling the Antoni A tissue seen in the neurilemmoma.

Treatment of the solitary neurofibroma consists of simple excision. Iatrogenic damage to the nerve fascicles is more likely than with resection of the neurilemmoma, due to the intertwined growth of the neurofibroma.

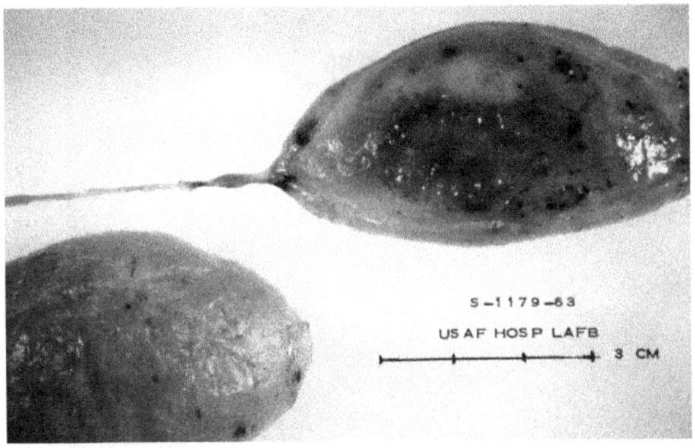

▲ **Figure 6–68.** Photographic appearance of a solitary neurofibroma.

C. Neurofibromatosis Type 1 (von Recklinghausen Disease)

von Recklinghausen disease is a familial dysplasia, inherited as an autosomal dominant trait, with an incidence of approximately 1 in every 3500 live births, approximately 50% of which are due to spontaneous mutations. The first noticeable clinical manifestations begin during the first few years of life with the emergence of small café-au-lait spots. Over time, these lesions grow in number and size. Unlike the lesions seen in fibrous dysplasia, the lesions in von Recklinghausen disease do not have rough edges. If a patient has more than six lesions that have smooth edges and are greater than 1.5 cm in diameter, the diagnosis of von Recklinghausen disease is certain.

Later in life, the patient develops multiple neurofibromas, each of which appears as a soft cutaneous nodule (Figure 6–69). This pedunculated skin lesion, which is called fibroma molluscum, can be large and pendulous. More pathognomonic of the disease is the plexiform neurofibroma, occurring in 25% of patients, which appears in larger nerves and can involve an entire extremity (see Figure 6–69). When the overlying skin of an extremity is loose and hyperpigmented, the condition is called elephantiasis neuromatosa, or "elephant man syndrome." (It is now thought that John Merrick, the so-called elephant man, was actually affected by Proteus syndrome.) Among the bony changes seen in von Recklinghausen disease are scoliosis in up to 20%, spinal meningocele, scalloping of the vertebra, osteolytic lesions in bone, congenital anterolateral tibial bowing, and pseudarthrosis of the tibia in 5%.

Sarcomatous transformation may occur in large and deep neurofibromas. This occurs at a later age in 3% to 5% of patients.

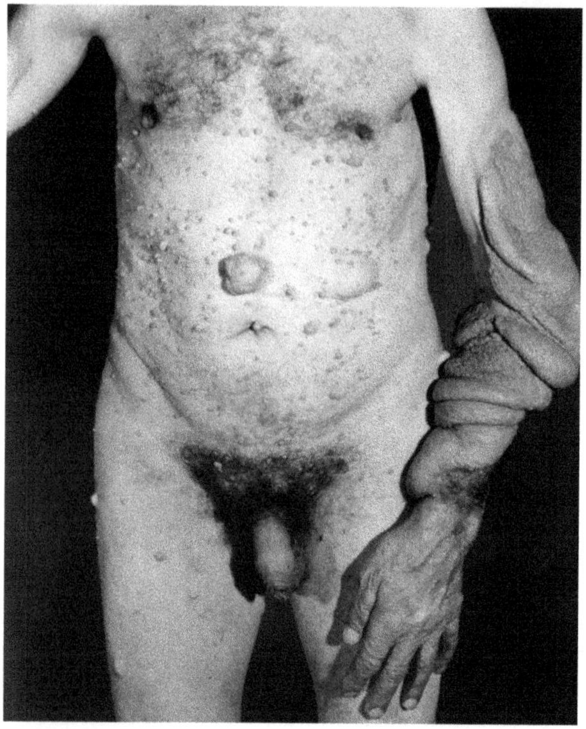

▲ **Figure 6–69.** Cutaneous manifestations of neurofibromatosis.

Essentials of Diagnosis

- *Neurilemomas are usually easily dissected off the associated nerve, whereas neurofibromas generally are far more intertwined in the nerve fascicles, making nerve-sparing resection more difficult.*
- *Patients with neurofibromatosis have a lifetime risk of secondary sarcoma of up to 5%.*

Intramuscular Myxomas

The intramuscular myxoma is a rare tumor seen most commonly in women 40 to 60 years of age and affecting the large muscles about the thighs, shoulders, buttocks, and arms. It is a slow-growing, well-marginated tumor that has the gelatinous physical quality of a ganglion cyst or myxoid liposarcoma. The intramuscular myxoma causes no pain and can grow to greater than 15 cm in diameter. Although it appears radiolucent on CT scan, MRI demonstrates an intermediate signal on the T1-weighted image and an extremely high signal on the T2-weighted image. Multiple myxomas are associated with polyostotic fibrous dysplasia in Mazabraud syndrome.

The intramuscular myxoma can be resected marginally. After this procedure, the recurrence rate is extremely low.

Essentials of Diagnosis

- *Many soft-tissue lesions have very characteristic findings on imaging studies, but those with nonspecific findings should be diagnosed with needle or incisional biopsy rather than excisional biopsy.*

Gounder MM, Mahoney MR, Van Tine BA et al. Sorafenib for advanced and refractory desmoid tumors. *N Engl J Med.* 2018;379(25):2417-2428. [PMID: 30575484]

Hirai T, Kobayashi H, Akiyama T. Predictive factors for complications after surgical treatment for schwannomas of the extremities. *BMC Musculoskelet Disord.* 2019;20(1):166. [PMID: 30975128]

Kasper B, Baumgarten C, Carcia J, et al. An update on the management of sporadic desmoid-type fibromatosis: a European Consensus Initiative between Sarcoma PAtients EuroNet (SPAEN) and European Organization for Resesarch and Treatment of Cancer (EORTC)/Soft Tissue and Bone Sarcoma Group (STBSG). *Ann Oncol.* 2017;28(10):2399-2408. [PMID: 28961825]

Lee HJ, Kim TW, Kim JM, et al. Percutaneous sclerotherapy using bleomycin for the treatment of vascular malformations. *Int J Dermatol.* 2017;56(11):1186-1191. [PMID: 28869282]

Liu D, Perera W, Schlicht S, et al. Musculoskeletal desmoid tumors: diagnostic imaging appearances. *J Med Imaging Radiat Oncol.* 2015;59(4):461-467. [PMID: 2594678]

Longo JF, Weber SM, Turner-Ivey BP, et al. Recent advances in the diagnosis and pathogenesis of neurofibromatosis type 1 (NF1) associated peripheral nervous system neoplasms. *Adv Anat Pathol.* 2018;25(5):353-368. [PMID: 29762158]

McGuaig CC. Update on classification and diagnosis of vascular malformations. *Curr Opin Pediatr.* 2017;29(4):448-454. [PMID: 28654575]

Najd MF, Shoushtarizadeh T, Mirzaei A. Intravascular glomus tumor of the wrist causing chronic wrist pain. *J Hand Microsurg.* 2018;10(2):113-115. [PMID: 30154627]

Panagopoulos I, Gorunoa L, Lobmaier I, et al. Karyotyping and analysis of GNAS locus in intramuscular myxomas. *Oncotarget.* 2017;8(13):22086-22094. [PMID: 28160572]

Seinen JM, Niebling MG, Bastiaanet E, et al. Four different treatment strategies in aggressive fibromatosis: a systematic review. *Clin Transi Radiat Oncol.* 2018;12:1-7. [PMID: 30069502]

Skorpil M, Ryden H, Berglund J, et al. Soft-tissue fat tumors: differentiating malignant from benign using proton density fat fraction quantification MRI. *J Clin Radiol.* 2019;74(7):534-538. [PMID: 31000331]

Smith CJ, Friedlander SF, Guma M. Infantile hemangiomas: an updated review on risk factors, pathogenesis, and treatment. *Birth Defects Res.* 2017;109(11):809-815. [PMID: 28402073]

Uusitalo E, Leppavirta J, Koffert A, et al. Incidence and mortality of neurofibromatosis: a total population study in Finland. *J Invest Dermatol.* 2015;135(3):904-906. [PMID: 25354145].

Yang S, Wang X, Jiang H, et al. Effective treatment of aggressive fibromatosis with celecoxib guided by genetic testing. *Cancer Biol Ther.* 2017;18(10):757-760. [PMID: 28881160].

MALIGNANT SOFT-TISSUE TUMORS

Sarcomas are capable of invasive, locally destructive growth with a tendency to recur and to metastasize. All sarcomas do not behave the same, however. Some sarcomas, such

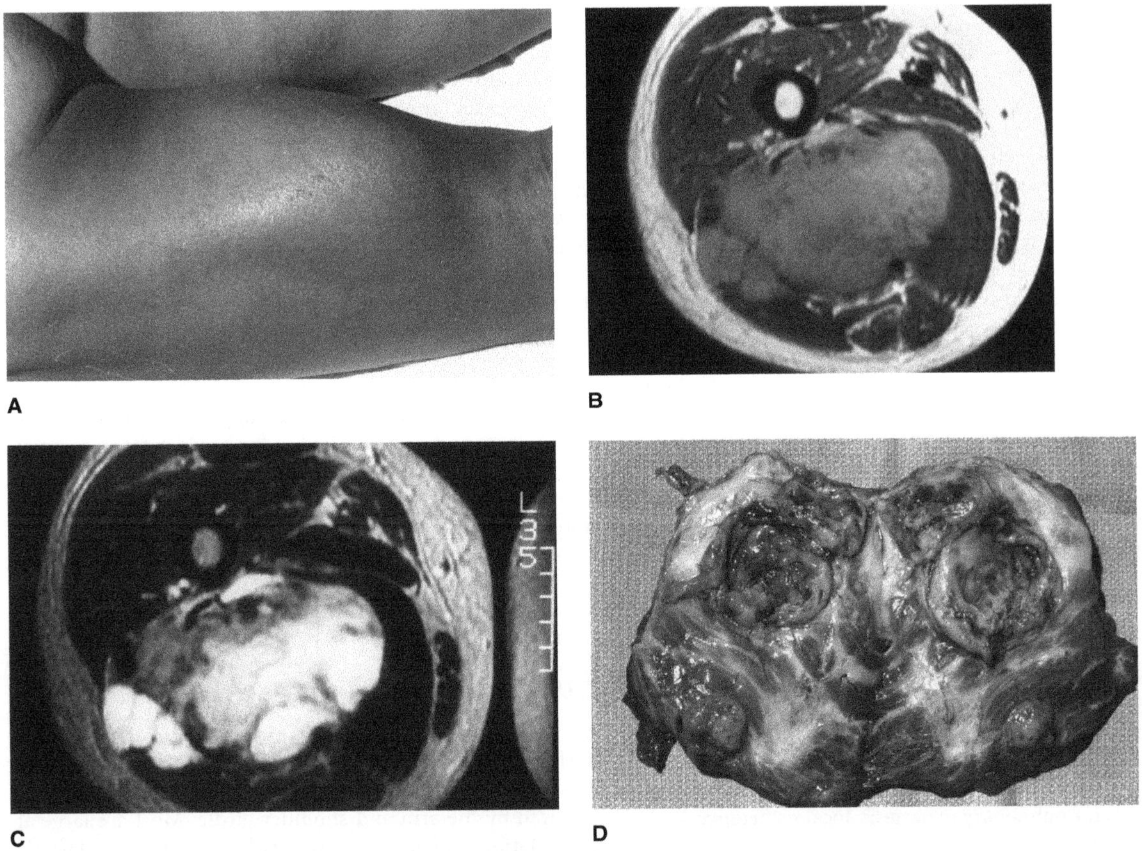

▲ **Figure 6–70.** Clinical appearance (**A**), T1-weighted MRI (**B**), T2-weighted MRI (**C**), and resected surgical specimen (**D**) of a large pleomorphic malignant fibrous histiocytoma in the posterior thigh of a 55-year-old man.

as dermatofibrosarcoma protuberans, rarely metastasize. Undifferentiated pleomorphic sarcoma, in contrast, does so with alacrity.

A. Fibrohistiocytic Tumors

Until recently, MFH was the most common soft-tissue sarcoma seen in adults (Figure 6–70). Strangely, although more frequently encountered than other adult soft-tissue sarcomas, the cell type(s) of origin remain unclear. However, ongoing developments in molecular diagnostics have allowed the determination of the origin of an increasing number of cases. The latest World Health Organization classification for sarcomas no longer includes MFH as a distinct entity. The current nomenclature for the majority of MFH is undifferentiated pleomorphic sarcoma.

1. Pleomorphic malignant fibrous histiocytoma/ undifferentiated high-grade pleomorphic sarcoma— Undifferentiated high-grade pleomorphic sarcoma occurs more frequently in men than in women by a ratio of 1.2:1, primarily affecting individuals between 50 and 70 years of age. Usually it is a deep lesion found in the large muscles about the thigh, hip, and retroperitoneal areas. The tumor may be asymptomatic.

On gross examination, the tumor appears multinodular and may demonstrate several separate satellite lesions in the same muscle belly, especially at the superior and interior poles. It may be necrotic and ranges in color from dirty gray to a reddish tan. Microscopy demonstrates that it is composed of malignant fibroblasts mixed with anaplastic and pleomorphic histiocytes.

The prognosis and treatment vary, depending on the size and location of the tumor. The overall local recurrence potential is 45%, with a 40% incidence of metastasis to the lung and with a 10% incidence of regional lymph node involvement. Tumors smaller than 5 cm in diameter and found in a subcutaneous location in the distal body parts carry a good prognosis, with a 5-year survival rate of 80%, whereas tumors that are 5 cm or more in diameter and located deep in a more proximal muscle group carry a poor prognosis, with a 5-year survival rate of only 55%.

Although the treatment depends on the clinical situation, it generally consists of an aggressive wide resection after careful preoperative staging, including an MRI of the primary tumor and CT scan of the chest. Amputation is rare, with limb salvage possible in the majority of cases.

The use of adjuvant radiation therapy is important in reducing the local recurrence rate. Many clinicians administer 50 to 55 Gy to a wide area, followed by a boost of 60 to 66 Gy aimed at the surgical site. An attempt is made to leave a longitudinal strip of tissue out of the field of radiation to reduce the chance of postirradiation edema distal to the treatment site. Some centers advocate preoperative and postoperative radiation with 50 Gy given before resection and approximately 15 Gy given postoperatively. Some institutions employ preoperative radiation exclusively. Local recurrence rates are generally between 5% and 25%.

The use of adjuvant chemotherapy is more controversial. Because limited data suggest that chemotherapy results in a significant improvement in survival and because most patients are older individuals who cannot tolerate the high-dose protocols, medical oncologists are divided on whether to advocate the use of chemotherapeutic agents in the treatment of undifferentiated pleomorphic sarcoma.

2. Giant cell malignant fibrous histiocytoma/undifferentiated pleomorphic sarcoma with giant cells—The giant cell type of MFH also affects older patients and is seen in large muscle groups. Histologically, multiple osteoclastic giant cells are seen, and there may be areas of hemorrhage. It carries a similar prognosis for pulmonary metastasis, local recurrence, and overall survival.

3. Inflammatory malignant fibrous histiocytoma/undifferentiated pleomorphic sarcoma with prominent inflammation—The inflammatory type of MFH affects the older age groups and is more common in the retroperitoneal areas. Histologically, it has prominent benign-appearing xanthomatous cells and mixed inflammatory cells including neutrophils, eosinophils, and occasional lymphocytes and plasma cells. There is some evidence that this entity may be a form of dedifferentiated liposarcoma. Although it has a similar rate of pulmonary metastasis, review of the literature suggests less favorable overall survival with an increased rate of disease-related mortality. This is probably related to the more frequent retroperitoneal location.

B. Fibrosarcoma

Historically considered the most common of the soft-tissue sarcomas, more accurate pathologic classification—MFH, certain liposarcomas, rhabdomyosarcoma, leiomyosarcomas, and malignant peripheral nerve sheath tumors were previously classified as fibrosarcoma—has demonstrated that fibrosarcomas are one of the least common soft-tissue sarcomas. The diagnosis is reserved for those tumors in which the histology demonstrates a uniform fasciculated growth pattern of spindle cells (malignant fibroblasts). It is clinically similar to MFH, occurs with nearly equal frequency in men and women, is found in patients between 30 and 55 years of age, and is sometimes slow growing and painless. This tumor tends to affect deep fascial structures of muscle about the knee and thigh most frequently, followed next by the forearm and leg.

On gross examination, fibrosarcoma appears as a firm and lobulated lesion that has a yellowish white to tan color. The lesion may demonstrate a few calcific or osseous deposits on radiographic exam. Microscopy reveals spindle, uniformly shaped fibroblasts oriented in a herringbone pattern. Cells show varying degrees of mitotic activity. Fibrosarcomas contain no malignant histiocytes.

The treatment and prognosis depend on the grade of tumor in a particular patient. Low-grade fibrosarcoma is nearly the same tumor as a benign desmoid tumor and has an extremely low rate of metastasis. However, high-grade fibrosarcoma requires an aggressive wide surgical resection, along with radiation therapy, and has a pulmonary metastasis rate of 50% to 60%. Lymph node involvement is rare. The use of chemotherapy is considered controversial in patients with fibrosarcoma, as it is in patients with MFH.

C. Myxofibrosarcoma

Also known as myxoid MFH, myxofibrosarcoma is a relatively common sarcoma in the elderly, seen in the 50- to 80-year age group. The thigh is the most common location followed by the arm and shoulder girdle. Most are large at presentation and may be low grade, with little metastatic potential, or high grade, with metastases occurring in 20% to 35% of cases. Larger tumors with increased necrosis exhibit an increased rate of metastasis. Local recurrence is seen in approximately one-half of cases after resection, and it is well described that lesions have the propensity to recur at a higher grade, having accumulated chromosomal aberrations. This property, combined with the fact that no specific cytogenetic abnormalities have been identified, highlights the role of genomic instability in the malignant degeneration of this entity. Largely because of the peak age group, chemotherapy is infrequently recommended; however, radiotherapy is routinely delivered either preoperatively or postoperatively.

D. Dermatofibrosarcoma Protuberans

Dermatofibrosarcoma protuberans, a low- to intermediate-grade fibrohistiocytic tumor, is unique because of its nodular cutaneous location. It is seen more commonly in males than females and occurs in young or middle-age (20-40 years) adults. It is typically located about the trunk and proximal extremities. Antecedent trauma is recorded in 10% to 20% of cases.

Dermatofibrosarcoma protuberans begins as a painless subcutaneous nodule or nodules and slowly develops into an elevated multinodular plaque (Figure 6–71). Microscopic

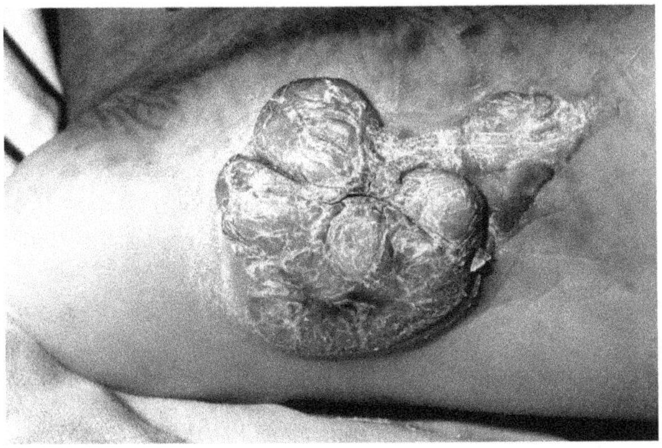

▲ **Figure 6–71.** Clinical appearance of dermatofibrosarcoma protuberans on the bottom of the heel of a 30-year-old man.

examination of the lesion reveals the same storiform or basket-weave pattern of a benign or malignant fibrous histiocytoma but with a very low mitotic index. The pattern tends to infiltrate extensively into surrounding subcutaneous fat and skin, which accounts for the high local recurrence rate, sometimes reported to approach 50%.

Characteristic cytogenetic abnormalities are described with characteristic features such as reciprocal t(17;22)(q22;q13) or, more commonly, supernumerary ring chromosomes containing sequences from chromosomes 17 and 22. The specific cytogenetic rearrangement may not be as critical as the resulting fusion product of collagen 1 alpha 1 and platelet-derived growth factor (COL1A1-PDGFB), which is detected in the vast majority of cases.

Surgical treatment, consisting of an aggressive resection, is associated with a lower recurrence rate of 20%. Because of the low mitotic index, radiation therapy is not usually indicated, and the chance of pulmonary metastasis is only 1%.

Essentials of Diagnosis

- *Malignant fibrous histiocytoma has recently been reclassified largely due to increased ability to determine cell lineage with modern molecular techniques.*

E. Liposarcomas

Liposarcoma is the second most common soft-tissue sarcoma after undifferentiated pleomorphic sarcoma. Like MFH, liposarcoma is a tumor of older (40-60 years) patients and can be large and deep seated. Four types of liposarcoma are discussed in the following sections. The well-differentiated type and the myxoid type are associated with a low chance for lung metastasis, whereas the round cell and the pleomorphic types tend to behave more aggressively.

1. Well-differentiated liposarcoma—This very low-grade tumor affects individuals who are 40 to 60 years of age and occurs more frequently in men than in women. It grows extremely slowly and reaches a large size without causing pain. The deep-seated tumor is found in the retroperitoneum, buttock, or thigh. In some cases of well-differentiated liposarcoma, findings include inflammation and sclerosis.

On gross examination, this tumor has a fatty lobulated appearance similar to a benign lipoma. Even under the microscope, many large areas of the tumor appear benign. However, with proper sampling, the pathologist will find a few areas of lipoblast activity to suggest the diagnosis of a liposarcoma. MRI findings are sometimes difficult to distinguish from a large deep lipoma (Figure 6–72).

In cases of well-differentiated liposarcoma, a conservative wide resection is performed to avoid local recurrence. Adjuvant radiation therapy is not helpful, and chemotherapy is never used. The chance of metastatic disease is very low, and the prognosis for survival is excellent.

2. Myxoid liposarcoma—Myxoid liposarcoma is the most common fat sarcoma, accounting for 40% to 50% of all

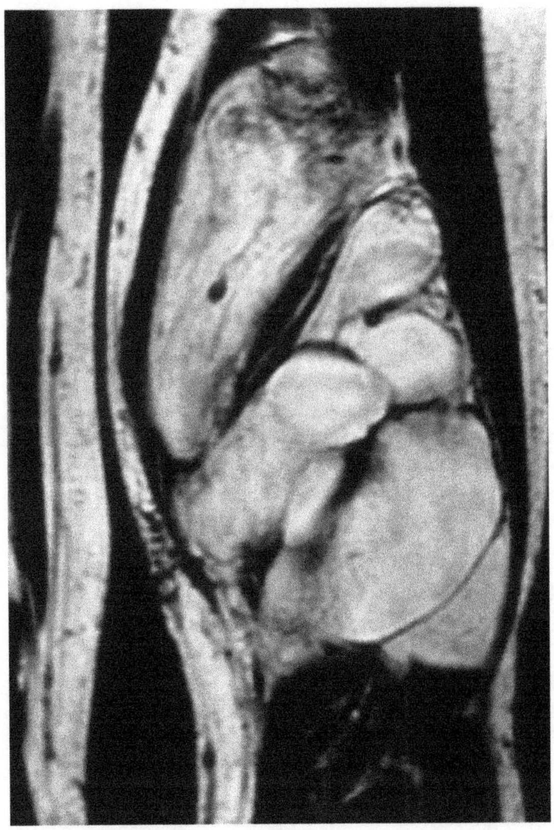

▲ **Figure 6–72.** T1-weighted MRI of a well-differentiated liposarcoma in the thigh of a 63-year-old man.

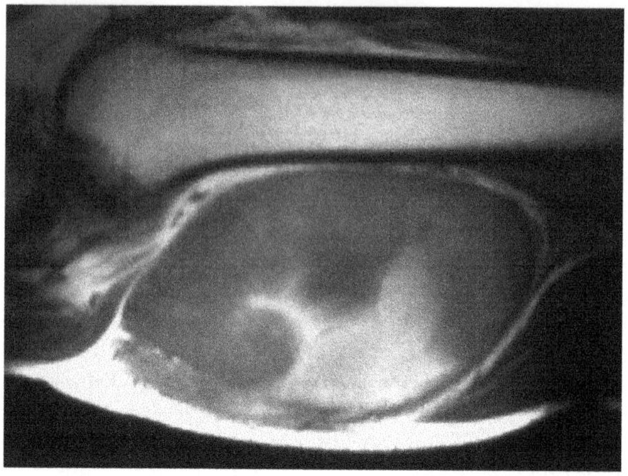

▲ **Figure 6–73.** Sagittal view T1-weighted MRI of a myxoid liposarcoma in the thigh of a 32-year-old man.

liposarcomas. The myxoid type is low to intermediate grade and seen in older patients (see Table 6–6). The clinical presentation is similar to the well-differentiated liposarcoma.

Gross examination of a myxoid liposarcoma reveals a lobulated pattern with some areas that appear similar to those of a lipoma but with other myxomatous areas. Microscopic examination shows myxoid tissue with areas of signet ring lipoblasts. It is common to find a delicate pattern of capillaries running through the myxoid areas. MRI frequently demonstrates a heterogeneous high- and low-signal pattern typical of myxoid liposarcoma but not present in cases of benign lipoma (Figure 6–73).

Characteristic translocations are also seen in myxoid liposarcoma. The predominant type is t(12;16)(q13;p11); however, t(12;22)(q13;q12) is also described. Multifocal myxoid liposarcoma is also described. Consideration for additional advanced axial imaging should be entertained with this histologic subtype. Although myxoid liposarcoma carries a very good prognosis, the tumor should be removed with wide margins. There is current debate over the use of neoadjuvant chemotherapy versus neoadjuvant radiotherapy, with this entity showing responsiveness to both. Adjuvant radiotherapy is still widely used today.

3. Round cell and pleomorphic liposarcoma—These high-grade liposarcomas are seen in the same locations and age group as the well-differentiated and myxoid subtypes. But unlike the latter, the round cell and pleomorphic types are fast-growing tumors that may be painful.

In cases of round cell or pleomorphic liposarcoma, the lesion does not have a fatty appearance on gross examination but instead looks more like an MFH or a fibrosarcoma. Moreover, on MRI, the lesion appears more like an MFH, with a low-signal pattern in the T1-weighted image and a high-signal pattern in the T2-weighted image. Microscopically, the round cell type of liposarcoma shows areas of uniformly shaped round cells similar to those found in Ewing sarcoma or lymphoma and also shows areas of myxoid tissue. In the pleomorphic type of liposarcoma, large and bizarre giant cells occur similar to those found in undifferentiated pleomorphic sarcoma and rhabdomyosarcoma.

In round cell and pleomorphic liposarcoma, there is an early and high rate of pulmonary metastasis. Accordingly, the prognosis for survival is poor. Thus, the treatment should include aggressive resection, adjuvant radiation therapy as necessary, and chemotherapy in selected patients.

Essentials of Diagnosis

- *CT scan of the abdomen and pelvis should be included in the staging and surveillance of liposarcomas due to the incidence of associated retroperitoneal tumors.*
- *Liposarcoma is particularly subject to sampling error with biopsy, so every effort should be made to sample the most aggressive-appearing portion of the tumor.*

F. Rhabdomyosarcomas

Rhabdomyosarcomas account for 20% of all soft-tissue sarcomas. The embryonal and alveolar types of rhabdomyosarcoma affect pediatric patients, and the rarer pleomorphic type affects adults.

1. Embryonal rhabdomyosarcoma—The embryonal type is seen in patients from birth to 15 years of age and encountered more frequently in boys than in girls. It is most common in the head and neck area. The so-called botryoid form is seen as a cluster of grapes under mucous membranes in the vagina, bladder, or retroperitoneal area. Histologically, it is a round cell tumor-like Ewing sarcoma, but some rhabdomyoblasts with cross striations are present in a few areas. The presence of anaplasia, or areas of cells containing enlarged, bizarre, hyperchromatic nuclei, is associated with a more aggressive phenotype.

Embryonal rhabdomyosarcoma is treated with local surgical resection plus preoperative and postoperative chemotherapy consisting of vincristine, dactinomycin, cyclophosphamide, and doxorubicin given in cyclic courses during a 2-year span. If the surgical margins are contaminated, local radiation therapy is used. With this program, the 5-year survival rate is 80%. Prior to the advent of chemotherapy, it was only 10%.

2. Alveolar rhabdomyosarcoma—This type of rhabdomyosarcoma affects individuals between 10 and 25 years of age and is found more commonly in males than in females. Besides affecting the head and neck, it can be seen in the extremities, especially the thigh and calf. Microscopic examination of the lesion reveals a typical alveolar pattern of round cells, with fewer rhabdomyoblasts seen in this type of rhabdomyosarcoma than in the embryonal type. This type of rhabdomyosarcoma is associated with the fusion genes *PAX3-FKHR* or *PAX7-FKHR*. Although not definitive, the presence of the translocation t(2;13)/*PAX3-FKHR* may be an adverse prognostic factor, with molecular screening being implemented in the future. Currently, the treatment is the same as for the embryonal type, but the prognosis is a bit worse.

3. Pleomorphic rhabdomyosarcoma—In the 1940s, pleomorphic rhabdomyosarcoma was a popular histologic diagnosis, and MFH was a rare one. Based on today's criteria, most of the old cases classified as pleomorphic rhabdomyosarcoma would now be classified as undifferentiated pleomorphic sarcoma. Currently, the pleomorphic type of rhabdomyosarcoma is the rarest type.

Pleomorphic rhabdomyosarcoma is a high-grade tumor that affects middle-age and older adults and is seen most commonly in the large muscle groups of the proximal extremities, usually the lower extremities. Microscopic examination of the tumor reveals large atypical giant cells, along with racket- or tadpole-shaped malignant rhabdomyoblasts that stain positive for glycogen, actin, and myosin. The tumor carries a poor prognosis and is associated with a high rate of metastasis to the lung. The treatment for pleomorphic rhabdomyosarcoma is similar to that for undifferentiated pleomorphic sarcoma and consists of a wide local resection and adjuvant radiation therapy. Chemotherapy is rarely indicated.

Essentials of Diagnosis

- *Alveolar rhabdomyosarcoma is associated with characteristic translocations t(1;13) or t(2;13), resulting in the PAX7-FKHR or PAX3-FKHR fusion products, respectively. This affects prognosis and may ultimately affect treatment protocols as well.*

G. Leiomyosarcoma

Leiomyosarcoma is a rare soft-tissue tumor whose cell type of origin is smooth muscle. It is seen in the middle-age adult (see Table 6–6) and is much more common in women than in men. Its usual locations, in order of frequency, are retroperitoneal, intraabdominal, cutaneous, and subcutaneous. In some cases, the lesion has a venous wall origin and is found in the vena cava or large vessels of the leg. On microscopic examination, leiomyosarcoma can demonstrate a palisading, orderly fascicular pattern similar to a malignant schwannoma. A specific immunohistochemical staining for actin may be helpful in the differential diagnosis.

The prognosis and treatment for leiomyosarcoma are similar to those for fibrosarcoma. However, leiomyosarcomas of venous wall origin have a worse prognosis because they are difficult to resect and have a high rate of pulmonary metastasis.

H. Synovial Sarcomas

Synovial sarcoma (Figure 6–74) is the fourth most common soft-tissue sarcoma. It is seen in young adults between 15 and 35 years of age and affects males slightly more than females. The name of this tumor suggests a synovial cell origin; however, their true cell of origin is currently thought to be primitive mesenchymal cells or myoblasts. Nevertheless, they frequently arise from juxtaarticular structures, especially around the knee, and they can also arise from tendon sheaths, bursal sacs, fascial planes, and deep muscles. Synovial sarcomas can be seen about the shoulder, arm, elbow, and wrist and are the most common soft-tissue sarcoma in the foot.

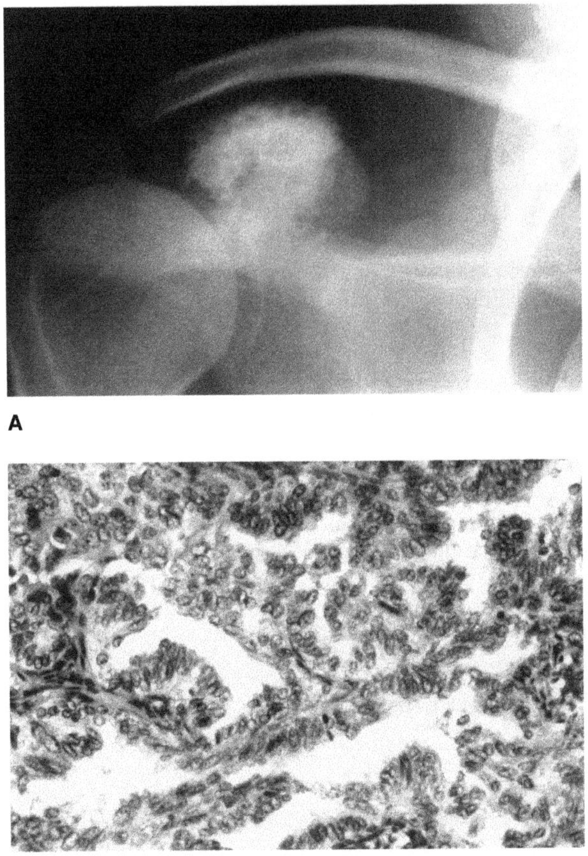

A

B

▲ **Figure 6–74.** Radiograph (**A**) and microscopic appearance (**B**) of a synovial sarcoma in the shoulder of a 20-year-old woman.

Synovial sarcomas initially grow slowly and cause pain in approximately half of affected patients. The tumors may appear after an injury, and because dystrophic calcification or even heterotopic bone formation is seen in half of the cases, the tumors are assumed to be a benign process for 2 to 4 years before a diagnostic biopsy is performed.

Microscopic examination of the tumor shows a typical biphasic pattern composed of epithelium-like cells that form nests, clefts, or tubular structures surrounded by malignant fibroblastic spindle cells. The epithelium-like cells produce a mucinous material that suggests a synovial cell origin, although this origin is unlikely. A monophasic form of synovial sarcoma is described and reported to consist of a dominant fibroblastic or epithelial cell pattern. If the lesion shows no biphasic component, however, it is difficult to confirm the diagnosis of synovial sarcoma.

Molecular characterization of this tumor reveals a particular translocation, t(X;18), representing the fusion of *SYT* (at 18q11) with either *SSX1* or *SSX2* (both at Xp11). Both *SYT* and *SSX* are transcription factors whose fusion product is seen in the majority of synovial sarcomas.

Despite the slow growth of synovial sarcoma, the 5- and 10-year survival rates are only 50% and 25%, respectively. In cases in which the tumors are heavily calcified, the 5-year survival rate is 80%. Because of the poor prognosis, the treatment plan should include aggressive wide resection, along with both radiation therapy and chemotherapy. Recent evidence shows that ifosfamide-based regimens are associated with improved patient outcomes. Lymph node involvement is seen in 20% of affected patients and may require a surgical excision followed by local radiation therapy.

Essentials of Diagnosis

- *Synovial sarcomas can present as small, calcified soft-tissue tumors in up to 50% of cases.*

I. Malignant Peripheral Nerve Sheath Tumor

A malignant peripheral nerve sheath tumor can arise from a preexisting benign solitary neurofibroma but more frequently arises from the multiple lesions of neurofibromatosis type 1. In both cases, the tumor mass is usually larger than 5 cm in diameter and may arise from a large deep neurogenic structure such as the sciatic nerve (Figure 6–75) or one of the spinal roots. Smaller nerves, even cutaneous branches, however, can give rise to these sarcomas. Malignant degeneration from a solitary neurofibroma usually occurs after 40 years of age with a 5-year survival rate of 75%. In contrast, patients whose tumor arose from the lesions of neurofibromatosis type 1 are generally younger and have a 5-year survival rate of 30%. Surgical treatment consists of a wide resection if possible. Adjuvant radiation and chemotherapy are used in selected cases.

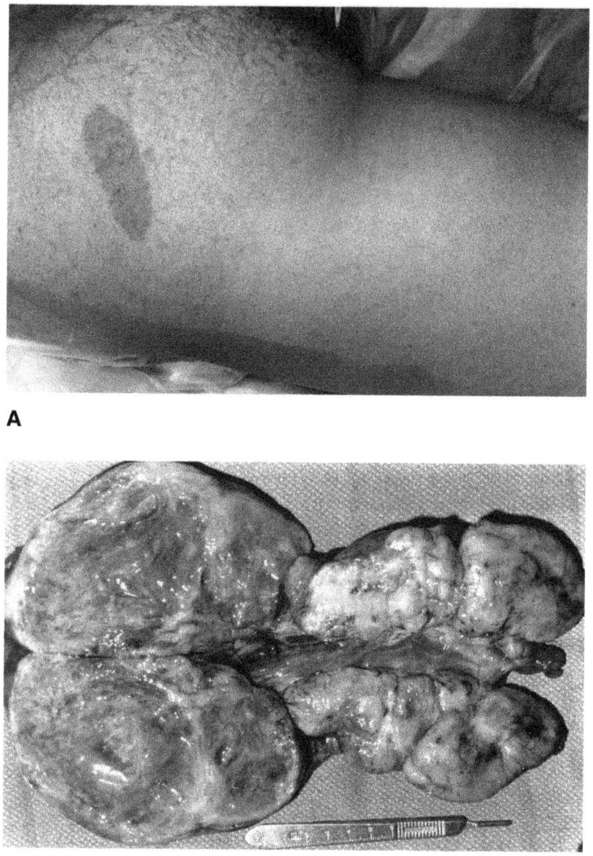

A

B

▲ **Figure 6–75.** Clinical appearance of a café-au-lait defect in the skin overlying a malignant schwannoma in the buttock area of a 42-year-old man (**A**), and gross appearance of the tumor in the resected sciatic nerve (**B**).

J. Malignant Vascular Tumors

1. Kaposi sarcoma—Of the malignant vascular tumors, Kaposi sarcoma is the most common with four specific subtypes: (1) chronic, (2) lymphadenopathic, (3) transplant associated, (4) acquired immunodeficiency syndrome (AIDS) related. Its pathogenesis is related to infection with Kaposi sarcoma–associated herpesvirus while in the immunocompromised state. It is found directly beneath the skin, generally in the lower extremity of adults, is seen more often in men than in women, and is endemic in central Africa. The cutaneous lesions seen frequently in the foot and ankle area are purplish in color and are nodular (Figure 6–76). Microscopic examination of Kaposi sarcoma shows an aggressive vascular pattern with rare mitosis. However, over a period of many years, the tumor progresses into a full-blown angiosarcoma or fibrosarcoma. Cytotoxic chemotherapeutic alternatives are limited due to the immunocompromised status of the host. With continued investigation in the field, antiviral medications will likely become a mainstay in the treatment of this disease. Although the behavior of Kaposi sarcoma is a function of the immunologic status of the patient and other variables, the overall mortality rate is 10% to 20%.

2. Angiosarcoma—Soft-tissue angiosarcoma is rare, accounting for less than 1% of all sarcomas. Although angiosarcomas are usually cutaneous lesions and tend to affect men more than women, they sometimes take the form of a deep

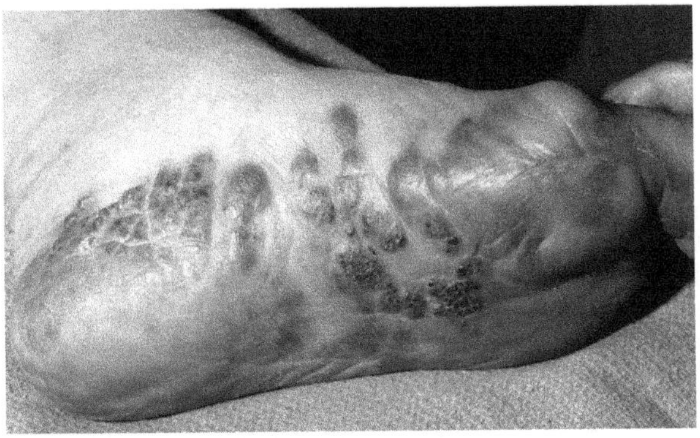

▲ **Figure 6–76.** Clinical appearance of Kaposi sarcoma of the foot.

tumor, and they are typically seen in the upper extremities of women who have chronic lymphedema following radical breast surgery and radiation therapy. Histologic examination of angiosarcoma shows anaplastic endothelial cells surrounded by reticulum fiber. Prognosis for the older patient is poor. Smaller lesions in younger (<50 years) patients have a distinctively better outcome. The treatment is wide resection, sometimes with radiation therapy.

3. Solitary fibrous tumor/hemangiopericytoma—The diagnosis of solitary fibrous tumor versus hemangiopericytoma is a topic of debate. It is now thought that many lesions previously characterized as hemangiopericytomas are actually extrapleural solitary fibrous tumors. Both may range from very low-grade to high-grade sarcoma. These rare perivascular tumors are thought to arise from pericytes. Pericytes are highly arborized perivascular cells that line capillaries and venules. The lesion, which affects male and female adults with equal frequency, is usually found deep in muscle bellies and generally located in the thigh or retroperitoneal area of the pelvis. Microscopic examination of the malignant solitary fibrous tumor reveals tightly packed cells with round nuclei with moderate amounts of cytoplasm with poorly defined borders. Bifurcating sinusoidal vessels that have a typical staghorn appearance are characteristic of the classic hemangiopericytoma. Cytogenetic analysis reveals multiple chromosome translocations including t(12;19) and t(13;22). Treatment consists of a wide surgical resection, followed by local radiation therapy. Some authors recommend preoperative embolization or afferent vessel ligation (or both) intraoperatively.

MISCELLANEOUS SOFT-TISSUE SARCOMAS

The remaining soft-tissue sarcomas are rare, and only a brief description of their clinical patterns is summarized.

A. Soft-Tissue Chondrosarcoma

There are three types of soft-tissue chondrosarcomas.

1. Myxoid chondrosarcoma—The myxoid chondrosarcoma is sometimes referred to as a chordoid sarcoma because it looks like a chordoma. It is a slow-growing tumor seen in adults, usually in deep structure of the leg. It has a myxoid appearance, does not calcify, and is low grade. Like the chordoma, the myxoid chondrosarcoma responds only to surgical removal.

2. Mesenchymal chondrosarcoma—This tumor affects individuals between 15 and 40 years of age, is found deep in the lower extremity and neck areas, is fast growing, and carries a poor prognosis because of the high risk of pulmonary metastasis. Calcification may be seen on radiograph, and microscopic examination reveals round cells scattered in a chondroid matrix. Treatment consists of a wide resection in conjunction with chemotherapy and radiation therapy.

3. Synovial chondrosarcoma—The conversion of a synovial chondromatosis to a malignant synovial chondrosarcoma is an extremely rare phenomenon. It can occur with lesions of the hip or knee region in older (>60 years) adults.

B. Ewing Sarcoma

Extraskeletal Ewing sarcoma can be found in individuals between 10 and 30 years of age and is usually located in the paravertebral area, thorax, or deep muscle area of the lower extremity. It is a fast-growing tumor with minimal pain symptoms. It carries the same prognosis as its counterpart in bone and is treated with the same combination of surgery, chemotherapy, and radiation therapy.

C. Alveolar Soft Part Sarcoma

This round cell sarcoma affects more females than males, is usually found in patients between 15 and 35 years of age, and arises in the deep muscle tissue of the lower extremity, usually the thigh. Alveolar soft part sarcoma is a slow-growing tumor but carries a poor prognosis because of early pulmonary metastasis. The tumor has increased vascularity and is thought to originate from a neurogenic stem cell. It derives its name from its alveolar pattern, which is seen on microscopic examination and can cause this tumor to be mistaken for an alveolar form of rhabdomyosarcoma. A cytogenetic, unbalanced abnormality, t(x;17)(p11.2;q25), is described. Treatment of alveolar soft part sarcoma consists of a wide surgical resection plus radiation therapy and chemotherapy.

D. Epithelioid Sarcoma

Although this superficial skin lesion is seen most commonly in the palm of the hand, it can also be found on the dorsum of the forearm or on the plantar aspect of the foot. It is a slow-growing tumor that affects patients between 20 and 30 years of age, causes minimal pain symptoms, and is associated with ulceration.

Because epithelioid sarcoma has a whitish color that under the microscope demonstrates cords of epithelium-like

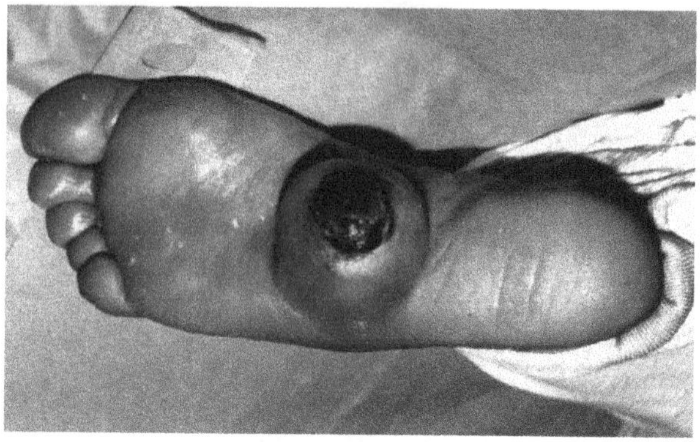

▲ **Figure 6–77.** Clinical appearance of epithelioid sarcoma on the plantar aspect of the foot of a 36-year-old man.

cells, it can be mistaken for a synovial sarcoma. Moreover, because of its firm multilobulated presentation, the epithelioid sarcoma may be mistaken for a plantar of palmar fibromatosis (Figure 6–77).

Epithelioid sarcoma spreads as a lumpy nodularity along tendon sheaths or fascial planes and frequently involves local lymph nodes. Local surgical resection is followed by a high local recurrence rate, and a late pulmonary metastasis is common. For this reason, early treatment should consist of an aggressive wide surgical resection.

E. Clear Cell Sarcoma

The clear cell sarcoma is thought to be a deep, noncutaneous variant of the well-known cutaneous melanoma. It is extremely rare, affects women more often than men, and commonly occurs between 20 and 40 years of age. It arises in tendon sheaths and fascial planes, most frequently in the foot and ankle but also in the knee and arm. Clear cell sarcoma starts slowly as a painless lump and has a high potential to spread to local lymph nodes. The lesion in many cases demonstrates evidence of melanin and melanosomes and may be of neural crest origin. The microscopic clear cell appearance can cause this sarcoma to be confused with epithelioid sarcoma and synovial sarcoma.

The prognosis is poor because of a high rate of pulmonary metastasis. This tumor may spread via lymphatics as well. Treatment consists of early aggressive wide resection and may include chemotherapy and local radiation therapy.

Essentials of Diagnosis

- *Although most mesenchymal malignancies do not usually metastasize to lymph nodes, synovial sarcoma, epithelioid sarcoma, and rhabdomyosarcoma are exceptions.*
- *Soft-tissue sarcoma in the adult is generally more sensitive to radiation therapy than chemotherapy.*

Blackadar CB. Historical review of the causes of Cancer. *World J Clin Oncol.* 2016;7(1):54-86. [PMID: 26862491]

Carvalho SD, Pissaloux D, Combe A, et al. Pleomorphic sarcomas: the state of the art. *Surg Pathol Clin.* 2019;12(1):63-105. [PMID:30709449]

Chowdhry V, Goldberg S, DeLaney TF, et al. Myxoid liposarcoma: treatment outcomes from chemotherapy and radiation therapy. *Sarcoma.* 2018;2018:8029157. [PMID: 15380587]

Crago AM, Brennan MF. Principles in management of soft tissue sarcoma. *Adv Surg.* 2015;49:107-122. [PMID: 26299493]

Crago AM, Dickson MA. Liposarcoma: multimodality management and future targeted therapies. *Surg Oncol Clin N Am.* 2016;25(4):761-773. [PMID: 27591497]

Cramer SL, Miller AL, Pressey JG, et al. Pediatric anaplastic embryonal rhabdomyosarcoma: targeted therapy guided by genetic analysis and a patient-derived xenograft study. *Front Oncol.* 2018;7:327. [PMID: 29376028]

Demicco EG, Boland GM, Brewer SK, et al. Progressive loss of myogenic differentiation in leiomyosarcoma has prognostic value. *Histopathology.* 2015;66(5):627-638. [PMID: 24889065]

Desar IM, Fleuren ED, van der Graaf WT. Systemic treatment for adults with synovial sarcoma. *Curr Treat Options Oncol.* 2018;19(2):13. [PMID: 29516254]

El Beaino M, Araujo DM, Lazar AJ, et al. Synovial sarcoma: advances in diagnosis and treatment identification of new biologic targets to improve multimodal therapy. *Ann Surg Oncol.* 2017;8:2145-2154. [PMID: 28397189]

Gurria JP, Dasgupta R. Rhabdomyosarcoma and extraosseous Ewing sarcoma. *Children (Basel).* 2018;5(12):165. [PMID: 30544742]

Hoefkens F, Dehandschutter C, Somville J, et al. Soft tissue sarcoma of the extremities: pending questions on surgery and radiotherapy. *Radiat Oncol.* 2016;11(1):136. [PMID: 27733179]

Ma S, Fan L, Liu Y, et al. MET-overexpressing myxofibrosarcoma frequently exhibit polysomy of chromosome 7 but not MET amplification, especially in high-grade cases: clinical and pathological review of 30 myxofibrosarcoma cases. *Diagn Pathol.* 2018;113(1):56. [PMID: 30126419]

Mukaihara K, Tanabe Y, Kubota D, et al. Cabozantinib and dasatinib exert anti-tumor activity in alveolar soft part sarcoma. *PLoS One.* 2017;12(9):e0185321. [PMID: 28945796]

Muratori F, Bettini L, Fresnos F, et al. Myxoid liposarcoma: prognostic factors and metastatic patterns in a series of 148 patients treated at a single institution. *Int J Surg Oncol.* 2018;2018:8928706. [PMID: 29977616]

Noujaim J, Thway K, Fisher C, et al. Dermatofibrosarcoma protuberans: from translocation to targeted therapy. *Cancer Biol Med.* 2015;12(4):375-384. [PMID: 26779374]

Paludo J, Fritchie K, Haddox CL, et al. Extraskeletal osteosarcoma: outcomes and the role of chemotherapy. *Am J Clin Oncol.* 2018;41(9):832-837. [PMID: 28622153].

Pan M, Merchant M. Risk factors including age, stage and anatomic location that impact the outcomes of patients with synovial sarcoma. *Med Sci.* 2018;6(1):21. [PMID: 29509716]

Ramey SJ, Yechieli R, Zhao W, et al. Limb-sparing surgery plus radiotherapy results in superior survival: an analysis of patients with high-grade, extremity soft-tissue sarcoma from the NCDB and SEER. *Cancer Med.* 2018;7(9):4228-4239. [PMID: 30030882]

Ridel RF, Jones RL, Italiano A, et al. Systemic anti-cancer therapy in synovial sarcoma: a systematic review. *Cancers (Basel).* 2018;10(11):417. [PMID: 30388821]

Tang Z, Zeng Q, Zhang X, et al. Predicting radiotherapy response for patients with soft tissue sarcoma by developing a molecular signature. *Oncol Rep.* 2017;38(5):2814-2824. [PMID: 29048650]

Tinkle CL, Fernandez-Pineda I, Sykes A, et al. Nonrhabdomyosarcoma soft tissue sarcoma (NRSTS) in pediatric and young adult patients: results from a prospective study using limited-0margin radiotherapy. *Cancer.* 2017;123(22):4419-4429. [PMID: 28759114]

MANAGEMENT OF CARCINOMA METASTASIZED TO BONE

Incidence and Natural History of Metastases

A. Common Metastatic Carcinomas and Areas of Skeletal Involvement

Metastatic involvement of the musculoskeletal system is one of the most significant clinical issues facing orthopedic oncologists. Skeletal metastasis is a common cause of severe morbidity, reduction in quality of life, and early mortality. As systemic treatment of cancer improves, patients are living longer and the prevalence of skeletal metastases is rising. The number of patients with metastasis to the skeletal system from a carcinoma is 15 times greater than the number of patients with primary bone tumors of all types. Approximately a third of all diagnosed adenocarcinomas include skeletal metastases, resulting in approximately 300,000 cases per year. Furthermore, 70% of patients with advanced terminal carcinoma demonstrate bone metastases at autopsy. The carcinomas that commonly metastasize to bone are prostate, breast, kidney, thyroid, and lung carcinomas. One study showed that nearly 90% of patients with these types of carcinoma had bone metastases. Among the carcinomas that less commonly metastasize to bone are cancers of the skin, oral cavity, esophagus, cervix, stomach, and colon.

The spine is the most frequent area of bone metastasis. Other common skeletal sites include the pelvis, femur, rib, proximal humerus, and skull, in that order. Metastatic lesions are rarely found distal to the elbow or knee. If lesions are found in these areas, so-called acral metastases, the lung is the most common source. Solitary bone lesions comprise only approximately 10% of cases of bone metastasis.

B. Clinical Course of Metastases

The mechanism of metastases is accounted for in a modified "seed/soil" theorem. Fewer than 1 in 10,000 neoplastic cells that escape into the circulation from the primary site are able to set up a metastatic focus, a complex multistep process by which the cell must first break free. This is a function of *degradative* enzymes such as collagenases, hydrolases, cathepsin D, and proteases. Once the cell invades the vascular channel, it circulates through the body. It is theorized that the cell is protected by a fibrin platelet clot. However, clinical trials with heparin do not show a significant change in metastatic outcome. Local factors such as integrins are instrumental in attracting the circulating metastatic cell to a particular remote tissue site. Once within the new tissue, the metastatic cell releases factors such as tumor angiogenesis factor, inducing neovascularization, which in turn facilitates growth of the metastatic focus.

Patients with advanced metastatic disease frequently experience dysfunction of their hematopoietic and calcium homeostasis systems. Patients may develop a normochromic, normocytic anemia with leukocytosis. In response to the anemia, the increased production of immature cells is noted on the peripheral blood smear. This is termed the *leukoerythroblastic reaction.* Hypercalcemia may result in up to 30% of cases with extensive metastases. This is most frequently seen in myeloma, breast cancer, and non–small cell lung cancer.

Blastic metastases are frequently painless and associated with a lower incidence of pathologic fracture because the bone is not as severely weakened (Figures 6–78 and 6–79).

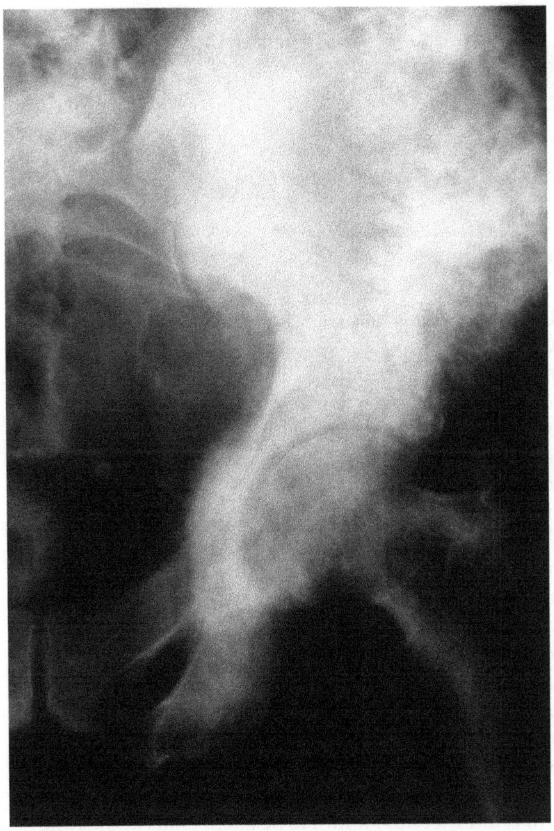

▲ **Figure 6–78.** Radiograph of a blastic carcinoma that metastasized from the prostate to the pelvis in an 85-year-old man.

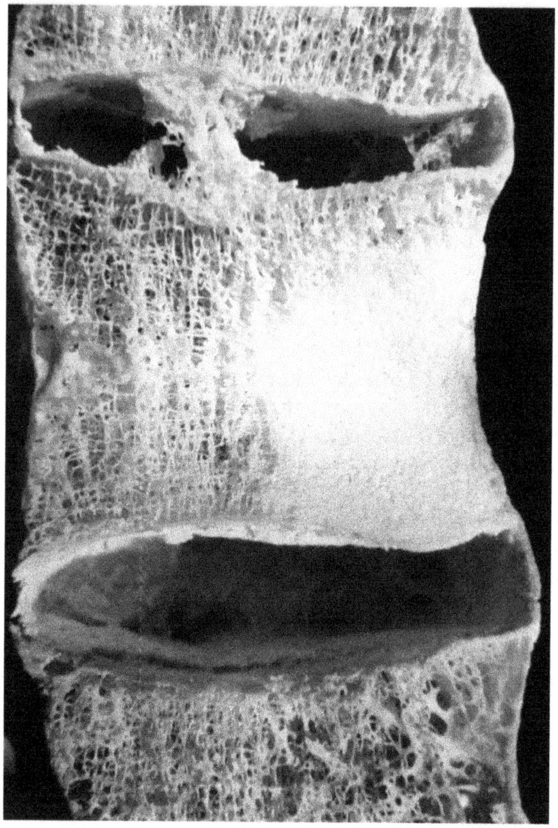

▲ **Figure 6–79.** Skeletal specimen of a blastic carcinoma that metastasized from the prostate to the lumbar spine.

Not all tumors that metastasize from the prostate to the bone are blastic. The lytic variants are painful and more likely to cause pathologic fractures.

Most tumors that metastasize from the breast to the bone are blastic, but some demonstrate mixtures of blastic and lytic areas in the same bone. By taking serial radiographs and noting the appearance of bone metastases, it is possible to follow the progress of treatment consisting of systemic therapy with hormones or chemotherapeutic agents plus local radiation therapy. A favorable response may show a gradual conversion from a lytic to a blastic appearance as the pain decreases.

Bone destruction in lytic lesions is a response by native osteoclasts to the tumor. Neovascularity is common. Among the tumors that are characteristic for this hemorrhagic response are thyroid carcinomas (Figure 6–80), renal cell carcinoma (Figure 6–81), and multiple myeloma. Before a surgical intervention, it is beneficial to perform a prophylactic embolization of the area to reduce perioperative bleeding. If a lesion is unexpectedly found to be aneurysmal at the time of surgical exploration, it is best to debulk the friable tumor mass rapidly down to normal bone and then pack the area until it can be stabilized with bone cement.

Diagnosis

A. General Approach

A methodical approach is mandatory in the workup of a patient with presumed metastatic disease to bone to locate the primary tumor. A thorough history and physical examination must be completed prior to laboratory and radiographic analysis. Eight percent of patients may have their primary carcinoma detected on physical exam. Laboratory analysis should include complete blood count, ESR, renal and liver panels, alkaline phosphate, and serum protein electrophoresis.

Radiographic examination should follow with a plain chest radiograph and radiographs of known involved bones. The entire bone should be visualized, because the presence of other lesions may impact treatment. Approximately 45% of primaries are detected in the lung on the chest radiograph. The workup should also include a whole-body technetium bone scan. Bone scan is more sensitive than plain radiographs in detecting early lesions. If myeloma, lymphoma, or renal carcinoma is suspected, a skeletal survey should be obtained as lesions may not be detected on bone scan. CT scans of the chest, abdomen, and pelvis should be performed. Lung CT can detect up to 15% of primaries missed on the plain radiograph.

These studies in conjunction with a well-planned biopsy detect the majority of cases. Routine radiographic screening studies in search of early metastatic disease are not very helpful (Figure 6–82). Lytic changes become evident on routine radiographs only when cortical destruction approaches 30% to 50% (Figure 6–83).

Treatment and Prognosis

A. Nonsurgical Treatment

Aside from symptomatic treatment, nonsurgical management of metastatic carcinoma to bone is comprised of chemotherapy, radiation treatment, and bisphosphonates. Radiation is used for both tumor control and palliation. Each patient must be carefully evaluated as a candidate for radiation therapy. The histologic type of disease, extent of disease, prognosis, marrow reserve, and overall constitution must be assessed. Lesions should be evaluated for pathologic fracture risk prior to the initiation of radiation therapy. If pain in the long bone is mechanical (arising from bone weakness or fracture), it is better treated with surgery, whereas pain from a tumoral source responds well to radiation. Preoperative radiation may eliminate the need for surgical intervention or identify radioresistant tumors that would benefit from surgical resection.

After sustaining a pathologic fracture secondary to metastatic carcinoma, the average survival time is 19 months. Each histologic type has varying lengths of survival (prostate, 29 months; breast, 23 months; renal, 12 months; lung, 4 months). Furthermore, each type of carcinoma exhibits

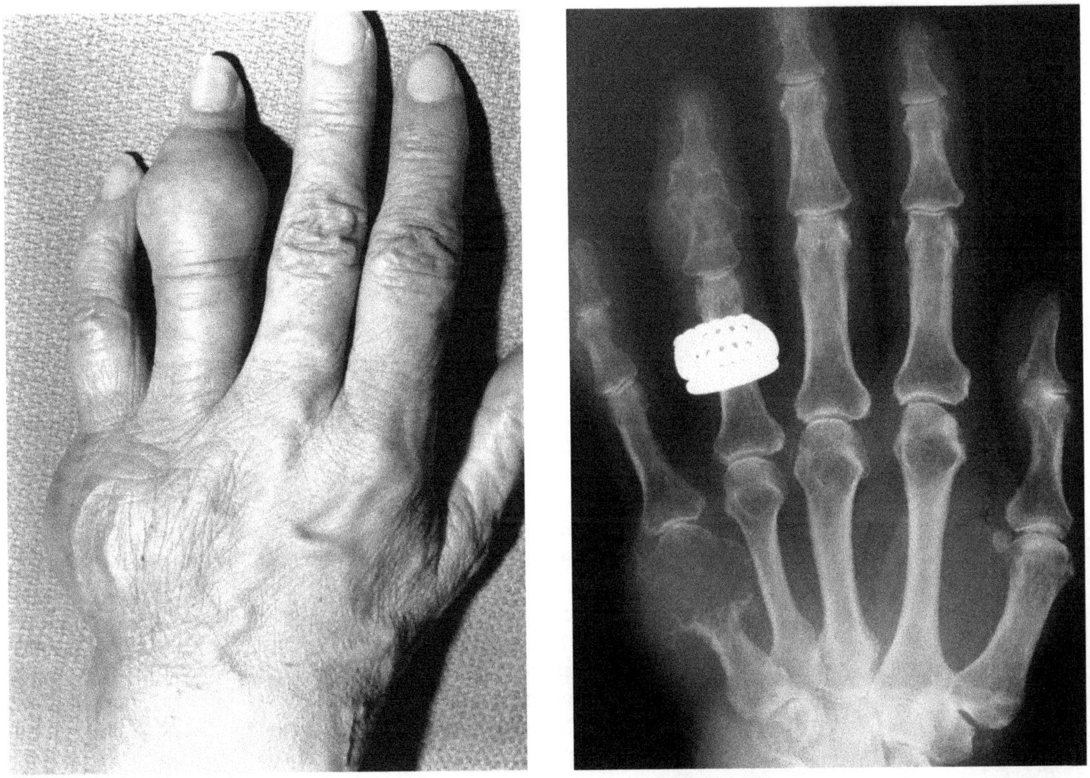

A B

▲ **Figure 6–80.** Clinical appearance (**A**) and radiographic appearance (**B**) of aneurysmal lesions in a case of carcinoma that metastasized from the thyroid to the hand.

varying radiosensitivity. Prostate, breast, and myeloma demonstrate excellent sensitivity, whereas kidney and lung are relatively radioresistant. When used appropriately, 90% of patients gain at least minimal relief, with up to two-thirds obtaining complete relief. Seventy percent of patients who

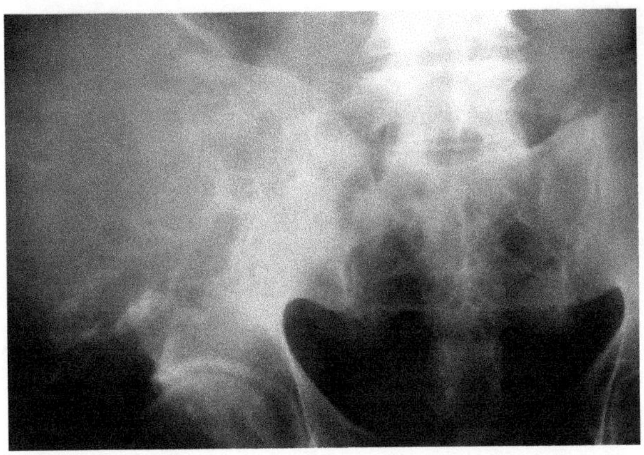

▲ **Figure 6–81.** Radiograph of a metastatic hypernephroma in the ilium.

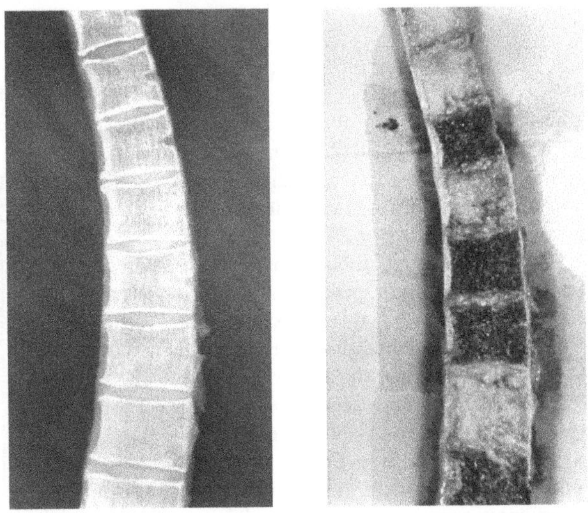

A B

▲ **Figure 6–82.** Radiograph (**A**) and gross appearance (**B**) of bone in a case of carcinoma that metastasized from the lung to the spine.

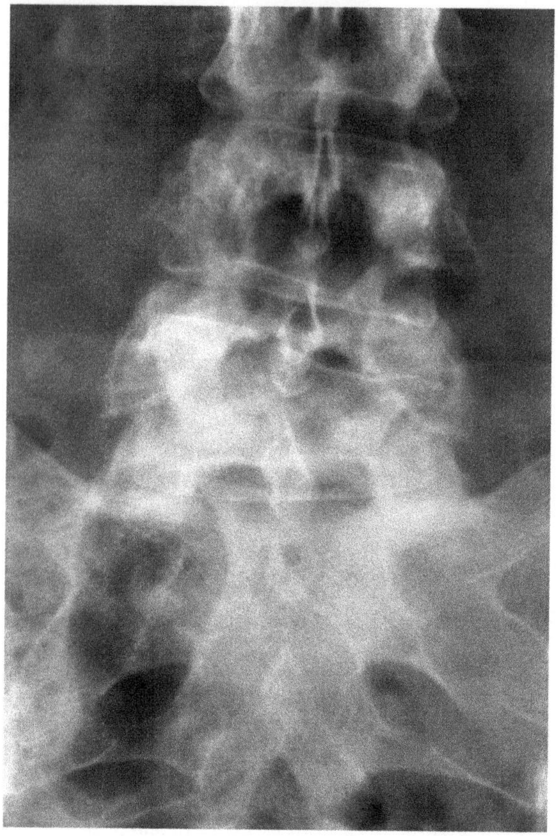

▲ **Figure 6–83.** Radiograph of the spine of a 45-year-old woman whose cancer had metastasized from the breast.

are ambulatory retain this function after radiation therapy to the lower extremities.

Chemotherapy is disease specific and is the mainstay of treatment for metastatic cancer. Hormonal therapy also has an important role in the management of metastatic breast and prostate cancer. Fortunately, these agents are easy to administer and have few side effects.

For breast cancer, medical hormonal manipulation can be done by use of antiestrogens, progestins, luteinizing hormone–releasing hormone, or adrenal-suppressing agents. Tamoxifen is effective in 30% of all breast cancer cases but increases to 50% to 75% of cases when the tumor is known to be estrogen receptor, progesterone receptor positive. Surgical ablation (oophorectomy) may also have a role in certain cases.

For prostate cancer, reduction in testosterone levels via bilateral orchiectomy or administration of estrogens or antiandrogens may produce dramatic results in certain cases. Estrogens are no longer used as first-line agents because of the risk of cardiovascular complications.

The use of agents aimed at decreasing bone turnover, including bisphosphonates, osteoprotegerin, and nuclear factor kappa B inhibitor, has also been introduced to limit progression of bone metastases, which is largely mediated by osteoclasts. Although the effect on overall tumor burden is unclear, there is evidence that bisphosphonates decrease skeletal-related events, which include fracture, need for surgical treatment, need for radiation, spinal cord compression, and hypercalcemia. Preclinical studies also suggest that when combined with cytotoxic agents, bisphosphonates may synergistically reduce the incidence of osseous metastases and prolong survival.

B. Surgical Treatment

The goals for surgical intervention in the patient with metastatic carcinoma to bone are relief of pain; prevention of pathologic fractures; stabilization of realized pathologic fractures; enhancement of mobility, function, and quality of life; and perhaps improvement of survival. It is generally agreed that a patient must have a life expectancy of at least 6 weeks to warrant operative intervention. Special considerations to surgical management include noting that bone quality is attenuated and healing will be delayed if even possible. Cancer patients, irrespective of their age, may have increased difficulty protecting their fixation device/prosthesis secondary to systemic debilitation. Accordingly, rigid fixation, with polymethylmethacrylate (PMMA) augmentation as needed, is mandatory. It is important that a diagnosis be established prior to any surgical intervention, as the planned intervention may change based on the diagnosis.

1. Hip—Seventy-five percent of all surgery for cancer that has metastasized to bone is performed in the hip area (Figure 6–84). The femur is the most common site of pathologic fracture, with femoral neck fractures accounting for 50% of pathologic fractures.

Resection and reconstruction with a cemented bipolar hemiarthroplasty are the mainstay of treatment for femoral neck fractures. Before these procedures are performed, it is

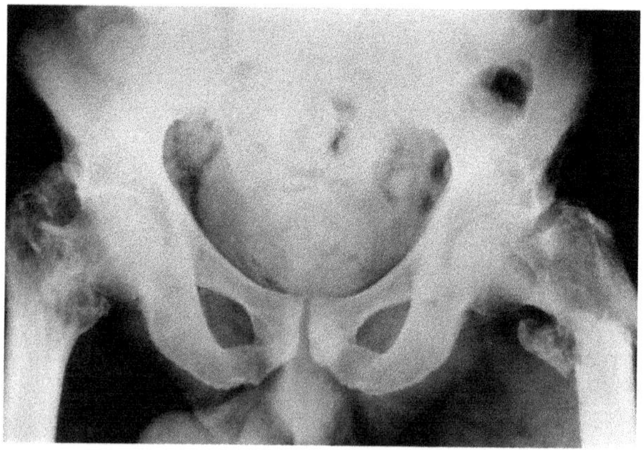

▲ **Figure 6–84.** Radiograph of the pathologic fractures of both hips in a 55-year-old man with lung carcinoma.

wise to evaluate the entire shaft of the femur and the supraacetabular area for other lytic lesions that might require a longer stem femoral component for the shaft or a modified cemented acetabular component with a total hip replacement for acetabular lesions.

In many cases, the diagnosis of metastasis to the proximal femur is made before a fracture occurs. In these cases, it is the responsibility of the orthopedic surgeon to decide whether the patient should receive some form of internal stabilization prior to radiation therapy. A CT scan of the involved area helps make this decision. Mirels criteria can be used to help guide whether or not a lesion without a fracture warrants prophylactic surgical treatment. Lesions are scored based on site, presence of pain, type of lesion (blastic, lytic, or mixed), and size of the lesion in relation to the size of the bone. A score greater than or equal to 8 predicts a higher risk of pathologic fracture and is therefore considered an indication for prophylactic surgical fixation. CT-based structural rigidity analysis is an imaging technique that measures the minimal cross-sectional rigidity of bones and is designed to monitor fracture risk associated with osteolytic lesions. It has been found to be more sensitive and specific than the Mirels score in predicting impending femoral pathologic fracture.

2. Supraacetabular area—In the case of a small supraacetabular lesion with intact cortical bone, a cemented cup with a total hip system is generally most appropriate. Augmentation of the fully cemented reconstruction with screws may be necessary in advanced cases (Figure 6–85). Percutaneous acetabuloplasty is an option for patients with a structurally compromised acetabulum. This involves aggressive intralesional curettage of the area back to healthy bone, followed by the placement of large (4.76 mm) threaded Steinmann pins into the sacroiliac area. The pins are placed with an initial foundation batch of cement, leaving them exposed for a second batch of cement, on top of which the cup is placed. A femoral component can then be placed, generally using a cemented technique.

3. Femoral shaft—Diaphyseal lesions that affect the femur but spare the peritrochanteric area are best handled with some form of intramedullary nail (Figure 6–86). Fixation of the entire femur, including the peritrochanteric area, with a reconstruction-type nail is preferable in the event the disease progresses within the bone. Current intramedullary fixation devices often do not need cement augmentation. However, in cases of severe bone deficiency, PMMA introduction, either directly into the defect or indirectly at the nail insertion site, is preferable.

4. Humerus—Humeral lesions account for most upper extremity metastatic disease. Because lesions of the humerus do not limit a patient's mobility to the same degree as lower extremity tumors, indications for surgical treatment should

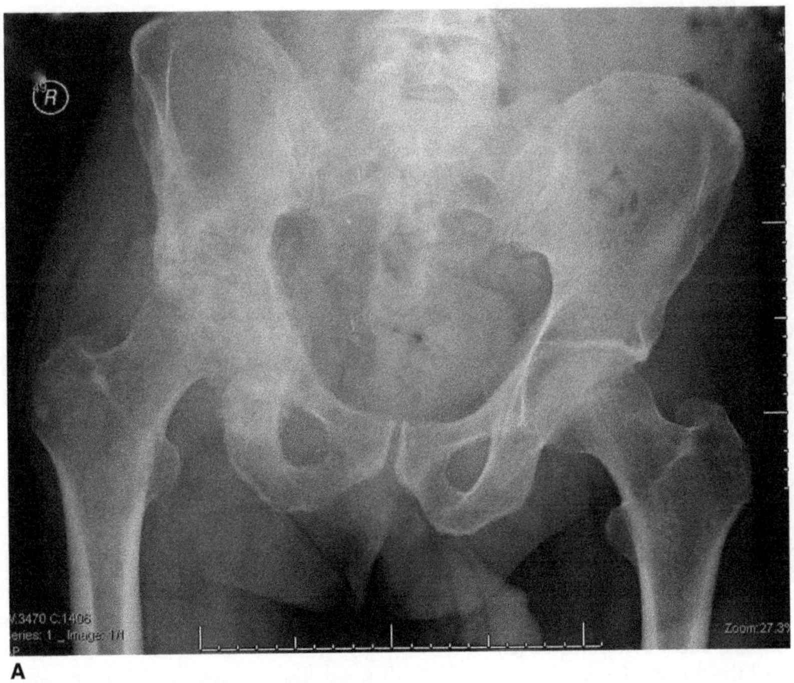

A

▲ **Figure 6–85.** Preoperative (**A**) and postoperative (**B**) radiographs of the pelvis of a 65-year-old man with metastatic transitional cell carcinoma to the right acetabular region.

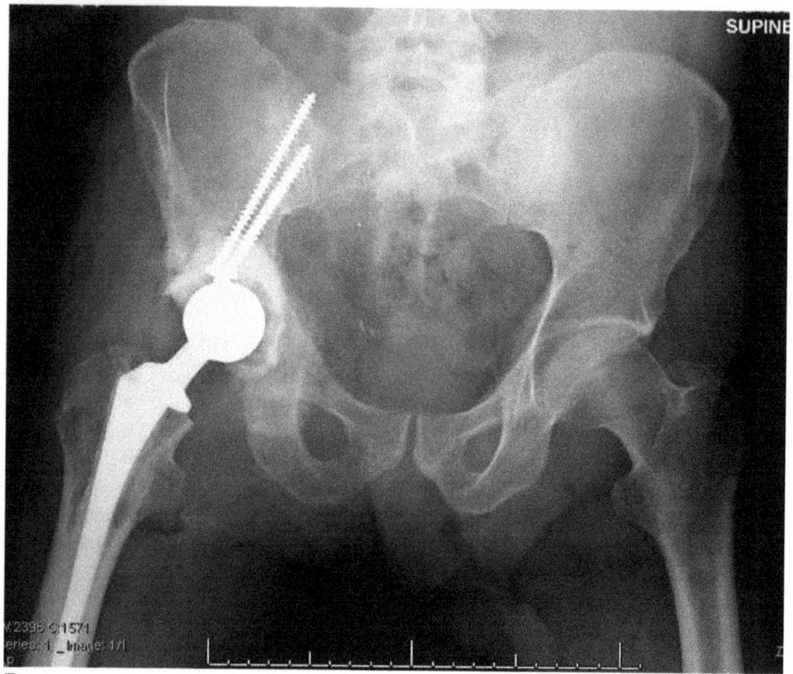

B

▲ **Figure 6–85.** (*Continued*)

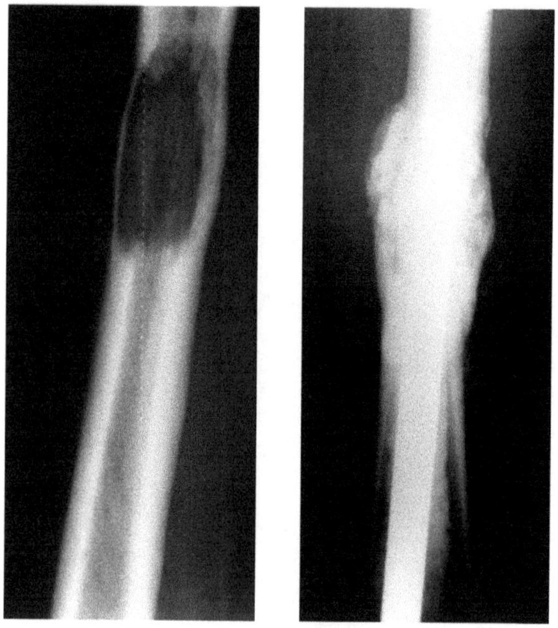

A B

▲ **Figure 6–86.** Preoperative (**A**) and postoperative (**B**) radiographs of the midshaft of the femur of a patient whose treatment involved fixation with a cemented intramedullary nail.

be tailored to the individual patient. Lesions of the proximal humerus can be treated with long-stemmed endoprosthetic reconstruction (Figure 6–87). Proximal humerus plating can also be used, followed by radiation. As in the lower extremity, diaphyseal lesions can be treated with intramedullary nail fixation.

5. Spine—In most cases of metastasis to the spine, the patient's pain can be managed adequately with local radiation therapy and medication. However, surgery is indicated in the cast of spinal instability, pathologic fracture with associated bony protrusion into the vertebral canal and cord compromise, failure to respond to radiation, or deterioration despite radiation. Prognosis of patients with spinal metastases can be predicted using the Tokuhashi score, which incorporates the patient's general condition, the number of metastases both in the spine and extraspinal, the primary malignancy, and whether or not there are neurologic changes present. This score can help guide the approach to treatment by predicting life expectancy.

The surgical approach and type of stabilization depend on tumor location. Anterior, posterior, or combined approaches may be needed depending on the type of decompression and stabilization required (Figure 6–88). En bloc spondylectomy can be performed as a potentially curative surgery in patients with good life expectancy. A scoring system known as the Spinal Instability Neoplastic Score (SINS) can be used to help predict the need for surgical stabilization. This score is

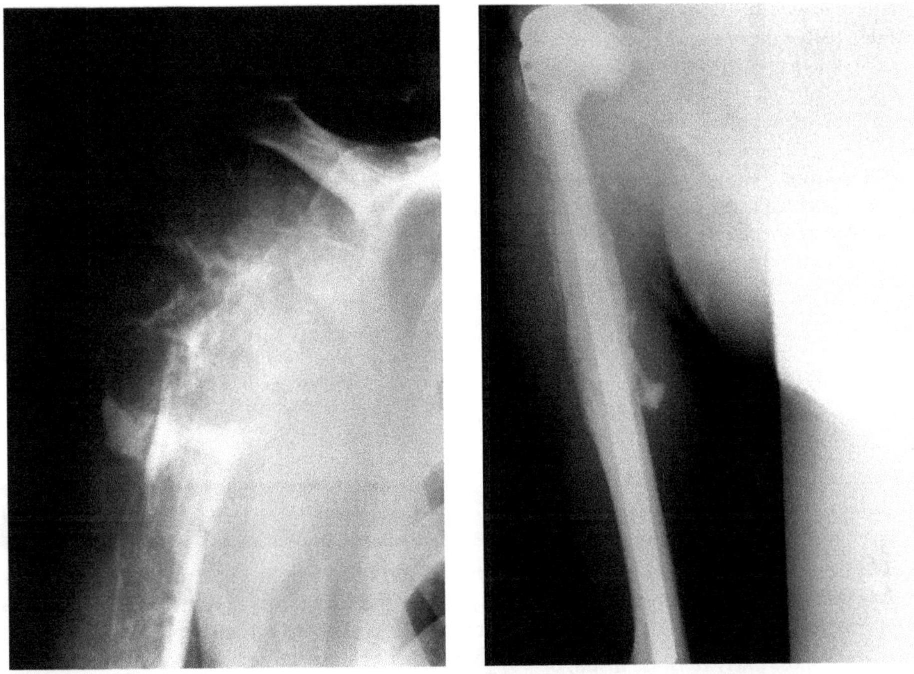

A B

▲ **Figure 6–87.** Preoperative (**A**) and postoperative (**B**) radiographs of the proximal humerus of a patient whose treatment involved the use of a long-stem Neer prosthesis.

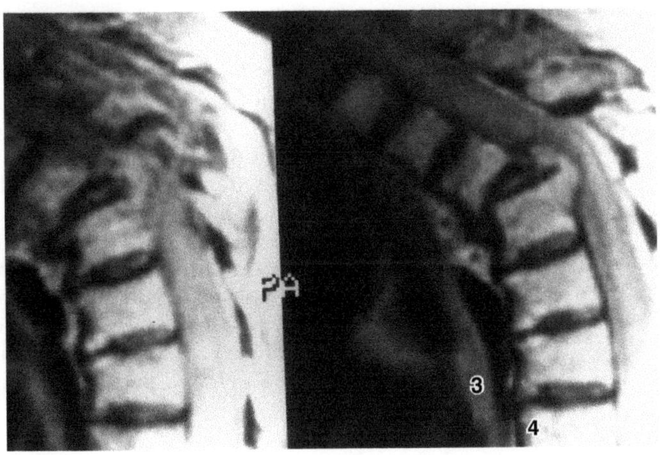

A

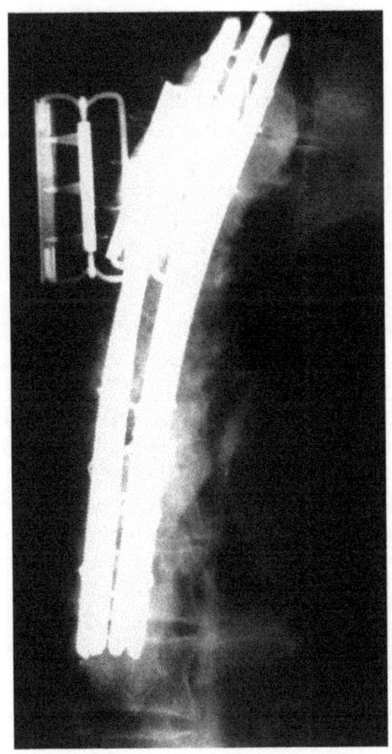

B

▲ **Figure 6–88.** Preoperative T1-weighted MRI (**A**) and postoperative radiograph (**B**) of the spine of a patient whose treatment involved the use of posterior rods and sublaminar wires for stabilization.

based on location of the lesion within the spine (junctional, mobile spine, or rigid spine), pain, type of lesion (lytic, mixed, or blastic), spinal alignment, the degree of vertebral body collapse, and whether or not the posterior column is involved. A patient with a score of 7 or higher should be considered for surgery.

In some patients with painful pathologic compression fractures, kyphoplasty or vertebroplasty can help relieve symptoms. The posterior wall of the vertebral body should be intact in order to avoid cement extravasation into the vertebral canal.

Essentials of Diagnosis

- *Prostate, breast, kidney, thyroid, and lung carcinomas are the most common to metastasize to bone.*
- *Surgical treatment of metastatic bone disease should focus on early return to function and maximization of quality of life.*
- *Ionized calcium should routinely be checked in metastatic bone disease due to the morbidity and mortality of hypercalcemia of malignancy.*
- *Carcinoma of the lung is the most likely to cause distal, or so-called acral, metastases.*

Damron TA, Nazarian A, Entezari V, et al. CT-based structural rigidity analysis is more accurate than Mirels scoring for fracture reduction in metastatic femoral lesions. *Clin Orthop Relat Res.* 2016;474(3):643. [PMID: 26169800]

Dea N, Versteeg AL, Sahgal A et al. Metastatic spine disease: should patients with short life expectancy be denied surgical care? *Neurosurgery.* 2020;87(2):303-311. [PMID: 31690935]

Fisher CG, DiPaola CP, Ryken TC, et al. A novel classification system for spinal instability in neoplastic disease: an evidence based approach and expert consensus from the Spine Oncology Study Group. *Spine.* 2010;35:E1221-E1229. [PMID: 20562730]

Gupta S, Gulia A, Kurisunkal V, et al. Principles of management of extremity skeletal metastasis. *Indian J Palliat Care.* 2019;25(4):580-586. [PMID: 31673216]

Mirels H. Metastatic disease in long bones. A proposed scoring system for diagnosing impending pathologic fractures. *Clin Orthop Relat Res.* 1989;249:256. [PMID: 2684463]

Mjelstad A, Zakariasson G, Valachis A. Optimizing antiresorptive treatment in patients with bone metastases: time to initiation, switching strategies, and treatment duration. *Support Care Cancer.* 2019;27(10):3859-3867. [PMID: 30759277]

Mossa-Baha M, Gerszten PC, Myrehuang S, et al. Spinal metastasis: diagnosis, management and follow-up. *Br J Radiol.* 2019;92(1103):20190211. [PMID: 31322920]

Park JS, Park SJ, Lee CS. Incidence and prognosis of patients with spinal metastasis as the initial manifestation of malignancy: analysis of 338 patients undergoing surgical treatment. *Bone Joint J.* 2019;101-B(11):1379-1384. [PMID: 31674246]

Seider MJ, Pugh SL, Langer C, et al. Randomized phase III trial to evaluate radiopharmaceuticals and zoledronic acid in the palliation of osteoblastic metastases from lung, breast, and prostate cancer: report of the NRG Oncology RTOG 0517 trial. *Ann Nucl Med.* 2018;32(8):553-560. [PMID: 30094545]

Thio QCBS, Karhade AV, Ognik PT, et al. Development and internal validation of machine learning algorithms for preoperative survival prediction of extremity metastatic disease. *Clin Orthop Relat Res.* 2020;478(2):322-333. [PMID: 31651589]

Tokuhashi Y, Matsuzaki H, Oda H, et al. A revised scoring system for preoperative evaluation of metastatic spine tumor prognosis. *Spine.* 2005;30(19):2186-2191. [PMID: 16205345]

Tomita K, Kawahara N, Baba H, Tsuchiya H, Fujita T, Toribatake Y. Total en bloc spondylectomy: a new surgical technique for primary malignant vertebral tumors. *Spine (Phila Pa 1976).* 1997;22(3):324-333. [PMID: 9051895]

DIFFERENTIAL DIAGNOSIS OF PSEUDOTUMOROUS CONDITIONS

In addition to benign, malignant, and metastatic neoplasms, a group of pseudotumors masquerade as bone and soft-tissue tumors. These lesions actually appear with greater frequency than either primary bone or soft-tissue tumors.

Stress-Reactive Lesions

The most common pseudotumors are those related to either bone or soft-tissue injury.

A. Stress Fracture of Bone

Stress fractures are common in young (<30 years) athletic individuals and can produce radiographic features that might suggest the diagnosis of a bone-forming sarcoma or Ewing sarcoma. It is important to obtain a careful history from patients regarding their physical activity both at work and at play. There will be no history of a single injury if the bone symptoms are caused by repetitive impact loading stress such as occurs with working out or cross-country running. The stress fracture usually occurs several weeks after a sudden increase in physical activity for which the patient is not properly conditioned. This is a common situation in the military, particularly during initial training.

Stress fractures are commonly located in the metaphyseal-diaphyseal areas of long weight-bearing bones. Early radiographs frequently appear normal before periosteal new bone begins to form. The most sensitive early diagnostic tool is a bone scan, which can appear hot or abnormal in the case of stress fractures, neoplasms, and infections. The MRI is sensitive to early fluid shifts in the periosteum overlying a stress fracture, but it is also sensitive to neoplastic and infectious conditions. One of the best methods to help rule out tumors and infection is to simply stop all physical stress to the injured bone for a period of 4 weeks. In patients with stress fracture, the pain should resolve spontaneously during this period, and a follow-up radiograph taken after this period reveals a typical fusiform circumferential periosteal callous formation. In patients with a tumor or infection, the pain persists, and the radiographic signs of permeative osteolysis predominate, in which case a biopsy and/or culture are indicated.

At times, the clinical picture of a stress fracture is confused by the preexistence of a benign stress raiser, such as a nonossifying fibroma or fibrous cortical defect (Figure 6–89).

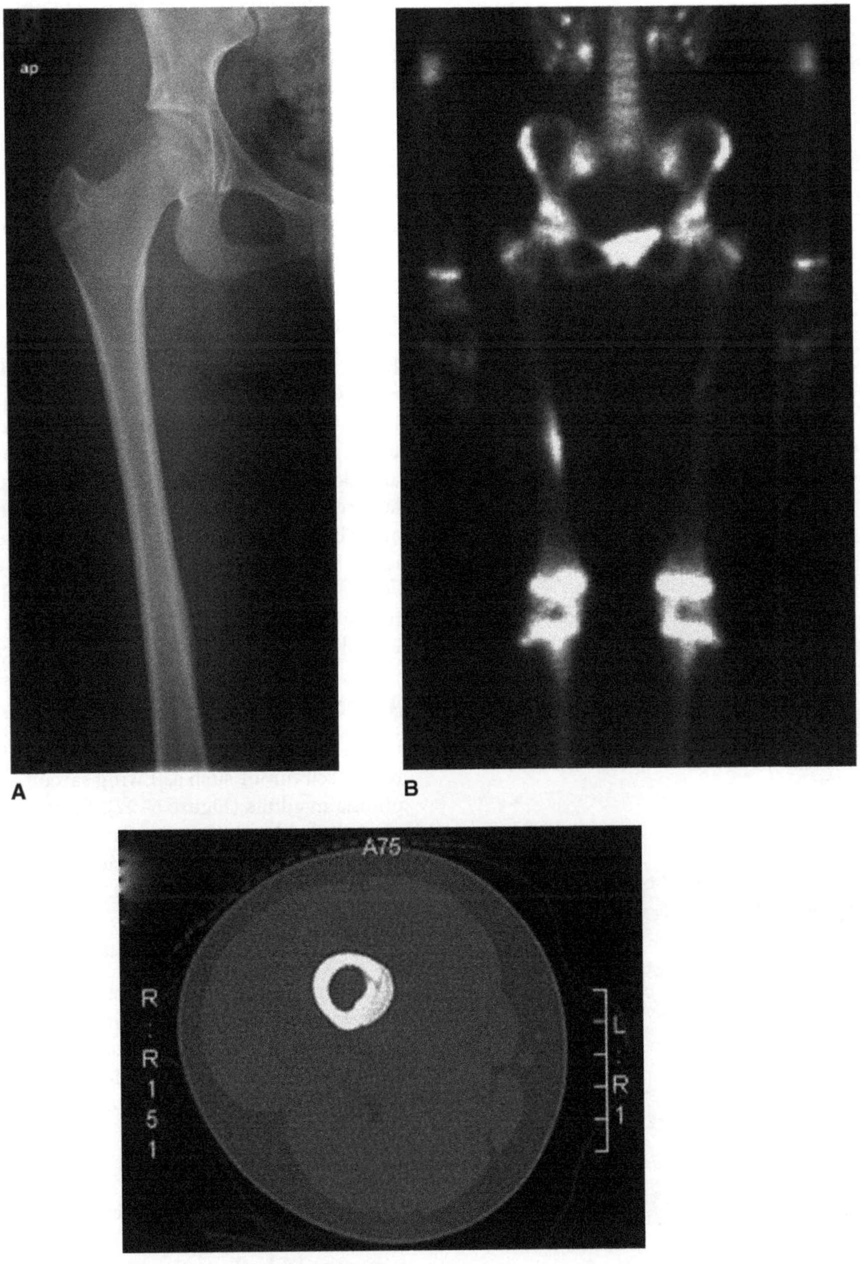

▲ **Figure 6–89.** Radiograph (**A**), isotope bone scan (**B**), and CT scan (**C**) of the femur of a 14-year-old girl with a stress fracture. Notice the subtle increased uptake in the contralateral femur in **B** and the absence of a nidus, which would be seen in osteoid osteoma, but rather a linear lucency in **C**.

In older patients, especially in postmenopausal women, stress fractures can occur with minimal physical activity. The circumstances under which the fracture occurred might not come out in a routine history. A common location of osteoporotic stress fractures is in the sacrum (Figure 6–90).

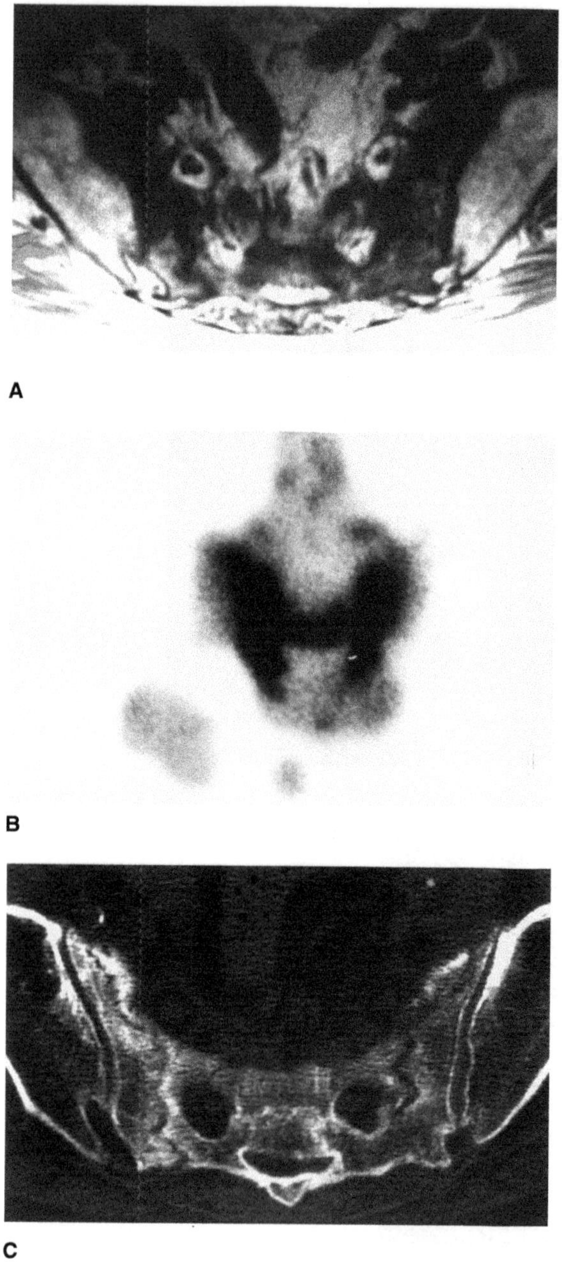

▲ **Figure 6–90.** T1-weighted MRI (**A**), isotope bone scan (**B**), and CT scan (**C**) of the sacrum in a 71-year-old woman with stress fracture.

B. Myositis Ossificans

Another common stress-reactive pseudotumor seen in the extremity is myositis ossificans, which occurs most frequently in the lower extremity in young men. The quadriceps muscle is commonly involved because of direct blows or tearing injury to this muscle. The pseudotumor mass may not arise for several months after the injury and may not be related to a specific injury. In older (>40 years), more sedentary patients, there may be no history of stress injury.

Early radiographs may not reveal soft-tissue calcification. With maturation, ossification occurs in the traumatized muscle fascial planes, which may suggest the diagnosis of a synovial sarcoma or other calcifying sarcoma. If the myositis pseudotumor is attached to the subjacent bone, it can mimic a parosteal osteosarcoma (Figure 6–91).

Infectious Diseases

Bacterial, viral, tuberculous, or fungal infections of the bone or soft tissue can frequently mimic a neoplastic process. This is particularly the case with infections that are not highly virulent, do not create systemic symptoms or a febrile response, and do not cause a large alteration in acute-phase reactant laboratory work. If a tender mass is present on examination and a bone or soft-tissue tumor is suggested by imaging studies, a biopsy may be indicated and should include a tissue culture to make the correct diagnosis. Inflammatory pseudotumors can be seen in any age group but are more common in children and frequently affect the lower extremity.

A. Bacterial Infection

Bacterial infections of bone can take on the appearance of a round cell tumor such as Ewing sarcoma in children or lymphoma in adults (Figure 6–92). In contrast, tuberculous and fungal infections are less inflammatory and thus have more localized, well-marginated lesions that take on the imaging appearance of a benign tumor.

B. Tuberculous or Fungal Infection

A tuberculous or fungal infection of the spine or extremity can present as a pseudotumor in children or young adults (Figure 6–93). The incidence of tuberculous and fungal infections, which are low-grade infections that typically have an insidious onset, is also increased in patients with AIDS.

C. Caffey Disease

Caffey disease can mimic a neoplastic process. It is an idiopathic form of periostitis that is seen in infants younger than 6 months and affects the extremities, shoulder girdle, and mandible (Figure 6–94). It may have a viral origin and is currently much rarer than it was 30 years ago. The bony changes are osteoblastic and could suggest the diagnosis of an

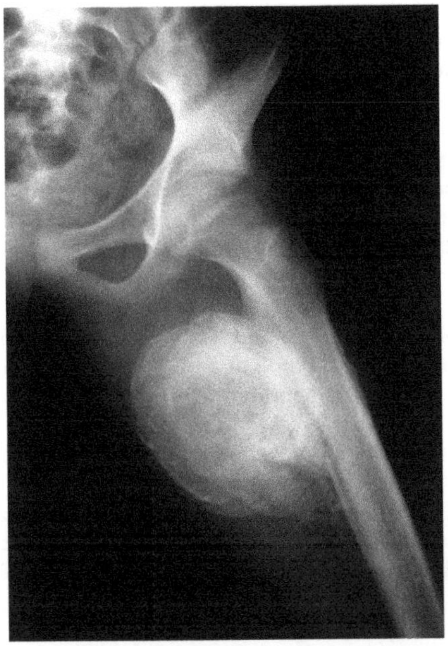

A

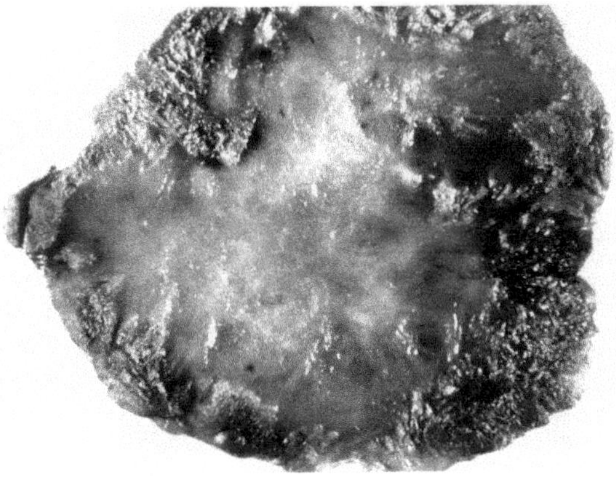

B

▲ **Figure 6–91.** Radiograph (**A**) and gross appearance of a resected specimen (**B**) of myositis ossificans in the adductor muscles of a 12-year-old girl.

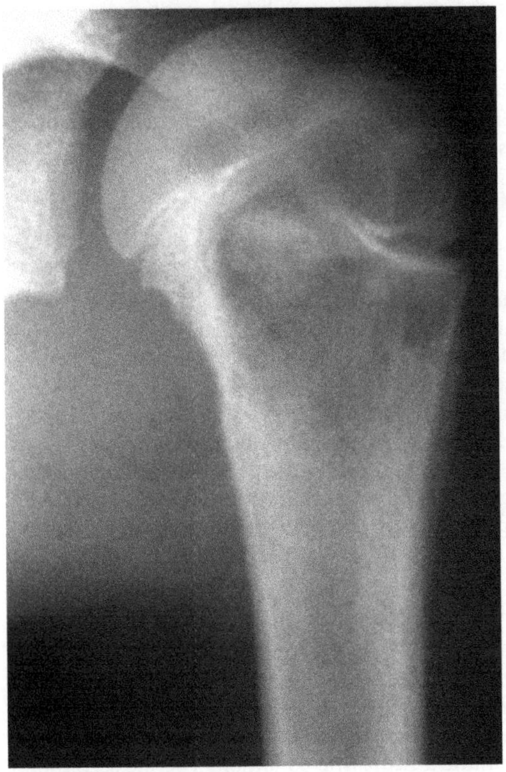

▲ **Figure 6–92.** Radiograph of acute osteomyelitis caused by *Staphylococcus aureus* in the proximal humerus of a 13-year-old boy.

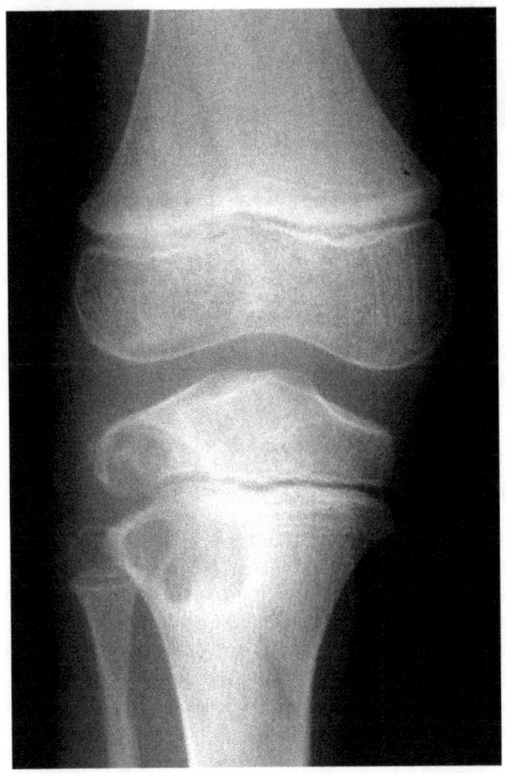

▲ **Figure 6–93.** Radiograph of tuberculous osteomyelitis in the proximal tibia of a 10-year-old girl.

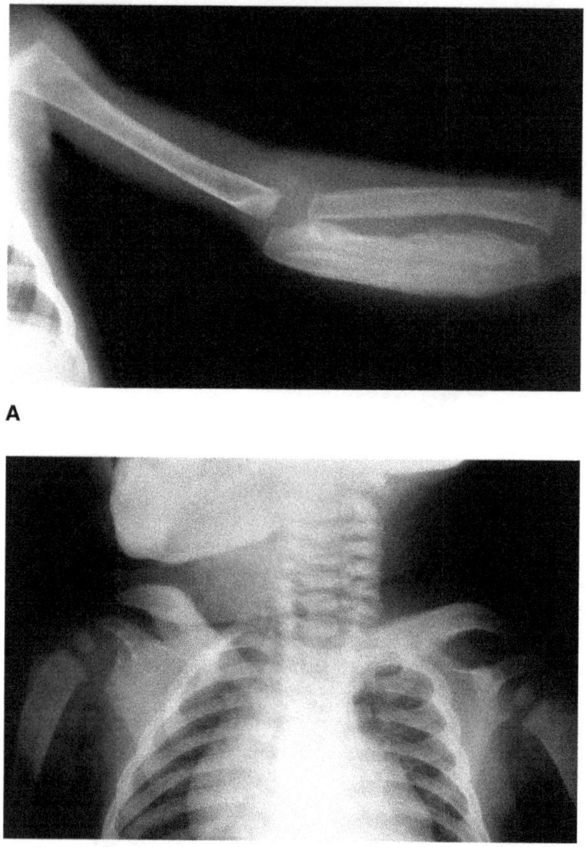

A

B

▲ **Figure 6–94.** Radiographs of the upper extremity (**A**) and the bilateral shoulders (**B**) of a 5-month-old infant with Caffey disease.

osteosarcoma, which is rare in infants. Caffey disease is self-limiting and usually clears spontaneously without disability.

Metabolic Disorders

A. Brown Tumor of Primary Hyperparathyroidism

Brown tumor is the most common metabolic disorder that mimics a neoplastic process in bone. The lytic giant cell lesions occur symmetrically in metaphyseal-epiphyseal bone as the result of increased parathyroid hormone production by a solitary parathyroid adenoma, by hyperplastic parathyroid glands, or by a solitary parathyroid carcinoma. Brown tumors occur three times more often in females than in males and are usually seen between 15 and 70 years of age. They are most common in the ends of the long bone, followed next in frequency in the pelvis, long bone diaphysis, maxillary bone, cranium, rib, and hand. Brown tumors are rarely seen in the spine. Symptoms of pain are related to the local bone destruction, but widespread pain may result from generalized osteomalacia. The hyperparathyroid condition can lead to weight loss, psychological disorders, gastrointestinal disorders, renal stones, polyuria, and polydipsia.

The radiographic features of the brown tumor in bone include a round lytic area that may be multicentric and may suggest the diagnosis of metastatic carcinoma, multiple myeloma, or histiocytic lymphoma (Figure 6–95). In the case of a solitary lesion, it may suggest the diagnosis of a nonossifying fibroma, fibrous dysplasia, giant cell tumor, or aneurysmal bone cyst. At the time of biopsy, the brown tumor has the reddish-brown appearance of a giant cell tumor. Microscopically, it looks like a giant cell tumor except that the background stromal cells are more fibroblastic and the bone trabeculae demonstrate abnormally thick and poorly mineralized osteoid seams. Because of the marked similarity between the brown tumor and the giant cell tumor, clinicians should routinely order an analysis of serum calcium, phosphorus, and alkaline phosphatase levels in all patients with bone lesions that produce giant cells.

In patients with brown tumors, the treatment consists of removing the source of the excessive parathyroid hormone. After this, the bony defects usually heal spontaneously. Bone grafting is rarely required. Although the secondary hyperparathyroidism seen in renal failure patients does not usually develop into brown tumors, it does produce pseudotumorous calcification in soft tissue, a condition similar to tumoral calcinosis, which is discussed later in this section.

B. Paget Disease

Paget disease is frequently included in discussions of metabolic bone disorders, although the demonstration of cytoplasmic and nuclear inclusion bodies in osteoclasts of pagetic bone similar to paramyxovirus infections may suggest a viral origin. Most clinicians are familiar with the late changes in Paget disease, which include the bowing of long bones and the finding of dense blastic changes on radiographic examination. However, many are unfamiliar with the early lytic phase of Paget disease when the radiographic findings are more suggestive of metastatic carcinoma, histiocytic lymphoma, primary sarcoma, or even primary hyperparathyroidism (Figure 6–96).

C. Gaucher Disease

Gaucher disease is a rare familial disorder in which accumulation of glucocerebroside causes enlargement of the liver, spleen, and marrow tissues. The marrow infiltration in children and young adults causes a gradual loss of bone that can mimic a neoplastic condition. The most common areas involved include the distal femur, tibia, humerus, vertebral column, skull, and mandible. Isolated focal destructive

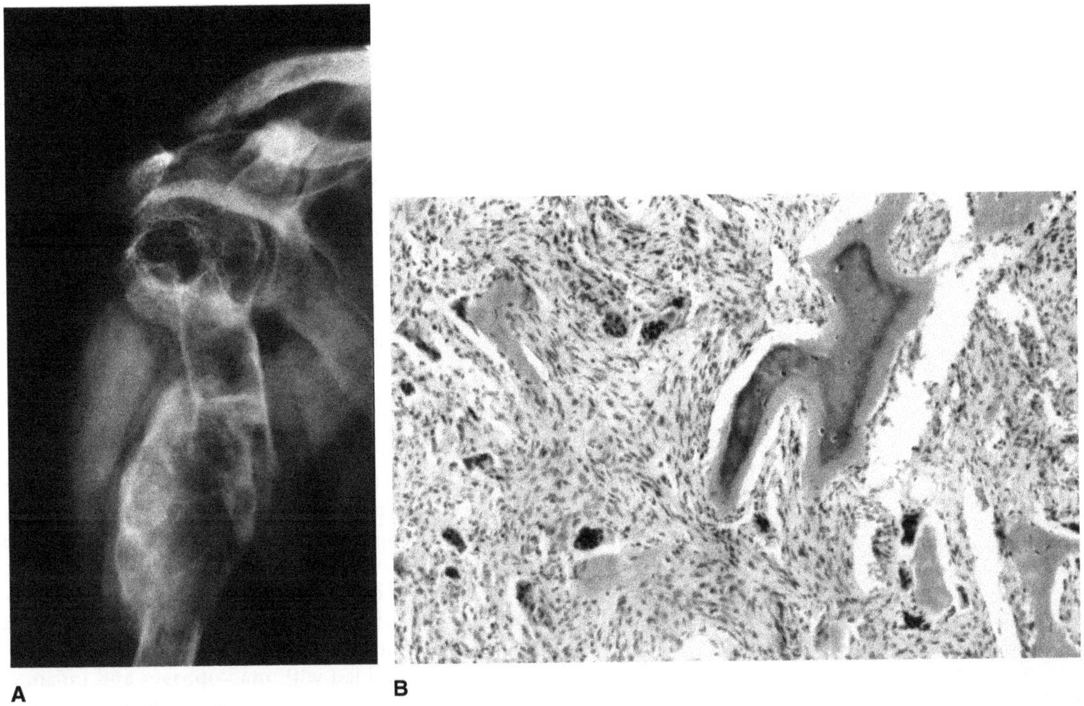

▲ **Figure 6–95.** Radiograph (**A**) and photomicrograph (**B**) of a brown tumor of hyperparathyroidism in the proximal humerus of a 40-year-old woman.

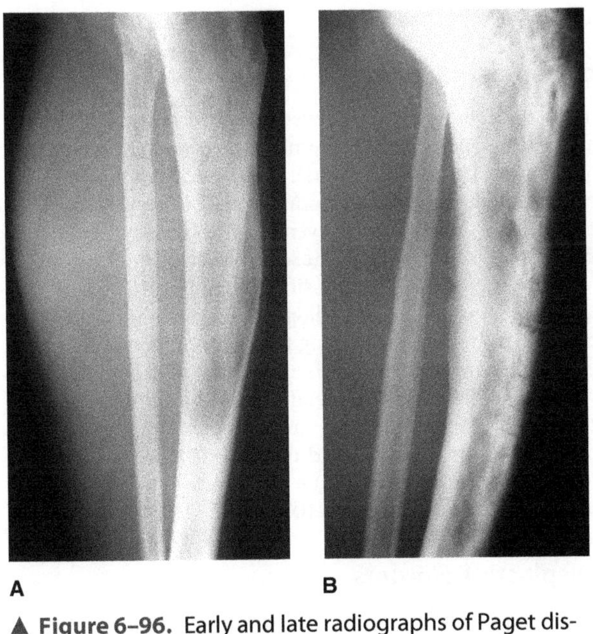

▲ **Figure 6–96.** Early and late radiographs of Paget disease of the tibia, taken when the patient was 45 years of age (**A**) and when he was 65 years of age (**B**).

changes with endosteal scalloping and moth-eaten patterns may suggest the diagnosis of metastatic disease, myelomatosis, primary sarcoma, or fibrous dysplasia (Figure 6–97).

Hemorrhagic Conditions

A. Pseudotumor of Hemophilia

A hematoma in the soft tissue or bone under the periosteum may be difficult to distinguish from a tumor. Hematoma formation is frequently precipitated by some form of trauma, and the bones most commonly involved are the femur, pelvis, tibia, and small bones of the hand. It is rare to see multiple lesions. The bony lesions can be central or eccentric. The finding of lytic destruction followed by sclerotic reaction at the periphery may mimic the radiographic picture of an aneurysmal bone cyst or a giant cell tumor. In the hand bones, the osseous pseudotumors take on the appearance of a giant cell reparative granuloma or an osteoblastoma. The subperiosteal lesions bulge into the surrounding soft tissue and show reactive periosteal new bone formation and subjacent cortical erosion that may mimic Ewing sarcoma or hemorrhagic osteosarcoma (Figure 6–98).

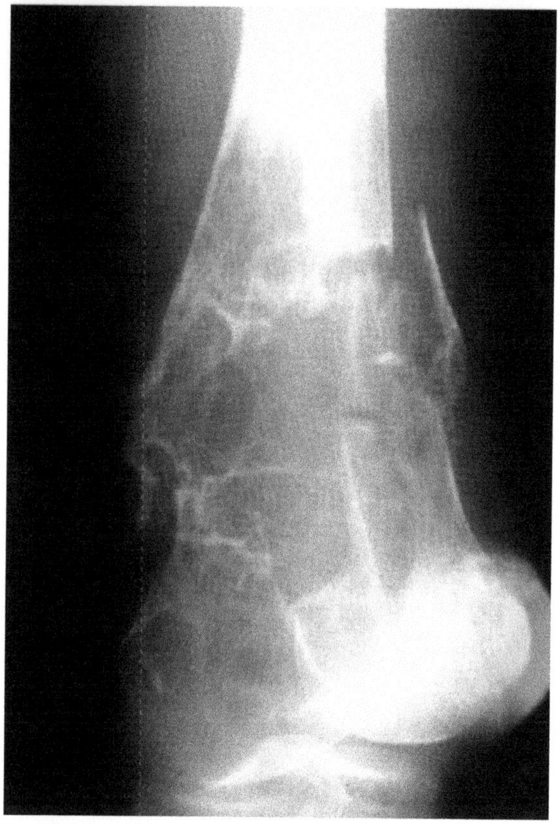

▲ **Figure 6–97.** Radiograph of a pathologic fracture secondary to Gaucher disease involving the distal femur in a 29-year-old man.

B. Intramuscular Hematoma

Another hemorrhagic disorder that can produce a pseudotumor of soft tissue is the intramuscular hematoma. It is similar to the soft-tissue pseudotumor of hemophilia but without a bleeding abnormality. Intramuscular hematomas are almost always related to blunt trauma, but they occasionally result from a traction injury that may subsequently produce myositis ossificans. There may be no superficial signs of bruising in the overlying skin, and sometimes the hematoma grows in size at a later date, even as long as several years after the initial injury. The radiographic examination is of little help because no calcification or bony abnormality is evident. The MRI is the best imaging study, but unfortunately, the appearance of an intramuscular hematoma on MRI can mimic that of a deep soft-tissue sarcoma such as a malignant fibrous histiocytoma (Figure 6–99).

Ectopic Calcification

Ectopic calcification in soft tissue has many causes, most of which are related to chronic degenerative disorders in collagenous structures such as tendons or ligaments about a joint. However, in cases in which the dystrophic calcification is associated with a soft-tissue mass, the clinician must rule out the diagnosis of a soft-tissue sarcoma such as synovial sarcoma.

A. Tumoral Calcinosis

Tumoral calcinosis, seen about the hip, shoulder, and elbow, is characterized by extensive calcium phosphate deposition in a benign fibrous mass. There is a familial form associated with a loss-of-function mutation in the *FGF23* gene. A gain-of-function mutation in the same gene results in autosomal dominant hypophosphatemic rickets. Otherwise, it is an idiopathic condition that affects patients between 10 and 30 years of age and occurs more frequently in males than in females. Multiple lesions occur, and the lesions cause minimal pain and tenderness.

In cases of tumoral calcinosis, the extensive central fluffy calcification might suggest the diagnosis of a synovial sarcoma, soft-tissue chondrosarcoma, or tuberculosis (Figure 6–100). At biopsy, a chalky white paste exudes from a spongelike fibrous mass. Microscopic findings include extensive amorphous calcium phosphate deposits in a fibrous stroma speckled with macrophages and inflammatory cells. If the pseudotumor is not completely removed, a recurrence is very likely.

A similar condition is seen in patients with renal osteodystrophy with secondary hyperparathyroidism, and the mechanism for the deposition in this case is a high level of calcium phosphorus production.

B. Compartment Syndrome

The ischemic calcification and even ossification that occur in traumatic compartment syndromes in the lower extremity can often mimic a tumor. The initial injury is usually a crushing type that causes increased compartment pressure from muscle swelling. This pressure eventually leads to ischemic necrosis of the compartment muscle, which several years later becomes calcific or even ossified. Because the muscle appears firm and calcified on radiographic examination, the clinician may not relate the finding to an old injury and may suspect a calcifying sarcoma such as synovial sarcoma. The most common place for this pseudotumor is in one of the muscle compartments of the leg, and it causes stiffness and muscle weakness at the ankle and foot area (Figure 6–101). This process can mimic soft-tissue calcifications secondary to a neoplastic process (Figure 6–102).

Dysplastic Disorders

Many developmental or dysplastic conditions can create bony abnormalities, which, on radiographic examination, can mimic a bone tumor. These are usually focal defects in endochondral bone formation that result from a failure to

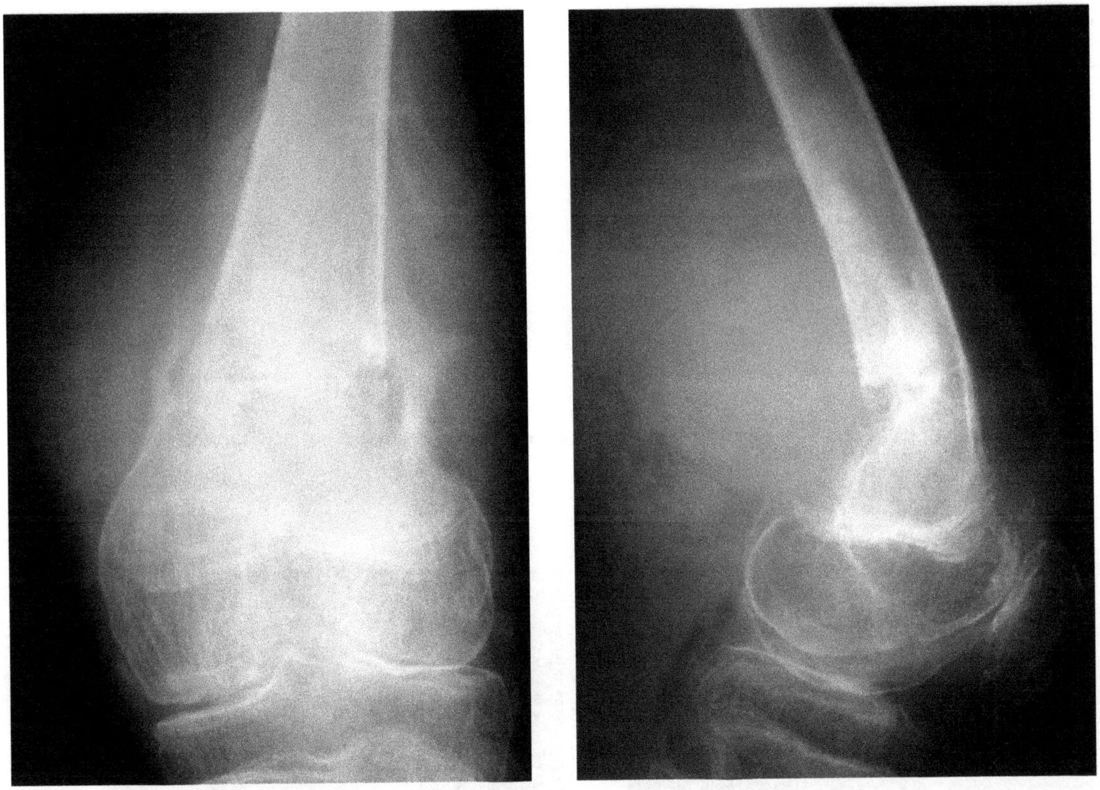

A B

▲ **Figure 6–98.** Anteroposterior (**A**) and lateral (**B**) radiographs of a pseudotumor of hemophilia in the distal femur of a 14-year-old boy.

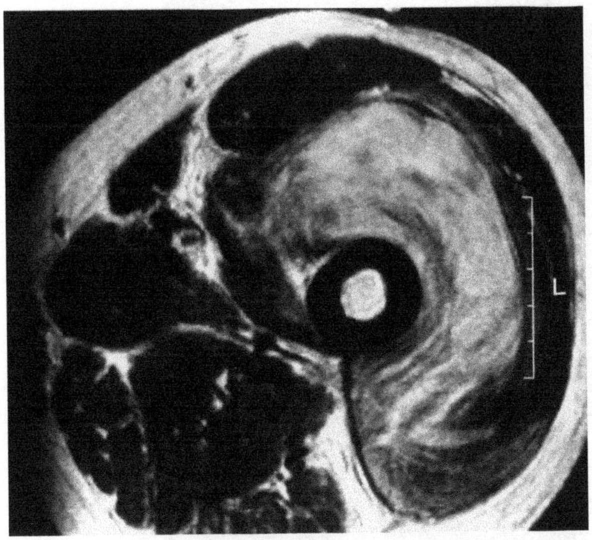

▲ **Figure 6–99.** Axial view T2-weighted MRI of a hematoma in the quadriceps muscles of a 46-year-old woman.

remodel primary woven bone forming at the metaphyseal end of the physis.

A. Osteoma

Osteoma commonly occurs in the skull or maxilla and is composed of dense unorganized woven bone seen just beneath the cortex. There is no lytic component in or around the dense bone, and no symptoms are associated with the presence of osteomas. Because the lesions are commonly seen in the metaphyseal areas about the knee, the clinician may become concerned about the diagnosis of an early osteosarcoma. However, the lack of periosteal response and minimal uptake on an isotope bone scan help rule out sarcoma (Figure 6–103). In such cases, there should be no concern about future problems from the lesion, and usually no intervention is necessary.

B. Bone Island

The bone island, or enostosis, is an even more sharply marginated dysplastic process than the osteoma. It is most

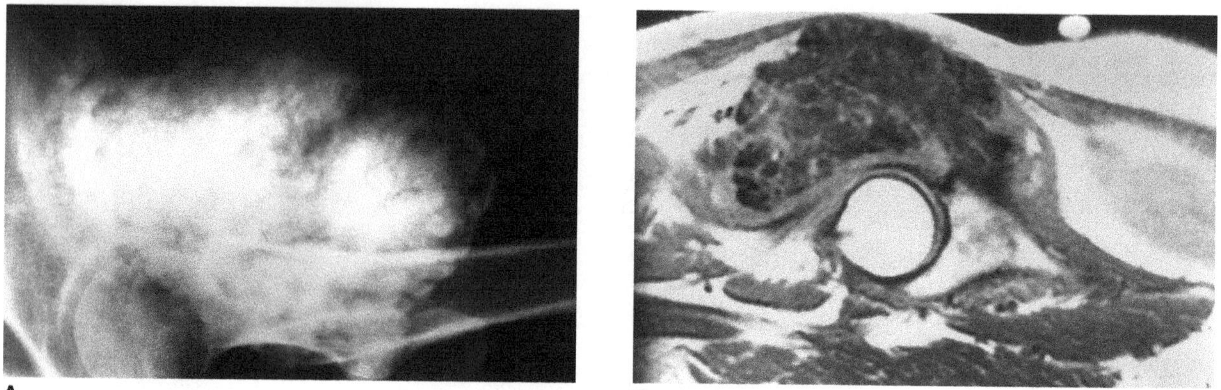

A B

▲ **Figure 6–100.** Radiograph (**A**) and T1-weighted MRI (**B**) of tumoral calcinosis in the hip of a 54-year-old woman.

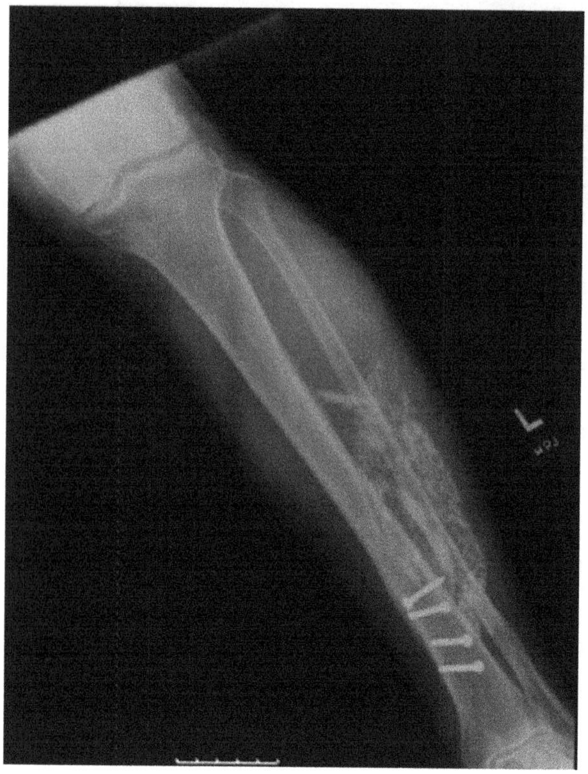

A

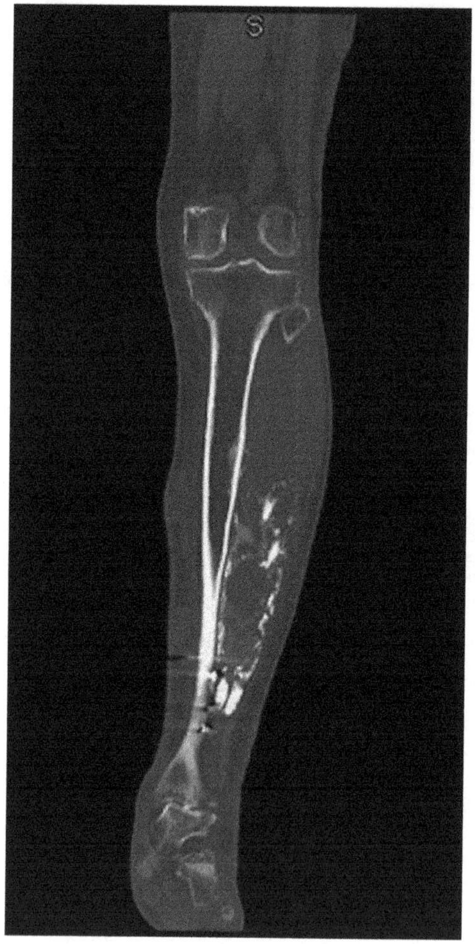

B

▲ **Figure 6–101.** Radiograph (**A**) and CT scan (**B**) of an old compartment syndrome of the anterior compartment of the leg of an 81-year-old woman who had a history of fracture treated with internal fixation 60 years prior.

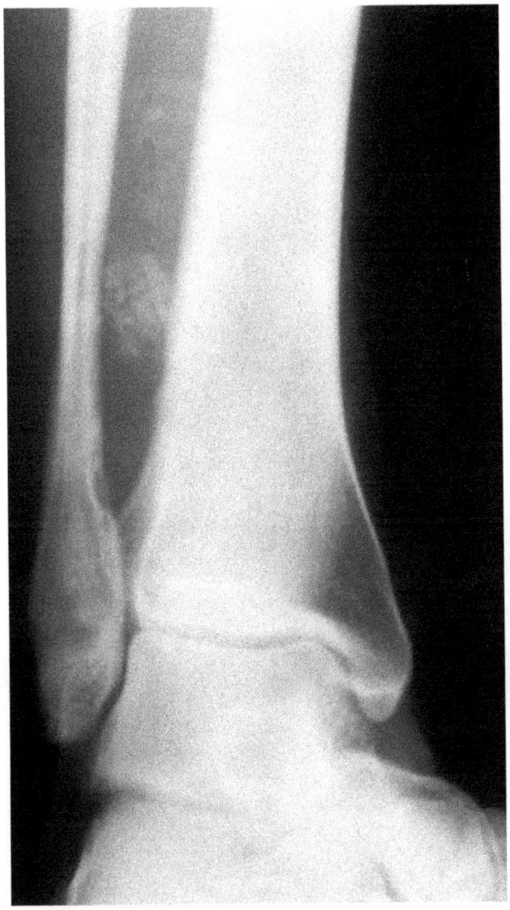

▲ **Figure 6–102.** Radiograph of calcification in synovial sarcoma of the leg.

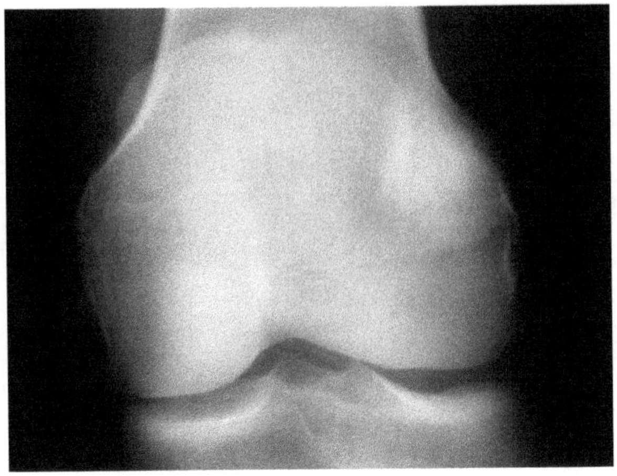

A

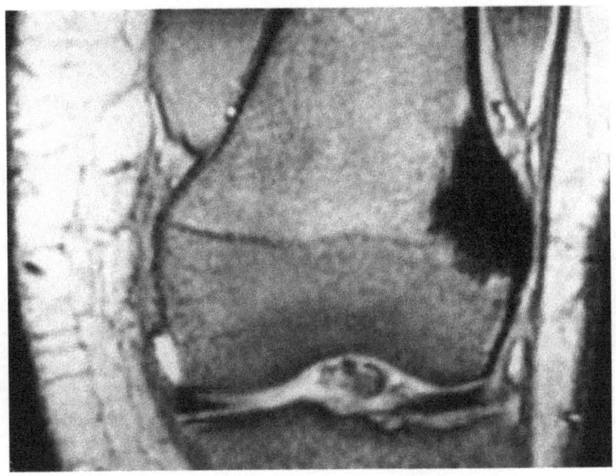

B

▲ **Figure 6–103.** Radiograph (**A**) and T2-weighted MRI (**B**) of a dysplastic process in the distal femur of a 64-year-old woman.

commonly located in the pelvis. It can mimic a blastic metastatic lesion in patients with prostate cancer. However, with a bone island, as with an osteoma, the bone scan shows minimal and very focal activity, and the CT scan and MRI show no reaction in the surrounding marrow. Figure 6–104 shows the findings of a bone island through the pelvis of a 35-year-old man.

Bone Infarcts

The two types of bone infarcts that can mimic bone tumors are the metaphyseal type and the epiphyseal type. They can be idiopathic in origin or secondary to increased alcohol consumption or corticosteroid use.

A. Metaphyseal Bone Infarct

The most common bone infarct is in the metaphyseal region, which is typically seen about the knee, hip, and shoulder in adults. Radiographically, the infarct can mimic a low-grade cartilaginous tumor such as an enchondroma. An infarct presents with a sclerotic honeycombed pattern (Figure 6–105), whereas a cartilaginous lesion presents with central flocculated calcification (Figure 6–106).

B. Epiphyseal Bone Infarct

Although epiphyseal bone infarcts have the same etiology as those in the metaphysis, these are most commonly found in the femoral condyles and the proximal femoral and humeral epiphyses. In these locations, the lytic change seen in the epiphyseal bone can mimic a chondroblastoma. The differential diagnosis can be difficult before the appearance

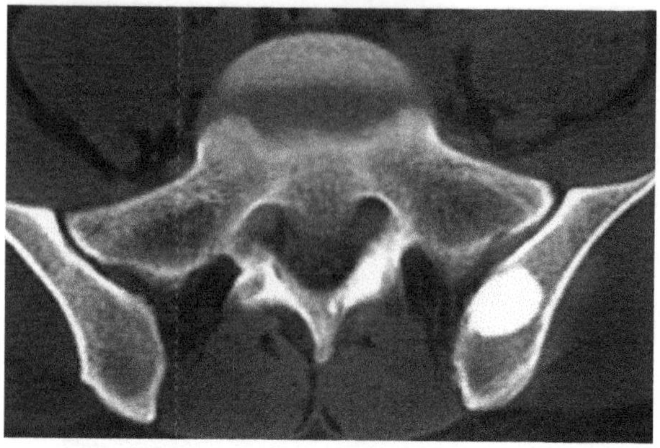

A

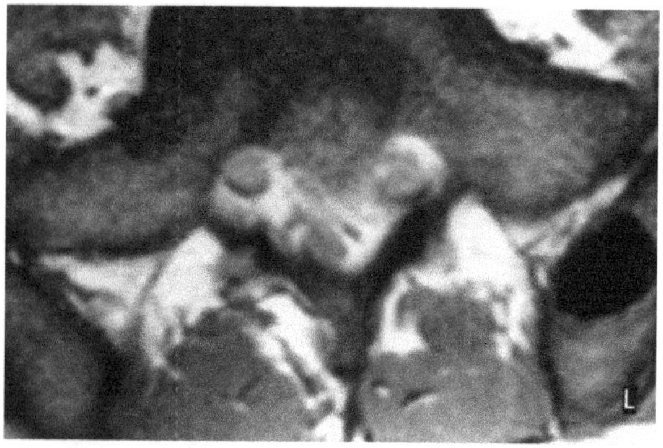

B

▲ **Figure 6–104.** CT scan (**A**) and T2-weighted MRI (**B**) of a bone island in the ilium of a 35-year-old man.

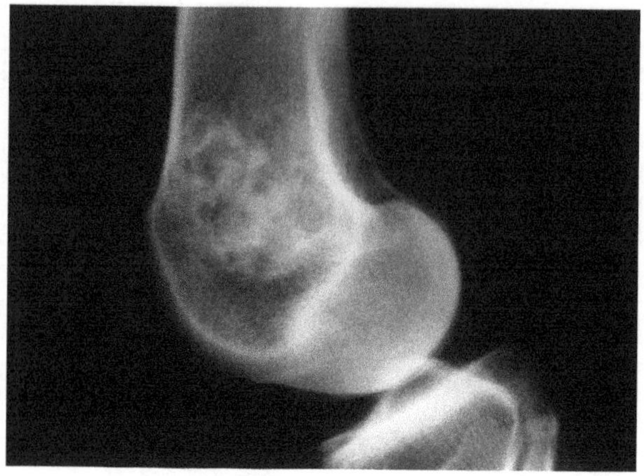

A

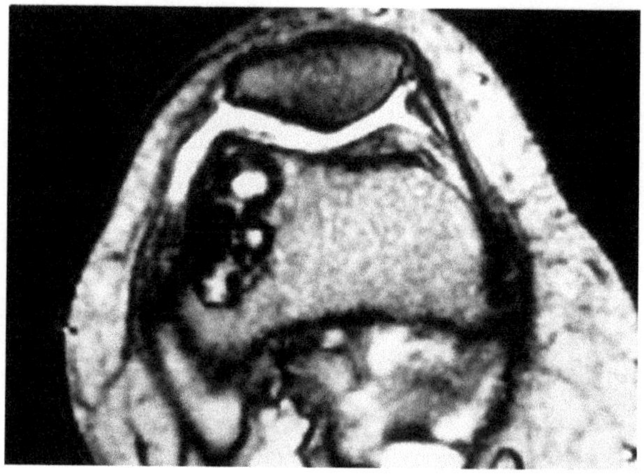

B

▲ **Figure 6–105.** Radiograph (**A**) and T1-weighted MRI (**B**) of a metaphyseal infarct in the distal femur of a 52-year-old woman.

of a crescent sign or other radiographic signs of subchondral collapse that usually rule out the chondroblastoma (Figure 6–107).

Histiocytic Disorders

A. Langerhans Cell Histiocytosis

Langerhans cell histiocytosis can present in a variety of ways. Previously considered distinct diseases, including eosinophilic granuloma, Hand-Schüller-Christian disease, and Letterer-Siwe disease, they are now considered part of the same spectrum of histiocytosis presentation. Of these, the localized granulomatous form, which is called eosinophilic granuloma or Langerhans cell granulomatosis, is the one that mimics a tumor radiographically. Eosinophilic granuloma is seen twice as often in boys as in girls and commonly occurs between 5 and 15 years of age. It is usually monostotic but in 10% of cases involves two or three separate areas. It is a histiocytic process of unknown cause but may have a viral origin. It causes local inflammatory pain and may result in low-grade fever associated with an elevated sedimentation rate. Although the most common location of eosinophilic granuloma is the skull, it is also seen in the rib, pelvis, maxilla, vertebral body (presenting as vertebra plana) (Figure 6–108), clavicle, and scapula, listed in order of frequency. Although more commonly affecting flat bones, it can arise in the diaphysis of long bones and, less commonly, in the metaphysis or the epiphysis.

Eosinophilic granuloma can be extremely permeative and destructive, especially in long bones (Figure 6–109) and vertebrae (Figure 6–110), thereby mimicking a more aggressive process, such as Ewing sarcoma, metastatic neuroblastoma, or osteomyelitis. It can also produce a so-called onionskin periostitis of the type seen in Ewing sarcoma. The

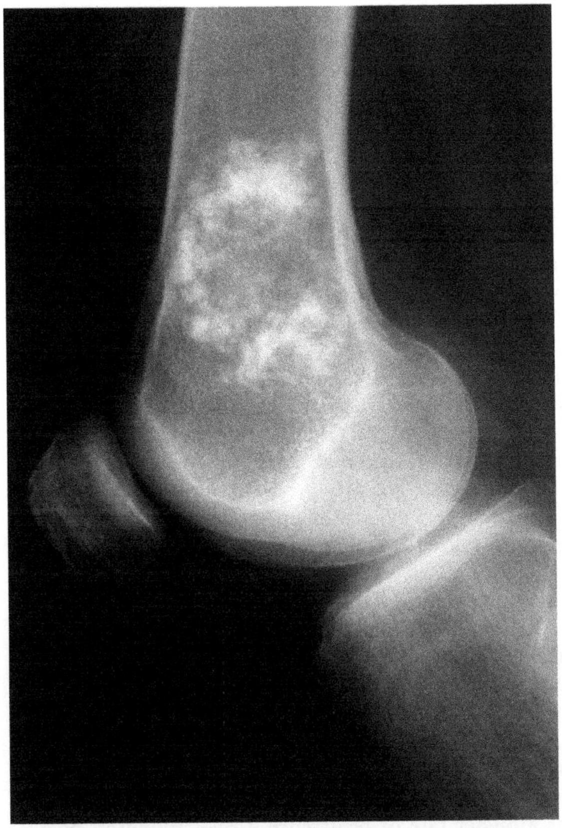

▲ **Figure 6–106.** Radiograph of a large enchondroma in the distal femur.

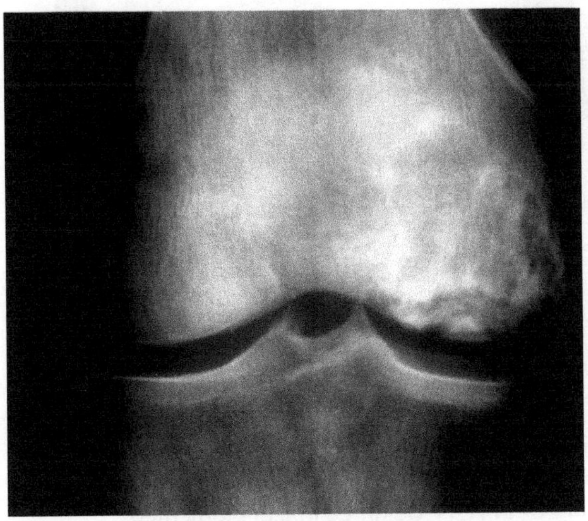

▲ **Figure 6–107.** Radiograph of an epiphyseal infarct in the femoral condyle of a 45-year-old woman.

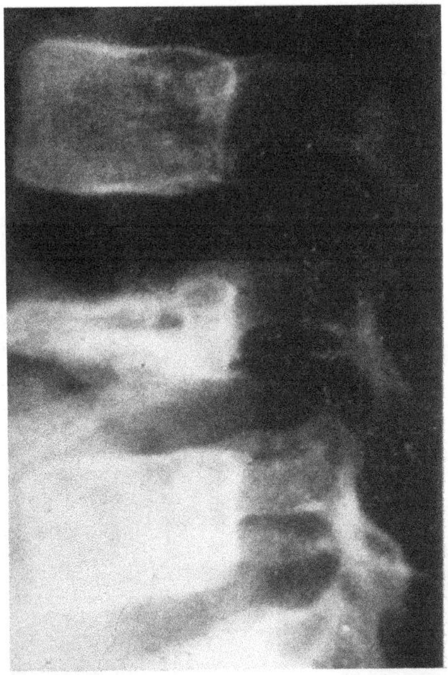

▲ **Figure 6–108.** Lateral radiograph of spine demonstrating characteristic vertebra plana of Langerhans cell histiocytosis.

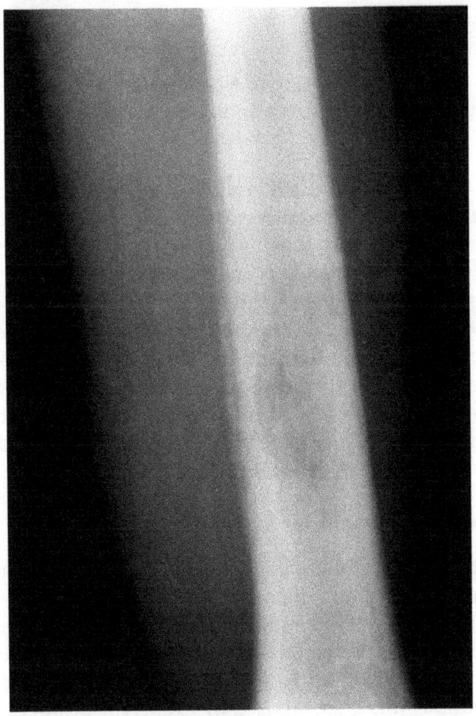

▲ **Figure 6–109.** Radiograph of a lesion of Langerhans cell histiocytosis of the humerus in a 12-year-old boy.

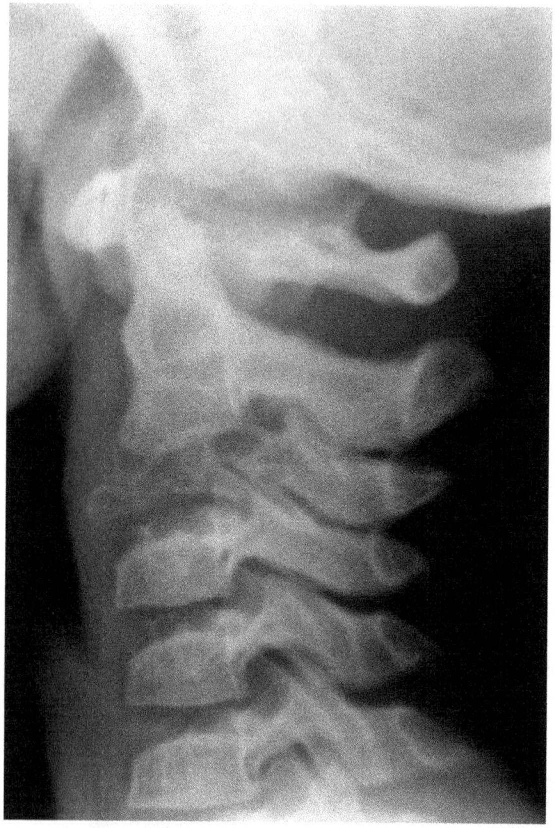

▲ **Figure 6–110.** Radiograph of a Langerhans cell histiocytosis in the body of the C3 vertebra in a 5-year-old girl.

lesion has a more aggressive pattern in younger children and later becomes more focal and granulomatous. Microscopic findings include large pale-staining histiocytes speckled with small bright-staining eosinophils and occasional giant cells.

Eosinophilic granulomas tend to involute spontaneously without treatment, and therefore, treatment should be conservative. Simple curettement and corticosteroid injections are beneficial. In difficult areas such as the spine or pelvis, low-dose radiation treatment (600-800 cGy) can be considered. In more disseminated cases that do not respond to simple treatment, low-dose chemotherapy is appropriate.

B. Pigmented Villonodular Synovitis

Although previously thought of as chronic inflammation or trauma-induced condition, pigmented villonodular synovitis (PVNS) is an idiopathic monoarticular synovial disease involving histiocytic proliferation that is now thought to be neoplastic in origin. PVNS is also known as tenosynovial giant cell tumor. It is characterized by exuberant proliferation of synovial villi and nodules and most frequently occurs in the tissue about major joints of the lower extremity in patients between 20 and 40 years of age. The knee joint is the most common site of involvement, followed next by the hip, ankle, and foot. Involvement of the upper extremity is rare. It can occur as an isolated intraarticular lesion, known as localized type, or present as a diffuse type, with extraarticular extension. Diffuse-type PVNS portends a worse prognosis. Giant cell tumor of the tendon sheath is related to PVNS and occurs along tendon sheaths of the hand and feet.

PVNS is associated with a 5q33 chromosomal rearrangement as well as increased expression of the *CSF1* gene. Histopathology will demonstrate characteristic hemosiderin-stained multinucleated giant cells.

PVNS usually presents with pain and swelling of the joint, as well as recurrent atraumatic hemarthrosis. The inflamed synovium can cause juxtaarticular erosion into bone at the point of attachment of the joint capsule, as is seen in any chronic proliferative synovitis, including hemophilia and coccidioidomycosis.

In fewer than 10% of cases, pigmented villonodular synovitis is more localized and presents as a focal soft-tissue mass high in the suprapatellar pouch or in the popliteal space, and no generalized swelling of the knee occurs. In these cases, the mass can mimic a soft-tissue sarcoma such as a synovial sarcoma (Figure 6–111). Cortical erosion with secondary bony changes can also be appreciated frequently (Figure 6–112).

Treatment for PVNS is open or arthroscopic synovectomy. Radiation treatment can be combined with surgery to decrease recurrence rate, although recurrence is still very common. Diffuse type can be difficult to treat surgically and has a higher rate of recurrence. CSF-1 inhibitors as a systemic treatment have shown promise in early phases for patients with diffuse or recurrent disease.

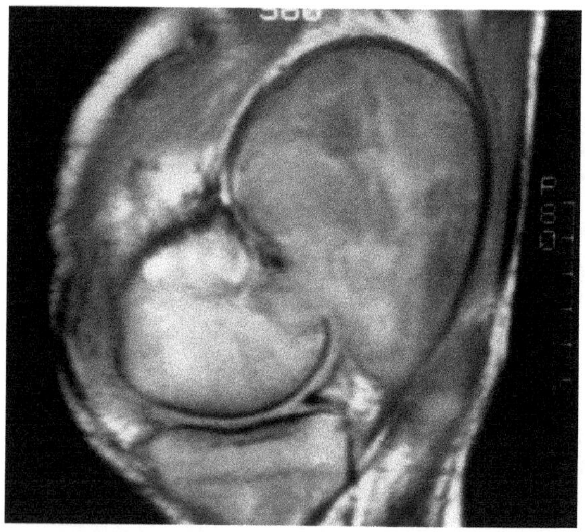

▲ **Figure 6–111.** T1-weighted MRI of pigmented villonodular synovitis in the popliteal space of a 50-year-old man.

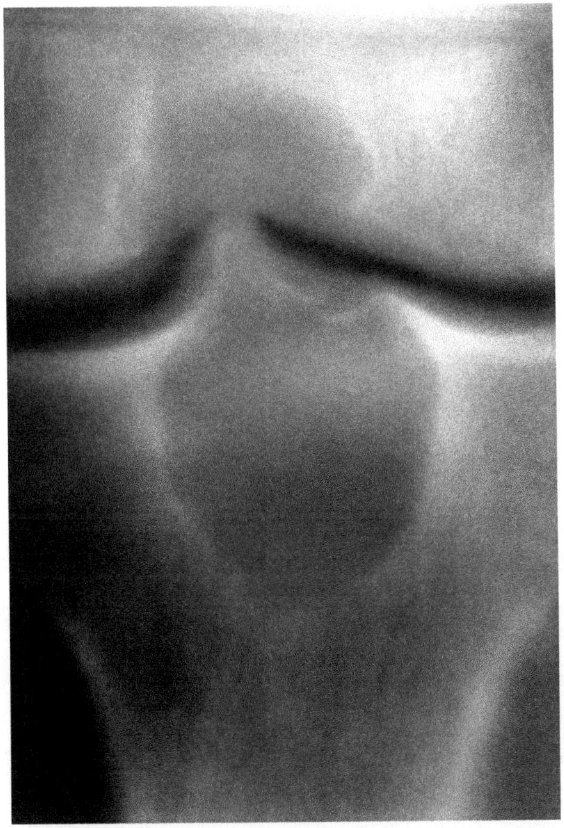

▲ **Figure 6–112.** Tomogram of pigmented villonodular synovitis in the proximal tibia of a young man.

Hip Arthroplasty-Related Pseudotumors

These lesions, which are nonneoplastic and noninfectious, are caused by the metallic wear of metal-on-metal total hip arthroplasty. They are well circumscribed, located near a total hip arthroplasty, and can be either cystic or solid. They can mimic an infectious or a neoplastic lesion and are associated with pain as well as bony erosion, although most are symptomatic and are discovered incidentally. Diagnosis is made on MRI with metal subtraction. These pseudotumors have a variable appearance ranging from thin-walled cystic lesions, to ill-defined solid masses. There is often associated synovial thickening, surrounding fluid, or debris. Serum metal ions (cobalt, chromium) can help confirm the diagnosis. Treatment for symptomatic lesions is revision arthroplasty, although observation should be considered if symptoms are mild as there is a propensity for poor outcomes following surgical intervention.

Essentials of Diagnosis

- *Myositis ossificans exhibits peripheral or centripetal calcification as opposed to calcifying soft-tissue malignancies.*
- *Infection of bone can take on many appearances, but clues to the diagnosis include violation of anatomic boundaries usually respected by tumors, such as the growth plate and the intervertebral disk.*

Corral-Gudino L, Tan AJ, Del Pino-Montes J, et al. Bisphosphonates for Paget's disease of bone in adults. *Cochrane Database Syst Rev.* 2017;12:CD004956. [PMID: 29192423]

Karaca L, Polat G, Sade R, et al. Nontraumatic tumoral calcinosis. *Joint Bone Spine.* 2017;84(4):491. [PMID: 27663758]

Meyes C, Lisiecki J, Miller S, et al. Heterotopic ossification: a comprehensive review. *JBMR Plus.* 2019;3(4):e10172. [PMID: 31044187]

Ralston SH, Corral-Gudino L, Cooper C, et al. Diagnosis and management of Paget's disease of bone in adults: a clinical guideline. *J Bone Miner Res.* 2019;34(4):579-604. [PMID: 30803025]

Stephen S, Shallop B, Lackman R, et al. Pigmented villonodular synovitis: a comprehensive review and proposed treatment algorithm. *JBJS Rev.* 2016;4(7):01874474-201607000-00005. [PMID: 27509331]

Sutphen SA, MacLaughlin LH, Madsen AA, et al. Prevalence of pseudotumor in patients after metal-on-metal hip arthroplasty evaluated with metal ion analysis and MARS-MRI. *J Arthroplasty.* 2016;31(1):260-263. [PMID: 26253484]

Tap WD, Wainberg ZA, Anthony SP, et al. Structure-guided blockade of CSF1R kinase in tenosynovial giant-cell tumor. *N Engl J Med.* 2015;373(5):428-437. [PMID: 26222558]

Thacker NH, Abla O. Pediatric Langerhans cells histiocytosis: state of science and future directions. *Clin Adv Hematol Oncol.* 2019;17(2):122-131. [PMID: 30845115]

Walczak BE, Johnson CN, Howe BM. Myositis ossificans. *J Am Acad Orthop Surg.* 2015;23(10):612-622. [PMID: 26320160]

Zinn DJ, Chakraborty R, Allen CE. Langerhans cell histiocytosis: emerging insights and clinical implications. *Oncology.* 2016;30(2):122-132. [PMID: 26888790]

7 Arthritis and Joint Preservation Surgery

Anton Plakseychuk, MD PhD
Harry B. Skinner, MD, PhD
Robert Tisherman, MD

The Arthritis Foundation reported that there are over 100 types of arthritis. And about 91.2 million adults either have physician-diagnosed arthritis and/or report joint symptoms consistent with a diagnosis of arthritis. This translates to almost one in three persons aged 18 to 64 years. After the age of 65, half of men and two-thirds of women have arthritis. The incidence is on the rise, and it is estimated that by 2040, almost half the population will have physician-confirmed arthritis. Arthritis and polyarticular arthritis, in particular, are more common in females and obese people. Age significantly increases the prevalence. One estimate puts the total costs related to arthritis (eg, medical care, earning losses, lost time) at 1% of US gross domestic product equaling about $304 billion for the 2013 fiscal year. Among people with arthritis, 33% have depression or anxiety, 25% have cardiac problems, 20% have respiratory conditions, and 16% have diabetes. It is likely that arthritis predisposes people to these comorbidities through physical inactivity.

The pathophysiology of noninflammatory arthritis is primarily mechanical but introduced cellular and biochemical processes will also change the normal slow cartilage remodeling process. There will be excess degeneration, less regeneration, and abnormal separation of the cartilage. Progressive cartilage loss, increased thickness of the subchondral plate, and cyst formation will happen. With time, the cartilage gets thinner, looser, and weaker; bone will rub against bone, causing remodeling of the bone and osteophytes formation. Friction will cause mild inflammation. All these changes will make the normal movement and gliding of the joint more difficult and uncomfortable, and eventually painful. The pathophysiology of inflammatory arthritis can be infectious, crystal-induced, reactive, or autoimmune. Inflammatory cytokines and autoantibodies create an inflammation cascade and pannus formation, which can invade the cartilage and bone and damage them. Diagnosis and treatment of multiple forms of arthritis will be discussed in this chapter, as well as surgical joint preservation options and techniques.

Jafarzadeh SR, Felson DT. Updated estimates suggest a much higher prevalence of arthritis in United States adults than previous ones. *Arthritis Rheumatol.* 2018;70:185-192. [PMID: 29178176]

Murphy L, Helmick CG. The impact of osteoarthritis in the United States: a population-health perspective: a population-based review of the fourth most common cause of hospitalization in U.S. adults. *Orthop Nurs.* 2012;31:85-91. [PMID: 22373741]

Pujalte GG, Albano-Aluquin SA. Differential diagnosis of polyarticular arthritis. *Am Fam Physician.* 2015;93:35-41. [PMID: 26132125]

ARTHRITIS AND RELATED CONDITIONS

Evaluation of Arthritis

To treat arthritic conditions of the joints appropriately, an understanding of the disease process is essential. This begins with accurate diagnosis and a history of the progression of the disease, so that the future progression can be predicted and appropriate decisions regarding treatment can be made. The physician must evaluate the possibility of traumatic, inflammatory, developmental, idiopathic, and metabolic causes of the arthritis (Table 7–1). Evaluation of the history, physical examination, imaging, and laboratory data is helpful in arriving at a diagnosis.

A. History

The history is very important in defining the disease process. The mechanism of injury and timing and duration of symptoms since onset are key factors. The mechanism of injury is most often insidious. The individual is often unable to recall a specific event that elicited the symptoms. However, when there was a sudden traumatic event in the past and especially when there was prior surgery, this information is important. The timing and severity of pain are valuable pieces of

Table 7–1. Causes of arthritic conditions.

Traumatic causes	Traumatic arthritis, osteonecrosis (posttraumatic)
Inflammatory causes	Infectious arthritis, gout, pseudogout, rheumatoid arthritis, systemic lupus erythematosus, ankylosing spondylitis, juvenile rheumatoid arthritis, Reiter syndrome
Developmental causes	Developmental dysplasia of the hip, hemophilic arthritis, following slipped capital femoral epiphysis, following Legg-Calvé-Perthes disease
Idiopathic causes	Osteoarthritis, osteonecrosis
Metabolic causes	Gout, calcium pyrophosphate deposition disease, ochronosis, Gaucher disease

information. Most often, symptoms are initially mild and gradually worsen. Constant pain, night and day, implies infection, cancer, or a functional disorder. Perception of pain differs among individuals, but pain that awakens the patient is considered severe and requires evaluation. Symptoms frequently alternatively worsen and improve over time, and the patient's recollection of this and especially of whether there has been swelling is an important sign; also important is the distribution of joints if more than one is involved. The degree of interference with activities indicates the seriousness of the disorder. Pain only with activity such as walking, standing, or running suggests that joint loading is the cause.

Pain location helps distinguish referred pain from joint pain. Hip pain, for example, is felt typically in the groin or in the lateral aspect of the hip or anterior thigh but seldom in the buttock. Patients may complain of pain being in the "hip," but questioning by the physician may reveal it to actually be pain in the buttock, and this most often arises from the spine. Acetabular pain or femoral head pain is frequently felt in the groin. Proximal femur pain is usually appreciated in the anteroproximal thigh. As another example of the importance of pain location, knee pain may be localized as anterior (patellofemoral), medial (medial compartment), or lateral (lateral compartment). Or, it may also be poorly localized by the patient. Pain in the back of the knee may result from a popliteal cyst (Baker cyst) or a torn meniscus. A swollen knee may be painful because of pressure, and this can be diffuse pain or may be posterior. Pain with any motion may indicate a septic joint or possibly a gouty joint. Arthritic pain in the elbow and shoulder is less clearly defined by patients, and in such cases, the physical examination is important. Shoulder pain may be caused by cervical, cardiac, or even diaphragmatic disorders.

Knowledge of the age distribution of the various arthritic disorders can be very helpful in diagnosing the disease. For example, a hip disorder in a patient under age 40 is unlikely to be osteoarthritis unless a predisposing condition is present, such as trauma. A more likely diagnosis is osteonecrosis.

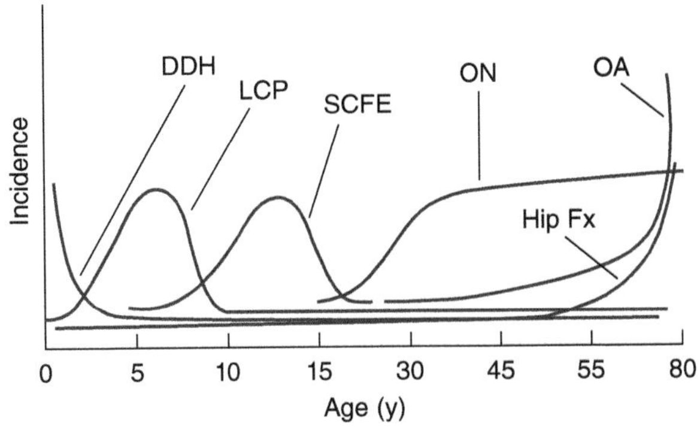

▲ **Figure 7–1.** The age distribution of hip disorders is given in a schematic representation. DDH, developmental dysplasia of the hip; Hip Fx, hip fracture; LCP, Legg-Calvé-Perthes disease; OA, osteoarthrosis; ON, osteonecrosis; SCFE, slipped capital femoral epiphysis.

Similarly, a chronic condition of the knee in a 45-year-old man is likely to be a degenerative meniscus tear, unless the patient had a meniscectomy in his early 20s. This concept applies to all of the common disorders of the hip and knee (Figures 7–1 and 7–2). Further, a history of one of these disorders at an earlier age predisposes a patient to earlier osteoarthrosis.

B. Physical Examination

1. Hip—The physical examination of the hip is important to verify that the reported pain arises from the hip joint and to determine the severity of the arthritis. This begins with visual

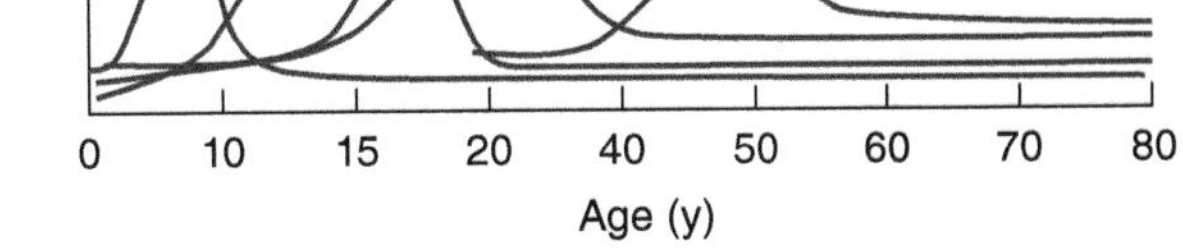

▲ **Figure 7–2.** The age distribution of knee disorders is given schematically as a function of age. Blount's ds, tibia vara; OA, osteoarthrosis; P-F ds, patellofemoral arthralgia. Meniscal tears can be either medial or lateral and are traumatic in the younger age group and degenerative in the older age group. Osteoarthrosis shows an earlier onset with the knee than with the hip because there is an incidence of medial gonarthrosis in the 40s and 50s caused by medial meniscectomy in the late teens and early 20s.

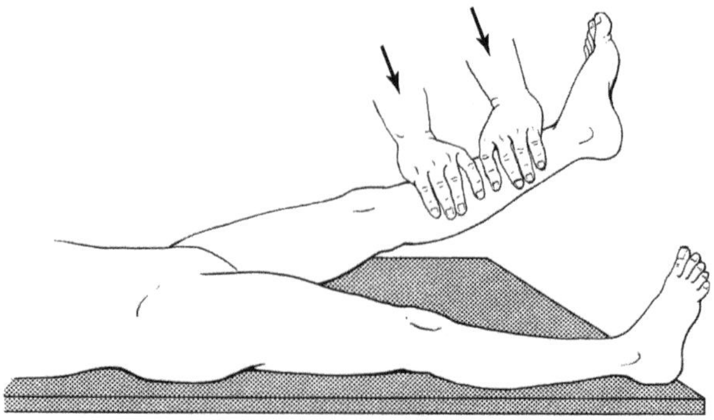

▲ **Figure 7–3.** Resisted straight leg raising test. The examiner asks the patient to actively raise the straight leg to approximately 30 degrees. This produces hip pain in severe arthritis. If no pain is produced, the examiner applies pressure to the thigh, which the patient resists. This increased joint loading uncovers mild to moderate hip pain.

inspection and palpation of the muscles, bones, and joints. Many muscles surround the hip joint and large portions of the bone, limiting this portion of the examination. Other causes of the pain must be sought, such as pain referred from the lumbar spine. It is useful to document range of motion (ROM), gait, leg-length discrepancy, and muscle weakness. Pain arising from the hip is typically elicited at the extremes of ROM. Active straight leg raising or resisted straight leg raising may produce hip pain (Figure 7–3). Log rolling (internal and external rotation of the hip in extension) usually elicits hip pain if the arthritis is severe. Frequently, internal rotation of the hip in flexion is limited; this condition is one of the first signs of osteoarthritis of the hip. Abduction of the hip against gravity loads the hip and may produce hip pain of arthritis but does not do so if pain in the buttock or thigh is referred from the spine. Increased loading may be achieved by applying resistance to abduction. In the young (under age 40) patient with groin pain, provocative maneuvers can be used to diagnose labral tears. Flexion of the hip with external rotation and abduction is followed by extension, adduction, and internal rotation. Clicking or catching is observed in patients with anterior labral tears. Posterior tears of the labrum are identified by moving the hip from extension, abduction, and external rotation to flexion, adduction, and internal rotation.

The ROM in flexion, extension (flexion contracture), abduction, adduction, and internal rotation and external rotation is measured. Decreased internal rotation is an early finding in osteoarthritis.

2. Knee—The physical examination of the knee localizes the pain to the knee and to the specific involved compartment. As with the hip, this begins with visual inspection and palpation of the muscles, bones, and joints. Because knee pain can be referred from the hip, evaluation of the hip should be routine. Ligamentous evaluation of the knee is performed to discern knee stability (see Chapter 4). Instability is not common in osteoarthritis but is often seen in rheumatoid osteoarthritis and results from bone loss rather than ligament injury. Alignment of the knee while standing is measured to evaluate for varus or valgus deformities. In the setting of existing osteoarthritis, varus or valgus malalignment increases the odds of progression of osteoarthritis in the medial or lateral compartments by four-fold and five-fold, respectively, over an 18-month period. ROM of the knee is measured, and any flexion contracture or extensor lag is noted. Flexion contracture is an inability to come to full extension passively, whereas an extensor lag indicates an inability to extend the knee actively as far as it will extend passively. The contracture is common in advanced osteoarthritis, whereas the lag is generally a quadriceps muscle or tendon problem. The medial and lateral compartments are loaded during flexion and extension with varus and valgus stress, respectively, to elicit pain arising from each compartment. The patellofemoral joint may be assessed for pain and bone-on-bone crepitation by flexion and extension with pressure on the patella. The presence of fluid, synovitis, and erythema is also important.

3. Shoulder—Because shoulder pain can be referred from the cervical spine, evaluation of both is often necessary. Examination of the shoulder begins with visual inspection for asymmetry of bone and muscle contours in comparison to the other side. Palpation of the muscle to evaluate tone and each of the three bones, including the humerus, clavicle, and scapula, follows. Not only the glenohumeral but also the acromioclavicular and sternoclavicular joints should be palpated. As with the hip, many muscles surround the portions of the shoulder, limiting this portion of the examination. However, tenderness over the anterolateral humeral head can often be found with rotator cuff disorders. Tendinitis of the long head of the biceps yields pain with palpation on the anteromedial shoulder, over the bicipital groove. Active ROM is then assessed in flexion and abduction. External rotation is reproducibly measured by keeping the elbow on the waist and rotating the hand away from the body. Internal rotation is best evaluated by the patient positioning the hand behind the back and then measuring the highest vertebral level of the spine that the thumb can be positioned. Most individuals can position the thumb to the midthoracic area (eg, T6 or T7). When internal rotation is limited, the thumb can be elevated to lower levels, for example, L5. If active ROM is at all limited, passive ROM should be assessed. Strength of the upper extremity muscle is then evaluated along with sensation and deep tendon reflexes. Decreased strength in external rotation with the elbow at the side indicates significant rotator cuff weakness. Provocative tests can help evaluate the cause of symptoms including instability, biceps tendon injuries, and rotator cuff injuries (see Chapter 3).

4. Elbow—Inspection of the elbow includes measurement of the "carrying angle," the normal being a 5- to 7-degree angle of valgus alignment between the humerus and forearm. Visual inspection for scars and obvious deformities, as well as swelling, is performed. The joint and bony prominences are palpated, including the medial and lateral epicondyles, radial head, and olecranon. Active and passive motions are recorded for both flexion and extension and pronation and supination followed by strength and provocative tests as described in Chapter 3. For example, the most common malady of the elbow is epicondylitis. Tenderness over the lateral epicondyle, exacerbated by resisted wrist dorsiflexion, is present with lateral epicondylitis (tennis elbow). Tenderness over the medial epicondyle with pain exacerbated by resisted wrist flexion is present with medial epicondylitis. As other examples, limitation of flexion and extension is seen not only with arthritis but also with post-traumatic stiffness.

C. Imaging Studies

The most fundamental data aiding in diagnosis of arthritis can be provided by plain radiographs with a minimum of two views. Views of the hip include a modified anteroposterior (AP) view of the pelvis (which clips the iliac wings to show the proximal femora) and a lateral view of the affected hip (either "frog," an AP view with the hip externally rotated and abducted, or a true lateral view). Views of the knee should include AP standing view of bilateral knees, a 10-degree down-angled beam posteroanterior radiograph of the knee bent in 30 to 45 degrees of flexion taken while the patient is standing (the flexion weight-bearing view), a lateral view, and a tangential patellar view with the knee bent 45 degrees (the Merchant view) (Table 7–2). Osteoarthritis of the hip and knee can be quantitated using the Kellgren-Lawrence five-level scale where 0 is normal, 1 is doubtful, 2 is mild or minimal, 3 is moderate, and 4 is severe. Views of the shoulder should include AP of the glenohumeral joint (Grashey view), axillary lateral, scapular Y, and acromioclavicular joint (Zanca view) views of the scapula. In patients with a history of shoulder dislocation, the West Point axillary and Stryker notch views may help to further assess for bone Bankart and Hill-Sachs lesions, respectively. Supraspinatus outlet views may be helpful in revealing acromial bone spurs and defining the classification of the acromion as flat, curved, or hooked, which can provide diagnostic information in patients with impingement syndrome. The elbow usually can be visualized with AP and lateral radiographs. Magnetic resonance imaging (MRI) is an additional imaging technique for diagnosing joint pathology. MRI has almost 100% sensitivity for defining avascular necrosis, a common cause of premature osteoarthritis of the hip. The addition of intraarticular contrast allows for improved definition of the extent of cartilage damage and the ability to see labral pathology.

Table 7–2. Radiographic findings in arthritis.

Disease State	Findings in Hip or Knee
Osteoarthritis	Joint space narrowing, subchondral sclerosis, osteophytes, subchondral cysts Hip: Superior or medial narrowing Knee: Early narrowing on Rosenberg views; flattening of femoral condyles
Rheumatoid arthritis or systemic lupus erythematosus	Uniform joint narrowing, erosion near joint capsule
Ankylosing spondylitis	Osteopenia, osteophytes, ankylosis of sacroiliac joints
Gout	Tophi, erosions
Calcium pyrophosphate deposition disease	Calcification of menisci and articular cartilage
Osteonecrosis	Crescent sign, spotty calcification
Gaucher disease	Erlenmeyer flask appearance, distal femora
Neuropathic joint	Four Ds: destruction, debris, dislocation, densification (sclerosis, hypertrophy)
Hemophilic arthropathy	Epiphyseal widening, sclerosis, cysts, joint space narrowing

D. Laboratory Findings

Basic blood testing should include a complete blood count, C-reactive protein (CRP), and erythrocyte sedimentation rate (ESR). A high level of CRP in the blood is a nonspecific marker of inflammation that will go up first in the case of acute infection. ESR is a marker of chronic inflammation and would be elevated in infection, lupus, rheumatoid arthritis, cancer, or other conditions. A normal white blood cell count may be helpful in the diagnosis of gout, especially if the inflamed joint is atypical (other than the first metatarsophalangeal joint).

Synovial fluid analysis is indicated in evaluation of infection, and it may also be quite helpful in the diagnosis of other arthritides. Aspiration of synovial fluid may reveal hemorrhagic fluid. If this is the result of a traumatic tap, it should be so noted and the fluid should be sent for analysis. If the fluid is grossly hemorrhagic, several diagnoses must be entertained, including hemophilia, neuropathic arthropathy, pigmented villonodular synovitis, hemangioma, or trauma. A finding of fat floating on the bloody fluid in the setting of a traumatic injury suggests the presence of an intraarticular fracture.

The combined history, physical examination, imaging, and appropriate laboratory studies should narrow the diagnoses to a relative few, if not the definitive one. It is helpful to consider diagnoses in categories, which, despite some overlap, provide a framework for further workup. Many of these arthritic conditions are described in the following sections.

Hall M, Bennell KL, Wrigley TV, et al. The knee adduction moment and knee osteoarthritis symptoms: relationships according to radiographic disease severity. *Osteoarthritis Cartilage.* 2017;25:34-41. [PMID: 27616685]

Parvizi J, Tan T, Goswani K, et al. The 2018 definition of periprosthetic hip and knee infection: an evidence-based and validated criteria. *J Arthroplasty.* 2018;33:1309-1314. [PMID: 29551303]

1. Noninflammatory Arthritis

The term **osteoarthritis** is a misnomer, because inflammation is not the primary pathologic process observed in this form of articular joint disruption. More accurately described as degenerative joint disease, the disease represents a final common pathway of injury to articular cartilage. Although the true nature and cause of osteoarthritis are unclear, radiographic findings and gross and microscopic pathologic features are fairly typical in most cases.

Categorization of primary and secondary forms of osteoarthritis, although still useful, is blurred. A designation of primary or idiopathic osteoarthritis was made when no identifiable predisposing conditions could be recognized. Osteoarthritis is considered secondary when an underlying cause such as trauma, previous deformity, or systemic disorder exists. Although many cases of hip osteoarthritis were considered idiopathic when the end-stage changes were observed, careful analysis indicated predisposing conditions such as slipped capital femoral epiphysis and mild acetabular dysplasia in many cases.

The joints most commonly involved include the hip; knee; distal interphalangeal, proximal interphalangeal, and first carpometacarpal joints of the hand; and cervical, thoracic, and lumbar spine.

Primary Osteoarthritis

A. Epidemiologic Features

Osteoarthritis is a widespread joint disorder in the United States, significantly affecting approximately 40 million people. Although autopsy studies show degenerative changes of weight-bearing joints in 90% of people older than 40 years, clinical symptoms are usually not present. The prevalence and severity of osteoarthritis increase with age.

When all ages are considered, men and women are equally affected. In those younger than 45 years, the disease is more prevalent in men; after age 55 years, women are more commonly afflicted. The pattern of joint involvement commonly includes the joints of the hands and knees in women and the hip joints in men. The risk of hip joint arthritis is significantly associated with increasing body mass index (BMI).

The incidence of hip osteoarthritis is higher in European and American white males than in Chinese, South African blacks, and East Indian persons. Primary hip osteoarthritis in Japanese persons is rare, but secondary osteoarthritis is common because of developmental dysplasia of the hip.

Some distinct forms of osteoarthritis may be inherited as a dominant trait with a Mendelian pattern. A primary generalized osteoarthritis of the interphalangeal joints, particularly the distal interphalangeal joints of the hand, is a prominent feature, and symmetric and uniform loss of articular cartilage of the knee and hip joints is evident. Other types of inherited osteoarthritis include familial chondrocalcinosis (with deposition of calcium pyrophosphate dihydrate crystals in cartilage), Stickler syndrome (characterized by vitreoretinal degeneration), hydroxyapatite deposition disease, and multiple epiphyseal dysplasias. Genetic mutation in the vitamin D and estrogen receptors have also been implicated in osteoarthritis, but their exact role remains unclear. However, epidemiologic studies have shown most osteoarthritis is inherited with a non-Mendelian pattern with multifactorial inheritance that may be further elucidated by genome-wide association studies.

B. Pathologic Features

Early features of osteoarthritis include focal swelling and softening of the cartilage matrix with increased water content. Early-stage osteoarthritis is characterized by mild inflammatory response within the synovium, mild loss of proteoglycans within the cartilage, and increasing disorganization of collagen fibers. Surface irregularities in the form of fibrillation also occur. Diffuse hypercellularity of the chondrocytes can be seen. The tidemark, an interface plane between articular cartilage and the zone of calcified cartilage, is thin and wavy early in osteoarthritis. During the second stage of articular cartilage degeneration with osteoarthritis, there is increased chondrocyte activity with proliferation and increased production of extracellular matrix. Simultaneously, there is an increase in catabolic activity with removal of damaged matrix to facilitate matrix remodeling. Chondrocyte repair response decreases with aging. Matrix degradation includes decreased proteoglycan production, less aggregation, and shorter glycosaminoglycan chains.

Later features of osteoarthritis include progressive loss of proteoglycans. Fibrillations in the surface progress to fissures and later into deeper clefts and the synovium becomes increasingly vascular and thickened. Chondrocyte cloning is seen along with reduplication of the tidemark, with discontinuous parallel lines indicating progression of calcification of the basal portion of the articular cartilage. Regions of eburnated bone represent complete loss of cartilage.

New bone formation occurs in a subchondral location as well as at margins of the articular cartilage. During later stages of osteoarthritis, areas of rarefaction of bone below eburnation are represented by "cysts" on radiographs and on gross inspection. Osteophyte formation can be seen at all stages of osteoarthritis and is caused by inappropriate activation of the endochondral ossification pathway mediated by Indian hedgehog signaling in response to mechanical stimuli.

C. Laboratory Findings

Specific diagnostic tests for osteoarthritis are currently not available. Routine blood tests, urinalysis, and even synovial fluid analysis do not provide useful information, except for exclusion of inflammatory or infectious arthritis. Experimental work on identification of markers of cartilage degradation in osteoarthritis may provide diagnostic tests in the future. These include sensitive and specific assays for synovial fluid cytokines, proteinases and their inhibitors, matrix components and their fragments, serum antibodies to cartilage collagen, and identification of proteoglycan subpopulations.

D. Imaging Studies

Typical radiographic features indicate late pathologic changes in osteoarthritis, specifically narrowing of the joint space, subchondral sclerosis, subchondral bone cysts, and marginal osteophytes. End-stage disease is complicated by bony erosions, subluxation, loose bodies, and deformity.

Heberden nodes are commonly seen in primary osteoarthritis, represented by bony and cartilaginous enlargement of the distal interphalangeal joints of the fingers. Similar enlargements of the proximal interphalangeal joints of the fingers are called **Bouchard nodes**.

Secondary Osteoarthritis

The term **secondary osteoarthritis** is applied when an underlying recognizable local or systemic factor exists. These include conditions leading to joint deformity or destruction of cartilage, followed by signs and symptoms typically seen with primary osteoarthritis. Examples of preexisting conditions leading to secondary osteoarthritic changes in joints include acute and chronic trauma, Legg-Calvé-Perthes disease, developmental dysplasia of the hip, rheumatoid arthritis (RA), bleeding dyscrasias, achondroplasia, infection, crystal deposition disease, neuropathic disorders, overuse of intraarticular steroids, and multiple epiphyseal dysplasias. Radiographic features of secondary osteoarthritis reflect the underlying pathologic changes plus the changes resulting from the primary osteoarthritis.

Jevsevar DS, Brown GA, Jones DL, et al. The American Academy of Orthopaedic Surgeons evidence-based guideline on treatment of osteoarthritis of the knee, 2nd edition. *J Bone Joint Surg Am.* 2013;95:1885-1886. [PMID: 24288804]

Jiang L, Rong J, Wang Y, et al. The relationship between body mass index and hip arthritis: a systematic review and meta-analysis. *Joint Bone Spine.* 2011;78:150-155. [PMID: 20580591]

van Meurs JB. Osteoarthritis year in review 2016: genetics, genomics and epigenetics. *Osteoarthritis Cartilage.* 2017;25:181-189. [PMID: 28100422]

2. Inflammatory Arthritis

Rheumatoid Arthritis

A chronic systemic progressive disorder, RA is the most common inflammatory arthritis. It characteristically affects several joints of the body symmetrically, often starting with the small joints of the hand and feet.

Although similar synovial histopathologic and joint abnormalities are identifiable in all patients, the articular and systemic manifestations, outcomes, and differences in genetic makeup and serologic findings vary widely in individual patients. The cause is unknown, although the disease probably occurs in response to a pathogenic agent in a genetically predisposed host. Smoking has been identified as an environmental risk factor. Other possible triggering factors include bacterial, mycoplasmal, or viral infections, as well as endogenous antigens in the form of rheumatoid factor, collagens, and mucopolysaccharides.

Diagnostic criteria for RA include morning stiffness for more than 1 hour, symmetric arthritis, rheumatoid nodules, swelling in three or more joints, arthritis of the hand (metacarpophalangeal joint, proximal interphalangeal joint, and wrist), radiographic changes of the hand including bony erosions and decalcification, and serum rheumatoid factor. In order to clinically confirm the diagnosis, the patient should have four or more of the criteria listed earlier for a 6-week period. The triad of arthritis, lymphadenopathy, and splenomegaly, known as Felty syndrome, is associated with anemia, thrombocytopenia, and neutropenia.

A. Epidemiologic Features

RA affects as much as 1% of the population in the United States. Women are two to four times more likely than men to get RA, and it occurs in all age groups but increases in incidence with advancing age, with a peak between the fourth and sixth decades.

Evidence for a genetic basis is provided by the association of RA with a certain haplotype of class II gene products of the major histocompatibility complex. Seventy-five percent of patients with RA carry circulating rheumatoid factors, which are autoantibodies against portions of the IgG antibody. In rheumatoid factor–positive patients, there is a high incidence of HLA-DR4 and HLA-DW4, except in black patients. Only a minority of individuals with HLA-DR4 develop RA, however.

B. Pathologic Features

RA is a T-cell (MHC type II)-mediated immune response against the patient's own tissue. Early rheumatoid synovitis consists of a local inflammatory response with accumulation of mononuclear cells. The antigen-presenting cell (macrophage) activates T lymphocytes, resulting in cytokine production, B-cell proliferation, and antibody formation. Chronic inflammation results in formation of a pannus, a thickened synovium filled with activated T and B lymphocytes and plasma cells, as well as fibroblastic and macrophagic types of synovial cells. Joint destruction begins with exposed bone at the margins of articular cartilage denuded of articular cartilage. Eventually, the cartilage itself is destroyed by inflammatory byproducts of the pannus. The synovial fluid, in contrast to the mononuclear cell infiltrate seen in the synovial membrane, has neutrophils forming 75% to 85% of the cells.

Rheumatoid factors are autoantibodies specific to antigens on the Fc fragment of native IgG. The antibodies include IgM, IgG, IgA, and IgE classes, but the IgM rheumatoid factor is typically measured. Immune complexes due to activated rheumatoid factor deposit in end tissues and can independently cause manifestations of the disease such as renal pathology. Rheumatoid factor may be a triggering factor for RA and may contribute to the chronic nature of the disease, but it is not found in all patients with RA. Rheumatoid factor is also frequently found in patients with other inflammatory diseases, however, as well as in 1% to 5% of normal patients.

C. Laboratory Findings

Anti–cyclic citrullinated peptide (anti-CCP) is the most sensitive and specific test for RA. Mutated citrullinated vimentin anti-MCV is another test, which may be more sensitive than anti-CCP but much less specific for RA. A high titer of rheumatoid factor (>1:160) is elevated in 75% to 80% of patients with RA. ESR and CRP levels would be elevated. Antinuclear antibodies are often positive in patients with severe RA (up to 37% in one study) but are not specific for the disease.

D. Imaging Studies

Early radiographic changes in rheumatoid osteoarthritis include swelling of the small peripheral joints and marginal bony erosions. Joint space narrowing occurs later and is uniform, unlike the focal narrowing seen in osteoarthritis. Regional osteoporosis occurs, unlike the sclerosis seen in osteoarthritis. Advanced changes include bone resorption, deformity, dislocation, and fragmentation of affected joints. For example, protrusio acetabuli may be seen in the hips, and ulnar subluxation is common in the metacarpophalangeal joints.

Aletada D, Smolen J. Diagnosis and management of rheumatoid arthritis: a review. *JAMA.* 2018;320:1360-1372. [PMID: 30285183]

McArdle A, Flatley B, Pennington SR, Fitzgerald O. Early biomarkers of joint damage in rheumatoid and psoriatic arthritis. *Arthritis Res Ther.* 2015;17:141. [PMID: 26028339]

Ankylosing Spondylitis

A seronegative (negative rheumatoid factor) inflammatory arthritis, ankylosing spondylitis consists of bilateral sacroiliitis with or without associated spondylitis and uveitis. An insidious disease, the diagnosis is often delayed because of vagueness of the early symptom of low back pain and late x-ray changes of sacroiliitis. Diagnostic clinical criteria include bilateral sacroiliitis assessed via MRI, HLA-B27 positivity, and uveitis, which may not be present in all patients. Clinical presentation of these individuals frequently involves low back pain, limited lumbar spine motion, decreased chest expansion, and sacroiliitis.

Joint involvement is primarily axial, including all portions of the spine, sacroiliac joint, and hip joints. Extraskeletal involvement includes dilation of the aorta, anterior uveitis, and restrictive lung disease secondary to restriction of thoracic cage mobility.

A. Epidemiologic Features

Ankylosing spondylitis affects approximately 0.2% of the population and is more prevalent in Caucasian populations. There is a male predominance (2-3:1 male to female), and ankylosing spondylitis typically presents during the third decade of life, but the juvenile subtype can be seen in younger patients. The association of HLA-B27 and ankylosing spondylitis is strong, with 90% of patients testing positive for this haplotype; however, only 2% of HLA-B27–positive patients develop ankylosing spondylitis. First-degree family members of a patient who has ankylosing spondylitis and is positive for HLA-B27 have a 20% risk of developing the disease.

B. Laboratory Findings

Active flares can lead to transient elevations in ESR and CRP. Testing for rheumatoid factor and antinuclear antibodies is negative.

C. Imaging Studies

Early in the course of ankylosing spondylitis, the sacroiliac joints may be widened, reflecting bony erosions of the iliac side of the joint. Later, the inflamed cartilage is replaced by ossification, resulting in ankylosis of the bilateral sacroiliac joints. Vertebrae of the thoracolumbar spine are squared off, with bridging syndesmophytes, forming a so-called "bamboo spine" that is pathognomonic for ankylosing spondylitis. Ankylosis of peripheral joints may be seen and is often asymmetric, with the shoulder and hip being the most frequently affected. MRI may provide early, sensitive, and specific imaging evidence of sacroiliitis and has become the most widely used diagnostic imaging test.

Sieper J, Poddubnyy D. Axial spondyloarthritis. *Lancet.* 2017;390: 73-84. [PMID: 28110981]

Taurog JD, Chhabra A, Colbert RA. Ankylosing spondylitis and axial spondyloarthritis. *N Engl J Med.* 2016;347:2563-2574. [PMID: 27355535]

Psoriatic Arthritis

A seronegative inflammatory arthritis associated with psoriasis, psoriatic arthritis was in the past considered a variant of RA. The discovery of rheumatoid factor led to the division of inflammatory arthritides into seropositive and seronegative diseases, separating psoriatic arthritis from RA.

Although psoriatic arthritis is characterized by a relatively benign course in most patients, up to 20% develop severe joint involvement. The distal interphalangeal joints of the fingers are commonly affected, but several patterns of peripheral arthritis exist, including an asymmetric oligoarthritis, a symmetric polyarthritis (similar to rheumatoid osteoarthritis), arthritis mutilans (a destructive, deforming type of arthritis), and a spondyloarthropathy (similar to ankylosing spondylitis, with sacroiliac joint involvement).

In addition to the dry erythematous papular skin lesions, nail changes include pitting, grooves, subungual hyperkeratosis, and destruction. Extraarticular manifestations of psoriatic arthritis include enthesitis, Achilles tendonitis, posterior tibial tendonitis, and plantar fasciitis.

A. Epidemiologic Features

In the United States, about 3.15% of the population is diagnosed with psoriasis, and 5% to 20% of patients with psoriasis have signs of psoriatic arthritis, with joint symptoms delayed as long as 20 years after onset of skin lesions. Both sexes are affected equally. HLA-B27 and the genes *IL12B* and *IL23R* have all been associated with psoriasis and psoriatic arthritis.

B. Laboratory Findings

There are no specific laboratory tests for psoriatic arthritis. Rheumatoid factor is usually negative but is present in up to 10% of patients. Nonspecific inflammatory markers may be elevated, including ESR and CRP.

C. Imaging Studies

Coexistence of erosive changes and bone formation is seen in peripheral joints, with absence of periarticular osteoporosis. Gross destruction of phalangeal joints (so-called "pencil-in-cup" appearance) and lysis of terminal phalanges are seen. Bilateral sacroiliac joint ankylosis and syndesmophytes of the spine are seen, as in ankylosing spondylitis.

Ritchlin C, Colbert R, Gladman D. Psoriatic arthritis. *N Engl J Med.* 2017;376:957-970. [PMID: 28273019]

Juvenile Idiopathic Arthritis

Juvenile idiopathic arthritis (JIA) is an inflammatory arthritic syndrome with a variety of symptoms and is a diagnosis of exclusion in children with arthritis onset before age 16. It was previously called juvenile RA but was renamed because it is not obviously related to adult RA. Early diagnosis is often difficult. Infection can present similarly in young patients and should be ruled out quickly. Criteria for JIA include distinction of mode of onset as systemic, polyarticular, or pauciarticular. Systemic onset (also known as **Still disease**) occurs in 20% of patients and is characterized by high fever, rash, lymphadenopathy, splenomegaly, carditis, and varying degrees of arthritis. Polyarticular onset occurs in 30% to 40% of patients and is notable for fewer systemic symptoms, low-grade fever, and synovitis of four or more joints. Pauciarticular onset develops in 40% to 50% of patients and involves one to four joints; there are no systemic signs, but there is an increased incidence of iridocyclitis. Iridocyclitis is an insidious complication that requires early ophthalmologic slit-lamp evaluation, if JIA is suspected, to prevent blindness.

A. Epidemiologic Features

The two peak ages of onset are between 1 and 3 years and between 8 and 12 years. Females are affected twice as often as males.

B. Laboratory Findings

Leukocytosis up to 30,000/mL is seen with systemic-onset JIA, with mild elevations in polyarticular-onset disease and normal values in pauciarticular-onset disease. White blood cell counts in synovial fluid range from 150 to 50,000/mL. The ESR and CRP are elevated.

Rheumatoid factor is typically negative in JIA, with less than 15% of patients having positive rheumatoid factor. As many as 50% of patients have positive antinuclear antibodies, a finding correlated with iridocyclitis and pauciarticular-onset disease.

C. Imaging Studies

Soft-tissue swelling and premature closure of physes may be seen early, as well as juxtaarticular osteopenia. Erosive changes are seen late and resemble those of rheumatoid osteoarthritis. Atlantoaxial instability should be ruled out with the use of flexion-extension radiographs in all patients presenting with JIA.

Crayne CB, Beukelman T. Juvenile idiopathic arthritis: oligoarthritis and polyarthritis. *Pediatr Clin North Am.* 2018;65: 657-674. [PMID: 30031492]

Palman J, Shoop-Worrall S, Hyrich K, McDonagh J. Update on the epidemiology, risk factors, and disease outcomes of Juvenile idiopathic arthritis. *Best Pract Red Clin Rheumatol.* 2018;32: 206-222. [PMID: 30527427]

Systemic Lupus Erythematosus

Systemic lupus erythematosus (SLE) is a chronic inflammatory disease that may affect multiple organ systems. It is an autoimmune disorder in which autoantibodies are formed, in most cases against cellular nuclear contents, known as antinuclear antibodies. The large variety of clinical appearances and laboratory findings may mimic many disorders. The diagnosis is based on the presence of four of the following 11 criteria: (1) malar rash; (2) discoid rash; (3) photosensitivity; (4) oral ulcers; (5) arthritis; (6) serositis; (7) renal disorders (proteinuria or casts); (8) neurologic disorders (seizures or psychosis); (9) hematologic disorders (hemolytic anemia, leukopenia, lymphopenia, thrombocytopenia); (10) immunologic disorders (positive lupus erythematosus [LE] cell preparation, anti-DNA antibody, anti-Sm antibody, false-positive serologic test for syphilis); and (11) abnormal titer of antinuclear antibody.

A. Epidemiologic Features

Females are affected eight times as often as males. An increased risk for SLE is noted for Asians and Polynesians over whites in Hawaii. Black females are also associated with an increased risk compared with white females. Genetic susceptibility is demonstrated with increased frequency (5%) among relatives of patients with the disease. An inherited complement deficiency is inferred from the absence, or near absence, of individual complement components, the most common being C2. Evidence of a statistical association of SLE with tobacco smoke exposure has been found.

B. Laboratory Findings

Antinuclear antibody determination is the most helpful screening test for SLE. In patients with untreated active disease, 98% have positive antinuclear antibody tests. The higher the titer of antinuclear antibodies, the more likely is the diagnosis of SLE or related rheumatic syndrome. A low value for the antinuclear antibody test is 1:320; values greater than 1:5120 are considered high.

If antinuclear antibody levels are positive, more specific tests may be performed, including testing for anti-DNA antibodies, antibodies to extractable nuclear antigens, and complement levels. High titers of antibodies to double-stranded DNA are highly suggestive for SLE. Low complement levels (C3, C4, and total hemolytic complement levels) are found in the disease but are also seen in related illnesses.

Anemia, leukopenia, and thrombocytopenia are seen, as well as elevations in the ESR. Renal function tests and muscle and liver enzyme tests are often abnormal, reflecting multiple organ system involvement.

C. Imaging Studies

The radiographic features of arthritis in SLE are similar to those of rheumatoid osteoarthritis. Osteonecrosis, particularly of the femoral and humeral heads, is frequently seen in SLE and may be related to autoimmune response or to the usage of corticosteroids.

Ceccarelli F, Perricone C, Cipriano R, et al. Joint involvement in systemic lupus erythematosus: from pathogenesis to clinical assessment. *Semin Arthritis Rheum.* 2017;47:53-64. [PMID: 28465078]

Nevskaya T, Gamble MP, Pope JE. A meta-analysis of avascular necrosis in systemic lupus erythematosus: prevalence and risk factors. *Clin Exp Rheumatol.* 2017;35:700-710. [PMID: 28240590]

Arthritis Associated With Inflammatory Bowel Disease

Peripheral arthritis and spondylitis are associated with ulcerative colitis and Crohn disease. Joint involvement is typically monoarticular or oligoarticular and often parallels the activity of the bowel disease. The arthritis, frequently migratory, is self-limiting in most cases, with only 10% of patients having chronic arthritis. The joints most commonly affected are the knees, hips, and ankles, in order of prevalence. Spondylitis associated with inflammatory bowel disease occurs in two forms. One is very similar to ankylosing spondylitis, including the increased incidence of the HLA-B27 haplotype. The other form has no identifiable genetic predisposition.

A. Epidemiologic Features

Up to 30% of patients with inflammatory bowel disease develop arthritis. There is no difference between the sexes in incidence.

B. Laboratory Findings

There is no specific diagnostic test. Synovial fluid analysis reveals an inflammatory process, with leukocyte counts of 4000 to 50,000/mL.

C. Imaging Studies

Peripheral arthritis is nonerosive, with juxtaarticular osteopenia and joint space narrowing. Spondylitis associated with inflammatory bowel disease resembles ankylosing spondylitis.

Greuter T, Vavricka S. Extraintestinal manifestation in inflammatory bowel disease: epidemiology, genetic, and pathogenesis. *Expert Rev Gastroenterol Hepatol.* 2019;13:307-317. [PMID: 30791773]

Reiter Syndrome

The classic triad of conjunctivitis, urethritis, and peripheral arthritis is known as **Reiter syndrome. Reactive arthritis** is becoming accepted as a more precise term because the initiating condition may be enteritis as well as a sexually transmitted disease. The peripheral arthritis is polyarticular and asymmetric, with knees, ankles, and foot joints most commonly affected.

A. Epidemiologic Features

Nongonococcal urethritis caused by *Chlamydia* accounts for the precipitating event in approximately 20% of cases. Patients who test positive for HLA-B27 are predisposed to developing arthritis after contracting nongonococcal urethritis. A reactive arthritis following enteric infection with *Salmonella, Shigella, Yersinia,* and *Campylobacter* is also noted. For enteric infections with *Shigella,* the risk of developing arthritis in individuals positive for HLA-B27 is close to 20%.

B. Laboratory Findings

There are no specific diagnostic tests for Reiter syndrome. Anemia, leukocytosis, and thrombocytosis occur, and the ESR is often elevated.

C. Imaging Studies

The radiographic features of Reiter syndrome are similar to those of ankylosing spondylitis, with calcifications of ligamentous insertions and ankylosing of joints. The sacroiliitis is unilateral, unlike in ankylosing spondylitis.

Garcia-Kutzback A, Chacon-Suchite J, Garcia-Ferrer H, Iraheta I. Reactive arthritis: update 2018. *Clin Rheumatol.* 2018;37:869-874. [PMID: 29455267]

Schmitt SK. Reactive arthritis. *Infect Dis Clin North Am.* 2017;31:265-277. [PMID: 28292540]

3. Metabolic Arthropathy

Gout

Deposition of monosodium urate crystals in the joints produces gout. Although most patients with gout have hyperuricemia, few patients with hyperuricemia develop gout. The causes of hyperuricemia include disorders resulting in overproduction or undersecretion of uric acid or a combination of these two abnormalities. Examples of uric acid overproduction include enzymatic mutations, leukemias, hemoglobinopathies, chemotherapy, and excessive purine intake.

The first attack involves sudden onset of painful arthritis, most often in the first metatarsophalangeal joint, but also in the ankle, knee, wrist, finger, and elbow. The intensity of the pain is comparable to that from a septic joint, and differentiation is necessary because the treatment is different. Coexistence of a septic joint is unusual but possible. Rapid resolution with colchicine or indomethacin is seen. Recurrent attacks are common in men aged 40 to 60 years. Chronic gouty arthritis is notable for tophaceous deposits, joint deformity, constant pain, and swelling.

A. Epidemiologic Features

Primary gout has hereditary features, with a familial incidence of 6% to 18%. It is likely that the serum urate concentration is controlled by multiple genes (most likely *SLC2A9* and *ABCG2*, which regulate urate excretion). Gout occurs in women, but at a later age, usually postmenopausal, and in association with hypertension and/or renal insufficiency, use of diuretics, and less alcohol consumption than men.

B. Laboratory Findings

The key diagnostic test is detection of monosodium urate crystals in white blood cells in synovial fluid. Negative birefringence of the needle-shaped crystals is seen by their yellow coloration on polarized light microscopy.

Hyperuricemia is usually seen, but up to a fourth of gout patients may have normal uric acid levels. Uric acid levels are elevated when they exceed 7 mg/dL. Elevated serum white blood cell count, serum ESR/CRP, synovial white blood cell count, and synovial polymorphonuclear leukocytes can be seen in acute gout, and thus, these tests cannot be used to differentiate between the septic arthritis and gout. Aspirates should be sent for culture to rule out coexisting infection.

C. Imaging Studies

Tophi may be seen when they are calcified but are not always visible. Soft-tissue swelling is seen, as well as erosions. Chronic changes consist of extensive bone loss, periarticular erosions, joint narrowing, and joint deformity.

Kuo CF, Grainge MJ, Zhang W, Doherty M. Global epidemiology of gout: prevalence, incidence, and risk factors. *Nat Rev Rheumatol.* 2015;11:649-662. [PMID: 26150127]

Lim SY, Lu N, Choi HK. Septic arthritis in gout patients: a population-based cohort study. *Rheumatology.* 2015;54:2095-2099. [PMID: 26170377]

Calcium Pyrophosphate Crystal Deposition Disease

Calcium pyrophosphate crystal deposition disease, a gout-like syndrome, is also known as pseudogout or chondrocalcinosis. Crystals of calcium pyrophosphate dihydrate are deposited in a joint, most commonly the knee and not the first metatarsophalangeal joint, as in gout. The diagnosis is made by demonstration of the crystals in tissue or synovial fluid and by the presence of characteristic radiographic findings.

Aging and trauma are associated with this disorder, as well as conditions such as hyperparathyroidism, gout, hemochromatosis, hypophosphatasia, and hypothyroidism. In patients over age 55, hyperparathyroidism should be considered as a cause.

A. Epidemiologic Features

Aging is the most common risk factor for chondrocalcinosis, and the prevalence is 7% to 10% of people at age 60 with equal sex distribution. Hereditary forms of calcium pyrophosphate dihydrate deposition disease are reported, with mutations in the ankylosis (*ANKH*) gene as the cause.

B. Pathologic Features

Calcification of multiple joint structures occurs, including articular cartilage and capsules, with heaviest deposition in fibrocartilaginous structures such as the menisci. The crystals are rhomboid-shaped, positively birefringent crystals that are more difficult to see on light microscopy than uric acid crystals.

C. Imaging Studies

Calcification of menisci and articular cartilage is seen as punctate or linear radiodensities, which delineate these normally radiolucent structures. Bursae, ligaments, and tendons may have calcifications as well. Bony signs include subchondral cyst formation, signs of carpal instability, sacroiliac joint erosions with vacuum phenomenon, and crowning of the odontoid process.

Kohn NN, Hughes RE, McCarty DJ Jr, et al. The significance of calcium phosphate crystals in the synovial fluid of arthritis patients: the "pseudogout syndrome." II. Identification of crystals. *Ann Intern Med.* 1962;56:738-745. [PMID: 14457846]

Rosenthal AK, Ryan LM. Calcium pyrophosphate deposition disease. *N Engl J Med.* 2016;374:2575-2584. [PMID: 27355536]

Ochronosis

A hereditary deficiency in the enzyme homogentisic acid oxidase is present in the disease known as **alkaptonuria.** The presence of unmetabolized homogentisic acid results in a brownish black color of the urine (thus the name of the disease). The term **ochronosis** describes the clinical condition of homogentisic acid deposited in connective tissues, manifested by bluish black pigmentation of the skin, ear, and sclera, and in cartilage.

The diagnosis is made when the triad of dark urine, degenerative arthritis, and abnormal pigmentation is present. Freshly passed urine is normal in color but turns dark when oxidized. Spondylosis is common, with knee, shoulder, and hip joint involvement also seen.

A. Epidemiologic Features

Alkaptonuria is caused by a rare recessive autosomal gene encoding homogentisate 1,2-dioxygenase. Genetic testing is available.

B. Imaging Studies

Spondylosis is seen, with calcification of intervertebral disks with few osteophytes. Joint involvement is similar in appearance to that of osteoarthritis, except for protrusio acetabuli.

Gil JA, Wawrzynski J, Waryasz GR. Orthopaedic manifestation of ochronosis: pathophysiology, presentation, diagnosis, and management. *Am J Med.* 2016;129(5):536.e1-6. [PMID: 26844634]

4. Osteochondroses

Osteonecrosis of the Femoral Head

A variety of conditions and diseases are associated with osteonecrosis, but the pathogenesis is unknown in most cases. Avascular necrosis of the femoral head (AVN) affects over 20,000 people in the United States annually and is the leading reason for total hip arthroplasty behind osteoarthritis. Direct injury to the blood supply of the femoral head is implicated in traumatic causes of femoral head avascular necrosis such as subcapital femoral neck fracture and dislocation of the hip. The disorder is bilateral in more than 60% of cases and affects other bones in approximately 15% of cases. The leading nontraumatic causes of osteonecrosis include alcoholism, idiopathic causes, and systemic steroid treatment. Relative risk of AVN is 3.3 with less than 400 mL of weekly alcohol intake, 9.8 with 400 to 1000 mL of alcohol per week, and 17.9 with greater than 1000 mL of alcohol per week. The mechanism by which steroids cause osteonecrosis is unknown, although theories include increased lipogenesis with increased size of intramedullary fat cells and increase in intraosseous pressure, which leads to intraosseous compartment syndrome and bone infarct.

Other associated conditions include hemoglobinopathies, Gaucher disease, caisson disease, hyperlipidemia, tobacco use, hypercoagulable states, irradiation, and diseases of bone marrow infiltration such as leukemia and lymphoma.

Table 7–3. Relations between the Marcus, Arlet-Ficat, Steinberg, and Pittsburgh classifications.

AVN Classification			
Marcus et al, 1973	**Arlet-Ficat, 1985**	**Steinberg, 1995**	**Pittsburgh, 2001**
Stage 1 Silent hip, increased density on radiograph Stage 2 Infarct demarcated by zone of increased density Stage 3 Crescent sign (subchondral radiolucency) Stage 4 Depression of lateral edge of infarct Stage 5 Flattening and compression of infarct Stage 6 Progressive compression and erosion, superimposed degenerative arthritis	Stage 0 Silent hip, normal radiograph Stage I Normal or minor changes on plain radiograph Stage II Sclerosis, or cysts of femoral head, diffuse porosis Transition stage Crescentic subchondral line, flattening Stage III Broken contour of the head, joint space normal Stage IV Collapse, flattened contour, decreased joint space, osteoarthrosis	Stage 0 Normal radiograph, bone scan, MRI Stage I Normal radiograph, abnormal MRI Stage II Cystic and sclerotic changes in the femoral head Stage III Subchondral collapse producing crescent sign Stage IV Flattening of the femoral head Stage V Joint narrowing with or without acetabular involvement Stage VI Advanced degenerative changes	Stage I Abnormal MRI, normal radiograph Stage II Abnormal MRI, abnormal radiograph (cystic, sclerotic changes, crescent sign) Normal contour of the head Stage III Abnormal MRI, abnormal radiograph, abnormal contour of the head (flattening, collapse, joint narrowing)

AVN, avascular necrosis; MRI, magnetic resonance imaging.

A. Pathologic Features

Regardless of underlying causes, the early lesions in femoral head osteonecrosis include necrosis of marrow and trabecular bone, usually in a wedge-shaped area in the region of the anterolateral superior femoral head. The overlying articular cartilage is largely unaffected because it is normally avascular, obtaining nutrition from the synovial fluid. The deep calcified layer of cartilage, however, does derive nutrition from epiphyseal vessels and also undergoes necrosis. Histologically, necrotic marrow and absence of osteocytes in lacunae are seen.

Leukocytes and mononuclear cells collect around necrotic and fibrovascular tissue and eventually replace necrotic marrow. Osteoclasts resorb dead trabeculae, and osteoblasts then attempt to repair the damaged tissue; during attempted repair, the necrotic trabeculae are susceptible to fracture. Grossly, a subchondral fracture forms, with deformation of overlying articular cartilage. With time, fragmentation of articular cartilage ensues, resulting in degenerative arthritis.

B. Imaging Studies

There are multiple classifications available for AVN. Marcus and Ficat created the original classification based on the plain radiographic appearance of femoral head osteonecrosis in progressive stages.

Classification was later based on extent of head involvement on MRI. The Pittsburgh classification of AVN was proposed to improve inter- and intraobserver reliability of prior classification. Table 7–3 compares existing classification systems. Many other classifications have been proposed to further delineate AVN lesions based on size and location of the lesion but have low interobserver reliability.

Ficat RP. Idiopathic bone necrosis of the femoral head- early diagnosis and treatment. *J Bone Joint Surg Br.* 1985;67:3-9. [PMID: 31557445]

Plakseychuk A, Shah M, Varitimidis S, Rubash HE, Sotereanos D. Classification of osteonecrosis of the femoral head: reliability, reproducibility, and prognostic value. *Clin Orthop Relat Res.* 2001;386:34-41. [PMID: 11347846]

Steinberg ME, Hayken GD, Steinberg DR. A quantitative system for staging avascular necrosis. *J Bone Joint Surgery Br.* 1995;77:34-41. [PMID: 7822393]

Wang A, Ren M, Wang J. The pathogenesis of steroid-induced osteonecrosis of the femoral head: a systematic review of the literature. *Gene.* 2018;671:103-109. [PMID: 29859289]

5. Other Disorders Associated with Arthritis

Hemophilia

Hemophilia A is a heritable bleeding disorder produced by deficiency of factor VIII. Hemophilia B is a disease caused by lack of clotting factor IX. Both hemophilia A (classic hemophilia) and hemophilia B (Christmas disease) are sex-linked recessive disorders, although 30% of patients may have no family history of the disease. Hemophilic arthropathy is secondary to repetitive minor traumas and primarily involves the knee joint, with the elbow and ankle joints affected less frequently.

A. Pathologic Features

Recurrent hemarthrosis produces deposits of hemosiderin and synovitis. In the acute phase, hypertrophy of synovium occurs, causing a higher risk of repeated bleeding. A pannus may form, as in rheumatoid osteoarthritis, with underlying cartilage destruction, possibly a result of the promotion of apoptosis of chondrocytes and cellular proliferation of the synovium by iron. With time, synovial fibrosis occurs, resulting in joint stiffness.

B. Imaging Studies

Soft-tissue swelling, seen early, is associated with hemarthroses. Later stages include widening of epiphyseal regions caused by overgrowth from increased vascularity. Skeletal changes are manifested as subchondral sclerosis and cyst formation early, with later loss of cartilage and secondary osteophyte formation. Squaring of the patella is seen, possibly resulting from overgrowth.

Wyseure T, Mosnier LO, von Drygalski A. Advances and challenges in hemophilic arthropathy. *Semin Hematol.* 2016;53: 10-19. [PMID: 26805902]

Gaucher Disease

A rare familial disorder, Gaucher disease is an inborn error of metabolism caused by a deficiency of the lysosomal hydrolase enzyme β-glucocerebrosidase. Accumulation of glucosylceramidase in phagocytic cells of the reticuloendothelial tissues occurs, including the liver, spleen, lymph nodes, and bone marrow.

The femur is the most commonly affected bone, but the vertebrae, ribs, sternum, and flat bones of the pelvis may also be affected. The manifestations of skeletal disease are the result of mechanical effects of infiltration of the abnormal cells, leading to erosion of cortices and interference with the normal vascular supply. Expansion of bone and areas of osteolysis predispose affected bones to pathologic fracture, and vascular interruption leads to avascular necrosis of the femoral hip.

A. Epidemiologic Features

Inherited in an autosomal recessive manner, Gaucher disease is the most common inherited disorder of lipid metabolism. The disease is especially common in the Ashkenazi Jewish community.

B. Pathologic Features

Histologic examination of involved reticuloendothelial tissues demonstrates foam cells, which are large lipid-laden macrophages.

C. Imaging Studies

Early stages of skeletal involvement in Gaucher disease include diffuse osteoporosis and medullary expansion. The distal femur may expand to form a characteristic Erlenmeyer flask deformity. Localized erosions and sclerotic areas are seen. Osteonecrosis may be seen in the femoral head, humeral head, and distal femur. Secondary degenerative changes follow collapse of necrotic articular bone. Treatment is now possible with enzyme replacement therapy using imiglucerase, but bone response is usually slower than soft-tissue response.

Piran S, Amato D. Gaucher disease: a systematic review and meta-analysis of bone complications and their response to treatment. *J Inherit Metab Dis.* 2010;33:271-279. [PMID: 20336376]

Stirnemann J, Belmatoug N, Camou F, et al. A review of Gaucher disease pathophysiology, clinical presentation, and treatments. *Int J Mol Sci.* 2017;18:e441. [PMID: 28218669]

Trochanteric Bursitis

Trochanteric bursitis is a term applied to pain elicited to palpation of the lateral side of the hip in the side-lying position. The tenderness is attributed to friction between the greater trochanter and the iliotibial band during motion. Repetitive activity like running or exercising on a Stairmaster can be an inciting cause. Trochanteric bursitis is one of several disorders that falls under the term *greater trochanteric pain syndrome*, which includes gluteus medius and minimus tears and "snapping hip." It affects about 1.8 patients per 100 per year. Risk factors include female gender, coexisting low back pain, iliotibial band tenderness, and obesity. It is diagnosed in the patient with a compatible history by point tenderness over the greater trochanter. A lack of tenderness suggests other sources of the pain, including referred lumbar pain.

Redmond JM, Chen AW, Domb BG. Greater trochanteric pain syndrome. *J Am Acad Orthop Surg.* 2016;24:231-240. [PMID: 26990713]

Speers CJ, Bhogal GS. Greater trochanteric pain syndrome: a review of diagnosis and management in general practice. *Br J Gen Pract.* 2017;67:479-480. [PMID: 28963433]

Hip Labral Tears

The hip has a cartilaginous extension of the bony acetabulum called the labrum that deepens the acetabulum and stabilizes the hip. Labral tears were newly rediscovered as a source of pain and a cause of osteoarthrosis, partially because of the relative ease of evaluating their presence and subsequently treating them. Labral tears are often seen in conjunction with acetabular dysplasia, thought to be due to overloading of the labrum. Arthroscopy can be used to repair the torn labrum or, in the case of defect, re-create a new labrum with an iliotibial band graft. Labral tear or defect is detrimental for the function of the normal hip joint. Anatomical and biomechanical studies demonstrated that acetabular labrum provides suction effect and stability to the hip joint. In an experimental study, 1 cm of labral resection caused significant displacement ("wobbling" effect) of the femoral head within the acetabulum with normal ROM. Successful labral repair could be crucial for restoration of the hip biomechanics and prevention of coxarthrosis. Labral tears can often be seen in asymptomatic individuals, and clinical assessment of labral pathology is key for identifying the labrum as a pain generator.

A. Pathologic Features

The normal labrum is triangular in shape and variable in circumferential rim length on average 15.8 and 13.7 cm for males and females, respectively. Labrum could be from 2 to 6 mm thick, with large labrum in dysplastic hips. The pathologic labrum is classified into types A and B, depending on whether the labrum is traumatic (triangular: A) or degenerative (thick and rounded: B), and three stages: (1) intrasubstance degeneration, (2) partial tear, and (3) complete tear. Labral tears most often occur along the anterosuperior edge.

B. Imaging Studies

MRI arthrography is the most sensitive and specific test for labral tears when compared to computed tomography (CT) arthrogram or plain MRI. Contrast is seen going into the tear, which is frequently in the weight-bearing area of the acetabulum.

Lertwanich P, Plakseychuk A, Kramer S, et al. Biomechanical evaluation contribution of the acetabular labrum to hip stability. *Knee Surg Sports Traumatol Arthosc.* 2016;24:2338-2345. [PMID: 25749654]

Register B, Pennock A, Ho C, et al. Prevalence of abnormal hip findings in asymptomatic participants: a prospective, blinded trial. *Am J Sports Med.* 2012;40:2720-2724. [PMID: 23104610]

Safran MR. The acetabular labrum: anatomic and functional characteristics and rationale for surgical intervention. *J Am Acad Orthop Surg.* 2010;18:338-345. [PMID: 20511439]

MEDICAL MANAGEMENT

Nonsteroidal Anti-inflammatory Drugs

The use of nonsteroidal anti-inflammatory drugs (NSAIDs) in the management of osteoarthritis is widespread but controversial. Because only minimal inflammatory changes are present in joints with osteoarthritis, the use of acetaminophen is advocated as a first-line drug. In a short-term study of patients treated for osteoarthritis, acetaminophen (4000 mg/d) was found to be as effective as ibuprofen (2400 mg/d).

The therapeutic effect of NSAIDs can be dramatic in the osteoarthritic patient, even with severe disease. The main problems with routine NSAID therapy are the gastrointestinal (GI) and renal complications and the inhibition of normal platelet function. Thus, alternative therapies should be carefully considered, and therapy should be closely monitored. Current NSAIDs work by altering prostaglandin synthesis through nonspecific inhibition of both cyclooxygenase isoforms 1 (COX-1) and 2 (COX-2). COX-1 inhibition can have deleterious effects on hemostasis and the GI tract.

Patients treated with NSAIDs have a three times greater relative risk of developing GI complications than nonusers. In one study, NSAIDs were associated with acute hospital admissions of 30% of elderly patients. Patients at high risk for developing ulcers with use of NSAIDs are those with any of the following characteristics: age older than 65 years, history of prior ulcer disease, use of multiple-dose or high-dose NSAIDs, or use of concomitant corticosteroids. The antiprostaglandin effects of NSAIDs can also reduce renal blood flow, leading to acute and chronic renal insufficiency. Patients at risk for acute renal insufficiency because of NSAIDs are elderly patients, those with atherosclerotic cardiovascular disease, and those with preexisting renal impairment. The platelet effects of these drugs are variable, depending on the NSAID half-life, on whether the NSAID inhibits thromboxane A, and on whether that inhibition is reversible. Aspirin, for example, is permanent for the life of the platelet. Many patients report increased bruising as a result of taking these drugs.

Table 7–4 compares the toxicities of currently available NSAIDs. Because the effects are not caused solely by the inhibitory effects on prostaglandin synthesis, the various chemical origins of these drugs may lead to slightly different clinical effects in different patients.

The chemical families of these drugs are noted in Table 7–5 with their half-lives and their dosing frequency. Dosing frequency is important because patient compliance with use of these drugs goes up with less frequent dosing, such as daily or twice daily.

COX-2–selective NSAIDs are now available. Most of the side effects attributable to NSAIDs are caused by inhibition of COX-1, an isoform that is normally present ("constitutive") in renal and GI tissues. COX-2–selective NSAIDs inhibit the isoenzyme that develops ("inducible") as a response to inflammation. By selectively inhibiting COX-2, the efficacy of NSAIDs is retained with much less side effects. Most NSAIDs have some effect on both enzymes, but in most cases, they largely affect either COX-1 or COX-2. Although COX-2–selective NSAIDs are purportedly safe, they are not without side effects. For example, rofecoxib (Vioxx), a COX-2-selective inhibitor that has been removed from the global health care market, was found to have cardiac toxicity not seen during safety trials. Additionally, celecoxib did not exhibit statistically significant decreased rates of complicated upper GI events in a randomized controlled trial.

Table 7–4. Toxicity profiles of currently available NSAIDs.

Generic Name	Proprietary Name	Gastrointestinal Toxicity	Renal Toxicity	Platelet Effects (days)[a]	Other Toxicity[b]
Diclofenac	Voltaren	Moderate	Moderate	1	Hepatitis
Etodolac	Lodine	Low[c]	Moderate	NA	—
Indomethacin	Indocin	High	Moderate	1	Headache
Nabumetone	Relafen	Low[c]	Moderate	NA	Hepatitis
Sulindac	Clinoril	Moderate	Low	1	Dermatitis
Tolmetin	Tolectin	Moderate	Moderate	2	—
Meclofenamate	Meclomen	Moderate	Moderate	1	Diarrhea
Piroxicam	Feldene	Moderate	Moderate	14	—
Fenoprofen	Nalfon	Moderate	Moderate	1	—
Flurbiprofen	Ansaid	Moderate	Moderate	1	—
Ibuprofen	Motrin	Moderate	Moderate	1	—
Ketoprofen	Orudis	Moderate	Moderate	2	—
Naproxen	Naprosyn	Moderate	Moderate	4	—
Oxaprozin	Daypro	Moderate	Moderate	NA	—
Ketorolac	Toradol	High	Moderate	1	—
Salicylsalicylic acid[d]	Disalcid	None	None	None	—
Sodium salicylate[d]	—	None	None	None	—
Aspirin	—	High	Moderate	10	Tinnitus
Diflunisal[e]	Dolobid	Low	Low	None	—
Celecoxib	Celebrex	Low	Low	None	Sulfa allergies
Meloxicam	Mobic	Low	Moderate	None	—

[a]Average time to normal platelet function after discontinuation of drug.
[b]Other NSAIDs may have similar toxicity, but the effects are more prevalent with these agents.
[c]Simultaneous efficacy comparisons in inflammatory disease not available.
[d]No prostaglandin inhibition.
[e]Weak prostaglandin inhibitor.
NA, data not available; NSAIDs, nonsteroidal anti-inflammatory drugs.

The choice of an appropriate NSAID should be based on the following factors: clotting problems, compliance of the patient, GI symptom history, renal function, drug cost, and the effect on the patient with previously used NSAIDs. Patients taking warfarin would probably be better treated with a drug having no platelet effect that is COX-2 specific. Patients with a poor response to one type of NSAID may benefit from a trial with one from another chemical family. A patient with a history of poor drug compliance with other medications would benefit from once-daily dosing, whereas a patient already taking another drug three times daily would probably find three-times-daily dosing more convenient. Obviously, a patient with renal disease should be treated with a drug having not only low renal toxicity, but also a short half-life to minimize the accumulation of the drug in the body because of lack of renal excretion. The COX-2–selective NSAIDs will not eliminate the need for the other drugs. The vast majority of patients tolerate the side effects of the older drugs, and the risk-benefit ratio for these drugs is quite favorable, especially for short courses of treatment.

Table 7–5. Dosage data of currently available NSAIDs.

Generic Name	Proprietary Name	Largest Unit Dose (mg)	Half-Life (h)	Dosing Frequency[a]	Family
Diclofenac	Voltaren	75	2	bid	Acetic acid
Etodolac	Lodine	300	6	qid	Acetic acid
Indomethacin	Indocin	50	4	tid	Acetic acid
Nabumetone	Relafen	500	20-30	2 qd	Acetic acid
Sulindac	Clinoril	200	8-14	bid	Acetic acid
Tolmetin	Tolectin	400	1-2	tid	Acetic acid
Meclofenamate	Meclomen	100	2	tid	Fenamates
Piroxicam	Feldene	20	30-86	qd	Oxicams
Meloxicam	Mobic	15	15-20	qd	Oxicams
Fenoprofen	Nalfon	600	2-3	qid	Propionates
Flurbiprofen	Ansaid	100	6	tid	Propionates
Ibuprofen	Motrin	800	2	qid	Propionates
Ketoprofen	Orudis	75	3	tid	Propionates
Naproxen	Naprosyn	500	14	bid	Propionates
Oxaprozin	Daypro	600	40-50	2 qd	Propionates
Ketorolac	Toradol	10	5	qid	Pyrrolo-pyrrole
Salicylsalicylic acid	Disalcid	750	1	qid	Salicylates
Sodium salicylate	—	650	0.5	q4h	Salicylates
Aspirin	—	325	0.25	2q4h	Salicylates
Diflunisal	Dolobid	500	10	bid	Salicylates
Celecoxib	Celebrex	200	11	bid	Sulfonamide

[a]Dosage required for treatment of inflammation.
bid, twice a day; NSAID, nonsteroidal anti-inflammatory drug; qd, each day; q4h, every 4 hours; qid, four times a day; tid, three times a day.

The advent of the COX-2–specific NSAIDs adds to their safety as analgesics for acute pain because the COX-2 inhibitors block the pain, fever, and inflammatory response while not affecting clotting. Thus, their use in the perioperative setting has significantly increased.

With the growing worldwide opioid epidemic, there has been movement toward increased utilization of NSAIDs and other nonaddictive pain management options. There is increasing evidence that multimodal pain management may be better than opioid-based pain management.

Surgical intervention is generally indicated for patients who have failed conservative therapy with NSAIDs. For patients who are not surgical candidates, a long-term regimen of narcotic medication may be considered.

Harrison RK, DiMeo T, Klinefelter R, et al. Multi-modal pain control in ambulatory hand surgery. *Am J Orthop (Belle Mead NJ).* 2018;47:1. [PMID: 29979803]

Jones P, Lamdin R. Oral cyclooxygenase 2 inhibitors versus other oral analgesics for acute soft tissue injury: systematic review and meta-analysis. *Clin Drug Invest.* 2010;30:419-437. [PMID: 20527999]

Silverstein FE, Faich G, Goldstein JL, et al. Gastrointestinal toxicity with celecoxib vs nonsteroidal anti-inflammatory drugs for osteoarthritis and rheumatoid arthritis: the CLASS study: a randomized controlled trial. Celecoxib Long Term Arthritis Safety Study. *JAMA.* 2000;284:1247-1255. [PMID: 10979111]

Sun F, Zhang Y, Li Q. Therapeutic mechanism of ibuprofen, prednisone and betamethasone in osteoarthritis. *Mol Med Rep.* 2017;15:981-987. [PMID: 28035387]

Disease-Modifying Agents in Rheumatoid Arthritis

Several new disease-modifying antirheumatic drugs (DMARDs) are now available for the medical treatment of RA, in addition to methotrexate and glucocorticoids. Although the experience of these new agents is limited, the mechanisms of their actions may guide orthopedic surgeons with respect to their potential effect on surgical procedures. Etanercept is an artificially bioengineered molecule that binds to the receptor of tumor necrosis factor (TNF), preventing activation of the inflammatory cascade. Infliximab is a chimeric antibody that also targets TNF. Both of these drugs have been shown to increase the risk for surgical site infection after arthroplasty and should be discontinued one full dosage cycle prior to major surgery. Rituximab targets the B cell, and tocilizumab inhibits interleukin-6, and both have shown significant improvements in RA. Leflunomide inhibits an enzyme, decreasing levels of pyrimidine nucleotides and inhibiting clonal expansion of T cells in RA. The number of DMARDs on the market is increasing, and the recommendations for when to discontinue prior to surgery to prevent surgical site infections varies based upon the mechanism of action.

Goodman S, Springer B, Guyatt G, et al. 2017 American College of Rheumatology/American Association of Hip and Knee Surgeons Guideline for the perioperative management of antirheumatic medication in patients with rheumatic diseases undergoing elective total hip or total knee arthroplasty. *Arthritis Rheumatol.* 2017;69:1538-1551. [PMID: 28620948]

OTHER THERAPIES

Nutritional Supplements

The nutritional supplements glucosamine sulfate and chondroitin sulfate are popular as nonprescription products for arthritis therapy. This popularity arises from the concept that these products may serve as substrate for the reparative processes in cartilage. Glucosamine sulfate is found as an intermediate product in mucopolysaccharide synthesis, and an elevated urinary excretion is seen in patients with osteoarthritis and rheumatoid osteoarthritis. Chondroitin sulfate is another glycosaminoglycan present in articular cartilage. American Academy of Orthopaedic Surgeons guidelines based upon available research and meta-analyses at this time recommend strongly against the use of chondroitin sulfate and glucosamine sulfate for osteoarthritis. These recommendations are based upon multiple randomized controlled trials, most of which do show slight improvements in pain and mobility in patients taking these supplements, but none of these differences met the level of being clinically significant for patients.

Brief AA, Maurer SG, Di Cesare PE. Use of glucosamine and chondroitin sulfate in the management of osteoarthritis. *J Am Acad Orthop Surg.* 2001;9:71-78. [PMID: 11281631]

Jevsevar DS. Treatment of osteoarthritis of the knee: evidence-based guideline, 2nd edition. *J Am Acad Orthop Surg.* 2013;21:571-576. [PMID: 23996988]

Injections

One of the mainstays of the treatment of osteoarthrosis and rheumatoid osteoarthritis is the cortisone injection, which can be used for joints, bursae, and trigger points. Generally, injections of shoulders, elbows, wrists, finger joints, knees, ankles, and joints of the foot can be given in the office without radiographic or ultrasound control. While more accurate injection of corticosteroid was obtained under ultrasound guidance, no significant difference was noted in the clinical outcome. Hips and some joints of the foot and hand are best done with radiographic or ultrasound control to ensure location of the injection. The injections can be therapeutic with steroids or diagnostic with local anesthetic. For example, differentiation between the amount of a patient's pain coming from the back and the proportion coming from the hip can be ascertained with a lidocaine injection into the hip. This reliably informs the patient as to the realistic expectations of pain relief after a hip replacement. Similarly, an ankle injection predicts pain relief after ankle fusion.

Hyaluronic acid is a long-chain polysaccharide responsible for the viscoelastic properties of synovial joint fluid. In pathologic states, such as osteoarthritis and rheumatoid osteoarthritis, both the concentration and the molecular size of hyaluronic acid are diminished. In animal experimental models, evidence indicates that hyaluronic injections may retard progression of osteoarthritis. Intraarticular administration of hyaluronic acid is now available for treatment of osteoarthritis of the knee with products of different molecular weight. The initial treatment protocols for these drugs called for weekly injections for 3 to 5 weeks to obtain a therapeutic effect. A single injection treatment is also available, but cost must always be factored in to patient decision-making. Serial injections of hyaluronic acid in patients with osteoarthritic knees are reported to reduce pain for up to 10 months, but the mechanism of action is uncertain and has been proposed to be chondroprotection, proteoglycan and glycosaminoglycan synthesis, anti-inflammatory, mechanical, subchondral, and analgesic actions. Because of the short half-life of hyaluronic acid, it is unlikely that the injections significantly boost lubrication of arthritic joints. Rather than being a disease-modifying therapy, the injectable hyaluronic acid products should be considered long-acting pain-relieving drugs. Questions about the efficacy of these products still remain, as studies and meta-analyses indicate a weak effect, if any, falling beneath the level of a minimally important difference in multiple metanalyses looking at patient-reported outcomes.

Concoff A, Sancheti P, Niazi F, et al. The efficacy of multiple versus single hyaluronic acid injections: a systematic review and meta-analysis. *BMC Musculoskeletal Disord.* 2017;18:542. [PMID: 29268731]

Juni P, Hari R, Rutjes AW, et al. Intra-articular corticosteroid for knee osteoarthritis. *Cochrane Database Syst Rev.* 2015;22:CD05328. [PMID: 26490760]

Leite VK, Daud Amadera J, Buehler A. Viscosupplementation for hip osteoarthritis: a systematic review and meta-analysis of the efficacy on pain and disability, and the occurrence of adverse events. *Arc Phys Med Rehabil.* 2018;99:574-583. [PMID: 28803906]

Platelet-Rich Plasma

Platelet-rich plasma (PRP) is an autologous blood product that is created through centrifugation of blood and activation of the platelets through calcium chloride. The activated platelets release multiple growth factors that have been proposed to improve healing including vascular endothelial growth factor (VEGF), transforming growth factor-β (TGF-β), platelet-derived growth factor (PDGF), insulin-like growth factor (IGF-1), and connective tissue growth factor (CTGF). Through the release of these growth factors, PRP is theorized to reduce joint inflammation, decrease the rates of cellular apoptosis, and increase the production of extracellular matrix. The preparation of PRP is proprietary in many cases, and the concentration of platelets, growth factors, cytokines, and inflammatory markers has been shown to vary widely with different preparations. There is now limited evidence for improvement in pain scores and improved return to play after PRP injections for lateral epicondylitis, but the evidence for the benefits of PRP in other pathologic conditions remains limited. Multiple randomized controlled trials have studied the effects of PRP injection in patients with knee osteoarthritis, and while most found some improvement, the results vary widely. Many studies showing some benefit to pain and function found that this improvement was not clinically significant. At the current time, injection of PRP is often not covered by US insurance companies, and the cost to the patient shoulder be weighed against the potential benefit with shared decision-making.

Dai W, Zhou A, Zhang H, Zhang J. Efficacy of platelet-rich plasma in the treatment of knee osteoarthritis: a meta-analysis of randomized controlled trials. *Arthroscopy.* 2017;33:659-670. [PMID: 28012635]

Laudy AB, Bakker EW, Rekers M, Moen MH. Efficacy of platelet-rich plasma injections in osteoarthritis of the knee: a systematic review and meta-analysis. *Br J Sports Med.* 2015;49:657-672. [PMID: 25416198]

Orthotic Treatment

The use of orthotics can ameliorate the symptoms of osteoarthrosis in the knee, the ankle, and possibly the elbow, but other joints are not really amenable to this treatment. The medial compartment of the knee is more commonly affected than the lateral, leading to, or resulting from, varus deformity. Thus, this disorder lends itself to orthotic treatment to remove the deformity. Heel wedges and valgus braces can be helpful in relieving the pain and improving the ambulatory function of patients with medial gonarthrosis. Similarly, orthotics to control varus and valgus forces at the ankle can be very helpful for ankle arthrosis.

Clouthier A, Hassan E, Brandon SCE, et al. Identification of good candidates for valgus bracing as a treatment for medial knee osteoarthritis. *J Orthop Res.* 2018;36:351-356. [PMID: 28755495]

Dadabo J, Fram J, Jayabalan P. Noninterventional therapies for the management of knee osteoarthritis. *J Knee Surg.* 2019;32:46-54. [PMID: 30477045]

SURGICAL MANAGEMENT

PROCEDURES FOR RESTORATION OF FUNCTION/IMPROVEMENT OF PAIN

Hip Arthroscopy

A. Femoroacetabular Impingement

Femoroacetabular impingement (FAI) is due to an incongruity of the hip joint. There are two types of FAI, cam and pincer impingement, although the two frequently coexist (Figure 7–4). Cam impingement results from abutment of an abnormally shaped femoral head into the acetabulum. The resultant shear forces are transmitted along the acetabular rim, causing injury to the labrum. Pincer impingement results from relative acetabular overcoverage. The labrum impinges on the femoral neck, which causes labral injury and subsequent ossification of the labrum, further deepening the socket and worsening the situation. Both cam and pincer types of impingement result in decreased clearance of the head–neck junction and labral injury.

Although in the past FAI was treated with an open procedure (surgical dislocation of the hip), arthroscopic techniques for FAI have become very popular due to quicker recovery and less morbidity. For pincer lesions, anterior and anterolateral portals are established in the hip joint. A burr is inserted through the anterolateral portal, and the rim of the acetabulum is resected. The labrum can be preserved by placing the burr behind and underneath the labrum and subsequently refixing it after the rim of the acetabulum is adequately resected. For the treatment of cam lesions, a femoral osteochondroplasty is performed. A burr is inserted through the anterior portal, and the femoral head–neck junction is progressively resected until it no longer impinges on the acetabulum. Care must be taken not to damage the blood supply to the femoral head. The deep branch of the medial

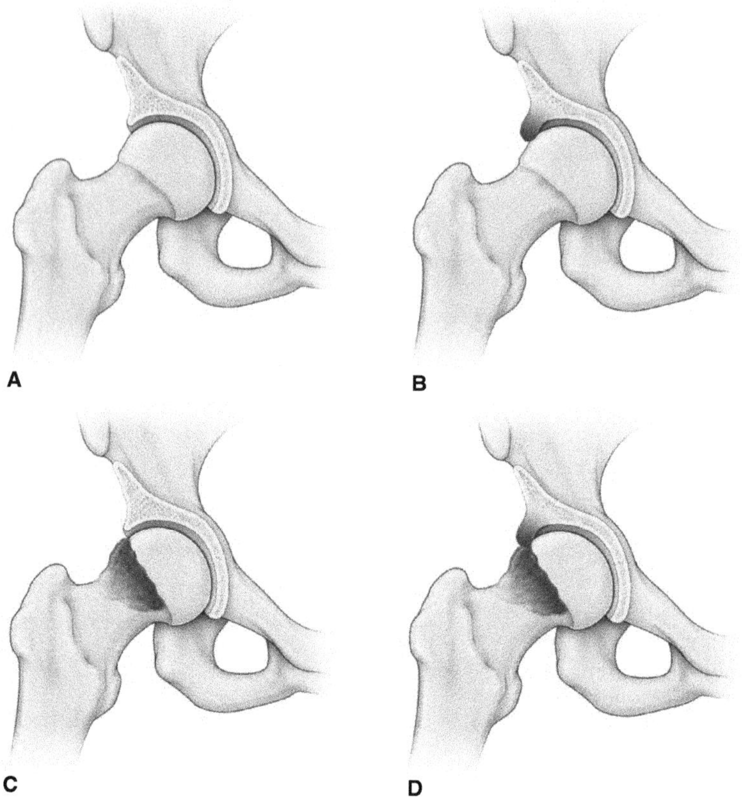

▲ **Figure 7–4. A:** Normal. **B:** Pincer. **C:** Cam. **D:** Combined.

femoral circumflex courses along the posterior aspect of the greater trochanter, posterior to the tendon of obturator externus, and anterior to the tendons of superior gemellus, obturator internus, and inferior gemellus. It perforates the capsule above the superior gemellus and distal to the tendon or piriformis, before dividing into two to four terminal retinacular branches. Maintaining the attachment of the external rotators maintains the blood supply to the femoral head. Additionally, the superior-lateral retinacular vessels must also be maintained during femoral neck osteoplasty.

Long-term outcomes of these arthroscopic techniques have been comparable to the open procedures for the treatment of FAI.

B. Labral Tears

The most common causes of acetabular labral tears are FAI and trauma. They are rarely an isolated event, with one study finding over 90% of patients undergoing hip arthroscopy for atraumatic labral tears having radiographic evidence of a bony abnormality such as dysplasia or FAI. Patients commonly complain of mechanical symptoms, such as clicking, catching, and/or a locking sensation.

Arthroscopic techniques for labral injury include debridement versus repair of the lesions. Repair of the labral tear, if feasible, has improved long-term survival compared with debridement alone. The goal of arthroscopic debridement of a torn hip labrum is to relieve pain by eliminating the unstable flap tear that causes the observed hip discomfort. Type I tears occur when there is detachment of the labrum at the zone of transition to the articular cartilage. These tears can be repaired with reattachment of the labrum to the acetabular rim, usually with a suture anchor. Type II tears are intrasubstance splits with one or more cleavage planes. These tears can be repaired with a suture lasso technique and a bioabsorbable suture. Good to excellent short-term results have been achieved in 67% to 93% of cases of arthroscopic partial labrectomy. Outcome data on labrum repairs are still lacking; however, some investigators have demonstrated the healing capabilities of the labrum in an ovine model, whereas others have shown the superior biomechanical properties of a repaired labrum in a cadaver model.

Microfracture

Microfracture is another arthroscopic technique that helps to restore function and decrease pain. It is used for the

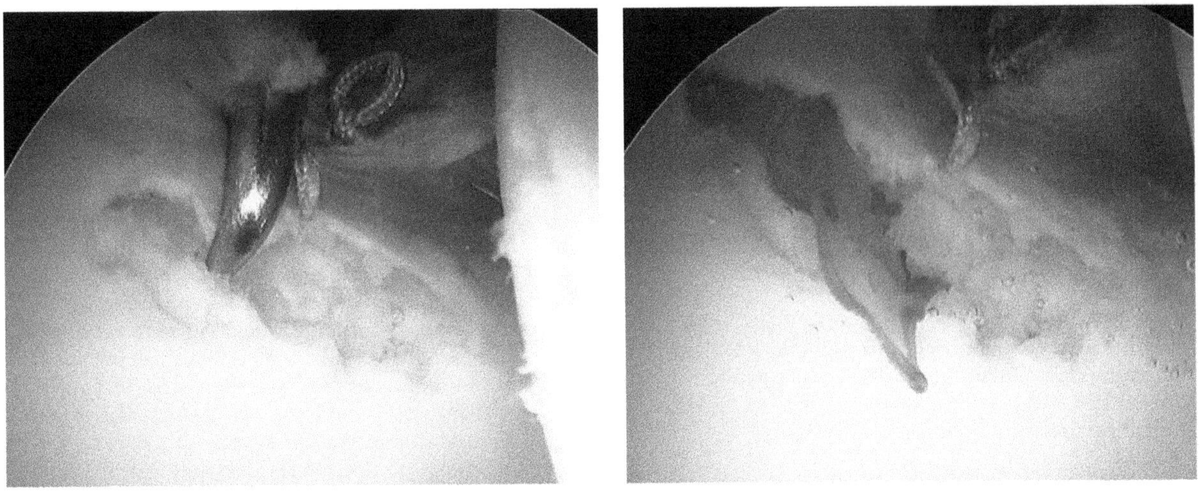

▲ **Figure 7–5.** Microfracture of an osteochondral defect in the hip joint.

treatment of small- to medium-sized osteochondral defects. Through the use of an awl, the surgeon creates tiny fractures in the subchondral bone plate (Figure 7–5). This causes a clot to develop, which eventually forms fibrocartilage. Recovery is quick, and short-term results show 95% to 100% defect coverage. Functional outcome data for this procedure are lacking in the hip, but it is well established with good outcomes in the knee.

Anwander H, Siebenrock K, Tannast M, Stappacher S. Labral reattachment in femoroacetabular impingement surgery results in increased 10-year survivorship compared with resection. *Clin Orthop Relat Res.* 2017;475:1178-1188. [PMID: 27744594]

Marquez-Lara A, Mannava S, Howse E, et al. Arthroscopic management of hip chondral defects: a systematic review of the literature. *Arthroscopy.* 2016;32:1435-1443. [PMID: 27117866]

Nwachukwu B, Rebolledo B, McCormick F, et al. Arthroscopic versus open treatment of femoroacetabular impingement: a systematic review of medium- to long-term outcomes. *Am J Sports Med.* 2016;44:1062-1068. [PMID: 26059179]

PROCEDURES FOR JOINT PRESERVATION

A joint can potentially deteriorate for many reasons. The wear and tear of many years may be most common. In addition, infection can result in articular cartilage damage that then progresses over the years. Trauma may distort the joint, cause instability, or result in abnormal muscle forces, as occurs, for example, with a rotator cuff tear leading to cuff arthropathy. Other causes include (1) synovitis, as occurs, for example, with hemophilia, which forces the joint to dispose of blood on multiple occasions, and RA, which causes a proliferation of the synovium, which may destroy the articular cartilage; (2) osteonecrosis, which may result in fatigue fractures and collapse of the joint, with subsequent incongruity; and (3) abnormal distribution of load in the joint that results, for example, from malalignment. Certain procedures can slow progression of the deterioration resulting from these three causes and prolong the useful service of the joint. These procedures include synovectomy, core decompression, and osteotomy.

Synovectomy

Synovectomy is a treatment that may prolong the life of the articular cartilage through removal of proliferative synovitis, which damages cartilage. Synovectomy is indicated for chronic but not acute synovitis. Chronic synovitis is a clinical entity characterized by proliferation of the synovium and may be monoarticular, as in pigmented villonodular synovitis, or polyarticular, as in RA or hemophilia. The term **synovitis** is relatively nonspecific, and the disorder is usually the result of a reaction to joint irritation.

A. Indications and Contraindications

The most common indication for synovectomy is RA, but the procedure may be beneficial in many other conditions, such as synovial osteochondromatosis, pigmented villonodular synovitis, and hemophilia, and occasionally following chronic or acute infection.

More specific indications for synovectomy include the following conditions:

1. Synovitis with disease limited to the synovial membrane with little or no involvement of the other structures of the joint
2. Recurrent hemarthroses in conditions such as pigmented villonodular synovitis or hemophilia

3. Infection when along with irrigation and debridement of the joint there is imminent destruction by lysosomal enzymes derived from white blood cells that may be liberated from the infection
4. Failure of conservative management

Contraindications include reduced ROM, significant degenerative arthrosis of the involved joint or other joint, or cartilage involvement.

B. Technique

Synovectomy is most commonly performed on the knee but also often on the elbow, ankle, and wrist. Three main techniques are available: open synovectomy, synovectomy with use of the arthroscope, and radiation synovectomy.

1. Open synovectomy—Open synovectomy is becoming less common because of pain that causes difficulty in obtaining full motion following surgery. Continuous passive motion may be beneficial in these cases. Open synovectomy may be necessary in cases of pigmented villonodular synovitis or synovial osteochondromatosis, although these diseases may also be treated by arthroscopy, which permits noninvasive complete removal of the synovium in many cases.

2. Synovectomy with use of arthroscope—Synovectomy with use of the arthroscope may be tedious, especially in large joints such as the knee, because complete treatment requires removal of the entire synovium in many cases.

A study of pigmented villonodular synovitis of the knee treated by total and partial arthroscopic synovectomy demonstrated that total synovectomy resulted in a low recurrence rate, whereas partial synovectomy resulted in symptomatic and functional improvement but a fairly high recurrence rate. Arthroscopic synovectomy was recommended only for localized lesions.

3. Radiation synovectomy—Radiation synovectomy is a technique that is becoming much more popular. It is used in knee joints affected by rheumatoid osteoarthritis. An injection of dysprosium-165-ferric hydroxide macroaggregates is given and leads to improvement in a significant percentage of patients. Proliferation of synovium decreases following this procedure, and there is less pain, blood loss, and expense than with more invasive procedures.

A similar technique is used in the knee joint in hemophiliacs. Phosphorus-32 chromic phosphate colloid is used and can be given on an outpatient basis.

Colman MW, Ye J, Weiss KR, Goodman MA, McGough RL 3rd. Does combined open and arthroscopic synovectomy for diffuse PVNS of the knee improve recurrence rates? *Clin Orthop Rel Res.* 2013;471:883-890. [PMID: 22996360]

Willimon SC, Busch MT, Perkins CA. Pigmented villonodular synovitis of the knee: an underappreciated source of pain in children and adolescents. *J Pediatr Orthop.* 2018;38:e482-e485. [PMID: 29917011]

Cartilage Repair Techniques

Defects of articular cartilage were long considered permanent injuries, and the irrevocable sequela was gradual deterioration over time. The treatment of cartilaginous diseases and injuries was limited by the slow and poorly understood metabolism of articular chondrocytes. Current cartilage repair procedures pertain only to focal full-thickness cartilage defects. Such injuries are typically found in young (<40 years) patients injured during athletic activities or in patients with osteochondritis dissecans. Cartilage repair techniques are contraindicated in smokers and patients with high BMI (>35 kg/m^2), malalignment, meniscal deficiency, ligamentous laxity, or inflammatory conditions.

Because articular cartilage is avascular, prior surgical treatment consisted of chondroplasty, where underlying subchondral bone was either drilled, burred, or microfractured to produce bleeding and an inflammatory response. Although multiple growth factors may be released with bleeding, the ensuing repair tissue is essentially fibrous scar tissue with inferior load-bearing capabilities compared with articular cartilage. As a result, the repair tissue eventually degrades, leaving the defect little better than if left alone. Microfracture is still an option, primarily for smaller lesions.

Larger lesions (>4 cm^2) can be treated with autologous or allograft cartilage transplant. Much enthusiasm followed autologous cartilage transplant in which viable articular chondrocytes are harvested from a patient with a focal cartilaginous defect and cultured in a laboratory. The population of chondrocytes is expanded and placed back in the patient at the site of the cartilage lesion. The cells are held in place with a flap of periosteum sutured to surrounding healthy cartilage. Although encouraging early clinical results were reported with this method, similar results are shown using only the flap of periosteum, and recent studies suggest that the evidence for the efficacy of this technique is inconclusive. Mosaicplasty, also known as osteochondral autograft transplantation, is another method of dealing with small- to medium-sized focal lesions of cartilage and includes transplantation of small osteochondral plugs of mature cartilage and bone from another region of the patient's joint or body. Small cylinders of cartilage and bone are removed from less important locations and transplanted into focal femoral lesions. Although encouraging short-term results are reported, whether the reconstructed cartilage endures is unknown. Larger lesions, such as those comprising an entire compartment of the knee, may be treated with bulk osteochondral allografts.

In contrast to these focal lesions, osteoarthritis with involvement of significant portions of a joint is a more prevalent affliction, affecting more than 40 million individuals in the United States. The early pathologic observations of osteoarthritis indicate structural degradation of the superficial layers of the cartilage architecture. Meaningful spontaneous repair of injuries limited to cartilage is not observed clinically, but a variety of experimental evidence suggests a latent ability to affect some degree of healing after injury and, possibly, osteoarthritis. These suppositions include observation of increased DNA synthesis and proteoglycan synthesis in chondrocytes during intermediate stages of osteoarthritis. The procedures just described for cartilage repair do not apply for osteoarthritics when there is involvement of significant portions of a joint.

Zellner J, Grechenig S, Pfeifer C, et al. Clinical and radiological regeneration of large and deep osteochondral defects of the knee by bone augmentation combined with matrix-guided autologous chondrocyte transplantation. *Am J Sports Med.* 2017;45:3069-3080. [PMID: 28777662]

Core Decompression

A. Indications and Contraindications

Core decompression with or without bone grafting is a surgical treatment primarily used for the femoral head because the hip is the joint most commonly affected by osteonecrosis. The knee and the shoulder are affected less commonly. Osteonecrosis results from loss of blood supply to the bone and is associated with a variety of conditions. Under repetitive stress, microfractures occur, are not repaired, and eventually lead to collapse of the necrotic bone and disruption of the joint surface.

Several factors have been examined as potentially predictive of progression in the patient with an asymptomatic osteonecrotic lesion of the femoral head. While lesion location, lesion stage, age, gender, and BMI have all been suspected as important, the size of the lesion, particularly when over one-third of the size of the femoral head, is probably the most significant risk factor for progression.

Spontaneous repair of the osteonecrotic lesion may occur when lesion size is less than 15% of the femoral head or the lesion is located more central and away from the articular surface. Core decompression with or without structural bone grafting is considered acceptable treatment for precollapse stages of AVN. Free vascularized fibula graft (FVFG) transplant has proven to have superior results compared to core decompression; however, this transplant is technically very demanding. Core decompression and FVFG have no role in treatment of AVN after collapse, and joint replacement is then best.

B. Technique

The goal of core decompression is to alleviate hypertension in the bone caused by obstructed venous egress from the affected area. The theory is that drilling a hole in an involved bony area diminishes pressure and permits the ingrowth of new blood vessels, which allow repair of the avascular bone and prevent joint destruction. Corticocancellous bone grafting is considered an alternative to simple core decompression because some evidence indicates this would place the femoral head at less risk of collapse in the postoperative period before new bone formation can occur. Core decompression or structural bone grafting is indicated in early osteonecrosis prior to collapse of the femoral head (Ficat stage I or II).

Core decompression is usually performed on the hip but may also be done on the knee or the shoulder. A lateral approach is used for the hip, and a pin is placed into the osteonecrotic area under fluoroscopic control. A reamer or core device is then passed over the pin to achieve decompression, and a sample of bone may be obtained for pathologic analysis. If structural bone grafting is to be performed, the graft may be placed over the pin (allograft or autograft fibula). Again, placement is performed under direct radiograph control.

The results of core decompression are mixed, possibly as a result of differences in technique, lack of standardization of staging, and different etiologies of the osteonecrosis. Complications include fracture from torsional failure resulting from stress concentration site in the lateral aspect of the cortex.

Fornell S, Ribera J, Mella M, et al. Effects of electrical stimulation in the treatment of osteonecrosis of the femoral head. *Hip Int.* 2018;38:434-441. [PMID: 29048692]

Plakseychuk AY, Kim SY, Park BC, et al. Vascularized compared with nonvascularized fibular grafting for the treatment of osteonecrosis of the femoral head. *J Bone Joint Surg Am.* 2003;85:589-596. [PMID: 12672831]

Sotereanos D, Plakseychuk A, Rubash HE. Free vascularized fibula grafting for the treatment of osteonecrosis of the femoral head. *Clin Orthop Relat Res.* 1997;344:243-256. [PMID: 9372775]

Osteotomy

Osteotomy should be considered part of the armamentarium of the orthopedic surgeon in the treatment of biomechanical disorders of the knee and the hip. Osteotomy of the hip for osteoarthritis is less frequently performed than osteotomy of the knee. Abnormal distribution of load may be alleviated by osteotomy. Femoral head coverage may be improved with osteotomy of the pelvis, orientation of the femoral head may be improved with osteotomy of the proximal femur, and realignment of the load on the medial and lateral condyles of the tibia may be improved with osteotomy of the femur and/or the tibia. The most common procedure is high tibial osteotomy, to correct varus malalignment of the knee with an opening wedge of bone on the medial site of the tibia. Other corrective osteotomies are performed for residual deformity from healed fractures. Either intraarticular osteotomes, such as condylar osteotomy of the medial compartment (Figure 7–6), or extraarticular osteotomies can be done to correct deformity (Figure 7–7).

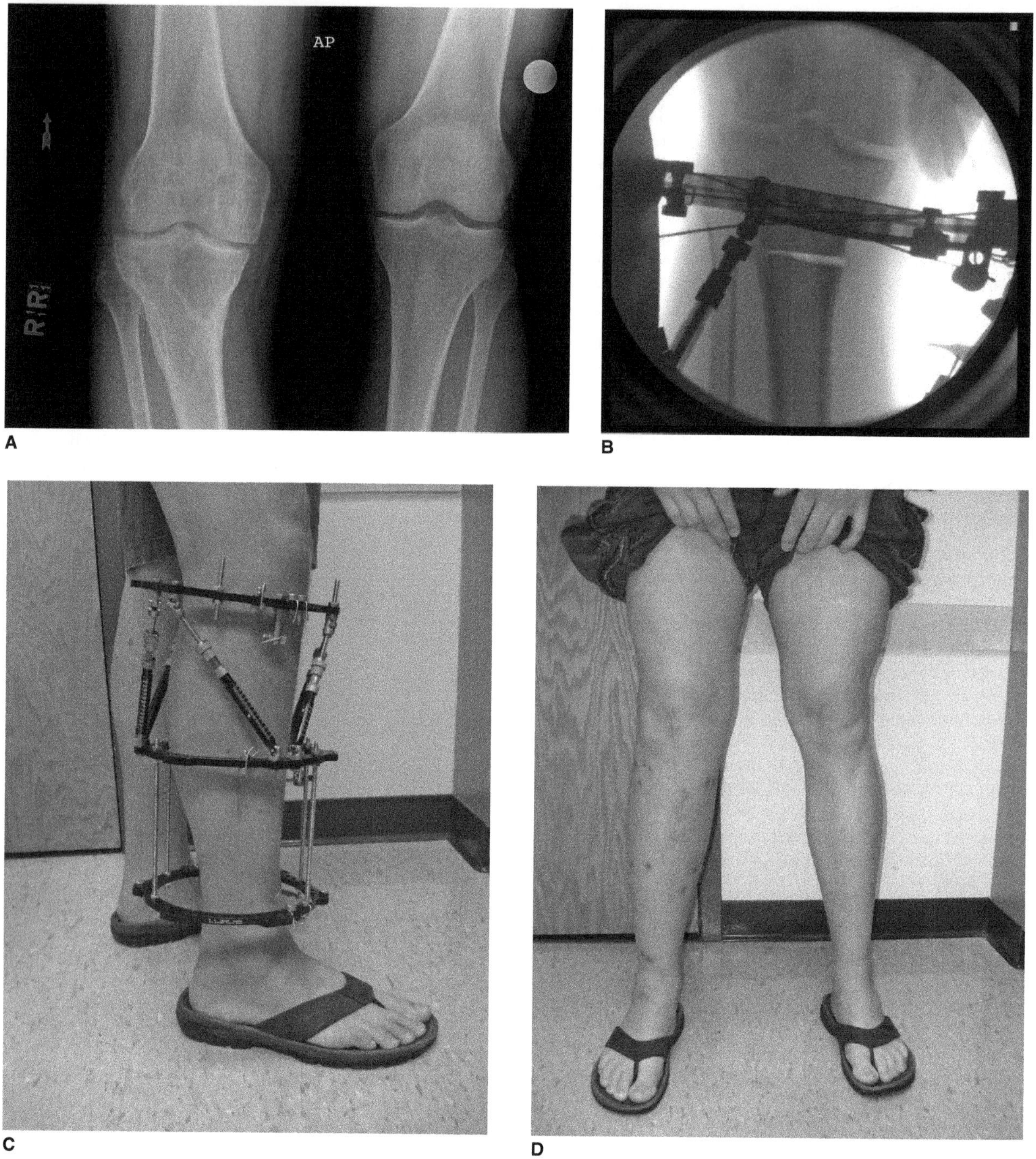

▲ **Figure 7–6.** High tibial osteotomy for posttraumatic deformity. **A:** Preoperative radiograph of proximal tibia deformity. **B:** Intraoperative x-ray after tibial osteotomy and external fixator application. **C:** External fixator. **D:** Deformity correction.

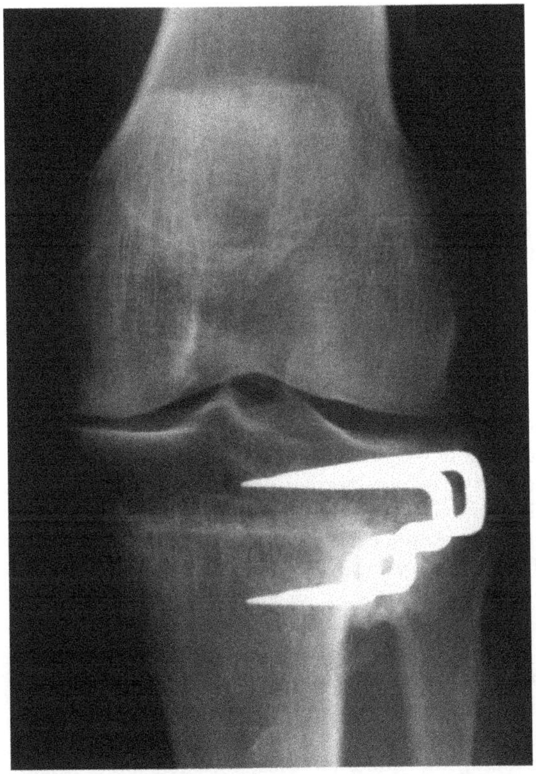

▲ **Figure 7–7.** High tibial osteotomy, showing staples holding the osteotomy in place.

A. High Tibial Osteotomy

High tibial osteotomy surgery has decreased and unilateral knee joint replacement has increased in recent years; however, high tibial osteotomy is still indicated when there is bone deformity that would compromise joint replacement. This procedure is indicated in relatively young (<55 years) patients with good ROM and no joint flexion contracture (Figure 7–6). Corrective osteotomy is usually performed at the apex of the deformity, and when large, the deformity can be gradually corrected with a circular external fixator. The patient may continue weight bearing as tolerated through the course of treatment.

B. Osteotomy of the Hip

Certain unusual conditions of the hip can be treated with osteotomy to prevent or retard coxarthrosis. These include osteochondritis dissecans and other traumatic conditions that produce localized damage to the surface of the hip. Various biomechanical theories have been proposed regarding the benefit of osteotomy of the pelvis and hip in decreasing the load on the hip. Although the theoretical arguments may be correct, in practical terms, the two reasons for performing this procedure are (1) to move a normal viable cartilage surface to the weight-bearing area where previously there was degenerated, thinned articular cartilage; and (2) to reduce the biomechanical loads on the joints that cause pain. These can be reduced either through alteration of moment arms for muscles or, alternatively, by releasing or weakening the muscles. Significantly lengthening or shortening a muscle reduces the force it can apply across a joint. In hip disorders, disease on one side of the hip joint cannot be addressed by an operation on the other side. For example, although it is tempting to use femoral osteotomy to treat acetabular dysplasia, only temporary relief may be obtained.

1. Treatment for acetabular dysplasia—Acetabular dysplasia, as occurs in developmental dysplasia of the hip, may be defined by the center edge angle. The normal center edge angle is 25 to 45 degrees; an angle of less than 20 degrees is considered dysplastic (Figure 7–8). The anterior center

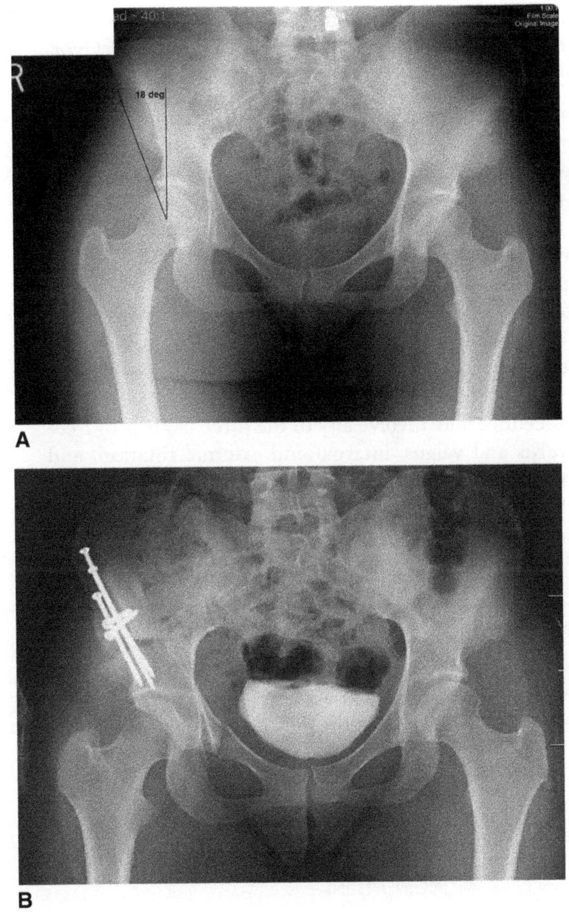

▲ **Figure 7–8. A:** Anterosuperior pelvis film demonstrating the center edge angle. **B:** Same patient after Ganz periacetabular osteotomy, with center edge angle improved.

edge angle can also demonstrate an acetabulum that is too open anteriorly; an angle of 17 to 20 degrees is considered the lower limit on the false profile view. There is also an increased acetabular index.

Numerous pelvic and femoral osteotomies have been developed to help restore proper joint biomechanics and delay the onset of osteoarthritis. Reinhold Ganz developed the Bernese periacetabular osteotomy in 1984 to address acetabular dysplasia. The Ganz osteotomy three-dimensionally reorients the acetabulum so that hip joint forces are more evenly distributed. Since then, the procedure has changed slightly in surgical approach and technique, but the fundamental osteotomies remain the same. Through a shortened ilioinguinal incision, four osteotomies and one controlled fracture around the acetabulum are performed and followed by fixation with multiple screws. The complication rate is relatively low despite the complexity of the procedure. The key point for a successful long-term outcome is an optimal reorientation of the acetabulum. With an optimal reorientation and a spherical femoral head, the cumulative survivorship of the hip after 10 years is 80% to 90%.

2. Treatment of femoral disorders—Osteotomy of the femur can safely and reliably be performed in the intertrochanteric region, with the expectation of union. Osteotomy of the femoral neck is likely to compromise the blood supply to the femoral head as the deep branch of the medial femoral circumflex courses along the posterior aspect of the greater trochanter.

Intertrochanteric osteotomies of the femur of various types are described. The goal of osteotomy is reorienting degenerated articular cartilage away from the weight-bearing dome so that there is more viable cartilage in this location. This procedure may involve any of the three degrees of freedom: varus and valgus, internal and external rotation, and flexion and extension. It is necessary when planning these procedures to be sure the osteotomy will provide an adequate ROM for the patient. These osteotomies are done around the world, and less so in the United States.

Sun H, Zhou L, Li F, Duan J. Comparison between closing-wedge and opening-wedge high tibial osteotomy in patients with medial knee osteoarthritis: a systematic review and meta-analysis. *J Knee Surg.* 2017;30:158-165. [PMID: 27218480]

York PJ, Wydra FB, Belton ME, Vidal AF. Joint preservation techniques in orthopaedic surgery. *Sports Health.* 2017;9:545-554. [PMID: 28632455]

JOINT SALVAGE PROCEDURES

1. Arthrodesis

Arthrodesis is the creation of a bony union across a joint, eliminating motion and relieving pain caused by arthritis. Although ankylosis may prevent observable motion, when incomplete, micromotion may be associated with significant pain. The creation of a fibrous union across a joint with no motion is ankylosis. Ankylosis or arthrodesis may occur spontaneously, as in infection or ankylosing spondylitis, or may be surgically produced. The functional results of spontaneous arthrodesis are not ideal because the patient typically holds the joint in the position that causes minimum pain, which frequently is an inappropriate position for function. Although surgical arthrodesis can be created in almost any joint, including the spine, the most common joints fused are the ankle, knee, shoulder, and hip. The technique used in any of the joints follows the same general pattern. The articular surfaces are denuded of remaining articular cartilage and then placed together in the optimal position of function after shaping to achieve maximum contact between the two opposing surfaces. Bone grafting is frequently used, and some form of fixation, either internal (plates, rods, or screws) or external (external fixators or a cast), is used to immobilize the arthrodesis site in the optimal position (Table 7–6).

Table 7–6. Optimal position of joints after arthrodesis.

Joint	Angle	Length	Other Consideration
Ankle	0° dorsiflexion 0-5° valgus of hindfoot 5-10° external rotation	Slight shortening	Talus displaced posteriorly
Knee	15° flexion 5-8° flexion	Slight shortening	—
Shoulder	20-30° flexion 20-40° abduction (lateral border of scapula) 25-40° internal rotation	—	Patient's hand should be able to touch the head and face
Hip	25° flexion 0-5° abduction (measured between the shaft and a line through the ischia) 0-5° external rotation	Slight shortening	Do *not* destroy abductor mechanism

After adequate healing, the rehabilitation process is begun. Multiple techniques of arthrodesis have been described for each joint.

Ankle Arthrodesis

Arthrodesis of the tibiotalar joint is generally considered to be a good operation for treatment of tibiotalar arthrosis. A well-done ankle arthrodesis results in freedom from pain and nearly normal walking ability. One reason that ankle arthrodesis has been highly regarded in the past was that other options, such as total ankle replacement, were less viable.

The indications for ankle arthrodesis are as follows:

1. Degenerative arthrosis
2. RA
3. Posttraumatic arthritis
4. Avascular necrosis of the talus
5. Neurologic disease resulting in an unstable ankle
6. Neuropathic ankle joint

The relative contraindications for tibiotalar arthrodesis include degenerative joint disease in the subtalar and midtarsal joints, but these patients may be considered for pantalar fusion.

The ankle arthrodesis can be performed through an anterior, lateral, or medial approach, and even posterior approaches are described. Arthroscopic techniques are now employed in patients with minimal deformity. The most common techniques are external fixation or internal screw fixation to achieve compression. Preparation of the ankle for arthrodesis is performed as mentioned earlier. Positioning of the ankle is important, with the talus in a neutral position or at an angle of 5 degrees of dorsiflexion. The midtarsal joints have a greater ROM in plantar flexion than in dorsiflexion, resulting in a more flexible foot. The talus is also displaced slightly posteriorly to make it easier for the patient to roll the foot over at the completion of the stance phase. A varus position is to be avoided because this restricts mobility at the midtarsal joints.

Kugan R, Aslam N, Bose D, McNally M. Outcome of arthrodesis of the hindfoot as a salvage procedure for complex ankle pathology using the Ilizarov technique. *Bone Joint J.* 2013;95:371-377. [PMID: 23450023]

Quayle J, Shafafy R, Khan MA, et al. Arthroscopic versus open ankle arthrodesis. *Foot Ankle Surg.* 2018;24:137-142. [PMID: 29409224]

Knee Arthrodesis

Knee arthrodesis is seldom done for primary problems and generally done as the last resort for other problems. Indications for the procedure include infection, a neuropathic joint secondary to syphilis or diabetes, complete loss of quadriceps function, or as a salvage procedure following a failed total knee arthroplasty. Quadriceps dysfunction or extensor mechanism incompetence is only a relative indication for arthrodesis because joint mobility can be maintained without quadriceps function, and joint stability can be obtained through use of an orthosis that holds the joint extended for standing and walking but can be unlocked for sitting. Although knee arthrodesis is usually successful and provides pain-free weight bearing, it is associated with other problems, especially in tall people. Sitting in airplanes, movie theaters, and even automobiles may be difficult. The most common indication for knee arthrodesis is failed total knee arthroplasty, usually because of infection. In a patient who wishes to maintain an active lifestyle, such as hunting on rough ground or performing manual labor, a knee arthrodesis is a viable alternative. Active infection is an absolute contraindication to knee arthrodesis. The relative contraindications include bilateral disease or an above-knee amputation of the other leg as it would then be extremely difficult to arise from a chair.

The technique of arthrodesis varies with the problem being treated. After infection, particularly when it is associated with total knee arthroplasty, bone loss is often moderate to severe. Severe cases of bone loss may require distraction osteogenesis to achieve enough bone to prevent disabling shortening. This technique can also be used to get fusion of the femur to the tibia. Cancellous bone from the distal femur and proximal tibia may be nearly nonexistent, and external fixation may be necessary to obtain adequate immobilization for arthrodesis. For less severe cases, intramedullary rod fixation works well, particularly if the infection is under control. Similarly, use of double plates at 90 degrees is a viable method of immobilization. Frequently, iliac crest bone grafting is necessary to stimulate healing. Although bone loss often makes it necessary to shorten the extremity, some shortening (2-3 cm) is desirable to ease ambulation by preventing a circumduction gait. The knee should be positioned at 10 to 15 degrees of flexion and at the normal valgus alignment of 5 to 8 degrees, if possible.

Bruno A, Kirieno A, Peccati A, et al. Knee arthrodesis by the Ilizarov method in the treatment of total knee arthroplasty failure. *Knee.* 2017;24:91-99. [PMID: 27876266]

Kuchinad R, Fourman MS, Fragomen AT, Rozbruch SR. Knee arthrodesis as limb salvage for complex failures of total knee arthroplasty. *J Arthroplasty.* 2014;29:2150-2155. [PMID: 25138614]

Elbow Arthrodesis

Elbow arthrodesis is an uncommon procedure because it causes disabling limitations from loss of elbow motion. To perform activities of daily living, a total flexion arc of 100 degrees from 30 degrees of extension to 130 degrees of flexion is required. A total range of 100 degrees for pronation and supination is also required. Painful arthritis in a patient who is willing to accept the trade-off between stability and loss of motion is the indication for arthrodesis. Salvage of infectious processes, such as tuberculosis or fungus or bacterial infections after joint replacement, is also an indication for arthrodesis.

Fixation with a plate and screws or an external fixator are effective for elbow arthrodesis, and resection of the radial head can aid in pronation and supination when needed. The position of fusion at 90 degrees is the best compromise for overall function.

Kovack TJ, Jacob PB, Mighell MA. Elbow arthrodesis: a novel technique and review of the literature. *Orthopaedics.* 2014;37:313-319. [PMID: 24810812]

Morrey BF, Askew LJ, Chao EY. A biomechanical study of normal elbow motion. *J Bone Joint Surg Am.* 1981;62:872-877. [PMID: 7240327]

Shoulder Arthrodesis

Shoulder arthrodesis is a stabilization procedure to optimize upper extremity function in patients in whom mobilization of the shoulder is not possible. Loss of the stabilizing muscles, permanent and severe brachial plexus nerve injury, multiple failed glenohumeral joint stabilization procedures, and sepsis after a total shoulder arthroplasty are indications for shoulder arthrodesis. Contraindications include contralateral shoulder arthrodesis, advanced patient age, and ipsilateral elbow and/or scapulothoracic arthrodesis. Paralysis of the scapular muscles is also a contraindication as the mobility of the shoulder afterward is dependent upon these muscles.

Rigid internal fixation with a plate and screws so that the axilla can be washed and the hand can reach the mouth is best (see Table 7–6). After surgery, exercises are begun to gently obtain scapular motion. Functional results are varied and depend on the position of fusion. Overhead work or work with the arm abducted is not possible, and excessive internal and external rotation must be avoided.

Puskas GJ, Lädermann A, Hirsinger S, Hoffmeyer P, Gerber C. Revision rate after screw of plate arthrodesis of the glenohumeral joint. *Orthop Traumatol Surg Res.* 2017;103:875-884. [PMID: 28669920]

Wagner ER, McLaughlin R, Sarfani S, et al. Long-term outcomes of glenohumeral arthrodesis. *J Bone Joint Surg Am.* 2018;100:598-604. [PMID: 29613929]

Hip Arthrodesis

Hip arthrodesis is rarely performed because of the success of total hip arthroplasty. Arthrodesis of the hip, as of other joints, does produce a relatively pain-free stable joint that allows the patient to perform heavy labor. The disadvantage of hip arthrodesis in a young person is that, over a period of time, degenerative disk disease of the lumbar spine and degenerative arthrosis of the ipsilateral knee frequently occur, even with optimal position of the arthrodesis. In fact, an indication for converting a hip fusion to a total hip arthroplasty is incapacitating back or knee pain.

The strongest indication for arthrodesis of the hip is tuberculosis. Chronic osteomyelitis is a relative indication. Contraindications to arthrodesis include limited motion of the ipsilateral knee, degenerative arthrosis of the ipsilateral knee, degenerative lumbar spine disease, and arthrosis of the contralateral hip. Perhaps the biggest problem in performing a hip arthrodesis in a patient with adequate indications is obtaining agreement from the patient. Because joint replacement offers mobility, early rehabilitation, and a less extensive operation, patients are reluctant to consider the potential problems of hip arthrodesis. This is particularly true when total hip arthroplasty is performed in professional athletes, permitting some of them to continue in sports. Because of these factors, hip arthrodesis is now a relatively uncommon operation.

Multiple techniques are described for performing hip arthrodesis. Truly rigid fixation is difficult to achieve, and immobilization after surgery is usually needed. During the fusion procedure, care should be taken to preserve the abductors, so future reconstructive procedures may be performed if desired. The crucial aspect of the operation is fusing the hip in the appropriate position. The optimal position is slight flexion (25 degrees) from the normal position of the pelvis and spine, slight external rotation (5 degrees), and neutral abduction and adduction. Previously, the hip was placed in abduction, producing a very abnormal gait with additional stress on the lumbar spine. A position of neutral to slight abduction minimizes this problem because the body's center of gravity when the patient is in a one-legged stance is moved closer to the foot. Too much flexion makes both walking and lying in bed difficult, and too little flexion makes sitting difficult. Too much external rotation forces uncomfortable knee motion. Conversion of hip arthrodesis to hip arthroplasty has been performed to increase functionality of the hip but has a high risk for complications and need for revision procedures.

Jaurequi JJ, Kim JK, Shield WP, et al. Hip fusion takedown to a total hip arthroplasty: is it worth it? A systematic review. *Int Orthop.* 2017;41:1535-1542. [PMID: 28349181]

Kliushin NM, Ababkov YV, Ermakov AM, Malkova TA. Modified Girdlestone arthroplasty and hip arthrodesis using the Ilizarov external fixator as a salvage method in the management of severely infected total hip replacement. *Indian J Orthop.* 2016;50:16-24. [PMID: 26955173]

2. Resection Arthroplasty

Resection arthroplasty, or excisional arthroplasty, is a procedure that is applied primarily to the hip, shoulder, elbow, and, more recently, the knee. Resection arthroplasty, or a modification called **fascial arthroplasty,** was a procedure used in the elbow for many years. Resection arthroplasty of the hip is also called **Girdlestone pseudoarthrosis** and dates back to 1923. It can be performed as an intervening and sometimes permanent treatment for infection following total hip arthroplasty.

Resection Hip Arthroplasty

Resection arthroplasty of the hip produces a relatively pain-free joint with reasonably good motion. It is indicated as a primary procedure when ankylosis would result in the hip being placed in an unsuitable position and total hip arthroplasty would result in a high risk for dislocation or infection. Spinal cord injury, head injury, and, perhaps, severe Parkinson disease may warrant primary resection arthroplasty. Disadvantages of the procedure result from lack of mechanical continuity between the femur and the pelvis; this causes an abnormal gait and the need for support with a cane or other device and shortening of the limb. In primary resection arthroplasty, the procedure is a reconstructive procedure in which the femoral head and neck are removed flush with the intertrochanteric line and the capsule is reconstructed to help provide some stability of the hip. Traction with a pin in the tibia can be used for variable periods to diminish leg shortening.

Hip resection arthroplasty can be used as a salvage procedure in patients who previously had infection following total hip replacement because they usually have the most stable hip joints because dense scar tissue has formed. The procedure can be very helpful in reambulating wheelchair-bound patients in whom peroneal care is very difficult. For infection compromising total hip replacement, resection arthroplasty is accomplished by removing all cement, the prosthesis, and any necrotic bone and soft tissue.

Resection Knee Arthroplasty

Resection arthroplasty of the knee has a much less satisfactory functional result. After removal of an infected knee prosthesis, there is usually significant bone loss and the knee is quite unstable. Bracing improves the condition only modestly, and the patient still requires crutches or a walker to ambulate. Knee fusion is a preferred technique over this in most patients as it allows for early, stable mobilization.

Resection Elbow Arthroplasty

Resection arthroplasty or fascial arthroplasty of the elbow is one means of managing painful arthritis after trauma or infection. Resection arthroplasty may also be performed for failure of total elbow arthroplasty resulting from sepsis or severe osteolysis. Resection arthroplasty in the patient with RA should be discouraged because one of the problems associated with the procedure is instability, and the rheumatoid patient frequently depends on the upper extremity to ambulate with walking aids. Interpositional arthroplasty, using fascia or split-thickness skin grafts, was thought to reduce resorption of bone, but the additional benefit of the interpositional tissue is doubtful. Although resection arthroplasty frequently relieves pain, instability is a major problem and bracing is sometimes needed. With the availability of elbow arthroplasty, this procedure is rarely performed but is still used in cases of failed elbow arthroplasty.

Malcolm TL, Gad BV, Elsharkawy KA, Hiquera CA. Complication, survival, and reoperation rates following Girdlestone resection arthroplasty. *J Arthroplasty.* 2015;30:1183-1186. [PMID: 25754256]

Rhee YG, Cho NS, Park JG, Song JH. Resection arthroplasty for periprosthetic infection after total elbow arthroplasty. *J Shoulder Elbow Surg.* 2016;25:105-111. [PMID: 26475639]

8 Adult Reconstructive Surgery

Richard L. McGough, III, MD
Patrick J. McMahon, MD

Introduction

Hip and knee arthroplasty have been a boon to mankind. Prior generations suffered mightily with end-stage arthritis, having no means of relieving pain and restoring function once joint cartilage was lost. Individuals struck with "rheumatism" lost their ability to meaningfully ambulate and engage in activity. Beginning in the 1960s, joint replacement offered these individuals the opportunity to restore their ambulatory ability and to resume their activities. These surgeries and the prostheses used in them were continuously modified in the ensuing 50 years, providing off-the-shelf availability to fit nearly any individual.

Although these procedures were very successful in appropriate individuals, they were initially undertaken with caution. Highly specialized individuals in highly specialized centers performed joint replacements on carefully selected patients. As medical procedures popularize and proliferate, more patients request them from more surgeons. Consequently, the indications for arthroplasty loosened, and the fear of complications lessened. This allowed more people to undergo joint replacement, but at a great cost not only to society, but to the individuals themselves, as periprosthetic infection is a devastating complication. Surgeons and hospital systems have therefore become increasingly selective with regard to patients, procedures, and the surgeons who perform them, as it became obvious that an infected or dysfunctional prosthetic joint is far worse than an arthritic joint.

Hip Hemiarthroplasty

Performing a hemiarthroplasty on the hip is a procedure whereby only the femoral portion of the joint is replaced. In this way, the femoral head is removed, and a prosthesis is placed in the remaining femoral bone and allowed to articulate with the acetabulum.

A. Indications

Hemiarthroplasty has a fairly small number of indications including displaced femoral neck fractures in elderly individuals, oncologic resections of the femur, and avascular necrosis (Figure 8–1). Contraindications to hemiarthroplasty include substantial arthritic changes of the acetabular cartilage and active infection.

The success of hemiarthroplasty depends greatly upon its indications. In elderly individuals who suffer displaced femoral neck fractures and who lack arthritic changes, hemiarthroplasty has traditionally provided lifelong relief from pain and allows the individual to ambulate. Functional success is strongly dependent upon preinjury function, as most individuals require more ambulatory assistance after this type of injury and surgery than they had at baseline before injury. The functional results in oncologic resections have rarely been studied, as the focus was oncologic success and mild pain or functional deficiencies were considered secondary issues. Use of hemiarthroplasty in avascular necrosis is controversial because many patients do not have complete pain relief. This is balanced by the risk of complications, especially prosthetic dislocation, being substantially higher after total hip arthroplasty (THA) being done for avascular necrosis.

Several controversies surround the use of hemiarthroplasty for fragility fractures of the femoral neck in older individuals. Deciding whether to fix the fracture or replace it can be challenging in people in their 50s and 60s, as medical comorbidities and osteoporosis begin to become more prominent in this age group. An individualized approach with careful discussion and patient counseling is often necessary. A second controversy exists regarding whether to cement the femoral stem or to use an uncemented technique. While uncemented hemiarthroplasty for fragility fractures can be successful, these injuries exist because the bone quality is substantially compromised. Periprosthetic fractures at the time of implantation are certainly at higher risk with

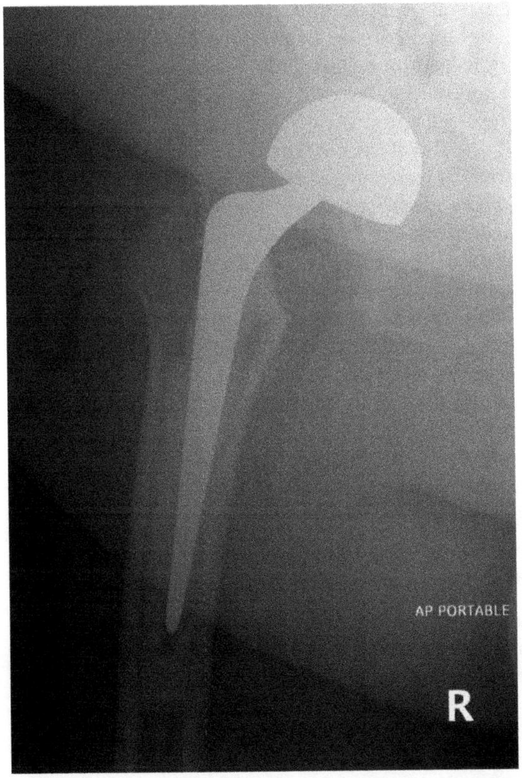

▲ **Figure 8–1.** An anteroposterior radiograph demonstrating a cemented hip hemiarthroplasty performed for a fracture of the femoral neck.

uncemented technique, and prosthesis subsidence and loosening are more common than with the cemented technique. Cemented hemiarthroplasty likely requires less revision surgery than prosthetic reconstruction without cement. A final controversy exists regarding *who* should have a hip hemiarthroplasty versus a total hip replacement, or even *whether* hemiarthroplasty should be used for these conditions. Some individuals will experience groin pain and progressive arthritis after hemiarthroplasty and may require conversion to total hip replacement. In the past, it was thought that function after total hip replacement was superior but there are unlikely to be significant differences in function or pain in ambulatory, older individuals who undergo hemiarthroplasty. Overall, total hip replacement seems to be the better alternative in those who are chronologically or physiologically younger, whereas hemiarthroplasty provides sufficient pain and functional outcomes with fewer complications and lower cost in older individuals.

Although hemiarthroplasty requires less surgery than total hip replacement, the complication profile is similar. Periprosthetic infections certainly can occur, and their risk when compared to elective total hip replacement is likely higher, as most of these procedures are done in older, sicker individuals who cannot be as medically optimized preoperatively because of the urgency of the surgery. Periprosthetic dislocation, while less common than in total hip replacement, can still occur and seems to be more frequent when low-cost "fracture stems" and posterior approaches are used. Low-cost fracture stems often lack the necessary hip offset to appropriately tension the soft tissues without undue limb lengthening. Posterior surgical approaches are more commonly used with hemiarthroplasty and have a higher risk of dislocation. Other complications include aseptic loosening, fracture, nerve injury, venous thrombosis, pulmonary emboli, and leg length discrepancies.

B. Clinical Results

The majority of patients undergoing hemiarthroplasty for fractures undergo a "step down" in their function despite technical surgical success and no complications. Many older individuals greatly fear falling after this event, with some refusing to ambulate. In general, a completely independent ambulator may resort to using a cane, and a cane ambulator may prefer a walker afterward. Walker ambulators who suffer this fracture often do not meaningfully walk afterward, and those who only transfer preoperatively rarely walk postoperatively. In those individuals, Girdlestone resection arthroplasty may be the better option, as it has reduced costs, fewer complications, and excellent pain relief.

Chammout G, Kelly-Pettersson P, Hedbeck CJ, Stark A, Mukka S, Sköldenberg O. HOPE-Trial: hemiarthroplasty compared with total hip arthroplasty for displaced femoral neck fractures in octogenarians: a randomized controlled trial. *JBJS Open Access.* 2019;4(2):e0059. [PMID: 31334466]

Ravi B, Pincus D, Khan H, Wasserstein D, Jenkinson R, Kreder HJ. Comparing complications and costs of total hip arthroplasty and hemiarthroplasty for femoral neck fractures: a propensity score-matched, population-based study. *J Bone Joint Surg Am.* 2019;101(7):572-579. [PMID: 30946190]

Veldman HD, Heyligers IC, Grimm B, Boymans TA. Cemented versus cementless hemiarthroplasty for a displaced fracture of the femoral neck: a systematic review and meta-analysis of current generation hip stems. *Bone Joint J.* 2017;99-B(4):421-431. [PMID: 28385929]

Total Hip Arthroplasty

THA has been a tremendously successful procedure, relieving pain and restoring function to millions worldwide. While this procedure has been one of the best that orthopedic surgery has to offer, it is not without its caveats, risks, and controversies.

A. Indications

There are several indications for hip replacement. The most common of these is osteoarthritis. Inflammatory arthritides, while much more common in the past, are better controlled medically at this time and do not come to hip replacement with as much frequency. When they do, they tend to have added complexity, with protrusio acetabuli, displacement of the medial wall of the acetabulum into the pelvis being more common, and dislocations being more frequent due to difficulties with stability from the soft tissues. Posttraumatic arthritis can produce special challenges due to femoral or acetabular malunion, scar formation, and prior orthopedic hardware. Lastly, some patients require conversion from hemiarthroplasty to THA, although this situation is unusual with careful patient selection.

A time existed when very few contraindications to THA (other than active infection) existed. As the recognition of the gravity of complications from THA grew, many surgeons developed stricter criteria for offering this complex, expensive procedure. Current contraindications to THA include, but are not limited to, active infection, obesity (although body mass index [BMI] definitions vary, many restrict THA to patients with a BMI <40), hepatitis C or B infection, uncontrolled diabetes mellitus (while there are varying hemoglobin A1c [HbA1c] thresholds, there is trivial increased infection risk with HbA1c <7), alcoholism, nicotine abuse, certain neuromuscular conditions, and inability or unwillingness to comply with postoperative rehabilitation.

B. Surgical Technique

Multiple surgical approaches can be used in THA. Initially, all THAs were done using a transtrochanteric approach. In this technique, the greater trochanter is osteotomized, allowing the abductors to be lifted above the acetabulum, providing excellent exposure. The trochanter is then fixed at the end of the procedure, wrapping wires or cables around it to restore the abductors. This approach is rarely done now, as nonunions can occur, leading to weakness and hip instability. Occasionally, it is necessary to perform this osteotomy for a *trochanteric advancement*, displacing it inferior, in revision surgery.

The most common approach for THA is the posterior or southern approach. This approach develops a plane behind the abductors by splitting the gluteus maximus muscle. The gemellus superior, gemellus inferior, obturator internus, obturator externus, and quadratus femoris muscles, known as the short external rotators, the piriformis muscle, and the hip capsule are then incised. The posterior approach is faster and has lesser blood loss, but correct component positioning is more difficult, as both acetabular and femoral anteversion are more difficult to attain. The rate of dislocation is therefore higher, but this may be ameliorated somewhat with a careful repair of the posterior soft tissues.

Direct lateral and anterolateral approaches develop a plane on the opposite side of the proximal femur. As the abductors proceed more anteriorly, a portion of them must be incised and reflected to gain access to the hip joint. These are later repaired using various techniques. This approach gives the most direct view of the acetabulum and is therefore preferred by some surgeons for revision surgery. It is not extensile, and excessive exposure can denervate the anterior gluteus medius and minimus, weakening the hip and yielding a permanent limp coined a Trendelenburg gait.

Direct anterior approaches have recently become more popular. This approach spares the abductors, potentially leading to more rapid recovery from surgery and less limping. Femoral exposure is more difficult, and release of the quadriceps femoris muscle origins is sometimes necessary in more muscular individuals.

Any of these approaches can yield a functional, complication-free technique, and much of the choice is surgeon preference and comfort.

C. Implants

Historically, all THA components were anchored to the bone using polymethylmethacrylate (PMMA) bone cement. The results of cemented femoral components were mostly very positive, while the results on the acetabular side were not as good, with substantial loosening by 15 years postoperative. Uncemented acetabular components were therefore developed to solve this problem and uncemented femoral fixation followed closely. Currently, most THAs in the United States are performed using uncemented components.

Uncemented fixation of THA components relies on osseointegration, the phenomenon by which bone grows into an implant and, with joint arthroplasty specifically, a metallic substrate. This generally provides a permanent bond, allowing the prosthesis to survive lifelong. Creating this bond relies on a tightly fitting prosthesis, with little to no micromotion. If motion exists, osseointegration will not occur. On the acetabular side, screw fixation can augment the initial press fit, whereas femoral integration relies upon precise matching of the prosthesis to either the metaphysis or diaphysis of the femur (Figure 8–2).

Because press-fit technique relies on precise, tight matching, it is often not suitable in a severely osteoporotic femur (Figure 8–3). As osteoporosis progresses, the bone itself widens to increase its bending strength. This renders precise shape matching less likely. As the bone is of poorer quality, PMMA cement is often used for fixation of the femoral components in osteoporotic bone, with a press-fit acetabulum used on the pelvic side. This "hybrid hip" was the most popular choice in the latter portions of the 20th century, with press-fit femoral fixation becoming dominant in the 21st century. Despite this, cemented femoral components still have a role, especially in severe osteoporosis, unusual femoral shapes, metabolic bone disease, and after

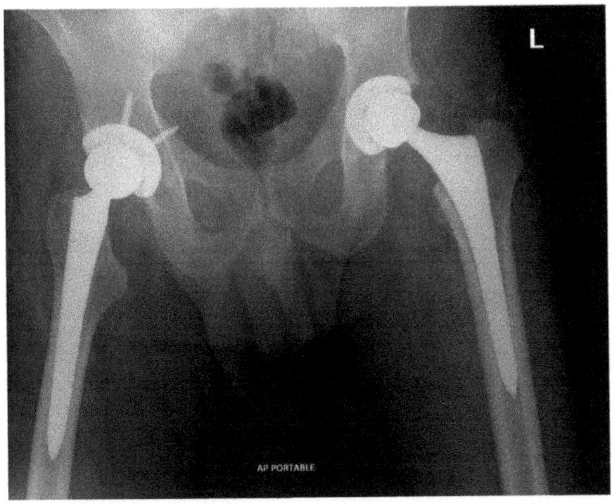

▲ **Figure 8–2.** Bilateral uncemented total hip replacements. The acetabular component on the patient's right has supplemental screw fixation.

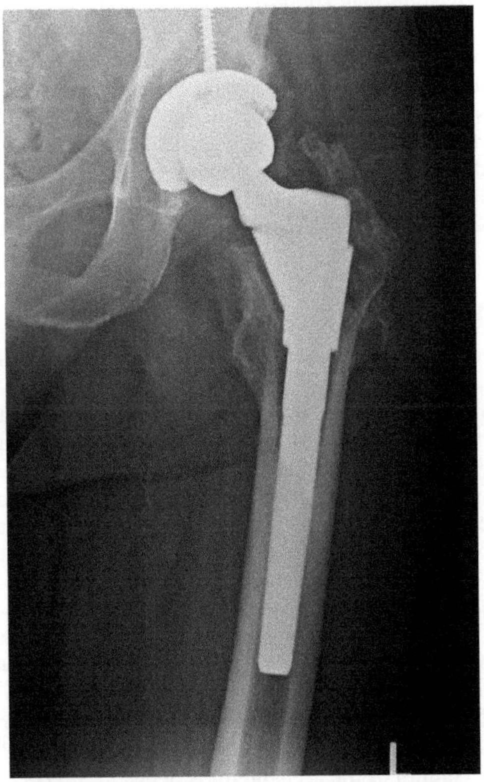

▲ **Figure 8–3.** An anteroposterior hip radiograph demonstrating a modular, press-fit hip replacement. This device has separate stem and metaphyseal components.

radiation therapy, which often destroys bone biology, inhibiting osseointegration.

D. Clinical Results

The results of THA have been very good overall. The overwhelming majority of patients are satisfied with their results, and complications generally occur in less than 5% of patients. With the advent of highly crosslinked polyethylene, wear-related osteolysis (bone destruction as a response to foreign microparticles shed from the surfaces of the prosthesis) has decreased, and wear-related component loosening is progressively decreasing as a cause for revision. The long-term survivorship of implants will likely increase.

The most common and dreaded complication is infection. Acute infections can generally be managed with debridement and antibiotics. While infection can occur anytime the skin is breached, the more common form of infection in arthroplasty is chronic. In this case, bacteria from some source (either the external world or the body itself) attach to the foreign prosthesis. These bacteria rapidly form biofilms, which are biologic scaffolds that effectively protect the bacteria from the immune system. These bacteria can then replicate safely, and a slow, progressive infection occurs. While its incidence decreases as the joint's life increases, infection is always a possibility, as hematogenous spread of bacteria never ceases lifelong. Patients are given antibiotic prophylaxis for procedures with high risk for bacteremia, such as dental procedures, for the first year or two postoperatively, and many surgeons continue prophylaxis lifelong for high-risk procedures. Chronic infection is very taxing on the patient, usually requiring prosthesis removal with possible later reimplantation, and long antibiotic regimens are often necessary for eradication.

Aseptic loosening was previously the most common reason for THA revision. The industrial process of sterilizing polyethylene in air produced free radical compounds within the material, causing oxidation and microscopic breakdown. This produced periprosthetic osteolysis via a RANKL pathway. RANKL (ligand) is secreted by osteoblasts and binds to the RANK receptor on osteoclast precursor and mature osteoclast cells stimulating osteoclastic bone resorption. In joint arthroplasty, this destroys the interface either between the bone and implant or surrounding cement. Loosening then happened mechanically.

Although hip instability is multifactorial, dislocation most commonly occurs due to component malposition or loss of abductor tension. This is managed nonoperatively with avoidance of hip positions known to elicit instability and braces and operatively with revision arthroplasty. The malposition of either the acetabular or femoral components can lead to impingement of the femoral neck on the rim of the acetabulum. This can cause levering of the head from the liner and resultant dislocation. Soft-tissue tension is obviously important. The abductor tension can be lessened due to surgical denervation, spinal problems, or tissue loss such as occurs due to metallic wear. Further, osteolysis, weakens the bone, and fracture of portions of the greater trochanter will allow the abductors to contract and lose tension. Without soft-tissue tension, even perfectly placed components can yield prosthetic dislocation. Constraint of the polyethylene liner is another option.

Other complications include deep venous thrombosis, pulmonary embolism, fracture, nerve injury, and leg length discrepancies. Prophylaxis of thromboembolic disease is oral administration of low-dose aspirin and sequential compression dressings on the legs of low-risk individuals. Those with prior deep venous thrombosis or pulmonary emboli or who are at higher risk for other reasons can usually be managed more aggressively with medications. Leg length discrepancies can be due to component malposition but may be inevitable because appropriate soft-tissue tension must be maintained for a stable hip. Patients are usually counseled regarding this preoperatively, and stable, symptomatic postoperative leg length discrepancies are managed with shoe lifts.

Cheng TE, Wallis JA, Taylor NF, et al. A prospective randomized clinical trial in total hip arthroplasty-comparing early results between the direct anterior approach and the posterior approach. *J Arthroplasty.* 2017;32(3):883-890. [PMID: 27687805]

Kiran M, Johnston LR, Sripada S, Mcleod GG, Jariwala AC. Cemented total hip replacement in patients under 55 years. *Acta Orthop.* 2018;89(2):152-155. [PMID: 29345170]

Maggs JL, Smeatham A, Whitehouse SL, Charity J, Timperley AJ, Gie GA. The Exeter contemporary flanged cemented acetabular component in primary total hip arthroplasty. *Bone Joint J.* 2016;98-B(3):307-312. [PMID: 26920954]

Meermans G, Konan S, Das R, Volpin A, Haddad FS. The direct anterior approach in total hip arthroplasty: a systematic review of the literature. *Bone Joint J.* 2017;99-B(6):732-740. [PMID: 28566391]

Miller LE, Gondusky JS, Bhattacharyya S, Kamath AF, Boettner F, Wright J. Does surgical approach affect outcomes in total hip arthroplasty through 90 days of follow-up? A systematic review with meta-analysis. *J Arthroplasty.* 2018;33(4):1296-1302. [PMID: 29195848]

Mjaaland KE, Svenningsen S, Fenstad AM, Havelin LI, Furnes O, Nordsletten L. Implant survival after minimally invasive anterior or anterolateral vs. conventional posterior or direct lateral approach: an analysis of 21,860 total hip arthroplasties from the Norwegian arthroplasty register (2008 to 2013). *J Bone Joint Surg Am.* 2017;99(10):840-847. [PMID: 28509824]

Revision Total Hip Arthroplasty

Revision THA has become substantially more common over the past 20 years. As more people are undergoing hip replacement, more are having complications necessitating revision.

A. Indications

The three most common indications for revision hip arthroplasty are infection, aseptic loosening, and hip instability, which are discussed earlier.

In contemplating hip revision, the cause of failure should be known. Attempting to revise a painful hip without accurate diagnosis will likely yield bone loss, substantial cost, and frustration of both the patient and surgeon. Having an accurate surgical plan for what needs to be removed and replaced will ease a difficult procedure.

B. Surgical Technique

Some special technical aspects need to be considered. As surgical exposure in any revision surgery is more difficult, a change in surgical approach may be warranted. Two types of trochanteric osteotomies can be considered. In a standard, transverse osteotomy, the proximal trochanter with its abductor attachment can be cut and reflected cephalad. This allows an increase in acetabular exposure, allowing specialized components to be implanted. The disadvantage to this is that the trochanteric fragment must then be stably fixed and heal. This is usually accomplished with claw plates and cables, but fixation may fail, leading to nonunion and loss of abductor tension. An extended trochanteric osteotomy can improve exposure but is generally performed to facilitate removal of the femoral prosthesis. This long, lateral osteotomy is easier to stably fix, but technically more difficult to perform without fracture. Other technical aids that should be considered preoperatively include the use of modular acetabular prosthesis augmentation and modular femoral prostheses (Figure 8–4). Both of these innovations allow for stable hip arthroplasty despite more extensive bone loss.

C. Implants

In choosing implants for revision hip replacement, careful attention should be paid to the remaining bone and soft tissues. A successful revision must yield stable implants, but also must yield a stable hip joint. For this reason, the use of specialized acetabular components is often chosen. These devices have multiple fixation points for screws, sometimes in both the dome of the component and the rim of the device. Having both types available allows orthogonal fixation of the socket within the remaining acetabulum. Certain revision components also have a "deep profile," as the acetabular center may have migrated medially. Returning it to its native location aids proper hip tensioning. Similarly, offset or thicker polyethylene liners may aid stability. Occasionally, bone loss in the acetabulum is so severe that acetabular cages or custom devices are required. These tools are useful if an entire column of the acetabulum is deficient, precluding stable acetabular cup placement. The anterior column is the anterior ilium, superior pubic ramus, anterior wall, and dome of the acetabulum. The posterior column is the greater

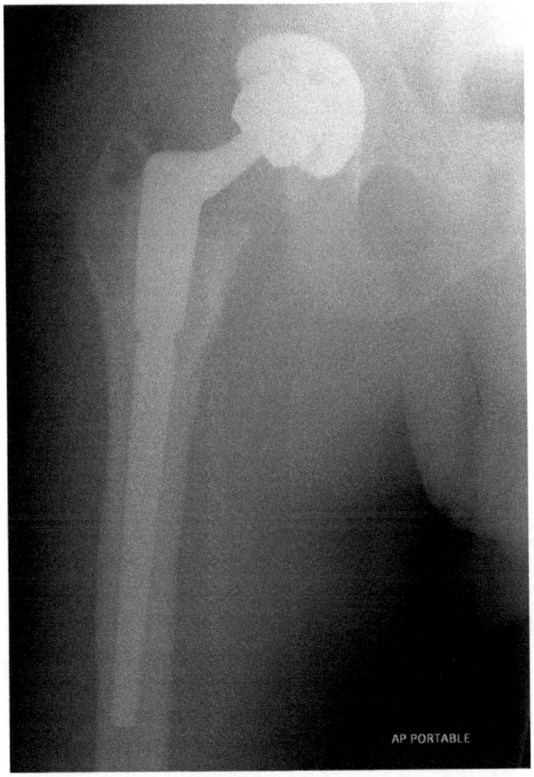

▲ **Figure 8–4.** A complex revision hip replacement. The femoral component is a modular proximal femoral replacement. A fully constrained liner is used to prevent dislocation.

and lesser sciatic notches, ischial tuberosity, posterior wall, and dome of the acetabulum. On rare occasions, custom-made "triflange" devices are used to attempt to stably fix the device to the remaining ilium, ischium, and pubis. Aside from component stability within the bone, stability of the hip joint must also be considered. While the overwhelming majority of revision surgeries can be performed using typical components, the risk of hip instability is at least an order of magnitude higher in revision than in primary THA. Various methods for coping with instability have been devised, including polyethylene liners that have elevated regions, liners that increase tension or change the angle of the hip, and liners that completely constrain the femoral head, holding it in place.

On the femoral side, revision implants were typically extensively coated, diaphyseal fit devices. These allowed for stable femoral fixation when metaphyseal bone was too deficient to support a more conventional prosthesis. There are now modular prostheses that allow a distal, diaphyseal stem to be placed with a proximal portion of variable diameter and length. This modularity aids in both prosthetic fit and hip stability. On unusual occasions, the proximal femoral bone has either fractured or is so deficient that no standard device can suffice for reconstruction. Proximal femoral replacements have been developed to replace any segment of deficient bone with a metallic prosthesis, allowing any length of bone to be removed and reconstructed (Figures 8–5 and 8–6).

D. Clinical Results

While revision hip replacement usually yields a stable, functional, pain-free reconstruction, the results lag far behind primary hip replacement, and complications are much more

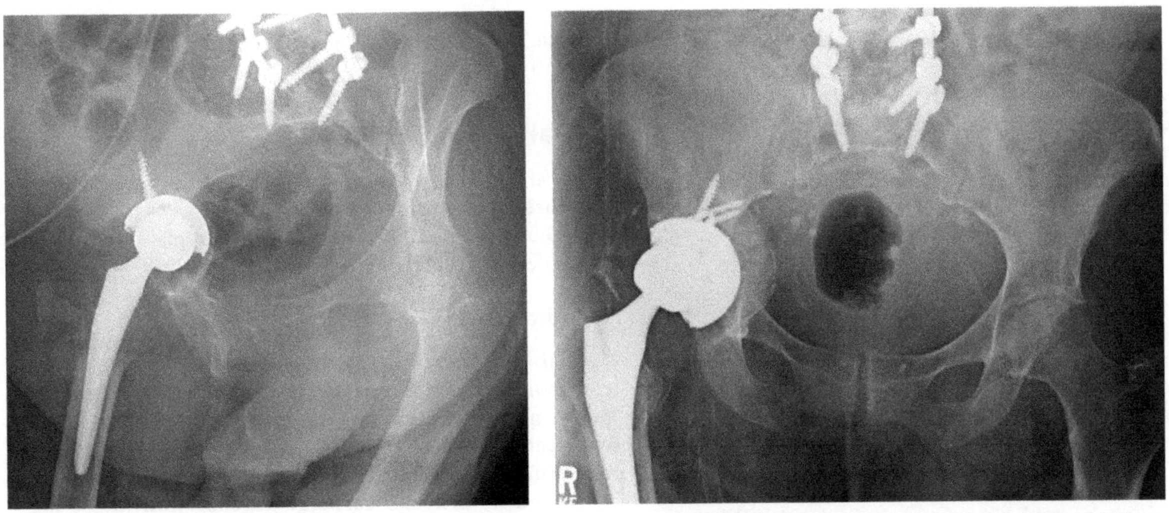

▲ **Figure 8–5.** Before and after. This patient's primary total hip arthroplasty underwent acetabular component loosening, with migration into the pelvis. This was reconstructed using a revision acetabular component with orthogonal screw fixation.

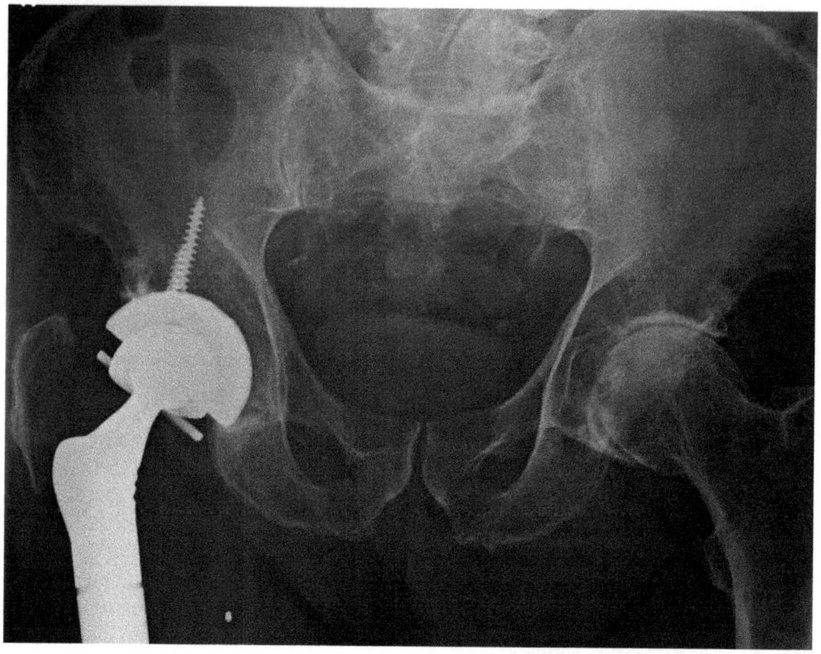

▲ **Figure 8–6.** A proximal femoral replacement done for complex hip revision. The entire proximal femur has been removed and replaced with a modular metallic prosthesis. The patient's native trochanter remains, providing a force couple between the abductors and quadriceps. Because of the innate instability of this reconstruction, a constrained acetabular liner was used.

frequent. As the volume of biological material is progressively replaced by foreign materials, the risk of infection increases, especially when the revision was done for infection. The generally stated risk of primary hip infection is slightly less than 1%. This rises to 3% to 5% in revisions and to 10% with megaprostheses. If prior infection occurred, rates as high as 50% have been recorded. The dislocation risk is also substantially higher, as more tissue needs to be removed, and the abductors are more frequently deficient. Because of this, the patient's leg more frequently needs to be lengthened for stability at the cost of a leg length discrepancy. Lastly, as more bone loss has occurred, prosthetic loosening is more frequent.

Boyer B, Bordini B, Caputo D, Neri T, Stea S, Toni A. What are the influencing factors on hip and knee arthroplasty survival? Prospective cohort study on 63619 arthroplasties. *Orthop Traumatol Surg Res.* 2019;105(7):1251-1256. [PMID: 31615748]

Fryhofer GW, Ramesh S, Sheth NP. Acetabular reconstruction in revision total hip arthroplasty. *J Clin Orthop Trauma.* 2020;11(1):22-28. [PMID: 32001979]

Gwam CU, Mistry JB, Mohamed NS, et al. Current Epidemiology of revision total hip arthroplasty in the United States: national inpatient sample 2009 to 2013. *J Arthroplasty.* 2017;32(7):2088-2092. [PMID: 28336249]

Ledford CK, Perry KI, Hanssen AD, Abdel MP. What are the contemporary etiologies for revision surgery and revision after primary, noncemented total hip arthroplasty? *J Am Acad Orthop Surg.* 2019;27(24):933-938. [PMID: 31805018]

Mehta N, Selvaratnam V, Alsousou J, Donnachie N, Carroll FA. Outcome of revision surgery in recurrent dislocation of primary total hip arthroplasty. *Hip Int.* 2020;11:1120700020911146. [PMID: 32157907]

Partial Knee Arthroplasty

There are three different compartments of the knee and partial knee replacements for each: medial unicompartmental replacements, lateral unicompartmental replacements, and patellofemoral replacements.

A. Indications

Medial unicompartmental replacements are the most common partial knee replacement (Figure 8–7). These are performed on varus knees and are an exacting procedure with careful inclusion criteria, including an intact anterior cruciate ligament (ACL), correctable varus less than 15%, and no articular cartilage degeneration in the lateral compartment and minimal to no degeneration in the patellofemoral joint. Rapid wear and failure will occur in the ACL-deficient knee.

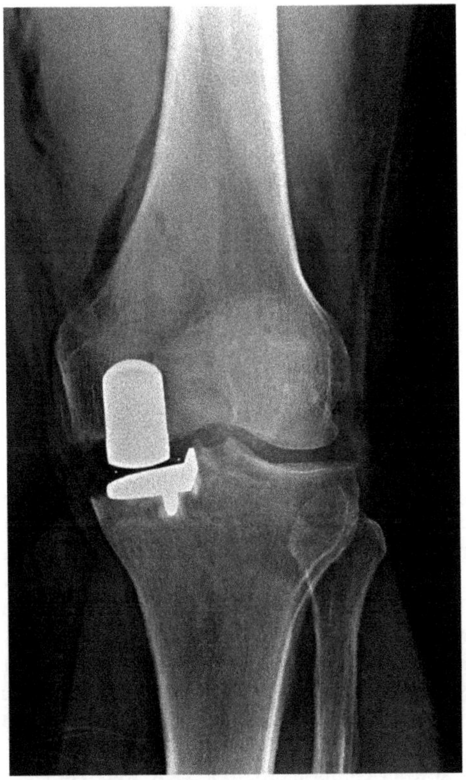

▲ **Figure 8–7.** A medial unicompartmental replacement.

Lateral unicompartmental replacements are much less common than medial, as valgus knees with isolated arthritis are uncommon. These follow the same inclusion criteria as medial unicompartmental replacements.

Patellofemoral replacements are the rarest of partial knee replacements. They should not be done for anterior knee pain unless substantial arthritis has occurred. They perform poorly when there is patellofemoral malalignment; then, a realignment procedure should be considered before contemplating arthroplasty. These replacements require full knee ROM preoperatively and are technically difficult to perform correctly.

B. Clinical Results

If the criteria for medial unicompartmental knee replacements are followed, medial unicompartmental arthroplasty should not be viewed as a bridging or temporary procedure, as patients will be unlikely to need future revision. Lateral unicompartmental knee replacements require conversion to total knee replacement more frequently than medial unicompartmental knee replacements. Patellofemoral replacements have a very mixed record of success. The first reason for this is a poor indication: anterior knee pain without arthritis is not an indication for patellofemoral replacement and replacement results are poor. A second major contraindication to patellofemoral replacement is patellar maltracking. If this is the primary symptom, a patellar realignment procedure (such as a tibial tubercle osteotomy or soft-tissue realignment) should be considered. Patellofemoral replacements should only be used in patients with end-stage degenerative joint disease, normal patellofemoral alignment, and an absence of arthritis in the other compartments of the knee.

Fiocchi A, Condello V, Madonna V, Bonomo M, Zorzi C. Medial vs lateral unicompartmental knee arthrroplasty: clinical results. *Acta Biomed.* 2017;88(2S):38-44. [PMID: 28657563]

Heaps BM, Blevins JL, Chiu YF, Konopka JF, Patel SP, McLawhorn AS. Improving estimates of annual survival rates for medial unicompartmental knee arthroplasty: a meta-analysis. *J Arthroplasty.* 2019;34(7):1538-1545. [PMID: 30954408]

Johal S, Nakano N, Baxter M, Hujazi I, Pandit H, Khanduja V. Unicompartmental knee arthroplasty: the past, current controversies, and future perspectives. *J Knee Surg.* 2018;3 1(10):992-998. [PMID: 29514367]

Mohammad HR, Strickland L, Hamilton TW, Murray DW. Long-term outcomes of over 8,000 medial Oxford phase 3 unicompartmental knees: a systematic review. *Acta Orthop.* 2018;89(1):101-107. [PMID: 28831821]

Remy F. Surgical technique in patellofemoral arthroplasty. *Orthop Traumatol Surg Res.* 2019;105(1S):S165-S176. [PMID: 30635231]

Total Knee Arthroplasty

Total knee arthroplasty (TKA) has also been extraordinarily successful. Crippling arthritis that formerly inhibited ambulation can now be treated with reconstruction, restoring the patients to function. Technically more difficult to do well than total hip replacements, knee replacements have changed substantially over the past four decades and are now one of the most popular procedures in orthopedic surgery.

A. Indications

Knee replacements are generally done for osteoarthritis of the knee. As opposed to partial knee replacements, total knee replacements can be performed for arthritis in multiple compartments and can be used to correct severe deformities. Other indications for total knee replacements include inflammatory and posttraumatic arthritides.

B. Surgical Technique

The surgical technique for knee replacement is more exacting than that of hip replacement. Care must be taken to preserve not only the extensor mechanism, but also the ligaments within the knee so that appropriate balancing can occur.

Multiple techniques exist for surgical exposure through the extensor mechanism. Overwhelmingly, the most common approach is the medial parapatellar approach, where the retinaculum is incised just medial to the patella. This allows complete joint visualization via a more moderately sized incision. Some surgeons will perform a lateral parapatellar approach in valgus knees, which is a slightly more demanding technique. Various midvastus and subvastus approaches also exist. A midvastus approach splits the medial quadriceps, preserving the entire quadriceps tendon. While interesting in its tendinous preservation, it is associated with increased bleeding postoperatively. Subvastus approaches preserve the entire quadriceps mechanism, allowing the knee replacement to be performed without altering the extensor mechanism. These approaches require much larger skin exposures to enable mobilization of the entire quadriceps mechanism.

Once the knee is entered, osteophytes, the infrapatellar fat pad, and the anterior menisci are removed. In a varus knee, the approach is carried around to the posteromedial corner, taking down the capsule while preserving the entire medial collateral ligament (MCL). This allows varus deformity correction. In a valgus knee, much of this capsule is left intact, and instead, the iliotibial band and lateral capsule are released. A decision must then be made regarding whether to preserve the posterior cruciate ligament (PCL). Nearly all knee replacements excise the ACL, but the PCL can often be retained. Another option is to remove it and substitute a PCL femoral design. Generally, the PCL is removed in situations of severe deformity to allow for better correction.

Once the soft-tissue releases have been completed, bony cuts can be made. The tibia is generally cut perpendicular to the anatomic axis of the tibia. Femoral cuts are made on the anterior and posterior condylar surfaces, allowing the creation of a flexion gap between the cut tibia and posterior femur. A distal femoral cut is also made, which creates an extension gap. These two gaps should be made to precisely match the inner surface of the chosen femoral component. The tibia is prepared by drilling into the metaphysis and often has a keel punched to create rotational stability. The patellar articular surface may also be removed if patellar resurfacing is desired.

Trial components are then placed within the knee, and the balance, ROM, stability, and patellar tracking are assessed. If these are judged to be appropriate, the final components are placed. Traditionally, all components were cemented into place using PMMA. Some newer designs allow all components to be press fit, with ingrowth surfaces for osseointegration (Figure 8–8).

C. Implants

The majority of TKAs retain both the medial and lateral collateral ligaments and remove the ACL and PCL. These *cruciate-sacrificing or -substituting* styles often have a polyethylene liner with a post between the femoral condyles to provide for the lack of cruciate ligaments. A *cruciate-retaining* TKA lacks that component stability because the patient's own PCL is retained. *Resurfacing hinge* knees have a mobile bearing mechanical hinge construct. These knees are generally used only when correction of deformity requires the sacrifice of the MCL or in cases where stability cannot be achieved using the patient's own collateral ligaments.

Traditionally, all components in a TKA were cemented into position using PMMA cement (Figure 8–9). Later designs allowed for a femoral component that was press fit onto the distal femur, having a surface for osseointegration.

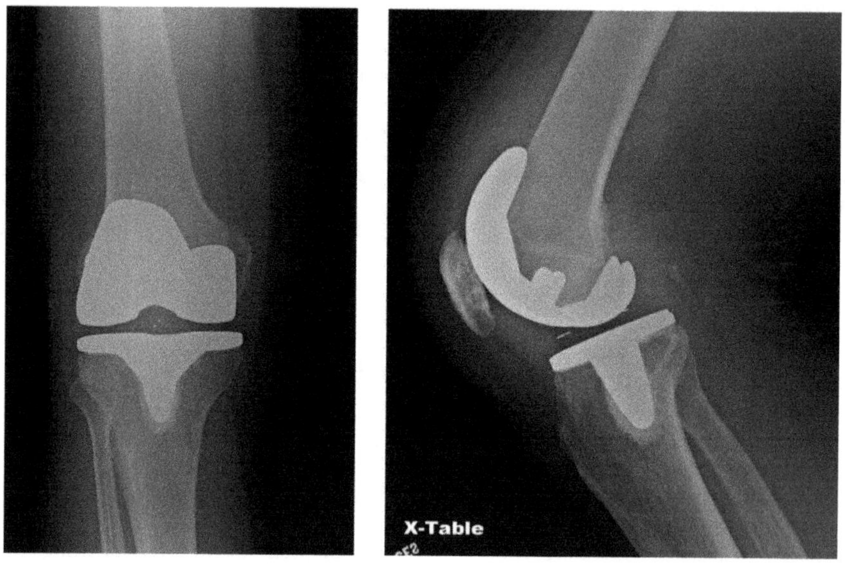

▲ **Figure 8–8.** Anteroposterior and lateral views of a cruciate-excising total knee replacement. The femoral component is press fit, and the tibial component is inserted with cement.

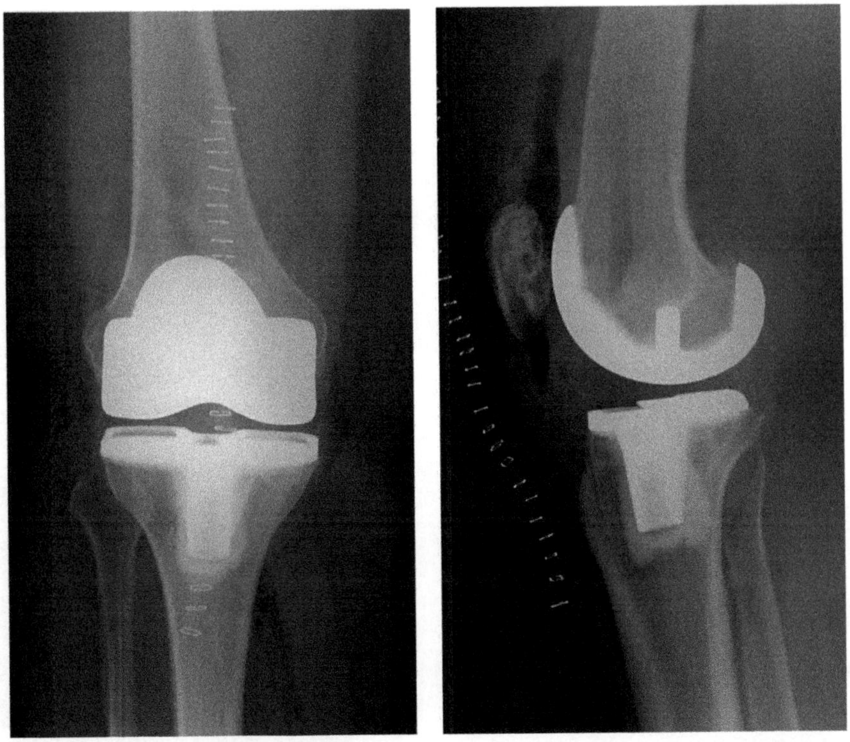

▲ **Figure 8–9.** Anteroposterior and lateral views of a fully cemented, cruciate-substituting total knee arthroplasty.

More recently, the tibial component was also modified to have press-fit/osseointegration fixation. One further choice is whether to resurface the patella. Patellar resurfacing versus leaving the native patellar articulation shows wide regional variations, with some surgeons routinely using press fit/osseointegration or cementing a patellar component in place after patellar articular surface resection has been performed and others never adding this component.

D. Clinical Results

Overall, the results of total knee replacement are very good. The majority of patients who undergo this procedure report improvements in pain, function, and quality of life. Most are able to rejoin daily and recreational activities previously too painful for them to perform. The biggest difficulty most patients have is regaining knee ROM. This is best attained with rigorous attention to detail in surgery and extensive rehabilitation. Because this recovery is painful, patients who present with poor motion "due to pain" are sometimes disappointed in their progress because they do not put in the effort needed for maximum knee flexion. Due to the mechanical constraints of TKA prostheses, few patients regain the same motion they had before becoming arthritic. Attaining a flexion greater than 115 degrees allows patients to sit in confined spaces, such as airplanes, and to ascend and descend stairs normally.

Although it is an excellent function-restoring procedure, TKA is not without complications. The most common serious complication is infection. As in other arthroplasties, infection after TKA is divided into acute or chronic infections. Acute infections occur at the time of surgery and may be amenable to debridement and antibiotic treatment if caught quickly. Chronic infections, however, are often hematogenous and present with a slow decrease in function with increasing pain. These infections are generally not amenable to simple debridement, and removal of the infected prosthesis, known as explantation either with immediate replantation (one-stage revision) or use of an antibiotic-laden spacer and later replantation (two-stage revision), is often necessary. Other common complications of TKA include thromboembolic disease and poor motion. In low-risk patients, thromboembolic prophylaxis can usually be done using oral administration of low-dose aspirin and sequential compression devices on the legs. Those with prior deep venous thrombosis or pulmonary embolism or who are at higher risk for other reasons can usually be managed more aggressively with medications.

Allen W, Eichinger J, Friedman R. Resurfaced versus non-resurfaced patella in total knee arthroplasty. *J Knee Surg.* 2019;32(7):611-615. [PMID: 30812045]

Assiotis A, To K, Morgan-Jones R, Pengas IP, Khan W. Patellar complications following total knee arthroplasty: a review of the current literature. *Eur J Orthop Surg Traumatol.* 2019;29(8):1605-1615. [PMID: 31302764]

Canovas F, Dagneaux L. Quality of life after total knee arthroplasty. *Orthop Traumatol Surg Res.* 2018;104(1S):S41-S46. [PMID: 29183821]

Gehrke T, Alijanipour P, Parvizi J. The management of an infected total knee arthroplasty. *Bone Joint J.* 2015;97-B(10 Suppl A):20-29. [PMID: 26430083]

Gunaratne R, Pratt DN, Banda J, Fick DP, Khan RJK, Robertson BW. Patient dissatisfaction following total knee arthroplasty: a systematic review of the literature. *J Arthroplasty.* 2017;32(12):3854-3860. [PMID: 28844632]

Longo UG, Ciuffreda M, Mannering N, et al. Outcomes of posterior-stabilized compared with cruciate-retaining total knee arthroplasty. *J Knee Surg.* 2018;31(4):321-340. [PMID: 28666292]

Wilson DG, Poole WE, Chauhan SK, Rogers BA. Systematic review of aspirin for thromboprophylaxis in modern elective total hip and knee arthroplasty. *Bone Joint J.* 2016;98-B(8):1056-1061. [PMID: 27482017]

Revision Total Knee Arthroplasty

Revision total knee replacement is a technically difficult procedure, and its necessity is unfortunately increasing.

A. Indications and Surgical Technique

The most common indication for revision TKA is infection. In the majority of circumstances, a two-stage revision, where the prior prosthesis is removed for some length of time and a new prosthesis is later inserted, is the most common method of treating this infection (Figure 8–10). The use of two-stage revision for infected TKA is generally effective but can compromise both the remaining bone and the soft tissues, as every surgery requires soft tissues to be manipulated and some bone is generally lost. Other indications for revision TKA are aseptic loosening (which also causes bone loss) and instability.

Instability can either be knee joint instability or patellofemoral instability. The etiology of knee joint instability is a flexion-extension mismatch; the space between the femur and tibia is different with the knee in full extension versus 90 degrees of flexion. This produces a knee that "feels loose" to the patient, causing pain, anxiety, and potential falls. Correcting a flexion-extension mismatch generally requires revising either the femoral component alone or both components. In severe cases, a hinge knee may be necessary if the mismatch cannot be resolved or the MCL is deficient. Patellofemoral instability causes anterior knee pain, limitations of flexion, and occasionally patellar dislocation. This is due to malrotation of the femoral and/or tibial components. Component revision is generally required unless a known soft-tissue problem allows soft-tissue reconstruction without revision.

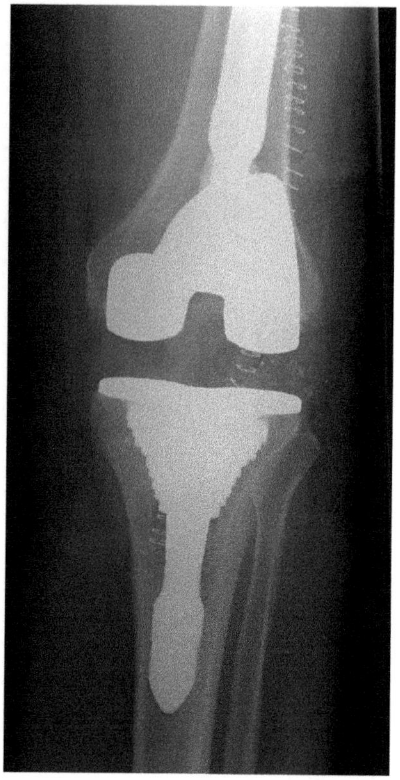

▲ **Figure 8–10.** A revision total knee arthroplasty demonstrating press-fit stems and a press-fit tibial sleeve for metaphyseal fixation.

With regard to soft tissue problems, two are of special note. The first is MCL deficiency, which has previously been discussed. This is higher risk in the revision setting (the MCL may tear off as exposure can be difficult) and often mandates the use of a hinge prosthesis. A second, more serious complication is extensor mechanism disruption. Because a knee without active extension is not functional, this can become a complication that is insurmountable. Because of the scar tissue that forms within a knee, extensive removal can cause either the quadriceps or patellar tendons to tear. To reduce this risk, a *quadriceps snip* may relieve pressure on these tissues and allow the patient to immediately rehabilitate the knee. A more extensive *V-Y turndown* or *tibial tubercle osteotomy* can have similar protective benefits but delays rehabilitation and may permanently reduce function.

B. Implants

Revision TKA systems generally have modular components that allow bone loss to be addressed. These can include diaphyseal stems to help support the prosthesis on compromised bone, metaphyseal cones or sleeves to utilize the remaining metaphyseal bone, and augments for the epiphyseal bone

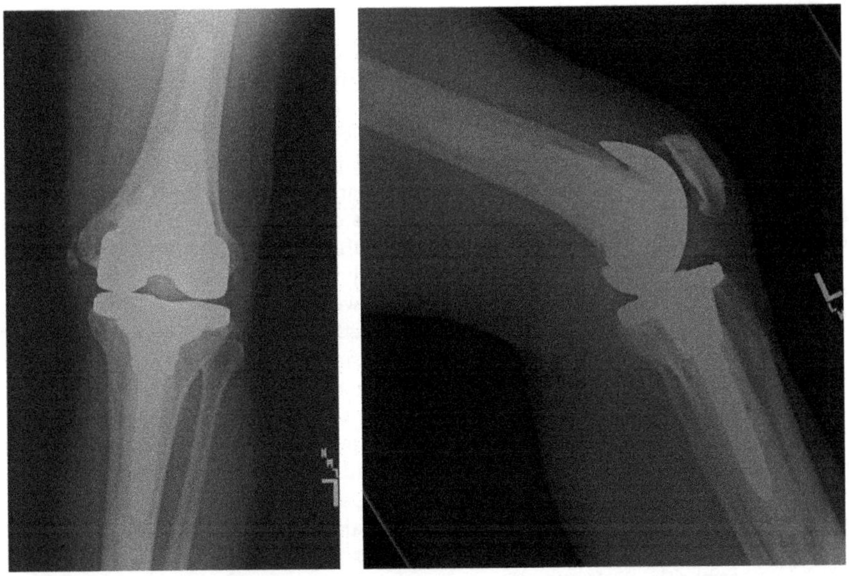

▲ **Figure 8–11.** Anteroposterior and lateral views of a revision total knee arthroplasty demonstrating cemented stems and press-fit tibial and femoral cones for metaphyseal fixation.

(Figures 8–11 and 8–12). These additions are often used in combinations to yield a stable construct. Stems can be either inserted with PMMA or press fit into the metadiaphyseal or diaphyseal bone. Cone or sleeve constructs are press fit into the metaphysis to allow biologic fixation.

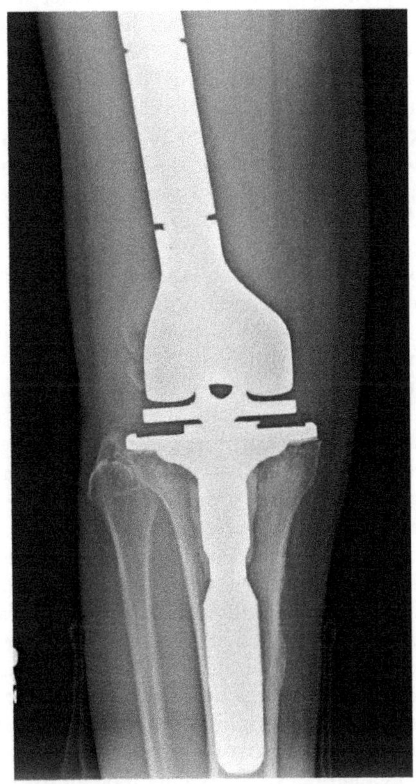

▲ **Figure 8–12.** A modular distal femoral replacement performed for extensive bone loss.

C. Clinical Results

Overall, the results of revision TKA are acceptable but are statistically inferior to primary TKA in most respects. The rate of reinfection, even after two-stage revision, is higher than that of primary TKA. This is organism dependent: Revisions for methicillin-resistant *Staphylococcus aureus* infections have a decreased cure rate than those for more sensitive organisms. Revisions for loosening or instability also have higher failure rates than in primary surgeries.

Complications for revision TKA are similar to those of primary TKA but occur more frequently. Instability and extensor mechanism problems are relatively rare in primary TKA and assume much more prominence in a revision setting due to soft-tissue compromise from multiple surgeries.

Assiotis A, To K, Morgan-Jones R, Pengas IP, Khan W. Patellar complications following total knee arthroplasty: a review of the current literature. *Eur J Orthop Surg Traumatol.* 2019;29(8):1605-1615. [PMID: 31302764]

Chen MJ, Hung JF, Chang CH, Lee SH, Shih HN, Chang YH. Periprosthetic knee infection reconstruction with a hinged prosthesis: implant survival and risk factors for treatment failure. *Knee.* 2020;27(3):1035-1042. [PMID: 32317140]

Delanois RE, Mistry JB, Gwam CU, Mohamed NS, Choksi US, Mont MA. Current epidemiology of revision total knee arthroplasty in the United States. *J Arthroplasty.* 2017;32(9):2663-2668. [PMID: 28456561]

Lei PF, Hu RY, Hu YH. Bone defects in revision total knee arthroplasty and management. *Orthop Surg.* 2019;11(1):15-24. [PMID: 30809942]

Zanirato A, Formica M, Cavagnaro L, Divano S, Burastero G, Felli L. Metaphyseal cones and sleeves in revision total knee arthroplasty: two sides of the same coin? Complications, clinical and radiological results-a systematic review of the literature. *Musculoskelet Surg.* 2020;104(1):25-35. [PMID: 30879231]

Total Shoulder Arthroplasty

A. Indications

The primary indication for shoulder arthroplasty is persistent pain resulting from the loss of articular cartilage and incongruent joint surfaces (ie, arthritis) that has failed nonsurgical management. The most common etiologies are osteoarthritis, rheumatoid osteoarthritis, posttraumatic arthritis, and cuff arthropathy. Shoulder arthroplasty is also done for severe comminuted proximal humeral fractures, especially in the elderly. Both total shoulder arthroplasty and hemiarthroplasty diminish pain. Total shoulder arthroplasty results in better pain relief than hemiarthroplasty. Hemiarthroplasty can be done with either a traditional stemmed humeral prosthesis or a humeral resurfacing prosthesis with similar outcomes. Less bone is removed with a humeral resurfacing prosthesis, but there are indications for a stemmed humeral prosthesis such as when humeral head bone loss prevents the resurfacing prosthesis from being well secured. Another reason that a hemiarthroplasty is done rather than a total shoulder arthroplasty is when there is significant erosion of the glenoid, such as beyond the base of the coracoids, that prevents the glenoid component from being secured. This can occur in osteoarthritis but is more common in rheumatoid osteoarthritis.

Decision-making in shoulder arthroplasty depends on many factors, including the integrity of the rotator cuff and the condition of the articular surfaces and the underlying bone, specifically the glenoid. Total shoulder arthroplasty, where the glenoid and humerus are replaced to simulate the normal anatomy, is not indicated in those with arthritis and who also have a torn rotator cuff that cannot be repaired at surgery. Most commonly, this is encountered in a patient who has tolerated a rotator cuff tear for many years and developed arthritis as a result. This occurs as the humerus comes to be positioned superior on the glenoid and the normal compression of the humeral head into the concavity of the glenoid, termed concavity compression, is lost. In the past, the resurfacing the glenoid with a glenoid prosthesis had unacceptably high rates of loosening thought to result from eccentric loading and a "rocking-horse effect." Shoulder instability is not usually corrected by anatomic total shoulder arthroplasty alone. In other words, a shoulder with intact articular surfaces that persistently dislocates will often dislocate after shoulder arthroplasty. This is because the total shoulder arthroplasty can correct damage to the articular surfaces but does not correct damage to the capsulolabrum.

The combination of a severe rotator cuff tear, joint osteoarthritis, and superior position of the humeral head on the glenoid is called cuff tear arthropathy and is usually associated with poor shoulder function. Surprisingly, there are some individuals with cuff arthropathy who have full ROM and little weakness. In these patients, a shoulder hemiarthroplasty is effective in diminishing pain. However, when the shoulder function is poor such that the individual is unable to lift the arm against gravity, termed "pseudoparalysis," a reverse total shoulder prosthesis is best. With this design, the socket is placed on the humerus, and the ball is placed on the glenoid. This not only diminishes pain but also improves function postoperatively.

Contraindications to shoulder arthroplasty include infection, neuropathic arthropathy, and the absence of a functional deltoid.

B. Surgical Technique

A deltopectoral surgical approach is performed, with careful retraction of the conjoined tendon medially to avoid injury to the musculocutaneous nerve. Current techniques of anatomic total shoulder arthroplasty require the subscapularis tendon to be detached, and this can be done in three different manners: incision of the tendon 1 cm lateral to the insertion, peeling the tendon off the lesser tuberosity, or detaching the tendon with osteotomy of the lesser tuberosity. Because there is often loss of external rotation motion in patients with shoulder arthroplasty, the subscapularis can be lengthened by attaching the tendon more medially on the lesser tuberosity. Likewise, a coronal Z-plasty of the tendon can be done to increase external rotation afterward. Many surgeons choose to incise the biceps tendon at the supraglenoid tubercle (ie, biceps tenotomy) to improve exposure. It can be tenodesed at the end if the surgeon chooses. The axillary nerve is palpated or exposed along the inferior border of the subscapularis to avoid injury. The anterior and inferior capsule is incised, and some surgeons choose to resect it to improve ROM in external rotation. The humeral head is dislocated anteriorly with extension and external rotation of the arm and is delivered out of the wound. The humeral head is osteotomized at the head–neck junction, while the remainder of the rotator cuff insertions remain intact. Preparation of the humeral intramedullary canal is followed by insertion of a trial stemmed humeral component to match the normal, about 30 degrees of retroversion. Attention then moves to the glenoid. The humeral stem may be left in place to tamponade bleeding and to diminish the chances of the humerus being damaged during glenoid preparation. The humerus is displaced posteriorly using a humeral head retractor for exposure of the glenoid.

Motorized reamers or a burr is used to remove a small amount of bone so that bleeding cortical bone remains for support of the glenoid component. With osteoarthritis, there is often posterior glenoid wear, and when mild, more anterior than posterior bone can be removed to restore normal glenoid version and provide an optimal surface for implanting the glenoid component. When larger, the posterior glenoid bone defect can be filled with a glenoid component that is thicker posterior than anterior. Using cement to fill a posterior glenoid defect is not recommended. Some surgeons have had success with bone grafts. Depending on the prosthesis to be used, holes are then drilled or a keel is burred for implantation of a cemented, all-polyethene glenoid component. Keeping the glenoid bone as dry as possible during cementing is a challenge. The appropriate diameter and thickness of the humeral head are then determined, and head components are trialed. The humeral component can be implanted with or without cement, and the subscapularis tendon is repaired. A biceps tenodesis may be done at this time as well. It is best to check that the axillary nerve is intact, and this can be done by palpating or exposing it again along the inferior border of the subscapularis and doing a tug test. This is done by the surgeon putting a finger laterally in the subdeltoid space and feeling for the branch of the axillary nerve while placing the other finger medially under the axillary nerve where it lies along the inferior border of the subscapularis. A gentle tug on the nerve with the subdeltoid finger is transmitted across the nerve and felt with the other finger.

C. Implants

There are four types of shoulder arthroplasty: humeral resurfacing hemiarthroplasty with either a very small stem or no stem at all, stemmed hemiarthroplasty, total shoulder arthroplasty, and reverse total shoulder arthroplasty.

Hemiarthroplasty can be done with a humeral resurfacing prosthesis that has survivorship similar to stemmed hemiarthroplasty. Humeral resurfacing prostheses necessitate sufficient humeral head bone stock for reaming and implantation. When there is severe humeral head deformity from large osteochondral lesions or sequelae of severe humeral head fractures, for example, resection of the humeral head and implantation with a stemmed hemiarthroplasty are best. Also, in the hands of most surgeons, the humeral resurfacing prosthesis does not allow adequate exposure for a glenoid component to be implanted.

Anatomic total shoulder arthroplasties have nonconstrained surfaces and stemmed humeral components. These prosthetic designs incorporate modular components and sufficient sizes to accommodate differences in anatomy found in the general population. Humeral stems are usually cementless designs. The glenoid components are all-polyethene and are pegged or keeled for cemented implantation. Some have metal pegs for ingrowth as well. Uncemented, metal-backed glenoid prostheses have failed at high rates.

In reverse total shoulder arthroplasty, the socket is placed on the humerus and the ball is placed on the glenoid, so that the surfaces are more constrained than in anatomic total shoulder arthroplasty. The glenoid components have cementless designs, and the humeral stem comes in both cemented and uncemented designs.

D. Clinical Results

Outcomes in survivorship and pain relief after shoulder arthroplasty are similar to those after hip and knee arthroplasty. Survivorship after reverse total shoulder arthroplasty that is done for cuff tear arthropathy, osteoarthritis, and irreparable rotator cuff tears without osteoarthritis is nearly or as good as that for anatomic total shoulder arthroplasty. Total shoulder arthroplasty alleviates about 90% of pain. There is not as much pain relief with hemiarthroplasty; pain is diminished by about two-thirds. Although easier for the surgeon to perform, surprisingly, revision is more common after hemiarthroplasty done for glenohumeral osteoarthritis than total shoulder arthroplasty. Primarily for this reason, hemiarthroplasty may not be as cost-effective as total shoulder arthroplasty. Outcomes after shoulder arthroplasty are similar for patients with osteoarthritis and rheumatoid arthritis.

Results after shoulder arthroplasty are not as good in younger patients as in the elderly. There are many possible reasons for this, but most likely, higher activity demands, higher expectations, and posttraumatic etiologies in younger patients result in less satisfactory results.

Improvements in function after shoulder arthroplasty are not as good as relief of pain. The best predictors of ROM and strength after shoulder arthroplasty are the ROM and strength present before surgery. Mild to moderate gains can be expected, but the patient with poor ROM and strength is likely to have persistent deficits postoperatively. Better improvements in ROM and strength can be expected in the patient with cuff arthropathy and pseudoparalysis who undergoes reverse total shoulder arthroplasty. Then, restoration of about two-thirds of normal ROM and strength in elevation is common.

Complications after shoulder arthroplasty are equal to or less than after hip or knee arthroplasty. Today, the most common "complication" of shoulder arthroplasty is a rotator cuff tear. This occurs because rotator cuff tears are common in patients in this age group; having had a shoulder arthroplasty does not diminish the chances of a rotator cuff tear occurring. Another complication is aseptic loosening, which occurs more commonly at the glenoid than the humeral prosthesis. Radiolucent lines occur around the all-polyethene glenoid component and depend on the type of prosthesis. It is more common in keeled than pegged designs. Radiolucent lines at the glenoid component are much more common than the rate of revision. Less common complications include fracture, nerve injury, instability, venous thrombosis, pulmonary emboli, and infection. Infection may be less than that after hip and knee arthroplasty (<0.5%) and may be due to the excellent blood supply and musculature surrounding the joint. Acromion fractures are a complication specific to reverse total shoulder arthroplasty, and other complications such as dislocation and heterotopic bone are higher than in anatomic total shoulder arthroplasty. Complications are higher for revision than primary shoulder arthroplasty.

Contraindications to total shoulder arthroplasty include active shoulder infection, poor bone stock that precludes fixation of the prosthesis, absence of deltoid function, and neuropathic arthropathy as occurs, for example, with a cervical syrinx.

Cuff DJ, Pupello DR, Santoni BG, Clark RE, Frankle MA. Reverse shoulder arthroplasty for the treatment of rotator cuff deficiency: a concise follow-up, at a minimum of 10 years, of previous reports. *J Bone Joint Surg Am.* 2017;99(22):1895-1899. [PMID: 29135662]

Deshmukh AV, Koris M, Zurakowski D, Thornhill TS. Total shoulder arthroplasty: long-term survivorship, functional outcome, and quality of life. *J Shoulder Elbow Surg.* 2005;14(5):471-479. [PMID: 16194737]

Hernandez NM, Chalmers BP, Wagner ER, Sperling JW, Cofield RH, Sanchez-Sotelo J. Revision to reverse total shoulder arthroplasty restores stability for patients with unstable shoulder prostheses. *Clin Orthop Relat Res.* 2017;475(11):2716-2722. [PMID: 28849539]

Neyton L, Kirsch JM, Collotte P, et al. Mid- to long-term follow-up of shoulder arthroplasty for primary glenohumeral osteoarthritis in patients aged 60 or under. *J Shoulder Elbow Surg.* 2019;28(9):1666-1673. [PMID: 31202630]

Nicholson GP. In older patients with proximal humeral fractures, reverse shoulder arthroplasty and nonoperative treatment did not differ for overall function or quality of life at 12 months. *J Bone Joint Surg Am.* 2020;102(10):906. [PMID: 32251140]

Sandow MJ, Tu CG. Porous metal wedge augments to address glenoid retroversion in anatomic shoulder arthroplasty: midterm update. *J Shoulder Elbow Surg.* 2020;29(9):1821-1830. [PMID: 32305149]

van Ochten JHM, van der Pluijm M, Pouw M, Felsch QTM, Heesterbeek P, de Vos MJ. Long-term survivorship and clinical and radiological follow-up of the primary uncemented Delta III reverse shoulder prosthesis. *J Orthop.* 2019;16(4):342-346. [PMID: 30996563]

Total Elbow Arthroplasty

A. Indications

Like other arthroplasties, the main indication for total elbow arthroplasty is persistent pain resulting from the loss of articular cartilage and incongruent joint surfaces (ie, arthritis) that has failed nonsurgical management. Etiologies include rheumatoid arthritis, osteoarthritis, and post-traumatic arthritis. However, total elbow arthroplasty is also done for distal humeral nonunions and severe comminuted distal humeral fractures, especially in the elderly. For young active patients, especially those with limited elbow motion, debridement using either an arthroscopic or open technique or interpositional arthroplasty may be best. However, it should be remembered that these are salvage procedures because they neither eliminate pain nor restore full function and are not indicated in those with preoperative instability. These procedures are for patients who are not ready to accept the limitations of a total elbow arthroplasty. Results after total elbow arthroplasty are best in elderly patients and those with rheumatoid arthritis, in part because these individuals are happy to once again use their elbows for activities of daily living.

B. Surgical Technique

Attention to the soft tissue, including the triceps insertion, collateral ligaments, and the ulnar nerve, is essential during total elbow arthroplasty. The Bryan posteromedial approach is often used for implantation of semiconstrained devices. The surgical plane is between the medial triceps and forearm flexors proximally and between the flexor carpi ulnaris and flexor carpi radialis distally. This allows direct visualization of the ulnar nerve and facilitates transposition of the nerve. With this approach, total elbow arthroplasty can be done without detachment of the triceps. Release of the collateral ligaments is required. Because integrity of the collateral ligaments is vital when a nonconstrained device is used, the Kocher posterolateral approach may be best because it allows preservation of the ulnar collateral ligament. This ligament provides the major restraint against valgus forces in the flexed elbow. The surgical plane is between the anconeus and extensor carpi ulnaris muscles distally and proximally between the triceps and brachioradialis muscles. The direct posterior approach can also be used but requires dissection of the posterior skin from the underlying tissue and detachment of the triceps tendon. Careful soft-tissue handling, especially when elevating the triceps from its insertion on the olecranon so that it remains in continuity with the forearm fascia, and then repair of the triceps tendon afterward are essential to avoid skin necrosis and weakness of the triceps muscle. A third possible approach is to use the triceps tongue technique. In this approach, a U- or V-shaped incision is made in the triceps tendon with its apex proximally. This allows the entire triceps enthesis to remain on the ulna. Dissection medially and laterally allows the collateral ligaments to be released, facilitating elbow exposure.

C. Implants

Total elbow arthroplasty designs have less constraint, permitting more normal elbow kinematics than in the past. Both unconstrained and semiconstrained prostheses diminish pain, and complications are similar. The two currently available types of total elbow arthroplasty include semiconstrained and resurfacing nonconstrained prostheses. Semiconstrained prostheses have stems on both the humerus and the ulna and a linked hinge that provides stability. Excision of the radial head is usual during implantation. They are not a simple hinge and, instead, have been called a "sloppy hinge" by some, hence their name *semiconstrained*. This lessened constraint has resulted in much better survivorship; highly constrained total elbow arthroplasty prostheses failed due to loosening. Dislocation is not a concern with semiconstrained prostheses. Semiconstrained prostheses are best when there is instability or loss of bone stock. In theory, nonconstrained implants load the prosthesis less and yield less aseptic loosening, but because there is much less stability from the prosthesis, they should not be used when there is ligamentous instability or loss of bone stock.

Radial head prostheses have long been available for severe fractures of the radial head. They may also be an aid in providing stability in the elbow with a comminuted radial head fracture. Short-term results are excellent and remain good over 10 years, although arthritis of the capitellum, radiolucencies along the stem, poor return to sports, and other problems occur; long-term follow-up is needed. Hemiarthroplasty is available, and early outcomes are encouraging for severe fractures of the distal humerus but less so for osteoarthritis.

D. Clinical Results

Total elbow arthroplasty has survivorship that may be as high as 85% at 10 years, but patient selection, compliance, and age are critical factors to success. In patients who have had a total elbow arthroplasty for posttraumatic arthritis, failure is much more common. Failure is also more common in younger patients, under 65 years of age. Outcome is similar in elderly patients who have had total elbow arthroplasty for treatment of osteoarthritis and rheumatoid osteoarthritis. Total elbow arthroplasty reliably improves functional ROM and strength in most patients. Even in those with ankylosis after posttraumatic arthritis, improvements of about 80 degrees of ROM occur in the flexion and extension arc.

Complications are more common than with other total joint arthroplasties, and the short-term complication rate (within the first year) may be as high as 10%. Complications include aseptic loosening, joint instability, fracture, ulnar neuropathy, wound complications, venous thrombosis, pulmonary emboli, and infection. Ulnar neuropathies do not usually require an additional procedure, paresthesias are usually transient, and motor weakness is rare. Many patients with rheumatoid arthritis have ulnar neuropathy before surgery, and the total elbow arthroplasty may not have contributed significantly to postoperative symptoms. Aseptic loosening, metallosis, severe wear of the polyethylene bushing in semiconstrained devices, instability in nonconstrained devices, and infection are reasons for revision. For aseptic loosening, revision with a longer stemmed prosthesis usually suffices. Impaction bone grafting into the endosteal canal of the distal humerus or proximal ulna is also an option. Polyethylene bushing wear is diagnosed from diminished space between the humeral and ulnar components on radiographs.

Contraindications to total elbow arthroplasty include active shoulder infection, poor bone stock that precludes fixation of the prosthesis, neuropathic arthropathy as occurs for example with a cervical syrinx, and the absence of biceps and triceps function.

Carbonell-Escobar R, Vaquero-Picado A, Barco R, Antuña S. Neurologic complications after surgical management of complex elbow trauma requiring radial head replacement. *J Shoulder Elbow Surg*. 2020;29(6):1282-1288. [PMID: 32284308]

Chang N, King GJW. Elbow hemiarthroplasty for the treatment of distal humerus fractures. *Orthop Clin North Am*. 2020;51(2):265-277. [PMID: 32138864]

Krukhaug Y, Hallan G, Dybvik E, Lie SA, Furnes ON. A survivorship study of 838 total elbow replacements: a report from the Norwegian Arthroplasty Register 1994-2016. *J Shoulder Elbow Surg*. 2018;27(2):260-269. [PMID: 29332662]

Lott A, Broder K, Goch A, Konda SR, Egol KA. Results after radial head arthroplasty in unstable fractures. *J Shoulder Elbow Surg*. 2018;27(2):270-275. [PMID: 29332663]

Siala M, Laumonerie P, Hedjoudje A, Delclaux S, Bonnevialle N, Mansat P. Outcomes of semiconstrained total elbow arthroplasty performed for arthritis in patients under 55 years old. *J Shoulder Elbow Surg*. 2020;29(4):859-866. [PMID: 31629652]

Werthel JD, Schoch B, Adams J, Steinmann S. Outcomes after hemiarthroplasty of the elbow for the management of posttraumatic arthritis: minimum 2-year follow-up. *J Am Acad Orthop Surg*. 2019;27(19):727-735. [PMID: 30789379]

9

Orthopedic Infections: Basic Principles of Pathogenesis, Diagnosis, and Treatment

Richard L. McGough, III, MD
Kwesi St. Louis, MD

ESSENTIALS OF DIAGNOSIS

Orthopedic infections are common entities. Although extremely uncommon, orthopedic infections can arise de novo, even in healthy hosts. Orthopedic infections are unfortunately one of the most common and most serious surgical complications as well. Infections, especially iatrogenic and nosocomial infections, are receiving increasing attention and visibility in the lay press. There is no shortage of popular media describing individual or institutional infectious complications, and there is a rapidly evolving movement by the Centers for Medicare and Medicaid Services (CMS) to not reimburse institutions for the treatment of nosocomial infection. For this reason, infection prevention, recognition, and prompt attention are of paramount importance.

The most essential element of diagnosis is an appropriate index of suspicion. Orthopedic infections are frequently subtle, and without a high level of suspicion, treatment will be delayed. Diagnosis is especially difficult for postoperative wounds for a variety of reasons. The first and most important reason for this difficulty is denial: the quality of our work becomes questioned, and the path of least resistance is to deny that a problem exists. This is especially dangerous in the postoperative situation and in compromised hosts. Primarily, prompt treatment may salvage the index procedure. Additionally, patients with decreased physiologic reserve may be able to mount a response to a developing infection but may not be able to clear an established one. A second difficulty with postoperative wounds is the overlapping qualities of subcutaneous hematomas, delayed wound healing, and frank infection. Many postoperative wounds can be slow to heal without being infected. Likewise, different individuals will demonstrate differing levels of swelling, erythema, and tissue warmth in an uncomplicated postoperative course based simply on body habitus, coagulation status, or skin complexion. Our mandate to "do no harm" becomes most difficult in the complex patient who is most threatened, as unnecessary returns to the operating room for unsubstantiated infectious concerns may subject the patient to further risk. Accurate diagnosis remains difficult, as most signs of infection are subjective.

In the first century AD, Celsus described the quartet of calor (warmth), dolor (pain), rubor (redness), and tumor (swelling) as the essential signs of infection. Two millennia later, these clinical clues are still the "vital signs" for this condition. Beyond this, infection should be suspected in patients who are "going the wrong direction" and are not improving with pain and swelling after treatment. More intensive investigations, as detailed later by general category, are warranted in these individuals.

Due to the breadth of orthopedic infections, any discussion of orthopedic infections varies tremendously based on etiology. Pediatric osteomyelitis, for example, is a very different entity than periprosthetic knee infections. Detailed discussions of specific infections are given in topical areas within this book. For the purposes of this chapter, different types of orthopedic infections will be discussed in various categories.

GENERAL CONSIDERATIONS

As alluded to earlier, orthopedic infections can be broadly divided into two categories. The first is spontaneous infection, where no trauma or surgical intervention has occurred, and some combination of factors contributes to the infection. This encompasses much of pediatric and adult osteomyelitis, as well as spontaneous soft-tissue infections. The second broad category is that of postoperative or posttraumatic infections. These occur when the soft-tissue envelope has been breached either deliberately (postoperative infections) or traumatically. In modern trauma care, infection can often be attributed to both, as can be seen after the surgical stabilization of open fractures.

Pediatric Osteomyelitis

Spontaneous osteomyelitis is not an uncommon entity in children. It may occur at any time from birth to adulthood but generally possesses a decreasing incidence into adolescence, after which it remains possible but becomes much rarer (see Clinical Corollary #1). The pathogenesis of pediatric osteomyelitis is thought to be due to the watershed nature of the metaphyseal vascularity, with a low-flow, centripetal system of vascularity. This grants normally encountered blood pathogens a microenvironment in which they may multiply isolated from most circulating lymphocytes, thereby evading initial immune surveillance. The most common pathogen is *Staphylococcus aureus,* followed by group A *Streptococcus* and *Haemophilus influenzae* in unvaccinated patients. Patients suffering from sickle cell anemia have an unusual propensity for *Salmonella* infections. In children under 4, *Kingella kingae* is a common cause of bone and joint infection. It has been reported as the cause of septic joint infections in up to 50% of cases in children 2 years and younger.

Montgomery NI, Rosenfeld S. Pediatric osteoarticular infection update. *J Pediatr Orthop.* 2015;35(1):74-81. [PMID: 24978126]

Upon multiplication, bacteria produce matrix metalloproteinases, which degrade the surrounding cancellous bone and allow abscess formation. The abscess further disrupts an already poor blood supply and shields bacteria from the immune response. This devascularization causes osteonecrosis and formation of a *sequestrum,* which is a radiographic hallmark of osteomyelitis. This sequestrum is seen as an area of hyperdense, necrotic bone surrounded by lysis on plain radiographs. The rate of progression depends on how robustly the host can respond to the infection. If the host is able to mount a response and surround the sequestrum, it will be encapsulated by a rim of living, immunocompetent bone called an *involucrum.* If, on the other hand, the infection spreads with enough vigor that the host bone cannot contain it, bacteria will continue to multiply. The abscess will enlarge and eventually destroy the surrounding cortex. This will cause a purulent response that will produce a very aggressive radiographic appearance, mimicking Ewing sarcoma (see Clinical Corollary #1). The purulent material will raise the surrounding periosteum, create a *Codman triangle,* produce a permeative appearance in the subjacent cortex, and may even form a soft-tissue mass.

Clinically, children with acute osteomyelitis typically appear ill. Many, if not most, will have a febrile response greater than 38.5°C. Nearly all will complain of localized pain and swelling and, in lower extremity cases, will present with an inability or unwillingness to ambulate. If the area of infection occurs beneath the adjacent joint capsule, an acute septic joint may occur with substantial pain, resistance to motion, and effusion. Radiographs may demonstrate the features described earlier and, in the case of joint sepsis, will have evidence of effusion. Laboratory analysis generally demonstrates leukocytosis with a left shift to greater than 70% neutrophils. Erythrocyte sedimentation rates (ESRs) will be elevated, as will C-reactive protein (CRP) levels. Laboratory results are especially important in the differential diagnosis of pediatric osteomyelitis because radiographs can easily be confused with pediatric sarcomas, especially Ewing sarcoma.

A. Clinical Corollary #1

Patient 1 is a healthy 15-year-old male student athlete who noted the onset of pain, swelling, and cramping in his left thigh 1 month before presentation. He denied any trauma. These symptoms gradually worsened to the point of his being unable to attend school. He also developed fevers, chills, night sweats, and malaise. Radiographs and a magnetic resonance imaging (MRI) scan were obtained by a community physician, and he was subsequently referred to a tertiary medical center.

Plain radiographs were essentially normal (Figures 9–1 to 9–5), but MRI scan revealed extensive bone marrow

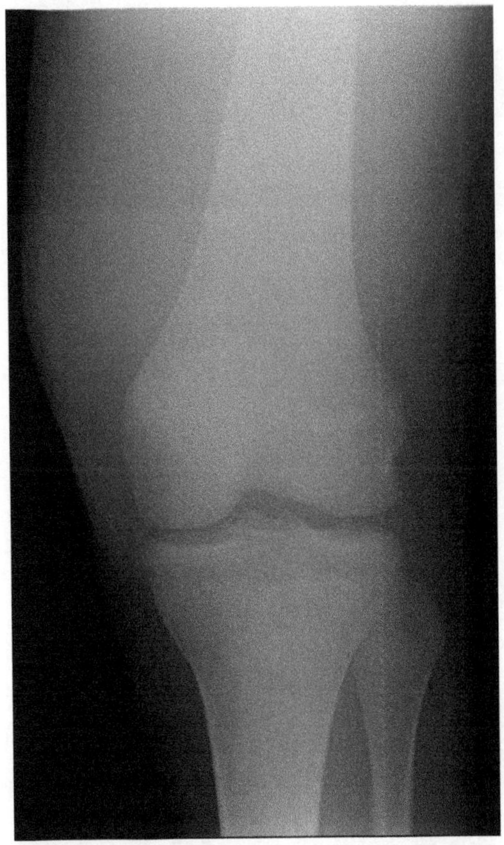

▲ **Figure 9–1.** Anteroposterior knee for Patient 1. Beside the suggestion of a soft-tissue mass, there are no obvious destructive changes to the bone.

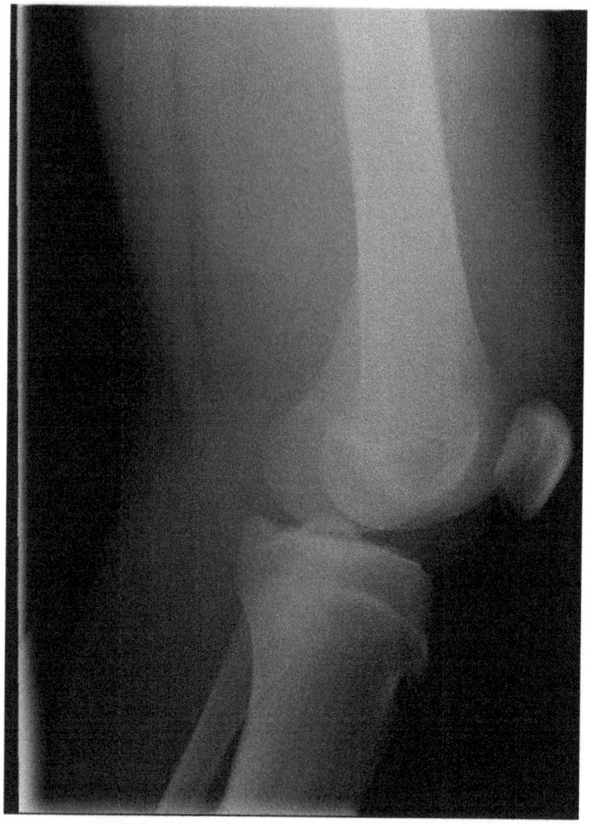

▲ **Figure 9–2.** Lateral knee for Patient 1.

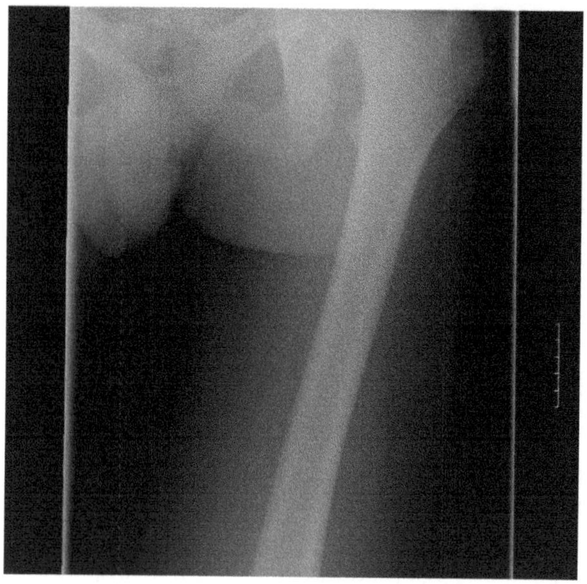

▲ **Figure 9–3.** Anteroposterior femur for Patient 1.

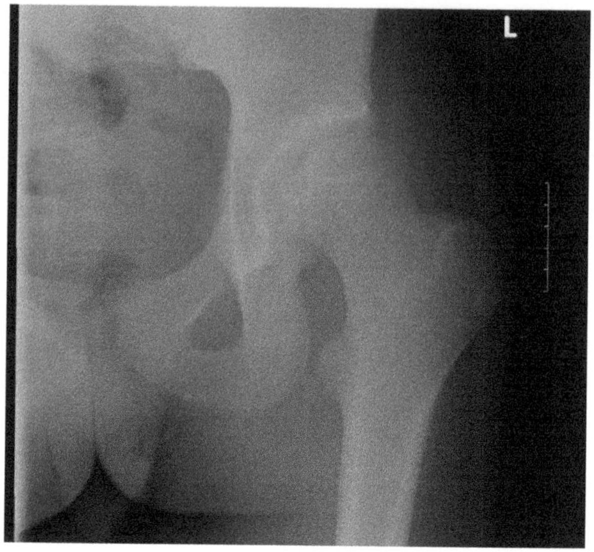

▲ **Figure 9–4.** Anteroposterior hip for Patient 1.

infiltration and a large soft-tissue mass involving nearly the entire circumference of the femur (Figures 9–6 to 9–10). The differential diagnosis at this point included bone neoplasm versus infection. The patient was sent for a computed tomography (CT) scan–guided biopsy. The CT scan suggested intramedullary abscess formation and showed air within the soft tissues (Figure 9–11). Laboratory evaluation showed a white blood cell count of 14.0×10^3 cells/mL with 79.4% neutrophils. ESR and CRP were 114 mm/h and 22.31 mg/dL, respectively, consistent with infection. Biopsy revealed acute inflammatory cells and bacteria, further substantiating the diagnosis.

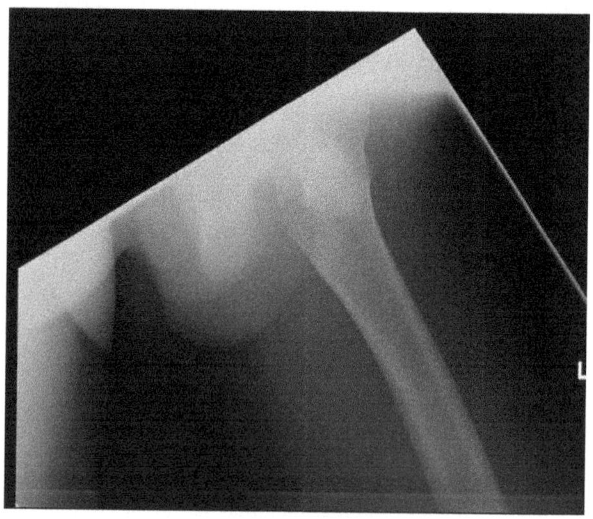

▲ **Figure 9–5.** Lateral femur for Patient 1.

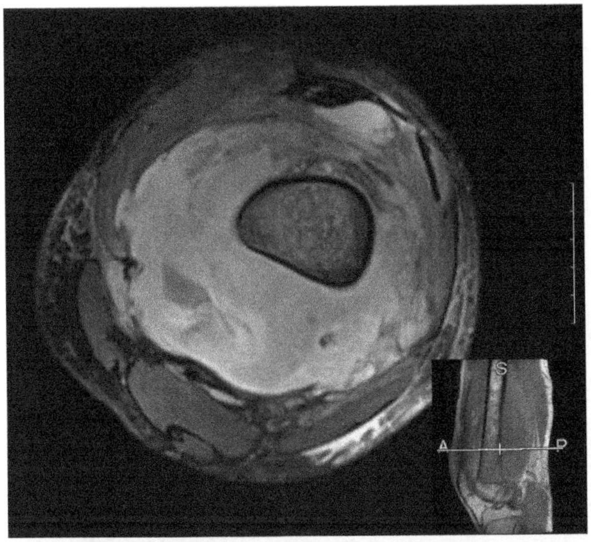

▲ **Figure 9–6.** Axial T2 MRI image of Patient 1. Note the extensive marrow involvement and nearly circumferential involvement of the femur.

The patient was taken to the operating room where a lateral approach to the femur was made. Copious amounts of purulent material were encountered, and the soft tissues were extensively irrigated and debrided. A 4-cm × 2-cm ovoid hole was made in the lateral cortex of the femur, and flexible reamers were passed into the proximal and distal femur. Antibiotic beads containing 1 g of tobramycin and 3 g of vancomycin per 40 g of polymethylmethacrylate (PMMA) were placed in the intramedullary canal (Figures 9–12 to 9–15). Operative cultures from the purulent material, soft tissue, and bone reamings were all positive for methicillin-sensitive *S aureus*, and the patient was placed on intravenous therapy with continuous-infusion oxacillin for 6 weeks under the supervision of a musculoskeletal infectious disease consultant.

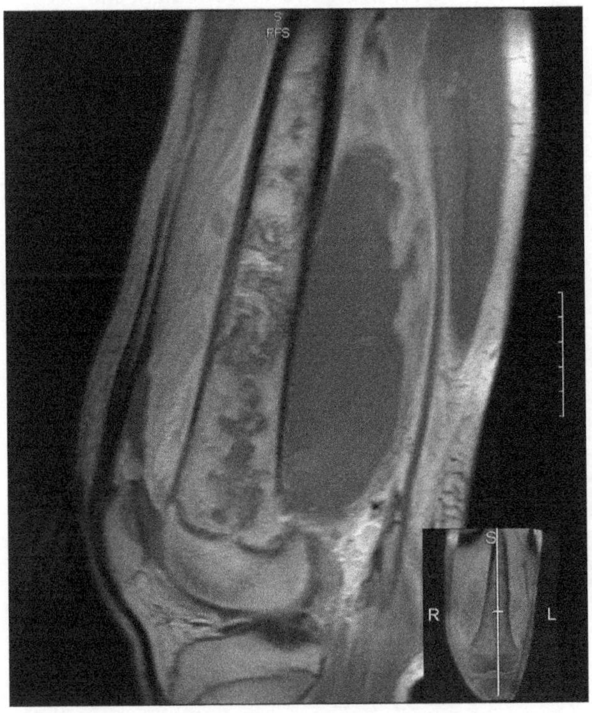

▲ **Figure 9–7.** Sagittal T1 MRI image of Patient 1.

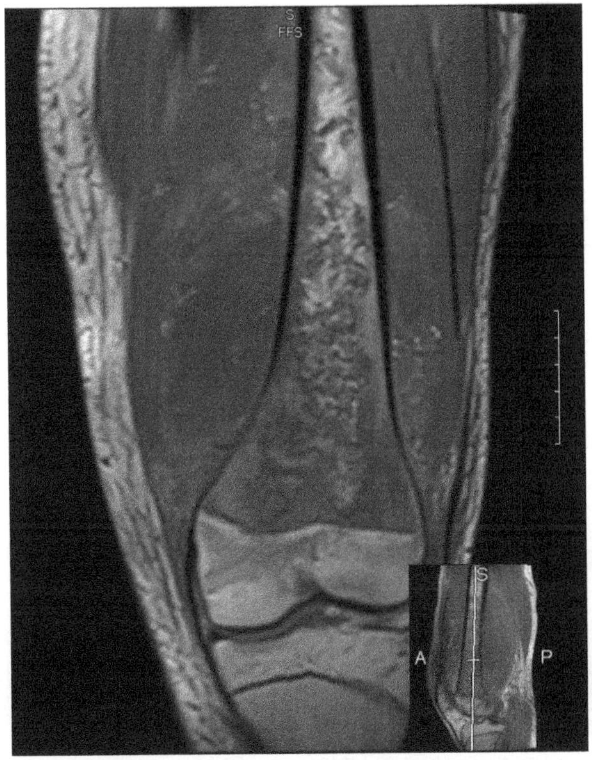

▲ **Figure 9–8.** Coronal T1 MRI image of Patient 1.

Subsequent to the completion of systemic antibiotic therapy, he was taken back to the operating room for removal of the antibiotic beads, irrigation, and repeat intraoperative cultures of the bone and soft tissues. These cultures were all negative. At the most recent follow-up, his knee motion was normal. The laboratory parameters had normalized with an ESR of 3 mm/h and a CRP of less than 0.1 mg/dL.

Adult Osteomyelitis

Adult osteomyelitis is fortunately rare. As the growing child reaches skeletal maturity, the metaphyseal bone vascularity changes, and the pediatric venous sinusoids are eliminated. This produces improved blood flow, decreasing the

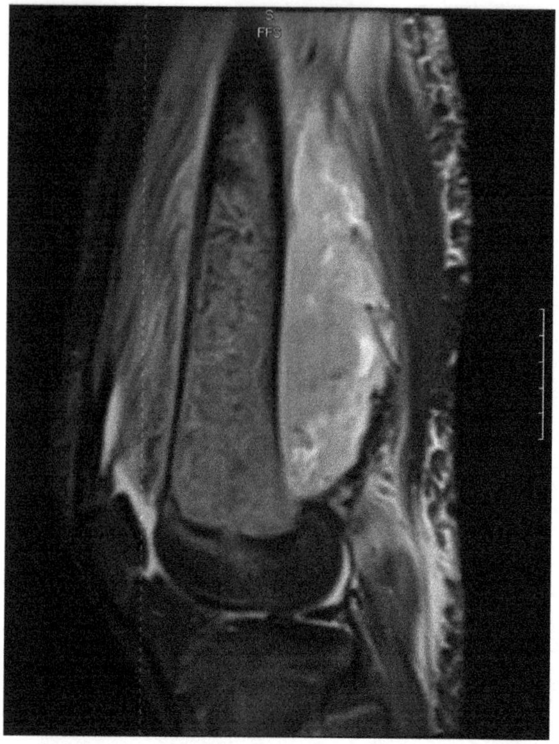

▲ **Figure 9–9.** Sagittal T2 MRI image of Patient 1. Note the extensive marrow involvement and nearly circumferential involvement of the femur.

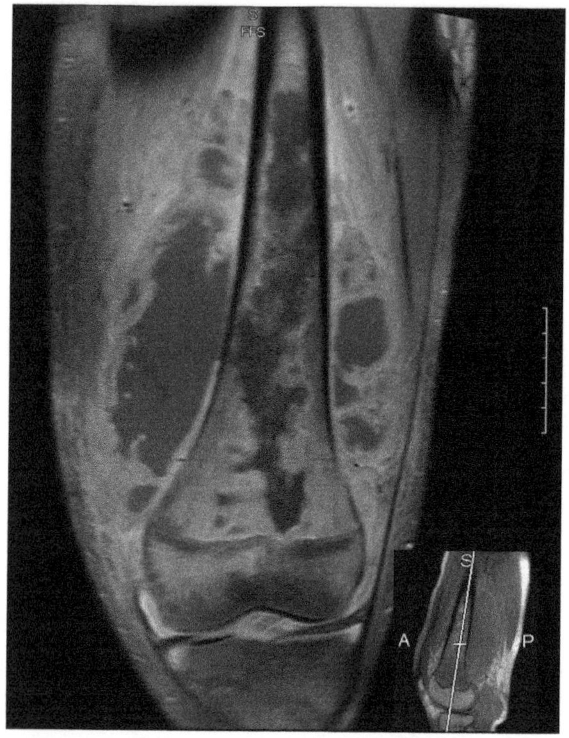

▲ **Figure 9–10.** Coronal fat-saturated MRI image of Patient 1. Note the extensive marrow involvement and nearly circumferential involvement of the femur.

prevalence of spontaneous osteomyelitis. Most cases of adult osteomyelitis are therefore a result of skin penetration, either deliberate or accidental. A few cases merit special mention.

Aside from accidental or surgical trauma, most cases of adult osteomyelitis occur in individuals who are unable to maintain a normal soft-tissue envelope over subjacent bone. This occurs with disturbing frequency in paraplegics and diabetics, as the normal protective sensation over bony prominences (sacrum, femora, ischial tuberosities, calcanei, and metatarsals) is impaired. This leads to pressure sores, which, if untreated, can progress to the bone. Once the bone is exposed to air, its vascularity is compromised, and osteomyelitis occurs. This form of osteomyelitis is much more chronic than that seen in children, and the symptomatology is quite different. Because many of these individuals are insensate, pain is not a prominent finding. Also, the acute purulent response found in the pediatric case is rarely present, instead manifesting as open, draining sinuses. Infectious indices (ESR/CRP) may demonstrate increased values, but a leukocytosis with left shift is generally absent. Individuals with this condition may persist for years or even decades with osteomyelitis, having no symptoms until developing squamous cell carcinoma (Marjolin ulcer) within the sinus tract.

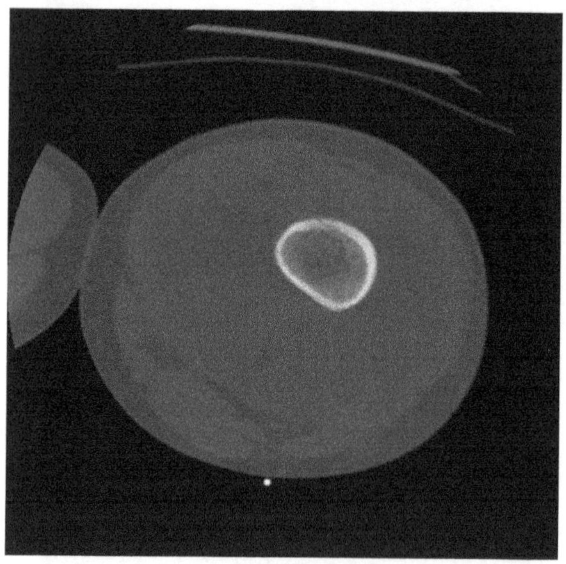

▲ **Figure 9–11.** This image was obtained at the time of Patient 1's CT-guided biopsy and shows an axial view of his thigh. There is a suggestion of air in the soft tissues, which supports the diagnosis of infection rather than tumor.

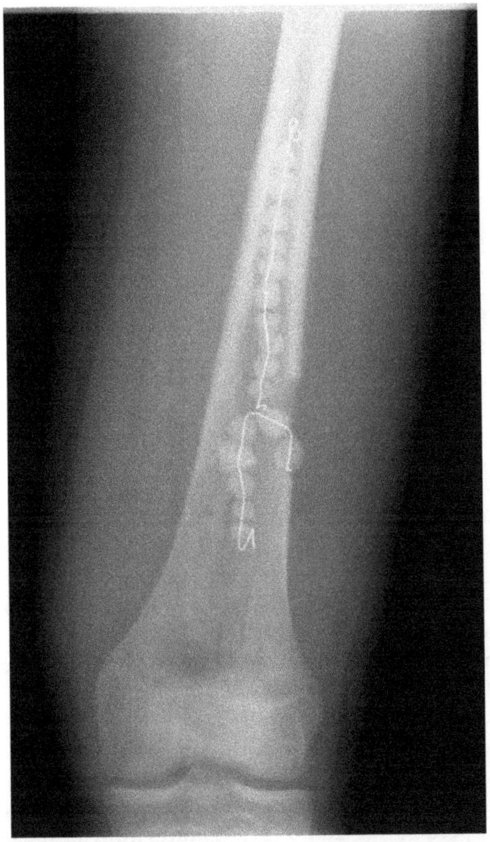

▲ **Figure 9–12.** Orthogonal view 1 of Patient 1's femur after debridement, irrigation, intramedullary reaming, and the placement of antibiotic beads. The beads were subsequently removed after 6 weeks of intravenous antibiotic therapy, and Patient 1's clinical examination improved tremendously. He has returned to limited participation in sports.

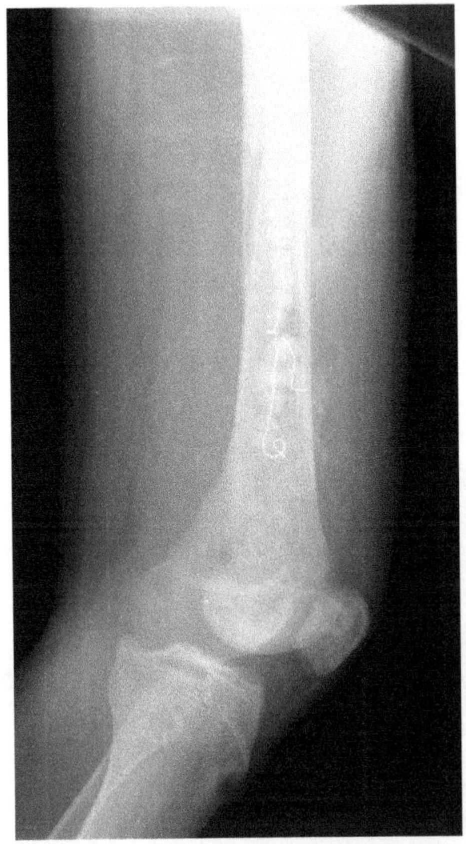

▲ **Figure 9–13.** Orthogonal view 2 of Patient 1's femur after debridement, irrigation, intramedullary reaming, and the placement of antibiotic beads. The beads were subsequently removed after 6 weeks of intravenous antibiotic therapy, and Patient 1's clinical examination improved tremendously. He has returned to limited participation in sports.

The situation is quite different in patients who are immunocompromised. Patients who are immunocompromised from human immunodeficiency virus (HIV) or acquired immunodeficiency syndrome (AIDS), who have undergone solid organ or bone marrow transplantation, or who are undergoing cytotoxic chemotherapy may develop acute osteomyelitis. The hallmark of this disease is pain without an obvious source, and this symptom may occur anywhere in the involved bone. This condition may also produce spontaneous joint sepsis, most commonly in the sternoclavicular and sacroiliac joints. Septic arthritis of other joints is rare at best. Immunocompromised individuals with osteomyelitis will present with pain and fever but will lack leukocytosis, as the dysfunctional immunity producing the osteomyelitis precludes an adequate immune response. Infectious indices are rarely useful, as many of these individuals have other causes of inflammation that will confound these nonspecific test parameters. A very high index of suspicion is required to make this diagnosis, as plain radiographs will likely only demonstrate osteopenia and MRI scanning shows only bony edema on T2-weighted sequences. Generally, no abscess forms within the bone. In this instance, prompt diagnosis can be critical because patients do not possess the immunologic reserve to fight a fulminant infection.

A. Clinical Corollary #2

Patient 2 is a 33-year-old man with a chief complaint of steadily increasing left thigh pain for 1 month. He denied any trauma or constitutional symptoms. He had a negative medical and surgical history but had a social history significant for heavy drug abuse. He was initially seen at a community hospital where radiographs suggested a permeative lesion in the lateral cortex of the left femur (Figure 9–16).

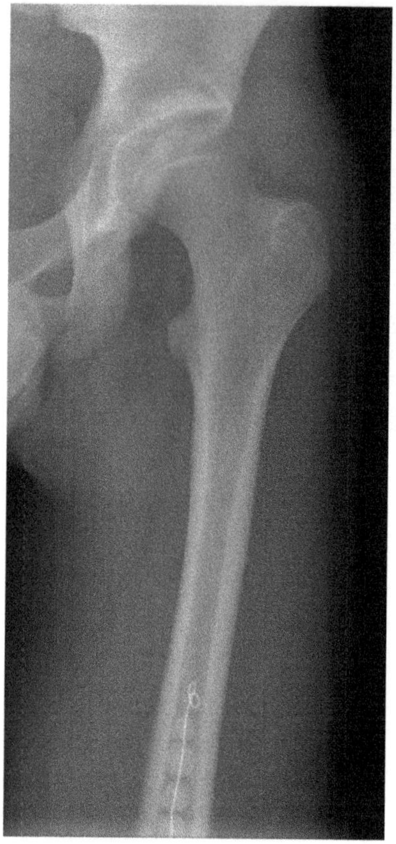

▲ **Figure 9–14.** Orthogonal view of Patient 1's femur after debridement, irrigation, intramedullary reaming, and the placement of antibiotic beads. The beads were subsequently removed after 6 weeks of intravenous antibiotic therapy, and Patient 1's clinical examination improved tremendously. He has returned to limited participation in sports.

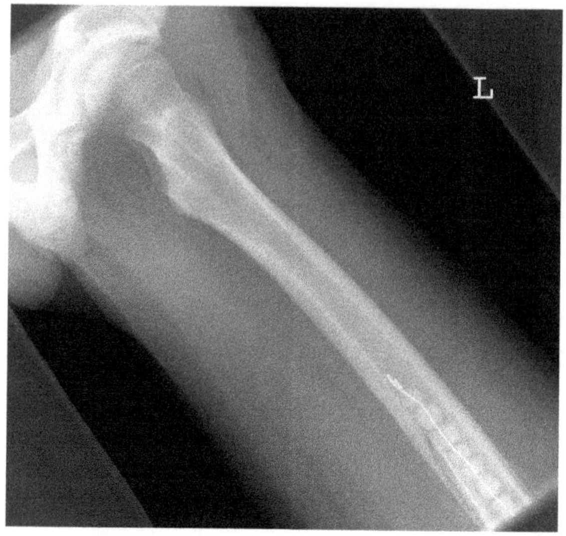

▲ **Figure 9–15.** Orthogonal view of Patient 1's femur after debridement, irrigation, intramedullary reaming, and the placement of antibiotic beads. The beads were subsequently removed after 6 weeks of intravenous antibiotic therapy, and Patient 1's clinical examination improved tremendously. He has returned to limited participation in sports.

He was subsequently transferred to a tertiary medical center for further management.

At the tertiary medical center, he was found to be afebrile with normal vital signs. Laboratory evaluation disclosed a white blood cell count of 12.4×10^9 cells/L with 70.5% neutrophils and a platelet count of 524×10^3 cells/mL. His ESR and CRP were both elevated at 66 mm/h and 1.96 mg/dL, respectively. CT scan and MRI scan were obtained. CT scan showed changes in the femur consistent with sequestrum formation, and MRI scan revealed intense soft-tissue edema around the lesion. A presumptive diagnosis of infection was made (Figures 9–17 to 9–20).

The patient was subsequently taken to the operating room where an open biopsy of the left femur and the surrounding tissues was performed. Pathology on frozen section was consistent with acute infection, and the diagnosis of osteomyelitis with soft-tissue involvement was made. The muscle around the femur was thoroughly debrided, and the femur itself was likewise debrided with rongeurs, curettes, and a high-speed burr (Figure 9–21). Cultures from the musculature, periosteum, bone, and intermedullary canal were all obtained. After copious irrigation, a strand of antibiotic beads containing 1 g of tobramycin and 3 g of vancomycin per 40 g of PMMA was made and placed next to the femur (Figure 9–22). The wound was closed in layers. Postoperative radiographs showed obliteration of the abnormal bone (Figure 9–23).

All operative cultures were positive for methicillin-resistant *S aureus* (MRSA). The patient was placed on oral antibiotic therapy with linezolid for 6 weeks with plans to remove his antibiotic beads and perform a repeat irrigation and debridement after the completion of antibiotic therapy.

Adult Spontaneous Soft-Tissue Infections

Soft-tissue infections are common. Admissions to medical services for cellulitis, a common skin infection, are frequent in most hospitals. These conditions may occur in the setting of medical comorbidities, such as venous stasis, diabetes, obesity, or immunocompromise. They are generally treated with antibiotics alone, and rarely is surgical intervention necessary.

Deep, abscess-producing skin infections in adults are usually the result of skin penetration. This occurs either due to trauma, iatrogenic skin penetration, or intravenous drug use.

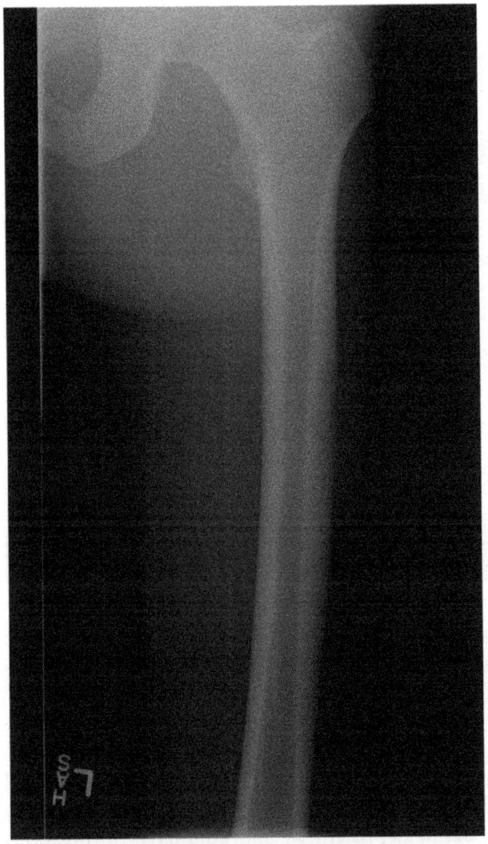

▲ **Figure 9–16.** Anteroposterior projection of Patient 2's femur. Note the poorly defined, permeative lesion in the lateral diaphyseal cortex. This was concerning for infection or a bone neoplasm.

The causative problems are sometimes obvious, as in the case of intravenous drug use, but may be difficult to ascertain, as in septic olecranon bursitis. Bursitis is often presumed to be due to trauma, as the extensor surface of the elbow is frequently traumatized. Surgical treatment of simple abscesses with irrigation and drainage as well as wound packing or vacuum-assisted closure generally yields satisfactory results. Occasionally, intravenous drug abusers can present with a mixed picture of both bone and soft-tissue infection (see Clinical Corollary #2).

Severe, spontaneous, deep soft-tissue infections, those occurring below the fascia, are decidedly rarer, and tend to occur in individuals with some form of immunocompromise. While the often publicized "flesh-eating bacteria" seen in necrotizing fasciitis may infect immunocompetent hosts, those with an immune-compromised comorbidity are at much greater risk. These individuals are generally as follows: patients who are neutropenic secondary to cytotoxic chemotherapy, those suffering from HIV/AIDS, or those with other,

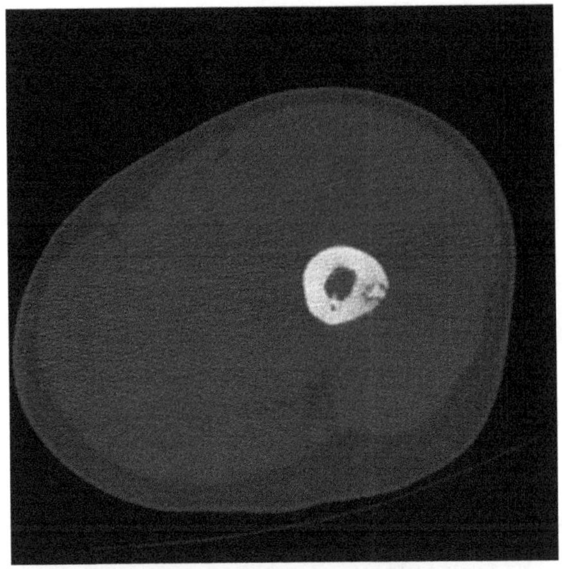

▲ **Figure 9–17.** Axial CT image suggests the presence of a sequestrum within the lateral cortex of the femur.

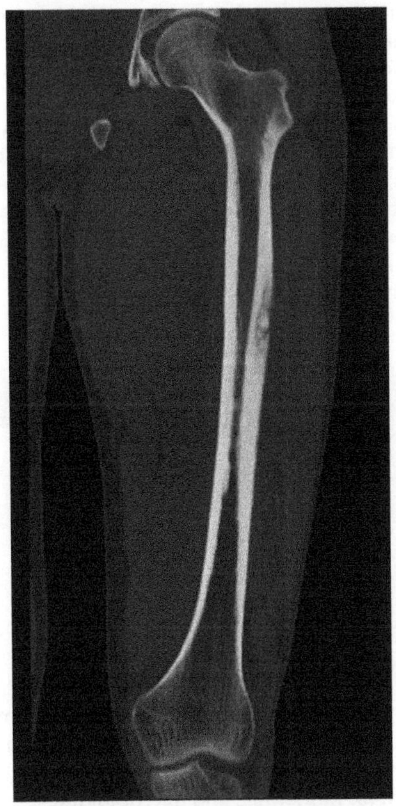

▲ **Figure 9–18.** Coronal CT image suggests the presence of a sequestrum within the lateral cortex of the femur.

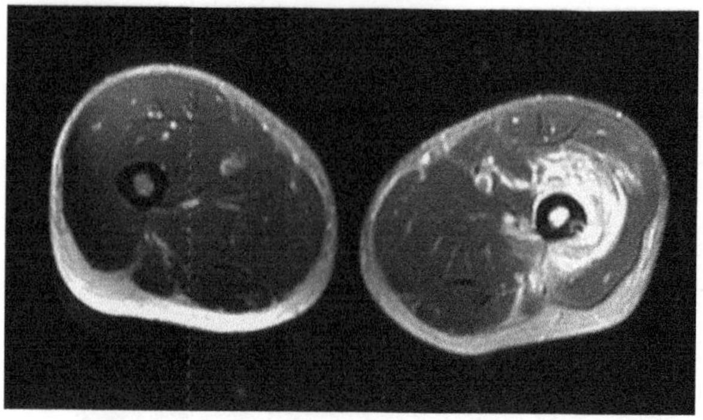

▲ **Figure 9–19.** Axial MRI image illustrating the dramatic difference between the affected and nonaffected limbs. The image also shows a substantial soft-tissue component to the process.

frequently autoimmune, diseases that render the normal tissues susceptible to bacteria in the environment. In immunocompromised individuals, the typical signs of infection may be absent, and the patient may simply manifest a high fever (>38.5°C), tenderness, and erythema. Advanced imaging with MRI may demonstrate only edema within the affected area because the patient often does not have adequate immunity to form an abscess. These patients are at great risk, and surgical debridement coupled with broad-spectrum antibiotics may be lifesaving.

Because of the vascular nature of muscle, pyomyositis in immunocompetent individuals is rare. Etiologically, pyomyositis is different than simple abscess formation; in pyomyositis, the bacteria occlude the small vascular inflow into the muscle, producing necrosis. This avascular bed is an ideal culture medium for bacteria, and liquefactive necrosis occurs. Treatment of pyomyositis is more extensive than many soft-tissue infections because all necrotic material must be thoroughly removed before the infection can be controlled. Serial debridement and adjunctive intravenous antibiotics are the mainstays of treatment, as initial debridement often fails to remove all necrotic material.

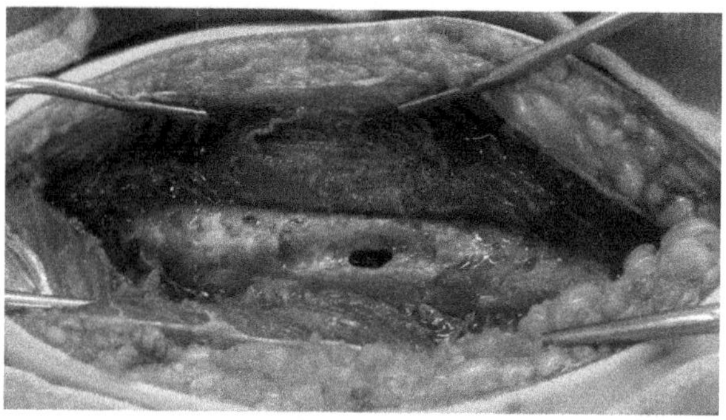

▲ **Figure 9–21.** Intraoperative view of Patient 2's femur after biopsy, culture, thorough curettage, and burring of the abnormal bone in the lateral cortex. Bone and soft tissue were sent for pathologic and microbiologic testing. All samples were positive for methicillin-resistant *Staphylococcus aureus* infection and negative for neoplasm.

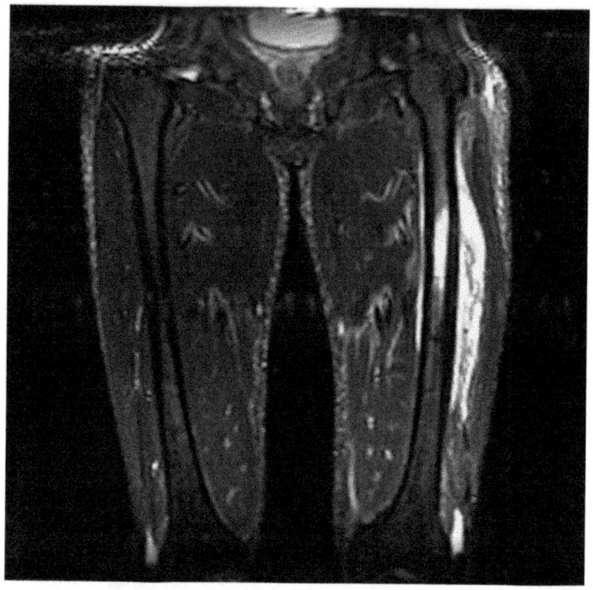

▲ **Figure 9–20.** Coronal MRI image illustrating the dramatic difference between the affected and nonaffected limbs. The image also shows a substantial soft-tissue component to the process.

Necrotizing fasciitis is the most dreaded deep soft-tissue infection. Classically caused by *Clostridium perfringens*, it can become a rapidly progressive, life-threatening event. Necrotizing fasciitis caused by other organisms may not present with as fulminant a course and may more closely mimic cellulitis or other soft-tissue infections. Necrotizing fasciitis is a clinical diagnosis: although MRI may demonstrate T2 enhancement of the fascia, this finding is extremely

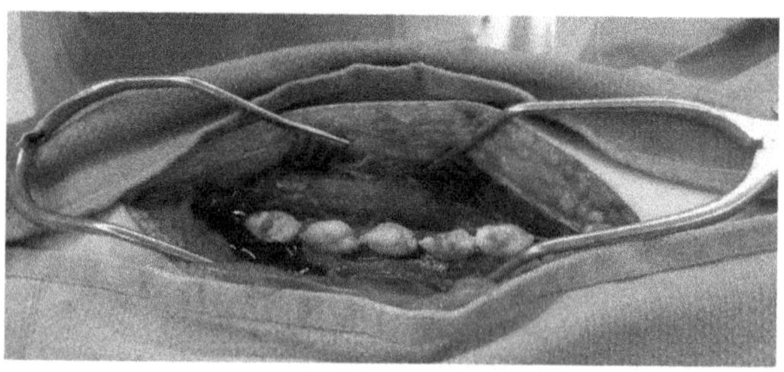

▲ **Figure 9–22.** A strand of antibiotic-impregnated beads were placed after copious irrigation with antibiotic-containing pulse lavage fluid.

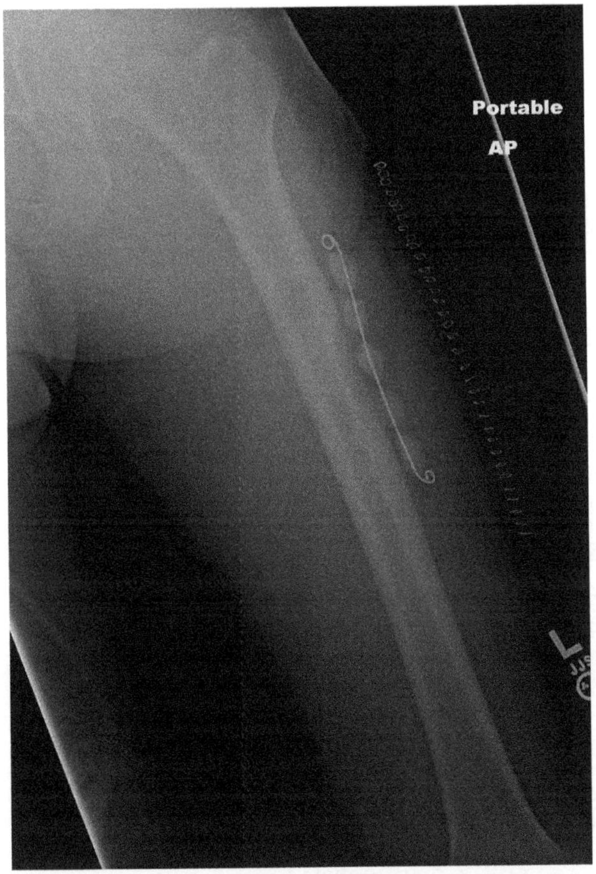

▲ **Figure 9–23.** Postoperative anteroposterior (AP) radiograph of Patient 2's femur. Note the removal of the permeative lateral bone (see Figure 9–17 for comparison).

nonspecific, and the clinician acting on the clinical findings will yield a much timelier diagnosis. Clinically, the patients are quite ill, with fever, malaise, and localized pain. Signs of systemic sepsis may be present, with mental status changes, tachycardia, or even hypotension. Palpation of the affected area demonstrates a swollen, boggy texture to the skin and soft tissues. The skin may also be hypermobile, similar to its character after a fasciocutaneous injury. Bullous changes may also occur.

Treatment of necrotizing fasciitis is time dependent. Time should not be wasted obtaining confirmatory diagnostic tests, as these are rarely specific enough to change the clinical diagnosis, and substantial delays may be limb or life threatening. Surgical treatment is extensive and requires debridement of *all* affected skin and fascia. In fulminant cases, soft-tissue reconstruction is generally required. Debridement to healthy, vascularized skin is mandatory, and debridement of the subjacent muscle may be required. The presence of myonecrosis may make amputation necessary, and the performance of a high amputation such as a hip disarticulation or forequarter amputation may be necessary as a lifesaving measure.

JOINT INFECTIONS

Prosthetic Joint Infections

Prosthetic joint infection (PJI) after arthroplasty is the most dreaded complication of total joint arthroplasty, which is performed with increasing frequency in our aging population. With the number of arthroplasties projected to increase dramatically, treating prosthetic infections may become a full-time profession for some orthopedic surgeons. The costs of this treatment are extensive and, when multiplied by our aging population, may become astronomical.

Prosthetic infections are divided into two categories. The first is an acute infection that develops within 3 to 6 weeks of surgery. In this case, the patient will demonstrate fever, increasing pain, erythema, and poor wound healing. Distinguishing a typical postoperative knee wound from an acutely infected postoperative knee wound is an art, and the gravity of ignoring the infection must be balanced with the morbidity of a return to the operating theater. Fortunately, acute sepsis following arthroplasty is rare (<1%).

The most common variety of prosthetic infection is a chronic infection occurring long after surgery. This occurs when a well-functioning joint of intermediate to long duration (>3 months, but perhaps years after the index procedure) becomes painful, warm, and effusive. Sinus tracts may form in the adjacent skin, leading to chronic drainage. In this situation, the infection has generally been present for weeks to years, and bacterial colonization and biofilm formation have organized on the joint surface.

The key to treating PJI is appropriate diagnosis and identification of the causative organism so that proper surgical treatment can be planned and ideal antibiotic regimens implemented. Starting in 2011, the Musculoskeletal Infection Society (MSIS) proposed criteria for the diagnosis of PJI using major and minor criteria. These criteria were updated and validated in 2018 (Table 9–1).

The culture of sonication of explanted components yields sensitivity of 97% and specificity of 90% in determining the causative organism.

Parvizi J, Tan TL, Goswami K, et al. The 2018 definition of periprosthetic hip and knee infection: an evidence-based and validated criteria. *J Arthroplasty*. 2018;33(5):1309-1314.e2. [PMID: 29551303]

Rothenberg AC, Wilson AE, Hayes JP, et al. Sonication of arthroplasty implants improves accuracy of periprosthetic joint infection cultures. *Clin Orthop Relat Res*. 2017;475(7):1827-1836. [PMID: 28290115]

The most common and effective treatment for known chronic knee PJI has been two-stage revision. This method

Table 9–1. MSIS PJI Scoring System, 2018.

Major criteria (at least one of the following)	Decision	
Two positive cultures of the same organism Sinus tract with evidence of communication to the joint or visualized prothesis	Infected	
Preoperative Diagnosis		
Minor Criteria	**Score**	**Decision**
Elevated serum CRP or D-Dimer	2	
Elevated serum ESR	1	≥6 Infected
Elevated synovial WBC count or leukocyte esterase	3	4-5 Inconclusive
Positive synovial alpha defensin	3	
Elevated synovial PMN (%)	2	≤3 Not infected
Elevated synovial CRP	1	
Intraoperative Diagnosis		
Inconclusive Pre-op Score or Dry Tap	**Score**	**Decision**
Preoperative score	–	≥6 Infected
Positive histology	3	
Positive purulence	3	4-5 Inconclusive
Single positive culture	2	≤3 Not infected

CRP, C-reactive protein; ESR, erythrocyte sedimentation rate; PJI, prosthetic joint infection; PMN, polymorphonuclear leukocytes; WBC, white blood cell.

Reprinted with permission, from Parvizi J et al. The 2018 definition of periprosthetic hip and knee infection: an evidence-based and validated criteria. *J Arthroplasty.* 2018;33(5):1309-1314.

is associated with substantial morbidity for the patient and cost to the health care system. As patients may develop these infections years after implantation, their immune systems may be senescent, and this factor combined with the comorbidities common with aging may preclude this type of care. Some have proposed single-stage revisions as viable options with good short-term outcomes in appropriate patients with susceptible organisms.

Srivastava K, Bozic KJ, Silverton C, Nelson AJ, Makhni EC, Davis JJ. Reconsidering strategies for managing chronic periprosthetic joint infection in total knee arthroplasty: using decision analytics to find the optimal strategy between one-stage and two-stage total knee revision. *J Bone Joint Surg Am.* 2019;101(1):14-24. [PMID: 30601412]

Traumatic Infections

Traumatic infections are unfortunately common, and their incidence corresponds directly to the energy imparted by the injury. The maxim that "an open fracture is a severe soft-tissue injury that happens to have a broken bone in it" is true, as devitalized tissue becomes rapidly colonized upon exposure to air, soil, or other materials. To minimize the risk of traumatic infection, all open fractures should be treated urgently with thorough debridement and skeletal stabilization. This allows devitalized tissues to declare themselves so that subsequent surgeries facilitate complete removal of all abnormal tissue. Despite the most meticulous care, open fractures may still become infected, and this problem is much more prevalent in certain anatomic locations. The tibia, a subcutaneous bone throughout much of its circumference, is the most at risk, and modern trauma care often combines soft-tissue reconstruction with bony stabilization to minimize the risk of osteomyelitis.

Septic Arthritis

Nonprosthetic septic arthritis is unusual in adults. Most commonly, a history of penetrating injury will be elicited. Septic arthritis can also be seen in immunocompromised individuals without trauma. Septic arthritis with a past history lacking trauma or immunocompromise is decidedly rare, and a more common crystalline arthropathy, such as gout, is more often the culprit.

Pathologically, a native joint is relatively resistant to infection. While cartilage itself is avascular, the synovium and joint capsule are richly vascularized and provide ample protection from infection. Children can develop septic arthritis from bacterial translocation from a nearby osteomyelitis due to the configuration of the joint capsule, allowing bacteria to enter the joint space. In adults, osteomyelitis in proximity rarely occurs. This is fortunate, as the sequelae of septic arthritis can be devastating and can lead to rapid joint destruction. Bacterial matrix metalloproteases can rapidly degrade the articular cartilage, leading to severe cartilage damage and end-stage arthrosis.

Clinically, patients present with severe pain, effusion, and resistance to joint motion. Warmth and redness of the surrounding skin may also be present. Unless an osteomyelitis in proximity is also present, both plain radiographs and MRI scanning will reveal only a joint effusion. Arthrocentesis demonstrates an exudative effusion, with a leukocyte count greater than 50×10^9 cells/L. Bacterial cultures are frequently positive, with *Staphylococcus* species being the most frequent causative organisms.

Treatment of septic arthritis is time dependent and demands a high index of suspicion. Awaiting final culture results in a patient with a purulent effusion may cause irreversible joint damage. Debate exists regarding the means of surgical treatment, with open synovectomy being the traditional procedure. Arthroscopic irrigation and debridement may allow more thorough visualization and lavage of all joint surfaces but is more technically demanding. All patients with septic arthritis are treated with antibiotics following surgery, frequently a short intravenous course. Results of this depend on both the cause of the infection and the amount of joint destruction that has occurred.

PATHOGENESIS

General

All clinical infections must be considered as a conflict between the attacking microbes' ability to cause disease and the host's immune defenses. Infections are more likely to occur if the organisms are more virulent and if the inoculum is larger. Conversely, an infection is less likely if the host has a greater ability to eradicate the pathogens or if the host has fewer deficits that encourage infection. Additionally, the pathogenesis of infection involving foreign materials and osteomyelitis are discussed.

Organisms

Although the musculoskeletal system may be infected by any infectious agent, the vast majority of infections are bacterial (Table 9–2). *S aureus*, *Streptococcus*, and *H influenzae* are the most common causes of acute hematogenous osteomyelitis in children. The most common causes of septic arthritis are *Neisseria gonorrhoeae*, *S aureus*, and group A *Streptococcus*. Septic arthritis is less often caused by gram-negative organisms, including *Escherichia coli*, *Pseudomonas aeruginosa*, *Klebsiella*, *Enterobacter*, *Serratia*, *Proteus*, and *Salmonella*. Uncommon bacterial organisms include *Borrelia burgdorferi* (Lyme disease), *Mycobacterium tuberculosis*, *Brucella*, and the anaerobes *Clostridium* and *Bacteroides*. Unusual organisms that may preferentially infect immunocompromised patients include fungi (*Blastomyces*, *Cryptococcus*, *Histoplasma*, *Sporotrichum*, and *Coccidioides*) and atypical mycobacteria (*Mycobacterium kansasii*, *M avium-intracellulare*, *M fortuitum*, *M triviale*, and *M scrofulaceum*).

Table 9–2. Common offending organisms in orthopedic conditions.

Disease	Offending Organism
Acute hematogenous osteomyelitis in children	*Staphylococcus aureus*, *Streptococcus*, and *Haemophilus influenzae*
Septic arthritis	Most common: *Neisseria gonorrhoeae*, *S aureus*, and group A *Streptococcus* Less common: *Escherichia coli*, *Pseudomonas aeruginosa*, *Klebsiella*, *Kingella*, *Enterobacter*, *Serratia*, *Proteus*, and *Salmonella* Uncommon bacterial organisms: *Borrelia burgdorferi* (Lyme disease), *Mycobacterium tuberculosis*, *Brucella*, and the anaerobes *Clostridium* and *Bacteroides*
Patients with immunocompromise	Fungi: *Blastomyces*, *Cryptococcus*, *Histoplasma*, *Sporotrichum*, and *Coccidioides* Atypical *Mycobacterium* species: *kansasii*, *avium-intracellulare*, *fortuitum*, *triviale*, and *scrofulaceum* *Campylobacter*, *Peptostreptococcus*, and *Propionibacterium*

Peterson MC. Rheumatic manifestations of *Campylobacter jejuni* and *C. fetus* infections in adults. *Scand J Rheumatol.* 1994;23:167-170. [PMID: 8091140]

The increase in the immunocompromised population due to the success of solid organ transplants and advancements in the treatment of HIV/AIDS and autoimmune disorders has increased the spectrum of bacteria that can cause musculoskeletal infection. Likewise, an increase in the number of antibiotic-resistant organisms presents a difficult, constantly evolving challenge in the eradication of infection. MRSA can infect bones, joints, soft tissues, and surgical implants. Other common bacterial species have become more resistant to a variety of drugs, delaying the proper treatment of infection and decreasing the number of antibiotics that can be used effectively. For instance, *Acinetobacter baumannii* is a pan-resistant bacterial strain that can cause severe lung and soft-tissue infections. Its role in clinically significant osteomyelitis is unknown, although some evidence suggests that it may be of limited importance.

Host Factors

A given host may have several factors that promote or defend against infection. Comorbid medical conditions and compromised immunity play a role in the establishment of infectious disease. The presence (or lack) of implanted devices affects infection risk and treatment strategies. Nutritional status and acute nutritional requirements also play a role.

A. Comorbid Diseases and Host Immunity

Comorbid diseases that are known to contribute to infection risk include diseases such as diabetes mellitus, obesity, peripheral vascular disease, chronic renal and liver disease, cancer, autoimmune diseases, and AIDS. Iatrogenic causes, often as a treatment for other diseases, include the use of cytotoxic chemotherapy, corticosteroids, and inhibitors of inflammatory molecules (eg, inhibitors of tumor necrosis factor-alpha). Diabetes mellitus has been shown to increase the risk of infection following surgeries, including total joint surgery, spinal surgeries, and foot and ankle surgery. The role that diabetes plays in infectious disease pathogenesis is related to vascular disease, as well as the effects of high glucose, which can cause granulocyte dysfunction. Obesity, often associated with diabetes, has also been shown in some studies to be an independent risk factor for infection.

B. Nutrition and Infection

Nutritional status must be thought of in terms of host requirements. In an adult with static requirements, poor nutrition may develop due to a variety of medical issues, including advanced age, alcoholism, renal disease, chronic diseases, cancer, malabsorption, and other infirmities. It is also necessary to consider the nutritional requirements of patients who have increased nutritional physiologic demand. These patients at baseline may have been well nourished. A significant event, however, such as trauma, may increase a patient's nutritional requirements and cause a relative nutritional deficiency. Laboratory testing for nutritional deficiency includes levels of transferrin (normal, 70-850 mg/dL), serum albumin (normal, 3.4-5.0 g/dL), total lymphocyte count (normal, 0.8-3.65 × 10^3 cells/μL), and prealbumin (normal, 18-38 mg/dL). Values below those shown may indicate malnutrition and consequent immunocompromise.

C. Foreign Material

All biomaterials commonly used for total joint arthroplasty increase the incidence of *S aureus* infections. In contrast, biomaterials appear to have no effect on *E coli* and *Staphylococcus epidermidis* infections except when PMMA is used, in which case the incidence rises markedly.

D. Biofilms

Adherence of bacteria to the surface of implants is promoted by a polysaccharide biofilm called glycocalyx that acts as a barrier against host defense mechanisms and antibiotics. In addition, this film makes culture of organisms difficult, even with the use of special techniques. Hence, other approaches must be taken for culture and treatment. Mixing antibiotics such as vancomycin and gentamicin into PMMA cement can theoretically lower the risk of infection from cemented metal joint replacements, presumably by killing surface bacteria before they produce glycocalyx. Before a glycocalyx is produced, the bacteria undergo a process referred to as quorum sensing. Quorum sensing dispersion is a technique under development that might allow clinicians to disrupt a biofilm, therefore making it susceptible to treatment. As stated, the formation of biofilm makes cultures unreliable. Other means, such as polymerase chain reaction, have been employed to diagnose infection. Biofilms dramatically reduce the efficacy of antibiotics, because only rifampin has the ability to readily penetrate the glycocalyx. The polysaccharides of this layer essentially isolate and protect bacteria from all other medical treatments. For this reason, removal of metallic devices is often performed when possible.

Lauderdale KJ, Malone CL, Boles BR, Morcuende J, Horswill AR. Biofilm dispersal of community-associated methicillin-resistant *Staphylococcus aureus* on orthopedic implant material. *J Orthop Res.* 2010;28:55-61. [PMID: 19610092]

PREVENTION

Overview

Prevention of perioperative infection starts long before the operative date, continues both during and after surgery, and is influenced by multiple factors and personnel. As discussed previously, medical comorbidities influence the pathogenesis of infection. It follows that the management and prevention of such comorbidities will contribute to infection prevention. Multiple physician and patient factors contribute to medical optimization of comorbidities before surgery. Preoperatively, factors such as nutrition, MRSA colonization, preoperative hygiene, and bathing can contribute to infection risk. Perioperative and intraoperative factors such as proper prepping, operative room sterility, appropriate use of antibiotics, closure material choice, and minimization of intraoperative time can help prevent infection. Finally, optimizing postoperative factors including postoperative antibiotics, management of blood glucose levels, and choices regarding blood transfusions can also positively affect infection rates.

In thinking about medical optimization for infection prevention, orthopedic surgeons have been forced to relearn quite a bit of medicine and to consider patient factors previously left to the patient's primary care physician. We have become medically involved with modifiable risk factors to the point of dictating diet regimens and optimizing diabetic control. This has required a complete change in attitude for us, as we can no longer stand by as passive technicians, but must understand these medical factors as never before. Further, we have needed to grow accustomed to having difficult lifestyle discussions. Smoking cessation programs, while always important, have become common referrals for our practices. Discussions of weight loss, while always difficult and requiring a modicum of sensitivity, have become easier as our entire field has moved away from offering elective surgery to everyone and, instead, has started risk-stratifying patients before doing what we do best.

Preoperative Optimization

A. Medical Comorbidities

Some medical comorbidities (and their necessary treatment) represent nonmodifiable risk factors for infection, whereas other present an opportunity for preoperative optimization. Rheumatoid arthritis (RA) provides an excellent example. Individuals with RA have an increased risk of infection, both from the disease and its treatment. Surgeons working in concert with the patient's rheumatologist can optimize the treatment of RA while decreasing the risk of poor operative outcomes, including infection. This approach to medical comorbidity management can be applied to other diseases as well.

Obesity, for instance, represents a modifiable risk factor that is becoming a more frequently encountered condition in developed countries, especially in the United States. In the total joint literature, obesity has been shown to be associated with an increased risk of infection. An increase of 5 points in body mass index (BMI) has been shown to be associated with a 50% increase in the odds ratio for acquiring a PJI. In the spine literature, obese patients have an odds ratio of 2.2 relative to nonobese patients. The surgeon must be aware of the association between obesity and infection and work with patients to decrease their risk of infection. Unfortunately, weight loss can be extremely difficult, especially in patients with orthopedic conditions. Gastric bypass therapy may be necessary before orthopedic intervention, especially in patients with a BMI greater than 45. This, unfortunately, produces relative malnutrition.

Bosco JA 3rd, Slover JD, Haas JP. Perioperative strategies for decreasing infection: a comprehensive evidence-based approach. *J Bone Joint Surg Am.* 2010;92:232-239. [PMID: 20048118]

Dowsey MM, Choong PF. Obese diabetic patients are at substantial risk for deep infection after primary TKA. *Clin Orthop Relat Res.* 2009;467:1577-1581. [PMID: 2674158]

Jämsen E, Varonen M, Huhtala H, et al. Incidence of prosthetic joint infections after primary knee arthroplasty. *J Arthroplasty.* 2010;25:87-92. [PMID: 19056210]

Moucha CS, Clyburn T, Evans RP, Prokuski L. Modifiable risk factors for surgical site infection. *J Bone Joint Surg Am.* 2011; 93:398-404. [PMID: 21325594]

B. Nutrition

The overall health of a given host's immune system influences susceptibility to infection. Indeed, malnutrition can lead directly to immune dysfunction. A recent review highlights the importance of recognizing and correcting patient nutrition. Testing for nutritional status should include albumin (normal, 3.4-5.0 g/dL), total lymphocyte count (normal, 0.8-3.65 × 10^3 cells/μL), and transferrin (normal, 70-850 mg/dL) levels. Supplementation to correct deficiency of both macro- and micronutrients should be accomplished preoperatively.

Katona P, Katona-Apte J. The interaction between nutrition and infection. *Clin Infect Dis.* 2008;46:1582-1588. [PMID: 18419494]

C. *Staphylococcus aureus* Decolonization/Preoperative Bathing

It has been clear for some time that certain organisms possess an increased potential to cause severe infections. *S aureus* is one such bacterium. Attempts to thwart infection with *S aureus* have led to the development of preoperative decolonization protocols designed to eradicate *S aureus* from the skin flora before the patient undergoes surgery. At certain institutions, adult reconstruction surgeons have begun to screen the nares of patients preoperatively. One protocol uses nasal cultures 2 to 4 weeks before surgery. If positive for *S aureus*, patients apply nasal mupirocin twice daily and take chlorhexidine baths for the 5 days immediately prior to surgery. This has been shown to decrease the rate of *S aureus* infections, as well as the overall rate of surgical site infections. Similar protocols have been used to prevent infections in other surgical disciplines, prompting the Cochrane group to conclude that nasal mupirocin is effective in preventing infections. Conversely, a separate Cochrane review demonstrated that chlorhexidine baths alone did not change the incidence of infection as compared to washing preoperatively with regular soap and water.

Rao N, Cannella B, Crossett LS, Yates AJ Jr, McGough R 3rd. A preoperative decolonization protocol for *Staphylococcus aureus* prevents orthopaedic infections. *Clin Orthop Relat Res.* 2008;466:1343-1348. [PMID: 2384036]

Rao N, Cannella BA, Crossett LS, Yates AJ Jr, McGough RL 3rd, Hamilton CW. Preoperative screening/decolonization for *Staphylococcus aureus* to prevent orthopedic surgical site infection prospective cohort study with 2-year follow-up. *J Arthroplasty.* 2011;26:1501-1507. [PMID: 21507604]

Perioperative and Intraoperative Factors

A. Prepping

Preparing the patient for surgery requires many steps once the patient has arrived in the operating theatre. The first decision in regard to infection control is whether or not to remove hair. The three options for hair removal are shaving, clipping, and depilatory creams. Alternatively, the hair can be left intact. Traditionally, it has been taught that shaving is inferior, a finding that is supported by a recent Cochrane review. However, no difference was found between removing the hair using the other two approaches and leaving the hair intact. The next step that influences infection control involves the selection of prepping solution. Options include iodophor or chlorhexidine gluconate–based solutions. These can be aqueous or alcohol based. Alcohol-based chlorhexidine gluconate solutions are superior to other preparation solutions when the outcome measure is simply positive cultures from the operative field. However, the extent to which these cultures correlate with an eventual surgical site infection is not clear. These alcohol-based solutions can also be difficult to use in certain facilities as they are flammable. While intraoperative fires are generally confined to procedures with an open airway and oxygen-enriched respiration (otorhinolaryngology and thoracic procedures), many institutions do not allow their use. Interestingly, in urologic surgery, other preparation solutions have been shown to be superior. This is ostensibly the result either of a statistical phenomenon or a different bacterial milieu in this patient population that responds differently to a given preparation solution. It is not clear that there are any significant differences between different preparation solutions.

Edwards PS, Lipp A, Holmes A. Preoperative skin antiseptics for preventing surgical wound infections after clean surgery. *Cochrane Database Syst Rev.* 2004;3:CD003949. [PMID: 15266508]

Ostrander RV, Botte MJ, Brage ME. Efficacy of surgical preparation solutions in foot and ankle surgery. *J Bone Joint Surg Am.* 2005;87:980-985. [PMID: 15866959]

Saltzman MD, Nuber GW, Gryzlo SM, Marecek GS, Koh JL. Efficacy of surgical preparation solutions in shoulder surgery. *J Bone Joint Surg Am.* 2009;91:1949-1953. [PMID: 19651954]

B. Antibiotics

The use of preoperative antibiotics within 1 hour of surgery is standard, routine, and required for adherence to national Surgical Care Improvement Project (SCIP) protocols. While this national protocol is no longer active, many of its precepts remain. Recommendations for antibiotic timing, duration, selection, and redosing include the following: administration of a first-generation cephalosporin within 1 hour of surgical initiation, use of clindamycin or vancomycin if the patient is allergic to cephalosporin, and maintenance of antibiotics for no more than 24 hours total unless infection is suspected or confirmed. A proposed adjunct to systemic antibiotics involves the use of local antibiotics, namely gentamicin. Two separate studies used a rat injury model to show improved bactericidal activity in vivo. Results are yet to be demonstrated in a human, randomized controlled trial.

C. Operating Room Sterility

Sterility in the operating theater is the responsibility of everyone who enters the room. This includes the surgical team, the anesthesiology team, the operating room staff, and the medical equipment team. Lapses in sterile technique can undoubtedly increase bacterial exposure to the patient. However, other factors also contribute, namely the sterility of the air in which the surgery is performed. Ultraviolet (UV) lighting has long been tried as an attempt to reduce the bacterial content of the air. A recent study demonstrated a decreased incidence of surgical site infections with use of UV light in the operating theater. In addition, the sterility of the air and the direction of the air flow are also controllable factors in the operating room. For many years, both vertical and horizontal airflow systems, combined with a variety of filters, have been employed to theoretically lower the risk of surgical site infections. Despite these efforts over many years, there is still no clear consensus on whether such systems decrease, make no difference, or actually increase the risk of airborne contamination.

Brandt C, Hott U, Sohr D, Daschner F, Gastmeier P, Ruden H. Operating room ventilation with laminar airflow shows no protective effect on the surgical site infection rate in orthopedic and abdominal surgery. *Ann Surg.* 2008;248:695-700. [PMID: 18948793]

D. Closure

The two main options for closure of a surgical wound are sutures and staples. Closure with staples may increase the risk of infection. When closing deep layers with suture, the nature of the filament can be considered. Traditional teaching is that monofilament closure decreases the risk of infection because theoretically, braided sutures provide a greater surface area for microbial contamination than monofilament sutures. This is likely merely anecdotal, however, as no studies have demonstrated superiority of one closure material over another regarding infection. Adherence to good surgical tissue handling techniques including atraumatic closure technique, maintenance of full-thickness fasciocutaneous flaps, and avoidance of excessive tissue undermining or devascularization are likely substantially more important than the choice of closure material.

E. Postoperative Blood Glucose Control

It is well known that diabetes is a risk factor for surgical site infections. The consequence of poor perioperative glucose control in terms of surgical site infection is somewhat less clear. Poor control of postoperative hyperglycemia substantially increases the risk of surgical site infection.

CLINICAL FINDINGS

Despite 2000 years of medical progress, the aforementioned cardinal signs of inflammation described by the Roman encyclopedist Celsus in the first century AD are still our primary means of diagnosing infection. In immunocompetent hosts, many, if not all, of the signs will be present if an acute infection is present. In the postsurgical setting, wound drainage, whether purulent, bloody, or clear, may also indicate that an infectious process is occurring. The postsurgical setting is more difficult, however, because the signs mentioned earlier are significant for inflammation in general and are not specific for infection. Distinguishing between a routine postoperative wound, a poorly healing postoperative wound, a hematoma, or an infection can be extremely difficult.

In the postoperative situation, infection may be diagnosed by a clinical scenario that does not improve with time. After surgery, pain, swelling, and erythema usually decrease over a period of days to weeks. If, instead of improving, the symptoms of inflammation increase, infection may be present.

Laboratory studies may help to distinguish infection from other diagnoses. The presence of a high white blood cell count, especially if the percentage of neutrophils is greater than 70% of the total, suggests infection. Leukocytosis is not sensitive for localized infection, however, and has greater sensitivity with systemic disease than with a localized problem. An increased ESR is another sensitive but nonspecific marker. The ESR will increase any time inflammation is present, dramatically reducing its utility in the postoperative situation or in any scenario wherein multiple inflammatory etiologies may be present. An increase in the serum CRP is somewhat more specific for infection, but not specific enough to act on in the absence of other signs or symptoms. The CRP generally increases very rapidly in the presence of infection and then begins to decrease after 48 to 72 hours. The ESR takes much longer to normalize, often peaking over a period of several days and decreasing much more slowly. Abnormalities in these lab values are corroborative of, but not diagnostic of, a musculoskeletal infection.

DIFFERENTIAL DIAGNOSIS

Infection, the great masquerader, generally is part of an extensive differential diagnosis. In fact, the diagnosis of infection is frequently confounded by many other medical conditions, most of them quite common.

Infection is frequently confused with trauma. In the early stages of a healing contusion, the soft-tissue hematoma mimics an abscess. Because hematomas may subsequently become infected, the clinical scenario may become further confused. The increasing prevalence of anticoagulation for a number of cardiac or other medical comorbidities renders even the most trivial trauma capable of producing substantial bleeding. Furthermore, metabolizing blood products may yield a febrile response, placing the clinician in a position of possibly operating on a hematoma in an anticoagulated patient, or ignoring a large soft-tissue infection in an individual who is substantially medically compromised.

Some musculoskeletal neoplasms may be confused with infections. Most soft-tissue sarcomas produce swelling and may produce pain to palpation. Their heterogeneous imaging characteristics on MRI scan have led numerous surgeons into a "simple irrigation and debridement" that unfortunately enters a sarcoma, thus producing substantial bleeding and possible oncologic compromise. Radiographically, osteosarcoma may look nearly exactly like osteomyelitis. Both can produce geographic or permeative bony changes with substantial new bone formation. Both are painful and produce swelling. Both can occur in the metaphyses of children. Similarly, Ewing sarcoma produces permeative bony changes mimicking those produced by purulence. Because Ewing sarcoma, lymphoma, and osteomyelitis are composed of small blue cells without matrix, all may resemble frank purulence at the time of debridement. The orthopedic oncologist's admonition to "send every infection to pathology and culture every tumor" was born of this confusion.

Fortunately, needle biopsy may assist in narrowing this differential diagnosis without undue potential for causing harm. Unless the patient is septic and in extremis, most suspected infections can be simply aspirated, either with or without radiographic imaging guidance. This approach has multiple advantages:

1. Infections composed of purulent material can be aspirated, and appropriate cultures can be obtained quickly, easily, and before the administration of antibiotics.
2. Needle aspiration is unlikely to cause bleeding complications, even in anticoagulated patients. Hemostasis is almost always achievable using direct pressure, and the patient's coagulopathy may be corrected before any necessary surgical interventions.
3. In cases where sarcoma enters the differential diagnosis, needle biopsy may not only obtain purulent samples (if infection is present), but will also allow pathologic diagnosis. Although there is current debate regarding whether needle tracks should be excised at the time of sarcoma surgery, excising a needle track is always easier than a surgical incision, and does not have the potential complication of an improperly placed incision.

Other inflammatory conditions also mimic infection. Because the physical signs of infection are the signs of inflammation, the two can present nearly identically. Aseptic myonecrosis, as seen in statin-induced myonecrosis, is remarkably similar to infection, with pain, inflammation, and swelling. Diabetic myonecrosis may behave like infection as well. Tumoral calcinosis, as seen in patients with renal insufficiency, produces soft-tissue masses with pain and skin changes, also mimicking abscesses.

COMPLICATIONS

The complications of infection may be truly grave. In situations of systemic sepsis, failure to adequately treat both the local and systemic manifestations of infection may lead to the patient's demise. Similarly, clostridial fasciitis may become rapidly progressive, causing massive tissue loss, loss of limb, or even death. If the patient's system fails to clear or suppress either prosthetic infection or osteomyelitis, amputation may be required to control local disease. Even with successful treatment, infection may lead to substantial loss of tissue, function, social status, and income for the affected patient.

One specific complication of chronic infection is the development of squamous cell carcinoma (a "Marjolin ulcer"). This occurs when any chronically (generally of >20 years' duration) draining infection causes enough irritation to the surrounding skin to cause the development of an invasive carcinoma. Because this becomes a potentially life-threatening situation in the face of limb salvage that has failed to control the baseline infection, amputation is often the treatment of choice.

TREATMENT

Treatment of orthopedic infections generally involves a multimodality and often multidisciplinary approach. Although simple skin infections such as cellulitis or folliculitis may respond completely with medical treatments alone, deep orthopedic infections generally require both surgical and medical intervention. The presence of inert materials, such as dead bone or metal prostheses, frequently mandates a more aggressive approach as the blood flow required for successful antibiotic treatment is obviously not present.

Pediatric Osteomyelitis

Pediatric osteomyelitis is primarily a surgical disease. The slow, sinusoidal blood flow within the metaphyses allows bacteria to multiply in the region (see General Considerations). Once a sequestrum has formed, this necrotic substrate provides a perfect medium for bacterial growth. Infection will progress until an involucrum forms or the bone is entirely destroyed.

Surgery consists of draining the infected bone and removing any sequestrum, if present. If no sequestrum is present, the bone may be opened with a high-speed burr, gouges, drill, or osteotome, and the purulent material drained. If the adjacent joint is also involved, it may be opened, drained, and irrigated. A deep drain is usually placed within the bone and/or joint and left until drainage ceases. Intravenous antibiotics are then instituted and tailored to the culture results, if positive. Four to 6 weeks of treatment are generally sufficient to produce a cure.

Adult Osteomyelitis

Treatment of adult osteomyelitis is often much more difficult than the pediatric variety. The comorbidities surrounding the orthopedic condition are chronic and may only be optimized rather than eliminated. Adult osteomyelitis also requires much more aggressive surgical and medical treatment than the pediatric condition.

Like pediatric osteomyelitis, treating adult osteomyelitis absolutely requires the removal of all necrotic bone. This is frequently much more difficult, as areas of necrosis may be extensive and removal of all dead bone may produce large, segmental bony defects. Similarly, extensive areas of poorly vascularized, fibrotic, or necrotic soft tissue may be present, requiring thorough debridement.

Careful preoperative planning is required. The extent of bony involvement can be estimated preoperatively using CT scanning, as necrotic bone is frequently sclerotic and hyperdense with this modality. If a segmental defect is anticipated or if circumferential debridement would yield a bone at substantial risk for pathologic fracture, stabilization will be necessary. For small defects or situations where a limited number of debridements is anticipated, stabilization using intramedullary nail or plate fixation may be ideal. For larger defects or situations where multiple debridements are necessary, external fixation either using standard or thin wire (Ilizarov) techniques may be ideal. This allows skeletal stabilization with access to the soft tissues. External fixation may ultimately be revised to internal fixation once the infection is eradicated or used as definitive fixation after grafting or bone transport.

Planning for soft-tissue reconstruction is also necessary. Draining sinuses, necrotic tissue, and poorly vascularized areas should be thoroughly and radically debrided. This generally yields soft-tissue defects that require plastic surgical reconstruction, either with local or free tissue transfers.

Adult osteomyelitis secondary to pressure phenomena provides a special case (see General Considerations). In this situation, patients are either mentally or physically inhibited from perceiving or responding to pressure. If the pressure sore extends to the bone, osteomyelitis occurs by definition. Bone biopsy is not necessary for diagnosis in this case but may be useful to tailor antibiotic treatment. Surgical treatment, if necessary based on patient wishes, life expectancy, and comorbidities, is often radical with removal of large portions of the sacrum, pelvis, or proximal femur. Plastic reconstruction is generally necessary.

Antibiotic treatment for adult osteomyelitis is often multimodal. Using two or even three agents in combination can facilitate penetration into involved tissues and can help to limit side effects and toxicities. Obtaining a culture from a deep source is very important for speciation, and patients with chronic draining sinuses are often given an antibiotic holiday for several days to weeks to allow deep cultures to grow. Deep tissue cultures are both more sensitive and specific than culture swabs. Culturing sinus tracts or purulent drainage is of no benefit and may cause harm and confusion.

Adult Soft-Tissue Infections

Soft-tissue infections that result from intravenous or subcutaneous drug abuse may be treated by incision and drainage, possibly with open packing and systemic antibiotics. More severe infections, especially in immunocompromised individuals, require much more aggressive treatment. All abscess cavities must be thoroughly opened, and all necrotic tissue removed. Broad-spectrum antibiotics are generally used, and multiple agents may be used in combination, depending on the clinical scenario. Successful treatment demands an immunocompetent host, so any immunomodulating agents should be discontinued. Leukocyte proliferation growth factors may be contemplated in neutropenic hosts.

Treatment of neutropenic myonecrosis is especially difficult. In this scenario, a neutropenic host presents with fever, severe pain, and cellulitis. MRI generally fails to reveal any abscess or other surgical condition, as the host does not possess enough immune function even to create an abscess. Broad-spectrum antibiotics are instituted, as in any neutropenic fever protocol, but will fail to reduce fevers or eliminate erythema. If the patient's condition continues to deteriorate without another source, the area of erythema should be opened, and the subjacent muscle examined surgically. Frequently, the muscle will be completely necrotic, but *without* the liquefactive necrosis encountered in the pyomyositis of immunocompetent individuals. Debridement must continue until adequate bleeding and viable muscle are appreciated. The entire necrotic portion of the compartment must be removed. In severe cases, the entire compartment will be necrotic, and all vessels leading into the muscle will have clotted due to bacterial thrombi. This appearance is not dissimilar to that found in advanced compartment syndrome, with patent major vessels and compromised muscular branches. Unlike in compartment syndrome, the entire compartment must be removed as a lifesaving measure.

Prosthetic Infections

As previously mentioned, the treatment of PJI depends on the acuity of the infection from the time of surgery or the inciting event. Early (within 4-6 weeks of surgery or within a few days of an invasive procedure) infections can be treated with surgical irrigation and exchange of the bearing surfaces. After this course of treatment, the surgeon must maintain a high level of vigilance, because this limited approach may not be successful. In chronic infections (over 6 weeks after implantation with no inciting event), the surgeon must assume that biofilm has contaminated the metal prosthesis and cannot be salvaged. If the patient is able to tolerate a staged revision and systemic antibiotics, this is the treatment with the greatest chance of success. If the patient cannot tolerate a staged revision due to comorbidities, the options include chronic antibiotic suppression and amputation. As the population ages, joint arthroplasties increase in frequency, and bacterial resistance continues to evolve, prosthetic infections will continue to challenge orthopedic surgeons.

Traumatic Infections

Traumatic infections are an especially difficult problem because they combine the infection risks inherent in any orthopedic surgery as well as the contamination of the traumatic event. The mainstays of modern treatment are prompt, thorough debridement of devitalized tissue and rigid fixation. Not surprisingly, the risk of infection is directly proportional to the degree of soft-tissue damage imparted by the injury. The patient's functional capacity, regenerative capacity, nutrition, and overall health also affect the risk of infection. Although the surgeon has no control over the magnitude of the trauma or the health of the individual, the surgeon has complete control over the quality of the debridement and fixation and therefore must maximize these. The optimal treatment of traumatic infections often involves a multidisciplinary team including orthopedic surgeons, plastic surgeons, and infectious disease specialists. Indeed, the literature suggests that patients treated with a multidisciplinary approach have better outcomes than those who are not.

Cierny G 3rd, DiPasquale D. Treatment of chronic infection. *J Am Acad Orthop Surg.* 2006;14:S105-S110. [PMID: 17003180]

Ziran BH, Rao N, Hall RA. A dedicated team approach enhances outcomes of osteomyelitis treatment. *Clin Orthop Relat Res.* 2003;414:31-36. [PMID: 12966273]

PROGNOSIS

It is virtually impossible to predict the prognosis of musculoskeletal infections as a whole because the ultimate success of treatment depends on enumerable variables, as we have indicated many times within this chapter. Host factors (age, nutrition, comorbidities, anatomic location), pathogen factors (organism type and virulence), and physician factors (index of suspicion, quality of technique, available resources) all impact tremendously on the patient's outcome. The principles of musculoskeletal infection treatment are the same in every instance. A high index of suspicion, correct interpretation of laboratory and clinical data, thorough surgery when indicated, optimization of host factors, and pathogen-specific antibiotic therapy are the pillars of treatment for musculoskeletal infections. In all instances, adherence to these principles will maximize the patient's prognosis.

10 Foot and Ankle Surgery

Kshitij Manchanda, MD
Steven D. K. Ross, MD
Dane K. Wukich, MD

BIOMECHANIC PRINCIPLES OF THE FOOT AND ANKLE

The primary role of the foot and ankle is locomotion. It is critical for those treating disorders of the foot and ankle to not only have knowledge and understanding of the anatomy but also the biomechanical principles of the foot and ankle. The following is a brief description of the biomechanics of the foot and ankle during the gait cycle. Understanding and being familiar with these principles aids in diagnosing problems that affect the anatomy and function of the foot and ankle.

Gait

Gait is the orderly progression of the body through space while expending as little energy as possible. The phases of gait are described in more detail in Chapter 13. As the body moves through a gait cycle, muscle forces are generated actively to counteract the passive effects of gravity on the body. To accommodate these forces, the foot is flexible at the time of heel strike to allow for absorption of impact of the body against the ground. However, at the end of stance phase, the foot becomes rigid at toe-off, when it must assist in propelling the body forward. The magnitude of the forces on the foot increases significantly as the speed of gait increases. For example, when an individual is walking, the initial force with which the foot meets the ground is approximately 80% of body weight. With jogging, the force increases to approximately 160%. The peak force against the foot during walking is 110% of body weight, and for jogging 240%. This marked increase in force contributes to some of the injuries seen in runners.

The Walking Cycle

An important component of the physical examination is observation of the patient during the walking cycle (Figures 10–1 and 10–2). This helps in determining the cause of a gait anomaly. For example, an equinus deformity from spasticity or contracture will cause the forefoot to make initial contact with the ground rather than the heel. Furthermore, at 7% of the gait cycle, the foot is usually flat on the ground, but spasticity or contracture of the Achilles tendon causes this to be delayed. At 12% of the cycle, the opposite foot toes off and the swing phase begins. Heel rise of the standing foot begins at 34% of the cycle as the swinging leg passes the standing limb. However, with spasticity, heel rise may occur earlier, whereas with gastrocsoleus weakness, heel rise will be later. Heel strike of the opposite foot occurs at 50% of the cycle, ending the period of single-limb support, and may occur sooner if there is weakness of the contralateral gastrocsoleus muscle. Toe-off of the opposite foot occurs at 62% of the cycle, at the beginning of the swing phase. These markers of the gait cycle should be kept in mind when observing gait, so pathologic conditions may be identified.

Motions of the Foot and Ankle

The majority of dorsiflexion and plantarflexion occurs through the ankle joint. The subtalar joint allows for inversion (varus) and eversion (valgus). Adduction, which is movement toward the midline, and abduction, which is movement away from the midline, occurs through the transverse tarsal joint (talonavicular and calcaneocuboid joints). Supination and pronation are used in describing combinations of movements, but unfortunately, these terms are sometimes used interchangeably with inversion/eversion. Supination is a combination of plantarflexion of the ankle joint, inversion of the subtalar joint, and adduction of the transverse tarsal joint. Pronation is the exact opposite movement: dorsiflexion of the ankle joint, eversion of the subtalar joint, and abduction of the transverse tarsal joint. The nomenclature may also be confusing when such terms as forefoot varus and forefoot valgus are used (Figure 10–3). Forefoot varus or valgus is an anatomic deformity that may be observed when the hindfoot is placed in neutral position.

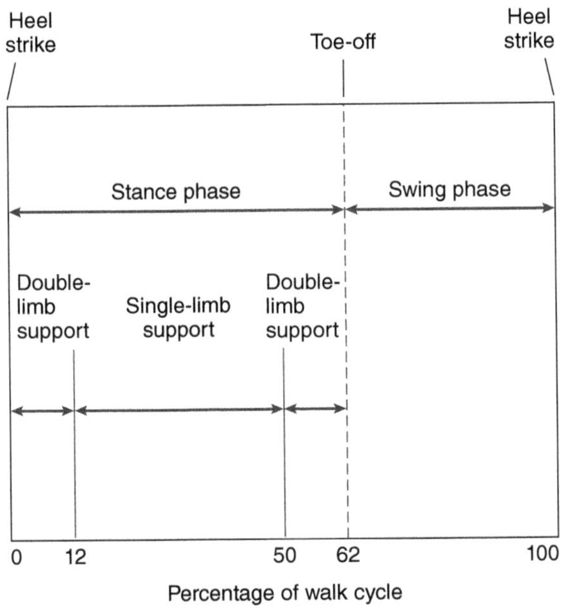

▲ **Figure 10–1. Phases of the walking cycle. Stance phase constitutes approximately 62% and swing phase 38% of the cycle.** (Reprinted with permission, from Mann RA, Coughlin MJ. *The Video Textbook of Foot and Ankle Surgery*. Medical Video Productions, 1991.)

Neutral position is achieved when the calcaneus is aligned with the long axis of the tibia and the head of the talus is covered with the navicular bone. Forefoot varus deformity is present when the lateral aspect of the forefoot is in greater plantarflexion than the medial aspect (ie, the medial column is elevated). With a flexible deformity, the foot lies flat on the floor during stance, but with a fixed deformity, excessive weight is borne on the lateral side of the foot. As a result, as the weight passes onto the forefoot, the calcaneus goes into a valgus position, and this may result in lateral impingement of the calcaneus against the fibula if severe. In forefoot valgus deformity, the medial side of the foot has greater plantarflexion than the lateral side and results in excessive weight bearing by the first metatarsal head. To accommodate for this deformity, the calcaneus assumes a varus position, which may result in a feeling of instability at the ankle joint.

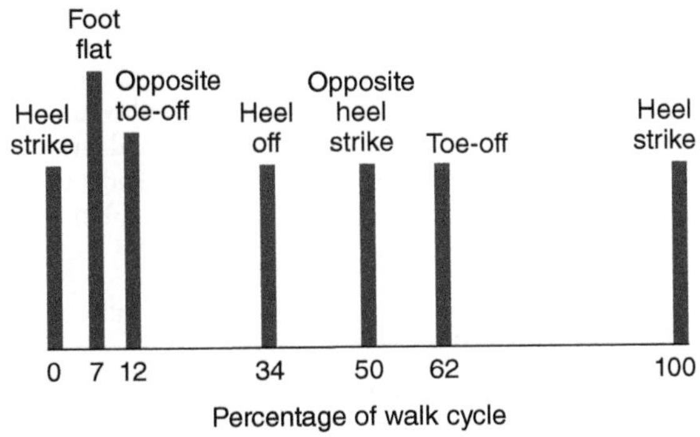

▲ **Figure 10–2. Events of the walking cycle.** (Reprinted with permission, from Mann RA, Coughlin MJ. *The Video Textbook of Foot and Ankle Surgery*. Medical Video Productions, 1991.)

Mechanisms of the Foot During Weight Bearing

During gait, the foot is flexible at heel strike to absorb the impact of striking the ground. As a result, the subtalar joint collapses into a position of valgus, causing internal rotation of the tibia and resulting in unlocking of the transverse tarsal (talonavicular and calcaneocuboid) joint. This allows the foot to be flexible. During heel strike, the anterior compartment muscles are the only muscles that are active and firing. The anterior compartment muscles control the initial rapid plantarflexion following heel strike by an eccentric or lengthening contraction (ie, decelerating plantarflexion). The flexibility of the foot is greatest at approximately 7% of the cycle. As the body passes over the foot in foot flat, the heel begins to rise and then forces the metatarsophalangeal joints into extension (dorsiflexion). As this occurs, the foot is converted into a rigid lever that supports the body at the time of toe-off. The mechanisms that bring about conversion of the foot from a flexible to a rigid structure are (1) the tightening of the plantar aponeurosis, the windlass mechanism; (2) the progressive external rotation of the lower extremity, which begins at the pelvis and is passed distally across the ankle joint into the subtalar joint; and (3) the stabilization of the transverse tarsal joint, which results from the progressive inversion of the subtalar joint.

Joints of the Foot and Ankle

A. Ankle Joint

The ankle joint is the articulation of the talus with the tibia and fibula and has a range of motion (ROM) of 15 degrees of dorsiflexion to 55 degrees of plantarflexion. There is also a small amount of motion in the transverse plane, approximately 15 degrees. The anterior compartment muscles of the leg, the tibialis anterior and the toe extensors, control the amount of plantarflexion of the ankle joint from the time point of heel ground contact to 10% stance. These muscles are responsible for dorsiflexion of the foot and ankle during swing phase. Any weakness or pathology affecting the anterior compartment may result in a footslap at heel strike and a dropfoot during swing phase. The greatest force across the ankle joint during walking is calculated to be approximately 4.5 times body weight, which occurs at 40% of the walking cycle.

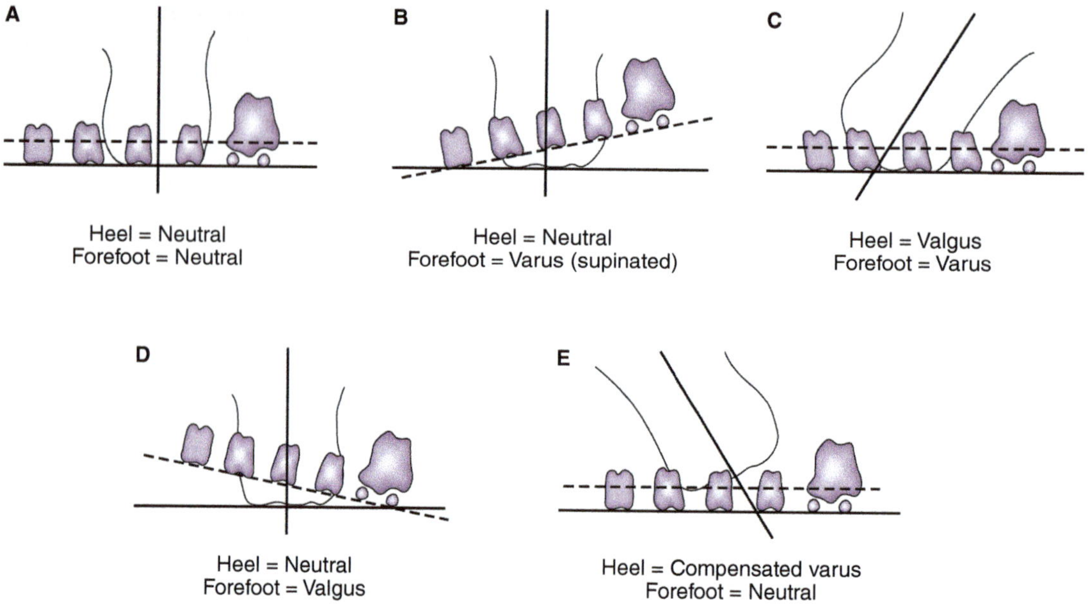

▲ **Figure 10–3.** Biomechanics of foot pressure. **A:** Normal alignment: forefoot perpendicular to heel. **B:** Forefoot varus (uncompensated): lateral aspect of forefoot plantarflexed in relation to medial aspect. **C:** Forefoot varus (compensated): with the forefoot flat on the floor, the heel assumes a valgus position. **D:** Forefoot valgus (uncompensated): medial aspect of forefoot plantarflexed in relation to lateral aspect. **E:** Forefoot valgus (compensated): with the forefoot flat on the floor, the heel assumes a varus position. (Reprinted with permission, from Mann RA, Coughlin MJ. *The Video Textbook of Foot and Ankle Surgery.* Medical Video Productions, 1991.)

B. Subtalar Joint

The subtalar joint is the articulation between the talus and the calcaneus and is comprised of three components: the posterior, middle, and anterior facets. The most important and largest of these facets is the posterior facet. Through the subtalar joint, there is inversion of approximately 20 degrees and eversion of approximately 5 to 10 degrees. These motions are brought about by the tibialis posterior muscle (inversion) and the peroneus brevis (eversion). During the walking cycle at initial ground contact, eversion is a passive mechanism and occurs because of the shape of the articulations and their ligamentous support. Inversion occurs both actively and passively at the time of toe-off. Active control is achieved by the gastrocsoleus and posterior tibial muscles, and passive inversion occurs by the action of the plantar aponeurosis, the external rotation of the lower extremity, and the oblique metatarsal break.

C. Talonavicular Joint and Calcaneocuboid Joint

The talonavicular and calcaneocuboid joints (also known as the transverse tarsal joint) functionally act as a single joint. The transverse tarsal joint is responsible for adduction and abduction, 15 degrees and 10 degrees, respectively. The head of the talus is firmly seated into the navicular at the time of toe-off, adding stability to the foot. The transverse tarsal joint also permits accommodation for supination and pronation. Also, the stability of the transverse tarsal joint is controlled by the position of the subtalar joint. When the subtalar joint is in an inverted position, the axes of these two joints are nonparallel, giving rise to increased stability of the hindfoot. When the calcaneus is in an everted position at the time of heel strike, these joints are parallel to one another, thereby giving rise to increased flexibility of these joints (Figure 10–4). Clinically, it is important to maintain the subtalar joint in 5 to 7 degrees of valgus during subtalar arthrodesis in order to maintain the foot's flexibility and ability to walk. If the subtalar joint is malpositioned into hindfoot varus, the transverse tarsal joint will be locked and the resulting foot will be stiff, causing difficulty with ambulation for the patient.

D. Metatarsophalangeal Joints

The metatarsophalangeal joint is the articulation of the metatarsal head and base of the proximal phalanx. The normal motion at this joint is 50 to 70 degrees of dorsiflexion (extension) to 15 to 25 degrees of plantarflexion (flexion). The importance of this joint in the walking cycle is discussed in detail in the following section on the first toe.

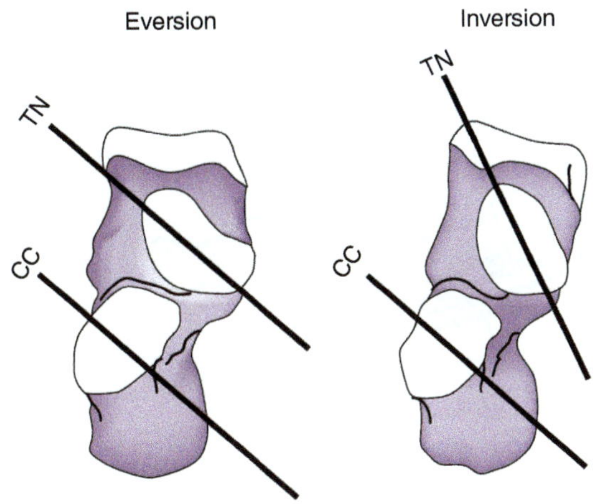

▲ **Figure 10–4.** The function of the transverse tarsal joint as described by Elftman demonstrates that when the calcaneus is in eversion, the resultant axes of the talonavicular (TN) and calcaneocuboid (CC) joints are parallel or congruent. When the subtalar joint is in an inverted position, the axes are incongruent, giving increased stability to the midfoot. (Reprinted with permission, from Mann RA, Coughlin MJ. *The Video Textbook of Foot and Ankle Surgery*. Medical Video Productions, 1991.)

E. The Plantar Aponeurosis

Although the plantar aponeurosis is not an articulation per se, it plays a predominant role in the overall stability of the foot. The plantar aponeurosis originates from the tubercle of the calcaneus and inserts on the base of the proximal phalanges (Figure 10–5). During gait, the metatarsophalangeal joints extend at the last half of the stance phase. The plantar aponeurosis forces the metatarsal heads into a plantarward direction, which raises the longitudinal arch, and this is known as the windlass mechanism. Additionally, the plantar aponeurosis increases the effect that a tensile force in the Achilles tendon has on the tensile force in the plantar fascia. The result is a rigid foot that allows for the body to push-off during gait. This mechanism also helps to invert the subtalar joint, thereby increasing the rigidity of the foot for push-off.

F. Gait Abnormalities

Common disorders of gait are described.

1. Pes planus deformity—Pes planus is a decreased longitudinal arch. This may occur when the patient has hypermobility of the joints and the foot is too flexible. As a result, the gait pattern is abnormal; there is excessive valgus of the hindfoot and, in severe cases, breaking down of the longitudinal arch. The forefoot becomes abducted at the beginning of the gait cycle, and there is increased weight bearing surface on the plantar aspect of the foot. This may cause easy fatigability because of the lack of adequate support of the longitudinal arch.

2. Cavus deformity—A cavus deformity is an excessive elevation of the longitudinal arch. Frequently, there is an associated decrease in the motion of the foot, and the hindfoot is in varus while the forefoot is in valgus. Also, the toes may assume a claw deformity. Clinical examples of this deformity are Charcot-Marie-Tooth disease, poliomyelitis, and sometimes chronic compartment syndrome of the leg. The overall effect is decreased surface area for weight bearing. Claw toe deformities may further reduce contact with the ground. As a result, the gait pattern is abnormal, and increased pressure on the heel at heel strike is seen. With the progression of gait, there is increased pressure of the lateral plantar aspect of the foot and the first metatarsal head.

3. Dropfoot gait—Weakness of the anterior tibialis muscle (ie, lumbar radiculopathy) or a common peroneal nerve palsy may result in a dropfoot gait. These patients lack ankle active dorsiflexion, and the ankle joint plantarflexors have no antagonist. These patients adopt a steppage-type gait, manifested by increased flexion of the hip and knee to enable the swinging leg to clear the ground. If this compensatory mechanism does not occur, the patient may catch the toes on the ground and fall.

4. Equinus gait—An equinus contracture can occur if there is anterior compartment weakness, which results in uncompensated pull of the gastrocsoleus complex. Equinus contractures may also be caused by a stroke or head injury, trauma to the lower extremity, or a congenital deformity, and it often is associated with tightness of the posterior capsule. The ankle is plantarflexed to varying degrees during the gait cycle, characterized by an increase in forefoot ground contact. Often, the heel does not touch the ground unless the patient assumes a foot forward posture with the knee extended. The anterior loading of the foot results in a back knee thrust, which may, over a long period of time, result in a hyperextension deformity of the knee. A weak quadriceps muscle may accentuate this problem.

Alazzawi S, Sukeik M, King D, et al. Foot and ankle history and clinical examination: a guide to everyday practice. *World J Orthop*. 2017;8(1):21-29. [PMID: 28144575]

Buldt AK, Levinger P, Murley GS, et al. Foot posture is associated with kinematics of the foot during gait: A comparison of normal, planus and cavus feet. *Gait Posture*. 2015;42(1):42-48. [PMID: 25819716]

Fukano M, Fukubayashi T, Kumai T. In vivo talocrural and subtalar kinematics during the stance phase of walking in individuals with repetitive ankle sprains. *J Biomech*. 2020;101:109651. [PMID: 32029243]

Kim HY, Shin HS, Ko JH, et al. Gait analysis of symptomatic flatfoot in children: an observational study. *Clin Orthop Surg*. 2017;9(3):363-373. [PMID: 28861205]

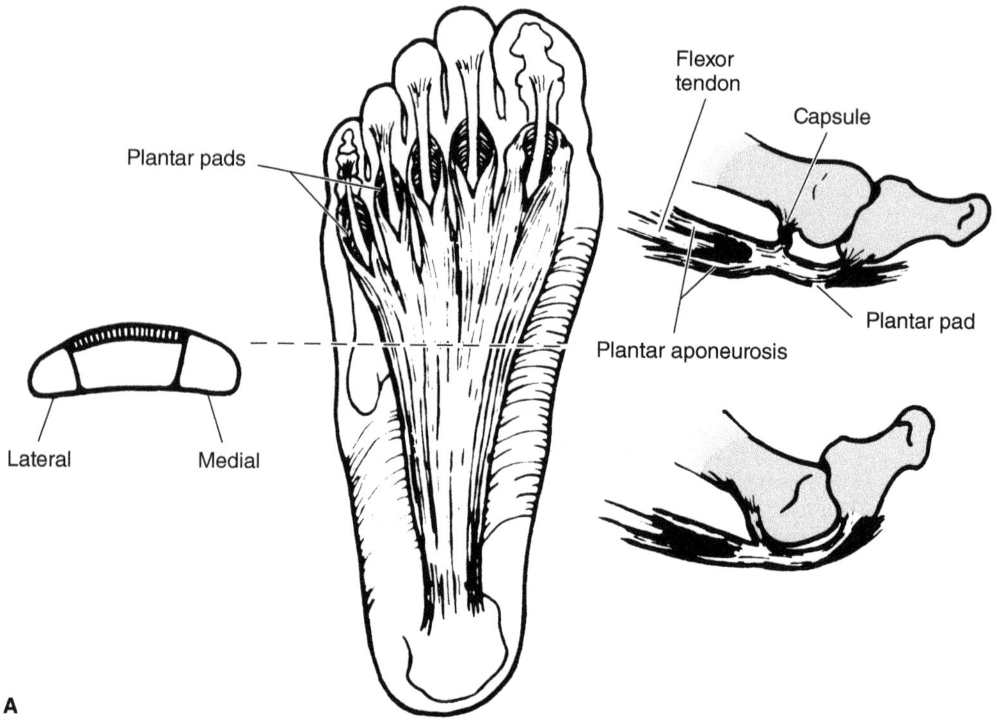

A

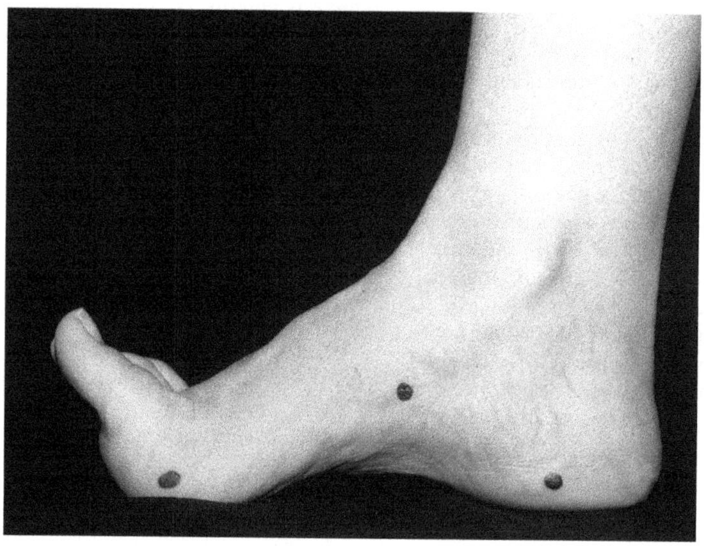

B

▲ **Figure 10–5.** Windlass mechanism. **A:** The plantar aponeurosis, which arises from the tubercle of the calcaneus, divides and inserts into the base of each of the proximal phalanges. **B:** Dorsiflexion of the metatarsophalangeal joints wraps the plantar aponeurosis around the metatarsal head, depressing the metatarsal heads and elevating the longitudinal arch. (Reprinted with permission, from Mann RA, Coughlin MJ. *The Video Textbook of Foot and Ankle Surgery.* Medical Video Productions, 1991.)

DEFORMITIES OF THE FIRST TOE

Biomechanical Principles

The first metatarsophalangeal joint functions mainly as a weight bearing structure and stabilizer of the medial aspect of the longitudinal arch. The static stability of the first metatarsophalangeal joint is provided by the collateral ligaments and the strong plantar plate, which consists of the plantar aponeurosis and the joint capsule. Added dynamic stability is provided by the abductor hallucis and adductor hallucis muscles, which insert along the medial and lateral sides of the metatarsal head, respectively. No muscle inserts into the metatarsal head per se, and therefore, it is suspended in a sling of muscles and tendons. This allows the metatarsal head to be pushed in a medial or lateral direction, depending on the deviation of the proximal phalanx.

The plantar aponeurosis forces the metatarsal heads into plantarflexion during the last third of the stance phase of the walking cycle. The hallux experiences greater pressure as it is transferred from the metatarsal heads to the lesser toes (Figure 10–5). If this windlass mechanism for the hallux is lost as occurs in a bunion deformity, pressure is no longer transferred to the toes but remains beneath the metatarsal heads. Metatarsalgia results from the transfer of this load, especially beneath the lesser metatarsal heads. The second metatarsal frequently bears the load because the weight-bearing ability of the first metatarsal is disrupted. Changes to the normal biomechanics of this joint may result in a transfer lesion, which is a hyperkeratotic lesion under the lesser metatarsal heads. Surgical procedures on the hallux can disrupt this mechanism. In the Keller arthroplasty, the base of the proximal phalanx is resected, thereby disrupting the insertion of the plantar aponeurosis into the hallux. Prosthetic replacement of the first metatarsal joint may also result in loss of this mechanism. Metatarsal osteotomy or first tarsometarsal arthrodesis with excessive shortening (>5-7 mm) or dorsiflexion of the first metatarsal may also contribute to this problem.

Normal Anatomy

The first metatarsophalangeal joint is complex. It is made up of the articular surface of the metatarsal head and the base of the proximal phalanx, along with the two plantar, sesamoid bones. The sesamoids are connected by an intersesamoidal ligament, separated by a bony crista, and lie within the dual tendons of the flexor hallucis brevis. Medially and laterally, the collateral ligaments stabilize the metatarsophalangeal joint, and toward the plantar surface, they blend with the adductor and abductor hallucis tendons along the lateral and medial sides of the joint. Further toward the plantar surface, the sesamoids are stabilized by the firm attachment of the encapsulating plantar aponeurosis, which inserts into the base of the proximal phalanx. Plantar to the sesamoids passes the flexor hallucis longus tendon. Dorsally, the extensor hallucis longus tendon is stabilized by a medial and lateral hood mechanism similar to that present in the hand, and the extensor digitorum brevis muscle inserts into the proximal phalanx along the lateral aspect of the joint. Normal motion of the metatarsophalangeal joint consists of dorsiflexion and plantarflexion.

1. Hallux Valgus

Hallux valgus is also known as a bunion deformity. It is a complex deformity that includes lateral deviation of the proximal phalanx and the resultant medially directed pressure exerted against the metatarsal head. The medial eminence becomes prominent as the proximal phalanx drifts into a valgus position and the first metatarsal into varus (metatarsus primus varus). With chronic bunion deformity, the medial joint capsule becomes attenuated, and the lateral joint capsule becomes contracted. Although radiographically the sesamoids appeared subluxated, often the sesamoids initially remain aligned within the crista. The radiographic appearance is due to pronation of the hallux. As the metatarsal head is pushed medially, the sesamoids, which are firmly anchored by the adductor hallucis tendon and transverse metatarsal ligament, can slowly erode the crista. This allows for lateral subluxation of the sesamoids from being directly plantar to the first metatarsal. With the lateral deviation of the hallux, the extensor hallucis longus and flexor hallucis longus assume a lateral position and contribute to the lateral forces on the hallux. With a severe deformity, both the extrinsic and intrinsic muscles lie lateral to the longitudinal axis of the first metatarsophalangeal joint, thereby further enhancing the deformity. As the deformity progresses, further pronation of the hallux occurs because attenuation of the weakest portion of the capsule (the dorsomedial aspect) allows the abductor hallucis tendon to slide beneath the metatarsal head and rotate the proximal phalanx into a position of pronation. More rapid progression of the deformity may occur in a small percentage of patients whose first metatarsocuneiform joint demonstrates a significant degree of instability. Over the past decade, much has been learned about hallux valgus. Traditionally thought of as a two-dimensional deformity (frontal and sagittal), we now recognize that hallux valgus is a multiplanar deformity. Pronation of the first ray is an important part of pathoanatomy, often leading to medial hallux pinch callus formation.

General Considerations

The incidence of hallux valgus deformity is 10 times greater in women than in men and is also significantly higher in shod populations than unshod ones. And because women do so more than men, the conclusion can be made that a major contributing cause of hallux valgus deformity is wearing constricting shoes. Other factors that may contribute to hallux valgus are familial history of bunions, bilateral involvement, a long first ray, an oval or curved metatarsophalangeal joint articular surface, spasticity, and systemic disease such as rheumatoid arthritis. Common coexisting findings may include chronic tightness of the Achilles tendon or gastrocnemius, increased first ray mobility, or pes planus.

Clinical Findings

A. Symptoms and Signs

The most common symptom is pain over the medial eminence. Patients also complain of pain in the joint and pain under the second metatarsal head (transfer lesion or metatarsalgia). The deformity may impact the type of shoewear that can be worn, and activity limitation may be part of the constellation of symptoms. The patient's occupation, sports activities, and typical shoewear should be noted.

A complete evaluation is performed on both lower extremities with the patient undressed from the knees to the toes. The patient is instructed to stand and walk. The posture of the foot is noted as well as the position of the hallux and lesser toes. The skin is evaluated for erythema, swelling, ulceration, or callosities. The ROM is checked at the ankle, subtalar, transverse tarsal, and metatarsophalangeal joints. The neurovascular status of the foot is carefully assessed, noting absent pulses and venous stasis changes. If there is compromise of the vascularity, then vascular studies may be obtained. Doppler studies are obtained if there is any question regarding the circulatory status of the foot. It is important to note the ROM of the first metatarsophalangeal joint in the deformed and corrected position. The amount of motion limitation will give the surgeon insight into the degree of surgical correction that can be obtained at the joint without impairing motion of the joint. In addition, compression of the metatarsophalangeal joint with the grind test may identify subtle arthritic changes. The sesamoid apparatus should also be examined for tenderness. The first metatarsocuneiform joint is examined for hypermobility by stabilizing the medial cuneiform and ranging the first metatarsal dorsomedially and plantolaterally.

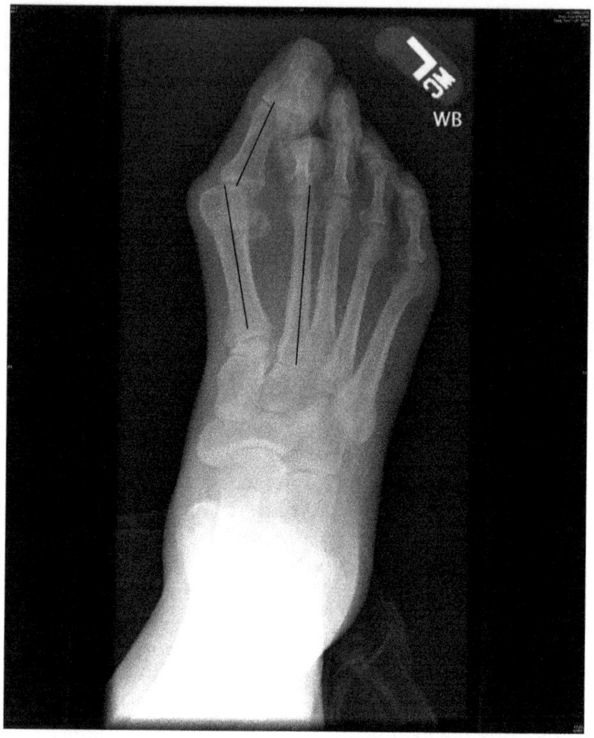

▲ **Figure 10–6.** Anteroposterior weight-bearing radiograph of a patient with a symptomatic hallux valgus deformity. Lines drawn show hallux valgus angle and first-second intermetatarsal angle.

B. Imaging Studies

Weight-bearing radiographs of the foot are important to evaluate the type and severity of the hallux valgus deformity. Axial sesamoid views are important as well. Radiographic evaluation of the first metatarsophalangeal joint includes:

1. The hallux valgus angle: The angle created by the intersection of the lines that longitudinally bisect the proximal phalanx and first metatarsal. A normal angle is less than 15 degrees (Figure 10–6).
2. The first-second intermetatarsal angle: The angle created by the intersection of the lines bisecting the first and second metatarsal shafts. A normal angle is less than 9 degrees (Figure 10–6).
3. The distal metatarsal articular angle: The angle of the distal articular surface of the first metatarsal to the long axis of the metatarsal. Normal is less than 10 degrees of lateral deviation.
4. Congruency of the first metatarsophalangeal joint: A congruent joint has no lateral subluxation of the proximal phalanx in relation to the first metatarsal head, and an incongruent joint has lateral subluxation of the proximal phalanx on the metatarsal head (Figure 10–7).
5. The first metatarsocuneiform joint: The angle is based on the distal articular surface of the medial cuneiform and the longitudinal axis of the first metatarsal. Excessive medial deviation may indicate that hypermobility may be present. Plantar gapping on the lateral x-ray also is indicative of hypermobility
6. Arthrosis of the metatarsophalangeal joint has joint space narrowing, osteophytes, subchondral sclerosis, and cysts.
7. The medial eminence: The characteristics are evaluated, especially size, as measured from the sagittal groove on the medial aspect of the first metatarsal shaft.

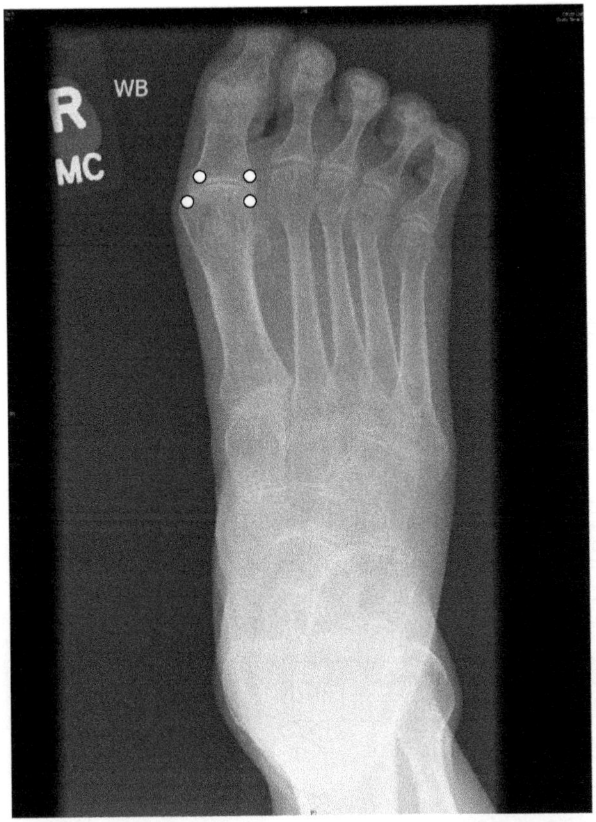

▲ **Figure 10–7.** Example of an incongruent first metatarsophalangeal joint, with mild lateral subluxation.

8. The hallux valgus interphalangeus angle is present when there is lateral deviation of the proximal or distal phalanx, or both, in relation to a line drawn across the base of the proximal phalanx. Normal is less than 10 degrees of lateral deviation.

Treatment

A. Nonoperative Treatment

As with all forefoot disorders, proper shoewear is important for successful conservative management. The patient should be encouraged to wear shoes of adequate size and shape. This simple form of management may relieve most symptoms. Padding is helpful to alleviate symptoms associated with the bunion deformity. Pads may be placed in the first web space or over the median eminence to help take pressure off a painful median eminence. Pads are also available that can be placed underneath the metatarsal heads to take pressure off painful calluses or sesamoids. In some patients, custom orthotic devices are helpful in decreasing pressure at symptomatic areas. Patients who fail these treatment options may consider surgical treatment to correct the deformity. Surgery is not recommended for cosmetic reasons or to allow patients to wear fashionable shoes, but rather to correct a symptomatic structural deformity.

Juvenile hallux valgus deformity is considered a different entity than adult hallux valgus. These patients may be challenging to treat, but as a general rule, nonoperative management should be continued until growth is completed, after which surgery may be considered. Extra care must be taken in juveniles as appearance may play a greater role in the patient's or parents' desire for surgery than in adults. Juvenile bunions are usually congruent deformities while adult bunions are often noncongruent deformities. Hallux valgus surgery is generally contraindicated in high-performance athletes or dancers until they are no longer able to perform at the level necessary to continue in their vocation or avocation. Premature surgery in these individuals may diminish their special abilities.

B. Surgical Treatment

1. Algorithm for surgical treatment—The patient's symptoms, the physical signs, and the radiographic findings must be taken into account when determining the best operation for that patient. It must be emphasized that there is not a single procedure appropriate for all hallux valgus deformities. Preoperative planning with all of these considerations is important.

The following factors need to be considered in the decision-making process:

1. Patient's chief complaint
2. Physical findings
3. Degree of hallux valgus angle and intermetatarsal angle
4. Distal metatarsal articular angle
5. Congruency or incongruency of the metatarsophalangeal joint
6. Presence of arthrosis of the joint
7. Degree of pronation of the hallux
8. Age of the patient
9. Circulatory status
10. Patient expectations for outcome of operation

The algorithm in Figure 10–8 divides hallux valgus deformities into three main groups: those with a congruent joint, those with an incongruent joint, and those associated with degenerative joint disease. The algorithm lists the operative procedure that may best correct the deformity within each classification. Although no one scheme is all inclusive, this algorithm is helpful in organizing the treatment plan.

The first step is to evaluate the first metatarsophalangeal joint for congruency. A congruent metatarsophalangeal joint generally requires excision of the large and symptomatic

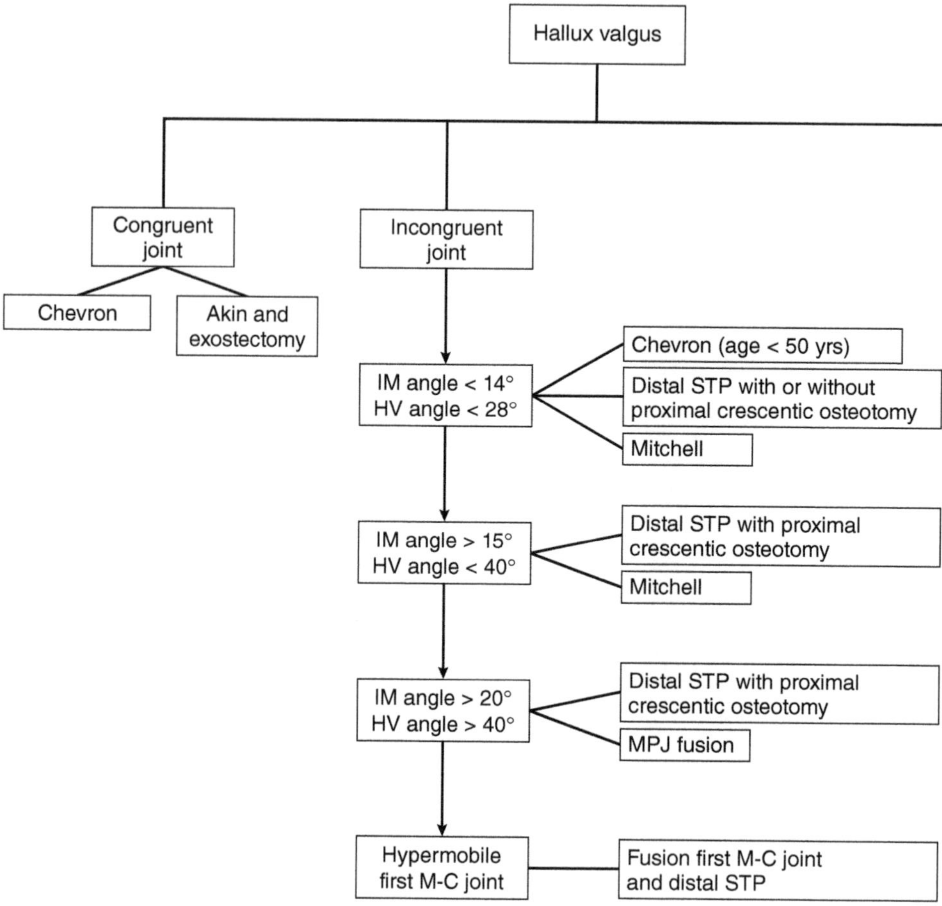

▲ **Figure 10–8. Algorithm for hallux valgus deformities. M-C, metatarsocuneiform; MPJ, metatarsal phalangeal joint; STP, soft-tissue procedure.** (Redrawn, with permission, from Mann RA, Coughlin MJ. *The Video Textbook of Foot and Ankle Surgery*. Medical Video Productions, 1991.)

medial eminence, and the joint does not require realignment. For a mild to moderate deformity, a biplanar chevron osteotomy with or without an Akin procedure yields good to excellent results.

With an incongruent joint, the proximal phalanx is subluxed laterally on the metatarsal head. The operative procedure necessitates that the proximal phalanx be reduced onto the metatarsal head. The procedure of choice depends on the severity of the deformity (Figure 10–8).

If the first metatarsocuneiform joint is hypermobile, a distal soft-tissue procedure with a metatarsocuneiform arthrodesis (Lapidus procedure) may be indicated. With a severe hallux valgus deformity, greater than 45- to 50-degree hallux valgus angle, and degenerative joint disease, arthrodesis of the metatarsophalangeal joint may be indicated. If routine hallux valgus repair is attempted in the patient with advanced arthrosis, stiffness of the metatarsophalangeal joint frequently results. Use of a prosthetic replacement, as a general rule, does not produce a satisfactory long-term result, particularly in active individuals.

2. Surgical procedures

A. Distal soft-tissue procedure—The McBride procedure was a commonly performed operation. It was modified by DuVries, followed by additional modifications, and is now called the distal soft-tissue procedure. The procedure used by itself is appropriate in mild hallux valgus deformities, where the intermetatarsal angle is less than 12 to 13 degrees and the hallux valgus angle is less than 30 degrees. Within this range of deformity, a satisfactory outcome can usually be anticipated from this procedure.

The distal soft-tissue procedure involves a medial incision to expose the metatarsophalangeal joint. The joint is inspected, and the medial eminence is removed 1 to 2 mm just medial to the sagittal sulcus and in line with the medial aspect of the metatarsal shaft. A second incision in the first interspace allows for releasing the soft-tissue contracture on the lateral side of the metatarsophalangeal joint. These structures include the lateral joint capsule, the adductor hallucis tendon, and the transverse metatarsal ligament (Figure 10–9). Once released, the medial side of the joint is plicated to hold the toe in correct alignment. Postoperatively, the patient is maintained in a firm compression dressing in the correct alignment, and the dressing is changed on a weekly basis for 8 weeks. During this period, the patient is permitted to ambulate in a postoperative shoe.

The most common complication of distal soft-tissue release is recurrence of the deformity, and this is usually because the deformity was too severe and a metatarsal osteotomy should have been added to the distal soft-tissue procedure. Other complications include paresthesias, instability, and overcorrection.

Hallux varus deformity is a medial deviation of the proximal phalanx on the metatarsal head, a complication that may occur in approximately 5% to 7% of cases. This deformity is usually a result of excessive excision of the medial eminence or fibular sesamoidectomy, which causes joint instability. Occasionally, the medial joint capsule is overplicated or the lateral joint capsule fails to attain adequate strength. Mild hallux varus deformity, up to 7 to 10 degrees, usually is of no clinical significance unless the joint is also hyperextended.

B. Distal soft-tissue procedure with proximal metatarsal osteotomy—A proximal metatarsal osteotomy will increase the correction of the distal soft-tissue procedure. Proximal metatarsal osteotomies address metatarsus primus varus (increased intermetatarsal angle), such as a deformity greater than 12 to 13 degrees, whereas the distal soft-tissue procedure alone cannot. Realignment of the fixed bony deformity present between the first and second metatarsals permits the combined procedure to be used for deformities with up to 50 degrees of hallux valgus and a 25-degree intermetatarsal angle.

The distal soft-tissue procedure is performed, as previously described. Another incision, based over the base of the first metatarsal, is made. A crescent-shaped saw blade is used to create a crescentic osteotomy, in which the concavity is directed proximally (Figure 10–10). This enables the surgeon to rotate the metatarsal head laterally as the metatarsocuneiform joint is pushed in a medial direction. This usually results in approximately 2 to 3 mm of lateral displacement of the osteotomy site. A single cancellous screw placed from the distal fragment into the proximal aspect allows for stable fixation. Other popular osteotomies include a chevron cut, Ludloff, scarf, and either opening or closing wedge osteotomies. Our preference when doing proximal procedures is to perform medial eminence excision after correction of the intermetatarsal angle. We have found that less medial eminence resection is then needed.

Postoperatively, the treatment is similar as for the distal soft-tissue procedure, with 8 weeks of dressing changes and immobilization in a postoperative shoe. Some surgeons use a controlled ankle motion boot or short leg cast.

The long-term results following the distal soft-tissue procedure with proximal osteotomy result in greater than 90% patient satisfaction. The addition of the osteotomy does create an increased risk of complications, but this risk is reported to be uniformly low. Dorsiflexion of the osteotomy site may occur but is usually not of clinical significance. Nonunion of the osteotomy is rare (<1% of cases). Excessive lateral displacement of the metatarsal head can result in hallux varus deformity, which is more resistant to treatment than when osteotomy is not included. Hallux varus is a potential for any proximal procedure since the power of correction, and even overcorrection, is greater than with distal procedures.

C. Chevron osteotomy—The chevron osteotomy is the most commonly performed bunion procedure in the United States. It is indicated for mild to moderate hallux valgus deformities, typically when the hallux valgus angle is less than 30 degrees and the intermetatarsal angle is less than 14 degrees. The distal metatarsal articular angle should be less than 12 degrees or complete correction will not be obtained. The operative procedure is based on lateral translation of the metatarsal head, along with plication of the medial joint capsule. The osteotomy is performed through a medial incision to allow removal of the medial eminence. Then, a chevron-shaped cut with the apex based distally is made with a small sagittal saw. The metatarsal head fragment is translated laterally approximately one-third of the width of the metatarsal head, or 3 to 4 mm. The medial bony prominence created by the shift of the metatarsal head is excised and the medial joint capsule plicated. The osteotomy site is fixed with a pin or a screw (Figure 10–11).

Postoperatively, the foot is firmly bandaged for 6 to 8 weeks in corrected alignment, and the patient is permitted to ambulate in a postoperative shoe. If a pin was used for fixation, it is removed after 4 to 6 weeks.

Radiographic improvement is seen with high patient satisfaction, and it is durable because there is consistent improvement with time. There is no difference in outcome between patients younger and older than 50 years. However, if the indications are stretched to include more severe deformities, higher rates of recurrence and unsatisfactory results are likely. The most serious complication, occurring in 0% to 20% of cases, is avascular necrosis of the metatarsal head, which is probably the result of extensive stripping of the soft tissue surrounding the head, especially if a lateral release is done concurrently. The major blood supply to the metatarsal head is from the plantar lateral corner of the metatarsal neck. Therefore, care must be used when performing the saw cut, and the saw should be removed once the osteotomy is completed so as to not injure the vessels on the lateral aspect of the metatarsal head. As with any type of osteotomy, the distal fragment is capable of migrating either too far laterally or medially, giving rise either to hallux varus deformity

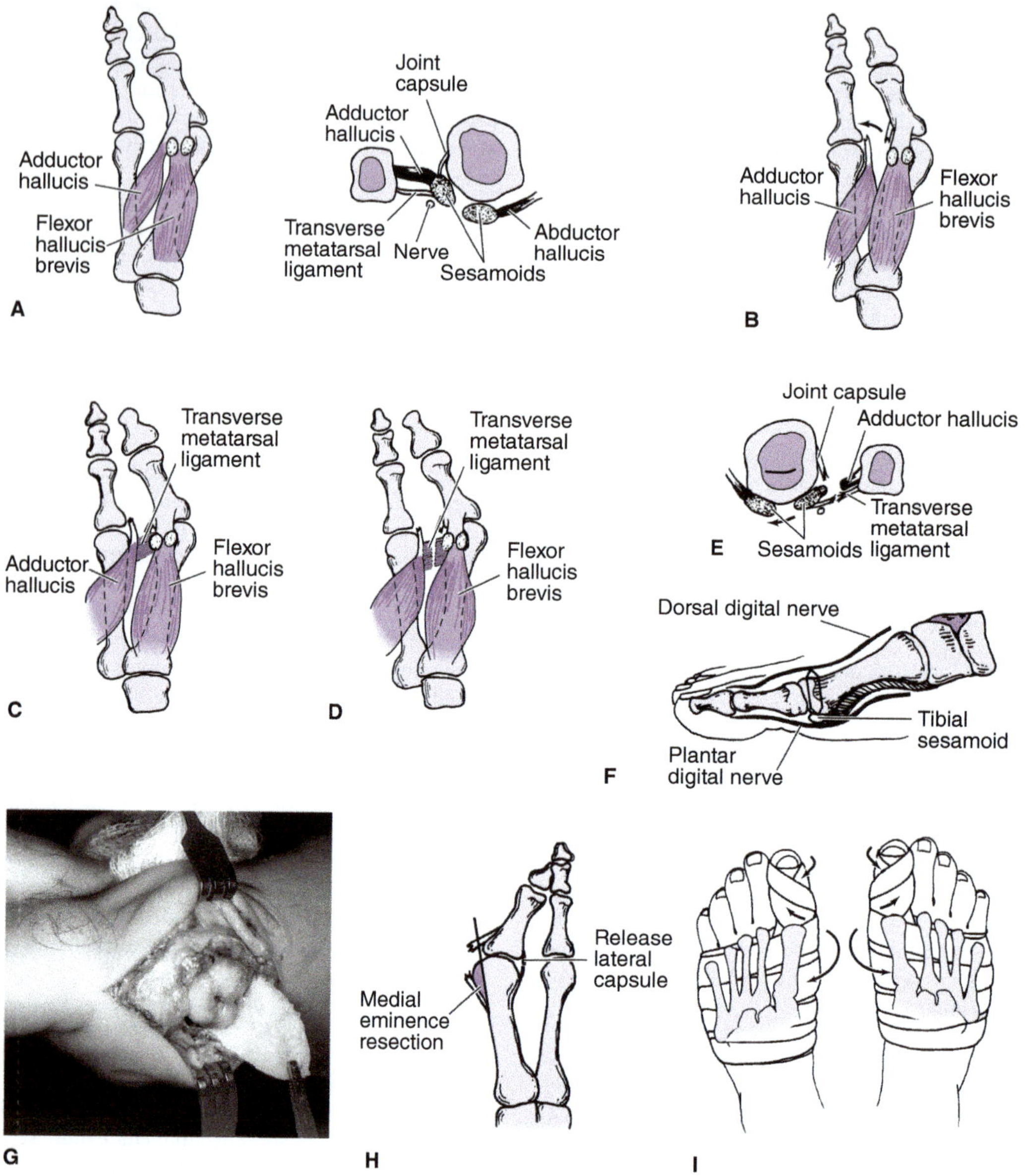

▲ **Figure 10–9.** Total soft-tissue procedure. **A:** The adductor tendon inserts into the lateral aspect of the fibular sesamoid and into the base of the proximal phalanx. **B:** The adductor tendon was removed from its insertion into the lateral side of the fibular sesamoid and base of the proximal phalanx. **C:** The transverse metatarsal ligament is passed from the second metatarsal into the fibular sesamoid. **D:** The transverse metatarsal ligament was transected. **E:** The three contracted structures on the lateral side of the metatarsophalangeal joint were released. **F:** The medical capsular incision begins 2 to 3 mm proximal to the base of the proximal phalanx, and a flap of tissue measuring 3 to 8 mm is removed. **G:** The medial eminence is exposed by creating a flap of capsule that is based proximally and plantarward. **H:** The medial eminence is removed in line with the medial aspect of the first metatarsal. **I:** The postoperative dressings are critical. Note that the metatarsal heads are firmly bound with the gauze, and the great toe is rotated so as to keep the sesamoids realigned beneath the metatarsal head. This necessitates dressing the right great toe in a counterclockwise direction and the left great toe in a clockwise direction when one is standing at the foot of the bed. (Reprinted with permission, from Mann RA, Coughlin MJ. *The Video Textbook of Foot and Ankle Surgery*. Medical Video Productions, 1991.)

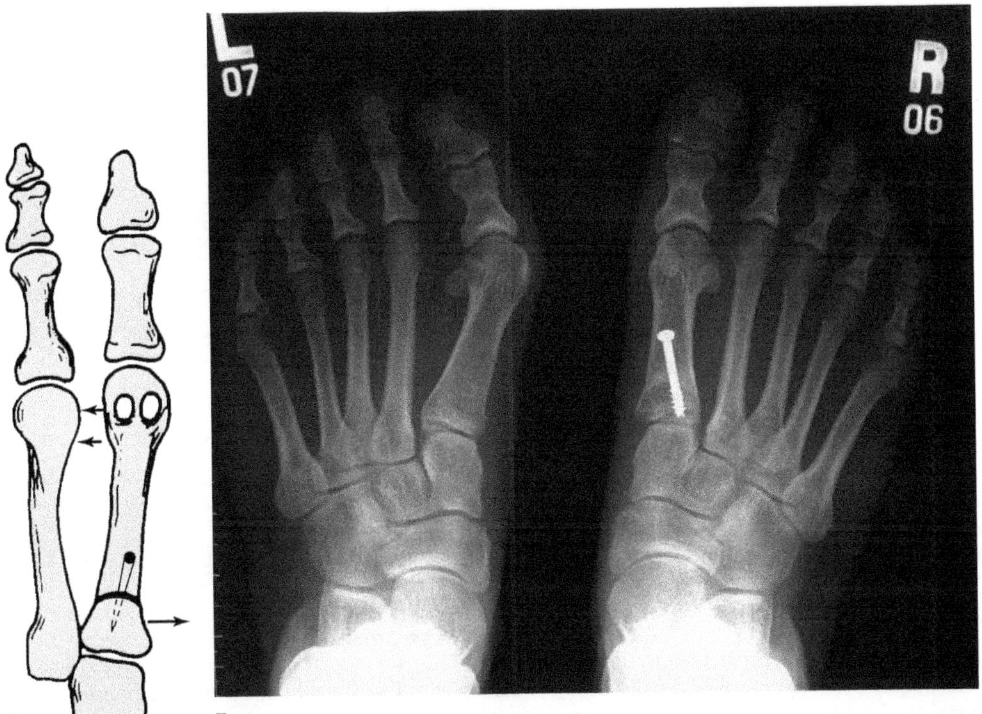

A B

▲ **Figure 10–10. A: The osteotomy site is reduced by pushing the proximal fragment medially with a small freer while pushing the metatarsal head laterally. This locks the lateral side of the osteotomy site so the internal fixation can be inserted.** (Reprinted with permission, from Mann RA, Coughlin MJ. *The Video Textbook of Foot and Ankle Surgery*. Medical Video Productions, 1991.) B: Anteroposterior postoperative radiographs of a case of proximal crescentic osteotomy. The patient underwent the same procedure to the contralateral foot.

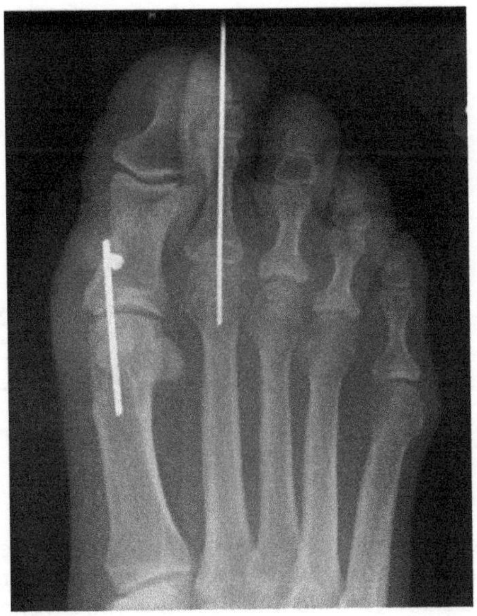

A

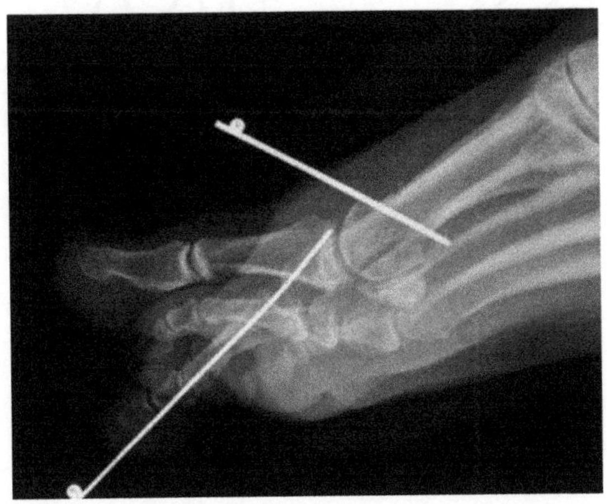

B

▲ **Figure 10–11. (A)** Anteroposterior and **(B)** lateral radiographs of a chevron osteotomy.

or recurrent hallux valgus deformity, respectively. Occasionally, arthrofibrosis of the joint is noted, resulting in significant joint stiffness.

D. Akin procedure—The Akin procedure is useful as an adjunct to a bunion procedure of the first metatarsal. It involves a medial closing-wedge osteotomy at the base of the proximal phalanx to correct the hallux valgus interphalangeus component of the deformity. It is commonly used with simple excision of the median eminence or with a chevron osteotomy to correct a mild to moderate hallux valgus deformity with a congruent joint. The Akin procedure is indicated for a hallux valgus deformity of less than 25 degrees with an intermetatarsal angle of 12 degrees or less.

Through a medial incision, the base of the proximal phalanx and the median eminence are exposed. After removing the median eminence in line with the metatarsal, a small sagittal saw is used to remove a wedge of bone from the medial aspect of the proximal phalanx. The osteotomy is closed down and stabilized internally with sutures, wires, staples, or screws (Figure 10–12). Dressings are applied for 6 to 8 weeks postoperatively. Patients may ambulate in a postoperative shoe until the osteotomy has healed.

E. Keller procedure—The Keller procedure is seldom indicated as a hallux valgus procedure and is usually used more for salvage purposes. It is reserved for elderly sedentary patients who are prone to skin problems and have arthritis. This procedure is contraindicated in an active person because of its known complications.

The procedure involves excision of the base of the proximal phalanx to decompress the metatarsophalangeal joint.

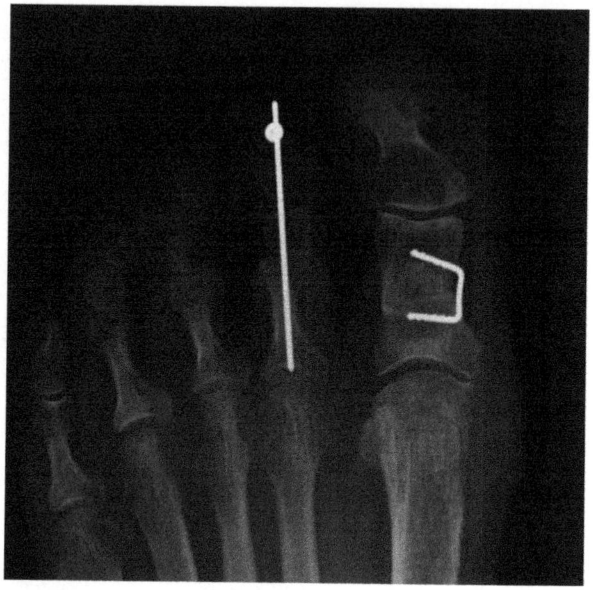

▲ **Figure 10–12.** Radiograph of an Akin osteotomy of the proximal phalanx.

Along with the procedure, the medial eminence is removed, and then the intrinsic muscle attachments are repaired to the remaining stump of bone (Figure 10–13). A Kirschner wire is drilled through the toe as a stabilizer until the toe heals and scar tissue forms, approximately 4 to 6 weeks. Postoperatively, the patient is permitted to ambulate in a postoperative shoe, and dressings are changed for 6 weeks.

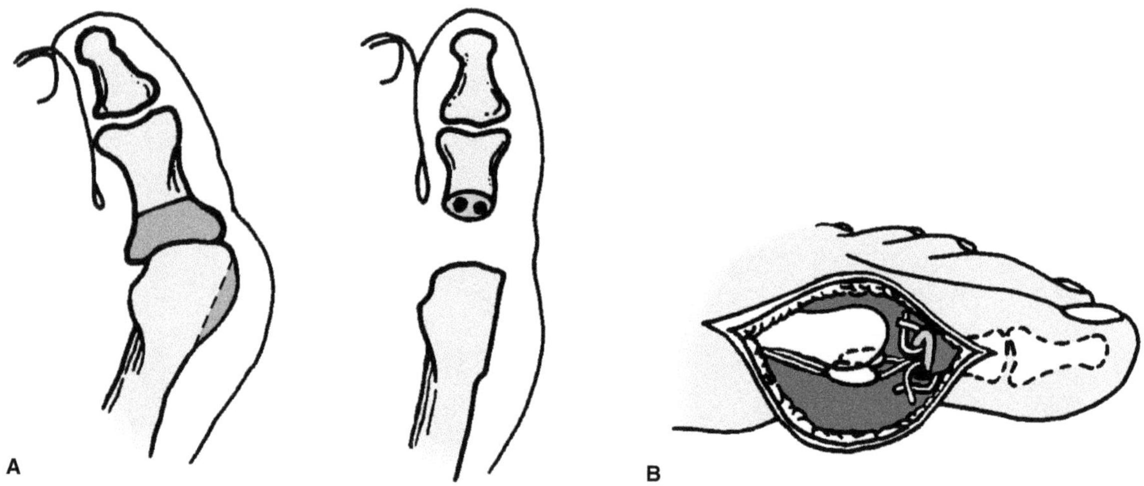

▲ **Figure 10–13.** Keller procedure. **A:** The medial eminence is removed in line with the medial aspect of the metatarsal shaft. The proximal third of the proximal phalanx is removed. **B:** An attempt is made to reapproximate the plantar and medial capsular structures to the remaining base of the proximal phalanx. (Reprinted with permission, from Mann RA, Coughlin MJ. *The Video Textbook of Foot and Ankle Surgery* Medical Video Productions, 1991.)

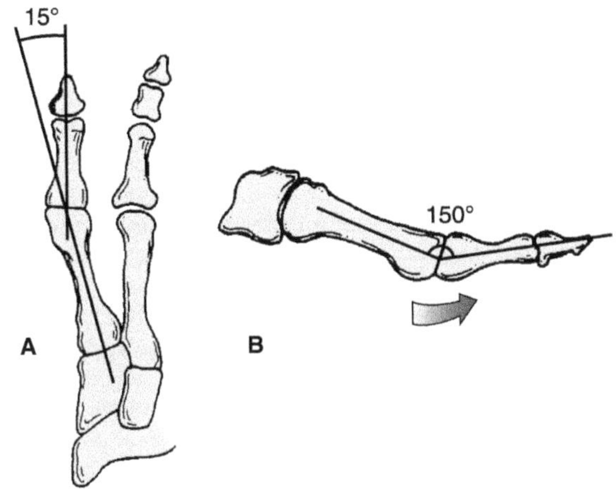

▲ **Figure 10–14.** Arthrodesis of the first metatarsophalangeal joint. **A:** The joint is placed into approximately 10 to 15 degrees of dorsiflexion in relation to the floor, which is approximately 25 to 30 degrees of dorsiflexion in relation to the first metatarsal shaft. (Reprinted, with permission, from Mann RA, Coughlin MJ. *The Video Textbook of Foot and Ankle Surgery.* Medical Video Productions, 1991.)

Results in the older (>65 years) patient with low functional demand are satisfactory. If the procedure is used in a younger patient, there is instability and loss of weight bearing by the first metatarsophalangeal joint because the base of the proximal phalanx was removed. There is significant loss of foot function, and a transfer lesion may develop beneath the second metatarsal head because the great toe no longer carries adequate weight. The metatarsophalangeal joint develops into a cocked-up deformity with some varus malalignment.

F. Arthrodesis of the first metatarsophalangeal joint—Arthrodesis of the first metatarsophalangeal joint is used in treatment of severe hallux valgus deformities with concomitant advanced degenerative arthrosis of the joint or as a salvage procedure following a previously failed surgical attempt to realign the metatarsophalangeal joint. Also, patients with deformities in which the proximal phalanx is subluxed more than 50% of the metatarsal head or who have significant stiffness of the metatarsophalangeal joint should be considered for fusion.

The procedure is performed through a dorsal longitudinal incision, and the joint surface is prepared. Some use a sagittal saw to yield two flat surfaces. Alternatively, a dome-shaped reamer may be used to create a ball-and-socket type of configuration. The arthrodesis site can be stabilized in several different ways to include crossed screws, an interfragmentary screw, and a dorsal plate or Steinmann pins if the bone quality is poor. As with any fusion, the position of the arthrodesis is critical; the joint should be placed in 15 degrees of valgus and 10 to 15 degrees of dorsiflexion in relation to the ground or the plantar aspect of the foot. In relation to the first metatarsal shaft, which is inclined plantarward approximately 15 degrees, it should be in approximately 30 degrees of dorsiflexion (Figures 10–14 and 10–15). Any pronation that is present must also be corrected.

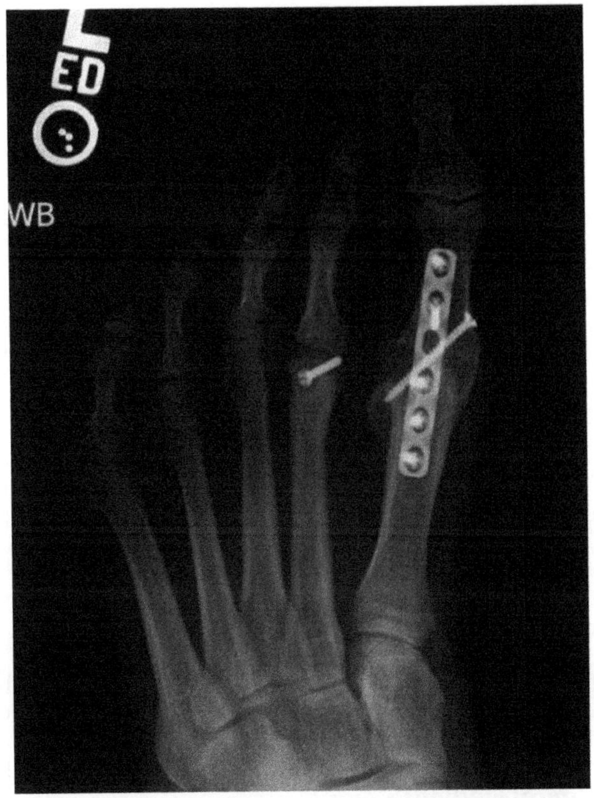

▲ **Figure 10–15.** Radiograph of a patient with a first metatarsophalangeal arthrodesis for degenerative arthritis and severe hallux valgus deformity.

The patient may ambulate on the heel while wearing a postoperative shoe or boot and progress to full weight bearing in the postoperative shoe until radiographic union is seen, generally in 12 weeks. The unreliable patient may be treated in a short leg walking cast.

The most common complication of arthrodesis of the first metatarsophalangeal joint is malposition. If the toe is not placed into adequate dorsiflexion or valgus, excessive stress occurs against the interphalangeal joint, which may result in a painful arthritic condition of the joint. The fusion rate is 90% to 95%. In cases of severe hallux valgus deformities, the arthrodesis will correct the hallux valgus angle as well as the increased intermetatarsal angle; thus, the need for a proximal osteotomy is unnecessary. Occasionally, the degree of valgus and dorsiflexion is correct but the toe is left in a pronated position, which results in pressure along the medial side of the interphalangeal joint and possible discomfort.

Following arthrodesis of the first metatarsophalangeal joint in proper alignment, the patient's gait is improved in propulsive power, weight-bearing function of the foot, and stability during gait. These patients are able to roll over the fusion site in an ordinary store-bought shoe, and they may expect to return to normal activities. Squatting is the only activity that is difficult because the toe must be in full dorsiflexion. Patients are able to return to most types of athletic activities, although at a somewhat slower pace. Well-done fusions in the correct patients are associated with high patient satisfaction.

2. Hallux Rigidus

General Considerations

Hallux rigidus describes degenerative osteoarthrosis of the first metatarsophalangeal joint. It is a common entity and frequently affects patients at a much younger age than arthritis of other joints, often seen in patients from their thirties onward. The reason why arthritis of this joint is seen in younger patients is unclear but may be associated with an unrecognized chondral injury to the metatarsal head. It is also associated with hallux valgus interphalangeus, bilateral involvement in those with a family history, and female gender.

Clinical Findings

A. Symptoms and Signs

Patients complain primarily of pain of the first metatarsophalangeal joint, especially with extension. Also, the dorsal eminence may prevent shoewear and have associated swelling and redness. Weight bearing and sports activities exacerbate the pain.

B. Imaging Studies

Weight-bearing radiographs of the foot demonstrate arthritic changes, including loss of joint space, subchondral sclerosis or cysts, and the presence of osteophytes, especially on the dorsal aspect of the metatarsal neck.

C. Conservative Management

Conservative treatment consists of nonsteroidal anti-inflammatory drugs (NSAIDs) and wearing a stiff-soled shoe with a deep toe box. An orthotic device with a Morton's extension or a carbon fiber plate would be beneficial. Both of the devices prevent extension in late stance phase. A rocker-bottom shoe can be helpful. In sedentary patients, these measures may be sufficient to treat symptoms; however, in more active individuals, surgical treatment is often indicated. Occasional corticosteroid injections can provide substantial relief in patients who are ready for surgery.

D. Surgical Treatment

There are multiple described surgical treatment options for hallux rigidus, including simple bone resection, arthroplasty, arthrodesis, and osteotomies. Of these, the simplest is a cheilectomy and is indicated in patients with mild to moderate arthrosis but who have a large dorsal osteophyte. Approximately one-fourth to one-third of the dorsal metatarsal head and proximal phalanx is excised (Figure 10–16). The medial and lateral osteophytes are also debrided, and a thorough synovectomy of the joint is performed. Postoperatively, patients regain up to 50% of their dorsiflexion and have improvement of their total motion. More than 90% of patients have improvement of pain, ability to wear shoes, and increased physical abilities. This procedure is less likely to have a favorable outcome on joints with advanced arthritis. A recent study, however, demonstrated favorable long-term results in patients with stage 1 to 3 hallux rigidus.

There has also been recent enthusiasm for implant arthroplasty for hallux rigidus. Implants range from a synthetic cartilage implant to metallic hemiarthroplasty and even total joint arthroplasty.

A Keller procedure is a resection arthroplasty and may be useful in older, less active patients, but it has a high rate of complications, as previously discussed. Prosthetic replacement of the arthritic first metatarsophalangeal joint can be used in older, lower demand patients but has high rates of failure in younger, more active individuals. Recently, synthetic cartilage implants and metallic arthroplasty have been reported with successful outcomes at short-term follow-up.

First metatarsophalangeal joint arthrodesis is a predictable and durable procedure. The drawback is lost motion at the joint. However, patients can remain quite active with a first metatarsophalangeal joint fusion as described previously. In general, patients with advanced hallux rigidus and little remaining motion have a very high satisfaction rate after metatarsophalangeal joint arthrodesis. Those patients with preserved motion who want to wear high heels generally are not satisfied with metatarsophalangeal joint arthrodesis.

3. Sesamoid Disorders

General Considerations

The sesamoid bones are plantar to the first metatarsal head and are part of the first metatarsophalangeal joint complex. Sesamoid disorders can be painful as they are in the weight-bearing part of the foot. Fractures, osteonecrosis, arthritis, and subluxation can affect the sesamoids. A puzzling entity is called sesamoiditis, which means inflammation of the sesamoids, but it encompasses painful sesamoids without an etiology.

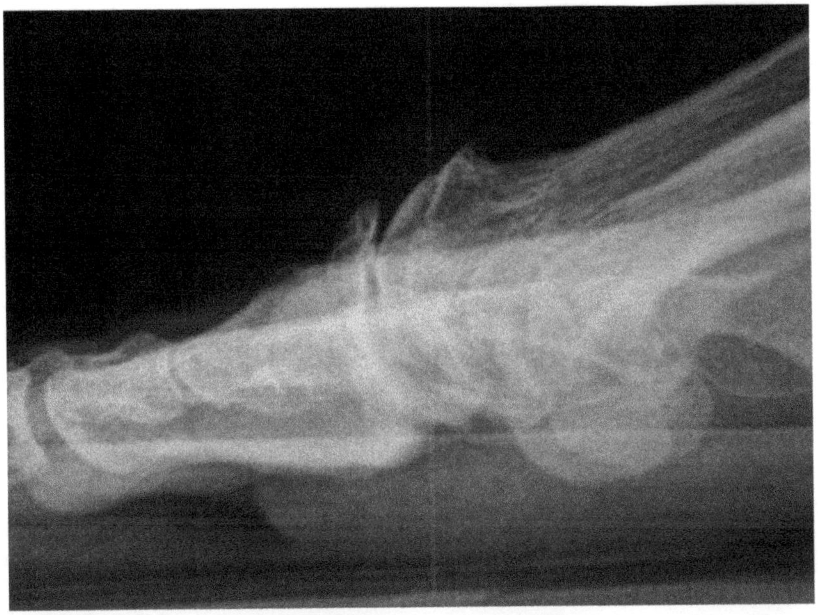

A

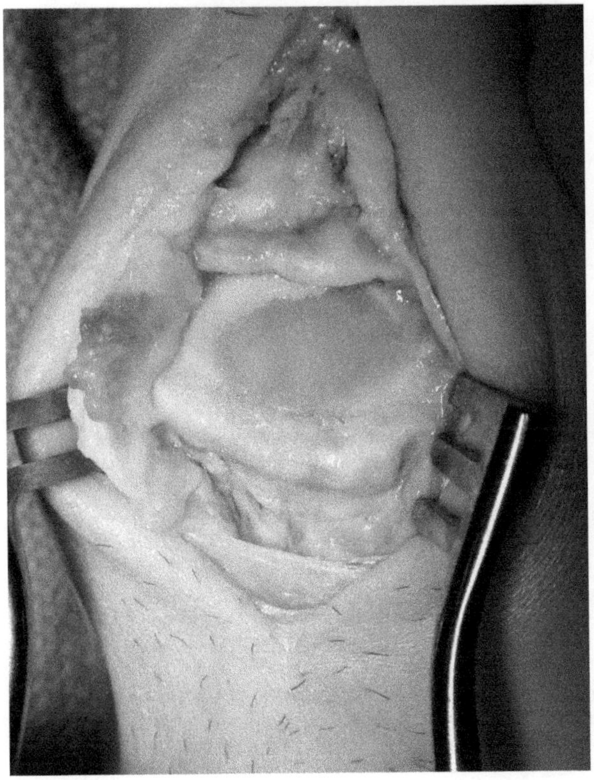

B

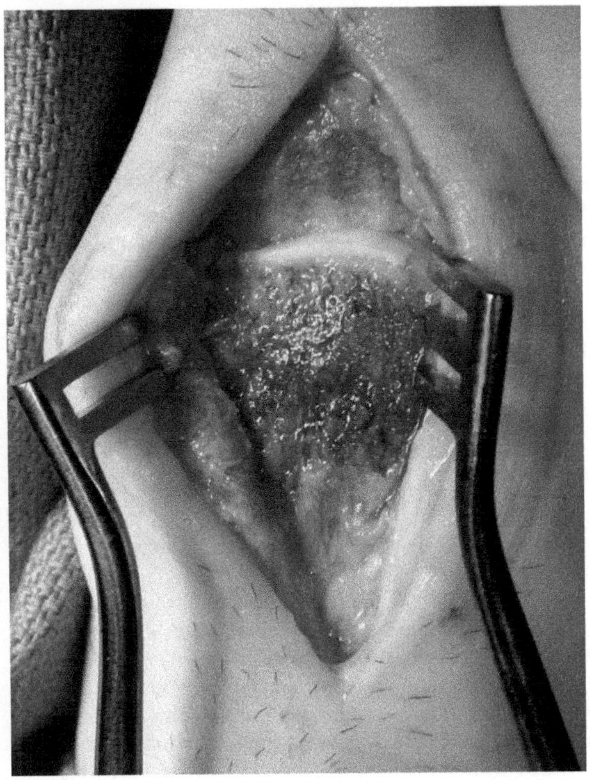

C

▲ **Figure 10–16.** **A:** Preoperative lateral radiograph of a patient with hallux rigidus. **B:** Intraoperative photograph of the dorsal osteophyte. **C:** Following removal of the osteophyte. **D:** Extension of the first metatarsophalangeal joint is 70 degrees and confirms adequate resection of the first metatarsal head.

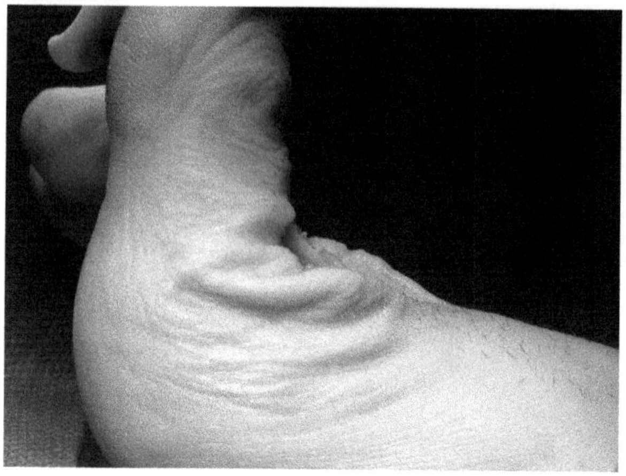

D

▲ **Figure 10–16.** (*Continued*)

Clinical Findings

A. Symptoms and Signs

The patient complains of pain directly under the first metatarsophalangeal joint that is worse with weight-bearing activities. The history may be significant for a trauma to the toe causing a fracture, but most commonly, the pain has an insidious onset.

Manual palpation of the area will reveal which sesamoid is affected, medial or lateral. Also, during the physical examination, postural abnormalities of the foot that may be contributing to the condition are evaluated. For example, hallux valgus deformity may cause a subluxation of the sesamoid from its normal articulation with the plantar aspect of the metatarsal head, causing pain, whereas pes cavus may result in greater pressure under the sesamoids, leading to symptoms.

B. Imaging Studies

Radiographs of the weight-bearing foot are taken and include a skyline or sesamoid view, which is a tangential view of the sesamoid metatarsal head articulation. On the anteroposterior view, subluxation of the sesamoids lateral to the first metatarsal head can be present with hallux valgus deformities. Occasionally it can be difficult to determine which sesamoid is symptomatic, and the use of a metallic marker on the anteroposterior view can assist in identifying which sesamoid is symptomatic. On the skyline view, fragmentation can be seen in cases with osteonecrosis, and joint space narrowing and osteophyte formation are seen with osteoarthritis. Displaced fractures are easy to determine, but nondisplaced fractures may be difficult to distinguish from a bipartite sesamoid that is a normal finding. A magnetic resonance imaging (MRI) or bone scan may be helpful in the case of normal radiographs to diagnose osteonecrosis or sesamoiditis.

C. Treatment

Acute injuries involving the sesamoid can be treated with a course of cast immobilization, sometimes non–weight bearing. A toe plate on the cast will provide greater immobilization and support. For chronic problems, a stiff-soled postoperative-type shoe may be used, and a soft felt pad can be placed just proximal to the sesamoids to take the pressure off the involved area. If needed, an orthotic device with a metatarsal pad or bar will relieve sesamoid pressure. Usually the majority of symptoms resolve in a matter of weeks, although some degree of discomfort may persist for several months. If 6 to 12 months of conservative treatment does not relieve the symptoms, the affected sesamoid can be removed. However, there is the possibility of transferring pain to the remaining sesamoid. In general, isolated sesamoidectomy in well-informed patients has a high satisfaction rate.

An TW, Cassinelli S, Charlton TP, et al. Radiographic and magnetic resonance imaging of the symptomatic synthetic cartilage implant. *Foot Ankle Int.* 2020;41(1):25-30. [PMID: 31538827]

Cassinelli SJ, Chen S, Charlton TP, et al. Early outcomes and complications of synthetic cartilage implant for treatment of hallux rigidus in the United States. *Foot Ankle Int.* 2019;40(10): 1140-1148. [PMID: 31195830]

Chien C, Alfred T, Freihaut R, et al. First metatarsophalangeal joint arthrodesis in hallux valgus versus hallux rigidus using cup and cone preparation compression screw and dorsal plate fixation. *Cureus.* 2017;9(10):e1786. [PMID: 29279812]

Dayton P, Feilmeier M, Kauwe M, et al. Relationship of frontal plane rotation of first metatarsal to proximal articular set angle and hallux alignment in patients undergoing tarsometatarsal arthrodesis for hallux abductor valgus: a case series and critical review of the literature. *J Foot Ankle Surg.* 2013;52(3):348-354. [PMID: 23473673]

Filippi J, Briceno J. Complications after metatarsal osteotomies for hallux valgus: malunion, nonunion, avascular necrosis, and metatarsophalangeal osteoarthritis. *Foot Ankle Clin.* 2020; 25(1):169-182. [PMID: 31997743]

Galois L, Hemmer J, Ray V, et al. Surgical options for hallux rigidus: state of the art and review of the literature. *Eur J Orthop Surg Traumatol.* 2020;30(1):57-65. [PMID: 31392522]

Glazebrook M, Blundell CM, O'Dowd D, et al. Midterm outcomes of a synthetic cartilage implant for the first metatarsophalangeal joint in advanced hallux rigidus. *Foot Ankle Int.* 2019;40(4): 374-383. [PMID: 30501401]

Goldberg A, Singh D, Glazebrook M, et al. Association between patient factors and outcome of synthetic cartilage implant hemiarthroplasty vs first metatarsophalangeal joint arthrodesis in advanced hallux rigidus. *Foot Ankle Int.* 2017;38(11): 1199-1206. [PMID: 28820949]

Kline AJ, Hasselman CT. Resurfacing of the metatarsal head to treat advanced hallux rigidus. *Foot Ankle Clin.* 2015;20(3): 451-463. [PMID: 26320559]

Moerenhout K, Chopra S, Crevoisier X. Outcome of the modified Lapidus procedure for hallux valgus deformity during the first year following surgery: a prospective clinical and gait analysis study. *Clin Biomech (Bristol, Avon)*. 2019;61:205-210. [PMID: 30594769]

Sidon E, Rogero R, Bell T, et al. Long-term follow-up of cheilectomy for treatment of hallux rigidus. *Foot Ankle Int*. 2019; 40(10):1114-1121. [PMID: 31307212]

DEFORMITIES OF THE LESSER TOES

The most common disorders of the lesser toes are mallet toe, hammer toe, and claw toe deformities. Understanding the etiology is important in effective treatment for these deformities. Some of the causes include inflammatory arthritis, trauma, congenital abnormalities, or neuromuscular disorders. Anatomic factors, such as a wide foot, a long second ray, or postural abnormalities of the foot may also contribute to deformities. However, the most common etiology is long-standing, ill-fitting shoewear. A narrow toe box with a high heel places abnormal forces on the lesser toes. Other disorders include hard and soft corns and metatarsophalangeal joint subluxation or dislocation. Patients may complain of pain and difficulty with shoewear. Importantly, patients with neuropathy may develop ulcerations over the bony prominences of these deformities, such as the proximal interphalangeal joint in a hammer toe or claw toe deformity.

General Considerations

The anatomic structures that stabilize the metatarsophalangeal joint on the plantar aspect are the plantar capsule, plantar aponeurosis (plantar plate), and medial and lateral collateral ligaments. On the dorsal aspect of the metatarsophalangeal joint, the extensor digitorum longus and brevis tendons and the extensor hood or sling make up the extensor mechanism that allows for dorsiflexion of the metatarsophalangeal joint. In addition, this mechanism can extend the distal interphalangeal and proximal interphalangeal joints if the proximal phalanx is in a neutral or plantarflexed position. On the plantar aspect, the interossei and lumbricals lines of action pass plantarward to the axis of the metatarsophalangeal joint and thus flex the metatarsophalangeal joint. The flexor digitorum brevis flexes the proximal interphalangeal joint, and the flexor digitorum longus muscle flexes the distal interphalangeal joint. When the metatarsophalangeal joint is hyperextended, the ability of the extensor hood to extend the distal interphalangeal and proximal interphalangeal joints is significantly diminished. Chronic hyperextension of the metatarsophalangeal joint eventually leads to fixed flexion deformities at the interphalangeal joints. A fixed deformity is significantly more symptomatic than a flexible deformity.

1. Mallet Toe Deformity

A mallet toe is a flexion deformity of the distal interphalangeal joint, and it may be fixed or flexible. In most cases, the second toe is involved, because it is the longest toe.

Clinical Findings

A. Symptoms and Signs

The patient complains of pain either on the dorsum of the distal interphalangeal joint or at the tip of the toe from striking the ground. The affected area may have a callus. Patients with peripheral neuropathy may present with an ulcer. The nail may develop a deformity with chronic trauma due to pressure from the shoe or ground.

Physical examination includes a complete evaluation of both feet, including the neurovascular status. To diagnose a flexible mallet toe, the ankle is brought into plantarflexion. If the deformity corrects and then recurs when the ankle is placed into dorsiflexion, the mallet toe is flexible. However, with a fixed deformity, ankle motion does not affect the deformity.

B. Imaging Studies

Weight-bearing radiographs of the foot are obtained to show the deformity of the distal interphalangeal joint.

Treatment

A. Conservative Management

The patient should be educated to wear a shoe with a wide toe box to accommodate the deformed toe. An extra-depth shoe may be needed to decrease pressure on the deformity. A small felt pad may be placed on the shoe liner, just proximal to the deformity, to prevent the tip of the toe from striking the ground.

B. Surgical Treatment

A flexible mallet toe can be treated by releasing the flexor digitorum longus tendon. This can be accomplished under a digital block, and a small incision on the plantar aspect of the toe at the level of the middle phalanx allows for releasing the flexor tendon. This treatment is usually effective.

With a fixed mallet toe deformity, the toe must be treated with a condylectomy. Under digital or ankle block anesthesia, a dorsal elliptical incision over the distal interphalangeal joint exposes the distal aspect of the middle phalanx. The head and neck of the middle phalanx are removed with a small bone cutter. A 0.045-inch K-wire typically is used to maintain the reduction for 4 weeks (Figure 10–17).

Generally, good resolution of symptoms and deformity results. Persistent deformity or recurrence may occur if contracture of the flexor digitorum longus tendon was not appreciated prior to surgery or insufficient bone was

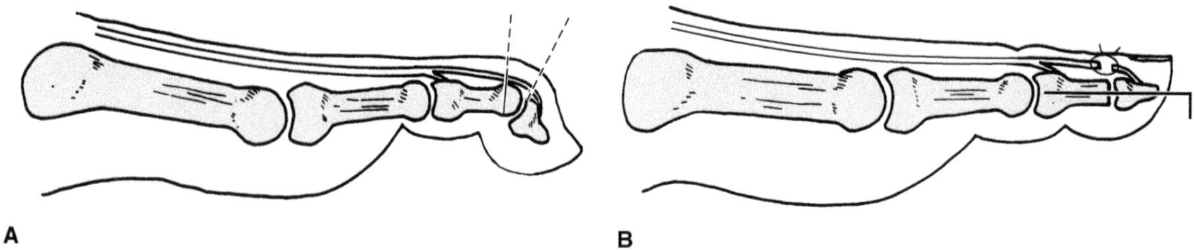

▲ **Figure 10–17.** Mallet toe repair. **A:** Resection of condyles of the middle phalanx. **B:** Intramedullary K-wire fixation. (Reprinted with permission, from Mann RA, Coughlin MJ. *The Video Textbook of Foot and Ankle Surgery.* Medical Video Productions, 1991.)

removed from the middle phalanx to decompress the deformity adequately.

2. Hammer Toe Deformity

A hammer toe involves a flexion contracture of the proximal interphalangeal joint, and it may be fixed or flexible. It is frequently associated with varying degrees of hyperextension of the metatarsophalangeal joint, and there may be an associated flexion deformity of the distal interphalangeal joint. Occasionally, the distal interphalangeal joint has an extension deformity.

Clinical Findings

A. Symptoms and Signs

Like the mallet toe, patients complain of pain and difficulty with shoewear. The pain is localized to the dorsal aspect of the proximal interphalangeal joint or on the plantar aspect of the affected metatarsal head. It is important with physical examination to evaluate both lower extremities and assess whether the deformity is fixed or flexible. The metatarsophalangeal joints commonly have hyperextension deformities. There may be a callus or an ulcer of the skin over the extensor surface of the proximal interphalangeal joint, where it rubs against the shoe. It is important to evaluate any deformity involving the hallux as a hallux valgus deformity may be part of the cause of a second hammer toe deformity. If this is the case, then the hallux valgus deformity requires correction to provide space for the second toe to be reduced into corrected alignment.

B. Imaging Studies

Weight-bearing radiographs of the foot will reveal arthrosis of the joint. The radiographs will confirm the clinical findings of the proximal interphalangeal flexion deformity, hyperextension deformity at the metatarsophalangeal joint, and hallux valgus deformity. It is important to fully evaluate the entire forefoot and all its joints when planning a procedure.

Treatment

A. Conservative Management

As with mallet toes, patients may benefit from shoewear that accommodates the deformity. The shoe should have a wide toe box and may be of extra depth. Over-the-counter toe sleeves and pads can alleviate pain in the affected areas, especially around skin callus. With more severe deformities, shoewear becomes more difficult. Hence, nonoperative management becomes more difficult. This is especially true with a severe hallux valgus deformity or claw toe deformity.

B. Surgical Treatment

The operative procedure to correct the hammer toe deformity depends on whether it is a fixed or flexible deformity. The deformity of the metatarsophalangeal joint needs to be corrected as well as the hallux deformity, if present. This will provide a space for the second toe to be placed in correct alignment.

1. Flexible hammer toe deformity—A flexible hammer toe deformity can be treated with a Girdlestone flexor tendon transfer. A small plantar incision is made to harvest the flexor digitorum longus. The tendon is split in half, and each portion is brought up subcutaneously on each side of the proximal phalanx through a dorsal longitudinal incision. The tendon segments are sutured into the extensor hood mechanism with the toe held in approximately 5 degrees of plantarflexion and the ankle in plantarflexion (Figure 10–18). This causes the long flexor tendon to act as an extensor of the interphalangeal joints and a flexor of the metatarsophalangeal joint, thereby correcting the deformity. A soft dressing is applied, and a postoperative shoe is worn for 4 weeks, after which ambulation is allowed. A small subset of patients may not be happy with the lack of active flexor digitorum longus flexion postoperatively and should be advised of this preoperatively.

2. Fixed hammer toe deformity—A fixed hammer toe deformity requires a bony procedure to correct the flexion contracture. This is accomplished with the DuVries

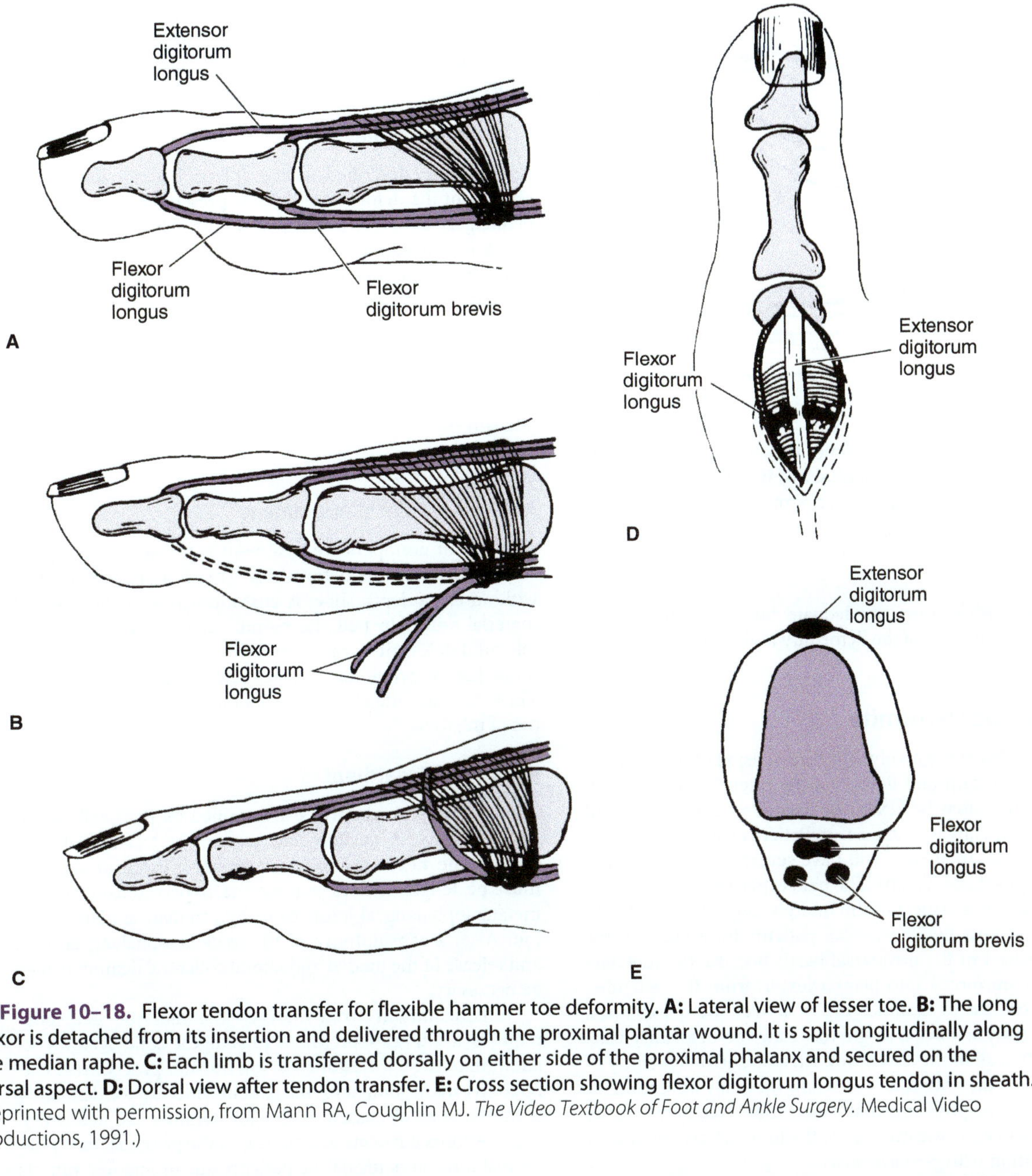

▲ **Figure 10–18.** Flexor tendon transfer for flexible hammer toe deformity. **A:** Lateral view of lesser toe. **B:** The long flexor is detached from its insertion and delivered through the proximal plantar wound. It is split longitudinally along the median raphe. **C:** Each limb is transferred dorsally on either side of the proximal phalanx and secured on the dorsal aspect. **D:** Dorsal view after tendon transfer. **E:** Cross section showing flexor digitorum longus tendon in sheath. (Reprinted with permission, from Mann RA, Coughlin MJ. *The Video Textbook of Foot and Ankle Surgery*. Medical Video Productions, 1991.)

proximal phalangeal condylectomy or arthrodesis of the joint. This procedure is identical to that described for treatment of the mallet toe deformity but occurs at the proximal interphalangeal joint instead of the distal interphalangeal joint (Figure 10–19). Surgeons debate on whether to strive for fusion of the interphalangeal joint or instead achieve an arthroplasty. Clinical results show a majority of patients are satisfied, and there is a low risk of recurrence of deformity. The interphalangeal joint can be temporarily stabilized with K-wires or with permanent implants. K-wires are much less expensive.

3. Complications—The main complication observed with either procedure is inadequate correction of the deformity, usually because of failure to appreciate a contracture of the flexor digitorum longus tendon at the time of surgery. In the

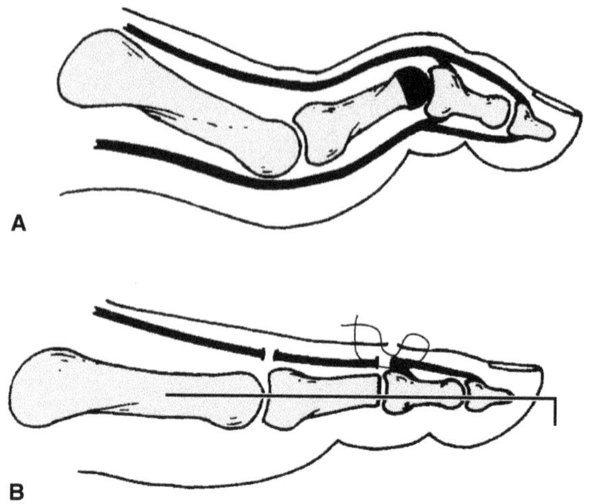

▲ **Figure 10–19.** Fixed hammer toe repair. **A:** Resection of the head of the proximal phalanx. **B:** Intramedullary K-wire fixation. (Reprinted with permission, from Mann RA, Coughlin MJ. *The Video Textbook of Foot and Ankle Surgery.* Medical Video Productions, 1991.)

DuVries condylectomy, inadequate bone may have been resected. Recurrence of the deformity is also one of the more common complications.

3. Claw Toe Deformity

A claw toe deformity involves hyperextension of the metatarsophalangeal joint and flexion of the interphalangeal joint. The deformity may be flexible or fixed. Patients complain of pain and difficulty with shoewear. Patients with a neuromuscular disorder frequently will have severe fixed deformities (ie, Charcot-Marie-Tooth). The pain experienced by patients is over the dorsal aspect of the interphalangeal joints due to pressure against the shoe. Also, patients have pain on the plantar aspect of the metatarsal heads because the metatarsal heads are forced into plantarflexion from the extended toe. In contrast to hammer toe or mallet toe deformities, which usually involve a single toe, claw toe deformity usually involves all of the lesser toes. An associated deformity of the great toe may occur as well. Claw toes may be secondary to neurological problems that cause imbalance between the intrinsic and extrinsic muscles of the foot and are often seen in association with pes cavovarus.

▶ Clinical Findings

A. Symptoms and Signs

Physical examination is performed in a similar manner to mallet and hammer toe deformities. With claw toe deformities, the metatarsal heads are prominent plantarly because the fat pad may be displaced distally and the skin beneath the metatarsal heads may be atrophic. Callosities may be present on the extensor surface of the proximal interphalangeal joints and on the plantar aspect of the metatarsophalangeal joints.

B. Imaging Studies

As previously described, radiographs of the foot confirm the severity of the deformity, which is present at the metatarsophalangeal and interphalangeal joints. The posture of the entire foot needs to be evaluated, looking for the presence of a cavus-type foot deformity, characterized by increased calcaneal pitch and increased plantarflexion of the first metatarsal. The calcaneal inclination angle, also known as the calcaneal pitch, is drawn on a weight-bearing lateral foot radiograph between the calcaneal inclination axis and the supporting horizontal surface and normally is approximately 20 degrees.

▶ Treatment

A. Conservative Management

The goal of nonoperative treatment is to decrease the pressure on the claw toe deformities. This is best accomplished with an extra-depth shoe. A custom orthotic device of soft material will help pad the painful metatarsal heads. Flexible mild deformities can be treated with shoe inserts placed immediately proximal to the metatarsophalangeal joints. These can have the effect of balancing the extensors and flexors of the toes.

B. Surgical Treatment

The operative procedure is determined by the flexibility of the deformity. A flexible claw toe can be treated with the Girdlestone flexor tendon transfer. The extensor tendons must be lengthened to correct the hyperextension of the metatarsophalangeal joints to realign to neutral plantarflexion. Also, a capsulotomy of the metatarsophalangeal joint and release of the medial and lateral collateral ligaments may be necessary.

A concomitant fixed claw or hammer toe deformity requires a DuVries proximal phalangeal condylectomy in addition to the Girdlestone tendon transfer procedure. Postoperative management for the patient with claw toe deformity is the same as discussed earlier for hammer toe deformity. Some authors advocate arthrodesis of the proximal interphalangeal joint in neuropathic patients due to ongoing muscle imbalance that could contribute to recurrence.

Following this surgical procedure, no active motion of the toes occurs. The toes are usually well aligned in a plantigrade position. The marked deformity of the proximal interphalangeal joints is relieved so they no longer strike the top of the shoe. The main problems that can occur after surgery are (1) failure to correct a fixed claw toe deformity adequately by use of the tendon transfer and (2) failure to release the fixed deformity adequately at the metatarsophalangeal joint, resulting in recurrence of the deformity.

4. Hard Corn and Soft Corn (Clavus Durum and Clavus Mollum)

A corn is a keratotic lesion that can develop over a bony prominence on the lesser toes from excessive pressure on the skin such as shoewear. A hard corn (clavus durum) frequently involves the dorsal and lateral aspect of the fifth toe, over the bony prominence of the lateral condyle of the proximal phalanx, whereas a soft corn (clavus mollum) presents in the web space, and it is so named because maceration results from moisture between the toes. The soft corn may occur anywhere along the toe where a bony prominence is present, but it is seen mostly in the fourth web space between the base of the proximal phalanx of the fourth toe and the medial condyle of the head of the proximal phalanx of the fifth toe. In a severe case, an ulceration or local infection may occur because of the extent of the maceration.

Treatment

A. Conservative Management

Decreasing the pressure on the affected toes will help improve symptoms. This can be accomplished with shoewear with a large toe box to relieve this pressure. Local debridement or shaving of the keratotic lesion reduces pain temporarily. This can be performed by the patient; however, it may be difficult in older patients because of decreasing flexibility and poor eyesight. Skin compromise, especially in the diabetic patient, must be avoided. At times, soft pads or lamb's wool can be placed around the toe to minimize pressure on the involved area, but the patient must wear a shoe with an adequate toe box to accommodate such modalities.

B. Surgical Treatment

1. Surgical treatment of the hard corn—A hard corn on the fifth toe can be simply treated surgically by excising the distal aspect of the proximal phalanx. Sometimes, the dorsolateral part of the proximal portion of the middle phalanx also needs to be removed. The operation is performed through a longitudinal incision dorsally to avoid a painful scar from chafing against the shoe. The extensor tendon is split, the collateral ligaments cut, and the condyle exposed. With a bone cutter, the distal portion of the proximal phalanx is generously removed and the edges smoothed with a rongeur. Following closure, a compression dressing is applied for several days. The toe is taped to the adjacent fourth toe for 8 weeks, and the patient may ambulate in a postoperative shoe. Long-term results show a high level of patient satisfaction and a low recurrence rate. Removal of excessive bone is the major complication, which causes the small toe to become too floppy, creating a nuisance for the patient.

2. Surgical treatment for the soft corn—Soft corns are treated surgically by making an incision over the lesion and using a small rongeur to remove the underlying bony excrescence. This is a simple procedure and almost invariably results in satisfactory resolution of the problem.

3. Syndactyly—Syndactylization is a procedure in which the fourth and fifth toes are connected by removing the web space skin and suturing the two toes together. This will eliminate the problem of a soft corn in the web space. Also, a soft corn can be treated with a condylectomy of the prominent part of the phalanx. However, this procedure can only be performed if there is no sign of significant maceration, ulceration, or infection. If there is compromise of the skin, then a syndactylization is indicated.

5. Subluxation and Dislocation of the Metatarsophalangeal Joint

In more severe deformities of the lesser toes, dorsal subluxation or dislocation of the metatarsophalangeal joint may occur. The plantar structures of the plantar plate, collateral ligaments, and plantar capsule become incompetent, and the toe assumes a dorsal position. A hammer toe or mallet toe may be associated with the subluxation or dislocation. Patients complain of pain over the dorsal interphalangeal joint from pressure from shoewear or on the plantar aspect of the metatarsal head. Keratosis can form under the plantar metatarsal head from increased weight-bearing pressure.

General Considerations

The most commonly affected toe is the second, and it is usually associated with a hallux valgus deformity. The pressure of the deformed hallux causes the second toe to sublux or dislocate. Less commonly, a nonspecific synovitis, isolated to the metatarsophalangeal joint and usually involving the second metatarsophalangeal joint, can result in a dislocation. The patient notes some discomfort and swelling around the metatarsophalangeal joint that eventually resolves, usually in 3 to 6 months. Then, an ensuing deformity is noted with subluxation and possibly dislocation of the joint. Other causes of subluxation and dislocation are direct trauma, rheumatoid or psoriatic arthritis, neuromuscular disorder, and repeated corticosteroid injections.

A somewhat more difficult multiplanar deformity is a medially or laterally deviated toe. The most common toe affected is the second because of its prevalence with hallux valgus deformities. With the bunion pressing on the second toe, it can sublux or dislocate and then deviate medially (crossover toe). This deformity may be the result of a steroid injection into the joint. With such a deformity, shoewear is problematic. Patients must wear sandals or an extra-depth shoe to accommodate the deformity.

Clinical Findings

A. Symptoms and Signs

Patients present with complaints of pain, deformity, difficulty with shoewear, and sometimes swelling. The pain is usually located directly at the joint, on the plantar aspect of the metatarsal head, or over the dorsal aspect of the interphalangeal joint. On physical examination, the patient is evaluated in both a standing and sitting position. The affected metatarsophalangeal joint is palpated for active synovitis, flexibility of the joint, and degree of subluxation. An anterior drawer test is performed on the affected joint to determine its stability. This is performed by holding the proximal phalanx between the examiner's fingers and moving it dorsally and plantarward, similar to a Lachman test of the knee. Also, the hallux is noted for any deformity, especially a hallux valgus deformity, as this is frequently associated with crossover of the second toe on the first toe.

B. Imaging Studies

Weight-bearing foot radiographs allow for evaluation of the severity of the subluxation or frank dislocation. Also, the hallux valgus deformity is evaluated, and changes about the articular surface of the joint are observed. Patients with rheumatoid arthritis usually have multiple joint abnormalities.

Treatment

A. Conservative Management

Patient education is an important first step to conservative management. A wide toe box shoe to accommodate the patient's deformity is often helpful. If needed, a total contact soft orthotic device will relieve pressure on the metatarsal head. The shoewear may need to be adjusted to accommodate an insert. For nonspecific synovitis, a cortisone injection may be beneficial; however, this should be used with caution because a steroid injection can lead to dislocation of the joint. If an injection is given, consideration for taping the toe in flexion to prevent dislocation should be considered. If the patient cannot be accommodated adequately with these modalities, surgical intervention may be indicated. A significant hallux valgus deformity indicates the need for correction to make a space for second toe correction. Failure to treat both problems results in recurrence of the deformity.

B. Surgical Treatment

The subluxed metatarsophalangeal joint with a flexible hammer toe is treated by releasing the dorsal contracture of the extensor tendons, joint capsule, and collateral ligaments. A Girdlestone flexor tendon transfer, as previously described, can maintain the correction. Also, tenodesis of the plantar plate may be a treatment option. Alternatively, after thorough extensor tendon lengthening and capsulotomy of the metatarsophalangeal joint, temporary fixation with a K-wire can maintain stability. If a fixed hammer toe is present, a proximal phalanx condylectomy is added to the procedure. A dislocation of the metatarsophalangeal joint is a more severe deformity and requires some bony correction. The soft tissues, including the extensor tendons, joint capsule, and collateral ligaments, are incised. In addition, a synovectomy of the metatarsophalangeal joint is performed, and finally, a shortening osteotomy of the metatarsal is performed to allow reduction of the joint. Accompanying hammer toe procedures are performed to correct the invariably present fixed hammer toe.

A 0.062-inch K-wire is used to stabilize the correction for 4 to 6 weeks. After pin removal, the toe is taped for several weeks. This procedure results in significant joint stiffness and possible resubluxation of the joint.

For severe deformities such as dislocation of the metatarsophalangeal joint, a bony procedure is added. This is achieved with an osteotomy at the level of the metatarsal neck or more proximal. The osteotomy is performed through a hockey stick incision over the dorsal joint, and the saw blade is placed at the dorsal aspect of the metatarsal head and aimed proximally. The saw blade is kept parallel to the plantar aspect of the foot to result in a long oblique osteotomy. A 1-mm saw blade is used for most osteotomies. A thicker saw blade, 2 mm, is used when more than 5 mm of shortening is required or with a plantar inclination of less than 19 degrees. Once the osteotomy is complete, the metatarsal head is allowed to slide proximally to the appropriate level that will allow the joint to reduce. The amount of shortening is usually between 4.0 and 6.0 mm. The osteotomy is then fixed with a single 2.5-mm or smaller diameter cortical screw.

If necessary, a hammer toe procedure may be added to fully correct the deformity. Good to excellent results have been reported. There can be reduction in pain, improvement of function, and resolution of intractable plantar keratosis, without the complication of joint stiffness as occurs with the previously described procedures. Complications from this procedure are stiffness, redislocation, plantar-penetrating hardware, and floating-toe deformity (extension contracture of the metatarsophalangeal joint causing the toe not to touch the ground).

A crossover toe is difficult to treat. Generally, the deformity is more severe and radiographs show a dislocated second or third metatarsophalangeal joint with medial or lateral deviation. The operative treatment realigns the toe with soft-tissue release of the contracted tendons and ligaments medially or laterally, depending on the deformity. For more severe deformities, a bony procedure is added. This can be accomplished with a closing-wedge osteotomy at the base of the proximal phalanx or an oblique distal metatarsal osteotomy, previously described for treatment of dorsally subluxated metatarsophalangeal joints. The technique is identical, but some soft-tissue balancing may need to be added to the procedure to correct the medial/lateral deviation.

Recently, repair of the plantar plate has been used to address multidirectional instability of the metatarsophalangeal joint. The indirect repair (dorsal approach) for plantar plate tears and instability has provided a reliable method of directly repairing the pathology. In addition, tendon transfer utilizing the extensor digitorum brevis and labral tape has been used.

Albright RH, Hassan M, Randich J, et al. Risk factors for failure in hammertoe surgery. *Foot Ankle Int.* 2020;41(5):562-571. [PMID: 32026702]

Albright RH, Waverly BJ, Klein E, et al. Percutaneous Kirschner wire versus commercial implant for hammertoe repair: a cost-effectiveness analysis. *J Foot Ankle Surg.* 2018;57(2):332-338. [PMID: 29478480]

Catena F, Doty JF, Jastifer J, et al. Prospective study of hammertoe correction with an intramedullary implant. *Foot Ankle Int.* 2014;35(4):319-325. [PMID: 24443491]

Coughlin MJ, Dorris J, Polk E. Operative repair of the fixed hammertoe deformity. *Foot Ankle Int.* 2000;21(2):94-104. [PMID: 10694020]

Jastifer JR, Coughlin MJ. Exposure via sequential release of the metatarsophalangeal joint for plantar plate repair through a dorsal approach without an intraarticular osteotomy. *Foot Ankle Int.* 2015;36(3):335-338. [PMID: 25288329]

REGIONAL ANESTHESIA FOR FOOT AND ANKLE DISORDERS

Regional anesthesia is an important component of foot and ankle surgery because most procedures are performed in the outpatient setting. Even when inpatient surgery is performed, regional anesthesia can minimize opioid use and facilitate discharge planning. The nerve block can be administered by the surgeon or anesthesiologists specializing in regional anesthesia. Many operations distal to the ankle can be performed without general anesthesia, which can eliminate the possible complications of central nervous system depression. In addition, the postoperative opioid requirements are significantly reduced.

Digital Block

A. Indications

A digital block is ideal for operations involving the toes. These may include procedures for nail disorders, correction of hammer toe or mallet toe, tendon releases, and some metatarsophalangeal joint procedures.

B. Technique

Short- and longer-term anesthesia is provided by digital block using a 1:1 mixture of 1% lidocaine hydrochloride and 0.25% bupivacaine. A short 25-gauge needle is used to inject approximately 1.5 mL on either side of the toe within the subcutaneous layer between the skin and deeper fascia. The needle is then passed toward the plantar aspect of the toe to anesthetize the digital nerves. Both sides of the toe should be anesthetized. Anesthesia should be administered before the operative site is prepared to allow the approximately 15 minutes necessary for the block to take effect before starting a procedure.

Ankle Block

A. Indications

Ankle block anesthesia is useful for forefoot and midfoot procedures. These can include bunionectomies, neuroma excision, metatarsal osteotomies, and tarsometatarsal arthrodeses. Also, ankle block anesthesia is preferred to multiple digital blocks for ipsilateral multiple toe procedures. Ankle block anesthesia is also appropriate for more proximal procedures, such as hindfoot arthrodesis or ankle arthroscopy.

B. Technique

An ankle block anesthetizes the posterior tibial nerve, deep peroneal nerve, sural nerve, saphenous nerve, and superficial peroneal nerve. The posterior tibial nerve requires a larger 3-cm, 22- or 25-gauge needle and approximately 7 to 10 mL of a 1:1 mixture of 1% lidocaine hydrochloride and 0.25% bupivacaine. The landmark for the posterior tibial nerve behind the malleolus is approximately two finger breadths proximal to the tip of the malleolus and along the medial border of the Achilles tendon (Figure 10–20). The needle is inserted perpendicular to the shaft of the tibia until the posterior cortex of the tibia is palpated with the tip of the needle. The needle is then withdrawn approximately 2 mm. Approximately 5 mL of anesthetic agent is injected into this area after aspiration is done to confirm that the needle is not in a vessel. The deep peroneal nerve is injected on the dorsal foot at the level of the navicular. The extensor hallucis and extensor digitorum longus tendons are palpated at this site, and the deep peroneal nerve is just lateral to the dorsalis pedis artery. The 25-gauge needle is inserted and advanced to bone and then withdrawn 1 to 2 mm, aspiration is attempted, and approximately 5 mL of anesthetic is injected. The saphenous nerve is identified one to two finger breadths proximal to the tip of the medial malleolus and just posterior to the saphenous vein. A 25-gauge needle is inserted and 5 mL of anesthetic injected. The sural nerve is blocked approximately 1 to 1.5 cm distal to the tip of the lateral malleolus and can often be palpated in the subcutaneous fat. A 25-gauge needle is inserted and approximately 5 mL of anesthetic injected. The superficial peroneal nerve is blocked, acknowledging it has branched, starting two finger breadths proximal and anterior to the tip of the lateral malleolus, and the injection is carried out below the subcutaneous veins but above the long extensor tendons in a ring-type block. Approximately 5 mL of anesthetic agent

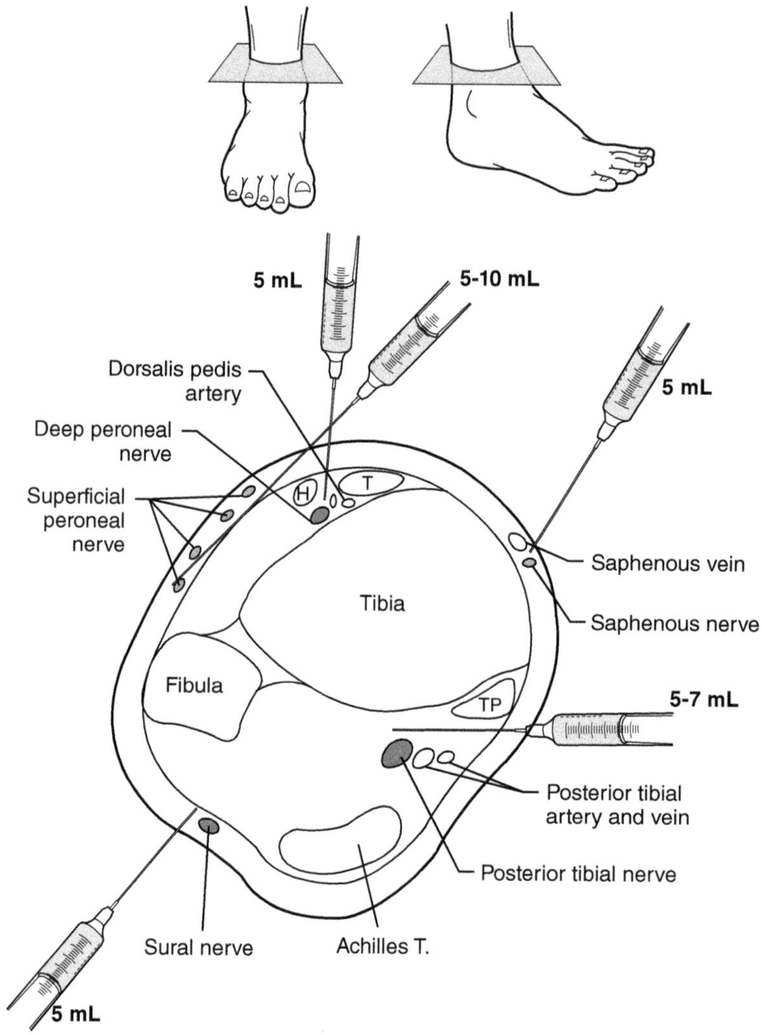

▲ **Figure 10–20. Anesthetic technique for ankle block. H, extensor hallucis longus tendon; T, tibialis anterior tendon; TP, tibialis posterior tendon.** (Reprinted with permission, from Delgado-Martinez AD, Marchal-Escalona JM. Supramalleolar ankle block anesthesia and ankle tourniquet for foot surgery. *Foot Ankle Int.* 2001;22:836.)

is used. The anesthesia for ankle block takes effect within 15 to 20 minutes, so it should be administered prior to the operative site being prepared so the block can take effect before starting a procedure.

Popliteal Block

A. Indications

The popliteal block can be used for most major foot or ankle procedures. These include ankle arthrodesis, hindfoot arthrodesis, calcaneal osteotomy, tarsometatarsal arthrodesis, posterior tibial tendon reconstruction, and surgical treatment of calcaneal or ankle fractures. The nerve block can be used with general anesthesia, sedation, or as the sole anesthetic technique. If a thigh tourniquet is required, then a general anesthetic may be added. The popliteal nerve block has low morbidity, high success rate, long analgesia, and can be administered by the orthopedic surgeon or anesthesiologist.

B. Technique

The patient is placed in the lateral decubitus position with a pillow between the knees. The landmarks to block the tibial nerve in the popliteal fossa are the lateral and medial epicondyles of the femur and the medial and lateral bellies of the

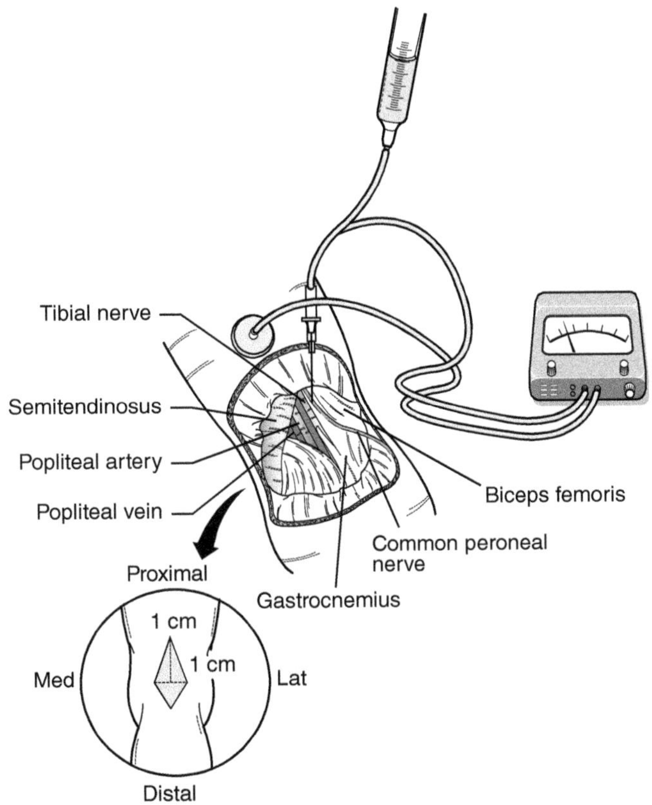

▲ **Figure 10–21. Anesthetic technique. The popliteal block is performed with the needle tip inserted 7 to 8 cm above the popliteal crease and 1 cm lateral to the midline.** (Reprinted with permission, from Rongstad KM, Mann RA, Prieskorn D, et al. Popliteal sciatic nerve block for postoperative analgesia. *Foot Ankle Int.* 1996;17:378.)

gastrocnemius. Ultrasound-guided popliteal block is quite helpful, not only to localize the vital structures, but also to avoid an intraneural injection. The puncture site with a stimulating needle is at the middle of the line connecting the epicondyles (Figure 10–21), and the nerve stimulator is set at 1.2 mA and is inserted vertically to locate the tibial nerve. At a penetration depth of 2 to 3 cm, a contraction is found, and the needle is advanced until plantarflexion and inversion occurs. The output of the stimulator is decreased gradually to 0.5 mA. Following aspiration, a test dose of 1 mL of 0.5% bupivacaine is placed. The test dose should cause a pause of muscle contraction, and the remaining 29 mL of 0.5% bupivacaine is injected with intermittent aspiration. The peroneal nerve is located at the head of the fibula, and the neurostimulator using an output of 1.2 mA causes dorsiflexion and eversion of the foot. The output is reduced to 0.5 mA to confirm the proximity of the nerve, and 3 to 5 mL of bupivacaine is injected. Finally, the saphenous nerve is located at the level of the tibial tubercle. The area infiltrated is between the tibial tubercle and the proximal gastrocnemius muscle. Approximately 3 to 5 mL of 0.5% bupivacaine is used. Alternatively, a more proximal sciatic nerve block can be performed as well.

The use of an indwelling perineural catheter can provide up to 72 hours of postoperative pain relief compared to 13 to 16 hours with a single-shot popliteal block. The stimulating needle is placed anterior to the biceps femoris tendon at the superior pole of the patella level, angling 45 degrees (Figure 10–22). The nerve stimulator is used to confirm placement, and a test dose of 1 mL of anesthetic is placed. Then a standard block of 20 mL of 0.5% bupivacaine is placed. The catheter is connected to a pain pump to infuse the local anesthetic dose depending on the patient's weight. The pain pump begins infusion at 6 hours postoperatively and then is removed by a visiting nurse at 72 hours. Another method for the sciatic popliteal block is localizing with ultrasound guidance and then inserting the needle at the separation of the tibial nerve and common peroneal nerve.

Regional blocks performed with multiple anesthetics may provide longer pain relief at the cost of prolonged sensory deficits compared to blocks performed with a single anesthetic.

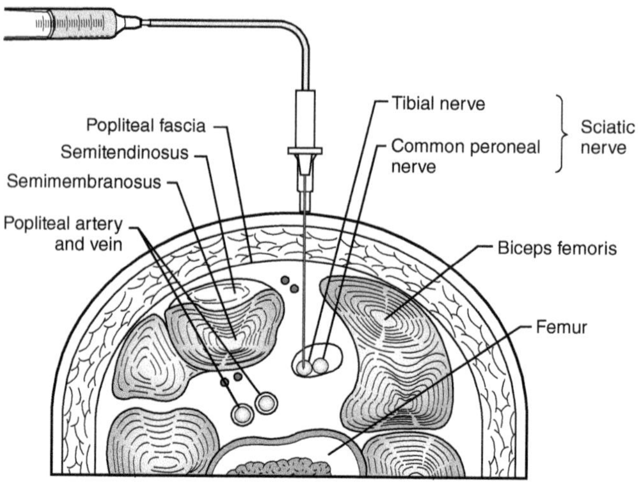

▲ **Figure 10–22. Anesthetic technique for the popliteal block. The needle top is positioned to localize the sciatic nerve, and aspiration ensures no vascular penetration.** (Reprinted with permission, from Rongstad KM, Mann RA, Prieskorn D, et al. Popliteal sciatic nerve block for postoperative analgesia. *Foot Ankle Int.* 1996;17:378.)

Dang DY, McGarry SM, Melbihess EJ, et al. Comparison of single-agent versus 3-additive regional anesthesia for foot and ankle surgery. *Foot Ankle Int.* 2019;40(10):1195-1202. [PMID: 31307211]

Vadivelu N, Kai AM, Maslin B, et al. Role of regional anesthesia in foot and ankle surgery. *Foot Ankle Spec.* 2015;8(3):212-219. [PMID: 25655517]

METATARSALGIA

Metatarsalgia is a general term for pain arising from the plantar metatarsal head region. The center of pressure during normal gait is initially applied to the heel, and this force progresses distally along the plantar aspect of the foot during the stance phase. For more than 50% of the stance time, the pressure is concentrated beneath the metatarsal head area. This extended period of pressure can be associated with pain. A precise diagnosis is necessary in metatarsalgia to direct treatment toward the specific cause.

Etiologic Findings

Metatarsalgia encompasses a broad spectrum of conditions. It may be associated with abnormalities of the metatarsal head, subluxation or dislocation of the metatarsophalangeal joints, systemic diseases, dermatologic lesions, soft-tissue disorders, or iatrogenic causes. Table 10–1 lists the various causes of metatarsalgia and the differential diagnoses that should be considered in evaluating these patients.

Clinical Findings

A. Symptoms and Signs

The clinical evaluation begins with a careful history directed toward delineating the precise location of the pain. The physical examination of the foot and lower extremity begins with the patient standing. Any deformities of the toes are noted, such as clawing of the toes, a long second ray, or swelling around any of the joints. The patient should be evaluated for a postural problem of the foot,

Table 10–1. Causes of metatarsalgia.

Causes of metatarsalgia
Bone causes
Prominent fibular condyle of the metatarsal head
Long metatarsal
Morton foot
Hypermobile first ray
Posttraumatic malalignment of metatarsals
Abnormal foot posture such as forefoot varus or valgus, cavus foot, or equinus deformity
Systemic disease, rheumatoid arthritis, psoriatic arthritis
Dermatologic lesions
Wart, seed corn, hyperkeratosis of the skin
Soft-tissue disorders
Atrophy of the plantar fat pad
Sequelae of a crush injury
Plantar scars secondary to trauma or surgery
Metatarsophalangeal joint disorders
Subluxed or dislocated joint
Freiberg infraction
Nonspecific synovitis
Iatrogenic causes
Residuals of metatarsal surgery
Transfer lesion due to previous surgery
Hallux valgus surgery (eg, shortening or dorsiflexion of the metatarsal)

such as a flatfoot or cavus foot. The plantar aspect of the foot is carefully evaluated for evidence of callus formation. The metatarsal heads are palpated individually to assess for generalized plantar fat pad atrophy, a prominent fibular condyle, synovitis, or possibly a transfer lesion beneath a metatarsal head resulting from previous forefoot surgery. Posterior muscle group tightness must be assessed to eliminate a contracture of the Achilles or gastrocnemius muscle. It is important to discriminate metatarsalgia from interdigital neuroma.

B. Imaging Studies

The radiographic evaluation includes weight-bearing anteroposterior, lateral, and oblique views of the foot. Occasionally, the so-called skyline view of the metatarsal heads (obtained with the metatarsophalangeal joints in dorsiflexion) is helpful to evaluate their overall alignment, particularly in cases resulting from previous surgery, by demonstrating the height of the metatarsal heads. MRI can be useful in the diagnosis of metatarsalgia, such as distinguishing among a neuroma, cyst, bursa, plantar plate rupture, or synovitis.

▶ Treatment

A. Conservative Management

Conservative management is directed at relieving the pressure beneath the area of maximum pain. This includes a shoe of appropriate style and adequate size to allow an orthotic device to be inserted. A lace-type shoe with a soft sole material and an adequate toe box is appropriate. High-heeled shoes, loafers, or tight shoes are inappropriate because they have decreased volume for the foot and may cause increased pressure against the involved area. As a general rule, the softer the orthotic device, the more comfortable the patient feels. A hard acrylic orthotic device is not particularly comfortable for the patient and should usually be avoided. Debridement of plantar calluses can reduce pressure and provide relief as well.

B. Surgical Treatment

The surgical management of metatarsalgia depends on the cause and is discussed in different sections of this chapter. In general, pain from a bony prominence can be relieved by a partial ostectomy or osteotomy, dermatologic lesions such as warts can often be burned off with liquid nitrogen or excised, and pain caused by a subluxated metatarsophalangeal joint can be corrected with tendon transfer. The outcome depends on the severity of the problem and the type of surgical intervention required for correction. Patients with posterior muscle group contracture and metatarsalgia can benefit from gastrocnemius recession or Achilles tendon lengthening.

KERATOTIC DISORDERS OF THE PLANTAR SKIN

Keratotic disorders of the foot usually manifest in plantar callosities and are also called intractable plantar keratosis. These occur as a result of friction (shear) and increased pressure over bony prominences. Some plantar callosity is normal, but if it becomes excessive, it can be painful and disabling. It also is a sign of abnormal biomechanics.

▶ General Considerations

Many of the intractable plantar keratoses arise from the bony abnormalities of the forefoot. These abnormalities are listed in Table 10–1.

▶ Clinical Findings

A. Symptoms and Signs

The patient's history will reveal the affected area of the foot and the severity of pain. In addition, the past medical history is important, as past operations and medical disorders may be part of the etiology. The patient's work, type of activities, shoewear, how often the callus needs to be trimmed, and the type of orthotic devices used are all important in a complete history. The physical examination, however, is the most important factor in the diagnosis of intractable plantar keratoses. First, the overall posture of the foot needs to be evaluated to determine whether the condition is the result of a postural abnormality. This is accomplished with the patient undressed from both knees down and standing. Findings can involve a rigid plantarflexed first metatarsal that could cause diffuse callus beneath the first metatarsal head, or a hypermobile first ray that fails to support the medial forefoot resulting in generalized callus formation beneath the second and third metatarsal heads. With varus deformity of the forefoot (the lateral aspect of the foot in greater plantarflexion than the medial aspect), there may be callus formation beneath the fifth metatarsal head. Also, the type of callus should be noted. Diffuse callus is usually associated with a long metatarsal. This callus may have arisen after trauma or surgery in which an adjacent metatarsal was dorsiflexed, thereby increasing the weight bearing load of the metatarsal. In contrast, a distinct well-localized lesion beneath the metatarsal head is often caused by a prominent fibular condyle of the metatarsal head of the second or third metatarsal. A callus on the bottom of the foot must be differentiated from a plantar wart, which can occasionally mimic a plantar callosity. Shaving the lesion reveals bleeding from end arteries in a plantar wart, whereas a keratotic lesion consists only of hyperkeratotic tissue.

B. Imaging Studies

Weight-bearing anteroposterior, oblique, and lateral radiographs of the foot will generally reveal abnormalities seen clinically. These include hallux valgus, hammer toe, claw toe, and varus deformity.

Treatment

A. Conservative Management

Debridement or trimming of the intractable plantar keratosis can provide some relief, albeit temporary. Directing the treatment to the underlying deformity will bring long-term benefit. This can be achieved by decreasing the direct pressure or friction from the callosities. A shoe that is made of soft material and accommodates the size and shape of the foot will provide some relief of pain and disability. This usually involves a lace-up type shoe with adequate padding. Inexpensive padding and soft inserts can be found over the counter and will benefit many patients. With some patients and deformities, however, a total contact orthotic device can be effective (Figure 10–23). It is usually made of soft material and redistributes the weight bearing from bony prominences that cause the callosities.

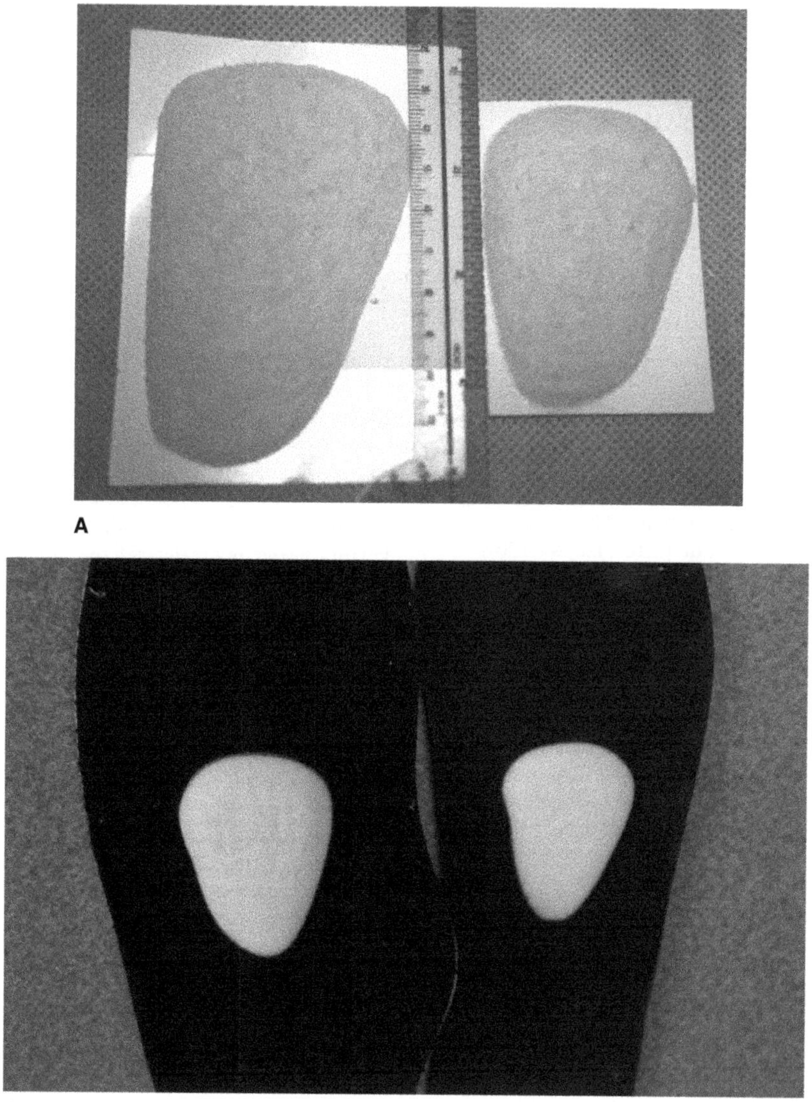

A

B

▲ **Figure 10–23. A:** A metatarsal pad may help redistribute weight bearing and relieve symptoms. **B:** Soft, over-the-counter, felt metatarsal pads are effective in decreasing pressure under the metatarsal heads. These can be adhered to a shoe insert to allow for use in multiple shoes. (Reprinted with permission, from Mann RA, Coughlin MJ. *The Video Textbook of Foot and Ankle Surgery*. Medical Video Productions, 1991.)

B. Surgical Treatment

Operative procedures for intractable plantar keratoses are determined by the underlying deformity. One of the most common problems is a prominent fibular condyle of the metatarsal head. It occurs most frequently underneath the second metatarsal but may also be found underneath the third and fourth metatarsals. The prominence is approached through a dorsal hockey stick incision over the metatarsophalangeal joint, and the toe is plantarflexed to expose the plantar aspect of the metatarsal head. An osteotome is used to excise 30% of the plantar condyle of the metatarsal head, thereby removing the sharp bony prominence (Figure 10–24). This procedure results in predictable pain relief of the affected toe, although 5% to 10% of patients develop a transfer lesion beneath the adjacent metatarsal head.

A diffuse callus beneath the second metatarsal that is the result of a dorsiflexed or hypermobile first metatarsal can be treated with dorsiflexion osteotomy done at the base of the second metatarsal. If the lesion is the result of an excessively long metatarsal, it may be shortened to the level of a line drawn between the adjacent metatarsal heads, thereby reestablishing a smooth metatarsal parabola. If the callus is a result of a dislocated metatarsophalangeal joint, such as in a claw toe deformity, the joint must be reduced, using one of the techniques previously described. Correction of the joint alignment will decrease the plantar stress against the metatarsal head. All of these surgical procedures to eliminate a callus are fairly successful, although the possibility of a transfer lesion developing is approximately 5% to 10%.

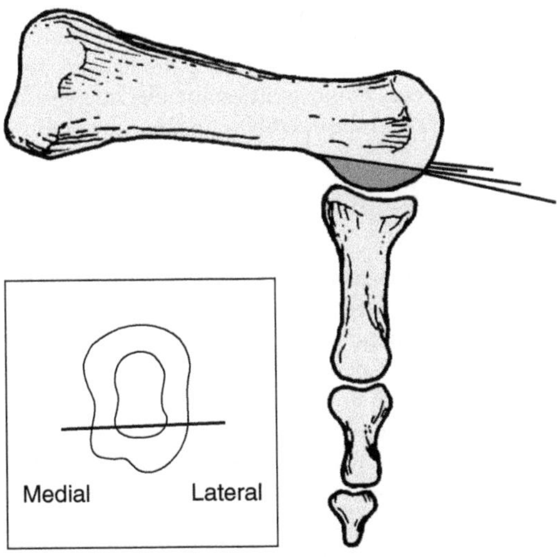

▲ **Figure 10–24. A plantar condylectomy is performed with resection of one-fourth to one-third of the plantar surface of the metatarsal head.** (Reprinted with permission, from Mann RA, Coughlin MJ. *The Video Textbook of Foot and Ankle Surgery.* Medical Video Productions, 1991.)

The tibial sesamoid can be prominent, and an underlying callosity can form. This is treated through a medial approach, and the plantar third of the sesamoid is shaved down. This alleviates the callus in almost all cases, with the only significant complication being caused by inadvertent disruption of the plantar medial cutaneous nerve during the surgical approach to the sesamoid.

Keratoses can occur about the fifth metatarsal head. If it occurs on the lateral aspect of the forefoot, the deformity may be a bunionette, also called tailor's bunion. A diffuse callus beneath the fifth metatarsal head can be treated with a midshaft metatarsal osteotomy to bring it out of its plantarflexed position, which usually alleviates the condition. Delayed healing of midshaft osteotomies is a possibility. It is unusual for a transfer lesion to occur beneath the fourth metatarsal head. If the bony prominence is on the lateral aspect of the foot rather than the plantar aspect, then an osteotomy of the fifth metatarsal head will correct this deformity. A chevron-type osteotomy can be made and the head is translated medially (Figure 10–25).

Finally, a subhallux sesamoid can cause a small callus on the plantar aspect of the interphalangeal joint of the great toe. Treatment is simply surgical excision of the sesamoid, and good results can be expected with little or no disability.

Slullitel G. Current concepts of treatment of metatarsalgia. *Foot Ankle Clin.* 2019;24(4):xiii-xiv. [PMID: 31653374]

DIABETIC FOOT

Approximately 30 million people in the United States have diabetes, and foot problems are one of the most common causes for hospitalization, accounting for 20% or more of all inpatient days in this population. More than half of all nontraumatic amputations are performed on diabetic patients. Treatment of the diabetic patient with foot problems can be complex and requires a team approach, involving the primary care physician, vascular surgeon, orthopedic surgeon, infectious disease specialist, orthotist, diabetic nurse specialist, and, whenever possible, the patient's family members.

▶ Pathophysiologic Findings

Diabetes is a metabolic disorder that involves all of the organ systems. Those of primary interest to the orthopedist are integumentary with the risk of ulceration, neurologic with the loss of protective sensation, vascular with diminished perfusion, and immunologic with limited ability to fight infection. The most frequent diabetes-related foot problem is breakdown of the skin of the foot, also known as a diabetic foot ulcer (Figure 10–26). The cause of foot ulcers is multifactorial, but they can be neuropathic, neuroischemic, or ischemic in origin. Peripheral neuropathy is very common, and unappreciated local stresses are applied to the skin by poorly fitting shoes and internally by skeletal deformity. Autonomic

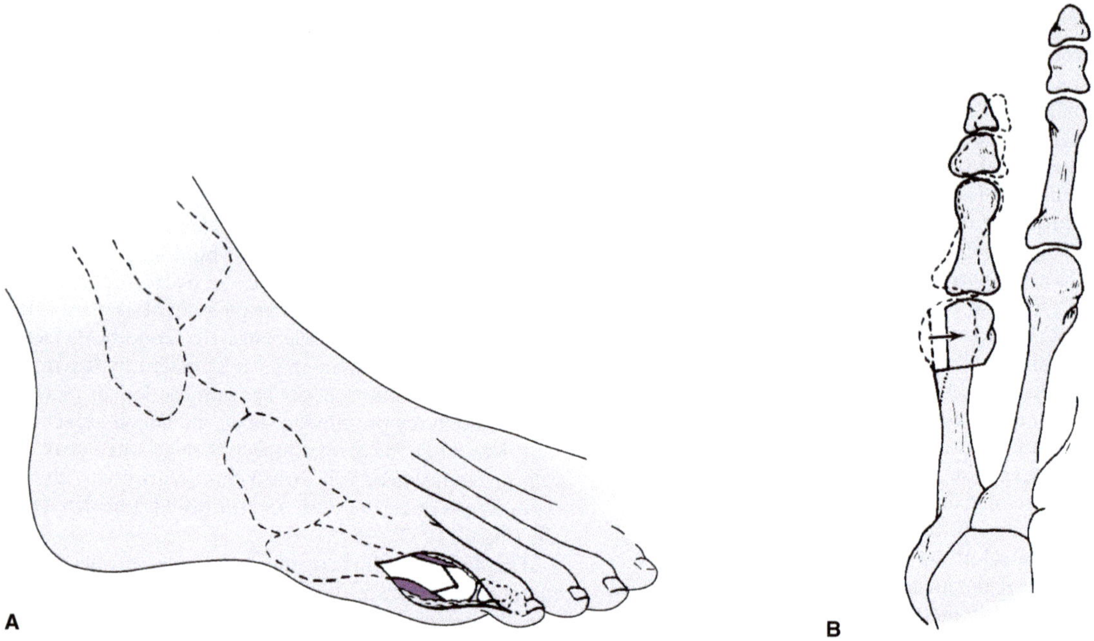

▲ **Figure 10–25. A:** Lateral view of chevron fifth metatarsal osteotomy. **B:** Diagram following completion of this procedure. (Reprinted with permission, from Mann RA, Coughlin MJ. *The Video Textbook of Foot and Ankle Surgery.* Medical Video Productions, 1991.)

neuropathy causes dry skin and cracks in the dermis, which may become portals of entry for infection. Reactive hyperemia, which normally helps to clear infections, is blunted by autonomic neuropathy. Motor neuropathy affects the intrinsic muscles of the foot and may lead to claw toe deformities with metatarsal heads and proximal interphalangeal joints becoming prominent and predisposing to ulcerations. Poorly controlled diabetes leads to impaired wound healing, stiff tendons, and blunted immune response. Atherosclerosis is also more common and more severe in patients with diabetes. As a result of these comorbidities, the diabetic foot is vulnerable to pressure and shear, which can have devastating consequences.

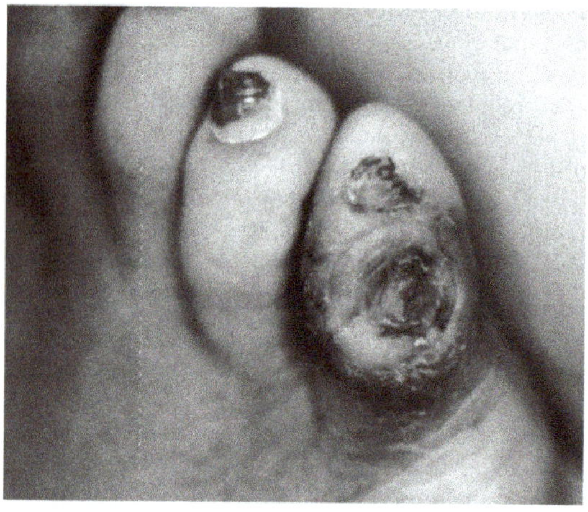

▲ **Figure 10–26.** Ulceration over the dorsolateral aspect of the fifth toe as the result of pressure from a shoe. (Reprinted with permission, from Mann RA, Coughlin MJ. *The Video Textbook of Foot and Ankle Surgery.* Medical Video Productions, 1991.)

History

Orthopedic surgeons, particularly those with a special interest in foot and ankle surgery, are especially well qualified to provide care across the diabetic foot spectrum. Routine screening evaluations can detect peripheral neuropathy, peripheral artery disease, and skeletal deformities that place patients in the high-risk category. The common pathway to major amputation begins with a wound that becomes infected. Preventing or reducing the rate of major amputation in diabetic patients should be the goal for every surgeon. This requires early intervention, prior to development of a wound. Appropriate shoewear and orthotics should be prescribed in high-risk patients. When a diabetic patient presents to an orthopedist, there are four areas of impact: ulcers and their prevention, amputations, Charcot arthropathy, and toenail abnormalities. With infected foot ulceration, it is essential to obtain a history that will help delineate why the ulcer occurred and how to optimize the patient's healing. A past history of foot surgery is sought, previous or current antibiotic usage is detailed, and any recent trauma to the foot is noted. A history is taken to document the severity of the patient's diabetes, including how long ago the diabetes was diagnosed, whether the patient is taking insulin, their recent level of glycemic control, what other organ systems are involved, and the degree of neuropathy that is present in the patient's feet.

Clinical Findings

A. General Examination

Examination of the diabetic patient should begin with inspection of the shoe for internal and external wear patterns. The leg and foot are inspected for overall appearance of the skin, hair growth, perfusion, pulses, and color.

B. Foot Examination

Any bony prominences are recognized as areas of potential skin breakdown. The most common prominences are located at the apex of deformities such as under the metatarsal heads, on the dorsum of the proximal interphalangeal joints, under the medial sesamoid, at the base of the fifth metatarsal, under the medial arch in the Charcot foot, and over the medial eminence of the hallux. ROM of the ankle should be assessed because ankle equinus increases the risk of forefoot ulcers and midfoot neuropathic arthropathy. Neurologic examination should test for the presence of protective sensation, as defined by the patient's ability to feel the 5.07/10-g Semmes-Weinstein monofilament as well as motor function. Any ulcers or preulcerative lesions should be carefully documented and evaluated for evidence of inflammation or infection in the adjacent soft tissues. Wounds should be measured for length, width, and depth, in addition to documenting their location. Open wounds should be probed with a sterile Q-tip or other appropriate instrument to evaluate the extent of involvement of deeper structures, such as tendons, joints, and bone. A positive probe to bone test may indicate the presence of osteomyelitis.

C. Vascular Findings

Vascular evaluation is essential to ensure that the patient has adequate perfusion to allow healing. A history of claudication is important to elicit. Documenting the presence or absence of hair growth as well as skin temperature are easy techniques for screening. Patients with palpable pedal pulses and normal capillary filling usually have adequate blood supply and do not require further vascular evaluation unless normal healing is not progressing. For patients with abnormal clinical findings, one method of assessing the overall potential for healing of foot lesions in a diabetic is the ankle-brachial index (ABI). This index is obtained by dividing the systolic blood pressure measurement in the dorsalis pedis and posterior tibial arteries by that in the brachial artery, as measured by Doppler ultrasound with an ankle cuff. Abnormal noninvasive testing should prompt vascular surgery consultation, particularly in delayed wound healing or prior to elective foot surgery. It must be kept in mind, however, that falsely elevated values of blood pressure (or noncompressible vessels) at the ankle may result from calcification of major blood vessels. In this case, measurement of the great toe pressure and toe brachial index is more reliable. Apparent vascular insufficiency in the light of an adequate ischemic index also warrants a vascular surgery consultation. A laser Doppler study can also be beneficial in assessing local skin perfusion. This information can be used to help predict the patient's response to surgical intervention. Normal arteries have triphasic waveforms, whereas monophasic waveforms are consistent with peripheral artery disease.

D. Imaging Studies

Radiographic studies should include weight-bearing radiographs of both feet and ankles as indicated. Plain radiographs can help identify bony prominences that predispose the patient to ulcer formation, and osteomyelitis or changes consistent with a neuropathic foot may be identified. Early Charcot (neuropathic) joint changes may be difficult to differentiate from osteomyelitis in the presence of an open wound. The four D's of neuropathic joints are helpful in delineating more advanced cases: debris, destruction, dislocation, and densification. Radiographs can also demonstrate vascular calcification of the tunica media (middle layer) of the ankle and pedal vessels.

The presence of bony infection may be delineated on serial radiographs as progressive osteolysis, realizing that changes on plain films are late findings and suggesting that the infection has been present for weeks. A technetium bone scan is sensitive in detecting early osteomyelitis but is quite nonspecific. MRI can demonstrate bony and soft-tissue changes, such as edema or the extent of an abscess cavity, and can be helpful in distinguishing Charcot changes from osteomyelitis. The recent addition of ring positron emission tomography (PET) scans is more effective in differentiating osteomyelitis from Charcot changes.

Classification and Treatment of Diabetic Foot Ulcers

The original Rancho Los Amigos Hospital Wagner classification of diabetic foot ulcers is based on the depth of tissue affected and extent of the foot involved. Treatment choice depends on the grade of ulcer (Figure 10–27). Table 10–2 shows treatment based on classification of foot ulcers. Meggitt and Brodsky have modified this classification, and it remains in widespread use. Other classifications have been used as well and include the University of Texas classification and the PEDIS Classification from the International Working Group for the Diabetic Foot.

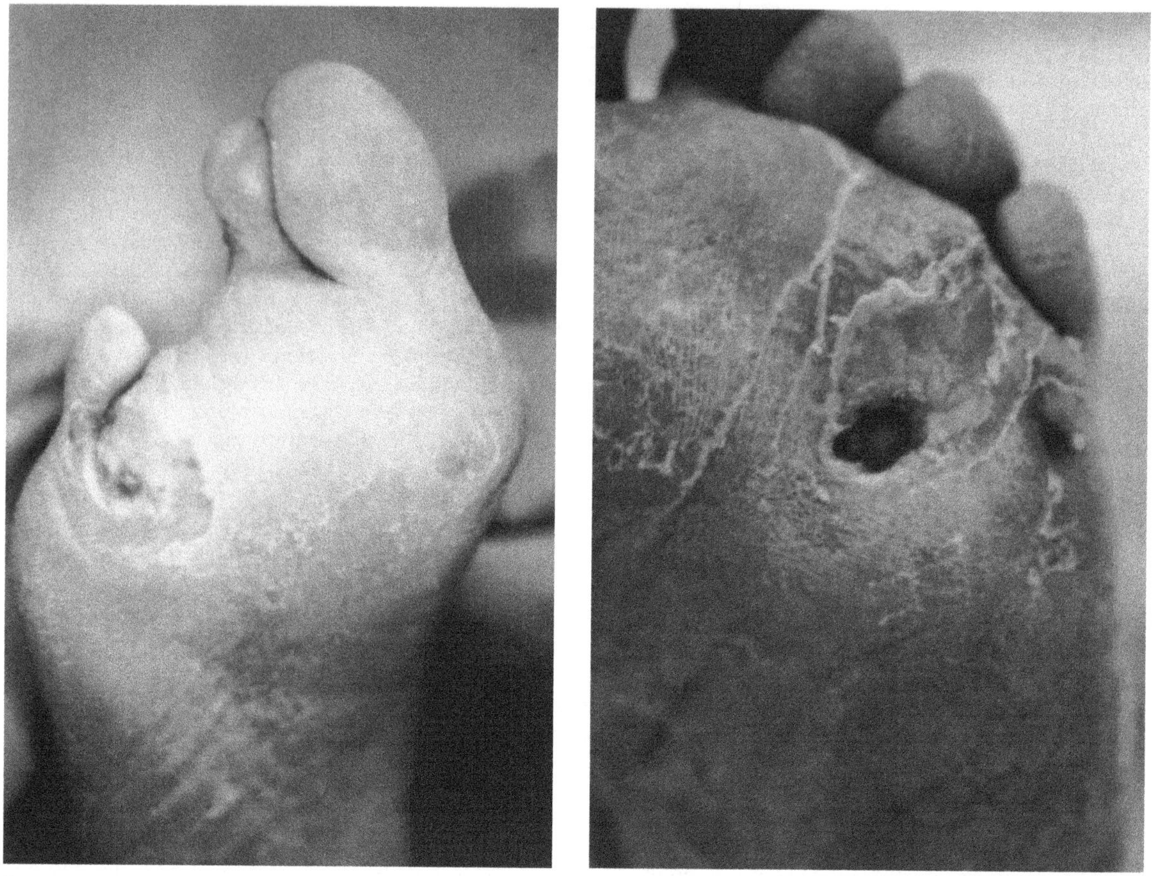

A B

▲ **Figure 10–27. Comparison of (A) grade 1 and (B) grade 2 ulcers (new depth and ischemia classification). Note the exposed deep tissues of the grade 2 ulcer.** (Reprinted with permission, from Brodsky JW. The diabetic foot. In Mann RA, Coughlin MJ, eds. *Surgery of the Foot and Ankle*, 6th ed. St. Louis: Mosby-Year Book; 1993.)

Expeditious healing of diabetic foot ulcers can prevent secondary infections and associated amputations. Important components in the initial treatment of diabetic foot ulcers include appropriate offloading, surgical debridement of devitalized tissue to convert chronic wounds into acute wounds, and moist wound healing. Specialized bioengineered tissue is available for advanced wound methods in patients who do not heal as expected. Early recognition of infection is critical to minimize tissue loss and preserves function. As a general rule in treating infections of the foot, a balance must be struck between salvage of tissue and foot function. A healed amputation at a more proximal level is more advantageous to the patient than leaving a marginally viable area of the foot that requires constant wound care.

Large surgical wounds heal slowly with the risk of secondary infection and, if possible, should not be left to heal by secondary intention. Split-thickness skin grafts, especially on the sole of the foot or over an amputation site, are prone to breakdown. Negative-pressure wound therapy has been a tremendous resource in treating diabetes-related soft-tissue wounds.

A. Surgical Treatment for Relieving Bony Prominences

As previously stated, a major goal of treatment in the ulcerated or at-risk foot is to relieve bony prominences that cause pressure on the skin. Treatment consists of measures to relieve the pressure. There are many appropriate measures to relieve pressure on the skin from the outside. Examples include extra-depth shoes for claw toes and accommodative foot orthoses with metatarsal pads to relieve pressure under a prominent metatarsal head. Debriding calluses in areas of weight bearing (ie, metatarsal heads) can reduce plantar pressure. If these measures fail or are inappropriate, the pressure should be relieved intrinsically by correcting the bony

Table 10–2. Classification and treatment of diabetic foot ulcers.

Grade	Classification	Treatment
0	Foot is "at risk" for developing ulcer. Skin remains intact, but underlying bone deformity places foot at risk for skin breakdown.	Proper footwear plus other preventive measures such as patient education and surgical correction as described in text.
1	Lesion affects skin only.	Outpatient dressing changes or total contact cast. Antibiotics usually not necessary.
2	Deep lesions that involve underlying tendons, bones, or ligaments (Figure 10–28).	Surgical debridement and hospitalization for aggressive wound care and intravenous antibiotics. Goal is conversion to grade 1 ulcer.
3	Abscess or osteomyelitis present as a complication of ulcer.	Emergency surgery for drainage of acute infection. Wound often left open, with dressing changes performed until definitive closure or amputation is done at a later date.
4	Gangrene is present in the toes or forefoot.	Appropriate amputation.
5	Entire foot is gangrenous.	Appropriate amputation.

deformity. These prominences are located at several common sites.

The hallux may have a prominence beneath the metatarsal head, on the plantar-medial aspect of the interphalangeal joint, or over the median eminence secondary to a bunion deformity. A prominence caused by the medial sesamoid can be relieved by complete or partial removal of the sesamoid. If this does not adequately relieve the prominence, a dorsiflexion osteotomy or resection of the metatarsal head can be performed. Ulcers found over the plantar-medial aspect of the interphalangeal joint can often be relieved by simple excision of the prominent medial condyles or by resection of the entire joint. If this ulcer is associated with limited metatarsophalangeal extension, then a cheilectomy or metatarsophalangeal arthroplasty may be appropriate to allow the toe to extend further during the toe-off phase of gait and thus decrease the pressure on the skin under the interphalangeal joint. The Keller procedure has been used with success for hallux interphalangeal joint ulcers associated with restricted metatarsophalangeal joint motion. A prominence over the median eminence can be addressed with a routine bunion procedure.

The diabetic patient is subject to claw toe deformities resulting from motor neuropathy, causing prominences under the metatarsal heads and over the dorsum of the proximal interphalangeal joints. Depending on the severity, treatment varies from reduction of the metatarsophalangeal joints and proximal interphalangeal arthroplasties to resection of the metatarsal heads and interphalangeal fusions.

A collapsed longitudinal arch from Charcot changes causes the classic rocker-bottom foot with prominences along the plantar and medial aspects of the midfoot. This can be addressed with a simple exostectomy for a mild deformity that is stable or with an appropriate osteotomy and arthrodesis for more complex deformities or progressive instability.

In addition to osseous procedures, tendon lengthening, release, or transfers may benefit patients with osseous deformity. Achilles tendon or gastrocnemius lengthening is a well-recognized treatment for ankle equinus. Patients with diabetes may have coronal and frontal malalignment as well. For example, patients with lateral column overload may benefit from release or lengthening of the posterior tibial tendon. In some cases, a split tibialis tendon transfer may be needed. Similarly, with severe valgus deformities, release of the peroneal tendons may be necessary.

B. Treatment of Osteomyelitis

Osteomyelitis is a common complication present in Wagner grade 3 diabetic foot ulcers. The infection is seldom eradicated without surgical debridement of the bone, although there is evidence that forefoot osteomyelitis can be treated without surgery. Other authors recommend conservative surgery in the forefoot. Frequently, more radical treatment than simple exostectomy is required. For example, infection of a proximal phalanx is usually treated by resection of the phalanx. Osteomyelitis of the metatarsal may require ray amputation if more than just the head is involved. If multiple metatarsals are infected, a transmetatarsal amputation is often the best treatment with the reminder to always consider lengthening the Achilles tendon to decrease load on the residual forefoot.

Osteomyelitis of the midfoot is often a complication of a collapsed Charcot foot. The treatment options for such an infection include wide local debridement with exostectomy or a more proximal amputation. Similarly, osteomyelitis of the calcaneus can be treated with a partial calcanectomy or a more proximal amputation.

Treatment of each ulcer is individualized and should make sense with the underlying physiology. A patient with a superficial wound with good blood supply, minimal infection, and protective sensation would be treated with topical wound care, a shoe to accommodate the dressing, and limited activity to control swelling. A patient with an infected deep wound with osteomyelitis and nonreconstructable dysvascularity would probably be best served with early amputation. Of course, each patient is unique and deserves an evaluation of all organ systems to develop an appropriate treatment plan.

The goal of wound dressings is to mimic skin. They should provide a healing environment that is bacteria free, warm, moist, strain free, nontoxic, and well oxygenated. There is nothing that will provide all of these. Dressings should be chosen based on the needs of the wound, possibly needing infection control and debridement in the initial phases but later requiring protection and absorption of wound drainage. The gold standard for treating plantar ulcers is a total contact or healing cast. This protective cast provides wound protection, edema control, and a moist environment, and has been shown to decrease plantar loading to the ulcer. When the wound is draining, they require frequent changing or the odor can be intolerable.

Biologic wound healing products that provide wound healing factors can be helpful in the patient with marginal healing potential. Larger wounds, especially those with considerable drainage, can benefit from vacuum-assisted closure where a constant negative suction pressure is applied to a sealed wound, thereby decreasing its size and pulling away wound drainage.

There are a small number of patients who are marginal wound healers who will benefit from hyperbaric oxygen treatment. When placed in pure oxygen at two atmospheres of pressure, the serum becomes supersaturated and has been shown to benefit some patients who receive serial treatments. Recently the use of topical oxygen has been found to be effective. Despite this, hyperbaric oxygen remains a topic that generates substantial debate in the diabetic foot arena.

C. Charcot Foot

A Charcot joint is also referred to as a neuropathic, neurotrophic, or neuroarthropathic joint. Diabetes is by far the leading cause of Charcot joints, although any disease associated with central or peripheral nervous system pathology can be implicated. A Charcot foot is characterized by destruction of joint surfaces and fractures often accompanied by dislocations of one or more joints in a patient with inappropriate pain response. The requirements are an active patient who has neuropathy and adequate blood supply. Approximately 50% of patients do not recall a specific inciting traumatic incident. The pathophysiology is not fully understood, but there are two theories. The neurotraumatic theory says that cumulative mechanical strains in a patient with inadequate sensory protection leads to stress fractures that are progressive because the patient does not have adequate sensory feedback to limit their activity. The neurovascular theory suggests that there is a neurally initiated vascular reflex that leads to juxtaarticular osteopenia weakening the bone in this area while glycation of the joint capsule causes stiffness. These factors, when combined with mechanical stress, can lead to the fracture dislocations that are commonly seen. There are probably elements of both of these theories that contribute to Charcot arthropathy.

There are three classic stages in Charcot arthropathy as defined by Eichenholtz. Stage 1 is the acute inflammatory phase where there is swelling, redness, and increased warmth. Radiographs would likely show fractures and dislocations, and the involved area would be unstable. The concern in this stage would be to rule out infection. If the patient is neuropathic with good blood supply and has an acute, red, hot, swollen foot without an ulcer or a history of an ulcer in that area, it is more likely Charcot arthropathy and not infection. Hematogenous osteomyelitis is very rare, and infections in the foot are usually introduced locally through the skin. Stage 2 is the subacute phase where there are signs of healing, less swelling and warmth, and radiographic signs of new bone formation. Stage 3 is the chronic phase with consolidation and resolution of inflammation. Typical locations include the midfoot, with the creation of the rocker-bottom foot deformity as the arch collapses, and the hindfoot and the ankle, with the risk of collapse into varus or valgus that can lead to pressure ulcers. Stage 0 Charcot, also known as Charcot in situ, is the stage prior to developing changes seen on radiographs. During this acute inflammatory stage, MRI or bone scan will identify neuropathic changes prior to breakdown. Charcot changes at this stage are reversible, and this is often misdiagnosed as cellulitis, gout, or deep vein thrombosis.

1. Principles of treatment—There are several important principles to follow in the treatment of Charcot joints. The primary goal is to limit joint destruction and preserve a stable plantigrade foot that will protect the soft tissues and prevent ulceration.

2. Treatment of acute phase—For a patient who presents in the acute phase of Charcot joint, the initial treatment should be offloading, immobilization, and elevation of the foot. This can best be achieved with a non–weight-bearing total contact cast for patients who can be placed in a plantigrade position. The use of crutches, walkers, boots, wheelchairs, and scooters may be appropriate in patients to assist with offloading. The goal is to maintain and preserve a plantigrade foot that will not be at increased risk for ulceration. The skin must be checked at weekly intervals initially to look for breakdown. Traditionally, surgery was rarely attempted on the acute Charcot foot, unless necessitated by the inability to obtain a stable plantigrade position. Recently, there has been a trend to treat these as any other neuropathic fracture dislocation would be treated, with reduction and stabilization. Even in patients who will require acute stabilization to obtain a plantigrade foot, offloading in a total contact cast is a very effective method to reduce swelling and inflammation prior to surgical intervention. Once the acute phase subsides and the fractures heal, immobilization can be accomplished by means of an ankle-foot orthosis (AFO) or other appropriate removable supports. Custom-made shoes with inserts can then be fitted to accommodate for the bony prominences. Resolution of the acute phase may take several months.

3. Treatment of subacute phase—In this phase, the foot has stabilized, and there is no ongoing bony destruction and inflammation. Operations address the bony prominences that have been created by Charcot destruction and collapse.

Often, simple removal of a prominence (exostectomy) is all that is required, and occasionally, fusion of one or several joints is necessary. One of the most common foot deformities is a collapsed arch and rocker-bottom deformity from subluxation of multiple joints in the midfoot. Usually, an exostectomy of the prominent bones on the plantar aspect of the midfoot is sufficient. Alternatively, an osteotomy and arthrodesis of the midfoot can be performed to realign the foot and reconstitute the arch in cases where a simple exostectomy is inadequate (Figure 10–28). There is usually a contracture of the ankle plantar flexors, and this deforming force may need to be released as part of this procedure. Charcot reconstruction has a high complication rate and an extended time to achieve union. In the case of Charcot involvement of the ankle joint, the goal is a stable and plantigrade foot, which often requires arthrodesis. Retrograde intramedullary nailing has been shown to be successful in achieving union but also has significant complication rates. Deformities of the ankle in the frontal and coronal plane are not well tolerated because of the subcutaneous position of the malleoli.

Aragon-Sanchez J, Lázaro-Martínez JL, Alvaro-Afonso FJ, et al. Conservative surgery of diabetic forefoot osteomyelitis: how can I operate on this patient without amputation? *Int J Low Extrem Wounds.* 2015;14(2):108-131. [PMID: 25256285]

Chuan F, Tang K, Jiang P, et al. Reliability and validity of the perfusion, extent, depth, infection and sensation (PEDIS) classification system and score in patients with diabetic foot ulcer. *PLoS One.* 2015;10(4):e0124739. [PMID: 25875097]

Cychosz CC, Phisitkul P, Belatti DA, et al. Preventive and therapeutic strategies for diabetic foot ulcers. *Foot Ankle Int.* 2016;37(3):334-343. [PMID: 26475457]

Frykberg RG, Franks PJ, Edmonds M, et al. A multinational, multicenter, randomized, double-blinded, placebo-controlled trial to evaluate the efficacy of cyclical topical wound oxygen therapy (TWO2) in the treatment of chronic diabetic foot ulcers: the TWO2 study. *Diabetes Care.* 2020;43(3):616-624. [PMID: 31619393]

Lazaro-Martinez JL, Aragón-Sánchez J, García-Morales E. Antibiotics versus conservative surgery for treating diabetic foot osteomyelitis: a randomized comparative trial. *Diabetes Care.* 2014;37(3):789-795. [PMID: 24130347]

Schneekloth BJ, Lowery NJ, Wukich DK. Charcot neuroarthropathy in patients with diabetes: an updated systematic review of surgical management. *J Foot Ankle Surg.* 2016;55(3):586-590. [PMID: 26810129]

Wagner FW Jr. A classification and treatment program for diabetic, neuropathic, and dysvascular foot problems. *Instr Course Lect.* 1979;28:143. [No PMID]

Wukich DK, Shen W, Raspovic KM, et al. Noninvasive arterial testing in patients with diabetes: a guide for foot and ankle surgeons. *Foot Ankle Int.* 2015;36(12):1391-1399. [PMID: 26194106]

Wukich DK, Sung W. Charcot arthropathy of the foot and ankle: modern concepts and management review. *J Diabetes Compl.* 2009;23(6):409-426. [PMID: 18930414]

Wukich DK, Sung W, Wipf SAM, et al. The consequences of complacency: managing the effects of unrecognized Charcot feet. *Diabet Med.* 2011;28(2):195-198. [PMID: 21219429]

DISORDERS OF THE TOENAILS

Toenail problems in young patients with diabetes usually involve trauma, such as stubbing the toe or, more frequently, improper nail care, which can contribute to ingrown toenails. This is usually the result of tearing off a toenail, which leaves the nail too short and predisposes it to becoming ingrown.

Toenail problems in the older age group are more varied, including an incurvating nail, a thickened hypertrophied nail associated with a chronic fungal infection, an ingrown nail resulting from improper nail cutting, and on rare occasions, a subungual exostosis.

Etiologic Findings

The anatomy of the toenail is demonstrated in Figure 10–29. The nail unit consists of four components: the proximal nail fold, the nail matrix, the nail bed, and the hyponychium. The area in which most of the problems occur is the lateral or medial nail groove, where an ingrown nail occurs at the level of the nail bed or hyponychium.

Clinical Findings

A. Symptoms and Signs

The history of most nail problems is not complex and usually quickly defines the nature of the problem.

1. Infection of the toenails—Infection of the toenails usually begins slowly, with erythema and swelling along the margin of the nail, followed by increasing pain and drainage, and finally the development of granulation tissue, usually in response to the foreign body reaction to the nail itself.

2. Mycotic nail—In the case of the mycotic (fungal) nail, there is usually a long, slow history of development of deformation of the nail, often with medial or lateral deviation of the nail, marked hypertrophy, and increased pain when wearing shoes. At times, an incurvated nail condition develops in which one or both edges of the nail slowly curve inward, resulting in pinching of the nail plate. This may cause a localized infection, or it may be that just the sheer pressure of the nail against the skin is the cause of the pain.

3. Subungual exostosis—The patient who develops subungual exostosis usually notes pain increasing beneath the toenail over a long period. Erosion of the nail from below occurs because of the pressure of the exostosis against the nail itself. Often, the patient does not seek help until there is breakdown of the tissue, giving rise to a rather ugly appearing lesion that seems much more ominous than the condition itself.

B. Imaging Studies

Radiographs are necessary when evaluating a toenail problem for subungual exostosis, which is clearly seen with a lateral view. In patients with long-standing infected ingrown toenails, a radiograph can be important to rule out underlying osteomyelitis.

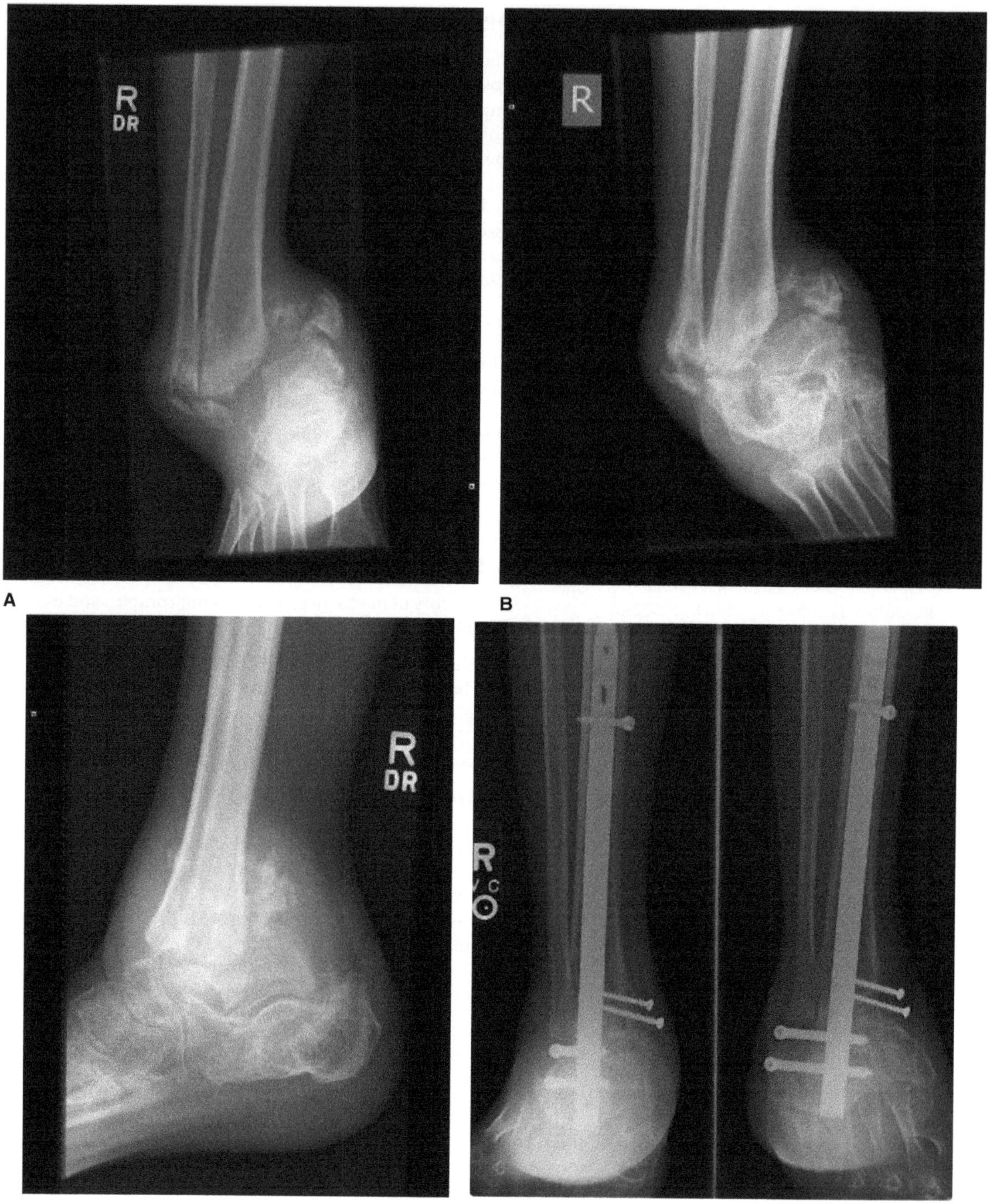

▲ **Figure 10–28. A-C:** This is a 35-year-old neuropathic insulin-dependent type 1 diabetic who complains of pain and instability of his ankle when walking. There is marked destruction of the ankle with severe instability and deformity that is not treatable with bracing. **D, E:** The ankle is stabilized with an arthrodesis using intramedullary fixation and returns the patient to an ambulatory status requiring a rocker-bottom shoe and an accommodative insert.

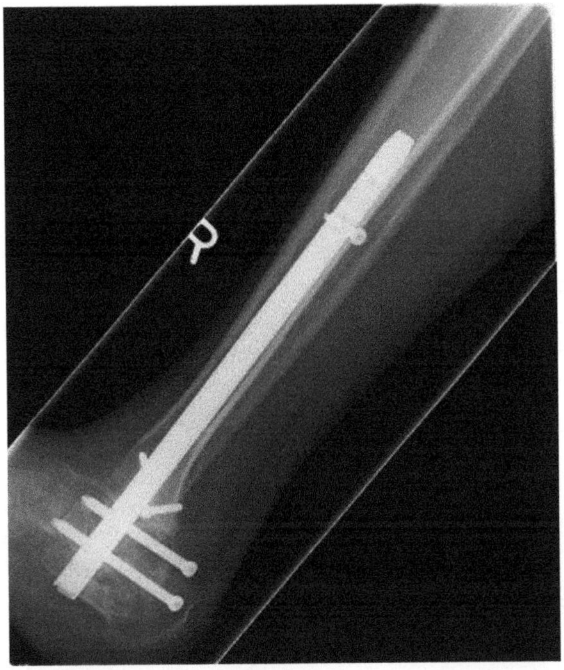

E

▲ **Figure 10–28.** (Continued)

Treatment

A. Conservative Management

1. Chronic ingrown toenail—For the chronic ingrown toenail, the margin of the nail is removed to relieve the pressure of the nail against the skin. This procedure, along with local care and occasionally systemic antibiotics, usually permits the condition to resolve. It is important, however, to explain to the patient the necessity of permitting the nail to grow out over the ungual labia to depress it and prevent the ingrown nail from recurring.

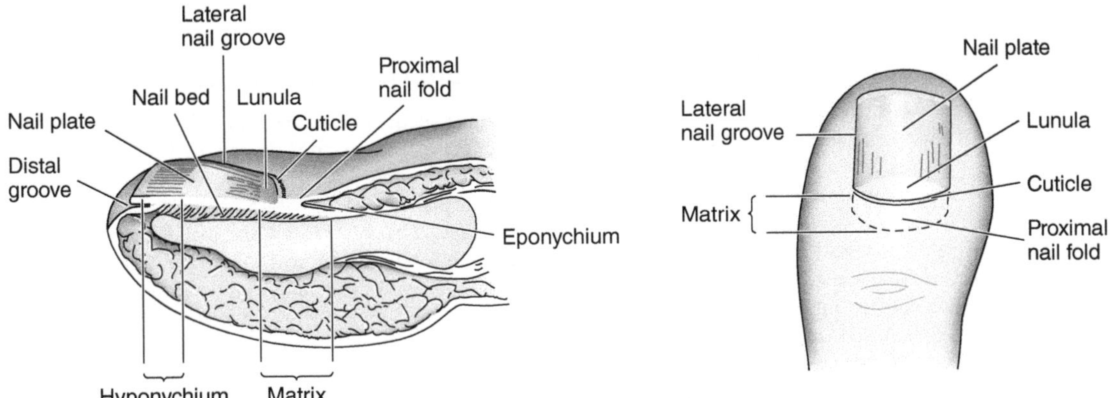

▲ **Figure 10–29. A:** Cross section of the toe demonstrates the components of the toenail and supporting structures. **B:** The proximal nail is covered by the proximal nail fold and cuticle. The lunula is the main germinal area. (Reprinted with permission, from Mann RA, Coughlin MJ. *The Video Textbook of Foot and Ankle Surgery.* Medical Video Productions, 1991.)

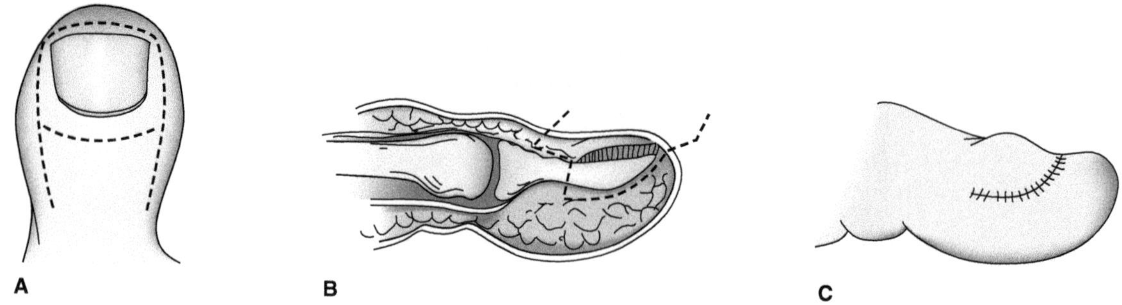

▲ **Figure 10–30.** Syme amputation of toenail. **A:** Elliptical or rectangular incision is centered over the nail bed and matrix. **B:** The distal half of the distal phalanx is resected. **C:** Excess skin is resected, and skin edges are approximated. (Reprinted with permission, from Mann RA, Coughlin MJ. *The Video Textbook of Foot and Ankle Surgery.* Medical Video Productions, 1991.)

2. Chronic onychophosis of the nail—Chronic onychophosis of the nail must be debrided. If an ingrown nail occurs, the margins must be trimmed to relieve the pressure against the skin.

3. Subungual exostosis—Subungual exostosis that is symptomatic is treated by excision.

B. Surgical Treatment

1. Ingrown toenail—The surgical management of the recurrent ingrown toenail consists of the Winograd procedure. In this procedure, the medial or lateral margin of the offending nail plate is removed along with the underlying nail matrix. The nail matrix is removed as thoroughly as possible to prevent the possible growth of a nail horn, which occurs in about 5% of cases. The nail matrix can be removed by sharp dissection or ablated with a laser or treated with phenol to kill the nail matrix.

2. Chronic infection—If there is severe distortion of the nail caused by chronic infection, the nail and the nail bed can be removed in their entirety. This usually results in a horny base where the nail existed, and this is often a satisfactory outcome. The terminal Syme amputation can be carried out to eliminate the nail and matrix completely (Figure 10–30). Although results are usually satisfactory, some patients do not like the appearance of the toe or absence of the toenail because of its somewhat bulbous appearance. The terminal Syme procedure can be carried out under digital block in most patients. An elliptical incision is made over the distal end of the toe, removing the nail and its matrix in their entirety. The distal portion of the distal phalanx is removed and the edges smoothed, thus shortening the toe. The tip of the toe is defatted and loosely sutured. In this manner, the nail is completely removed, and soft tissue covers the area of the former nail bed. The major significant complication associated with this procedure is the regrowth of residual nail matrix beneath the healed flap, which will result in an inclusion cyst that must be drained and the residual nail matrix excised.

3. Subungual exostosis—Surgical management of subungual exostosis requires lifting the nail, identification of the exostosis, and complete removal of the exostosis and its stalk. The dissection must be carefully carried out and the entire exostosis removed to prevent recurrence. The nail bed is repaired to cover the defect.

Baran R, Dawber RPR. *Diseases of the Nails and Their Management.* Oxford, United Kingdom: Blackwell Scientific Publications, Osney Mead; 1984.

Cho SY, Kim YC, Choi JW. Epidemiology and bone-related comorbidities of ingrown nail: a nationwide population-based study. *J Dermatol.* 2018;45(12):1418-1424. [PMID: 30264897]

Geizhals S, Lipner SR. Review of onychocryptosis: epidemiology, pathogenesis, risk factors, diagnosis and treatment. *Dermatol Online J.* 2019;25(9):13030/qt9985w2n0. [PMID: 31738836]

Mayeaux EJ Jr, Carter C, Murphy TE. Ingrown toenail management. *Am Fam Physician.* 2019;100(3):158-164. [PMID: 31361106]

NEUROLOGIC DISORDERS OF THE FOOT

1. Interdigital Neuroma (Morton Neuroma)

An interdigital neuroma is a painful affliction involving the plantar aspect of the forefoot. It usually involves the third interspace and is characterized by a well-localized area of pain on the plantar aspect of the foot that radiates into the web space. The symptoms are usually aggravated by ambulation and relieved by rest. As a rule, wearing a tight-fitting shoe aggravates the pain, and walking barefoot often relieves it.

▶ Etiologic Findings

The precise cause of interdigital neuroma has not been determined. It occurs in women about 10 times more frequently than men, and as a result, high-fashion shoewear has been implicated. Several studies demonstrate that the changes in

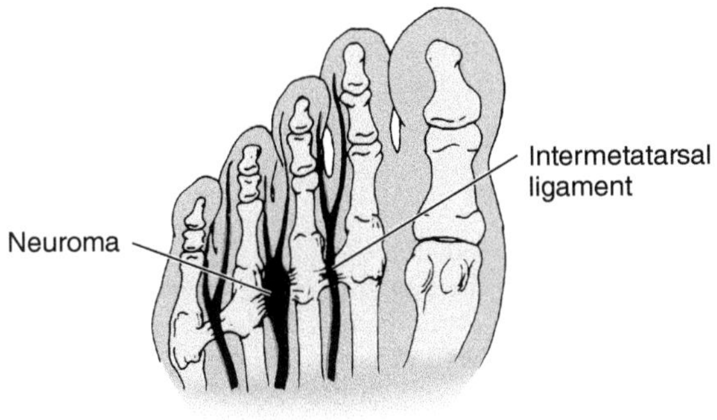

▲ **Figure 10–31. An interdigital neuroma impingement occurs beneath the intermetatarsal ligament.** (Reprinted with permission, from Mann RA, Coughlin MJ. *The Video Textbook of Foot and Ankle Surgery*. Medical Video Productions, 1991.)

the nerve appear to occur just distal to the transverse metatarsal ligament. This finding has given rise to the hypothesis that the neuroma results from the constant traction of the nerve against the ligament as the toes are brought into a dorsiflexed position, a theory that would explain the higher incidence in women wearing high-heeled shoes. Although this condition is called interdigital neuroma, it is not a true neuroma. The pathologic changes involve actual degeneration of the nerve fibers associated with deposition of amorphous eosinophilic material that is felt to be consistent with an entrapment neuropathy (Figure 10–31).

Clinical Findings

A. Symptoms and Signs

Patients with an interdigital neuroma usually present with a complaint of localized pain in the metatarsal head region that is increased by walking and relieved by rest and removing the shoe. Palpation of the involved interspace produces sharp pain that often radiates into the toes. There can be a palpable mass, and squeezing the forefoot, thereby narrowing the intermetatarsal space while compressing the mass, often reproduces the patient's symptoms. If this maneuver produces a snapping sensation, it is referred to as a Mulder click. The third interspace is more frequently involved than the second, and it is extremely rare to have involvement of the first or fourth web space. Pain over the metatarsophalangeal joint itself is caused by disease involving the metatarsophalangeal joint, and it is important to distinguish pain in the interspace from pain associated with pathology in the metatarsophalangeal joint. The differential diagnosis of metatarsalgia includes avascular necrosis (ie, Freiberg disease), synovitis due to mechanical instability, synovial cysts, or even referred pain from tarsal tunnel compression or lumbar disk disease. It is not uncommon for plantar plate problems to be misdiagnosed as interdigital neuromas.

B. Imaging Studies

Radiographs are not helpful in the diagnosis of an interdigital neuroma but may reveal pathology at the metatarsophalangeal joint as the cause of the patient's symptoms. There are several reports regarding the use of ultrasound to evaluate the presence of nerve enlargement, but this is very user dependent. MRI can be used effectively but is rarely necessary.

Treatment

A. Conservative Management

Conservative management begins with wearing a wider, soft-soled shoe to accommodate the foot without mediolateral compression and lowering the heel. A soft metatarsal support is placed in the shoe proximal to the area of the neuroma, thereby spreading the metatarsal heads and lifting them. Approximately one-third of the patients will respond to this treatment. Steroid injection into the web space can be helpful in resolving the symptoms but is not without the hazard of local fat atrophy, which can lead to diminished padding under the metatarsal heads or local skin thinning and discoloration. Injection of local anesthetic alone appears to be equivalent to injection of a corticosteroid and local anesthetic.

B. Surgical Treatment

Surgical excision of the nerve is indicated if conservative treatment fails. A dorsal incision is made in the midline of the involved web space and carried down to the transverse metatarsal ligament, which is divided. The nerve is noted to lie just beneath the transverse metatarsal ligament. A nerve that is quite thickened is reassuring evidence that the correct diagnosis has been made; however, a nerve of normal thickness should still be removed if the clinical diagnosis of neuroma has been made from other evidence. The nerve is delivered into the interspace by plantar pressure and is freed up distally and proximally, transected proximal to the metatarsal head, and then dissected out distally, where it is cut just past its bifurcation. Care is taken not to disrupt the surrounding fatty tissue or intrinsic muscles. A compression dressing is used and ambulation is permitted in a postoperative shoe. Decreased sensation in the toes on either side of the web space is expected postoperatively. Approximately 80% of patients are totally satisfied with the results of the procedure, whereas 20% obtain little or no relief. The precise cause of this failure rate is a bit of an enigma. Obviously in some patients, the diagnosis was incorrectly made and the metatarsophalangeal joint was actually involved.

C. Recurrent Neuroma

A recurrent neuroma is indeed a true surgical bulb neuroma that has resulted following the transection of the common digital nerve on the plantar aspect of the foot. True neuritic symptoms occur when the transection was not proximal enough or the nerve became adherent and trapped beneath the metatarsal head. Careful percussion of the plantar region of the symptoms to elicit the Tinel sign can frequently localize the cut end of the nerve (bulb neuroma). If the severed nerve can be clinically well localized, reexploration for the neuroma is carried out either through a dorsal or plantar approach. The neuroma is identified and transected to a more proximal level or implanted into muscle, and symptoms are relieved in 60% to 70% of patients.

2. Tarsal Tunnel Syndrome

Tarsal tunnel syndrome is a compressive or traction neuropathy of the posterior tibial nerve as it passes posterior to the medial malleolus. The tarsal tunnel is formed by the fibro-osseous tunnel extending from the flexor retinaculum as it wraps around the posterior aspect of the medial malleolus (Figure 10–32). Tarsal tunnel syndrome causes poorly localized dysesthesias on the plantar aspect of the foot. Symptoms are often aggravated by activity and relieved by rest. Some patients complain mainly of nocturnal dysesthesias.

Etiologic Findings

Tarsal tunnel syndrome may arise from a space-occupying lesion within the tarsal tunnel (eg, a ganglion, synovial cyst, or lipoma) or distally against one of the two terminal branches: the medial or lateral plantar nerve. It occasionally follows severe trauma to the lower extremity probably because of edema or scarring. Other causes are severe venous varicosities, tenosynovitis, or a tumor within the nerve. Traction neuropathy can occur in patients who have an excessively valgus hindfoot position, especially those that are unstable. As the patient walks, the posterior tibial nerve may be stretched as it courses around the convex side of the deformity. In more than half of the cases, however, the precise cause cannot be determined.

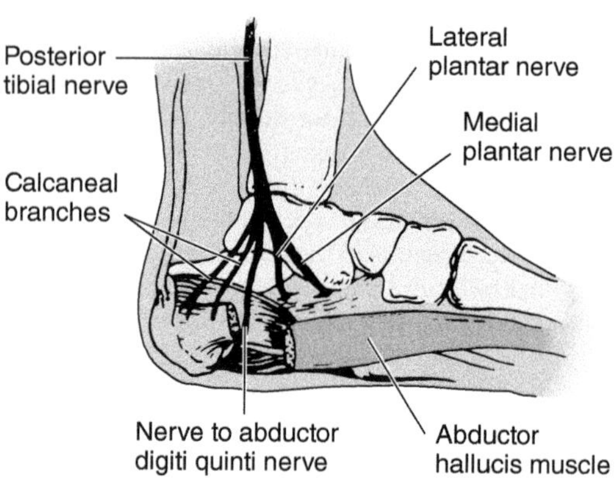

▲ **Figure 10–32.** Posterior tibial nerve and major branches. (Reprinted with permission, from Mann RA, Coughlin MJ. *The Video Textbook of Foot and Ankle Surgery.* Medical Video Productions, 1991.)

Clinical Findings

A. Symptoms and Signs

The diagnosis is entertained after obtaining a history of paresthesias or burning in the posterior tibial nerve distribution. Careful evaluation of the patient in the standing and sitting positions is necessary to check posture and increased fullness, thickening, or swelling in the involved tarsal tunnel area. Careful percussion may elicit a Tinel sign over the posterior tibial nerve in the tarsal tunnel or distally along the divisions of the posterior tibial nerve (the medial calcaneal nerve and medial and lateral plantar nerves).

Muscle weakness is usually not observed, but loss of sensation and two-point discrimination may be occasionally detected.

Electrodiagnostic studies should be carried out to help confirm the diagnosis of tarsal tunnel syndrome. Nerve conduction velocities along the medial plantar nerve to the abductor hallucis muscle (latency <6.2 ms) and of the lateral plantar nerve to the abductor digiti quinti (latency usually <7 ms) should be within 1 ms of each other, otherwise indicating nerve compression in the tarsal tunnel. Motor-evoked potentials that demonstrate a decreased amplitude and increased duration are also felt to be indicative of tarsal tunnel syndrome. The most accurate study for tarsal tunnel syndrome appears to be sensory nerve conduction velocity, although this is also the least reproducible study.

The definitive diagnosis of tarsal tunnel syndrome should be based on (1) the clinical history of ill-defined burning, tingling pain in the plantar aspect of the foot; (2) positive physical findings of Tinel sign along the course of the nerve; and (3) electrodiagnostic studies. If all three factors are not positive, the diagnosis of tarsal tunnel syndrome should be the suspect. MRI can be quite useful in demonstrating space-occupying lesions.

Treatment

A. Conservative Management

Tarsal tunnel syndrome should be managed with anti-inflammatory medications and an occasional steroid injection into the tarsal tunnel area. Aspiration and injection of a cyst or ganglion may be attempted but are rarely successful. Immobilization in a polypropylene AFO may also be useful, especially in the patient with unstable valgus who is suffering from a traction injury to the nerve. Compression hose may benefit patients with varicose veins, as distention of the veins within the tarsal tunnel can contribute to symptoms.

B. Surgical Treatment

Surgical intervention can be considered if conservative management fails. Approximately 75% of patients operated on for tarsal tunnel syndrome are satisfied with the result. The other 25% of patients may continue to have varying degrees of discomfort. The surgical release employs an incision behind the medial malleolus that is carried distally to about the level of the talonavicular joint. The investing retinaculum is exposed and released. The posterior tibial nerve is identified proximal to the tarsal tunnel area and carefully traced distally behind the medial malleolus. The division into its three terminal branches is identified. Because the medial calcaneal branch passes from the posterior aspect of the lateral plantar nerve, the dissection should be carried out along its dorsal aspect. There may be one or more medial calcaneal branches. The medial plantar nerve should be traced distally until it passes through the fibro-osseous tunnel in the abductor hallucis muscle. The lateral plantar nerve should be traced behind the abductor hallucis muscle until it passes toward the lateral aspect of the foot. A preoperative Tinel sign distal to the tarsal tunnel area requires that the area be carefully explored to determine whether there is a ganglion or cyst within the tendon sheath as a cause of the tarsal tunnel syndrome.

Postoperatively, a compression dressing is applied and weight bearing is restricted for 3 weeks, before progressive ambulation is permitted.

The results following tarsal tunnel release depend on the pathology that is found at the time of surgery. Removal of a space-occupying lesion usually relieves all of the symptoms. Involvement of a single nerve branch, such as the medial or lateral plantar nerve, also portends good results after surgery. If more diffuse pain is felt throughout the foot before surgery and no definite constriction on the nerve is found at exploration, only one half to two-thirds of the patients can be expected to experience pain relief. Patients with traction neuropathy due to the unstable valgus foot are treated by correction of the instability, usually with arthrodesis, and not with isolated soft-tissue tarsal tunnel release.

3. Traumatic Neuromas About the Foot

A traumatic neuroma about the foot presents a difficult problem in management because footwear can cause constant irritation of the neuroma. The most frequent cause of traumatic neuroma in the foot is previous surgery. Despite caution in making incisions about the foot, many lesser and occasionally major nerve trunks can be injured. The dorsal aspect of the foot is most frequently involved (Figure 10–33).

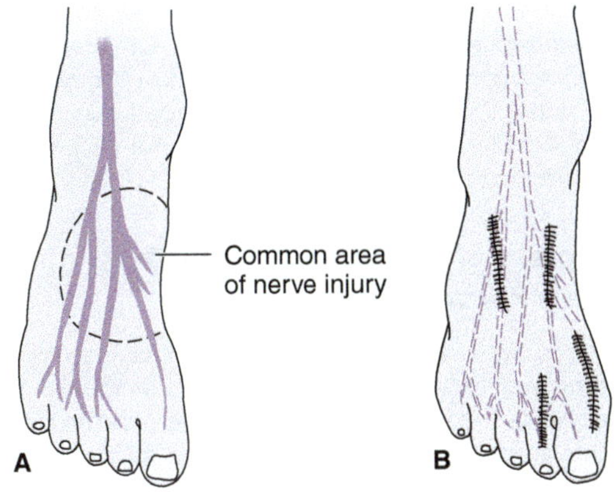

▲ **Figure 10–33. A:** Common area of traumatic nerve entrapment. **B:** Frequent incisions that may lead to entrapment of dorsal sensory nerves. (Reprinted with permission, from Mann RA, Coughlin MJ. *The Video Textbook of Foot and Ankle Surgery.* Medical Video Productions, 1991.)

Clinical Findings

The clinical evaluation begins with a careful history of the problem and an evaluation of the area involved determining the precise location of the neuroma, which is essential for proper treatment. Rarely is any type of electrodiagnostic study indicated, and radiographs are not usually necessary.

Treatment

A. Conservative Management

Attempts to relieve pressure on the neuroma with a large shoe or a carefully designed pad may be of benefit. Occasionally a steroid injection into the area may help, particularly when a small nerve is involved. Serial injections of long-acting local anesthetic without steroid may also provide relief and are not subject to the complications of repeated steroid injections. Surgical intervention is indicated if conservative measures fail.

B. Surgical Treatment

Careful planning must be undertaken prior to the excision of a traumatic neuroma. Findings that suggest surgery as an option include a positive Tinel sign and dramatic temporary relief from a local anesthetic injection. The exact location of the neuroma and the area of sensitivity proximal to it must be determined. The incision must be made as precisely as possible to identify the neuroma and trace the nerve proximally into an area that would not be affected by pressure from shoes and boots. The neuroma is excised, leaving enough nerve to bring the cut end into an area of minimal pressure. The cut end is buried into an excavation in bone, if possible, or beneath a muscle such as the extensor digitorum brevis muscle. When carrying out a resection of the sural nerve, it is important, particularly in an individual who wears heavy work boots, that the end of the nerve is brought proximally enough so that the top of the boot will not press upon the nerve, resulting in continued symptoms.

The results following resection of a traumatic neuroma are quite variable. Initial relief from removing the traumatic neuroma is routine, but unless the nerve is buried where it will not be exposed to pressure, the symptoms may recur in time. It is therefore preferable to bury the end of the nerve into bone, if possible. Resection of most neuromas will accentuate a sensory deficit, but this is usually not a significant clinical problem.

4. Entrapment of the Sensory Branch of the Deep Peroneal Nerve

Osteophyte formation at the talonavicular or metatarsocuneiform joint may entrap the sensory branch of the deep peroneal nerve as it passes beneath the extensor retinaculum. Patients complain of dysesthesias on the foot or difficulty in wearing shoes, depending on the location of the entrapment.

The sensory branch of the deep peroneal nerve passes onto the dorsum of the foot between the extensor hallucis longus and extensor digitorum longus tendons. It continues beneath the extensor retinaculum, coursing along the dorsal surface of the talus and navicular, and more distally across the metatarsocuneiform joints. Osteophyte formation at any point along the course of the nerve may cause sufficient pressure against the nerve to cause an entrapment problem.

Clinical Findings

A. Symptoms and Signs

The clinical evaluation begins with a careful history regarding the patient's complaint of dysesthesias over the dorsum of the foot. The physical examination demonstrates tingling along the course of the sensory branch of the deep peroneal nerve, which radiates into the first web space. Often the precise location of the nerve entrapment can be identified by careful palpation and by rolling the nerve across the involved bony prominence.

B. Imaging Studies

Radiographs usually reveal the offending osteophytes, often along the area of the talonavicular or metatarsocuneiform joints. Placing a radiographic marker at the area of maximum tenderness can help to identify the offending bony prominence.

Treatment

A. Conservative Management

Conservative management consists of attempting to keep the pressure off the involved area, either by padding the tongue of the shoe or by trying to create a pad that will not put pressure directly on the nerve. If these measures fail, decompression of the nerve will usually bring about satisfactory resolution of the condition.

B. Surgical Treatment

Depending on the area of entrapment (talonavicular or metatarsocuneiform), a slightly curved incision is made and carried down through the retinaculum to expose the nerve. Great caution must be taken during the approach so that the nerve is not inadvertently damaged. The nerve is carefully lifted off of its bed, exposing the osteophytes, which are removed with a rongeur. The bony surfaces are coated with bone wax prior to laying the nerve back on its bed. After wound closure in layers, the foot is immobilized for approximately 3 weeks in a postoperative shoe.

The results following release of the sensory portion of the deep peroneal nerve are usually satisfactory. Because the nerve itself usually is not damaged by the entrapment, a favorable outcome is expected.

Lizano-Diez X, Ginés-Cespedosa A, Alentorn-Geli E, et al. Corticosteroid injection for the treatment of Morton's neuroma: a prospective, double-blinded, randomized, placebo-controlled trial. *Foot Ankle Int.* 2017;38(9):944-951. [PMID: 28617064]

RHEUMATOID FOOT

The foot is involved in 90% of patients with long-standing rheumatoid arthritis, and the involvement is usually bilateral. The forefoot is most commonly involved and often contains the first joints to be affected, but deterioration of the subtalar joint has been noted in about 35% of patients and of the ankle joint in about 30%. Due to the pharmacologic advancements in inflammatory arthritis, severe foot disease is less common than several decades ago.

Etiologic Findings

The changes in the forefoot are caused by chronic synovitis, which destroys the supporting structures about the metatarsophalangeal joints. The joint capsules are distended and the ligaments injured. When these structures no longer function to provide stability for the joint, progressive dorsal subluxation and eventual dislocation of the metatarsophalangeal joints occur. As the metatarsophalangeal joints progress from subluxation to dislocation, the plantar fat pad is drawn distally, and the base of the proximal phalanx eventually comes to rest on the metatarsal head. Thus, the metatarsals are forced into a position of plantarflexion, which results in significant callus formation beneath the metatarsal heads. The changes at the metatarsophalangeal joints result in imbalance of the intrinsic muscles, and severe hammer toe and claw toe deformities usually result.

Significant midfoot and hindfoot pathology is also commonly seen in patients with rheumatoid arthritis. Rheumatoid arthritis is a potential cause of isolated, nontraumatic arthritis of the talonavicular joint. A severely flattened longitudinal arch can result from long-standing subtalar joint and/or talonavicular involvement with subluxation.

Clinical Findings

A. Symptoms and Signs

The clinical evaluation of the rheumatoid patient begins with a careful history of the disease, the medications the patient is taking, and an attempt to ascertain whether the disease process is currently in an active or a quiescent stage. It is important to obtain some indication of the patient's wound-healing capacity in the foot and elsewhere in the body.

The vascular status of the foot and quality of the skin are noted. The feet are assessed with the patient standing, which will often demonstrate marked deformities of multiple joints or localized involvement of only one or two joints. The patient is then seated, and a careful evaluation of all the joints about the foot and ankle is carried out to determine precisely the degree to which they are affected. Careful palpation of the metatarsophalangeal joints will often demonstrate the amount of synovitis as well as the degree of joint stability. The plantar aspect of the foot is inspected for the callus formation and past or present ulcerations. Flattening of the longitudinal arch and any hindfoot valgus are evaluated with a careful assessment of joint stability to determine the risk of deformity progression.

B. Imaging Studies

Radiographs help to assess the number and severity of the joints involved. Bilateral involvement is frequently symmetric. Standing radiographs are beneficial in assessing the effect of joint stability on the severity of deformity.

Treatment

A. Conservative Management

Conservative management includes medical management, usually carried out by the patient's rheumatologist. The patient with sufficient deformity should wear an extra-depth shoe with a soft accommodative liner to reduce pressure on the metatarsal heads and the toes, which may be severely contracted dorsally. Frequently, the patient is quite comfortable in this shoe and does not require further treatment. With significant ankle and hindfoot involvement, an ankle-foot orthosis may be required to help relieve pain by providing adequate stabilization.

B. Surgical Treatment

The main goal of surgical management of the forefoot is to create a stable foot that will alleviate the pain beneath the metatarsal heads (Figure 10–34). Preoperative consultation with the patient's rheumatologist is important to discuss what medications need to withheld during the perioperative period. Biologics such as adalimumab and etanercept are held, but long-term steroid use cannot be discontinued, potentially increasing the risk of delayed healing and

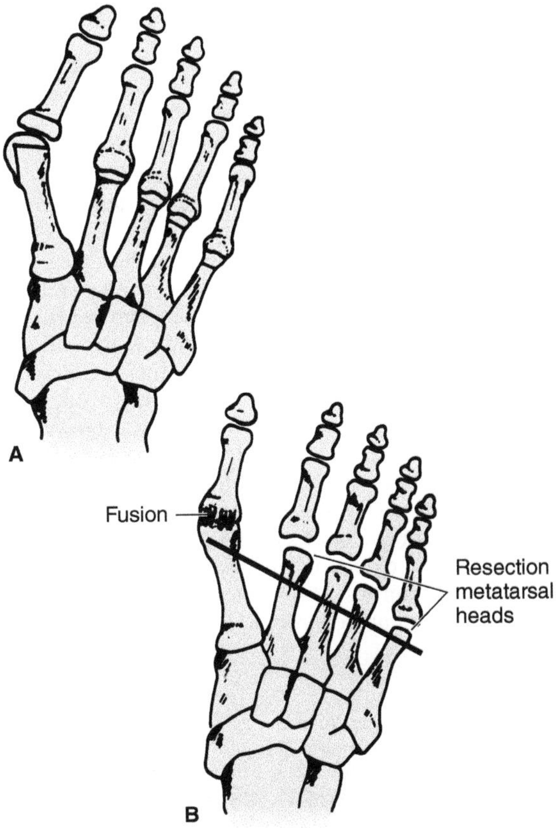

▲ **Figure 10–34. A:** Resection of metatarsal heads. **B:** Symmetric resection of metatarsal heads minimizes recurrence of intractable plantar keratoses. (Reprinted with permission, from Mann RA, Coughlin MJ. *The Video Textbook of Foot and Ankle Surgery.* Medical Video Productions, 1991.)

infection. Methotrexate can be continued throughout the perioperative period without a significantly increased risk of complications. Arthrodesis of the first metatarsophalangeal joint is the procedure most commonly used, with the joint placed in approximately 15 degrees of dorsiflexion in relation to the floor and approximately 15 degrees of valgus position. The lesser metatarsophalangeal joints are corrected by release of the soft-tissue contracture and resection arthroplasty. The metatarsal heads are excised to decompress the metatarsophalangeal joints, and the fat pad is brought back down onto the plantar aspect of the foot by realigning and securing the plantar plates of the joints under the residual metatarsals. The hammer toes can then be corrected by closed osteoclasis, which often results in satisfactory realignment. Open hammer toe procedures are also very effective in correcting residual deformities. The toes and metatarsophalangeal joint area are stabilized with longitudinal Kirschner wires postoperatively for approximately 4 weeks.

The results of this rheumatoid forefoot repair are gratifying, and about 90% of patients will be satisfied with the results. There are few complications; however, the blood supply to the toes is always of concern because the procedure is extensive. Occasionally, wound healing is delayed, particularly if the patient is taking high dosages of corticosteroids or a biologic medication.

Hindfoot and ankle disease is usually managed medically unless there is instability, progressive deformity, and/or recalcitrant pain. Orthotic support or bracing can be beneficial, but if the deformity is increasing and the patient's thin skin cannot tolerate further pressure, then surgical stabilization with arthrodesis is necessary. If only a single joint is involved with rheumatoid arthritis, a less extensive procedure is carried out. For isolated talonavicular rheumatoid arthritis with no significant deformity of the arch, an isolated talonavicular fusion is adequate. If significant deformity is present because of subtalar joint subluxation, a triple arthrodesis is required. Ankle joint involvement is treated with ankle joint fusion or total ankle arthroplasty. Details of the surgical procedures are described elsewhere in this chapter.

Ortega-Avila AB, Moreno-Velasco A, Cervera-Garvi P, Mrtinez-Rico M, Chicharro-Luna E, Gijon-Noqueron G. Surgical treatment for the ankle and foot in patients with rheumatoid arthritis: a systematic review. *J Clin Med.* 201;9(1):42. [PMID: 31878151]

HEEL PAIN

Heel pain can be caused by several distinct entities. When evaluating the patient for heel pain, the clinician must attempt to define as precisely as possible the location and, hence, the cause of the pain.

The causes of heel pain are presented in Table 10–3. The causes are quite variable and need to be carefully defined, so that proper treatment can be chosen.

Table 10–3. Causes of heel pain.

Causes of plantar heel pain
Plantar fasciitis
Atrophy of heel pad
Posttraumatic (eg, calcaneal fracture)
Enlarged calcaneal spur
Neurologic conditions such as tarsal tunnel syndrome or entrapment of nerve to abductor digiti quinti
Degenerative disk disease with radiation toward heel
Systemic disease (eg, Reiter syndrome, psoriatic arthritis)
Acute tear of plantar fascia
Calcaneal apophysitis
Causes of posterior heel pain
Retrocalcaneal bursitis
Achilles tendinitis
Haglund deformity
Degeneration of Achilles tendon insertion

Clinical Findings

A. Symptoms and Signs

Clinical evaluation begins with a careful history of the onset and location of the pain, the patient's activities, and types of footwear that aggravate and relieve the pain. Specific inquiry regarding radiation of pain proximally in the lower extremity may suggest lumbar disk disease as the cause. Patients active in sports should be questioned regarding significant changes in their level of activity because heel pain often is the result of increased stress on the foot. Bilateral symptoms may indicate seronegative arthritis.

The cause of the patient's heel pain can usually be determined by palpating the location of maximum tenderness.

Plantar fasciitis, the most common cause of plantar heel pain, usually has maximum tenderness along the plantar medial aspect of the heel, corresponding to the origin of the plantar fascia at the medial calcaneal tuberosity. In most cases, the pain is most severe with the first steps of the morning. The pain is usually aggravated by dorsiflexion of the toes—the so-called windlass stretch—because this applies more tension to the damaged plantar fascia. The pain may be exacerbated by passive ankle dorsiflexion in patients with contracture of the gastrocnemius muscle.

Achilles tendonitis/tendinosis typically occurs at one of two discreet sites: at the calcaneal insertion or centered 3 to 4 cm proximal to the insertion. Insertional Achilles tendonitis/tendinosis is characterized by pain and swelling that is increased by activity. There is usually tenderness in the posterior midline with local increased warmth. Noninsertional Achilles tendonitis/tendinosis is usually associated with a thickened tendon and is often severely tender to palpation at the thickened area in the midportion of the tendon. Both of these are more degenerative than true inflammatory processes and more properly referred to as tendinosis.

Heel pain can also be caused by inflammation of the retrocalcaneal bursa, between the tendoachilles and the posterior calcaneus and is often associated with the Haglund heel deformity.

Tarsal tunnel syndrome with involvement of the medial calcaneal branches should be investigated by careful percussion of the posterior tibial nerve. Evidence of degenerative disk disease requires careful testing of motor function and sensation more proximally in the calf.

B. Imaging Studies

Radiographs may demonstrate calcaneal spur formation or calcification at either the insertion of the Achilles tendon or the origin of the plantar fascia. Alternatively, the posterosuperior aspect of the calcaneus may be too prominent and protrude into the Achilles tendon, a condition known as Haglund disease or Haglund deformity, with the symptoms coming from the inflamed retrocalcaneal bursa. A bone scan will sometimes reveal increased activity diffusely about the calcaneus, as may be seen in systemic diseases such as Reiter syndrome, or a discreet area of uptake, as in a stress fracture. MRI scan may help to delineate the degree of the Achilles tendon degeneration present in cases of Achilles tendinosis and can help to identify rupture of the tendon if this is in question.

Treatment

A. Conservative Management

The conservative management of heel pain depends on the specific cause. Because many causes are related to abnormal stress on the foot, the basic principles involve reducing the stress on the involved area. Activity modification, footwear with a softer, more resilient heel, and use of a soft orthotic device under the longitudinal arch to relieve some of the pressure on the region of pain can be helpful. NSAIDs are often useful, as is physical therapy to teach stretching exercises of the Achilles tendon and plantar fascia. Plantar fasciitis is treated initially with stretching exercises, soft-cushioned heel shoes, NSAIDs if they are tolerated, and avoidance of strong toe-off activities such as running and jumping. The use of a night splint to help keep the Achilles tendon and plantar fascia stretched often relieves the acute pain patients experience when they first get up in the morning. Patients who are refractory to treatment may benefit from a steroid injection into the plantar fascia origin, although there is a risk of plantar fascia rupture. Cast immobilization has also been shown to benefit these refractory patients. Injection of platelet-rich plasma or extracorporeal pulse-activated therapy may also be of benefit to these refractory patients. Injection of platelet-rich plasma may be more effective than corticosteroid injection.

In general, the treatment of heel pain is often prolonged, requiring a great deal of patience on the part of the physician and patient. It is important to explain to the patient the nature of the problem and the fact that it is often a chronic condition that requires many months to resolve.

Achilles tendinosis is treated with stretching exercises, activity modification, NSAIDs, and a heel lift. If these modalities are inadequate, then bracing or casting will provide more relief to the damaged tissue.

B. Surgical Treatment

Patients with plantar fasciitis, in whom symptoms cannot be controlled after 9 to 12 months of conservative management, may become candidates for surgery. The options include orthotripsy or surgical release of the medial half of the plantar fascial origin. With surgical release, the success rate is approximately 75%. Caution must be exercised with the approach to the medial side of the heel to avoid damage to the medial calcaneal branch of the posterior tibial nerve. Disruption of this nerve will cause an area of heel numbness and possibly a troublesome neuroma along the medial side of the heel. An endoscopic approach for plantar fascia release has been described in patients who do not have a plantar heel spur that requires removal. Orthotripsy, while less invasive, still has conflicting literature as to its effectiveness.

Surgical treatment of Achilles tendinosis is offered if 6 to 9 months of conservative measures do not help to eliminate symptoms. Insertional Achilles tendinosis is treated with debridement of degenerative tendon and excision of bone spurs with repair of the Achilles insertion. If a Haglund deformity is present, it is also resected. Noninsertional Achilles tendinosis is treated with debridement of degenerative tendon. In either case, if the majority of the tendon is nonviable, it must be repaired, often requiring a graft such as the flexor hallucis longus tendon transfer.

Peerbooms JC, Lodder P, den Oudsten BL, et al. Positive effect of platelet-rich plasma on pain in plantar fasciitis: a double-blind multicenter randomized controlled trial. *Am J Sports Med.* 2019;47(13):3238-3246. [PMID: 31603721]

Thong-On S, Bovonsunthonchai S, Vachalathiti R, et al. Effects of strengthening and stretching exercises on the temporospatial gait parameters in patients with plantar fasciitis: a randomized controlled trial. *Ann Rehabil Med.* 2019;43(6):662-676. [PMID: 31918529]

Xu D, Jiang W, Huang D, et al. Comparison between extracorporeal shock wave therapy and local corticosteroid injection for plantar fasciitis. *Foot Ankle Int.* 2020;41(2):200-205. [PMID: 31744313]

ARTHRODESIS ABOUT THE FOOT AND ANKLE

General Considerations

A. Goals of Arthrodesis

Arthrodesis is surgical fixation of a joint to obtain fusion of the joint surfaces. Arthrodesis about the foot and ankle can be effective in achieving the following goals:

1. Elimination of joint pain
2. Correction of deformity
3. Stabilization of the foot or ankle when adequate muscle function or ligamentous support is lacking, as in residual poliomyelitis or the acquired flatfoot due to peritalar instability
4. Restoration of function by salvaging a situation in which no reasonable reconstructive procedure is available, as in fusion of the first metatarsophalangeal joint after failed hallux valgus repair

B. Principles of Arthrodesis

An arthrodesis about the foot and ankle requires adherence to these general principles:

1. To be effective, the arthrodesis must produce a plantigrade foot.
2. Broad, cancellous bony surfaces must be placed into apposition.
3. The arthrodesis site should be stabilized with rigid internal fixation, preferably with interfragmentary compression.
4. When correcting malalignment of the foot, it is imperative that the hindfoot be placed into 5 to 7 degrees of valgus and the forefoot in neutral position with regard to abduction, adduction, pronation, and supination.
5. The surgical approaches should be carried out in such a way as to minimize the risk of damage to the nerves.

C. Effects of Arthrodesis on Joint Motion

Following ankle arthrodesis, residual dorsiflexion and plantarflexion movement occurs within the subtalar and transverse tarsal joints, and additional, compensatory motion may develop over time. Arthritic changes in these joints may become symptomatic following ankle arthrodesis, and in time, extension of the fusion may be required.

The subtalar joint and transverse tarsal joints must be viewed as a joint complex similar to the universal joint of a car. Movement in these joints is interrelated. After subtalar arthrodesis, inversion and eversion are lost, but transverse tarsal joint motion in dorsiflexion and plantarflexion remains. Arthrodesis of the talonavicular joint, however, will eliminate most of the subtalar joint motion because rotation must occur around the head of the talus for subtalar motion to occur.

A triple arthrodesis eliminates the subtalar and transverse tarsal joint motion, causing increased stress on the ankle joint and the midtarsal joints distal to the fusion site. A small percentage of patients will develop degenerative changes in the ankle joint following triple arthrodesis. It is imperative, therefore, to carefully evaluate the ankle joint prior to carrying out a triple arthrodesis.

Arthrodesis of the medial three tarsometatarsal joints will not significantly affect motion of the foot and ankle, but a certain degree of stiffness is noted through the midtarsal area following this fusion. Fusion of the first metatarsophalangeal joint places added stress on the interphalangeal joint of the great toe, particularly with poor alignment. Although up to 40% of patients may develop degenerative changes in this joint, they are rarely of clinical significance.

D. Disadvantages of Arthrodesis

Although arthrodesis is an effective reconstructive tool, the resulting loss of motion places increased stress on the surrounding joints, making them more prone to developing arthritis (adjacent segment disease) or worsening preexisting degenerative changes. Thus, correction of a problem without arthrodesis is preferable whenever possible, such as with an osteotomy, tendon transfer, or both.

Ankle Fusion

A. Indications

The main indications for ankle arthrodesis are the following:

1. Arthrosis of the ankle joint usually secondary to a previous ankle fracture, although primary arthrosis does occur
2. Arthritis secondary to rheumatoid disease
3. Instability with malalignment of the ankle joint as the result of an epiphyseal injury or previous fracture

B. Technique

The surgical approach preferred by the authors is a transfibular approach (Figure 10–35). The incision begins along the fibula, approximately 10 cm proximal to the tip of the fibula, and is carried distally along the shaft of the fibula and then curves toward the base of the fourth metatarsal. In this way, the incision avoids the sural nerve posteriorly and the superficial peroneal nerve dorsally. The flaps that are created are full thickness, to lessen the possibility of wound-healing problems. The dissection is carried across the anterior aspect of the ankle joint, to the medial malleolus and along the lateral aspect of the neck of the talus. Posteriorly, the fibula

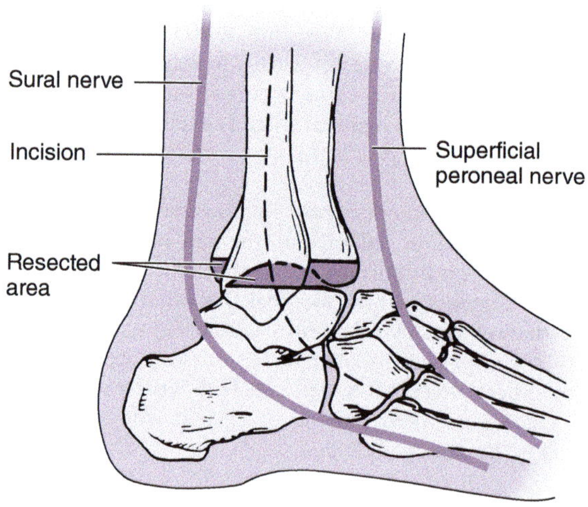

▲ Figure 10–35. Technique for ankle arthrodesis. Skin incision is laced between superficial peroneal nerve and sural nerve. (Reprinted with permission, from Mann RA, Coughlin MJ. *The Video Textbook of Foot and Ankle Surgery*. Medical Video Productions, 1991.)

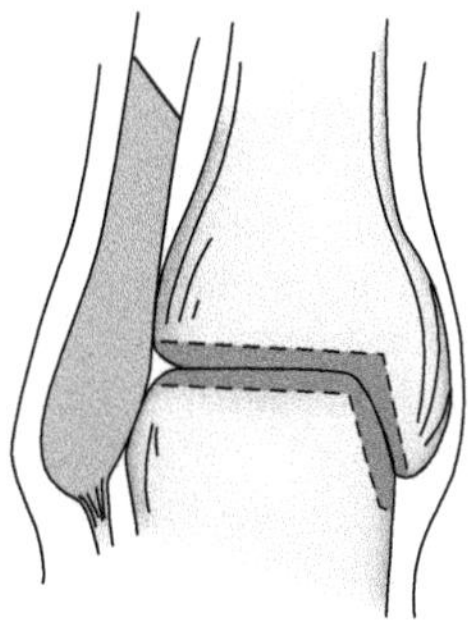

▲ **Figure 10–36.** **The fibula is excised approximately 2 to 2.5 cm proximal to the ankle joint, and the distal portion of the tibia is cut, producing a flat cut perpendicular to the long axis of the tibia.** (Reprinted with permission, from Mann RA, Coughlin MJ. *The Video Textbook of Foot and Ankle Surgery*. Medical Video Productions, 1991.)

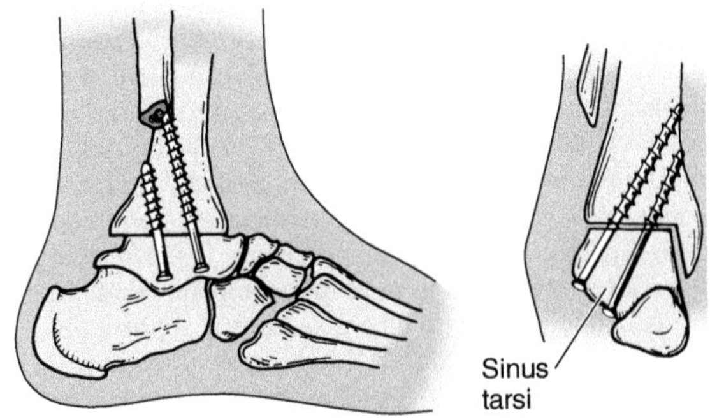

▲ **Figure 10–37.** **Diagram demonstrating placement of the 6.5-mm screws across the arthrodesis site.** (Reprinted with permission, from Mann RA, Coughlin MJ: *The Video Textbook of Foot and Ankle Surgery*. Medical Video Productions, 1991.)

and the posterior aspect of the ankle joint are exposed, while distally, the subtalar joint and sinus tarsi area are exposed. The fibula is removed approximately 2 cm proximal to the joint, after which the residual cartilage and subchondral bone are removed from the distal tibia (Figure 10–36). In some cases, resection of cartilage permits reduction, and in other cases, tibial osteotomy is necessary. A tibial osteotomy should be made as perpendicular as possible to the long axis of the tibia and should extend to the medial malleolus but not through it. The foot is placed into a plantigrade position and a cut made in the dome of the talus parallel to the cut in the tibia, thereby creating two flat surfaces and correcting any malalignment. At this point, the ankle should be aligned in neutral dorsiflexion and at about 5 degrees of valgus. The degree of rotation should be equal to that of the opposite extremity, which is usually 5 to 10 degrees of external rotation. If the two joint surfaces do not easily oppose each other, it is due to the medial malleolus being too long. The malleolus should then be exposed through a dorsomedial incision and the distal centimeter removed. Surgeons who perform ankle fusion must be familiar with various approaches because often patients have had multiple surgical procedures prior to the fusion.

The two articulating surfaces should now be in maximum apposition, with little or no pressure being exerted. Temporary fixation is obtained by inserting two 0.062-inch K-wires. Interfragmentary compression is gained with at least two large (≥6.5 mm) cancellous screws. These screws should be placed to gain adequate interfragmentary compression (Figure 10–37). Following insertion of the screws, there should be rigid fixation of the arthrodesis site. Because the joint surfaces are fully opposed, there may be no room for bone grafting. In the immediate postoperative period, a firm compression dressing incorporating plaster splints is applied. After swelling is decreased, a short leg cast is applied and weight bearing is not allowed for 6 weeks. Weight bearing is then allowed with the short leg cast in place for another 6 weeks. Arthrodesis generally occurs following 12 weeks of immobilization.

C. Complications

Nonunion of the ankle joint, although uncommon, does occur. Using the surgical technique described earlier, a fusion rate of 90% can be anticipated. If nonunion occurs, bone grafting and further internal fixation may be required.

Malalignment of the ankle joint with the foot in too much internal rotation is poorly tolerated and often requires revision surgery. Excessive plantarflexion causes a back knee thrust and eventually some knee discomfort, while excessive dorsiflexion causes increased stress on the heel (that can usually be treated with adequate padding). Varus ankle deformity may cause subtalar joint instability, and excessive valgus causes stress on the medial aspect of the knee joint.

During fixation, it is extremely important not to place any pin or screw across the subtalar joint for fear of damaging the posterior facet, which may lead to arthrosis.

D. Special Considerations

Avascular necrosis of the talus requires excision and tibiocalcaneal fusion or a fusion that bypasses the necrotic bone. Bone grafting may also be necessary when attempting to carry out a fusion after a severely comminuted pilon fracture because there are often defects that affect stability due to the previous crushing of cancellous bone.

Total Ankle Arthroplasty

Total ankle arthroplasty is an alternative to ankle arthrodesis for painful arthrosis of the ankle joint. Advantages include maintenance of some ankle joint motion with a more normal gait and thus less stress on adjacent joints. Unfortunately, the disadvantages of the procedure are that it is technically difficult with a steep learning curve, there are complications such as loosening of the prosthesis and impingement that do not exist with arthrodesis, and the long-term survival is unknown. Total ankle arthroplasty has relatively higher revision surgery with longer follow-up periods, and the intermediate-term survival rate and outcomes are good and are durable in select patients. The procedure is performed through an anterior incision in most of the implants that are currently available in the United States (ie, the Agility, the Eclipse, the Salto-Talaris, and the INBONE), all of which are two-part implants (Figure 10–38). The Zimmer Trabecular Metal Total Ankle uses a transfibular approach. There are several other prostheses, including the STAR, the Mobility, and the Hintegra, used primarily in Europe, that have promising early results; these are three-part implants with a polyethylene mobile bearing. Ankle arthroplasty implants are advancing rapidly, and there is the expectation that newer designs will continue to be approved by the US Food and Drug Administration (FDA) and become available in the United States. There is no advantage to the mobile bearing implants, although there is the possibility of less polyethylene wear; however, the disadvantage is the potential for instability of the mobile bearing. The ideal patient is older, thin, and less active, but there are no clinical data that specifically support this. Proponents of arthroplasty have suggested that their patients may be able to have a more active lifestyle than those with arthrodesis, but there are no studies that actually look at this. There are studies that show that patients after arthroplasty have a greater ability to perform light recreational activities such as swimming, biking, and hiking than they did before surgery. It is generally recommended that arthrodesis patients participate in low-impact sports.

Subtalar Arthrodesis

A. Indications

The main indications for subtalar arthrodesis are the following:

1. Arthrosis of the subtalar joint, usually following a calcaneal fracture, but occasionally for primary arthrosis of the joint
2. Varus or valgus deformity secondary to rheumatoid arthritis
3. Varus deformity secondary to residual clubfoot or possibly following compartment syndrome
4. Unstable subtalar joint secondary to poliomyelitis, a neuromuscular disorder, or tendon dysfunction such as posterior tibial tendon dysfunction
5. Symptomatic talocalcaneal coalition without secondary changes in the talonavicular or calcaneocuboid joints

B. Technique

The incision for subtalar arthrodesis begins at the tip of the fibula and is carried distally toward the base of the fourth metatarsal. As the incision is deepened, the sural nerve or one of its branches should be carefully noted and retracted. Small twigs of nerve may be present that unfortunately may be cut and give rise to a painful neuroma. The sinus tarsi area is exposed by reflecting the extensor digitorum brevis muscle distally. The use of a lamina spreader in the subtalar joint will enhance the exposure.

The articular cartilage is removed from the joint surfaces, including the middle and posterior facets. The bony joint surfaces are then deeply feathered or scaled using a small osteotome. These cuts through the subchondral bone greatly enhance the possibility of fusion. The area around the floor of the sinus tarsi and anterior process region can be carefully shaved to obtain local bone graft for the fusion.

The alignment of the subtalar joint is critical. It must be aligned into approximately 5 to 7 degrees of valgus position, producing a supple transverse tarsal joint. If it is placed in varus position, the foot is stiff and the patient will walk on the lateral side of the foot.

Rigid fixation of the subtalar joint is typically achieved by using large cannulated interfragmentary screws starting at the posterior tip of the calcaneus and passing into the body or neck of the talus. The guide pin is first placed up into the posterior facet, the subtalar joint is then manipulated into proper alignment, and the guide pin is passed into the talus. The alignment of the screw is verified on radiograph, and the screw inserted. An anteroposterior view of the ankle should also be obtained to verify the screws are not impinging in the lateral or medial gutter.

Following adequate internal fixation, the local bone graft is packed into the sinus tarsi area at the surgeon's discretion. Additional bone may be obtained from the area of the medial malleolus, the proximal tibia, or occasionally the iliac crest, although the latter site significantly adds to the morbidity of the procedure. Recently, the use of recombinant growth factor has been employed with success.

Postoperatively, a firm compression dressing incorporating plaster splints is applied. A short leg cast is applied, and weight bearing is not allowed for 6 weeks. The cast is changed, and weight bearing is not allowed for another 6 weeks. Immobilization for 12 weeks generally achieves an arthrodesis.

C. Complications

Nonunion of the subtalar joint is uncommon, although it can occur. Careful surgical technique and heavy scaling of the joint surfaces can help to prevent this complication. If nonunion occurs, bone grafting and added fixation are required to attempt to achieve a solid union.

Malalignment of the subtalar joint may also be a complication. Excessive valgus deformity following subtalar fusion may result in impingement laterally against the fibula or peroneal

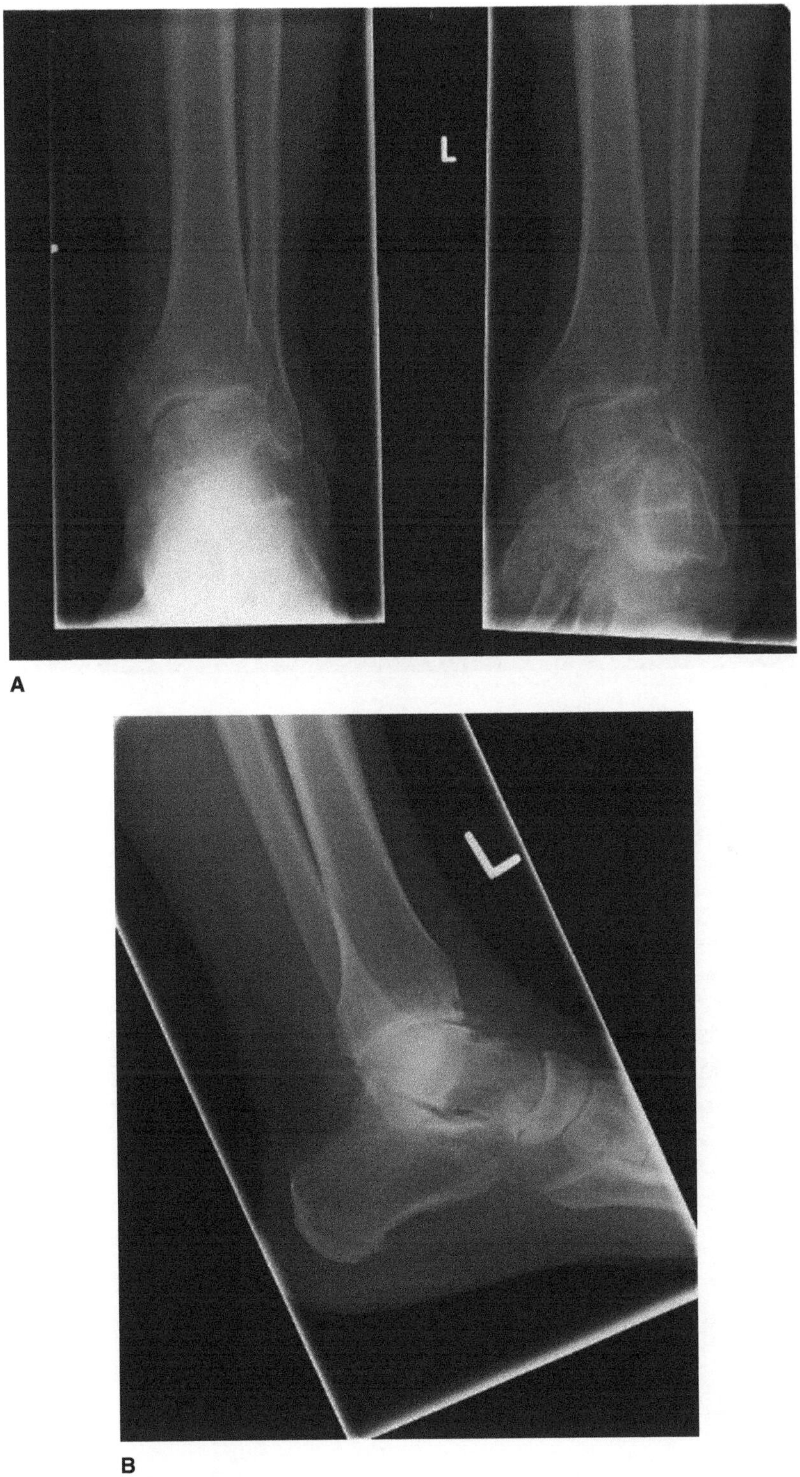

▲ **Figure 10–38.** **A, B:** This is a 60-year-old man with progressive ankle arthritis associated with instability. **C, D:** The same patient after ankle arthroplasty and ligament reconstruction.

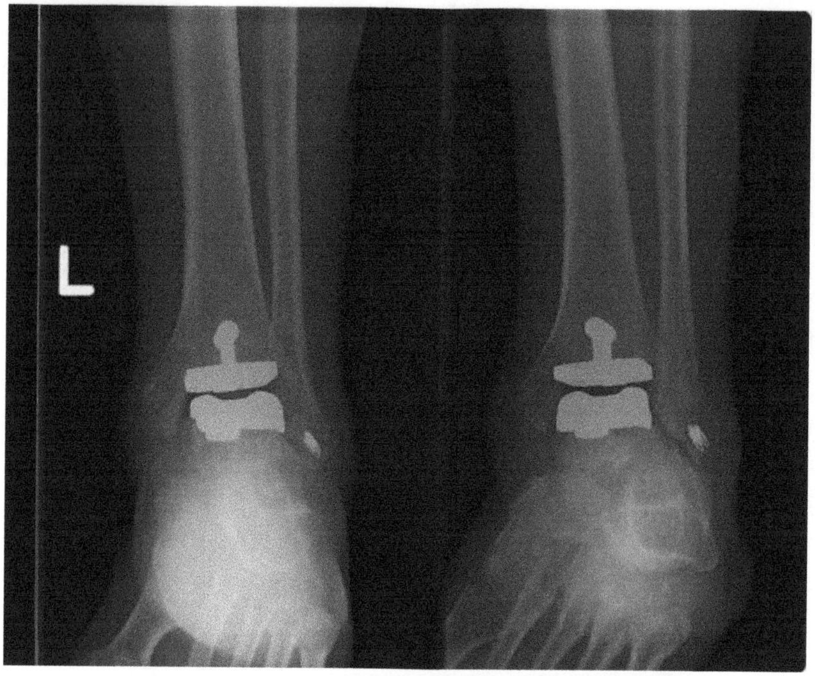

C

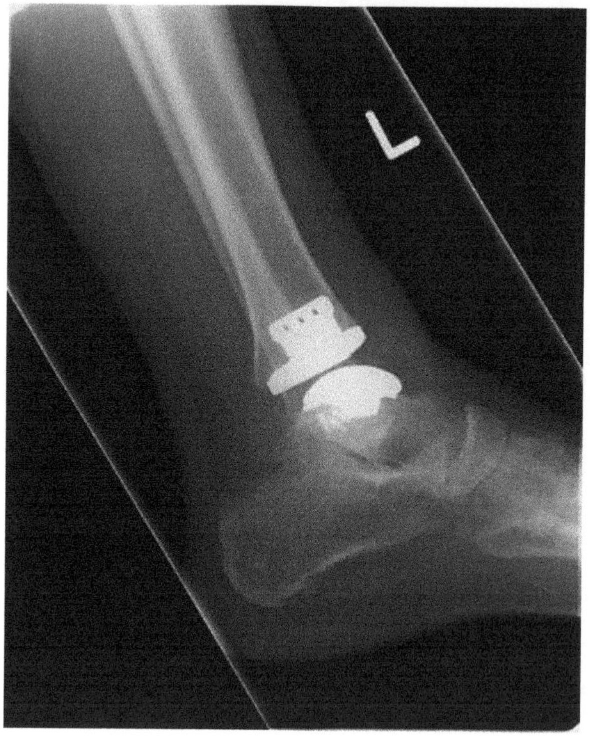

D

▲ **Figure 10–38.** (Continued)

tendons. It will also cause excessive stress along the medial aspect of the midfoot and occasionally the knee joint. A varus deformity of the subtalar joint imparts rigidity to the transverse tarsal joint, resulting in stiffness of the forefoot. This also increases pressure along the lateral aspect of the foot, particularly in the area of the base of the fifth metatarsal.

D. Special Considerations

The patient with rheumatoid arthritis or posttraumatic complications may have lateral subluxation of the calcaneus in relation to the talus, which usually requires computed tomography (CT) scanning for identification. The calcaneus must therefore be displaced medially at operation to align it with the lateral aspect of the talus and place it under the tibia in a proper weight-bearing position. If the calcaneus is fused with significant lateral deviation, the abnormal alignment places added stress on the ankle and midfoot region.

Special attention to the peroneal tendons is necessary when a subtalar arthrodesis is done to correct an old calcaneal fracture. Protrusion of the lateral wall of the body of the calcaneus from the healed fracture results in impingement of the peroneal tendons beneath the fibula. This protrusion must be carefully excised when the subtalar fusion is carried out, so that the lateral aspect of the talus and calcaneus are in line. Further, the peroneal tendon sheath should be dissected subperiosteally off the calcaneus to provide a tendon sheath and to protect the peroneal tendons from the raw, bony surface of the calcaneus.

Occasionally, a bone block distraction arthrodesis of the subtalar joint is performed in cases of severe deformity after a calcaneus fracture. If the talus has assumed a horizontal position because of flattening of Böhler's angle, this can cause limited ankle joint dorsiflexion. Placing a tricortical block of iliac crest into the posterior facet of the subtalar joint will help to improve the overall alignment of the hindfoot and regain ankle joint dorsiflexion.

Talonavicular Arthrodesis

A. Indications

Talonavicular arthrodesis is indicated in the following conditions:

1. Posttraumatic injury, rheumatoid arthritis, or primary arthrosis
2. Unstable talonavicular joint secondary to rupture of the posterior tibial tendon and the peritalar ligaments and rheumatoid arthritis
3. In conjunction with double or triple arthrodesis of the hindfoot

B. Technique

The talonavicular joint is approached through a medial or dorsomedial incision that starts in the region of the naviculocuneiform joint and extends to the neck of the talus. The soft tissues are stripped from around the joint and the articular cartilage removed with a curet or curved osteotome. Distraction of the joint by placing a towel clip into the navicular often facilitates exposure and debridement of the joint. Correct alignment of the talonavicular joint is extremely critical because this fusion essentially eliminates motion in the subtalar joint. The fusion position of the subtalar joint is 3 to 5 degrees of valgus with the forefoot in a plantigrade position (Figure 10–39). After the foot has been properly aligned to correspond to the opposite foot, fixation of the joint is carried out. Proper alignment of this joint is particularly critical when treating the laterally subluxed talonavicular joint in the patient with a ruptured posterior tibial tendon. The internal fixation is carried out by using interfragmentary compression with either large or smaller screws. Ideally, screws in more than one plane provide better stability.

Postoperatively, the patient is immobilized in a non–weight-bearing cast for 6 weeks followed by a weight-bearing cast for an additional 6 weeks.

The talonavicular joint has a relatively high incidence of nonunion, which is probably the result of the difficulty in exposing the joint. If the joint is also approached medially to gain additional exposure, the surfaces can be well scaled, and the fusion rate should approach 90%.

C. Complications

Complications of nonunion and misalignment are similar to those discussed for subtalar joint arthrodesis.

D. Special Considerations

An isolated talonavicular joint fusion will usually produce a satisfactory result, particularly in relatively sedentary patients older than 50 years. In younger, more active individuals with no other affliction (eg, rheumatoid arthritis), consideration should be given to including the calcaneocuboid joint at the same time to obtain a more stable transverse tarsal joint and enhance the fusion of the talonavicular joint through added stability.

Double Arthrodesis (Calcaneocuboid and Talonavicular Joints)

A. Indications

In recent years, double arthrodesis has evolved as a procedure that provides the same degree of stability to the foot as a triple arthrodesis (Figure 10–40). By locking the transverse tarsal joint (calcaneocuboid and talonavicular), further subtalar motion is prevented because these three joints function together. This procedure is also indicated in the younger, active patient in whom an isolated talonavicular fusion is contemplated because it gives added stability to the foot.

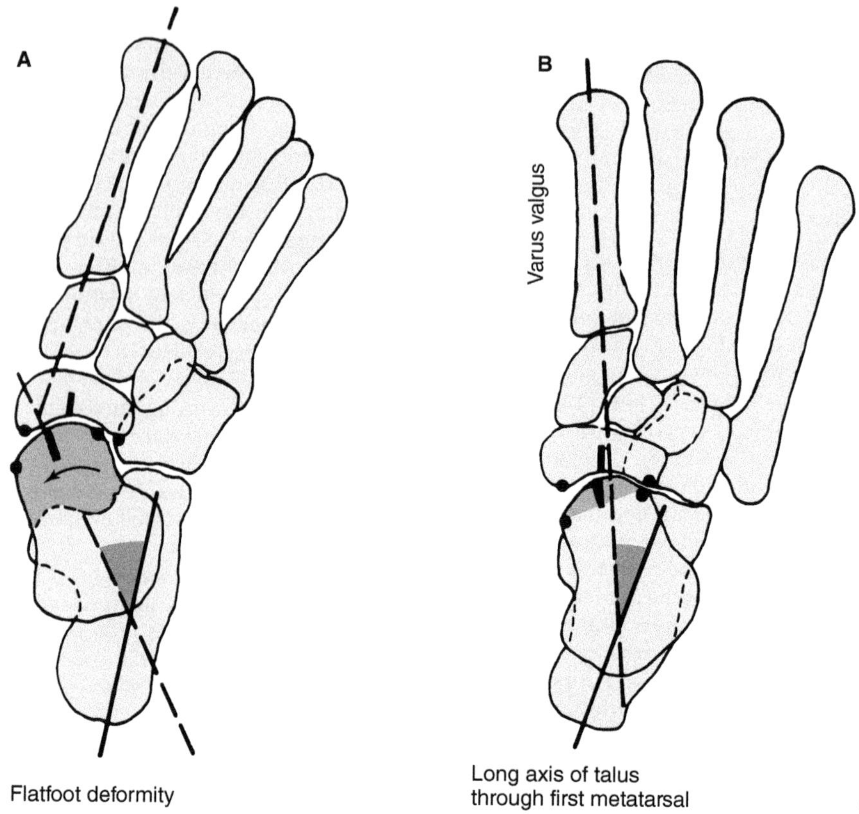

▲ **Figure 10–39.** Talonavicular fusion. **A:** Changes that occur in the talonavicular joint with a flatfoot deformity. Note that the head of the talus deviates medially as the forefoot deviates laterally into abductions. **B:** The forefoot was brought into adduction so the navicular is once again centered over the head of the talus. (Reprinted with permission, from Mann RA, Coughlin MJ. *The Video Textbook of Foot and Ankle Surgery*. Medical Video Productions, 1991.)

Indications for double arthrodesis are as follows:

1. Arthrosis of the talonavicular and calcaneocuboid joints (eg, following trauma)
2. Unstable talonavicular and calcaneocuboid joint following rupture of the posterior tibial tendon or neuromuscular disease when a flexible subtalar joint is present
3. Arthrosis of the talonavicular joint or calcaneocuboid joint in an active individual, usually younger than 50 years of age, to give the midfoot a greater degree of stability

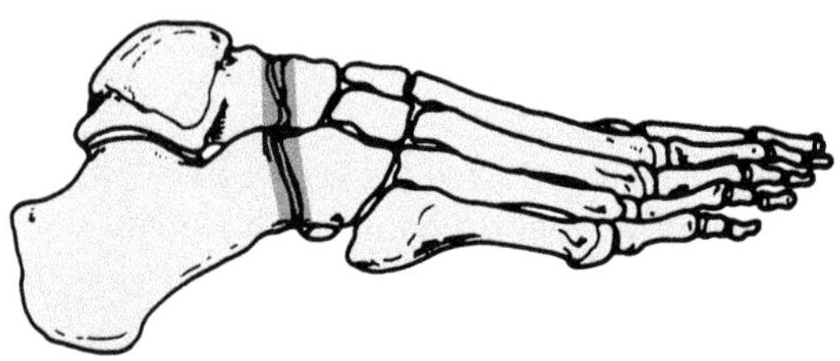

▲ **Figure 10–40.** Double arthrodesis consisting of a talonavicular and calcaneocuboid fusion. (Reprinted with permission, from Mann RA, Coughlin MJ. *The Video Textbook of Foot and Ankle Surgery*. Medical Video Productions, 1991.)

B. Technique

The talonavicular joint is approached through a medial or dorsomedial incision, as previously described, and the calcaneocuboid joint is approached through the same lateral approach used for subtalar fusion. Once these joints are exposed, the joint surfaces are denuded of articular cartilage and the subchondral bone is heavily feathered.

The alignment when carrying out a double arthrodesis is extremely critical because once this fusion has been achieved, the subtalar joint or the transverse tarsal joints no longer move. Therefore, the foot must be placed into a plantigrade position prior to the fixation of the arthrodesis site.

The desired position is 5 degrees of valgus of the calcaneus, neutral abduction and adduction of the transverse tarsal joint, and correction of any forefoot varus that is present. This alignment creates a plantigrade foot. The fixation of the talonavicular joint is done first with the insertion of a screw (6.5 mm) or screws (4 mm) or possibly the use of multiple staples. The calcaneocuboid joint is then fixed the same way. Postoperative care is the same as for other foot fusions.

C. Complications

Complications include nonunion and malalignment and are similar to those discussed for subtalar joint fusion.

Triple Arthrodesis

The triple arthrodesis is a fusion of the talonavicular, calcaneocuboid, and subtalar joints (Figure 10–41). In the past, it was the procedure of choice for all hindfoot problems, before isolated fusions became more accepted. Now, this procedure is still commonly used when limited fusions are inadequate.

A. Indications

Indications for triple arthrodesis are as follows:

1. Arthrosis secondary to trauma involving the subtalar, talonavicular, or calcaneocuboid joints
2. Arthrosis or instability of the talonavicular or calcaneocuboid joints in association with a fixed deformity of the subtalar joint
3. Instability of the foot secondary to posterior tibial tendon dysfunction with a fixed subtalar joint that cannot be realigned by a double arthrodesis
4. Unstable hindfoot secondary to poliomyelitis, nerve injury, or rheumatoid arthritis
5. Symptomatic, unresectable calcaneonavicular bar
6. Malalignment of the hindfoot secondary to trauma such as a crush injury or compartment syndrome

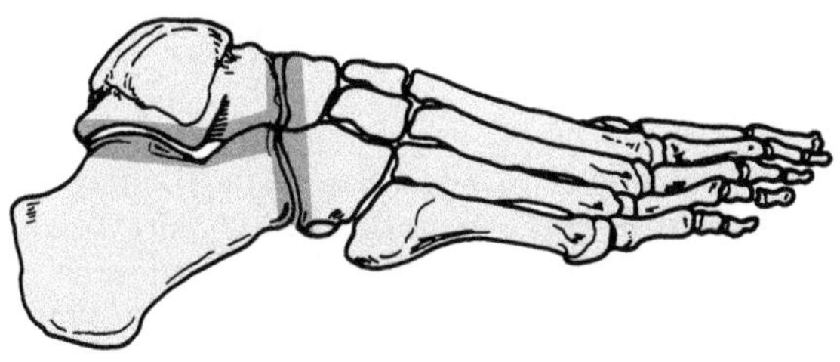

▲ **Figure 10–41.** Diagram of a triple arthrodesis. (Reprinted with permission, from Mann RA, Coughlin MJ. *The Video Textbook of Foot and Ankle Surgery*. Medical Video Productions, 1991.)

B. Technique

The triple arthrodesis is carried out as previously described for subtalar fusion and talonavicular fusion. The foot is fixed after manipulation back into a plantigrade position (3-5 degrees of valgus of the subtalar joint), neutral abduction and adduction of the transverse tarsal joint, and correction of forefoot varus. Postoperative care is the same as for subtalar fusion.

C. Complications

The main complication is failure of fusion of one of the joints, but this is uncommon, as the successful fusion rate exceeds 90%. The talonavicular joint is most likely to have nonunion. Malalignment of the foot or forefoot may require revision and technically is a difficult procedure. The sural nerve may become entrapped or disrupted through the lateral approach.

Tarsometatarsal Arthrodesis

Arthrodesis in the tarsometatarsal area may involve a single tarsometatarsal joint, usually the first joint, or multiple joints. The fusion mass commonly will extend proximally to include the intertarsal bones and sometimes even the naviculocuneiform joints. A careful determination of the involved joints is important when considering a tarsometatarsal fusion for a patient with posttraumatic disorders. At times, in addition to the plain radiographs, a CT scan and bone scan may be necessary to help in precisely defining the involved area.

A. Indications

The indications for a tarsometatarsal fusion are as follows:

1. Hypermobility of the first metatarsocuneiform joint associated with a hallux valgus deformity in a small percentage of patients with a bunion deformity
2. Arthrosis involving one or more of the tarsometatarsal joints either resulting from trauma or as a primary disease process
3. Arthrosis associated with a deformity resulting from an old Lisfranc fracture-dislocation

B. Technique

The surgical approach to the first metatarsocuneiform joint is through a dorsomedial longitudinal incision to expose the joint. If multiple joints are involved, the second incision is centered over the second metatarsal, through which the lateral side of the first and all of the second and third metatarsocuneiform joints can be adequately viewed (Figure 10–42). The incision must be sufficiently long to permit adequate exposure of the joints and must be extended proximally if the naviculocuneiform joints are going to be fused as well. Cautious dissection is necessary, as there are numerous

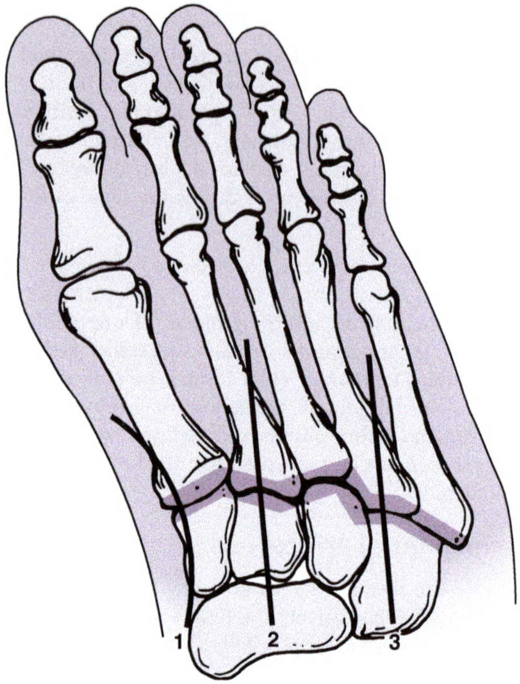

▲ **Figure 10–42. Longitudinal incisions used for a tarsometatarsal arthrodesis.** (Reprinted with permission, from Mann RA, Coughlin MJ. *The Video Textbook of Foot and Ankle Surgery*. Medical Video Productions, 1991.)

superficial nerves as well as the neurovascular bundle (dorsalis pedis and superficial branch of the deep peroneal nerve) passing over the area of the second metatarsocuneiform joint in this approach. If the fourth and fifth metatarsocuboid joints are to be fused, then a third longitudinal incision is made over this area to enable adequate exposure. Arthrodesis of the fourth and fifth joints significantly limits supination and pronation, and preservation of these lateral two joints is recommended. Interpositional arthroplasty has been used to preserve these joints. The articular cartilage is carefully removed from the tarsometatarsal and intertarsal joints, depending on the extent of the fusion mass. The bones are heavily feathered to create a good environment for healing. If a deformity is present (usually an abduction deformity of the foot or possibly dorsiflexion), it should be corrected concurrently. The first metatarsocuneiform joint is aligned and fixed using 4-mm cancellous screws or a dorsomedial plate. Interfragmentary longitudinal compression of the other joints is obtained to prevent possible nonunion. The screw pattern found to be most useful for the first metatarsocuneiform joint is crossing the joint with one brought from the dorsal aspect of the cuneiform directed distally and a second screw from the dorsal aspect of the metatarsal base directed proximally. Care must be taken to also correct any dorsiflexion or abduction deformity that is present.

Postoperatively, the joint is placed in a short leg, non-weight-bearing cast for 6 weeks and then in a weight-bearing cast for another 6 weeks.

C. Complications

The possibility of nonunion exists, but with interfragmentary compression and stable fixation, this risk is minimized. If nonunion occurs, bone grafting may be required as well as improved internal fixation. When multiple tarsometatarsal joints are fused, there is a moderate amount of swelling and tension placed against the incisions. It is critical postoperatively to use a compression dressing to minimize the risk of swelling and prevent possible wound sloughing. If sloughing occurs, it must be treated appropriately, and occasionally, skin grafting is required.

A tarsometatarsal fusion involving multiple joints may cause a plantar callus because one of the metatarsals has been placed in a position of too much plantarflexion. Osteotomy at the base of the metatarsal may be necessary to realign the metatarsal.

Staples should be avoided as a means of internal fixation of the tarsometatarsal joints because they have a tendency to cause dorsiflexion of the metatarsals, which could result in transfer pressure problems under the uninvolved metatarsal heads.

▶ First Metatarsophalangeal Joint Arthrodesis

See the discussion of hallux valgus at the beginning of this chapter.

▶ Interphalangeal Joint Arthrodesis (Hallux Arthrodesis)

A. Indications

Interphalangeal joint arthrodesis is usually indicated for the following problems:

1. Arthrosis, usually secondary to trauma or occasionally following a first metatarsophalangeal joint arthrodesis
2. Stabilization of the interphalangeal joint when carrying out a transfer of the extensor hallucis longus into the neck of the first metatarsal (first toe Jones procedure)

B. Technique

The interphalangeal joint is approached through a dorsal transverse incision centered over the joint. Usually, an ellipse of skin is removed, exposing the ends of the involved joints. Using a small power saw, the end of the distal portion of the proximal phalanx and the proximal portion of the distal phalanx are removed, placing the distal phalanx into approximately 5 to 7 degrees of plantarflexion and 3 to 4 degrees of valgus position. Internal fixation is achieved by using a longitudinal screw (4 mm) or crossed K-wires, or both.

A postoperative shoe is used, with weight bearing allowed but avoiding the toe-off phase of gait until fusion occurs, usually in 8 weeks.

C. Complications

Nonunion of interphalangeal joint fusion is uncommon. If it does occur, it often is asymptomatic and does not require treatment. If it is symptomatic, usually the fusion will need to be revised because the area is too small for adequate bone grafting.

Clough T, Bodo K, Majeed H, et al. Survivorship and long-term outcome of a consecutive series of 200 Scandinavian Total Ankle Replacement (STAR) implants. *Bone Joint J.* 2019;101-B(1):47-54. [PMID: 30601052]

Deleu PA, Besse JL, Naaim A, et al. Change in gait biomechanics after total ankle replacement and ankle arthrodesis: a systematic review and meta-analysis. *Clin Biomech.* 2020;73:213-225. [PMID: 32044672]

DiGiovanni CW, Lin SS, Baumhauer JF, et al. Recombinant human platelet-derived growth factor-BB and beta-tricalcium phosphate (rhPDGF-BB/beta-TCP): an alternative to autogenous bone graft. *J Bone Joint Surg Am.* 2013;95(13):1184-1192. [PMID: 23824386]

Jeyaseelan L, Si-Hyeong Park S, Al-Rumaih H, et al. Outcomes Following total ankle arthroplasty: a review of the registry data and current literature. *Orthop Clin North Am.* 2019;50(4): 539-548. [PMID: 31466669]

Lawton CD, Butler BA, Dekker RG 2nd, et al. Total ankle arthroplasty versus ankle arthrodesis-a comparison of outcomes over the last decade. *J Orthop Surg Res.* 2017;12(1):76. [PMID: 28521779]

Norvell DC, Ledoux WR, Shofer JB, et al. Effectiveness and safety of ankle arthrodesis versus arthroplasty: a prospective multicenter study. *J Bone Joint Surg Am.* 2019;101(16):1485-1494. [PMID: 31436657]

Nunley JA, Adams SB, Easley ME, et al. Prospective randomized trial comparing mobile-bearing and fixed-bearing total ankle replacement. *Foot Ankle Int.* 2019;40(11):1239-1248. [PMID: 31561727]

Sokolowski M, Krähenbühl N, Wang C, et al. Secondary subtalar joint osteoarthritis following total ankle replacement. *Foot Ankle Int.* 2019;40(10):1122-1128. [PMID: 31327242]

Veljkovic AN, Daniels TR, Glazebrook MA, et al. Outcomes of total ankle replacement, arthroscopic ankle arthrodesis, and open ankle arthrodesis for isolated non-deformed end-stage ankle arthritis. *J Bone Joint Surg Am.* 2019;101(17):1523-1529. [PMID: 31483394]

CONGENITAL FLATFOOT

Congenital flatfoot is the term used to describe a flatfoot present since birth. The condition may not be apparent during the early years of life but is usually identified toward the end of the first or during the second decade. The typical asymptomatic flexible flatfoot is probably a normal variant of the longitudinal arch. This deformity must be differentiated from the symptomatic flexible or more rigid flatfoot, which usually will become symptomatic in the early teen years and is often caused by a tarsal coalition. A tarsal coalition is the union of two or more tarsal bones, usually occurring between the calcaneus and the navicular or between the talus and the calcaneus. This process is a congenital failure of segmentation between the bones of the hindfoot. Coalitions are usually not symptomatic until adolescence, with symptoms brought on by increasing stiffness of the hindfoot as the cartilaginous coalition begins to ossify. These individuals have a fairly flexible foot until adolescence, when the foot often becomes more rigid and symptomatic.

The patient with a tarsal coalition will frequently present with a peroneal spastic flatfoot, usually around the age of 10 to 12 years. The theory is that the foot is locked in a valgus position by the peroneal muscle spasm that is trying to immobilize the painful peritalar joints. The navicular bone usually forms from three ossification centers inside the original cartilage, and occasionally, the medial center fails to coalesce with the main body, leaving a synchondrosis that is called an accessory navicular. Flatfoot associated with an accessory navicular bone usually becomes symptomatic in the early to mid-teenage years and may be unilateral or bilateral.

Residual congenital deformity from conditions such as clubfoot or congenital vertical talus is present from birth and is discussed in Chapter 12.

The patient with generalized ligamentous laxity such as Marfan syndrome or Ehlers-Danlos syndrome may present with flatfoot. Generalized ligamentous laxity will be present from the time of birth, and the diagnosis is usually already known.

Clinical Findings

A. Symptoms and Signs

The clinical evaluation begins with the patient in a standing position. In all cases of congenital flatfoot, the longitudinal arch flattens when the patient is standing. In the case of tarsal coalition with peroneal spastic flatfoot, the calcaneus is in a severe fixed valgus position. A tarsal coalition or an accessory navicular may be unilateral, as well as the residuals of a congenital deformity such as clubfoot or congenital vertical talus. The symptomatic and asymptomatic flexible flatfoot and the defects associated with generalized ligamentous laxity are present bilaterally.

Physical examination of these patients is extremely important. The asymptomatic flexible flatfoot will usually demonstrate a satisfactory ROM and no contracture of the Achilles tendon. The symptomatic flexible flatfoot, however, will almost invariably have an equinus contracture. To adequately test for tightness of the Achilles tendon, the forefoot is adducted so that the head of the talus is first covered with the navicular, after which the ankle is dorsiflexed with the knee extended. If the foot is simply dorsiflexed, permitting lateral subluxation of the talonavicular joint, the examiner often is fooled into thinking that ankle dorsiflexion is adequate when indeed it is not.

The patient with tarsal coalition usually demonstrates restricted hindfoot motion secondary to peroneal spasm and to the cartilaginous or bony bar. The peroneal tendons can be felt to be bowstrung behind the fibula, not permitting passive or active inversion of the subtalar joint to occur. On occasion, clonus can be elicited. As a rule, stressing of these joints causes the patient increased discomfort. In flatfoot associated with an accessory navicular, pain is present over the prominence. Frequently, stressing of the posterior tibial tendon aggravates the condition. The patient with residual congenital deformity often demonstrates a certain degree of stiffness of the foot and, not infrequently, varying degrees of deformity of the remainder of the foot. The patient with generalized ligamentous laxity demonstrates marked hypermobility of all the joints, with no contractures whatsoever.

B. Imaging Studies

The radiographic evaluation is useful in differentiating the various types of flatfoot. In almost all cases, the lateral view shows a lack of normal dorsiflexion alignment of the calcaneus, which is approximately 20 degrees or more. In symptomatic flexible flatfoot, the calcaneus may even be in a mild degree of equinus position. On the lateral radiograph, a line drawn through the long axis of the talus and first metatarsal (Meary's angle) will demonstrate an angle of more than 30 degrees in severe flatfoot, 15 to 30 degrees in moderate flatfoot, and 0 to 15 degrees in mild flatfoot (Figure 10–43).

The calcaneonavicular coalition is best observed on an oblique radiograph and is identified as a bridge from the anterior process of the calcaneus to the inferior lateral aspect of the navicular. The subtalar or talocalcaneal bar is best demonstrated on a CT scan taken in the coronal plane. MRI can identify nonosseous coalitions. Flatfoot associated with an accessory navicular demonstrates the accessory bone along the medial side of the navicular, but occasionally, a medial oblique view is necessary to outline the size of the fragment. In a patient with a residual congenital deformity, such as a clubfoot or congenital vertical talus, the changes about the foot will often be sufficient to make the diagnosis fairly obvious. The patient with generalized ligamentous laxity often demonstrates complete collapse of the longitudinal arch.

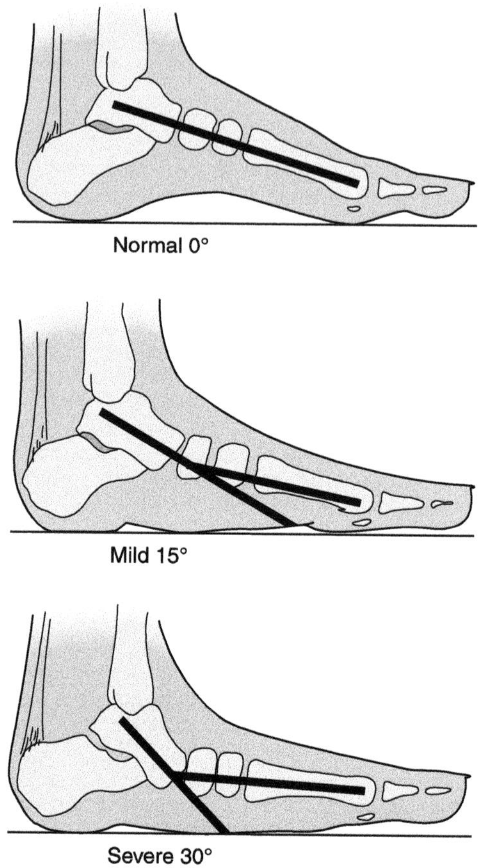

▲ Figure 10–43. Measurement of flatfoot deformity by using the lateral talometatarsal angle: 0 degrees, normal; 1 to 15 degrees, mild; 16 to 30 degrees, moderate; and >30 degrees, severe. (Reprinted with permission, from Bordelon RL. Correction of hypermobile flatfoot children by molded insert. *Foot Ankle.* 1980;1:143.)

Treatment

A. Conservative Management

Conservative management is undertaken for congenital flatfoot deformities. A longitudinal arch support may benefit the patient but is usually not necessary for the asymptomatic flexible flatfoot. For symptomatic flexible flatfoot, a semirigid longitudinal arch support and Achilles stretching exercises may be of some benefit.

The tarsal coalition can be treated conservatively with a short leg walking cast, followed by a polypropylene ankle-foot orthosis or a University of California Biomechanics Laboratory (UCBL) insert. If adequate pain relief is achieved, further treatment is not necessary. Flatfoot with an accessory navicular may respond to modification of the shoe to relieve some of the pressure from the involved area. Occasionally, the use of a longitudinal arch support will relieve the pressure.

Residual flatfoot resulting from congenital problems can be treated with an AFO or UCBL insert if symptomatic. The patient with generalized ligamentous laxity usually does not require any treatment at all.

B. Surgical Management

Surgical procedures are never appropriate for asymptomatic flatfoot. Symptomatic flexible or semiflexible flatfoot occasionally is treated surgically, particularly if equinus contracture is observed after age 5 or 6 years. A significant equinus contracture may benefit from lengthening of the Achilles tendon. A lateral column lengthening procedure, such as an Evans calcaneal osteotomy, is indicated in cases of symptomatic flexible flatfoot that have failed conservative management. This procedure helps to correct heel valgus and forefoot abduction and should be done as late into growth as possible to avoid disturbing open growth centers. Rarely should a triple arthrodesis be carried out because this leaves a young patient with a very stiff foot.

A tarsal coalition that does not respond to conservative management may require resection. The surgical approach to the calcaneonavicular bar is identical to that of the subtalar joint. The bar is carefully outlined and then resected in its entirety. Talocalcaneal coalitions are resectable throughout the adolescent years, if less than 20% of the posterior facet of the subtalar joint is involved or if the coalition is confined only to the middle facet. More extensive involvement of the subtalar joint in an adolescent or any bar in an adult patient is an indication for subtalar arthrodesis. The approach is through a medial incision centered over the middle facet, and caution is taken to carefully reflect the tendons and posterior tibial nerve. The extent of the coalition is identified, and it is resected to expose the area of normal-appearing articular cartilage. Bone wax is applied to the edges, or a free fat graft is inserted to prevent re-formation of the bar. Flatfoot associated with an accessory navicular may require excision of the accessory navicular and plication of the posterior tibial tendon (Kidner procedure). This fairly successful operation is usually carried out during the late adolescent years.

Residual congenital deformity or generalized ligamentous laxity will not usually require surgical management. In severe cases, a triple arthrodesis is indicated after the foot has matured.

Coleman S. *Complex Foot Deformities in Children*. Philadelphia, PA: Lea and Febiger; 1983.

Yildiz KI, Misir A, Kizkapan TB, et al. Functional and radiological outcomes after tarsal coalition resections: a minimum 5-year follow-up. *J Foot Ankle Surg*. 2019;58(6):1223-1228. [PMID: 31679676]

Zaw H, Calder JD. Tarsal coalitions. *Foot Ankle Clin*. 2010;15: 349-364. [PMID: 20534361]

ACQUIRED FLATFOOT DEFORMITY

Acquired flatfoot deformity is a condition affecting a foot that at one time had a normal functioning longitudinal arch. Over time, the arch progressively flattens, often causing the foot to become symptomatic. This deformity is different from congenital flatfoot deformity, which is present since birth. Acquired flatfoot deformity in the adult may be caused by the following conditions:

1. Posterior tibial tendon dysfunction
2. Arthrosis of the tarsometatarsal joints, which may be primary or secondary to a previous Lisfranc fracture or dislocation
3. Charcot changes in the midfoot resulting from a peripheral neuropathy
4. Talonavicular collapse resulting from trauma or rheumatoid arthritis

Acquired flatfoot deformities are complex deformities that affect different areas of the midfoot and hindfoot. The deformities may include dorsal subluxation of the talonavicular joint and tarsometatarsal joints, abduction of the forefoot, valgus deformity of the hindfoot, or all three. The extent of the deformity varies widely and is usually progressive. Depending on the etiology, acquired flatfoot deformity may affect a patient bilaterally.

Clinical Findings

A. Symptoms and Signs

A careful history is important to help distinguish among differing causes of acquired flatfoot deformity. Usually, no specific traumatic event is recalled by the patient who presents with dysfunction of the posterior tibial tendon. Approximately half of patients with tarsometatarsal joint arthrosis had a prior Lisfranc fracture-dislocation, whereas the other half has primary arthrosis. The patient with Charcot foot usually gives a relevant history of the cause of the peripheral neuropathy, such as diabetes. The patient with collapse of the talonavicular joint gives a history of prior trauma to the talus or navicular or has rheumatoid arthritis, which causes disruption of the spring ligament complex.

The physical examination begins by observing the foot with the patient standing, observing for unilateral or bilateral flattening of the longitudinal arch. Varying degrees of abduction of the forefoot and hindfoot valgus should also be evaluated.

The patient with posterior tibial tendon dysfunction demonstrates little or no active inversion strength in the weight-bearing position. Usually, the posterior tibial tendon is thick and swollen, and there is increased warmth and pain to palpation over the tendon sheath. When the patient is asked to stand on tiptoe, the involved calcaneus remains in valgus position rather than inverting, as normally occurs. When the patient is viewed from the posterior aspect, more toes are visible laterally on the involved foot than the uninvolved foot, commonly known as the too many toes sign.

Arthrosis of the tarsometatarsal joints creates a deformity of abduction of the forefoot with varying degrees of dorsiflexion, giving rise to a rather prominent medial cuneiform.

Not infrequently, palpable osteophytes are present on the dorsal and plantar aspect of the tarsometatarsal joints.

A Charcot foot presents with varying degrees of swelling and deformity. In the early stages, the foot demonstrates generalized swelling and increased warmth, with loss of sensation in a stocking-glove distribution. Deformity may vary from a mild flatfoot to a severe rocker-bottom deformity. It is important to palpate for bony prominences on the medial and plantar aspects of the foot that make it at risk for ulcerations.

In the patient with rheumatoid arthritis, most of the changes occur within the talonavicular joint. In this case, the head of the talus is often palpable on the plantar medial aspect of the foot. When the subtalar joint is more involved, a fixed hindfoot valgus deformity is usually present as well.

Posttraumatic deformities may vary, depending on precisely which joints are involved. If trauma led to a collapse of the navicular, the longitudinal arch is flattened with little forefoot abduction, and the head of the talus is often palpable on the plantar medial aspect of the foot. There is usually little or no motion in the hindfoot and midfoot joints.

B. Imaging Studies

Radiographs of the foot usually differentiate the cause of the problem. Hindfoot alignment views are particularly helpful in addition to ankle films. In the patient with posterior tibial tendon dysfunction, there is sagging of the talonavicular joint and abduction of the navicular on the head of the talus. The patient with tarsometatarsal joint arthrosis demonstrates typical degenerative changes at the affected joints, along with varying degrees of lateral and dorsal subluxation of the joints. Patients with Charcot foot demonstrate characteristic changes seen in a neuropathic joint, including dramatic bone destruction and joint dislocations (Figure 10–44). The patient with rheumatoid arthritis demonstrates the typical destructive changes observed with this disease process, with joint space narrowing but little osteophyte formation.

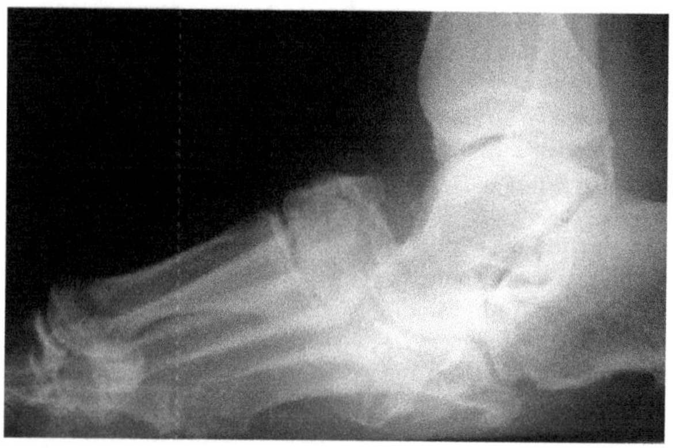

▲ **Figure 10–44.** Charcot midfoot changes resulting in joint dislocations and a rocker-bottom deformity of the foot.

Treatment

A. Conservative Management

Conservative management is aimed at providing support to the longitudinal arch. This can range from off the shelf noncustom inserts to custom above ankle orthoses such as a polypropylene AFO or Arizona brace. The orthosis must be shaped to accommodate any prominences that might be present. Unfortunately, these prominences present the potential for skin breakdown, particularly in the neuropathic foot. A rocker-bottom–type shoe with an adequate toe box is sometimes indicated to give the patient a smoother gait pattern. Targeted muscle strengthening exercises about the ankle can provide some relief in less active individuals.

B. Surgical Treatment

The surgical management of these various conditions is specific for each problem. Posterior tibial tendon dysfunction with a satisfactory ROM of the joints of the hindfoot and midfoot can be treated with reconstruction of the posterior tibial tendon, using a flexor digitorum longus tendon transfer. A calcaneal osteotomy is performed as well if a significant valgus deformity of the heel is present. Alternatively, a lateral column lengthening (anterior calcaneal osteotomy or calcaneal-cuboid distraction arthrodesis) can be used to correct a flexible flatfoot with significant abduction of the forefoot. Over the past decade, Z-osteotomy has been used to correct both hindfoot valgus and peritalar subluxation through a single incision. When a fixed deformity is present in the hindfoot or forefoot, arthrodesis is indicated. This may include isolated talonavicular arthrodesis, double arthrodesis, or triple arthrodesis.

The patient with Charcot foot is treated in a short leg cast until the acute process subsides, after which a polypropylene AFO is used. Occasionally, a bony prominence that continues to cause skin breakdown may be excised to permit the patient to use an AFO. In extreme rocker-bottom deformities, midfoot correction with an osteotomy may be required. The rheumatoid patient usually requires stabilization of the involved area with an isolated talonavicular fusion if little deformity is present or a triple arthrodesis if there is a hindfoot or midfoot deformity.

The posttraumatic foot with involvement of the talonavicular joint requires a triple arthrodesis. The fusion may need to be extended distally to include the naviculocuneiform joints if arthrosis is present at these joints.

The patient with arthrosis of the tarsometatarsal joints responds well to surgical management by realigning the foot and carrying out arthrodesis of the involved joints.

Chadwick C, Whitehouse SL, Saxby TS. Long-term follow-up of flexor digitorum longus transfer and calcaneal osteotomy for stage II posterior tibial tendon dysfunction. *Bone Joint J.* 2015;97-B(3):346-352. [PMID: 25737518]

Deland JT. Adult-acquired flatfoot deformity. *J Am Acad Orthop Surg.* 2008;16:399-406. [PMID: 18611997]

Ebaugh MP, Larson DR, Reb CW, et al. Outcomes of the extended z-cut osteotomy for correction of adult acquired flatfoot deformity. *Foot Ankle Int.* 2019;40(8):914-922. [PMID: 31088118]

So E, Reb CW, Larson DR, et al. Medial double arthrodesis: technique guide and tips. *J Foot Ankle Surg.* 2018;57(2):364-369. [PMID: 29254850]

CAVUS FOOT

Cavus foot deformity is characterized by an abnormal elevation of the longitudinal arch, with resulting decrease in the plantar weight-bearing area and stress concentrated on the metatarsal heads. The condition may be aggravated by clawing of the toes, further reducing the forefoot weight-bearing area. Generalized stiffness of the joints is common, causing the patient to avoid prolonged use of the foot.

Etiologic Findings

The various causes of cavus foot deformity include the following:

1. Anterior horn cell disease, such as poliomyelitis, diastematomyelia, and spinal cord tumor
2. Nerve disorders, such as Charcot-Marie-Tooth disease and spinal dysraphism
3. Muscular diseases, such as muscular dystrophy
4. Long tract and central diseases, such as Friedreich ataxia and cerebral palsy
5. Idiopathic conditions, such as residual clubfoot, arthrogryposis, and cavus foot of undetermined cause
6. Posttraumatic disorders following injuries, such as compartment syndrome or crush injury

Anatomy

Cavus foot deformity is extremely variable in its presentation, from mild to extremely severe degrees of cavus. The types of deformities can be classified based on localizing the area of deformity.

A. Posterior Cavus Deformity

Posterior cavus deformity is mainly of the calcaneus, when the calcaneal pitch is greater than 40 degrees measured on a weight-bearing lateral radiograph. Some degree of varus deformity of the heel is usually present as well.

B. Anterior Cavus Deformity

In anterior cavus deformity, there is a forefoot equinus deformity with the hindfoot in a neutral position. The anterior cavus may be localized, mainly involving the first and second metatarsal, or it may involve the entire forefoot positioned in plantarflexion. Some degree of adduction of the forefoot is usually present.

C. Combined Cavus Deformity

In a combined cavus deformity, which is the most severe, there are both anterior and posterior components.

Clinical Findings

A. Symptoms and Signs

A careful history regarding the onset of the condition and progression is important. A detailed family history should also be obtained because idiopathic cavus deformity does tend to run in families. Progression of deformity should be ascertained, particularly in the adolescent, because it may indicate a spinal cord abnormality or neoplasm. Activity level and ambulation should also be carefully evaluated as markers of progression of neural or muscular disease. A unilateral cavus deformity should be viewed with suspicion and may represent findings of spinal cord pathology.

The degree of deformity of the foot must be examined with the patient in a standing position. This also reveals any evidence of atrophy of the calf muscles, as seen in Charcot-Marie-Tooth disease, clubfoot, or arthrogryposis. The active and passive ROM of the joints of the foot and ankle should be carefully measured. The strength of each muscle must be carefully evaluated, especially if considering a tendon transfer. The degree of deformity and flexibility of the hindfoot, forefoot, metatarsophalangeal joints, and lesser toes must be ascertained. The presence of a tight plantar fascia should also be noted. The lateral ankle ligaments must be evaluated for integrity because they often become stretched with long-standing varus heel deformity. The Coleman block test is used to discriminate between forefoot-driven cavus and combined cavus. The Coleman block test is performed by placing the patient's foot on a wood block, 2.5 to 4 cm thick, with the heel and lateral border of foot on the block and the rest of the foot allowed to hang freely. If the varus corrects while the patient is standing on the block, the hindfoot and forefoot are considered flexible.

B. Imaging Studies

Weight-bearing radiographs of the foot and ankle are obtained to help classify the type of cavus deformity and formulate a treatment plan. Any degree of arthrosis or varus tilting of the talus in the ankle mortise is also evaluated.

Treatment

A. Conservative Management

Conservative care is tailored to the severity of the cavus deformity. Mild deformities may only require a softer-soled shoe. Significant clawing of the lesser toes may require an extra-depth shoe. A custom-made Plastazote liner with a built-in arch support helps decrease the stress on the metatarsal heads. A significant motor deficit may require an AFO to stabilize the ankle. Most cases of cavus foot can be managed with conservative modalities.

B. Surgical Treatment

Surgical treatment for the cavus foot is aimed at correcting the site of the deformity. The most frequent pattern consists of plantarflexion of the first metatarsal, contracture of the plantar fascia, and varus deformity of the calcaneus. If the hindfoot varus corrects with the Coleman block test, calcaneal osteotomy is not necessary. In this case, the deformity responds to release of the plantar fascia and dorsiflexion osteotomy of the first metatarsal. If the hindfoot varus does not correct, a lateralizing calcaneal osteotomy or closing-wedge osteotomy (Dwyer procedure) of the calcaneus is necessary. Fusion of the joints is avoided to maintain as much flexibility of the foot as possible, especially in adolescents and young adults (Figure 10–45).

A more severe deformity involving dorsiflexion of the calcaneus can be treated with sliding osteotomy of the calcaneus (Samilson procedure), correcting any varus deformity with a lateral closing-wedge osteotomy and releasing the plantar fascia (Figure 10–46). Forefoot deformity is treated with osteotomy of the first and sometimes second metatarsal. In some patients, transfer of the peroneus longus tendon into the brevis and lengthening of the posterior tibial tendon provide dynamic muscle balance for the foot.

Severe deformities not amenable to procedures that retain joint motion require triple arthrodesis. A Siffert beak-type triple arthrodesis corrects the deformity because the navicular is mortised under the head of the talus to help reduce the elevation of the longitudinal arch (Figure 10–47). A first metatarsal osteotomy may need to be added to the procedure as well.

The lesser toes may have either fixed or flexible claw toe deformities. Flexible deformity often responds to release of the extensor tendons and a Girdlestone flexor tendon

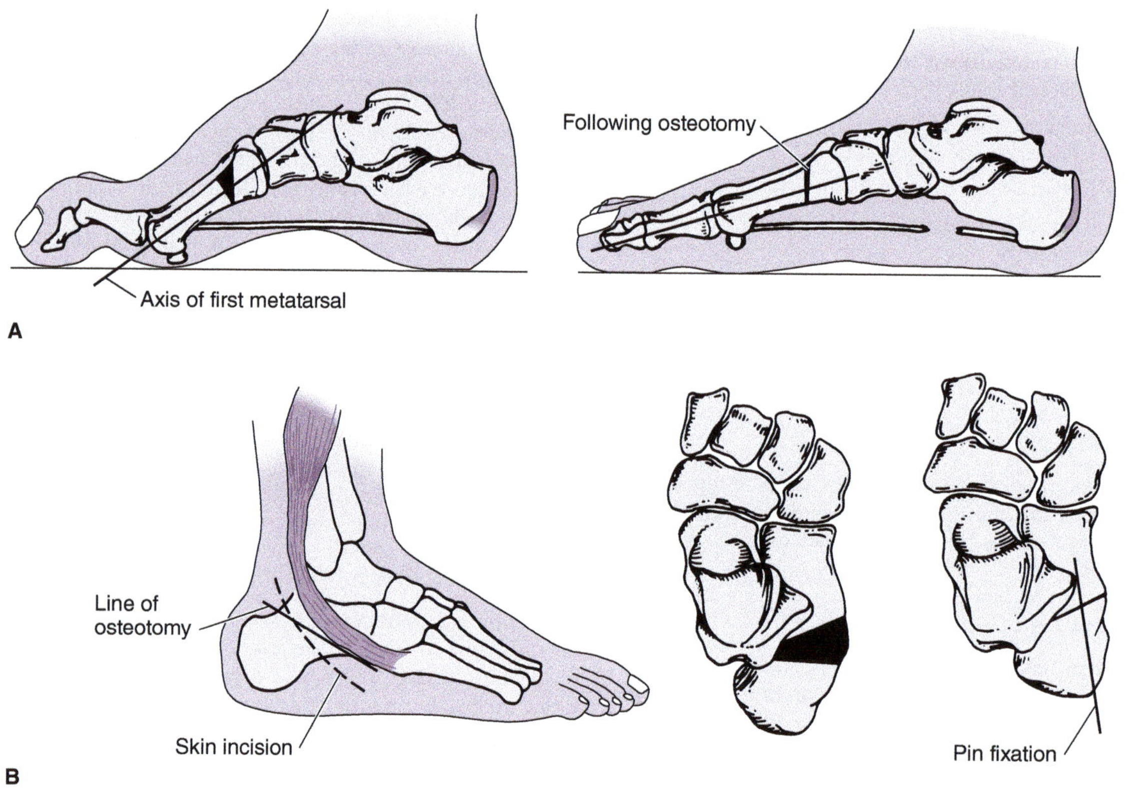

▲ **Figure 10–45.** Technique for correction of cavus foot. **A:** For first metatarsal osteotomy, a dorsally based wedge of bone was removed approximately 1 cm distal to the metatarsocuneiform joint. The plantar fascia was released. Dorsiflexion of the osteotomy site helps correct the cavus deformity by flattening the arch. **B:** Heel varus is corrected by a closing-wedge calcaneus osteotomy. (Reprinted with permission, from Mann RA, Coughlin MJ. *The Video Textbook of Foot and Ankle Surgery.* Medical Video Productions, 1991.)

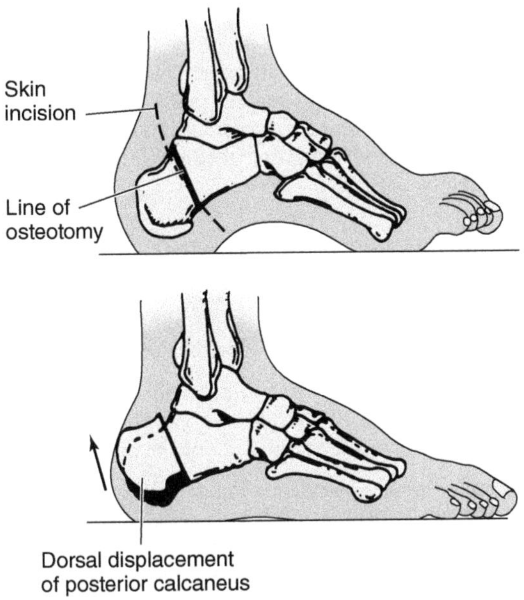

▲ **Figure 10–46.** Techniques of calcaneal osteotomy. In the treatment of pes cavus, the osteotomy permits the calcaneus to be moved into a more dorsal position and, if necessary, to be closed laterally to correct heel varus. (Reprinted with permission, from Mann RA, Coughlin MJ. *The Video Textbook of Foot and Ankle Surgery*. Medical Video Productions, 1991.)

transfer. If a fixed deformity is present, a DuVries phalangeal condylectomy corrects the hammer toe, followed by extensor tendon release and the Girdlestone procedure.

Hyperextension of the first metatarsophalangeal joint is corrected by interphalangeal arthrodesis of the hallux and transfer of the extensor hallucis longus tendon into the neck of the first metatarsal (Jones procedure).

Kroon M, Faber FWM, van der Linden M. Joint preservation surgery for correction of flexible pes cavovarus in adults. *Foot Ankle Int.* 2010;31(1):24-29. [PMID: 20067719]

Tennant JN, Carmont M, Phisitkul P. Calcaneus osteotomy. *Curr Rev Musculoskelet Med.* 2014;7(4):271-276. [PMID: 25186724]

ORTHOTIC DEVICES FOR THE FOOT AND ANKLE

Orthotic devices are used to redistribute stresses on the foot as it makes contact with the ground and to accommodate for abnormal function of defective muscles or ligaments. This is achieved by controlling the posture of the foot and padding certain areas to relieve pressure and provide increased comfort for the foot. Orthoses are also used to limit motion in arthritic joints, making them less painful. The orthotic device may be attached to the sole of the shoe, may be inserted inside the shoe as an insole, may cup the foot (UCBL insert), or may extend across the ankle to hold the entire foot and ankle in place (AFO).

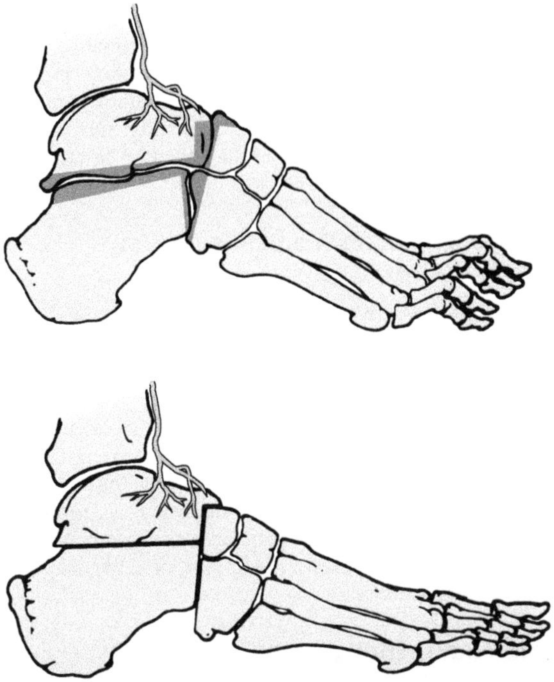

▲ **Figure 10–47.** A diagram of a beak-type triple arthrodesis. This mortises the navicular underneath a portion of the head of the talus to allow rotation of the distal portion of the foot, permitting flattening of the longitudinal arch and correction of the cavus deformity. (Reprinted with permission, from Mann RA, Coughlin MJ. *The Video Textbook of Foot and Ankle Surgery*. Medical Video Productions, 1991.)

Orthotic Shoe Sole Devices

A variety of heel and sole corrections are available to accommodate foot postural abnormalities. A medial or lateral heel or sole wedge (or a combination of both) can help control excessive pronation or supination from weak tendons, ligamentous instability, or fixed deformities. A wide heel is used to increase the stability of the subtalar joint. A rocker sole helps stabilize the forefoot in the case of a fracture or arthritis and also aids a patient with an ankle fusion to allow a more normal gait pattern.

Orthotic Insole Devices

Insole orthotic devices can be used for flexible deformities to alter the posture of the foot and for fixed deformities to redistribute stress. The simplest device is a soft liner for a shoe or boot made from a high-density foam material. Other simple orthoses include a soft felt pad to relieve pressure on the metatarsal heads or a combination of materials to produce a more rigid support to help control a forefoot deformity such as forefoot varus or valgus deformity. Orthotic devices take up space in the shoe, and the patient may need a larger or deeper shoe.

University of California Biomechanics Laboratory Insert

The principle of the UCBL insert is to correct a foot deformity such as flatfoot by stabilizing the calcaneus in neutral position and molding the orthosis to block abduction of the forefoot. Posting along the medial aspect may compensate for forefoot varus. In theory, this orthotic device is excellent for controlling the rearfoot and forefoot, but two caveats apply to the use of this device. The first is that the foot must be flexible because correction of a rigid deformity is impossible. The second is that a bony prominence can chafe against the polypropylene material, resulting in pain or skin breakdown over the prominence.

Ankle-Foot Orthosis

An AFO is a molded polypropylene device that passes along the posterior aspect of the calf and then onto the plantar aspect of the foot to the metatarsal heads. Alterations are made in a variety of ways to accommodate the patient's specific problem. Ankle problems such as arthrosis or dorsiflexion weakness require adequate rigidity to eliminate ankle joint motion. An orthosis for a subtalar joint problem should have enough flexibility to provide ankle joint motion but must be rigid enough to immobilize the subtalar joint. When the problem involves the transverse tarsal joint, the AFO can be fabricated to permit some ankle joint motion (so-called articulating AFO) but maintain immobilization of the transverse tarsal joint area, usually by blocking abduction of the forefoot. When managing tarsometatarsal arthritis, the footpiece is carried to the tips of the toes. Again, a significant fixed bony deformity results in pressure points, making fitting of the device difficult. If the patient has loss of sensation, careful construction and padding are essential to minimize the risk of ulcers forming over a bony prominence. In cases of marked instability or discomfort, an anterior shell can be added to the AFO, and the brace is extended proximally to create a patellar tendon bearing surface.

Double Upright Orthosis

The double upright orthosis with a hinged ankle may be used when individuals require stability but are engaged in physically demanding activities. The double upright orthosis is somewhat more cumbersome than the AFO but provides rigid immobilization. The hinge mechanism of the ankle joint may be changed, depending on the nature of the patient's problem. The ankle joint can be free, allowing dorsiflexion and plantarflexion to occur, or it can be fixed to prevent plantarflexion past 90 degrees. This brace can be modified with a spring load to provide dorsiflexion for the patient with dropfoot resulting from paralysis but should not be used for the patient with spasticity because it may accentuate the spasticity.

Prescriptions for Orthotic Devices

The following are typical prescriptions for orthotic devices.

A. Metatarsalgia or Atrophy of Plantar Fat Pad

1. Treatment—A full-length well-molded orthosis for metatarsal arch support is used to relieve pressure under the metatarsal heads. Soft insole material should be used.

2. Explanation—In the treatment of metatarsalgia or atrophy of the plantar fat pad, a full-length orthosis is needed that is molded to the plantar aspect of the foot and built up just proximal to the metatarsal heads to relieve pressure on them. The material should be soft to provide extra cushioning for the foot.

B. Ruptured Posterior Tibial Tendon With Moderately Severe Flexible Flatfoot Deformity

1. Treatment—AFO with trim-line cut to permit 30% ankle joint motion is molded to reestablish the longitudinal arch and built up on the lateral aspect of the footpiece to block abduction of the forefoot.

2. Explanation—With a moderately advanced flexible flatfoot deformity, an in-shoe orthotic device alone does not provide sufficient support; the AFO is needed to provide adequate stability. Some ankle joint motion is included, which makes ambulation more comfortable for the patient. The longitudinal arch is molded to support the foot in a plantigrade position, and the lateral aspect of the AFO is built up to prevent the forefoot from moving into an abducted position. By blocking abduction, the amount of pressure needed beneath the longitudinal arch to prevent it from collapsing is decreased.

C. Posterior Tibial Tendon Insufficiency With Mild Flatfoot Deformity and 5 Degrees of Forefoot Varus Deformity

1. Treatment—Use a well-molded longitudinal arch support, with a 5-degree varus post and a 3-degree medial heel lift.

2. Explanation—Insufficiency of the posterior tibial tendon that has not produced a significant foot deformity can be treated with a well-molded longitudinal arch support. The 5-degree varus forefoot post compensates for the fixed forefoot varus, and the 3-degree heel lift likewise helps tilt the hindfoot from valgus deformity closer to neutral position.

D. Dropfoot Secondary to Peroneal Nerve Injury

1. Treatment—An AFO with a full footpiece is molded to the longitudinal arch.

2. Explanation—A dropfoot secondary to a peroneal nerve injury responds well to an AFO with a full footpiece. The footpiece supports the toes so they do not drop and makes it easier for the patient to put on shoes.

E. Diabetic Neuropathy With Clawfoot Deformity

1. Treatment—An extra-depth shoe with a molded Plastazote liner is backed with a Pelite material.

2. Explanation—The patient with clawfoot deformity requires a shoe that has extra height in the toe box to provide enough room for the toes, so they do not chafe against the top of the shoe. The molded Plastazote liner is an excellent means of providing full contact to the plantar aspect of the foot. Plastazote has a tendency to bottom out, as it were, and by backing the material with a Pelite liner or some comparable material, the life expectancy of the Plastazote is extended significantly.

Forghany S, Bonanno DR, Menz HB, Landorf KB. An anatomically-based masking protocol for the assessment of in-shoe plantar pressure measurement of the forefoot. *J Foot Ankle Res.* 2018;11:31. [PMID: 2998374]

Liu XC, Embrey D, Tassone C, et al. Long-term effects of orthoses use on the changes of foot and ankle joint motions of children with spastic cerebral palsy. *PM R.* 2018;10(3):269-275. [PMID: 28867667]

Moulodi N, Kamyab M, Farzadi M. A comparison of the hallux valgus angle, range of motion, and patient satisfaction after use of dynamic and static orthoses. *Foot (Edinb).* 2019;41:6-11. [PMID: 31675599]

Williamson P, Lechtig A, Hanna P, et al. Pressure distribution in the ankle and subtalar joint with routine and oversized foot orthoses. *Foot Ankle Int.* 2018;39(8):994-1000. [PMID: 29696991]

LIGAMENTOUS INJURIES ABOUT THE ANKLE JOINT

Ankle ligament injuries are the most common musculoskeletal injury; therefore, accurate assessment and treatment of these injuries are important. The lateral collateral ligament complex is most commonly injured, but damage to other important structures around the ankle joint should not be overlooked.

Functional Anatomy

The lateral collateral ligament structure of the ankle consists of three distinct ligamentous bands: the anterior and posterior talofibular ligaments (ATFL and PTFL) and the calcaneofibular ligament (CFL).

When the ankle joint is in plantarflexion, the ATFL is positioned in line with the fibula and therefore placed under stress with an inversion injury and will be damaged. Conversely, when the ankle joint is in dorsiflexion, the CFL is positioned in line with the long axis of the fibula and is therefore subject to injury. If the applied stress is severe, both the ATFL and the CFL may be torn, no matter the position of the ankle joint. The syndesmosis ligament complex tethers the tibia and fibula together and is injured by an external rotational force to the foot. The deltoid ligament is the sole medial stabilizer of the ankle joint. An isolated deltoid ligament injury can occur with an eversion or external rotation force on the foot. The deltoid ligament can also be injured with syndesmosis ligament injuries, lateral ankle sprains, or fibula fracture (known as a Maisonneuve fracture). Syndesmotic injuries (so-called high ankle sprains) have increasingly become recognized.

Clinical Findings

A. Classification

Lateral collateral ankle ligament injuries are divided into three degrees of severity. A grade I sprain is confined to the ATFL and demonstrates no instability. A grade II sprain involves injury to both the ATFL and CFL, with mild laxity of one or both ligaments. A grade III sprain involves injury and significant laxity of both the ATFL and CFL.

B. Symptoms and Signs

A past history of injuries of the ankle and problems with chronic ankle ligament instability should be ascertained. A careful physical examination is important to evaluate the degree of involvement of each ligament and to rule out injury to any adjacent bony or soft-tissue structures. The ATFL, PTFL, CFL, and syndesmosis ligaments are palpated for tenderness. To evaluate for fractures, the proximal and distal fibula, the anterior process of the calcaneus, the lateral process of the talus, and the base of the fifth metatarsal should be palpated to evaluate for tenderness. Other areas where an injury must be ruled out include the subtalar joint and the peroneal tendon sheath.

A patient with significant medial joint pain with or without lateral ligament pain should be evaluated for an injury to the deltoid ligament complex, the posterior tibial tendon, and the medial talar dome. Assessment of ankle ligament stability requires clinical and radiographic stress examinations. To perform an anterior drawer maneuver, in order to test stability of the ATFL, the ankle is placed in 30 degrees of equinus, and the ankle is pulled in an anterior and slightly internally rotated direction (Figure 10–48). A feeling of subluxation is present if a significant ligament injury has occurred. A talar tilt maneuver is performed by placing an inversion stress on the heel. With the foot in plantarflexion, this tests the stability of the ATFL. With the foot in neutral

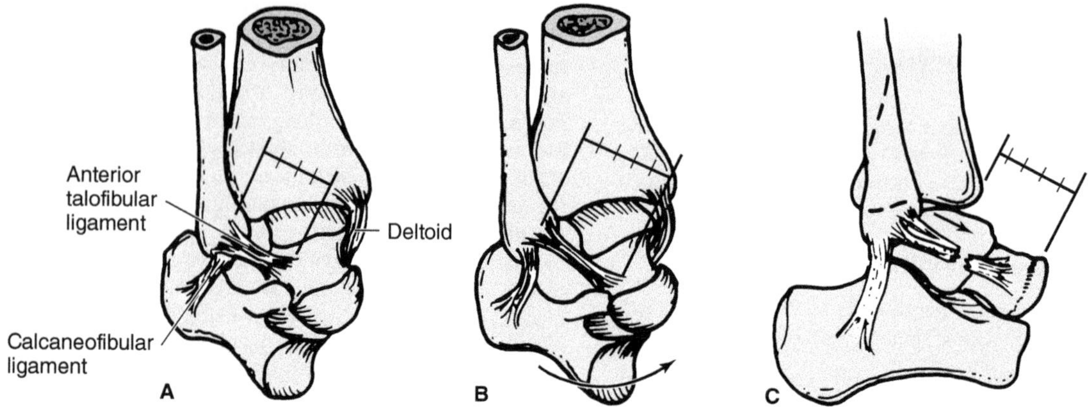

▲ **Figure 10–48.** Mechanics of carrying out a stress test of the lateral ankle ligaments. **A:** Normal anatomic alignment, which demonstrates the checkrein effect of the anterior talofibular ligament on the talus. **B:** The stress test for the calcaneofibular ligament is carried out by firmly inverting the calcaneus. **C:** The anterior talofibular ligament is tested by placing the ankle joint in neutral position and applying an anterior pull with slight medial rotation. (Reprinted with permission, from Mann RA, Coughlin MJ, eds. *Surgery of the Foot and Ankle*, 6th ed. St. Louis: Mosby-Year Book; 1993.)

or dorsiflexion, a talar tilt maneuver tests the stability of the CFL. If clinical instability is suggested by either maneuver, radiographic confirmation can be performed, with comparison to the unaffected ankle.

Deltoid ligament insufficiency may cause a feeling of instability and giving way, affecting the medial aspect of the ankle joint. Stress examination is performed by pulling the foot laterally and into valgus while stabilizing the distal tibia.

Injury to the syndesmosis ligament complex is suspected if the region between the distal anterior tibia and fibula is tender to palpation. If extensive swelling is present more than 2 cm proximal to the ankle joint, syndesmosis rupture is a strong possibility. Pain elicited by squeezing the tibia and fibula together in the midcalf is diagnostic of a syndesmosis ligament tear. A syndesmosis ligament injury is also suspected if external rotation of the foot is painful or if lateral translation of the talus in the ankle mortise occurs with direct lateral force on the foot.

C. Imaging Studies

Standard anteroposterior, lateral, and oblique radiographs of the ankle should be obtained to rule out a fracture of the fibula, talus, or calcaneus. If ligament laxity is suggested on clinical examination, stress radiographs should be obtained. An anteroposterior view is taken while a talar tilt maneuver is performed, and a lateral view is taken while an anterior drawer maneuver is performed. More than 10 degrees of tilt and more than 5 to 7 mm of anterior drawer are considered abnormal.

If a syndesmosis ligament injury is suspected, careful attention must be paid to the joint spaces to rule out widening of the ankle mortise. If instability is suspected, a stress radiograph is performed by externally rotating the foot with the tibia held still.

MRI or CT scan may be helpful in some instances if there is a high index of suspicion for an accompanying injury. Osteochondral injuries to the talus should be ruled out with an MRI scan. If a talus or calcaneus fracture is suspected, either MRI or CT scan may be of benefit.

Treatment

A. Conservative Management

Acute grade I ligament tears are treated with a lateral stabilizing ankle brace, ice, and avoidance of painful activities. Immediate full weight bearing is allowed, as are non–weight-bearing physical activities, such as bicycling and swimming. The brace can be discontinued in 1 month.

Grade II ligament tears are treated with protected weight bearing and a lateral stabilizing ankle brace. The patient can begin non–weight-bearing exercise (stationary bicycle) after 7 days, along with peroneal strengthening exercises. Weight-bearing exercise (jogging) may resume after 2 to 4 weeks.

In a grade III ligament tear, the ankle is immobilized with a removable walking cast for 3 to 4 weeks. This is followed by a period of physical therapy consisting of ROM exercises, peroneal strengthening, and proprioception training using a biomechanical ankle platform system (BAPS) board.

Treatment of isolated deltoid ligament sprains depends on the severity of the injury and is similar to lateral ligament injuries. Mild injuries can be treated with immediate mobilization and rapid return to activity, whereas more severe injuries should be casted for 3 to 4 weeks.

Syndesmosis ligament tears, if mild, can be treated with weight bearing in a cast or brace and close follow-up to assess for widening of the ankle joint mortise. If the interosseous membrane is damaged, as evidenced by massive swelling of the leg proximal to the ankle joint, treatment depends on the radiographic appearance of the ankle. If the mortise has not widened, the patient is kept on a non–weight-bearing regimen in a cast for 6 weeks, with close radiographic follow-up. If initial or follow-up radiographs show a widened mortise, the patient requires surgical repair of the syndesmosis ligaments. Screws and thick synthetic sutures have been used to stabilize the tibiofibular joint.

B. Surgical Treatment

The surgical treatment of an acute ligamentous injury is indicated only for the occasional elite athlete. Most ligamentous injuries, even grade III sprains, heal sufficiently with no significant disability if properly treated. However, even less severe ankle sprains may cause chronic pain or functional instability if left untreated.

The indication for a lateral ligament reconstruction is functional and/or mechanical ligament instability. A patient with ligament instability complains of recurrent sprains that occur with sports activities or even with activities of daily living, despite 4 to 6 months of physical therapy and use of a lateral stabilizing brace. A patient with functional ligament instability also complains of difficulty walking on uneven ground. This history must be found in conjunction with physical examination findings of ligament instability.

Although many lateral ankle reconstruction procedures are described for chronic lateral ankle ligament instability, a Broström repair is generally the procedure of choice. The Broström procedure is a soft-tissue ligamentous repair in which the ATFL and CFL are plicated and reattached to their anatomic positions (Figure 10–49). The repair is reinforced by bringing up a portion of the inferior extensor retinaculum. The Broström procedure is highly effective and has lower morbidity than other procedures that harvest the peroneus brevis tendon. In patients who have severe and long-standing laxity or have failed a Broström repair, revision surgery with an allograft or autograft tendon is indicated.

Chronic lateral ankle pain following an ankle sprain may be caused by a previously undiagnosed condition rather than chronic ankle instability. The differential diagnosis for chronic ankle pain is similar to that following an acute injury and also includes subtalar joint instability, subtalar joint chondral damage or synovitis, and dislocating or torn peroneal tendons. Impingement of scar tissue in the lateral gutter between the talus and fibula may also cause chronic lateral

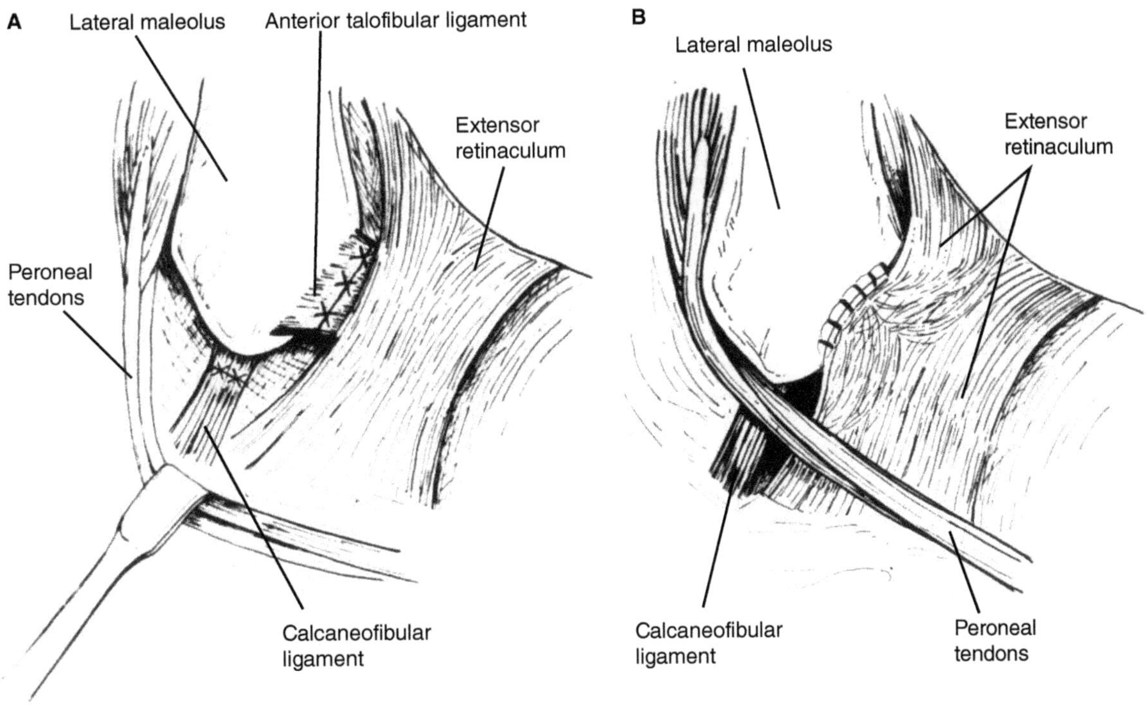

▲ **Figure 10–49. Modified Broström anatomic reconstruction. A: Imbrication of anterior talofibular and calcaneofibular ligaments. B: Imbrication of inferior extensor retinaculum to reinforce the repair.** (Reprinted with permisson, from Coughlin MJ, Mann RA, eds. *Surgery of the Foot and Ankle*, 7th ed. St. Louis: Mosby; 1999; Renstrom PA, Trevino S, eds. *Operative Techniques in Sports Medicine*, Vol. 2. New York: W.B. Saunders; 1994.)

ankle pain. In addition to a careful physical examination, an MRI or CT scan may be helpful for distinguishing among these possible causes of pain.

Surgical treatment may help relieve symptoms of chronic lateral ankle pain once an accurate diagnosis is made. Chondral or osteochondral fractures involving the ankle or subtalar joints can be treated with arthroscopic or open debridement or pinning. Subtalar joint instability is addressed with a Broström procedure. A fracture of the anterior or lateral process of the talus is either removed if it is small or fixed if it is a large fragment. Tears or dislocations of the peroneal tendons are repaired or stabilized. Scar tissue in the lateral gutter can be treated with arthroscopic debridement.

Chronic instability of the deltoid ligament or syndesmosis ligament is uncommon but can occur after an untreated injury. Diagnosis of either condition is made with stress radiographs. Treatment usually requires a free tendon graft to reconstruct the damaged ligament, with the addition of internal fixation for chronic syndesmosis tears.

Akoh CC, Phisitkul P. Anatomic ligament repairs of syndesmotic injuries. *Orthop Clin North Am.* 2019;50(3):401-414. [PMID: 31084843]

Clanton TO, Whitlow SR, Williams BT, et al. Biomechanical comparison of 3 current ankle syndesmosis repair techniques. *Foot Ankle Int.* 2017;38(2):200-207. [PMID: 27672016]

Hadadi M, Abbasi F. Comparison of the effect of the combined mechanism ankle support on static and dynamic postural control of chronic ankle instability patients. *Foot Ankle Int.* 2019;40(6):702-709. [PMID: 30808178]

Shimozono Y, Hurley ET, Myerson CL, et al. Suture button versus syndesmotic screw for syndesmosis injuries: a meta-analysis of randomized controlled trials. *Am J Sports Med.* 2019;47(11):2764-2771. [PMID: 30475639]

ARTHROSCOPIC EXAMINATION OF THE FOOT AND ANKLE

Arthroscopy is an important tool for use in the diagnosis and treatment of foot and ankle disorders. With developments in instrumentation, more ankle joint conditions can be treated arthroscopically. Arthroscopy of the subtalar joint is also now an accepted method for diagnosing and treating some subtalar joint abnormalities.

Advantages of Ankle Arthroscopy Over Ankle Arthrotomy

Arthroscopy of the ankle joint offers distinct advantages over open exploration of the ankle. The entire joint can be visualized using the arthroscope, including the lateral and medial gutters and the posterior aspect of the joint. Dynamic studies can be performed to stress ligaments or identify areas of soft-tissue or bony impingement. Furthermore, the low morbidity of arthroscopy allows rapid rehabilitation.

Table 10–4. Proven indications for ankle arthroscopy.

Loose body removal
Irrigation and debridement for infection
Shaving of small osteophytes
Debridement of localized general synovitis
Debridement of osteochondral fractures
Debridement of osteochondritis dissecans lesions
Debridement of soft-tissue impingement

Indications

Table 10–4 lists the indications for ankle joint arthroscopy. In addition, arthroscopic examination can be used as a diagnostic tool in some instances when the precise cause of ankle pain remains in question.

A. Therapeutic Indications

1. Loose bodies—Intraarticular loose bodies are generally easy to identify and remove arthroscopically. These bony or cartilaginous fragments may occur as a result of a single incident or repetitive trauma. They may also represent a fragment of an osteochondritis dissecans lesion. These can cause pain or locking symptoms of the ankle and are diagnosed on plain radiographs, CT, or MRI scan.

2. Ankle joint infection—Arthroscopic irrigation, drainage, and synovectomy is an excellent method of treating ankle joint infections.

3. Synovitis—Synovitis may be present as a result of inflammatory arthritis (rheumatoid arthritis) or neoplastic diseases (pigmented villonodular synovitis), following trauma, or for unknown reasons (idiopathic). Whether the synovitis is localized or diffuse, arthroscopic debridement of inflamed synovium often relieves symptoms. Synovectomy is more easily and thoroughly performed arthroscopically.

4. Osteophyte formation—Repetitive trauma or early osteoarthritis can lead to osteophyte formation on the anterior lip of the tibia and the neck of the talus. These lesions can cause pain with limited ankle joint dorsiflexion and can be removed arthroscopically with a high-speed burr.

5. Other lesions within the joint—Chondral or osteochondral lesions, whether caused by trauma or osteochondritis dissecans, can be treated arthroscopically. This may involve debridement of loose cartilage flaps, drilling of subchondral bone, or pinning of large osteochondral fragments.

Patients who present with ankle pain over the anterolateral joint line and a history of a severe ankle sprain or recurrent sprains may have impingement of scar tissue in the lateral gutter between the talus and fibula. This entity responds well to arthroscopic debridement of scar tissue from the lateral gutter.

6. Ankle arthrodesis—The technique causes less morbidity and allows a shorter time to fusion than open methods of ankle fusion. But this is a technically demanding procedure and cannot be used to correct any joint deformity.

7. Ankle arthritis—Arthroscopic debridement of the arthritic ankle joint is not beneficial for generalized arthritis but may help for localized degenerative changes accompanied by early osteophyte formation.

8. Ankle fractures—Arthroscopically assisted fixation of ankle fractures is described and potentially allows for a more accurate realignment of the joint surfaces and identification of chondral lesions that might otherwise be missed. However, the use of arthroscopy in the treatment of most routine ankle fractures is probably not indicated.

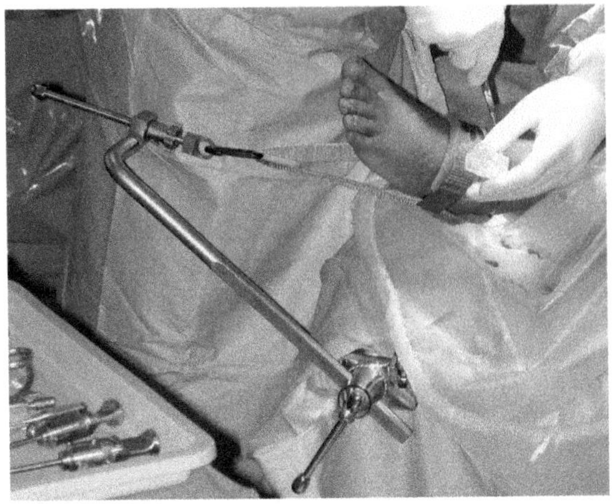

▲ **Figure 10–50.** Soft strap type of distractor used during ankle arthroscopy.

B. Diagnostic Indications

Ankle arthroscopy can be a valuable diagnostic tool when the cause of symptoms remains unclear (Table 10–5). Chronic ankle pain or swelling that remains refractory to conservative measures and was not diagnosed by conventional imaging studies may warrant arthroscopic exploration to help make a diagnosis. Chondral damage and inflamed synovium are examples of symptomatic lesions that may not be demonstrated on imaging studies including MRI. Patients with episodes of locking, stiffness, or instability for which a cause cannot be found may be aided by diagnostic ankle arthroscopy. Loose bodies, cartilage flaps, or arthrofibrosis may be contributing to such symptoms, all of which can be treated arthroscopically (Table 10–5).

Technique of Ankle Arthroscopy

The patient is placed supine on the operating table with the foot positioned to allow access from all directions. This can be achieved with the foot placed off the edge of the bed or with the thigh held flexed in a well-padded thigh holder (Figure 10–50). General or spinal anesthesia is necessary for full relaxation of the extremity.

The use of distraction greatly enhances arthroscopic procedures, providing better views of the structures of the joint and allowing instruments to be introduced into the joint. Noninvasive distractors with padded straps over the foot and heel are most commonly used (Figure 10–50). Invasive distractors require placement of pins or screws through the tibia proximally and the calcaneus or talus distally. Stronger distraction forces can be obtained in this manner, but the morbidity is higher when using an invasive distractor.

Most ankle arthroscopies are performed using two anterior portals: anterolateral and anteromedial. A posterolateral portal may be helpful for use as outflow or to access the posterior aspect of the joint. Thorough knowledge of the anatomy of the tendons, nerves, and vessels is essential to prevent damage to any of these structures with portal placement. The anterolateral portal is placed just lateral to the tendon of the peroneus tertius muscle, taking care to avoid branches of the superficial peroneal nerve. The anteromedial portal is placed just medial to the anterior tibial tendon, taking care to avoid the saphenous nerve and vein. The posterolateral portal is placed just lateral to the Achilles tendon to avoid damage to the sural nerve.

Initially, the entire joint is explored systematically to ensure that abnormalities are not overlooked. The cartilaginous surfaces of the talus and tibia are thoroughly examined for osteochondral defects, unstable cartilage flaps, and areas of softening. The medial and lateral gutters are explored, paying special attention to the tibiotalar and talofibular articulations. The synovium is inspected for inflammation. Ligamentous structures are identified, specifically the deltoid and talofibular ligaments, which are observed closely for signs of

Table 10–5. Refractory conditions diagnosed by arthroscopy.

Chondromalacia
Synovitis
Locking of the joint
Chronic stiffness
Instability
Loose bodies
Cartilage flaps
Arthrofibrosis

laxity while varus and valgus forces are applied. Loose bodies are carefully searched for, especially in the anterior and posterior recesses of the joint. The presence of osteophytes on the distal tibia and talar neck is also evaluated.

After a thorough diagnostic examination of the entire joint, surgical procedures are then performed. These include synovial biopsy or synovial resection, removal of loose bodies, debridement of abnormal cartilaginous surfaces with subchondral drilling, and removal of bone spurs.

Postoperatively, a compression dressing is applied with a posterior splint for 5 to 7 days to allow the portals to heal. Weight bearing is then progressed as tolerated, and activities are advanced to normal.

Complications

Although several complications are reported, the most common after ankle arthroscopy is nerve damage in the form of hypesthesias or neuroma formation associated with portal placement. Postoperative joint infection, draining sinuses, arterial or tendon damage, and infections at the sites of distraction pins are all described but are very uncommon complications of ankle arthroscopy.

Subtalar Joint Arthroscopy

The subtalar joint is technically challenging for arthroscopy, given its complex shape and the difficulty distracting the joint. Subtalar joint arthroscopy is indicated for several conditions involving the subtalar joint. Talocalcaneal interosseous ligament tears, chondral lesions, synovitis, and focal degenerative changes may respond to arthroscopic debridement of the subtalar joint.

For subtalar joint arthroscopy, the patient can either be placed supine with a bump under the ipsilateral hip or in the lateral decubitus position. Two portals are used over the anterolateral subtalar joint, approximately 1.5 cm apart. The anterior and lateral portions of the posterior facet and the interosseous ligament can be visualized from these portals. A third portal is placed posterolaterally, for outflow and for visualization of the posterior aspect of the joint. The references here provide additional details about the technique of subtalar joint arthroscopy.

Braunstein M, Baumbach SF, Urresti-Gundlach M, Borgmann L, Böcker W, Polzer H. Arthroscopically assisted treatment of complex ankle fractures: intra-articular findings and 1-year follow-up. *J Foot Ankle Surg.* 2020;59(1):9-15. [PMID: 31882154]

Phisitkul P, Akoh CC, Rungprai C, et al. Optimizing arthroscopy for osteochondral lesions of the talus: the effect of ankle positions and distraction during anterior and posterior arthroscopy in a cadaveric model. *Arthroscopy.* 2017;33(12):2238-2245. [PMID: 28807507]

Vega J, Dalmau-Pastor M, Malagelada F, et al. Ankle arthroscopy: an update. *J Bone Joint Surg Am.* 2017;99(16):1395-1407. [PMID: 28816902]

TENDON INJURIES

Tendon injuries about the foot and ankle are common causes of disability because large forces are acting on these tendons in a repetitive fashion during walking, running, and athletic activities. The tendons cross the ankle joint at an acute angle, further predisposing them to injury. Tendon injury may be caused by acute trauma, such as in Achilles tendon ruptures, or by chronic strain, such as in posterior tibial tendon dysfunction.

ACHILLES TENDON INJURIES

Achilles tendon abnormalities are extremely common, especially among active men and women between 30 and 50 years of age. The primary disorders are Achilles tendinitis, either insertional or noninsertional, and Achilles tendon ruptures. Achilles tendinitis was previously discussed in the section on heel pain.

1. Achilles Tendon Rupture

Pathogenesis

The mechanism of acute injury is usually mechanical overload from an eccentric contraction of the gastrocsoleus muscle complex. This occurs as a sudden, forceful dorsiflexion of the foot as the gastrocsoleus is contracted. The tear usually occurs 3 to 6 cm proximal to the insertion of the Achilles tendon, at the site of its poorest blood supply (watershed area). At times, a prodromal history of intermittent pain in the tendon is elicited, suggestive of a prior tendinitis. The typical patient is between 30 and 50 years of age and a recreational athlete. These factors suggest that insufficient conditioning of the musculotendinous unit plays a role in many injuries. The most common sports activities leading to Achilles tendon ruptures are basketball, racket sports, soccer, and softball.

Clinical Findings

A. Symptoms and Signs

The patient describes sudden pain in the calf after attempting a pushing-off movement, often accompanied by an audible pop. Immediate weakness is noted in the affected leg. On physical examination, a palpable defect is often present in the tendon. Ankle plantarflexion is markedly weak compared with the unaffected side. A positive Thompson test, diagnostic of complete Achilles tendon rupture, is performed with the patient prone and the affected knee bent 90 degrees. Squeezing the calf causes plantarflexion of the foot if the Achilles tendon is intact or partially torn but not if there is complete rupture of the tendon.

B. Imaging Studies

Plain radiographs are not helpful in diagnosing Achilles tendon tear, unless there is an avulsion off the calcaneus

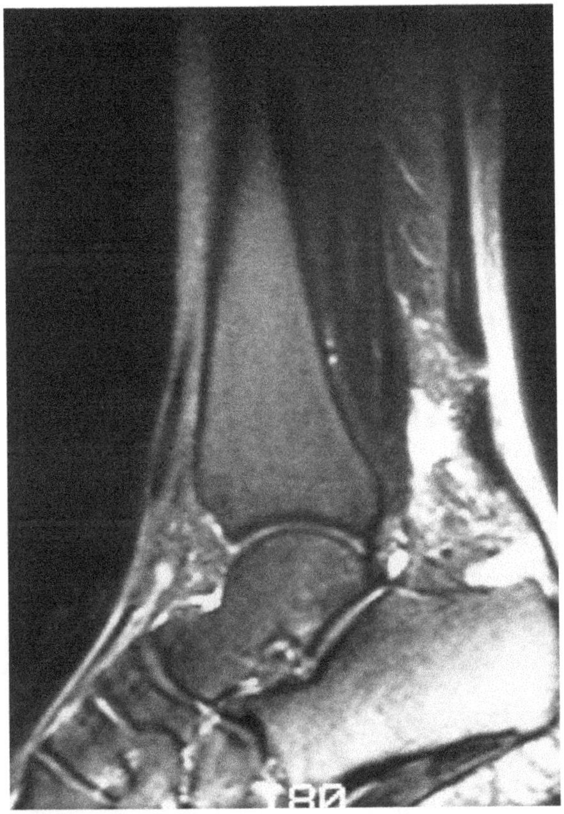

▲ **Figure 10–51.** MRI of Achilles tendon rupture.

with a fragment of bone, an uncommon condition. MRI is extremely sensitive in diagnosing this disorder and in determining if some tendon remains in continuity (Figure 10–51). However, MRI is rarely needed because physical exam is usually diagnostic of Achilles tendon rupture.

Treatment

Methods for treating Achilles tendon rupture include primary repair, using open or percutaneous techniques, or functional nonsurgical treatment. Multiple recent studies have demonstrated similar outcomes in randomized trials comparing surgery to nonsurgical treatment. The key to successful nonsurgical treatment is early recognition and functional treatment. Surgical repair is generally recommended for elite athletes, reruptures, or delayed recognition of the injury.

Nonsurgical treatment for Achilles tendon ruptures traditionally has been recommended for sedentary individuals, patients who are at increased risk of developing wound problems, or high-risk surgical patients. However, as previously mentioned, recent studies indicate that nonsurgical treatment has equivalent outcomes, even in active patients. The primary risk of nonsurgical treatment is a higher chance of rerupture. For the vast majority of patients, either treatment method results in a good outcome.

A. Nonsurgical Treatment

Traditionally, once an acute rupture is diagnosed, the patient was placed in a gravity equinus cast. If there is a question of whether the tendon edges are properly apposed in the cast, an MRI scan can be done, although this is not routine. After 4 weeks, the cast is changed, with correction of approximately half of the previous equinus. Over the next 4 weeks, the patient is brought down to neutral with serial casts. Once at neutral, the patient is given a removable walking cast for 4 weeks. Supervised strengthening activities then begin. A recent study from the United Kingdom demonstrated that traditional casting did not offer any benefit over early weight bearing in a functional brace.

B. Surgical Treatment

The surgical treatment of Achilles tendon ruptures may include traditional open techniques versus limited incision percutaneous techniques. Regardless of the method of repair, robust nonabsorbable sutures are woven through 3 to 4 cm of each tendon edge

Postoperatively, the foot and ankle are splinted in gravity equinus until the wound is healed. Over the next 2 to 3 weeks, the joint should be gradually brought out of equinus. Active dorsiflexion can be performed with gravity plantarflexion to reduce contracture. Weight bearing is then allowed, and ROM exercises are begun. Functional rehabilitation can begin at 6 to 8 weeks. The most concerning risk of surgical repair is wound healing problems, which occur in approximately 5% of patients.

C. Treatment of Chronic Ruptures or Reruptures

Chronic Achilles tendon ruptures, more than 6 weeks old, or reruptures of previously treated injuries can be challenging reconstruction problems because of retraction and degeneration of the tendon ends. A number of different procedures are described to address this problem, including a variety of synthetic and interpositional grafts.

Small defects can be repaired by using a gastrocnemius recession or by turning down a strip of gastrocnemius fascia, which is sutured into the distal tendon stump. Larger defects can be treated by using a V-Y lengthening of the gastrocnemius aponeurosis. If the deficit is too large for V-Y lengthening, transfer of the flexor hallucis longus tendon can be performed. Traditionally, the tendon of the flexor hallucis longus is transected distally in the foot, and the distal segment is tenodesed to the flexor digitorum longus to maintain flexion of the great toe. Recently, techniques have evolved to permit harvest of the tendon through the posterior ankle incision, obviating the need for a foot incision.

The transferred tendon is secured to the calcaneus through a drill hole or by using anchors or screws. A portion of the Achilles tendon can be used to reinforce the repair by securing it to the flexor hallucis.

The postoperative course for these procedures includes 6 weeks of non–weight bearing and a total of 3 months of protection in a cast or boot.

POSTERIOR TIBIAL TENDON INJURIES

This topic is covered in the section on acquired flatfoot deformities.

PERONEAL TENDON INJURIES

Peroneal tendon injuries fall into the categories of peroneal tendinitis, peroneal tendon tears, and peroneal tendon subluxation or dislocation.

1. Peroneal Tendonitis

Pathogenesis

Inflammation of the peroneal tendons may be caused by acute trauma, degenerative tendinosis, inflammatory arthropathy, or repetitive motion. Traumatic events that may induce tendinitis include a direct blow to the posterolateral ankle, a fracture of the calcaneus or fibula, or a severe inversion sprain of the ankle. Most tendinitis is caused by repetitive motion injury from recurrent rubbing of the peroneal tendons on the distal end of the fibula. Often there is an abnormal bony contour of the distal fibula or the peroneal tubercle. Tendinitis of the peroneus longus may be associated with abnormality of the os peroneum, a small sesamoid bone located in the tendon where it curves around the lateral border of the cuboid.

Clinical Findings

A. Symptoms and Signs

The patient complains of pain over the lateral aspect of the ankle, made worse with activity and improved with rest and NSAIDs. The onset may be insidious, or it may be associated with an acute injury. Physical examination usually demonstrates pain located along the course of the peroneal tendons. Pain and weakness are noted with resisted eversion of the foot.

B. Imaging Studies

An MRI scan may help distinguish between tendinitis and a tendon tear, although small tears may not be identified on an MRI.

Treatment

A. Nonsurgical

If symptoms are mild, the recommended treatment includes NSAIDs, activity modification, and an ankle brace. Four to 6 weeks of cast immobilization are used for more advanced symptoms or for patients who do not respond to initial treatment. Occasionally, a diagnostic injection with bupivacaine is given into the tendon sheath.

B. Surgical

Operative intervention is recommended for patients who fail conservative treatment. The tendon sheath is explored, inflamed synovium is removed, and the tendons are carefully explored to look for tears or degenerative lesions. Postoperatively, early ROM is encouraged.

2. Peroneal Tendon Tears

Pathogenesis

The majority of peroneal tendon tears are attritional in nature, caused by mechanical irritation within the fibular groove. The peroneus longus tendon, which lies posterior, places pressure on the brevis tendon. Also, a sharp lateral edge of the fibula may predispose to a longitudinal split of the tendons. Laxity of the tendon sheath and subluxation of the tendons out of the fibular groove may contribute to tears as well. Acute tears of the peroneal tendons may occur with a sudden, severe stress to the ankle, but usually, there is some degree of preexisting degeneration within the tendon.

Clinical Findings

Clinical presentation is similar to that of peroneal tendinitis, but with a more acute onset of pain and swelling along the tendon sheath.

Treatment

A. Nonsurgical

Initial treatment is similar to that of peroneal tendinitis, but it is less likely to result in resolution of symptoms if a tear is present.

B. Surgical

Surgical repair of a peroneal tendon tear is indicated when nonoperative treatment fails to relieve symptoms. During surgery, both tendons are carefully examined, the fibula is explored for sharp edges, and the tendon sheath is evaluated for laxity. Small areas of the tendon that demonstrate significant degeneration are removed. The remainder of the tendon is repaired with nylon or polypropylene suture. Postoperatively, the ankle is immobilized for 4 weeks; then weight bearing and gentle ROM are allowed. In some cases, side-to-side tenodesis of the brevis to longus is performed if the tendon is not amenable to repair.

3. Peroneal Tendon Subluxation and Dislocation

Pathogenesis

Peroneal tendon dislocation is caused by a sudden forceful dorsiflexion motion of the ankle combined with a simultaneous strong contraction of the peroneal musculature. This mechanism injures the superior peroneal retinaculum, which holds the peroneal tendons in place along the posterior border of the distal fibula. The retinaculum is either stripped off the fibular periosteum or avulsed with a small piece of fibular cortex. This permits the creation of a false pouch and laxity of the retinaculum, allowing the peroneal tendons to dislocate anteriorly. If this condition goes unrecognized, either the tendons remain dislocated or they relocate with the propensity for recurrent subluxation or dislocation.

Clinical Findings

A. Symptoms and Signs

The patient usually recalls an acute episode of trauma and frequently the sensation of the tendon dislocating. Pain and swelling are localized to the peroneal tendon sheath around the tip of the fibula. With recurrent subluxation or dislocation, the tendons are felt to pop out of place. On examination, resisted eversion of the ankle elicits pain and may cause the tendons to subluxate. Unfortunately, many acute peroneal tendon dislocations go unrecognized as lateral ankle sprains.

B. Imaging Studies

Radiographs may show a small piece of bone lateral to the distal fibula, indicative of avulsion of the retinaculum. MRI scan usually details the injury well if careful attention is paid to this area.

Treatment

A. Nonsurgical

Treatment of acute peroneal tendon dislocations consists of casting in plantarflexion and inversion for 4 weeks, followed by a walking cast for an additional 2 weeks. Cast treatment has at least a 50% failure rate. Once a tendon is chronically dislocated or recurrently subluxates, only surgical treatment will keep it in position.

B. Surgical

Surgical repair is recommended for an athletic individual following an acute dislocation of the peroneal tendons. It is also recommended for patients with recurrent dislocation if their physical activities are significantly restricted. The procedure consists of repairing the superior peroneal retinaculum to the fibula, either through drill holes or with suture anchors. In the case of attenuated retinaculum caused by chronic dislocations, the repair can be reinforced with a strip of Achilles or by rerouting the calcaneofibular ligament over the tendons. At the time of surgical repair, the tendons are inspected for tears and the contour of the posterior fibular groove is evaluated. If a shallow groove is noted, a bony procedure to deepen the groove is necessary to prevent recurrent dislocations. Postoperatively, the patient is immobilized in a cast for 6 weeks.

ANTERIOR TIBIAL TENDON RUPTURE

Pathogenesis

Rupture of the anterior tibial tendon occurs infrequently and most often in patients older than 60. The mechanism of injury is due to either chronic rubbing against the inferior edge of the extensor retinaculum or rubbing against an exostosis at the first metatarsocuneiform joint. The rupture usually occurs at the distal 2 to 3 cm of tendon. Nondegenerative traumatic ruptures of the anterior tibial tendon are rare. They may also occur secondary to synovitis in patients with inflammatory arthritis.

Clinical Findings

A. Symptoms and Signs

Patients with a degenerative rupture present with complaints of pain and swelling over the anterior ankle and a gait abnormality. They sense the foot slapping down, or they may be catching their toes on the ground when they walk. Patients frequently present after the symptoms have been bothersome for several months. Physical exam is notable for weakness of ankle dorsiflexion, often with a palpable mass over the anterior ankle joint.

B. Imaging Studies

If the diagnosis is in doubt, MRI scan can accurately determine if the tendon is ruptured.

Treatment

A. Nonsurgical

In the case of a less active patient, nonsurgical treatment appears to give equal functional results to surgical repair. Cast immobilization is followed by long-term use of an AFO.

B. Surgical

Acute tendon rupture in an active individual should be surgically repaired. A recent meta-analysis reported that surgical intervention provided better functional results than nonsurgical treatment. Surgical options include the use of an ipsilateral split/turn-down ipsilateral tibialis anterior tendon graft, semitendinosus autograft, direct repair, or extensor hallucis longus autograft. The most common postoperative complaint was mild dorsiflexion weakness, which did not appear to result in subjective functional limitation. Good functional results were found to occur regardless of patient age at the time of intervention. Chronic ruptures that are symptomatic usually require reconstruction using an extensor tendon graft or tendon transfer because the distal stump is usually too degenerated to perform a primary repair.

Costa ML, Achten J, Marian IR, et al. Plaster cast versus functional brace for non-surgical treatment of Achilles tendon rupture (UKSTAR): a multicentre randomised controlled trial and economic evaluation. *Lancet.* 2020;395(10222):441-448. [PMID: 32035553]

Glazebrook M, Rubinger D. Functional rehabilitation for nonsurgical treatment of acute Achilles tendon rupture. *Foot Ankle Clin.* 2019;24(3):387-398. [PMID: 31370992]

Reda Y, Farouk A, Abdelmonem I, El Shazly OA. Surgical versus non-surgical treatment for acute Achilles' tendon rupture. A systematic review of literature and meta-analysis. *Foot Ankle Surg.* 2019;pii:S1268-7731(19)30053-0. [PMID: 31027878]

Soroceanu A, Sidhwa F, Aarabi S, et al. Surgical versus nonsurgical treatment of acute Achilles tendon rupture: a meta-analysis of randomized trials. *J Bone Joint Surg Am.* 2012;94(23):2136-2143. [PMID: 23224384]

Stenson JF, Reb CW, Daniel JN, et al. Predicting failure of nonoperative treatment for insertional Achilles tendinosis. *Foot Ankle Spec.* 2018;11(3):252-255. [PMID: 28884594]

Tickner A, Thorng S, Martin M, et al. Management of isolated anterior tibial tendon rupture: a systematic review and meta-analysis. *J Foot Ankle Surg.* 2019;58(2):213-220. [PMID: 30554867]

OSTEOCHONDRAL LESIONS OF THE TALUS

Osteochondral lesions of the talus (OLTs) are defects of cartilage and subchondral bone in the talar dome. More sophisticated imaging techniques allow for precise diagnosis of OLTs, and advanced arthroscopic and open methods are available to treat this difficult problem.

Pathogenesis

OLTs, also known as osteochondritis dissecans lesions, are most commonly located in one of two areas on the talar dome: either posteromedial or anterolateral. The more common posteromedial lesions are usually deeper lesions involving subchondral bone. Their origin is thought to involve ischemia, often with an episode of trauma exacerbating the underlying condition. Anterolateral lesions are a result of a single traumatic episode or repetitive trauma from lateral ankle sprains. These lesions tend to be purely cartilaginous.

Clinical Findings

A. Symptoms and Signs

Patients usually present with several months of ankle pain following a routine ankle sprain. Sometimes patients recount a history of recurrent sprains to the ankle. The pain is usually located over the anterior aspect of the ankle on the side of the lesion, but it may be diffuse. Occasionally, there is a sensation of locking in the ankle when a loose flap of cartilage is present. A high index of suspicion is necessary because OLTs can be misdiagnosed as a chronic ankle sprain, as discussed in the section on ligamentous injuries about the ankle joint.

B. Imaging Studies

Radiographs are often normal in OLTs. MRI scan is the imaging procedure of choice for determining the size, location, and extent of bony or cartilaginous involvement (Figure 10–52).

Treatment

A. Nonsurgical

A 6-week trial of immobilization is warranted if the MRI scan shows no evidence of a displaced bone or cartilage fragment.

B. Surgical

The surgical treatment method depends on the type of lesion. Acutely displaced lesions can be reduced and stabilized with

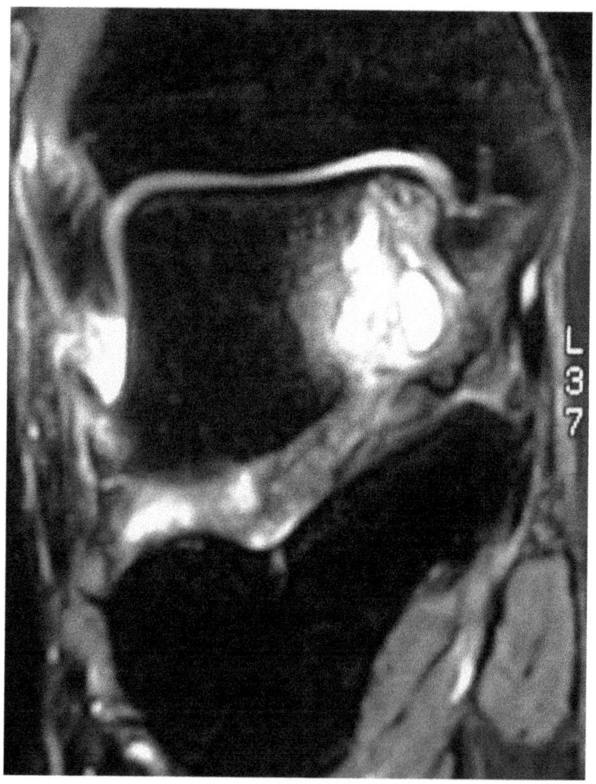

▲ **Figure 10–52.** MRI scan of extensive osteochondral lesion of the talus.

an absorbable pin by either open or arthroscopic methods. Purely cartilaginous lesions are curetted to a stable rim and drilled to stimulate vascular ingrowth and fibrocartilage formation. Arthroscopic microfracture provides good functional outcomes and improved quality of life with maintenance of satisfactory outcomes at a mean follow-up of 6.7 years. Therefore, arthroscopic microfracture seems to be reliable as a first-line treatment for OLT at an intermediate-term follow-up. Second-look arthroscopic results revealed that approximately one-third of lesions were incompletely healed and had inferior quality of repair tissue compared with that of native cartilage, despite the fact that arthroscopic microfracture provided functional improvements. OLTs with significant bony involvement require bone grafting in addition to drilling and curettage. A medial malleolar osteotomy is required to access a posteromedial lesion. If a bony lesion has intact overlying cartilage, retrograde drilling and bone grafting can be performed under radiographic guidance through the talus, thereby sparing the overlying cartilage. Postoperatively, patients are kept non–weight bearing for 4 weeks, but early ROM is encouraged.

New techniques were developed for larger lesions or ones that fail curettage and drilling. Osteochondral autograft or allograft plugs can be used to replace bone and cartilage defects. Autograft plugs are generally harvested from the ipsilateral knee. Intermediate-term follow-up data show good results in most patients following this technique. Autologous chondrocyte implantation is also used to a limited extent for OLTs. Matrix-associated autologous chondrocyte implantation is an area of research and potentially can provide long-term improvement of pain and functional impairment caused by focal full-thickness chondral and osteochondral talus lesions.

Choi SW, Lee GW, Lee KB. Arthroscopic microfracture for osteochondral lesions of the talus: functional outcomes at a mean of 6.7 years in 165 consecutive ankles. *Am J Sports Med.* 2020;48(1):153-158. [PMID: 31877099]

Ramponi L, Yasui Y, Murawski CD, et al. Lesion size is a predictor of clinical outcomes after bone marrow stimulation for osteochondral lesions of the talus: a systematic review. *Am J Sports Med.* 2017;45(7):1698-1705. [PMID: 27852595]

Yang HY, Lee KB. Arthroscopic microfracture for osteochondral lesions of the talus: second-look arthroscopic and magnetic resonance analysis of cartilage repair tissue outcomes. *J Bone Joint Surg Am.* 2020;102(1):10-20. [PMID: 31596800]

11 Hand Surgery

Dimitrios V. Papadopoulos, MD
Michael S. Bednar, MD
Anthony Davidson, BS
Christopher C. Schmidt, MD

GENERAL CONSIDERATIONS

The hand is essential to the human body, as for most of us it is our main way to interact with the environment and fulfill our daily needs. The functional capabilities of the hand are numerous since the hand is an end organ of the human mind. The hand's enormous capacity for adaptability allowed us to make stone tools in the past and now to pilot complex aircraft.

The human hand is capable of prehension, which involves approaching an object, grasping it, modulating and maintaining grasp, and ultimately releasing the object. When a power grasp is used, the object is pushed by the flexed fingers against the palm while the thumb metacarpal and proximal phalanx stabilize the object. When an object is held with precision pinch, the object is secured between the pulps of the thumb and index fingers or index and middle fingers.

The hand can touch objects or other human beings while sensing temperature, vibration, and texture. This quality of tactile gnosis is sophisticated enough to allow blind individuals to read the pattern of small elevations that distinguish one Braille letter from another.

Deep knowledge of the normal anatomy and its common variations is mandatory for the treatment of the hand pathologies. The main goal of treatment is usually restoration of the normal anatomy, but when that is not feasible, the attempt should aim on restoration of maximal function. The aesthetic appearance of the hand is vital because the hand is usually uncovered and exposed to the scrutiny of others and to the owner. Imperfections are often a source of embarrassment. Effective treatment requires a mature balancing of the need for optimal function and normal appearance of the hand. Complex reconstruction that restores prehension but results in a hideous appearance of the hand is ineffective if the patient is so reluctant to expose the hand that he or she avoids using it. Conversely, a functionless stiff finger leading to awkward motion of an otherwise supple hand may cause the patient more embarrassment than amputation.

DIAGNOSIS OF HAND DISORDERS

History

When a patient seeks evaluation of a hand disorder, the physician should ask many general questions as well as questions specific to hand function and injury. The chief complaint as perceived by the patient should be summarized in one or two sentences. The patient's hand dominance, age, gender, and occupation should be noted, as well as any hobbies that require hand dexterity or strength. The approximate date of onset of symptoms should be recorded. If injury is the cause of discomfort, the exact date and mechanism of injury should be noted and whether the injury occurred at the workplace. The patient should be questioned about prior treatment and his or her perception of its effectiveness.

Complaints should then be further detailed, such as the nature of pain (sharp, aching, dull, or burning), location, onset and progression of pain, whether night symptoms are present, aggravating and relieving factors, and whether the pain is worse upon awakening in the morning or after a full day of work. The patient should be asked whether symptoms include numbness or tingling, which would indicate a neurologic problem rather than a mechanical one, and also about skin coloration changes and sensitivity to cold indicating vascular conditions. Specific motor difficulties, such as difficulty in writing or unscrewing jar tops, should be noted. If the patient complains principally of unilateral symptoms, the examiner should ask whether similar symptoms are occurring on the opposite side. Finally, because the hand is an exposed area of the body, the impact of altered appearance should be discussed.

The medical history should include any prior hand injuries and any systemic diseases such as rheumatoid arthritis (RA) or other inflammatory arthropathies, diabetes, other endocrine disorders, renal disease, or vascular disease. Women of childbearing age should be questioned about recent pregnancies. A careful history suggests the correct diagnosis in approximately 90% of patients with hand problems.

Examination of the Hand

A. Inspection

Examination of the hand should begin with inspection. Vascular conditions can be assessed by noting the color of the fingers. Some information about nerve function can be obtained by observing sudomotor function (from the autonomic nerves that control sweating) as revealed by sweatiness of the finger pulps. Other signs that can be evaluated during inspection include swelling or lumps, lacerations, scars from injuries or previous surgeries, and any hand deformity. The posture of the digits and the wrist may signal tendon or bone disruption. Normally, a cascade of increased digital flexion is noted when ulnar digits are observed next to radial digits (Figure 11–1). Control of digital posture requires a complex balance of extrinsic and intrinsic muscle forces. Extrinsic muscles have their origin outside of the hand and their insertion on the hand or carpus, whereas intrinsic muscles have both origin and insertion within the hand. Extrinsic muscles are either flexors or extensors, and intrinsic muscles contribute to both digital flexion and extension. Do not forget to look at the nails as they may show signs of atrophy or disease; for example, psoriasis, which is sometimes associated with a typical arthropathy, or a "grooved" nail, which is a telltale feature of a ganglion cyst at the nail bed.

B. Palpation

Next, the hand, wrist, and forearm are gently palpated. The temperature and texture of the hand should be noted. Circulation is assessed by capillary refill; when the skin is blanched adjacent to the nail, circulation should return within 2 seconds. Swelling or thickening may be in the subcutaneous tissue, a tendon sheath, a joint, or one of the bones. If a nodule is felt, the underlying tendon should be moved (by flexing and extending the relevant finger) to discover if the nodule is attached to the tendon or its sheath. Areas of tenderness on palpation are carefully noted and linked with the underlying soft tissue or bony structures.

C. Range of Motion

The passive and active range of motion (ROM) of the shoulder, elbow, forearm, wrist, and hand are evaluated. The normal ROM of the wrist and fingers is summarized in Table 11–1. It is convention that in documenting ROM, active extension is to left and active flexion to right, and when the ranges of passive extension and flexion are different from those of active motion, the passive ROM values are noted in parentheses so that the ROM of a stiff proximal interphalangeal (PIP) joint would be recorded as 20/70 (15/80). This indicates an arc of active motion from 20 to 70 degrees and a passive arc of motion from 15 to 80 degrees.

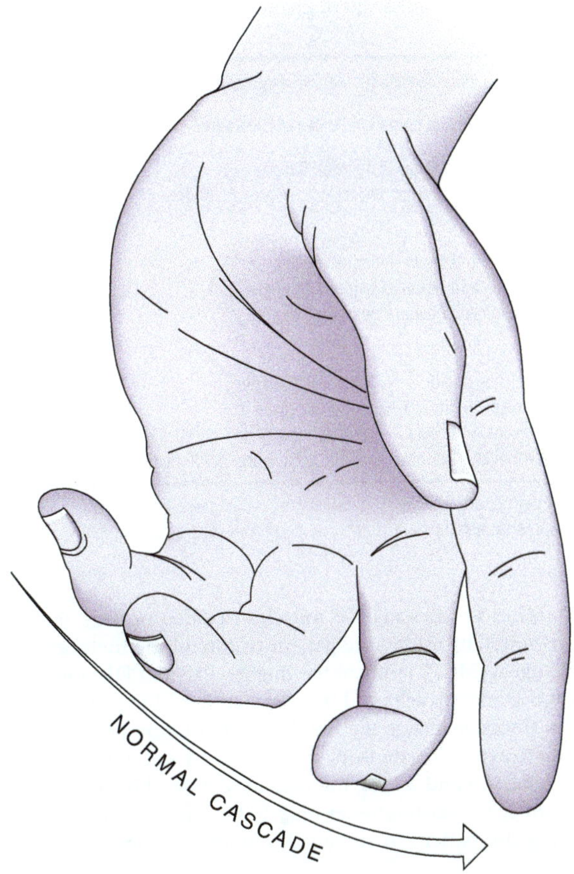

▲ **Figure 11–1.** **Normal cascade of digital flexion posture. When the wrist is in slight extension and the fingers are at rest, there is progressively less flexion from the little finger to the index finger.** (Reprinted with permission, from Carter PR. *Common Hand Injuries and Infections*. New York: WB Saunders; 1983.)

D. Motor Function

Motor function can be impaired due to either tendon (or muscle) injury or nerve dysfunction. The integrity of individual tendons (and/or muscles) should be documented. The tenodesis effect during wrist flexion/extension is helpful to evaluate tendon rupture. The flexor digitorum profundus to each finger is tested by holding the PIP joint in extension and asking the patient to flex the distal interphalangeal (DIP) joint (Figure 11–2). The flexor digitorum superficialis of each finger is tested by keeping all fingers except the one to be tested in full extension and then asking the patient to flex the finger being evaluated at the PIP joint (Figure 11–3). The function of the flexor pollicis longus is tested by asking the patient to flex the interphalangeal joint of the thumb.

Table 11–1. Normal range of motion in joints of arm and hand.

Elbow: Extension and flexion 0 degree/135 degree
Forearm: Supination and pronation 90 degree/90 degree
Wrist: Flexion and extension 80 degree/70 degree Radial deviation and ulnar deviation 20 degree/30 degree
Finger MP: Extension and flexion 0 degree/90 degree PIP: Extension and flexion 0 degree/110 degree DIP: Extension and flexion 0 degree/65 degree
Thumb CMC: Extension and flexion 50 degree/50 degree Abduction and adduction 70 degree/0 degree MP: Extension and flexion—variable, up to 0 degree/90 degree IP: Extension and flexion—variable, up to 0 degree/90 degree

CMC, carpometacarpal; DIP, distal interphalangeal; IP, interphalangeal; MP, metacarpal phalangeal; PIP, proximal interphalangeal.

Extension of the extrinsic muscles (located outside the hand) is tested by asking the patient to extend the metacarpophalangeal (MCP) joints of the fingers. PIP and DIP joint extension is mainly achieved by contraction of the intrinsic muscles (location inside the hand); therefore, the best way to evaluate extrinsic extensors' function is by holding MCP joints in flexion and asking the patient to extend his or her MCP joints. Dorsal interossei muscle function is screened by asking the patient to spread the fingers for abduction.

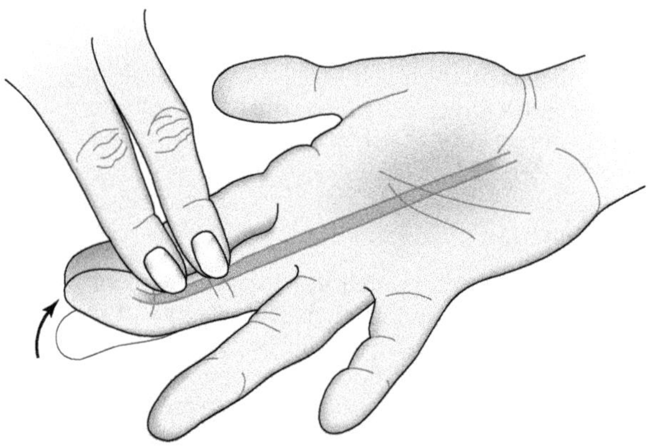

▲ **Figure 11–2. Testing of flexor digitorum profundus integrity. If the distal interphalangeal joint can be actively flexed while the proximal interphalangeal joint is stabilized, the profundus tendon is not severed.** (Reprinted with permission, from American Society for Surgery of the Hand. *The Hand: Examination and Diagnosis,* 2nd ed. Philadelphia: Churchill Livingstone; 1983.)

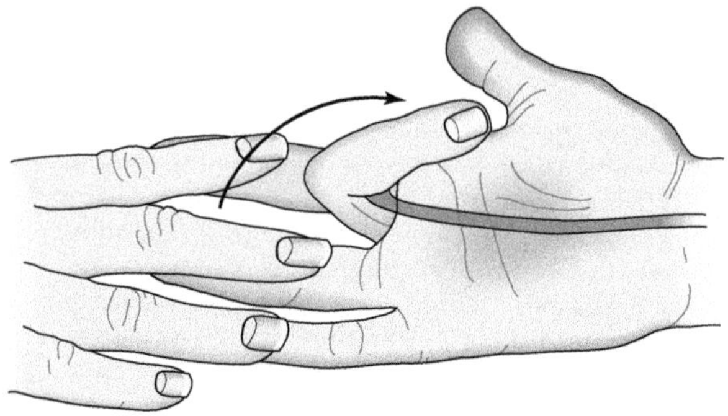

▲ **Figure 11–3. Testing of flexor digitorum superficialis integrity. If the proximal interphalangeal joint can be actively flexed while the adjacent fingers are held completely extended, the sublimis tendon is not severed.** (Reprinted with permission, from American Society for Surgery of the Hand. *The Hand: Examination and Diagnosis,* 2nd ed. Philadelphia: Churchill Livingstone; 1983.)

The examiner assesses the strength of muscle force while palpating the contraction of the hypothenar and the first dorsal interosseous muscles. Palmar interossei muscle function is evaluated by asking the patient to cross the fingers.

Assessment for nerve function may be organized by considering groups of muscles innervated by specific nerves and testing the muscles within each group (Table 11–2). Proximally, the median nerve innervates the pronator teres, flexor carpi radialis, palmaris longus, and flexor digitorum superficialis muscles. The anterior interosseous nerve branch of the

Table 11–2. Innervation of the hand and forearm.

Median nerve Proximal median nerve: pronator teres, flexor carpi radialis, flexor digitorum superficialis Anterior interosseous nerve: flexor pollicis longus, index and middle flexor digitorum profundus, pronator quadratus Distal median nerve: index and middle lumbrical, opponens pollicis, abductor pollicis brevis, flexor pollicis brevis
Ulnar nerve Proximal ulnar nerve: flexor carpi ulnaris, ring and small flexor digitorum profundus Distal ulnar nerve: flexor digiti minimi, abductor digiti minimi, opponens digiti minimi, volar and dorsal interossei, flexor pollicis brevis, adductor pollicis, ring and small lumbricals
Radial nerve: brachioradialis, extensor carpi radialis longus, supinator, anconeus
Posterior interosseous nerve: extensor carpi radialis brevis, extensor digitorum communis, extensor indicis proprius, extensor digiti minimi, extensor carpi ulnaris, abductor pollicis longus, extensor pollicis longus, extensor pollicis brevis

median nerve innervates the flexor digitorum profundus of the index and middle fingers, flexor pollicis longus, and pronator quadratus muscles. The motor branch of the median nerve to the thenar musculature innervates the opponens pollicis, abductor pollicis brevis, and superficial portion of the flexor pollicis brevis. The index and long finger lumbricals are innervated by median motor fibers running with the sensory nerve branches of the median nerve to the index and middle fingers.

The ulnar nerve innervates the flexor carpi ulnaris and flexor digitorum profundus of the ring and little fingers proximally. Within the hand, the ulnar nerve innervates the hypothenar musculature, flexor digiti quinti, and abductor digiti quinti. The deep motor branch of the ulnar nerve innervates the dorsal and palmar interosseous muscles, lumbricals to the ring and little fingers, deep portion of the flexor pollicis brevis, and adductor pollicis muscles.

The radial nerve innervates the triceps, brachioradialis, extensor carpi radialis longus and brevis, supinator, and anconeus muscles. The posterior interosseous division of the radial nerve then distally innervates the extensor digitorum communis, extensor indicis proprius, extensor digiti minimi, extensor carpi ulnaris, abductor pollicis longus, and extensor pollicis longus and brevis.

Muscle strength should be graded according to the Medical Research Council of Great Britain grading system based on a scale of 0 to 5, with 5/5 being normal strength, 4/5 less than normal strength but with ability to resist a fair amount of resistance, 3/5 resistance against gravity, 2/5 resistance with gravity eliminated, and 1/5 only a trace or flicker of contraction without significant motion.

E. Sensory Function

Examination of sensory function requires evaluation of the integrity of the median, ulnar, and radial nerves as well as the component proper digital nerves to each side of each finger. Each of the major nerves has an autogenous sensory zone: an area of the hand supplied predominantly by that nerve (Figure 11–4). The autogenous zone of the median nerve is the pulp of the index finger, whereas the ulnar nerve exclusively carries sensory fibers from the pulp of the little finger. The skin on the dorsum of the first web space is innervated by the superficial branch of the radial nerve.

The integrity of each digital nerve may be evaluated using either a blunt-tipped caliper or an unfolded paper clip to test two-point discrimination. The two points of the testing instrument are held apart at a measured distance. The examiner alternates between touching the skin with one or two points. The points may be either touched (static two-point discrimination) or longitudinally moved (moving two-point discrimination) against the skin on either the radial or ulnar side of the finger. The points should be pressed against the finger until the skin just begins to blanch. The two-point discrimination value is the smallest distance between the two points that the patient can correctly detect in two out of three trials. Because of the increased sensory cues provided by movement, moving two-point discrimination has a value less than or equal to static two-point discrimination. Static two-point discrimination is normal if the distance is less than 7 mm, impaired if 7 to 14 mm, and absent if 15 mm or greater.

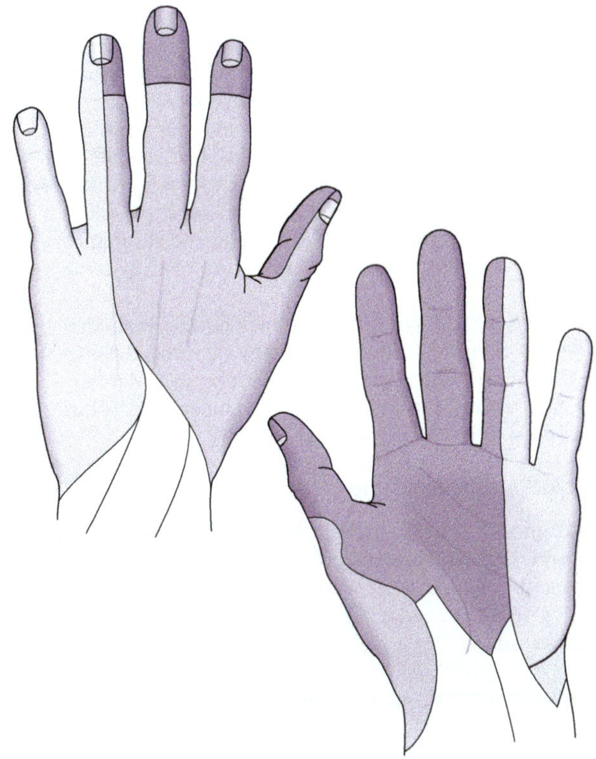

▲ **Figure 11–4. Sensory distribution in the hand. Light shading, ulnar nerve; medium shading, radial nerve; darkest shading, median nerve.** (Reprinted from Way LW, ed. *Current Surgical Diagnosis and Treatment*, 10th ed. Stamford, CT: Appleton & Lange; 1994.)

Diagnostic Studies

A number of studies may be helpful in establishing the proper diagnosis in a patient with hand or wrist pain or disorders. The choice of technique should be based on a careful history and physical examination.

A. Imaging Studies

In most instances, radiographic evaluation includes posteroanterior (PA) and lateral films. The importance of obtaining a true lateral radiograph of the finger and wrist cannot be overemphasized because many disorders, particularly interphalangeal joint subluxation and carpal instability, are not evident on oblique views. Oblique views may be useful in defining phalangeal fracture patterns. Tangential views are useful in assessing a carpometacarpal (CMC) boss (a mass of dorsal bone). The carpal tunnel view may allow visualization of a fracture of the hook of the hamate.

Stress views allow assessment of ligamentous stability. This is particularly useful in the evaluation of collateral ligament stability of the thumb MCP joint. However, they are rarely used nowadays due to the high sensitivity and specificity of other modalities such as magnetic resonance imaging (MRI) or ultrasound for evaluation of soft-tissue injuries.

Ligamentous stability of the wrist may also be evaluated by radial and ulnar deviation views and by clenched-fist grip views. Grip views and ulnar deviation views may demonstrate a gap between the scaphoid and the lunate that is not apparent on simple PA and lateral studies.

B. Electrodiagnostic Studies

Electrodiagnostic studies include both nerve conduction studies and electromyography (EMG). Nerve conduction studies measure both motor (proximal to distal) and sensory (distal to proximal) conduction. EMG allows evaluation of muscle function.

C. Computed Tomography Scan

A computed tomography (CT) scan allows excellent three-dimensional views of the osseous structures of the hand and wrist and is critical to evaluation of joints such as the distal radioulnar joint. The relationship of the distal ulna to the sigmoid notch should be viewed in pronation, neutral, and supination. CT scanning may be helpful in evaluating displacement as well as healing of scaphoid fractures and in surgical planning of distal radius fractures.

D. Magnetic Resonance Imaging

MRI provides visualization of soft-tissue structures such as ligaments and tendons. The integrity of the transverse carpal ligament may be evaluated, which is particularly helpful in patients with persistent symptoms following carpal tunnel release. Evaluation of tumors and avascular necrosis is also facilitated by MRI. MRI scans also allow visualization of many triangular fibrocartilage complex (TFCC) and intercarpal ligament tears.

E. Ultrasound

The applications of ultrasound for diagnosis of musculoskeletal conditions have been significantly expanded over the past years. While ultrasound was first used as a diagnostic tool for detection of foreign bodies following trauma, nowadays, it is mostly used as a diagnostic modality for tendon or ligament lesions, such as thumb ulnar collateral ligament ruptures. Another application of ultrasound that has been recently proposed is in patients with nerve compression neuropathies. Specifically, in cases of carpal tunnel syndrome, ultrasound can be used as a confirmation study in patients with equivocal signs, having a good sensitivity and specificity. Although musculoskeletal ultrasound serves as an excellent imaging modality with several advantages, including low cost, dynamic nature of exam, and easy use, its main disadvantage is that its diagnostic capacity is operator dependent.

F. Bone Scan

The technetium-99 methylene diphosphonate (MDP) bone scan is a useful physiologic test in the evaluation of unexplained hand or wrist pain. This test can rule out bone involvement and can be used to localize inflammatory processes for further study with CT or MRI scans (Figure 11–5).

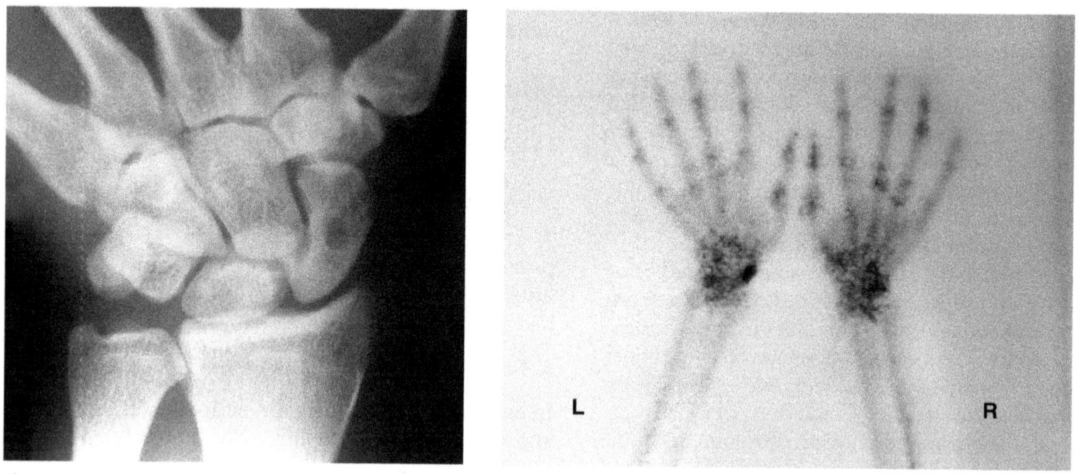

A B

▲ **Figure 11–5.** Radiograph **(A)** and bone scan **(B)** demonstrating increased activity in the region of the scaphoid in a woman with a symptomatic cyst.

G. Wrist Arthroscopy

Arthroscopic examination of the wrist allows for direct visualization of articular surfaces, carpal and intercarpal ligaments, and the TFCC. The effect of stress maneuvers on intercarpal kinematics may be directly observed. Wrist arthroscopy is particularly helpful in the debridement or repair of the TFCC tears. Partial tears of either the scapholunate or lunotriquetral ligaments may be debrided. Intraarticular fracture of the distal radius may be anatomically aligned and pinned under direct observation.

Ahsan ZS, Yao J. Complications of wrist and hand arthroscopy. *Hand Clin.* 2017;33(4):831-838. [PMID: 28991593.]

Dy C. What's new in hand surgery. *J Bone Joint Surg.* 2019;101(6): 479-485. [PMID: 30893228]

Fowler J, Munsch M, Tosti R, Hagberg W, Imbriglia J. Comparison of ultrasound and electrodiagnostic testing for diagnosis of carpal tunnel syndrome: study using a validated clinical tool as the reference standard. *J Bone Joint Surg Am.* 2014;96(17):e148. [PMID: 25187592]

Hoel RJ, Mittelsteadt MJ, Samborski SA, Bohn DC. Preoperative antibiotics in wrist arthroscopy. *J Hand Surg Am.* 2018;43(11):987-991.e1. [PMID: 29778348]

Moser TP, Martinez AP, Andoulsi S, Jeantroux J, Cardinal É. Radiographic/MR imaging correlation of the wrist. *Magn Reson Imaging Clin N Am.* 2019;27(4):601-623. [PMID: 31575396]

Tiegs-Heiden CA, Howe BM. Imaging of the hand and wrist. *Clin Sports Med.* 2020;39(2):223-245. [PMID: 32115082]

DISORDERS OF THE MUSCLES AND TENDONS OF THE HAND

DISRUPTION OF EXTENSOR TENDONS APPARATUS

Anatomy of Extrinsic Extensor Muscles

The extrinsic extensors run through six different fibroosseous retinacular compartments at the wrist level (Figure 11–6A). The first (most radial) compartment contains the abductor pollicis longus and the extensor pollicis brevis. The abductor pollicis longus has multiple slips that insert at the base of the thumb metacarpal and radially abducts the thumb, whereas the extensor pollicis brevis inserts on the dorsum of the proximal aspect of the proximal phalanx of the thumb and actively extends the MCP joint of the thumb.

The second extensor compartment contains the extensor carpi radialis longus and the extensor carpi radialis brevis. The extensor carpi radialis longus, inserting on the index metacarpal, dorsiflexes and radially deviates the wrist, and the extensor carpi radialis brevis, inserting into the base of the middle metacarpal, provides balanced wrist dorsiflexion.

The third compartment contains the extensor pollicis longus, which runs longitudinally down the forearm through the third compartment and turns abruptly radially over Lister tubercle, a dorsal prominence on the distal radius. Because its insertion is on the distal phalanx, the extensor pollicis longus provides forceful extension of the thumb interphalangeal joint. The oblique course of the extensor pollicis longus tendon provides a substantial adduction component to the pull of the extensor pollicis longus.

The fourth extensor compartment contains the extensor indicis proprius lying deep to the four tendons of the extensor digitorum communis, whereas the fifth compartment contains the extensor digiti quinti. These three muscles each have a role in digital extension at the MCP, PIP, and DIP joints of the fingers. The principal bony insertion of the extrinsic digital extensors is on the dorsal proximal aspect of the middle phalanx. MCP joint extension is provided by extrinsic extensor force transmitted through the sagittal bands. DIP and PIP joint extension is achieved through the conjoined lateral bands that are composed of tendinous slips from the extrinsic and intrinsic tendons.

The extensor indicis proprius inserts on the index finger ulnar to the extensor digitorum communis. The extensor digitorum communis inserts on the index, middle, ring, and, in some cases, little fingers. The extensor digiti quinti tendon inserts on the little finger ulnar to the extensor digitorum communis insertion.

The extensor carpi ulnaris tendon runs through the sixth compartment and inserts at the base of the little finger metacarpal. It provides wrist extension and ulnar deviation.

The extensor digitorum communis tendons of the middle, ring, and little fingers are tethered together by juncturae tendinum over the dorsum of the hand proximal to the MCP joint (Figure 11–6B). The extensor indicis proprius tendon may be recognized at the wrist level as possessing the most distal muscle belly of any of the digital extensor tendons.

The digital extensor tendons are stabilized over the midline of the MCP joint by their attachment to sagittal band fibers (Figure 11–7). The sagittal band fibers insert onto the volar proximal phalanx and onto the lateral borders of the volar plate. The sagittal band fibers form a sling that allows proximal extrinsic extensor tension to be transmitted to the proximal phalanx, permitting MCP joint extension without a tendinous insertion onto the proximal phalanx. By holding the extrinsic extensor tendon balanced over the prominence of the metacarpal head, the sagittal bands normally keep the extrinsic extensor as far as possible away from the center of rotation of the MCP joint, thereby giving it the greatest mechanical efficiency. With rupture or attenuation of the sagittal band fibers, the extrinsic extensor tendon can sublux to the ulnar side of the metacarpal head causing ulnar deviation of the finger.

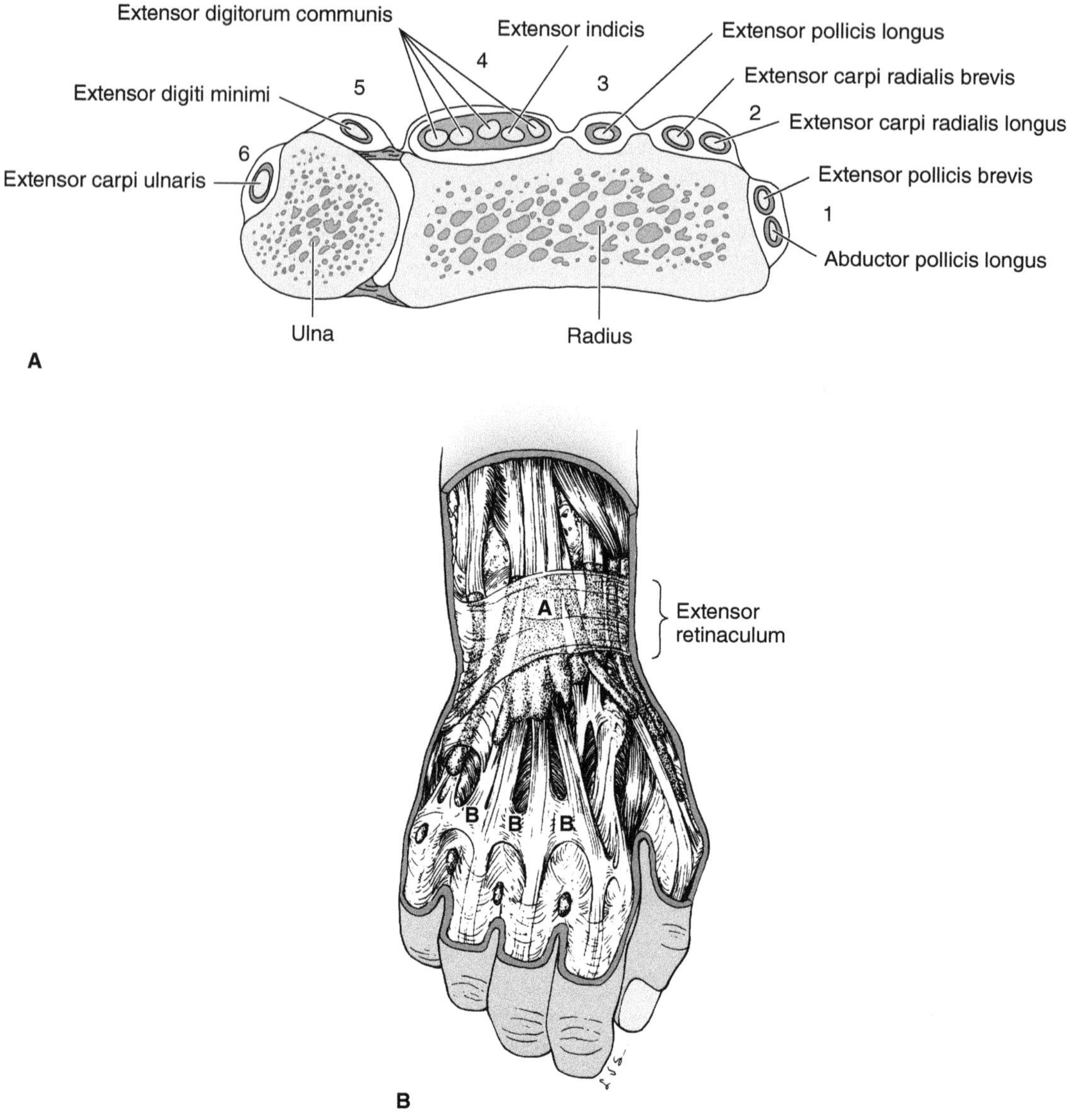

▲ **Figure 11–6. The six dorsal compartments of the wrist. A: Cross-section of pronated right wrist viewed from distal to proximal.** (Reproduced, with permission, from Reckling FW, et al. *Orthopaedic Anatomy and Surgical Approaches*. St. Louis: Mosby-Year Book; 1990.) **B: Dorsal view. A, extensor retinaculum over the compartments; B, juncturae tendinum (conexus intertendineus).** (Reprinted, from Way LW, ed. *Current Surgical Diagnosis & Treatment*, 10th ed. Stamford, CT: Appleton & Lange; 1994.)

Anatomy of the Dorsal Hood Apparatus

The dorsal hood apparatus, frequently referred to as the extensor mechanism, is the confluence of intrinsic and extrinsic tendon insertions on the dorsal aspect of the finger (see Figure 11–7). The extrinsic extensor tendon trifurcates at the base of the proximal phalanx to give origin to the central slip and the lateral bands. The central tendon inserts on the dorsal aspect of the middle phalanx. The lateral bands are joined by contributions from the extensor hood, the interossei, and lumbrical muscles to form the conjoined lateral bands. Through dorsal hood attachments, the extrinsic extensor muscles extend the MCP joint, the intrinsic muscles flex the MCP joint, and both the intrinsic and extrinsic muscles extend the PIP and DIP joints.

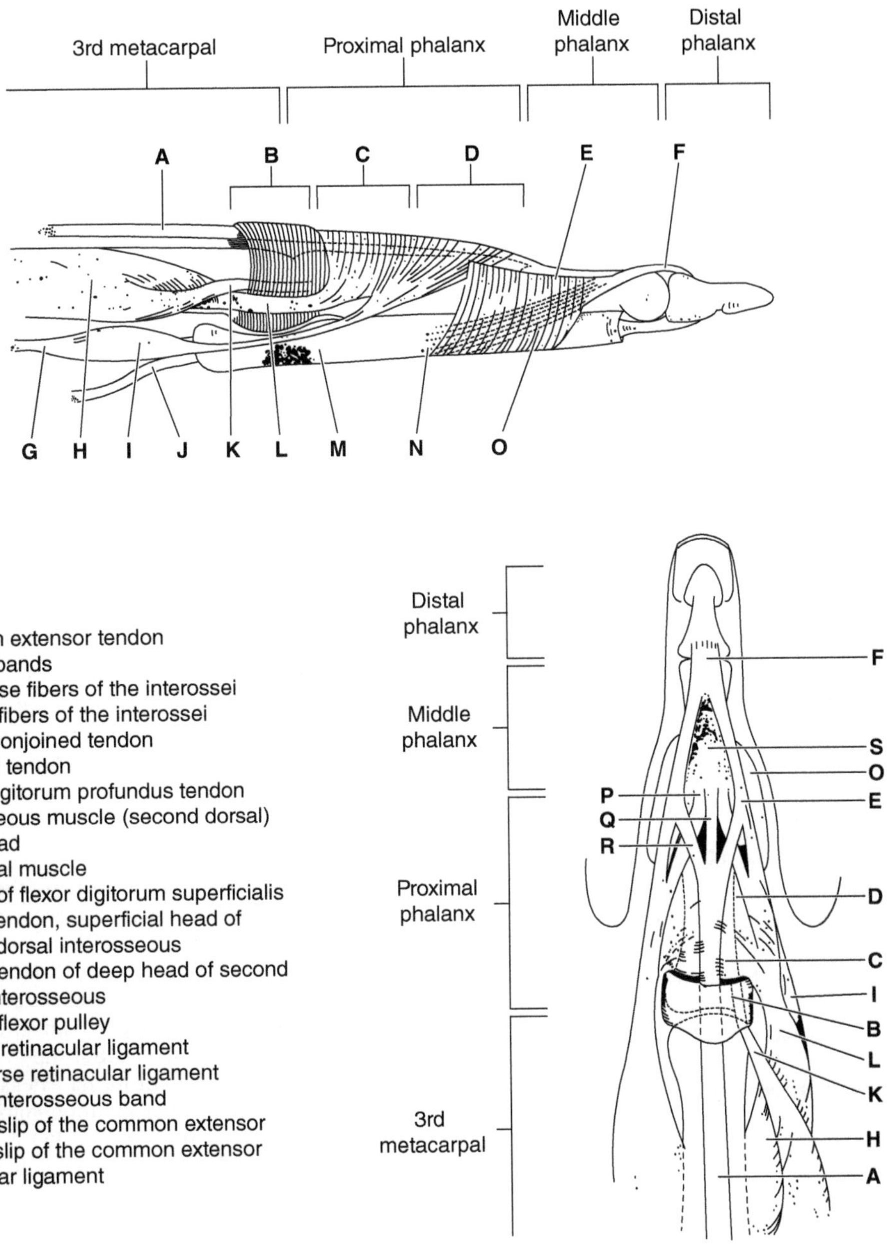

A. Common extensor tendon
B. Sagittal bands
C. Transverse fibers of the interossei
D. Oblique fibers of the interossei
E. Lateral conjoined tendon
F. Terminal tendon
G. Flexor digitorum profundus tendon
H. Interosseous muscle (second dorsal) deep head
I. Lumbrical muscle
J. Tendon of flexor digitorum superficialis
K. Medial tendon, superficial head of second dorsal interosseous
L. Lateral tendon of deep head of second dorsal interosseous
M. Fibrous flexor pulley
N. Oblique retinacular ligament
O. Transverse retinacular ligament
P. Medial interosseous band
Q. Central slip of the common extensor
R. Lateral slip of the common extensor
S. Triangular ligament

▲ **Figure 11–7. Extensor hood mechanism. The dorsal hood apparatus provides points of insertion of both extrinsic extensors and intrinsic muscles of the hand.** (Reprinted from Way LW, ed. *Current Surgical Diagnosis & Treatment*, 10th ed. Stamford, CT: Appleton & Lange; 1994.)

Extension of the MCP joint is achieved by the action of the extrinsic extensor tendons that pulls and lifts up the proximal phalanx through a sling mechanism facilitated by the sagittal band. Extension of the PIP joint is achieved through the action of the central slip and the intrinsic muscles through their contributions to the lateral bands. DIP extension is achieved through both intrinsic and extrinsic muscles that contribute to form the radial and ulnar conjoined lateral bands, which merge to form the terminal tendon insertion.

1. Sagittal Band Disruption

Anatomy and Clinical Findings

The sagittal band fibers originate from the MCP volar plate and the intermetacarpal ligament. Their function is to stabilize the extrinsic extensor tendons to transmit their extensor power and prevent tendon bowstring. They can be ruptured by trauma (boxer's knuckle) or become chronically attenuated due to synovitis of the MCP joint, as in RA. The middle finger is most commonly involved (48%), and usually the radial side of the sagittal band is injured or attenuated (9:1). As a result, the extensor tendon may dislocate into the gully between the adjacent metacarpal heads and become mechanically less effective at extending the MCP joint. The patient may be able to hold the MCP joint in extension once placed there but cannot initiate extension of the joint.

Treatment

An acute tear of the radial sagittal band within 1 week may be treated by extension splinting for 4 to 6 weeks. An alternative way of immobilization to the classic method of immobilization in full MCP joint extension is the relative motion splint. This splint is based on the relative motion concept that applies to injured tendons that share the same muscle belly with adjacent tendons. According to this concept, free flexion-extension at the MCP joint minus 15 to 20 degrees compared to the adjacent MCP joints is allowed because this difference in the ROM between the joint with the injured tendon and the adjacent joints results in markedly less force applied to the injured tendon. Compared to the classic extension splinting, patients wearing this brace feel much less awkward when performing their daily and work activities. Usually in chronic injuries, the band is irreparable, and a recentralizing procedure with sagittal band reconstruction is required. There are several techniques for reconstruction of the sagittal band utilizing capsular flaps or tendon slips.

2. Boutonnière Deformity

Clinical Findings

In cases when the central slip is lacerated or avulsed from the middle phalanx or when synovitis of the PIP joint leads to capsular distension, the extension force on the PIP joint is lost and active PIP joint extension is lacking. The finger is rapidly drawn into a position of PIP joint flexion as the unopposed motion of the flexor digitorum superficialis and profundus draws the finger into flexion (Figure 11–8). The triangular ligament is attenuated, and the lateral bands migrate apart and are drawn into a progressively more volar position, eventually coming to lie palmar to the axis of flexion of the joint. In the subluxed position, the lateral bands become a deforming force contributing to the tendency of the finger to flex at the PIP joint.

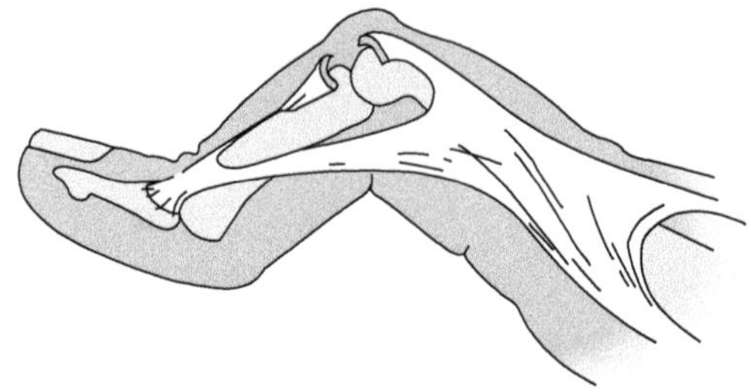

▲ **Figure 11–8.** Boutonnière deformity caused by loss of active proximal interphalangeal extension secondary to loss of the central slip insertion on the proximal dorsal middle phalanx. (Reprinted from Way LW, ed. *Current Surgical Diagnosis & Treatment,* 10th ed. Stamford, CT: Appleton & Lange; 1994.)

With central slip disruption, the extension force that normally is applied on the middle phalanx through both extrinsic extensor and intrinsic muscles bypasses the PIP joint and is refocused on the DIP joint, amplifying the force of extension of this joint and hyperextending it. Because the DIP joint is relatively resistant to active flexion, contraction of the flexor digitorum profundus muscle primarily flexes the PIP joint and is relatively ineffective in flexing the DIP joint, unless the PIP joint is supported in maximal extension. The digit eventually assumes the boutonnière deformity posture of PIP joint flexion and DIP joint hyperextension.

Treatment

Because the PIP joint is at the center of the complex balance of the intrinsic and extrinsic forces, restoration of proper balance and tension on the central slip may be technically difficult. When the central slip is acutely lacerated, it should be directly repaired and the joint should be pinned in full extension for 3 to 6 weeks to protect the integrity of the repair. In acute closed injuries of the central slip (<4 weeks), 6 weeks of splinting of the PIP joint in full extension is the recommended treatment. During the immobilization period, the DIP joint should remain free, and ROM exercises for prevention of joint stiffness are recommended. When diagnosis is delayed, a fixed flexion contracture of the PIP joint usually occurs.

Surgical treatment of chronic central slip ruptures in a finger is frequently disappointing. Restoration of full ROM is mandatory before addressing the deformity. During the surgical procedure, release of the contracture on the palmar aspect of the joint is performed before augmenting PIP joint extension on the dorsal aspect. An alternative strategy employs prolonged splinting to diminish the extent of the fixed PIP joint flexion contracture before surgery. Among the variety of splints available for this, the Capener splint and the Joint Jack splint are particularly useful. Serial casting of the finger with a circumferential digital cast that is changed every few days may also be helpful in bringing the PIP joint into extension. During the period of splinting, the patient should be instructed to carry out active flexion of the DIP joint, with the middle phalanx supported in extension. Care should be taken to assure that splints and casts allow DIP joint flexion. Once full PIP joint extension is achieved, splinting should be continued full time for an additional 6 to 12 weeks. In many instances, this achieves sufficient tightening of the central slip to permit satisfactory active PIP joint extension.

In chronic injuries of the central slip, three main operative interventions can be considered: terminal tendon tenotomy, lateral band dorsal relocation, and central slip reconstruction. The first, a Fowler type of tenotomy, obliquely divides the dorsal hood apparatus over the middle phalanx, proximal to the terminal tendon insertion. This diminishes DIP joint hyperextension and may improve active PIP joint extension by refocusing intrinsic and extrinsic forces at the more proximal joint. Regarding the two latter techniques, although they may increase active extension of the joint, they often do so at the loss of full PIP joint flexion.

3. Mallet Finger

Clinical Findings

The mallet finger deformity is characterized by a loss of active DIP joint extension with full passive ROM evident due to disruption of the terminal extensor tendon (Figure 11–9). The usual mechanism of injury involves sudden passive flexion of the actively extended DIP joint during traumatic impaction blow to the tip of the finger. More rarely, it can be caused by dorsal laceration. Disruption of the terminal tendon may be entirely confined to the tendon (soft-tissue mallet finger) or may involve an avulsed fracture fragment from the dorsal lip of the distal phalanx proximal articular surface (bony mallet finger).

Because the avulsed fragment includes the terminal tendon insertion, the clinical appearance of soft tissue and bony mallet fingers is similar. The distal joint rests in flexion, a posture that cannot be actively changed. Full passive extension of the DIP joint is possible.

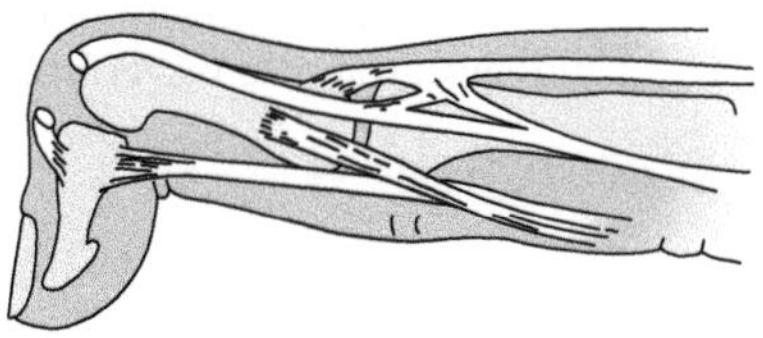

▲ **Figure 11–9.** Mallet finger deformity is secondary to loss of terminal tendon insertion on the distal phalanx. (Reprinted, from Way LW, ed. *Current Surgical Diagnosis & Treatment*, 10th ed. Stamford, CT: Appleton & Lange; 1994.)

Treatment

A radiograph should be obtained to determine whether a fracture is present and, if the dorsal fragment is large, whether the distal phalanx is subluxed palmarward. In most cases, these injuries can be treated conservatively, and surgical treatment is only rarely indicated. Surgical treatment is associated with a high rate of complications (53%-76%) such as joint incongruity, nail deformity, and infection; therefore, surgeons should be strict on the indications for the surgical treatment of a mallet finger. If the joint is congruent, splinting is recommended even if a small articular surface fracture site gap persists. The DIP joint should be splinted in extension continuously for 6 to 8 weeks, with free movement of the PIP joint. In bony mallet fingers with volar subluxation or with a fragment greater than 50% of the articular surface, closed reduction and percutaneous pinning are recommended. In chronic injuries lasting greater than 12 weeks with no arthritic changes, tendon advancement, tenodermodesis, or spiral oblique retinacular ligament reconstruction is recommended, but the results are poor.

Bruner S, Wittemann M, Jester A, et al. Dynamic splinting after extensor tendon repair in zones V to VII. *J Hand Surg.* 2003;28:224-227. [PMID: 12809652]

Merritt W. Relative motion splint: active motion after extensor tendon injury and repair. *J Hand Surg Am.* 2014;39(6): 1187-1194. [PMID: 24862114]

INTRINSIC PLUS AND INTRINSIC MINUS POSITIONS

Anatomy of the Intrinsic Muscles

The intrinsic muscles that control finger posture are the dorsal and palmar interossei, lumbricals, thenar, and hypothenar muscles. These muscles are responsible for MCP joint flexion, finger abduction and adduction, and extension of the PIP and DIP joints. The interossei muscles originate from the metacarpal shafts and pass dorsal to the deep transverse intermetacarpal ligament but volar to the axis of MCP joint rotation.

The index finger is abducted by the first dorsal interosseous muscle and adducted by the first palmar interosseous muscle. The middle finger is radially abducted by the second dorsal interosseous muscle and ulnarly abducted by the third dorsal interosseous muscle. The ring finger is adducted by the second volar interosseous muscle and abducted by the fourth dorsal interosseous muscle. The little finger is adducted by the third volar interosseous muscle and abducted by the abductor digiti quinti muscle.

The dorsal interossei are bipennate and have both superficial and deep muscle bellies. The superficial belly gives rise to a tendon that inserts on the lateral tubercle of the proximal phalanx and is responsible for finger abduction. The deep muscle belly inserts into the transverse fibers of the hood of the extensor apparatus and therefore contributes to MCP joint flexion. The volar interosseous muscles are unipennate and insert into the extensor apparatus, contributing to MCP joint flexion and finger adduction (see Figure 11–7).

The lumbricals originate from the radial side of the index, middle, ring, and little fingers in the palm from the flexor digitorum profundus tendon of the corresponding finger. These four lumbrical muscles insert into the radial lateral band of the dorsal hood aponeurosis of each finger. They are volar to the interosseous muscles, and they course palmar to the transverse intermetacarpal ligament. The lumbrical muscles extend the PIP and DIP joints and modulate flexor and extensor digital tone. The lumbrical muscles are the only muscles that relax their "antagonists," which are the flexor tendons, because their origin is into these tendons. Contraction of the profundus muscle belly draws the profundus tendon proximally and shifts the lumbrical origin proximally, thereby increasing tension on the dorsal hood fibers that extend the PIP and DIP joints. Contraction of the lumbrical muscle draws the proximal profundus distally and reduces tension on the flexor digitorum profundus at the DIP joint, so that DIP joint extension is facilitated.

The abductor digiti quinti, like the dorsal interossei, has two tendons of insertion. One of these tendons inserts directly onto the bone of the abductor tubercle along the ulnar aspect of the proximal phalanx, and the other insertion is into the dorsal hood apparatus. The flexor digiti quinti inserts onto the ulnar tubercle at the base of the proximal phalanx but does not insert into the dorsal hood apparatus. The primary function of the flexor digiti quinti is flexion of the MCP joint.

The thenar muscles are the abductor pollicis brevis, flexor pollicis brevis, opponens pollicis, and adductor pollicis.

1. Intrinsic Plus Position

Together, the interossei and lumbricals flex the MCP joints and extend the PIP and DIP joints. Hence, the posture of the hand in which the MCP joints are flexed and the PIP and DIP joints are extended is known as the intrinsic plus position (Figure 11–10). This is an ideal position for splinting the hand because the collateral ligaments of the MCP and interphalangeal joint are taut, and because it is also ideal for immobilization of most hand injuries, it is termed the *position of safety* or *position of advantage*.

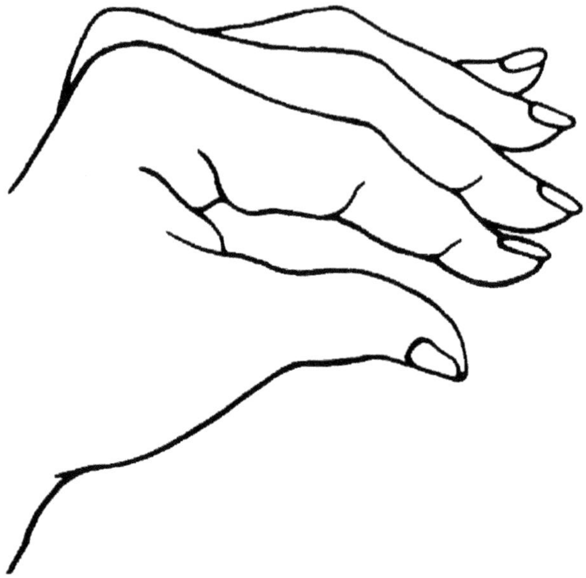

▲ **Figure 11–10.** Intrinsic plus position.

2. Intrinsic Minus Position

Clinical Findings

When the intrinsic muscles are paralyzed, the hand tends to assume the intrinsic minus posture, sometimes referred to as a claw hand. The normal length of the intrinsic muscles and tendons allows simultaneous full passive MCP joint extension and interphalangeal joint flexion; therefore, the intrinsic minus position requires full excursion of the relaxed intrinsic muscles (see Figures 11–10; Figure 11–11).

Although the extrinsic extensors have fibers that can provide PIP and DIP joint extension in the hand with competent intrinsic muscles, with intrinsic minus deformity, their excursion is expended in unopposed MCP joint hyperextension. Thus, the hand devoid of intrinsic power is unable to achieve active extension of the PIP and DIP joints, unless the MCP joint is flexed by other means.

Treatment

Surgical correction of the intrinsic minus hand must either prevent passive hyperextension of the MCP joint or restore active control of MCP joint flexion. The first can be achieved by either tenodesis or capsulodesis across the MCP joint, while the second is achieved by an active tendon transfer. Once MCP joint hyperextension is prevented, the extrinsic extensors usually can effectively open the hand by extending the PIP and DIP joints (positive Bouvier test). If active PIP joint extension is not possible through the extrinsic extensors when the MCP joint is flexed (negative Bouvier test), then tendon transfer to the digital lateral bands for MCP joint flexion and interphalangeal joint flexion should be performed.

INTRINSIC MUSCLE TIGHTNESS

Clinical Findings

When the lumbricals and interossei become contracted and overly tight, the limitation of their excursion does not permit full simultaneous MCP joint extension and interphalangeal joint flexion. The intrinsic tightness test was

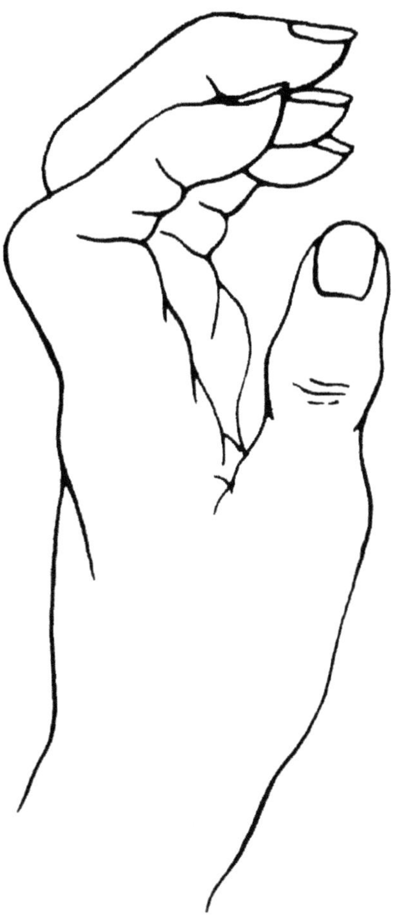

▲ **Figure 11–11.** Intrinsic minus position secondary to low median and ulnar nerve palsies.

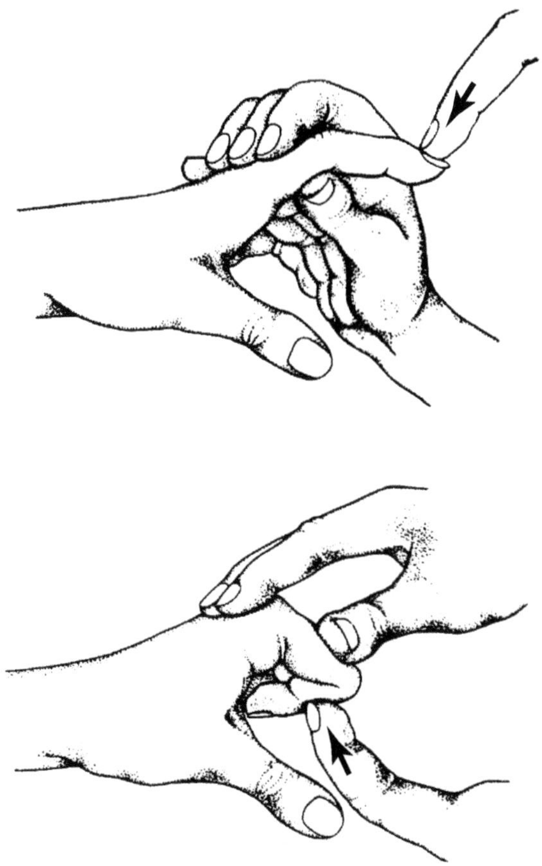

▲ **Figure 11–12. Intrinsic tightness test is performed by flexing the proximal interphalangeal joint with the metaphalangeal joint extended and flexed. Tightness to proximal interphalangeal flexion occurs with the metaphalangeal joint extended.** (Reprinted with permission, from Green DP, ed. *Operative Hand Surgery*, 2nd ed. Philadelphia: Churchill Livingstone; 1988.)

originally described by Finochietto and later by Bunnell (Figure 11–12). It is accomplished by first determining that the MCP and interphalangeal joints each have a full range of passive joint motion in a reduced position. The MCP joint is then passively held in an extended position while the examiner attempts to flex the PIP and DIP joints passively. If full passive flexion of the PIP and DIP joints is not possible in this position, the intrinsic muscles are deemed tight.

Causes of intrinsic muscle tightness include conditions as diverse as RA (due to MCP joint dislocation), neurological pathologies such as brain injury or cerebral palsy, and trauma (crush injuries, compartment syndrome, or vascular injuries).

Treatment

In mild cases, passive stretching exercises may be successful. Surgical treatment of intrinsic tightness may be carried out as an isolated procedure or in combination with MCP joint reconstruction. The intrinsic force can be diminished either by proximal muscle slide with subperiosteal elevation of the muscles (in less severe deformities with remaining intrinsic function) or by distal release with resection of one or both lateral bands (in severe cases when both MCP and interphalangeal joints are affected). The intrinsic tightness test may be used intraoperatively to judge the adequacy of intrinsic muscle release.

SWAN-NECK DEFORMITY

Clinical Findings

Swan-neck deformity is characterized by hyperextension of the PIP joint and flexion of the DIP joint (Figure 11–13). The pathophysiology of swan-neck deformity involves either volar plate incompetence or force imbalance on the PIP joint

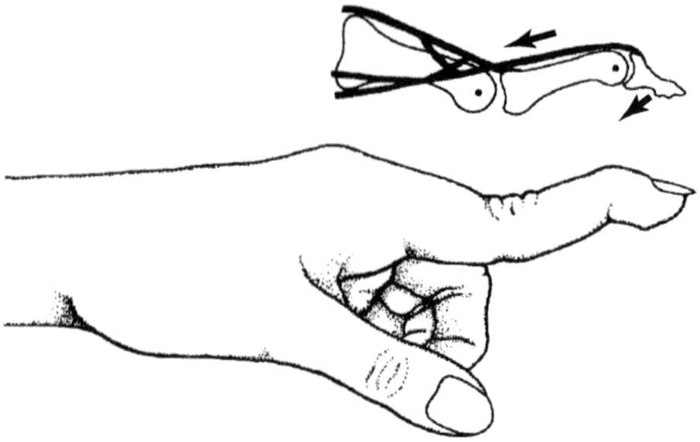

▲ **Figure 11–13.** **Swan-neck deformity.** (Reprinted with permission, from American Society for Surgery of the Hand. *The Hand: Examination and Diagnosis,* 2nd ed. Philadelphia: Churchill Livingstone; 1983.)

(extension force greater than flexion force). Synovitis of the PIP joint in patients with RA may distend the joint and attenuate the volar plate, which becomes ineffective in preventing PIP joint hyperextension. Force imbalance occurs with overly forceful intrinsic muscle contraction (as occurs with an intrinsic plus deformity), which transmits an abnormally high extension force on the PIP joint. Other common causes of force imbalance are mallet finger (the extension force is transmitted from the DIP joint to the proximal joint) and flexor digitorum superficialis lacerations.

In some fingers, a fixed extension contracture or ankylosis of the PIP joint may occur as a consequence of swan-neck deformity. In other fingers, the PIP joint remains supple, but the finger is locked in a hyperextended posture.

Treatment

The attenuated volar plate can be addressed with volar plate advancement. The force imbalance on the PIP joint can be restored with any of the following three procedures: (1) flexor digitorum superficialis tenodesis with rerouting over the A3 pulley, (2) spiral oblique retinacular ligament reconstruction in which one of the lateral bands is rerouted volar to the center of rotation of the PIP joint, or (3) central slip tenotomy (Fowler tenotomy).

FLEXOR TENDON INJURY

Following injury, the flexor tendon heals through both extrinsic and intrinsic mechanisms. Extrinsic tendon healing is stimulated by the surrounding synovial fluid, bringing inflammatory cells and fibroblasts to the site of repair by ingrowth of capillaries; this type of healing is responsible for adhesion formation at the repair site. Intrinsic healing occurs from tenocytes within the tendon. The goal of flexor tendon repair and postoperative care is to encourage both intrinsic and extrinsic healing without the formation of thick adhesions, which limit tendon excursion and ultimately result in restricted motion of the finger.

Anatomy and Clinical Findings

The extrinsic finger flexors are the flexor digitorum profundus and the flexor digitorum superficialis. Although the extrinsic flexors provide MCP joint flexion, this occurs only after most of their excursion is expended flexing the interphalangeal joints.

The flexor digitorum profundus originates from the proximal ulna and the interosseous membrane. In the forearm, it divides into two muscle groups: the most radial group goes to the index finger and the ulnar group goes to the middle, ring, and little fingers. The flexor digitorum profundus and the flexor pollicis longus muscles form the deep compartment of the volar forearm and their tendons occupy the floor of the carpal tunnel.

The tenosynovial sheath of the flexor pollicis longus is continuous with the radial bursa; the tenosynovial sheath to the little finger is continuous with the ulnar digital bursa. In some patients, these two bursae communicate, allowing a so-called horseshoe abscess to spread between the thumb and little finger if infection occurs in the flexor tendon sheath of either one of these digits.

The profundus tendon passes through the bifurcation of the flexor digitorum superficialis before inserting into the proximal palmar base of the distal phalanx. The innervation of the flexor digitorum profundus of the index and middle fingers is through the anterior interosseous branch of the median nerve, whereas the profundus of the ring and little fingers is innervated by the ulnar nerve. The flexor digitorum profundus provides digital flexion at both the PIP and DIP joints.

The flexor digitorum superficialis has two heads: the radial head originates from the proximal shaft of the radius, and the humeral ulnar head originates from the medial humeral epicondyle and coronoid process of the ulna. Each digit has a corresponding independent superficialis muscle. As the superficialis tendons pass through the carpal tunnel, the tendons of the middle and ring fingers are more superficial and central than those of the index and little fingers. In the proximal aspect of the finger, the flexor digitorum superficialis tendon bifurcates around the flexor digitorum profundus at the beginning of the A2 pulley to form the Camper's chiasm. The radial and ulnar slips rotate 180 degrees and insert into the proximal metaphysis of the middle phalanx. The entire flexor digitorum superficialis muscle receives innervation from the median nerve. The primary function of the superficialis is digital flexion at the PIP joint.

The flexor pollicis longus originates from two heads: the radial head takes origin from the proximal radius and interosseous membrane, and an accessory head originates from the coronoid process of the ulna and from the medial epicondyle of the humerus. In the palm, the flexor pollicis longus

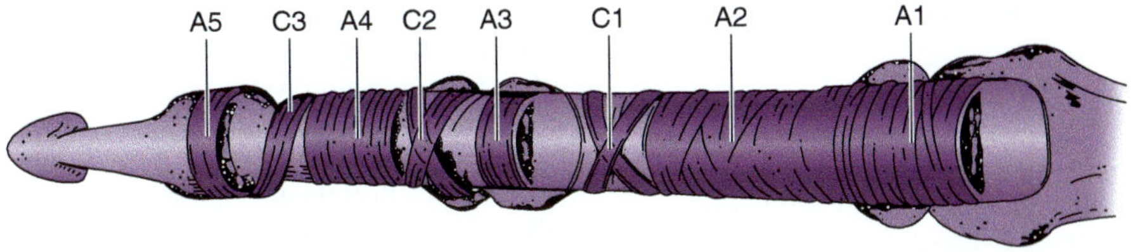

▲ **Figure 11–14.** Annular (A) and cruciate (C) pulley locations.

tendon transverses between the abductor pollicis brevis and the flexor pollicis brevis. The flexor pollicis longus inserts into the proximal base of the thumb distal phalanx and is innervated by the anterior interosseous branch of the median nerve. The flexor pollicis longus flexes both the interphalangeal and MCP joints of the thumb.

As the flexor tendons pass distal to the metacarpal neck, they enter the fibroosseous tunnel, consisting of the phalangeal bones and the flexor fibrous sheath. The fibroosseous tunnel extends distally to the proximal aspect of the distal phalanx. The fibrous sheath consists of annular pulleys, which provide mechanical stability, and cruciate pulleys, which provide flexibility (Figure 11–14). The first, third, and fifth annular pulleys (A1, A3, and A5) are located over the MCP, PIP, and DIP joints, respectively, and the second and fourth pulleys (A2 and A4) are situated over the middle portion of the proximal and middle phalanges. The A2 and A4 pulleys are the most essential in maintaining the mechanical advantage of the flexor tendons and preventing bowstringing.

Apart from the fibrous sheath, there is the synovial sheath (tenosynovium) that lines the tendons and supplies both nutrition and lubrication to the poorly vascularized flexor tendons. Proximal to the sheath, the tendons are well vascularized by the peritenon. Distal to the MCP joints, nutrition supply comes mainly through diffusion from the synovial sheath and through direct vascular supply from the vincular system: the vinculum longus and brevis.

The time since injury and the mechanism of injury (sharp, laceration, open injury vs avulsion, closed injury) should be noted in the history. On physical examination, the normal posture of the hand should be noted and presence of the tenodesis effect should be evaluated. Each tendon in each finger must be individually examined.

A. Normal Cascade of Fingers

The resting posture of the fingers should be observed. Disruption of the normal cascade of increasing flexion in the relaxed fingers from the index finger to the little finger should arouse suspicion of tendon disruption (Figure 11–15).

B. Normal Tenodesis Phenomenon

Tendon integrity may also be evaluated by taking advantage of the normal tenodesis positioning of the digits, which occurs as the wrist is passively brought through a ROM. Normally, as the wrist is extended, the digital extensors relax and the finger flexors become taut, passively flexing the fingers in the normal cascade pattern. When the muscles of the proximal forearm are squeezed, the fingers normally flex involuntarily.

C. Testing of Individual Tendons

Isolated testing of the superficialis and profundus tendons determines the integrity of each tendon (see Figures 11–2 and 11–3). Because the flexor digitorum superficialis of the little finger is not independent of the ring finger in many individuals, either because of cross connections between the two tendons or because of congenital absence of the tendon, it may be impossible from clinical examination to detect injury to the flexor digitorum superficialis tendon of the

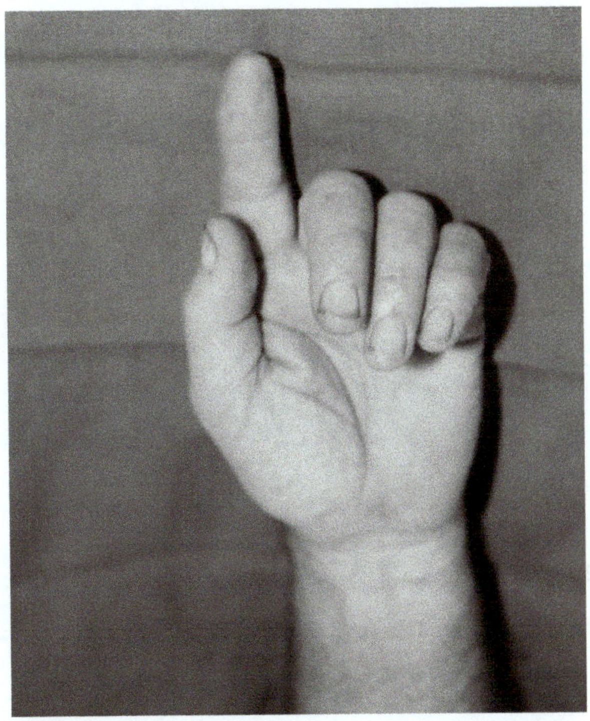

▲ **Figure 11–15.** If the index finger remains extended when the hand is at rest, its flexor tendons are severed.

little finger. The strength of flexion should be noted as each of the tendons is tested.

D. Partial Tears

Partial flexor tendon injuries are more difficult to diagnose because in this case patients retain a normal cascade of the fingers on inspection and they demonstrate a normal tenodesis phenomenon. Moreover, isolated active flexion of the interphalangeal joints is usually possible. However, if the patient is able to flex the finger but experiences pain with flexion and is unable to generate full power against resistance or if triggering is felt along the course of the tendon during flexion, a partial flexor tendon injury should be suspected.

Treatment

Traditionally, repair of flexor tendon injuries is performed under regional anesthesia. However, wide-awake surgery with local anesthetic, no tourniquet, and no sedation (WALANT) has gained ground over the past years. This method has the benefit that the patient is able to actively flex the digit, so surgeons can visualize the repair site to assess for any tendon gapping at the repair site and ensure smooth gliding through the A2 and A4 pulleys. In cases of partial tears of less than 50% of tendon width, conservative treatment with wound care and early ROM can be applied, although triggering commonly occurs.

Functional outcomes are equivalent if the repair is done the day of injury (primary repair) or within the first 7 to 14 days after the injury (delayed primary repair). Direct surgical repair can be performed within 3 weeks of injury, and afterward, flexor tendon reconstruction is needed.

Because repair requires proper visualization of both tendon stumps, the wound may need to be electively extended. The tendon ends must be gently retrieved because trauma to the flexor tendon sheath creates adverse scarring. Tendons should not be grasped along their tenosynovial surfaces. The A2 and A4 pulleys should be preserved. A maximum of 1 cm may be debrided from the tendon ends without compromising eventual digital extension. The core suture (suture crossing the repair site) should be either 3-0 or 4-0 of braided synthetic material (Figure 11–16).

The flexor tendon repair should be performed with four to six strands of suture crossing the repair site, rather than

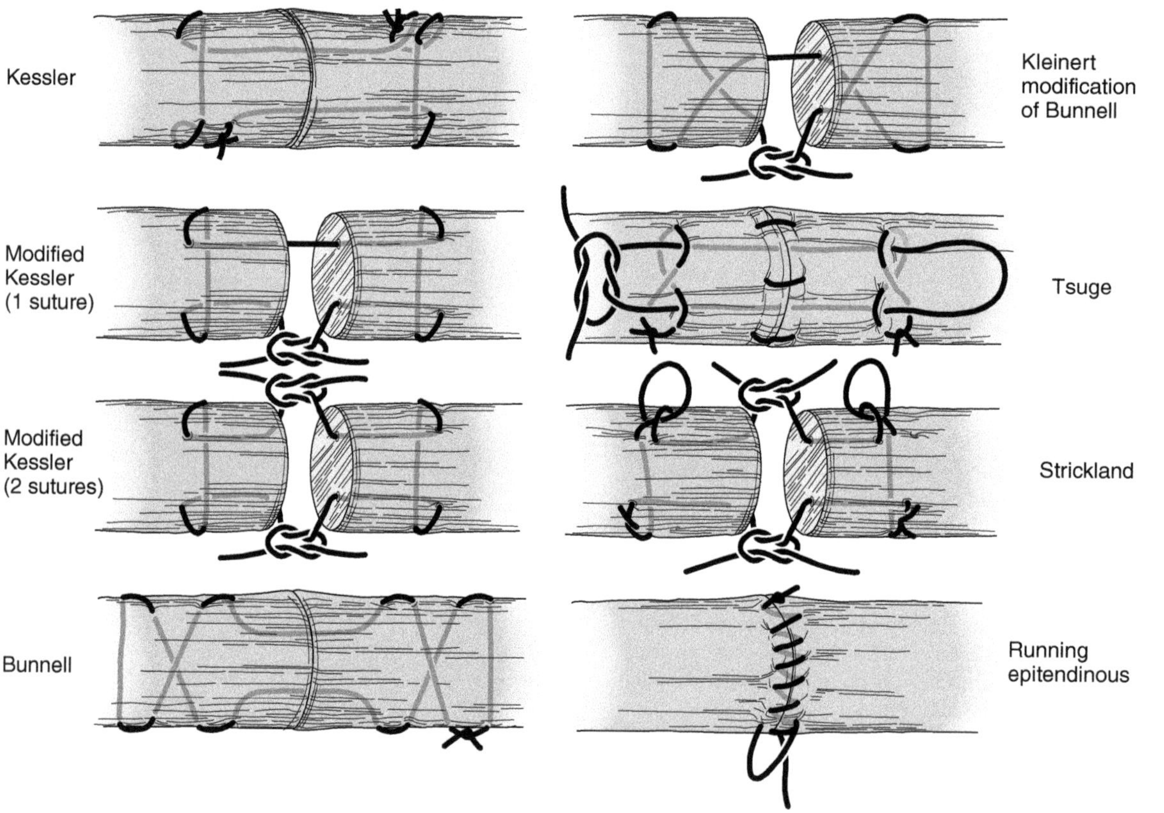

▲ Figure 11–16. Kessler sutures and other types of sutures for flexor tendon repair. (Reprinted with permission, from Green DP, ed. *Operative Hand Surgery,* 2nd ed. Philadelphia: Churchill Livingstone; 1988.)

two. Minimal gap between the stumps and smooth juncture of the tendon ends are essential. A running 6-0 nylon epitendinous suture strengthens the repair by 20% and facilitates gliding of the repair site. The role of flexor tendon sheath repair remains controversial. Regarding pulley management, studies have shown that incision of 25% of the A2 pulley and complete incisions of the A4 pulley do not result in functional deficits.

Because the results and complications of flexor tendon repair vary by level of injury, five zones of injury are defined (Figure 11–17). Zone I extends from the insertion of the profundus on the distal phalanx to the insertion of the flexor digitorum superficialis on the middle phalanx. The tendon may be directly repaired if the distal stump is large enough, or it may be reinserted to bone. Care must be taken not to advance the tendon more than 1 cm; otherwise, quadrigia effect with flexion lag in the adjacent digits (due to the common muscle belly of flexor digitorum profundus of small, ring, and long fingers) can occur.

Zone II, which extends from the proximal portion of the A1 pulley to the insertion of the superficialis tendon, is the most problematic region of injury because it contains both the profundus and superficialis tendons in a relatively avascular region. Repair in this zone has been historically linked with poor results due to high rate of adhesion formation and

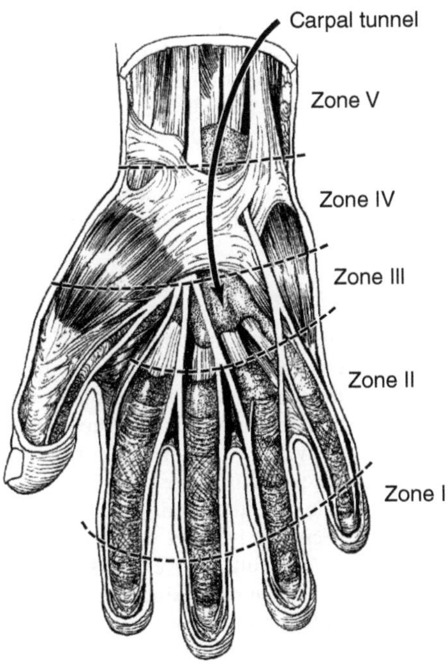

▲ **Figure 11–17. Flexor tendon injury zones.** (Reprinted from Way LW, ed. *Current Surgical Diagnosis & Treatment*, 10th ed. Stamford, CT: Appleton & Lange; 1994.)

stiffness. Care must be taken to preserve the vincular blood supply. When both the superficialis and profundus tendons are divided, it is preferable to repair both tendons because greater digital independence of motion may be achieved with a somewhat lower risk of tendon rupture during the rehabilitation period. Some authors recommend repair of only one slip of the superficialis to improve gliding. Repair of the superficialis tendon as well as the profundus tendon also diminishes the likelihood of PIP joint hyperextension deformity.

Zone III injuries are located between the proximal edge of the A1 pulley and the distal edge of the transverse carpal ligament.

In zone IV injuries, the area beneath the transverse carpal ligament, a step-cut release and repair of the transverse carpal ligament should be performed to prevent flexor tendon bowstringing. Like zone II, repair in this area is also associated with adhesion formation due to close proximity of the synovial sheaths. Zone V injuries are proximal to the transverse carpal ligament.

Zone I and II injuries of the thumb are handled similarly to those of analogous finger zones. In zone III of the thumb, it is difficult to access the flexor pollicis longus tendon as it passes through the thenar musculature. Options for treatment of injuries at this level include either primary tendon grafting or step-cut lengthening of the tendon in the forearm, so the repair is distal to the obscuring thenar muscles.

Improved results of flexor tendon surgery in recent years are substantially a result of the changes in postoperative rehabilitation protocols. Immobilization of the finger after tendon repair is appropriate only in very young or otherwise uncooperative patients. Following flexor tendon injury, the wrist should be immobilized at approximately 30 degrees of flexion, the MCP joints at approximately 45 degrees of flexion, and the interphalangeal joints at 0 to 15 degrees of flexion. Early passive ROM protocols are most commonly used today. Early initiation of passive ROM exercises decreases the adhesions at the repair site and enhances intrinsic tendon repair. Passive motion may be achieved either through rubber band splinting to flex the finger passively (Kleinert protocol) or by having the patient move the finger passively (Duran protocol). At 4 to 6 weeks following repair, active flexion and extension exercises are allowed as splinting is discontinued. At 6 to 8 weeks, passive extension exercises and isolated blocking are encouraged. After 8 weeks, the patient may begin flexion against resistance.

Early active motion protocol can also be applied with four- to six-strand repairs. Active assisted motion is begun within the first 2 weeks, and the wrist is extended and the fingers are passively flexed. The patient is then asked to flex the fingers actively to hold this position. In properly motivated and cooperative patients, an active hold program is begun during the first week. The therapist passively brings the hand into flexion, and the patient is asked to maintain the position.

Flexor Tendon Avulsion Injuries

The flexor tendon may be avulsed from its bony insertion, usually by forced extension of the finger while the finger is simultaneously actively flexed. An estimated 75% of flexor digitorum profundus avulsion injuries involve the ring finger. Such injuries occur in football and rugby, when the athlete grabs an opponent's jersey and a finger is involuntarily extended as the opponent attempts to elude tackle, and is then known as "jersey finger."

Flexor digitorum profundus avulsion injuries may be classified according to the level of profundus tendon retraction (Leddy classification). In type 1 injuries, the tendon retracts proximally from the sheath into the palm and vascular supply to the tendon is completely disrupted. Repair of these injuries should be performed within 7 to 10 days to avoid myostatic contracture, which will limit the ability to bring the tendon to its normal insertion without undue tension. In type 2 injuries, the tendon retracts to the level of the PIP joint. The tendon may be reinserted into the distal phalanx within several weeks after injury. Type 3 injuries involve an osseous distal phalangeal avulsion fragment that is so large it blocks retraction of the flexor digitorum profundus proximal to the A4 pulley. These injuries also may be repaired within several weeks after injury. In type 4 injuries, there is a bony fragment with simultaneous avulsion of the tendon from the fragment. In these cases, open reduction and internal fixation (ORIF) of the fragment should be performed first, followed by reattachment of the tendon to the osseous fragment. In all types, the tendon can either be repaired directly or be reinserted with a dorsal button. Missed or neglected profundus avulsion injuries, if symptomatic, may be treated by staged tendon reconstruction, DIP joint arthrodesis, or tenodesis.

Flexor Tendon Reconstruction

Direct repair of a disrupted flexor tendon is not possible if there is loss of the tendon substance, in chronic cases that are greater than 3 weeks old, or when there is myostatic contracture. If the flexor digitorum superficialis tendon is intact with a full active range of PIP joint motion, arthrodesis or tenodesis of the DIP joint may be elected, creating a so-called superficialis finger. If the patient requires active motion at the DIP joint, tendon reconstruction is necessary. Tendon reconstruction is usually indicated when neither flexor digitorum superficialis nor flexor digitorum profundus tendons can be repaired.

Primary tendon reconstruction may be performed only when the annular pulley system is pristine and full ROM of the joints is present. Otherwise, a two-stage reconstruction is recommended. In stage 1, the tendon remnants are excised from the sheath, and joint contractures are released. At a minimum, the A2 and A4 pulleys are reconstructed using a flexor tendon remnant, a tendon graft, or a strip of the wrist extensor retinaculum. A silicone rod similar in size to the anticipated tendon graft is secured to the distal phalanx and threaded through the sheath. Early passive ROM stimulates the development of a pseudosheath surrounding the silicone tendon rod.

The second stage of the procedure occurs at least 3 months after the initial procedure. Prior to the second stage, a satisfactory skin coverage and sensation, full passive range of MCP and interphalangeal joint motion, adequate digital circulation, and at least one intact digital nerve are required. Stage 2 tendon reconstruction can be performed either with tendon graft (Hunter's procedure) or by using the flexor digitorum superficialis that has been previously (during the first stage) sutured to the proximal stump of flexor digitorum profundus in the palm (Paneva-Holevich technique). The silicone tendon rod is replaced with a tendon graft. The donor tendon is secured to the distal phalanx, and in case of tendon grafting, the proximal attachment of the donor tendon to the profundus motor is performed either with a tendon weave or an end-to-end repair. Possible donor tendon sources for tendon grafting include the palmaris longus, plantaris, or toe extensor tendons. The palmaris longus and plantaris tendons are absent in a significant minority of individuals (15% for palmaris longus and 19% for plantaris tendon).

Establishing appropriate tension on the tendon graft is critical. If insufficient tension is placed on the tendon graft, a lumbrical plus deformity occurs. With this condition, as the patient pulls the proximal portion of the profundus tendon proximally, the lumbrical is placed under tension, and all of this tension is transmitted to the dorsal hood apparatus rather than to the flexor tendon graft. As a result, as the patient attempts to flex the finger, the finger paradoxically extends both the PIP and DIP joints. If the tendon graft tension is too tight, full extension is impossible. The results of primary tendon grafting are inferior to primary repair in similar circumstances.

A. Complications

1. Adhesions—The most common complication following flexor tendon surgery is formation of adhesions between the repair site and the surrounding fibroosseous tunnel, which may occur despite an appropriate therapy program. Although physical therapy can be attempted, surgical treatment with tenolysis is required in more than 50% of flexor tendon repairs. Tenolysis should be considered when there is a discrepancy between passive and active ROM, with restricted active flexion and full passive ROM. Soft-tissue stabilization (usually at least 3 months since repair or reconstruction) is a prerequisite for tenolysis.

Ideally, tenolysis should be performed under local anesthesia with intravenous sedation. Elevation of skin flaps allows wide exposure of the sheath. Care is taken to preserve the annular pulleys while adhesions are released between the tendon and the sheath and between the tendon and the phalanges. Evaluation of the adequacy of lysis may be obtained by asking the patient under local anesthesia to flex the finger actively. If regional or general anesthesia is employed, the tendon must be identified at a more proximal level and traction applied to the tendon at this level to confirm the improvement in joint motion.

Active ROM exercise is begun within the first 24 hours after surgery. Electrical stimulation of the proximal muscle belly may facilitate early motion.

2. Tendon repair rupture—The second major postoperative complication of flexor tendon repair is rupture of the repair (15%-25%). When the rupture is promptly diagnosed, a second repair should be attempted because success rates approach those of uncomplicated primary repair. If rupture is not promptly diagnosed, management is based on the length of the scar. If the scar is less than 1 cm, it is resected and primary repair is performed. In cases with a scar greater than 1 cm, either free tendon grafting (when annular pulley system is not collapsed) or staged tendon reconstruction (when the sheath is collapsed) is recommended.

3. Failure of staged reconstruction—If staged reconstruction fails, arthrodesis or amputation of the digit may be considered, particularly when accompanied by neurovascular compromise.

4. Joint contracture—This complication can occur in up to 17% of the cases.

Giesen T, Reissner L, Besmens I, Politikou O, Calcagni M. Flexor tendon repair in the hand with the M-Tang technique (without peripheral sutures), pulley division, and early active motion. *J Hand Surg Eur Vol.* 2018;43(5):474-479. [PMID: 29458310]

Gil JA, Skjong C, Katarincic JA, Got C. Flexor tendon repair with looped suture: 1 versus 2 knots. *J Hand Surg Am.* 2016;41(3):422-426. [PMID: 26787411]

Piper SL, Wheeler LC, Mills JK, Ezaki M, Oishi SN. Outcomes after primary repair and staged reconstruction of zone I and II flexor tendon injuries in children. *J Pediatr Orthop.* 2019;39(5):263-267. [PMID: 30969257]

Reissner L, Zechmann-Mueller N, Klein HJ, Calcagni M, Giesen T. Sonographic study of repair, gapping and tendon bowstringing after primary flexor digitorum profundus repair in zone 2. *J Hand Surg Eur Vol.* 2018;43(5):480-486. [PMID: 29554845]

Strickland JW, Schmidt CC. Repair of flexor digitorum profundus lacerations: the Indiana method. *Oper Tech Orthopaed.* 1998;8:73-85. [No PMID]

TENOSYNOVITIS

Tenosynovitis may develop in any of the extrinsic flexor or extensor tendons, either throughout their course or, more commonly, at points of constraint by fibrous pulleys or retinacular sheaths.

1. de Quervain Tenosynovitis

Clinical Findings

In this type of tenosynovitis, the extensor retinaculum over the first dorsal compartment becomes thickened, causing friction of the abductor pollicis longus and extensor pollicis brevis tendons as they glide beneath the retinacular pulley at the radial styloid region. Overuse, posttraumatic, and postpartum conditions are risk factors. Radial-sided wrist pain is provoked by lifting activity in which the thumb is adducted and flexed while the hand is ulnarly deviated. Activities such as inflating a blood pressure cuff, picking up an infant out of a crib, or lifting a heavy frying pan off the stove may provoke pain along the radial aspect of the wrist.

Physical examination reveals tenderness directly over the first extensor compartment. A provocative maneuver, the Finkelstein test, is helpful in diagnosing this disorder (Figure 11–18).

Treatment

First line of treatment includes rest, nonsteroidal anti-inflammatory drugs (NSAIDs), and splinting. Immobilization limits extensor pollicis brevis tendon excursion using a forearm-based thumb spica splint, which prevents both wrist deviation and thumb CMC and MCP motion while allowing interphalangeal joint motion. Steroid injection into the first extensor compartment along the course of the extensor pollicis brevis is usually the second step in conservative management and overall is superior to splinting in alleviating symptoms. However, multiple corticosteroid injections or a single high-dose corticosteroid injection can result in

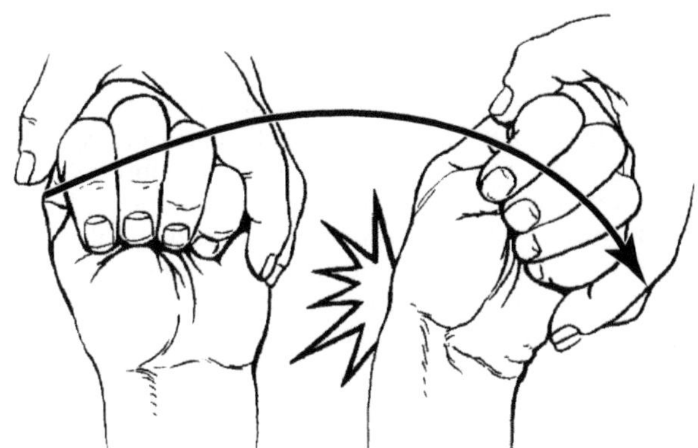

▲ **Figure 11–18.** Finkelstein maneuver. The patient's thumb is enclosed in the palm. The wrist is then abruptly deviated ulnarward by the examiner. In a positive test, pain is produced on the radial border of the wrist. (Reprinted with permission, from Lister G. *The Hand: Diagnosis and Indications*, 3rd ed. Philadelphia: Churchill Livingstone; 1993.)

marked fat atrophy over the radial styloid and skin discoloration. Although skin discoloration usually resolves after 1 year, fat atrophy does not resolve, and it leads to permanent irritation in this area. These complications are far more likely when the steroid is injected over the sheath into the subcutaneous fat and not directly into the sheath.

If de Quervain tenosynovitis is unresponsive to conservative care, surgical release of the overlying retinaculum may be elected. Because most patients with symptomatic disease have more than one abductor pollicis longus slip, the extensor pollicis brevis tendon must be identified and decompressed. In some cases, the first extensor compartment is divided by a septum, creating two separate tendon sheaths. In such cases, the more dorsal component sheath must also be opened to allow unconstrained extensor pollicis brevis tendon gliding.

Extreme caution must be exercised in carrying out the skin incision and subcutaneous dissection in this region because injury to the sensory branch of the radial nerve as it runs over the first compartment is a troublesome complication that may overshadow any benefit from tendon decompression. Moreover, the compartment should be incised dorsal in order to prevent volar subluxation of the tendons.

2. Flexor Stenotic Tenosynovitis (Trigger Finger)

Clinical Findings

Flexor tenosynovitis or tenovaginitis is caused by mechanical inhibition of smooth tendon gliding at the level of the A1 pulley, due to fibrocartilaginous metaplasia of the tendon and/or pulley. Occasionally, a pathologic nodule on the tendon may cause the mechanical block. It affects 2% to 3% of the population, and most commonly, the ring and long fingers are involved. The condition is characterized by pain and tenderness in the palm at the proximal edge of the digital A1 pulley (Figure 11–19). Patients frequently note catching or triggering of the affected finger or thumb after forceful flexion. In more severe cases, the opposite hand must be used to force the finger or thumb passively into extension. In the most severe cases, the finger becomes locked in a flexed position. Triggering is often more pronounced in the morning than later in the day. Stenosing tenosynovitis is more common in diabetic patients. When multiple digits are involved, the possibility of diabetes should be considered. In addition, in 60% of the cases, flexor tenosynovitis is associated with EMG findings consistent with carpal tunnel syndrome.

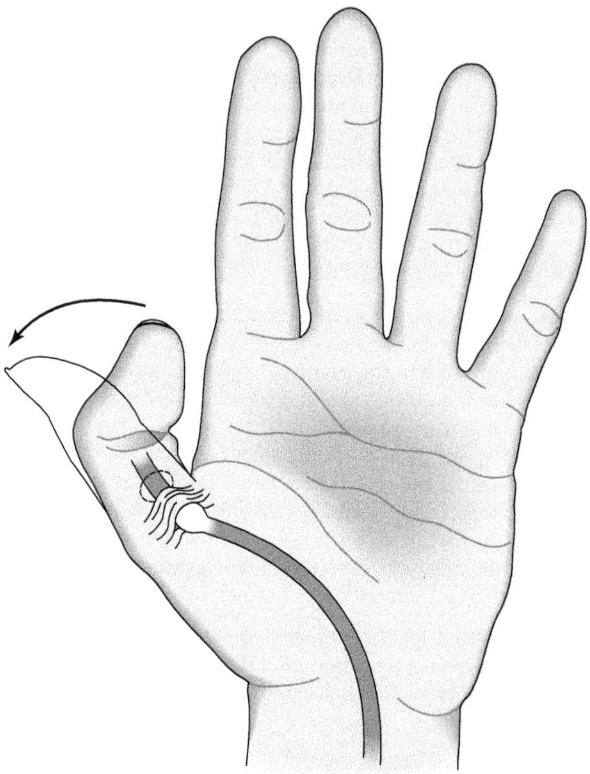

▲ **Figure 11–19.** Trigger thumb. (Reprinted with permission, from American Society for Surgery of the Hand. *The Hand: Examination and Diagnosis*, 2nd ed. Philadelphia: Churchill Livingstone; 1983.)

Treatment

A long-acting steroid injection into the flexor sheath is successfully in 60% to 90% of patients, although diabetics are less likely to respond. To inject a trigger finger, the needle is inserted at the proximal palmar crease for the index finger and the distal palmar crease for the middle, ring, and small fingers. The needle enters the flexor tendon, and pressure is applied to the plunger. The needle is slowly backed out until the needle is between the tendon and the tendon sheath, discerned by loss of plunger resistance. One milliliter of a combination of a short-acting anesthetic and steroid is given. The injection may be repeated if symptoms recur after an initially positive response to injection.

Surgical release of the A1 pulley is curative in digits refractory to steroid injection in more than 90% of the cases. Release is accomplished by directly exposing the pulley and incising its transversely oriented fibers longitudinally. The fibers of the A2 pulley must be spared to preserve effective digital flexion. In patients with RA, the entire annular pulley system should be preserved to minimize further ulnar drift of the fingers at the MCP joint. Triggering in these patients is treated by tenosynovectomy and excision of the ulnar slip of the flexor digitorum superficialis. Resection of one slip of the flexor digitorum superficialis may be also performed in recurrent triggering after A1 pulley release.

3. Flexor Carpi Radialis Tenosynovitis

Clinical Findings

Flexor carpi radialis tenosynovitis is uncommon. Inflammation of the tendon can be primary as a stenosing tenosynovitis throughout its fibroosseous tunnel or secondary to scaphoid fracture, distal radius fracture, or scaphotrapeziotrapezoidal (STT) or CMC arthritis. This condition is characterized by pain in the volar radial aspect of the wrist that is aggravated by active wrist flexion or passive wrist dorsiflexion. Marked tenderness is elicited on palpation along its course over the distal palmar wrist crease.

Treatment

Conservative care includes splinting the wrist in flexion and administration of oral anti-inflammatory medication. If these measures are ineffective, a long-acting steroid may be injected in close proximity to the tendon, but not into the tendon. Steroid injection is successful in primary tendinitis, but not in secondary tendinitis when there is an anatomic cause for inflammation.

Surgical release of the flexor carpi radialis sheath is rarely needed but can be considered when conservative measures fail. During surgical decompression, the tendon sheath is incised in the distal forearm up to the trapezial crest as it enters its fibroosseous tunnel. At this point, the fibroosseous sheath is further incised along its ulnar margin with caution not to injure the tendon.

Mangukiya HJ, Kale A, Mahajan NP, Ramteke U, Manna J. Functional outcome of De Quervain's tenosynovitis with longitudinal incision in surgically treated patients. *Musculoskelet Surg.* 2019;103(3):269-273. [PMID: 30600438]

Schwaiger K, Ensat F, Neureiter D, Wechselberger G, Hladik M. Trigger finger caused by extraskeletal chondroma. *J Hand Surg Am.* 2017;42(1):e51-e55. [PMID: 27817941]

Shultz KJ, Kittinger JL, Czerwinski WL, Weber RA. Outcomes of corticosteroid treatment for trigger finger by stage. *Plast Reconstr Surg.* 2018;142(4):983-990. [PMID: 29994845]

Wu F, Rajpura A, Sandher D. Finkelstein's test is superior to Eichhoff's test in the investigation of de Quervain's disease. *J Hand Microsurg.* 2018;10(2):116-118. [PMID: 30154628]

VASCULAR DISORDERS OF THE HAND

Anatomy

The blood supply to the hand is predominantly through the ulnar and radial arteries contributing to the superficial and deep palmar arches. The ulnar artery is larger than the radial artery and provides the primary arterial contribution to the hand. In most hands, the ulnar artery, which lies lateral to the ulnar nerve in the wrist, mainly supplies the superficial palmar arch. The superficial palmar arch provides the principal blood supply to the common and proper digital arteries. At the wrist, the radial artery bifurcates into a branch to the superficial palmar arch and a branch that passes dorsally around the scaphoid and trapezium deep to the flexor carpi radialis, the abductor pollicis longus, and extensor pollicis brevis tendons on the floor of the anatomic snuffbox, and then dives palmarward between the two heads of the first dorsal interosseous muscle to contribute to the deep palmar arch. Before entering the first dorsal interosseous muscle, it gives off the superficial radial branch, which contributes to the superficial palmar arch. Supplemental arteries include the anterior and posterior interosseous arteries. The median artery, a remnant of the embryologic vascular supply to the developing upper limb, contributes to the superficial palmar arch in 10% of patients.

The superficial palmar arch is located about 1 cm distal to the deep palmar arch. The superficial palmar arch is complete in 80% of individuals and incomplete in the other 20%. The deep palmar arch is located at the level of metacarpal bases and gives branches to the common digital arteries. The deep arch is complete, giving branches to all common digital arteries in 97% of individuals. The princeps pollicis artery is derived from the deep palmar arch in 98% of patients. The deep palmar arch also supplies the deep metacarpal arterial branches, which provide secondary blood flow to the digital arteries.

Clinical Findings

Patients with vascular insufficiency frequently complain of pain and cold intolerance. In some cases, symptoms of ulnar nerve compression may also present. On physical examination, inspection may reveal color changes. Paleness or whiteness of the fingers is more suggestive of loss of inflow, whereas redness or bluish discoloration suggests inadequate venous return. Ulcerations of the tips of the fingers may also be noted, denoting ischemia. A pulsatile mass indicating arterial aneurysm can also be seen or palpated. Physical examination should always include the Allen test, as described in the next section.

The duration of vascular symptoms should be noted. If the abnormality is congenital in origin, changes in symptoms over time should be documented. The occupational history should be recorded because workers who use vibrating tools, such as carpenters, machinists, and mechanics, are at high risk of developing vascular occlusion disorders. Also, occupations requiring outdoor work in all seasons (construction) or in a cold, indoor environments (butchering) are noted. A history of trauma may suggest arterial or periarterial damage. Any sports activities that involve repeated trauma to the hand should be recorded; golfers, baseball catchers, and handball players are particularly at risk of closed vascular injury. Exposure to vasoconstrictive drugs such as beta-blockers and tobacco abuse should also be noted, as should other diseases with known vascular effects such as scleroderma and diabetes. Pulses are palpated, noting thrills or bruits.

A. Provocative Tests

The Allen test allows assessment of the extent of connection between the radial and ulnar arteries through the palmar arches. The examiner compresses both the radial and ulnar arteries at the wrist and then asks the patient to squeeze and release the hand repetitively. After the hand blanches, pressure is released from the radial artery while compression is maintained on the ulnar artery. The examiner observes how long it takes for each of the fingers to regain its pink color. The initial step is repeated with both vessels compressed, and the ulnar artery occlusion is then released while pressure is maintained on the radial artery. Again, examination of the reperfusion of the fingers reveals which digits are primarily supplied through the ulnar artery. In this fashion, the extent of interconnections between the radial and ulnar arteries may be assessed.

Cold stress testing is a technique that evaluates the effect of cold on arterial spasm. During this test, the hand is submersed in ice water for 20 seconds. In cases of arterial disease, return to preexposure temperatures occurs in greater than 20 minutes, compared with normal subjects, who require approximately 10 minutes.

B. Diagnostic Studies

Noninvasive vascular diagnostic studies include color duplex ultrasonography, which detects the presence of flow, and plethysmography, which records the pulse volume difference between brachial and digital arteries. Invasive diagnostic procedures include arteriography, which is the gold standard, digital subtraction arteriography, and three-phase bone scan, during which phase 2 images may show decreased flow indicating vasospastic disorders.

ARTERIAL OCCLUSION

1. Arterial Trauma

Clinical Findings

Partial or complete disruption of an artery may occur as the result of lacerations, acute injection trauma, or cannulation injuries. Hemorrhage from arterial disruption should initially be treated with direct pressure. Total arterial disruption must be repaired if distal vascularity is inadequate. Partial arterial injuries may bleed profusely because the lacerated vessel ends are tethered to one another and are unable to retract, constrict, and occlude further flow. Partial arterial injury may require resection with or without reconstruction to prevent the formation of aneurysms or arteriovenous fistulas. Injection injury may produce either spasm or occlusion.

Treatment

The primary objective in treating arterial injuries is the restoration of adequate distal blood flow. Before the anastomosis of the artery, any clots in the vascular lumen should be removed. Fogarty catheters may be helpful in larger arteries, and if this is unsuccessful or in smaller vessels, anticoagulants or clot-dissolving agents such as heparin or urokinase may be injected. In case of suspected vascular spasm that blocks the blood flow, local or systemic vasodilators can be administered, or a stellate ganglion block can be employed. Care must be taken when using multiple agents to ensure they do not interfere with one another. For instance, use of urokinase after an axillary block may produce axillary artery hemorrhage, thereby compounding the problem.

2. Occlusive Vascular Disease

Etiologies include thrombosis due to blunt or penetrating arterial trauma, atherosclerosis, emboli, and a variety of systemic diseases. Systemic diseases include small-vessel occlusive diseases such as Buerger disease, systemic lupus erythematosus (SLE), RA, Sjögren syndrome, and dermatomyositis.

Clinical Findings

The most common occlusive vascular disease in the hand is hypothenar hammer syndrome. In these patients, the ulnar artery is thrombosed as a result of repetitive trauma to the hypothenar area of the hand. Patients with hypothenar hammer syndrome may complain of a tender pulsatile mass on the ulnar side of the palm. In some instances, presenting symptoms are that of a low ulnar nerve palsy because of compression of the ulnar nerve by the aneurysm at the level of Guyon's canal. Distal vascular insufficiency may be evident in the ring and little fingers.

Treatment

Surgical treatment of hypothenar hammer syndrome is based on whether evaluation demonstrates that all the fingers are well perfused by the radial artery alone. In such cases, excision of the segment of the ulnar artery containing the aneurysm or thrombosed segment and ligation of the vessel ends are curative. Sympathectomy through simple division of the sympathetic fibers that surround the vessel may confer a modest sympathectomy effect to the residual ulnar artery, alleviating symptoms. If, however, digital perfusion is inadequate after a vessel segment is resected and the tourniquet deflated, a segmental vein graft is required to reconstitute the ulnar artery. In cases of embolic disease in small vessels, thrombolytic agents including tissue plasminogen activator (TPA), streptokinase, or urokinase should be administered if diagnosis is made within 36 hours.

3. Aneurysm

A distinction should be made between true and false aneurysms. In a true aneurysm, all layers of the arterial wall are involved. These aneurysms are usually caused by blunt trauma but may also be secondary to degeneration or infection. False aneurysms are characterized by partial wall involvement, with periarterial tissues forming a false wall lined by endothelium. False aneurysms most commonly occur following penetrating trauma, or they can result from iatrogenic trauma, as in cases of radial artery injury during harvest of distal radius vascularized bone grafts for the treatment of scaphoid nonunions.

Both true and false aneurysms should be treated with resection. If, however, digital perfusion is inadequate after a vessel segment is resected and the tourniquet deflated, a segmental vein graft is required to reconstitute the artery.

VASOSPASTIC CONDITIONS

In these conditions, exposure to cold turns fingers initially white due to vasospasm, then blue due to venous stasis, and finally red from rebound hyperemia. Raynaud phenomenon (or Raynaud syndrome) and Raynaud disease are often confused. Raynaud phenomenon is a condition associated with another underlying cause such as connective tissue disorders such as SLE, neurologic disorders, arterial occlusive disorders, or blood dyscrasias or hematologic diseases. Raynaud disease (primary Raynaud) is present when Raynaud phenomenon occurs without another associated or causative disease. As opposed to Raynaud phenomenon, Raynaud disease most commonly occurs in young women less than 40 years old and is often bilateral. Patients with Raynaud disease usually do not present with severe symptoms leading to gangrene or atrophic changes, whereas this is more common in patients with Raynaud phenomenon.

Lifestyle modification including smoking cessation and avoidance of cold are the first line of treatment. Protection of the hands from cold with the use of gloves or mittens is also recommended. Medical treatment attempts to diminish occlusive phenomena. Alpha-receptor blocking agents, nitroglycerin ointment, nifedipine, and other calcium channel blockers are effective in decreasing spasm, whereas other vasodilators such as dipyridamole, pentoxifylline, and sildenafil can also be used. Botulinum toxin type A (Botox) injection around the neurovascular bundles in the palm can also help in patients who do not respond to medication. Digital artery sympathectomy, the surgical stripping of the periarterial tissue of the common digital artery over a short segment at the distal palmar level, may improve circulation to ischemic digits.

Karapolat S, Turkyilmaz A, Tekinbas C. Effects of endoscopic thoracic sympathectomy on Raynaud's disease. *J Laparoendosc Adv Surg Tech A*. 2018;28(6):726-729. [PMID: 29327980]

Lee ZH, Cohen JM, Daar D, Anzai L, Hacquebord J, Thanik V. Quantifying outcomes for leech therapy in digit revascularization and replantation. *J Hand Surg Eur Vol*. 2019;44(4):414-418. [PMID: 30636508]

Letamendia A, López-Román J, Bustamante-Munguira J, Herreros J. Digital periarterial sympathectomy in the management of post-traumatic Raynaud syndrome. *J Vasc Surg*. 2016;63(2):459-465. [PMID: 26506940]

DISORDERS OF THE NERVES OF THE HAND

PERIPHERAL NERVE INJURY

Nerve injuries may be stretching injuries, crushing injuries, or lacerations.

Anatomy

Peripheral nerves consist of a mixture of myelinated and unmyelinated axons. Motor, sensory, and sympathetic fibers often travel together in a single nerve. Axons are grouped in bundles termed *fascicles,* which are surrounded by perineurium. The fine connective tissue between axons within a fascicle is called endoneurium. Fascicles are held together as a nerve by the epineurium. Nerves are considered monofascicular, oligofascicular, or polyfascicular, depending on the number of fascicles. The relationship between fascicles changes along the longitudinal course of the nerve. The degree of fascicular change decreases distally. The mesoneurium, which is the connective tissue surrounding the epineurium, facilitates longitudinal gliding of the nerve.

After a nerve is injured, a number of changes occur. The somatosensory brain cortex reorganizes that the area innervated by the injured nerve is diminished. The cell body of the lacerated axon increases in size. The production of materials for repair of the cytoskeleton is increased, and the production of neurotransmitters decreases. At the proximal segment of the injured axon, further proximal degeneration occurs based on the severity of the injury. In the axon distal to the laceration, the so-called Wallerian degeneration occurs. The axoplasm and the myelin are degraded by phagocytes. Following this degradation, Schwann cells start to proliferate and form endoneurial base membrane. The proximal end starts to sprout axons that use the neural matrix that was formed by the Schwann cells in the distal segment and connect with the distal segment. The nerve regeneration through axonal migration propagates 1 mm/day.

Changes also occur at the neuromuscular junction. The muscle fibers can develop atrophy over time because endplates start to degenerate after a certain period of absence of afferent nerve signals. Muscle reinnervation occurs only if the axon reaches the muscle within a year. In contrast, sensory receptors may be effectively reinnervated years after the injury. Strength recovery is greater after primary nerve repair, less vigorous after repair with nerve grafting, and weakest after direct implantation of the nerve end into muscle.

Based on Seddon classification, nerve injuries are classified into three types. (1) Neurapraxia (same as Sunderland first degree) is a conduction block due to focal temporary demyelination, but the axons remain intact. Recovery is usually complete within days to a few months. (2) Axonotmesis (same as Sunderland second to fourth degree) describes an injury in which axonal disruption occurs, with the endoneurial tube remaining in continuity. The intact endoneurial tube provides the regenerating sprouting axons with a well-defined path to the end organs. Because axonal growth occurs at approximately 1 mm/day, recovery is good but slow. In some cases, though, neuroma-in-continuity can be formed. (3) Neurotmesis (same as Sunderland fifth degree) refers to complete transection of the nerve. Unless the nerve is repaired, the regenerating axons cannot find a suitable path and recovery does not occur. The frustrated sprouting axons form a neuroma at the distal end of the proximal segment of the lacerated nerve.

Clinical Findings

Patients complain of sensory deficits such as paresthesias or complete loss of sensation, pain, and weakness. Neurological physical examination of the hand includes assessment of motor and sensory function. This evaluation includes quantitative measurement of pinch and grip strength, static and moving two-point discrimination, and vibration and pressure measurements. Two-point discrimination reflects innervation density, whereas vibration and pressure measurements gauge innervation threshold.

Diagnostic Studies

Nerve conduction studies including EMG and conduction velocity studies are usually recommended to assess the location and the severity of the nerve injury. EMG may reveal fibrillations, positive sharp waves, and fasciculations, whereas conduction velocity study may reveal increased latencies, decreased velocities, and decreased motor and sensory action potentials.

Treatment

Observation with sequential EMG at 3 months is indicated in cases of neuropraxia or minimal axonotmesis (second degree based on Sunderland classification). Nerve repair should be carried out with magnification and microsurgical technique in more severe cases of axonotmesis or in case of neurotmesis. A tension-free repair provides the ideal environment for nerve regeneration. Tension at the repair site may be diminished by advancement of the nerve (ie, anterior transposition of the ulnar nerve for proximal forearm ulnar nerve laceration) or by limitation of joint motion. Repair yields better results when performed within 7 to 14 days of the injury. Epineurial repair is usually performed under magnification, using 8-0 or 9-0 suture (Figure 11–20A). When a

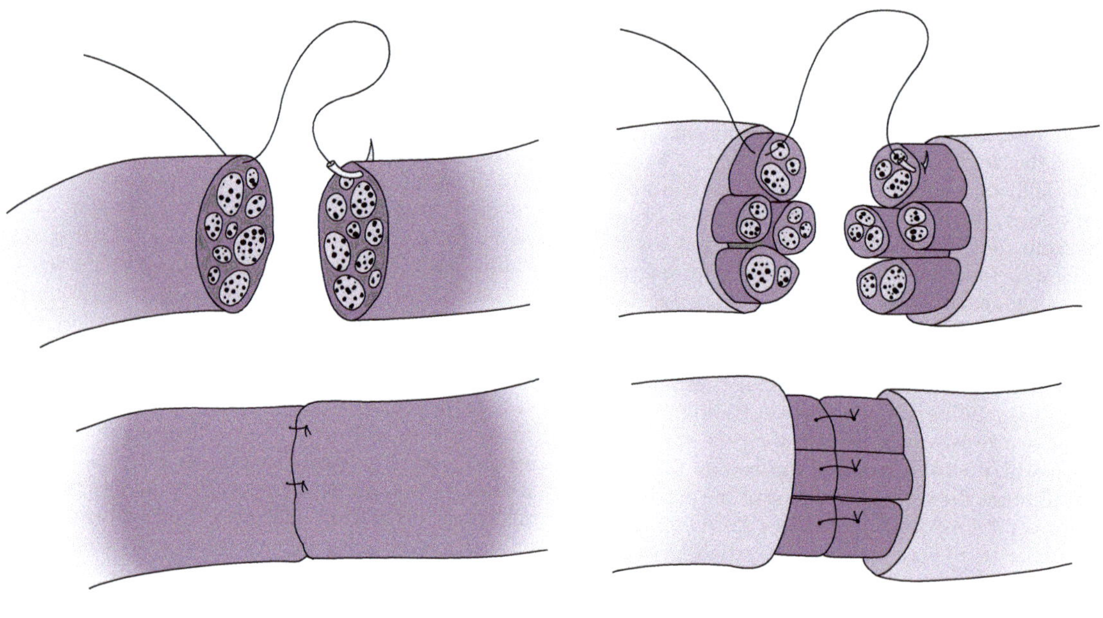

A. Epineurial repair

B. Group fascicular repair

▲ **Figure 11–20. A:** Schematic diagram of epineurial repair technique. **B:** Group fascicular repair technique. (Reprinted with permission, from Mackinnon SE, Dellon AL. *Surgery of the Peripheral Nerve.* New York: Thieme; 1988.)

particular fascicular group (eg, motor branch of the median nerve) is recognized as mediating a specific function, it may be repaired separately (Figure 11–20B). Fascicular and epineural repair have similar outcomes. Postoperative therapy may include motor and sensory reeducation to maximize the clinical result.

If a tension-free repair is impossible due to a large gap between the nerve ends, nerve grafting with autografts or allografts is necessary to bridge the defect. Frequently used autografts include the sural nerve, the anterior branch of the medial antebrachial cutaneous nerve, and the lateral antebrachial cutaneous nerve. Nerve defects up to 20 mm can be also managed by placing and securing the severed ends of the nerve within a conduit (synthetic or vein) that permits the uninterrupted regeneration of axons from the proximal nerve end.

Primary nerve repair is indicated after a sharp nerve division occurs. After avulsion injuries, repair even by nerve grafting cannot be performed until the proximal and distal extent of injury is known. When closed nerve injury occurs, sensory and motor function is closely monitored. If no recovery is seen within 3 months, electrodiagnostic studies are carried out. If no electrical evidence of recovery is documented, the nerve is explored, and neurolysis, secondary nerve repair, or nerve grafting is accomplished.

COMPRESSIVE NEUROPATHIES

Compressive neuropathies are a group of nerve injuries that have common etiological factors and occur at predictable sites of normal anatomic constraint. Nerve dysfunction is the result of neural ischemia in the compressed segment. Symptoms may resolve after release of the anatomic structures producing pressure on the nerve, particularly when compression is neither severe nor long standing.

1. Median Neuropathy

Carpal Tunnel Syndrome

A. Anatomy and Clinical Findings

Median nerve compressive neuropathy within the carpal tunnel is the most common compressive neuropathy in the body. The carpal tunnel is an osteoligamentous tunnel along the palmar aspect of the wrist anatomically defined by the scaphoid tubercle and the trapezium radially, the hook of the hamate and the pisiform ulnarly, the capitate dorsally, and the transverse carpal ligament palmarly (Figure 11–21). Carpal tunnel syndrome is most often idiopathic, and the most common cause in idiopathic carpal tunnel syndrome is pathologic and inflamed synovium. Risk factors for carpal

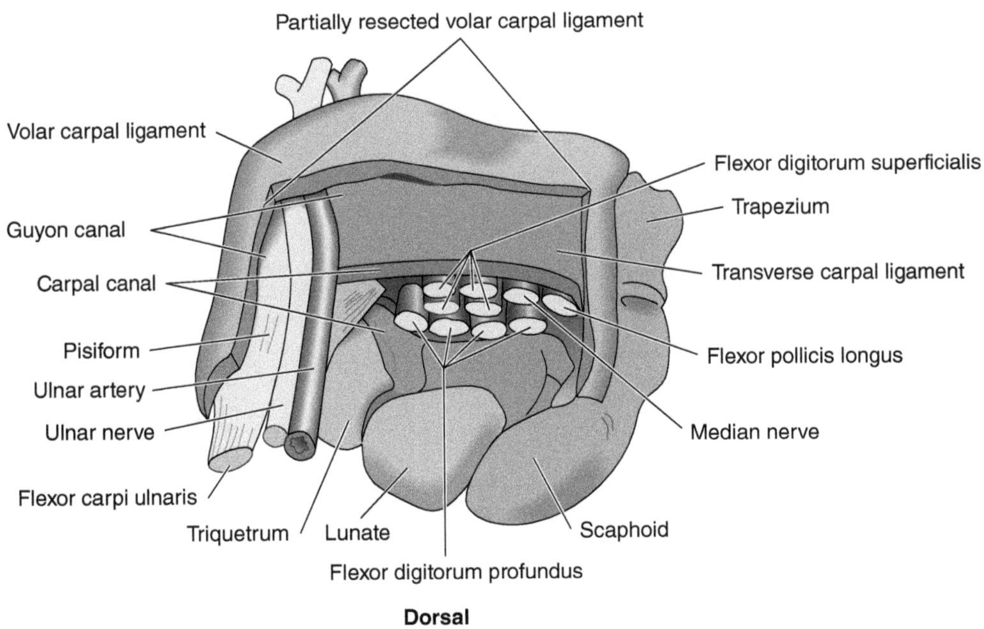

▲ **Figure 11–21.** **The Guyon canal and carpal tunnel and contents. (Cross section of supinated right wrist, viewed from proximal to distal.) Note the relationship between the transverse carpal ligament and the volar carpal ligament (partially resected).** (Reprinted with permission, from Reckling FW, Reckling JB, Mohn MP. *Orthopaedic Anatomy and Surgical Approaches*. St. Louis: Mosby-Year Book; 1990.)

tunnel syndrome include pregnancy, amyloidosis, acute or chronic inflammatory conditions, traumatic disorders of the wrist, endocrine disorders (diabetes mellitus and hypothyroidism), and tumors within the carpal tunnel.

It should be differentiated from other compressive median nerve neuropathies in the arm and from cervical radiculopathy. Diabetic neuropathy may produce symptoms similar to those of carpal tunnel syndrome, and patients with diabetic neuropathy may develop concomitant carpal tunnel syndrome.

1. Symptoms and signs—Most patients complain of numbness and tingling in the thumb and index and middle fingers, although many note that the entire hand feels numb. Pain rarely prevents the affected individual from falling asleep but characteristically awakens the patient from sleep after a number of hours. Often patients feel the urge to shake their hands and move their fingers to alleviate symptoms and return to sleep. Atypical symptoms include finger stiffness upon arising in the morning and clumsiness.

Discomfort or numbness, or both, may be incited by activities in which the wrist is held in a flexed position for a sustained period of time (eg, holding a steering wheel, telephone receiver, book, or newspaper). Discomfort and pain may radiate from the hand up the arm to the shoulder or neck. The patient may complain of clumsiness when trying to perform tasks such as unscrewing a jar top and may experience difficulty in holding on to a glass or cup securely.

Atrophy of muscles innervated by the median nerve is visible in severe long-standing cases but is uncommon in most cases of recent onset. Weakness of the abductor pollicis brevis muscle may be detected by careful manual muscle testing.

2. Provocative tests—Three provocative tests are helpful in establishing the diagnosis of carpal tunnel syndrome, and they are the Tinel sign, the Phalen maneuver, and the wrist compression test.

A. TINEL SIGN—The Tinel sign is elicited by percussing the skin over the median nerve just proximal to the carpal tunnel. When it is positive, the patient complains of an electric or tingling sensation radiating into the thumb, index, middle, or ring fingers.

B. PHALEN MANEUVER—The Phalen wrist flexion sign, or Phalen maneuver, is usually positive in patients with carpal tunnel syndrome and is thought by many to be even more diagnostic than the Tinel sign. When this maneuver is performed, the elbow should be maintained in extension while the wrist is passively flexed (Figure 11–22). The time is then measured from initiation of wrist flexion to onset of symptoms; onset within 60 seconds is considered supportive of the diagnosis of carpal tunnel syndrome. Both the time to onset and the location of paresthesias should be recorded.

C. WRIST COMPRESSION TEST (DURKAN'S TEST)—Pressure over the median nerve proximal to the wrist provokes

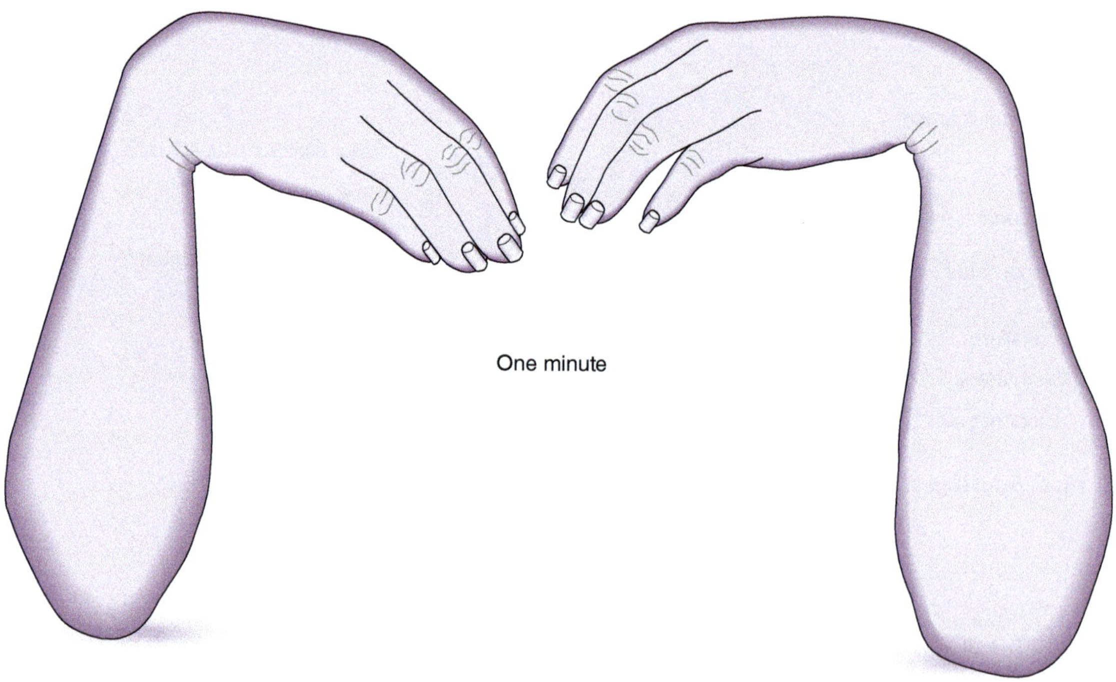

▲ **Figure 11–22.** Phalen maneuver. (Reprinted with permission, from American Society for Surgery of the Hand. *The Hand: Examination and Diagnosis,* 2nd ed. Philadelphia: Churchill Livingstone; 1983.)

symptoms within 30 seconds and is considered the most sensitive test. It is also confirmatory to other physical signs.

3. Two-point discrimination test—Two-point discrimination is often diminished in the finger pulps of patients with carpal tunnel syndrome. Sensation in the radial aspect of the palm should be normal, however, because the palmar cutaneous branch of the median nerve does not pass through the carpal tunnel.

4. Semmes-Weinstein monofilament test—This test evaluates a single nerve fiber that innervates group of receptors over a defined area and is the most sensitive test for early detection of sensory dysfunction.

5. Electrodiagnostic studies—Nerve conduction velocities and EMG help localize nerve compression to the wrist and evaluate residual neural and motor integrity. Electrodiagnostic studies are not needed to establish the diagnosis and usually are ordered in patients who have failed conservative care and are considered candidates for surgery. A distal motor latency greater than 3.5 to 4.0 ms is the best indicator of carpal tunnel syndrome. Patients with normal findings or with severe findings on these studies tend to have worse surgical outcomes compared to patients with moderate findings.

6. Ultrasound—Ultrasound as a diagnostic modality in carpal tunnel syndrome has been proposed as an alternative confirmatory study to nerve conduction studies. During examination, the ultrasound probe should be positioned perpendicular to the long axis of the forearm, and the cross-sectional area of the median nerve is measured at the carpal tunnel inlet just proximal to the level of the pisiform. The margins of the median nerve are defined as the margins within the hyperechoic nerve sheath. A threshold of 10 mm^2 or greater for the cross-sectional area of the nerve has been found to have a sensitivity and specificity of 89% and 90%, respectively, for the diagnosis of carpal tunnel syndrome.

B. Treatment

1. Conservative measures—Because the pressure within the carpal tunnel increases if the wrist is held in sustained flexion (usual sleep posture) or sustained extension, the first line of treatment includes a night splint that maintains the wrist in a neutral position, NSAIDs, and avoidance of aggravating activities. Clinical improvement with this simple measure adds further support to the diagnosis of carpal tunnel syndrome. Activities that provoke symptoms may be modified with simple measures such as adjustment of keyboard height and rotation of repetitive job activities.

Injection of steroids into the carpal tunnel often decreases the inflammatory response around the flexor tendons and diminishes symptoms. To inject the carpal tunnel, a 25-gauge 1.5-inch needle is placed at the palmar wrist crease just ulnar to the palmaris longus tendon. If the palmaris longus is absent, a line along the radial border of the ring finger is drawn to the wrist crease. Before placing the needle, patients are told they may experience an electric shock sensation in the fingers. If this sensation occurs, the needle may be in the median nerve, and the injection should not be given. The needle is withdrawn and placed a few millimeters ulnar. When inserting the needle, first the skin is punctured, and then a pop is felt as the needle passes through the transverse carpal ligament. A mixture of a short-acting anesthetic and steroid is injected. Transient relief of symptoms after injection suggests a greater likelihood of a favorable result after surgical decompression. Steroid injections have an 80% success rate in temporary relief of symptoms, although symptom relief continues at 1 year in only 20% of cases. Poor response to steroid injection is related to poor surgical outcome.

2. Surgical treatment—Patients unresponsive to conservative measures may benefit from surgical division of the transverse carpal ligament. This division may be accomplished through either direct open exposure or through an endoscopic approach. The open incision is made in the palm over the transverse carpal ligament, staying ulnar to the axis of the palmaris longus, along the longitudinal axis of the radial border of the ring finger. This incision avoids injury to the palmar cutaneous branch of the median nerve. After incising the palmar fascia longitudinally, the transverse carpal ligament is identified and sectioned longitudinally under direct observation. Endoscopic division of the transverse carpal ligament avoids a potentially tender palmar incision with either a single wrist portal proximal to the palm or with a combined proximal portal and short midpalmar portal along the axis of the open incision. Although some studies noted an earlier return to work activities after endoscopic release, the incidence of iatrogenic nerve and tendon injuries and late recurrence of symptoms from incomplete ligament division may be higher with endoscopic release than with open release. Both types of procedures are effective ways of treating carpal tunnel syndrome. The decision of which technique to use is based on the surgeon's experience. Endoscopic carpal tunnel release should not be used for treatment of recurrent carpal tunnel syndrome.

Patients are encouraged to actively move their fingers from the first postoperative day. Wrist motion is begun within the first week. Incisional tenderness often prevents patients from fully using their hands and returning to unrestricted work for the first 4 to 8 weeks. If patients have difficulty with hand function 3 to 4 weeks after surgery, a therapy program is prescribed consisting of desensitization, ROM, and strengthening. In 2% to 20% of cases, patients report ongoing symptoms at 1 year after surgery. The most common cause for failure is incomplete division of the transverse carpal ligament.

Pronator Syndrome

A. Anatomy and Clinical Findings

Median nerve compressive neuropathy can occur at the level of the proximal forearm. The anatomic structures that may compress the median nerve at this level include the ligament of Struthers (between the supracondylar process and the medial epicondyle), lacertus fibrosus (between the two heads of pronator teres muscle), and the proximal fibrous arch on the undersurface of the flexor digitorum superficialis muscle.

Patients with pronator syndrome complain of pain that is usually more severe in the volar forearm than in the hand and fingers. Complaints of numbness in the thumb, index, middle, and ring fingers may initially suggest the possibility of carpal tunnel syndrome. As opposed to carpal tunnel syndrome, patients with pronator syndrome may complain of numbness or other dysesthesias such as pain, tingling, or burning in the palm innervated by the last branch of the median nerve in the forearm, the palmar cutaneous branch. In addition, night symptoms are unusual in cases of pronator syndrome, whereas they are common in cases of carpal tunnel syndrome.

Examination may reveal sensory and motor deficits similar to carpal tunnel syndrome, but there may be sensory loss not only in distribution of the medial nerve in the fingers but also in the palm. The Tinel sign is positive at the forearm level rather than at the wrist. The Phalen maneuver does not provoke symptoms. Patients may experience pain with resistance to contraction of the pronator teres or flexor digitorum superficialis muscles tested by resistance to forearm pronation or to isolated flexion of the PIP joints of the long and ring fingers. In addition, resisted elbow flexion may reproduce symptoms when the nerve is compressed by the bicipital aponeurosis.

B. Treatment

First line of treatment includes immobilization and activity modification. If conservative treatment fails after 3 to 6 months, surgical treatment with generous decompression of all potentially constricting sites is recommended.

Anterior Interosseous Syndrome

A. Anatomy

The anterior interosseous nerve branch arises from the median nerve 4 to 6 cm below the elbow. This branch of the nerve innervates the flexor pollicis longus, flexor digitorum profundus of the index and middle fingers, and the pronator quadratus muscle. The anterior interosseous nerve may be compressed by the deep head of the pronator teres, the flexor digitorum superficialis aponeurotic arch, and an aberrant palmaris profundus. In addition, accessory muscles connecting the flexor digitorum superficialis to the flexor digitorum profundus proximally and the Gantzer muscle (the accessory head of the flexor pollicis longus) may cause compression of the anterior interosseous nerve.

B. Clinical Findings

Patients affected with anterior interosseous nerve syndrome present with sole motor deficits, and in contrast to those with pronator syndrome, they do not complain of numbness or pain. Typically, they present with inability to flex either the thumb interphalangeal joint or the index finger DIP joint.

C. Treatment

In the vast majority of patients, activity modification, splinting, and time result in improvement. Decompression of the anterior interosseous nerve may be indicated when it does not improve after conservative treatment. All potentially compressing structures must be exposed and released.

2. Ulnar Neuropathy

Cubital Tunnel Syndrome

A. Anatomy and Clinical Findings

Ulnar neuropathy is the second most common compression neuropathy in the body. The ulnar nerve may be compressed at the cubital tunnel, along the medial side of the elbow. The most common sites for compression are between the ulnar and humeral origins of the flexor carpi ulnaris, between the Osborne ligament and the medial collateral ligament, or at the arcade of Struthers that travels between the medial intermuscular septum and the medial head of the biceps. Less common sites are at the medial intermuscular septum, at the medial epicondyle, or by the anconeus muscle, an aberrant muscle from the medial epicondyle to the medial olecranon (Figure 11–23).

Patients affected with cubital tunnel syndrome most often complain of paresthesia and numbness involving the ring and little fingers. Because symptoms may be aggravated or provoked by sustained elbow flexion, patients may complain of increased symptoms while talking on the telephone. Many patients complain of being awakened at night by the symptoms, most often when sleeping with the elbows flexed. Patients whose exam demonstrates weakness of muscles innervated by the ulnar nerve may note clumsiness and lack of dexterity. On physical examination, inspection may reveal atrophy on the interosseous muscles between the metacarpals and clawing of the small and ring fingers. There is decreased sensation over dorsal and volar surfaces of the small and ulnar side of the ring fingers, while grasp and pinch strength may also be decreased due to extrinsic (flexor digitorum profundus of the little finger) and intrinsic (adductor pollicis) muscles weakness. Finger abduction and adduction strength is also decreased due to interossei weakness.

1. Provocative tests

A. Tinel sign—A positive Tinel sign is noted when percussion over the ulnar nerve at the elbow provokes paresthesias along the ulnar forearm and hand. The nerve may be noted to sublux over the medial epicondyle as the arm is brought into flexion.

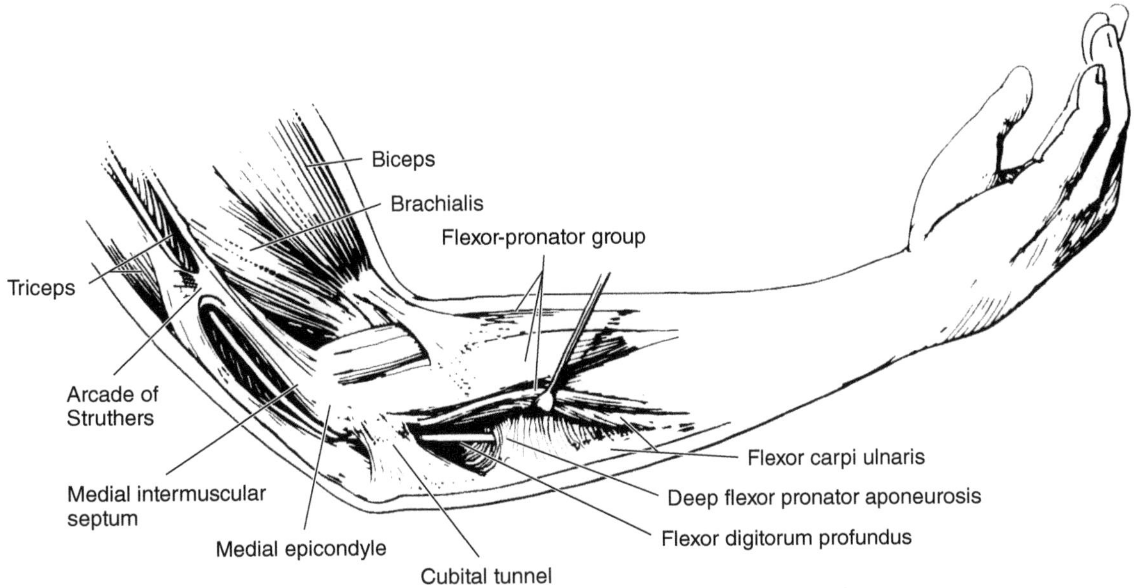

▲ **Figure 11–23. Points of constriction of the ulnar nerve at the elbow.** (Reprinted with permission from Amadio PC. Anatomic basis for a technique of ulnar nerve transposition. *Surg Radiol Anat*. 1986;8:155-61.)

B. FROMENT SIGN—With weakness of the ulnar nerve–innervated adductor pollicis muscle, a positive Froment sign may be observed. As the patient tries to hold a piece of paper placed between the thumb and the index finger, the thumb interphalangeal joint flexes in an attempt to substitute flexor pollicis longus activity for inadequate adductor pollicis strength.

C. JEANNE SIGN—The Jeanne sign is similar to the Froment sign, but the patient compensates for the inadequate adductor pollicis strength during pinch with MCP joint hyperextension.

D. ELBOW FLEXION TEST—The ulnar nerve may be rendered symptomatic by fully flexing the elbow with the wrist in the neutral position. The elbow flexion test, a provocative maneuver, is considered positive if paresthesia is elicited in the ring and little fingers within 60 seconds. The location of the paresthesia and the time between initiation of elbow flexion and the onset of symptoms should be recorded.

B. Treatment

1. Conservative treatment—Conservative measures constitute the first line of treatment, including nighttime splint that limits elbow flexion by holding the elbow at approximately 45 degrees of flexion, avoidance of aggravating activities, and NSAIDs. Conservative treatment is successful in about 65% of cases.

2. Surgical treatment—Several different techniques have been described to address ulnar nerve compression at the cubital tunnel. These include in situ decompression of the ulnar nerve within the cubital tunnel or decompression with anterior transposition of the nerve subcutaneously, intramuscularly, or submuscularly into the flexor pronator mass. Although in situ decompression was historically considered to be associated with persistent symptoms due to remaining tension on the nerve during elbow flexion or due to nerve irritation over the medial epicondyle, outcomes are similar between in situ decompression and anterior transposition, but with shorter recovery period and fewer complications with in situ decompression. The in situ decompression can be combined with medial epicondylectomy when there is visible anterior subluxation of the ulnar nerve.

When the nerve is transposed, great care must be taken to excise the medial intermuscular septum proximally and to release the aponeurosis between the humeral and ulnar origins of the flexor carpi ulnaris distally to avoid creating a new area of impingement. After surgery, initial rehabilitation focuses on regaining elbow ROM. Strengthening begins at 4 to 6 weeks, and the patient is usually able to return to unrestricted work at 8 to 12 weeks.

▶ Ulnar Tunnel Syndrome

A. Anatomy

The ulnar nerve travels from the forearm into the hand through the Guyon canal (see Figure 11–21), which is approximately 4 cm long. The anatomic borders of Guyon's canal are the pisiform and pisohamate ligament ulnarly and the hook of the hamate radially, which is the insertion of the volar carpal ligament that forms the roof of the tunnel and the transverse carpal ligament that forms the floor of the tunnel. Common causes for compression include ganglion cyst, lipoma, ulnar artery thrombosis or aneurysm, and hook of hamate fracture.

B. Clinical Findings

Examination should document ulnar nerve sensory and motor integrity. Patients with ulnar tunnel syndrome may present with pure motor, pure sensory, or mixed symptoms depending on the site of compression within the Guyon tunnel. Symptoms and signs are similar to cubital tunnel syndrome, with some differences. In contrast to the findings with cubital tunnel syndrome, the Tinel sign is positive at the wrist rather than at the elbow; the extrinsic motor function is normal, which may lead to more prominent clawing; and there are no sensory deficits in the dorsum of the hand as the dorsal sensory branch of ulnar nerve arises proximal to the wrist. The region of compression should be delineated by electrodiagnostic studies. In some cases, MRI studies demonstrate a space-occupying lesion such as a ganglion compressing the nerve within the Guyon canal.

C. Treatment

When splinting is ineffective, surgical decompression should be considered. When symptoms exist in tandem with carpal tunnel syndrome, release of the transverse carpal ligament favorably alters the shape and size of the Guyon canal. Postoperative care is the same as following carpal tunnel release.

3. Radial Neuropathy

Radial Tunnel Syndrome

A. Anatomy

Radial tunnel syndrome is a compression neuropathy of the posterior interosseous nerve in the region of the radial tunnel with pain and no motor or sensory deficits. The radial tunnel extends from the level of radiocapitellar past the proximal aspect of the supinator muscle, and some consider the radial tunnel to go to the distal aspect of the supinator muscle. Common sites of compression at the level of the proximal radius include fibers spanning the radiocapitellar joint, the radial recurrent vessels, the extensor carpi radialis brevis, the tendinous arch of the supinator (arcade of Frohse), and the point at which the nerve emerges from beneath the distal edge of the supinator.

B. Clinical Findings

Because radial tunnel syndrome often occurs in combination with lateral epicondylitis, the two diagnoses are frequently confused. Patients with radial tunnel syndrome experience pain over the midportion of the mobile wad (brachioradialis, extensor carpi radialis longus, and extensor carpi radialis brevis muscles), whereas the pain experienced by patients with lateral epicondylitis is located at or just distal to the lateral epicondyle. The diagnosis can be difficult. A long finger extension test is indicative of radial tunnel syndrome and is positive when, with the elbow extended, there is pain when simultaneously extending the wrist and fingers while the long finger is passively flexed by the examiner. Patients with radial tunnel syndrome often also experience pain with resisted forearm supination and resisted middle finger extension with elbow and wrist extended. The MRI and electrodiagnostic studies are usually inconclusive, whereas radial tunnel injection with local anesthetic is the most sensitive test and considered positive if it results in temporary nerve palsy and alleviation of pain.

C. Treatment

Conservative treatment of radial tunnel syndrome includes measures to avoid forceful extension of the wrist and fingers, wrist splinting in dorsiflexion, and corticosteroid injection. Persistent symptoms despite splinting may be treated by surgical decompression of the radial nerve. Concomitant lateral epicondylitis should be treated surgically at the same time that the radial nerve is decompressed.

Posterior Interosseous Nerve Syndrome

A. Anatomy

The radial nerve splits into the posterior interosseous nerve and the superficial sensory branch of the radial nerve after passing anteriorly to the radiocapitellar joint. The posterior interosseous nerve then passes beneath the origin of the extensor carpi radialis brevis, radial recurrent artery, and arcade of Frohse and travels between the two heads of supinator muscle. The posterior interosseous nerve is most commonly compressed at the same sites as in radial tunnel syndrome.

B. Clinical Findings

In contrast to the radial tunnel syndrome, patients with posterior interosseous nerve syndrome experience extrinsic extensor weakness. Pain may be less than that of patients with radial tunnel syndrome and is located over the dorsal forearm and wrist.

Paralysis may be either partial or complete. Because the brachioradialis, extensor carpi radialis longus, supinator, and often extensor carpi radialis brevis are innervated by the radial nerve proximal to the posterior interosseous nerve branch, these muscles are spared. MCP joint extension is the main deficit due to extensor digitorum communis, extensor indicis proprius, and extensor digiti quinti paralysis. Usually there is radial deviation with wrist extension due to functional extensor carpi radialis longus and absent extensor carpi radialis and extensor carpi radialis brevis. Pain with resisted supination is common in these patients.

The differential diagnosis in a patient with spontaneous loss of digital extension should include the possibility of multiple tendon ruptures in addition to possible radial neuropathy, particularly in patients with RA. The tenodesis effect, in which the fingers extend as the wrist is passively flexed, is preserved in posterior interosseous nerve syndrome but absent if the extensor tendons are ruptured. Electrodiagnostic studies are helpful to confirm diagnosis and identify the location of the compression.

C. Treatment

First line of treatment includes rest, activity modification, stretching exercises, and NSAIDs. A lidocaine/corticosteroid injection is also useful. Surgical decompression of the posterior interosseous nerve is recommended after 3 months of failed conservative treatment. If motor recovery does not occur, tendon transfers restore digital extension.

4. Thoracic Outlet Syndrome

Anatomy and Clinical Findings

This neurovascular syndrome results from compression of the brachial plexus and the subclavian vessels as they pass from the base of the neck to the axilla. The thoracic outlet is composed of three different spaces: the interscalene triangle, the costoclavicular space, and the retro-pectoralis minor space. The anatomic boundaries of the first space (interscalene triangle) are the scalenus anterior muscle anteriorly, the scalenus medius muscle posteriorly, and the first rib inferiorly. Thoracic outlet syndrome usually results from irritation of the of lower brachial plexus, the C8- and T1-derived nerves. It may be caused by osseous structures such as a cervical rib, prominent C7 transverse process, or a hypertrophic clavicle fracture callus. Soft-tissue causes are more common and include fibromuscular bands from the scalenus anterior to the scalenus medius, anterior hypertrophy, or tumors such as Pancoast tumor of the lung. Poor posture with slumping shoulders and prolonged military brace position, with the shoulders back, are both implicated as contributing factors.

The symptoms of thoracic outlet syndrome are often vague and variable and can be neurogenic or vascular. Neurogenic symptoms include pain over the neck, trapezius, shoulder, and distal arm with wide anatomic distribution from irritation of the lower brachial plexus. There is a variable degree of intrinsic muscle weakness, and numbness and paresthesia are also common. Physical examination should document C8 and T1 nerve root function by assessing sensation along the inner border of the hand and forearm and hand intrinsic muscle strength.

A. Provocative Tests

Provocative tests have a high rate of false-positive results.

1. Elevated stress test (Roos test)—Physical examination of the patient with suspected thoracic outlet syndrome should include an elevated stress test, in which the patient's shoulders are kept abducted at 90 degrees with elbows flexed and the arms externally rotated at 90 degrees. The patient is then asked to open and close the hands with the arms elevated for 3 minutes. Reproduction of symptoms is suggestive of thoracic outlet syndrome.

2. Other tests—The Adson sign and the Wright test may be helpful in detecting vascular compression. In a positive Adson test, the radial pulse can no longer be detected when the patient holds a deep breath with the arm extended, the forearm supinated, and the head turned toward the affected side. In the Wright test, the pulse can no longer be detected when the shoulder is abducted and externally rotated and the head is turned away from the involved shoulder. In addition, these maneuvers should reproduce the patient's symptoms.

B. Diagnostic Studies

Workup of the symptomatic patient should include radiographs of the cervical spine and chest to rule out a cervical rib, a prominent C7 transverse process, or a Pancoast tumor. In addition, electrodiagnostic studies, Doppler (in varied positions), and angiography are useful to assess the function of the lower nerve roots and to detect compression of the subclavian or axillary artery.

Treatment

Initial treatment includes postural exercises, activity modification, pain management, and anterior scalene blocks. Patients who are unresponsive to conservative treatment or have meaningful weakness may benefit from surgical resection of a cervical rib, resection of the first rib, or scalenotomy.

5. Cervical Root Compression

Cervical spine root compression may result in complaints of hand pain or weakness. It is useful to inquire routinely about pain or limitation of motion of the cervical spine. If the patient was involved in an accident involving sudden neck flexion and extension, this should be noted. Cervical root compression may occur from a herniated cervical disk, cervical spondylosis, intervertebral foraminal osteophytes, or, rarely, a cervical cord tumor.

Patients with cervical root compression most often complain of pain in a radicular rather than a peripheral nerve distribution. Despite symptoms involving the hand, most patients, when carefully questioned, are able to distinguish pain that begins in the neck and radiates to the hand from pain that begins in the hand and radiates proximally to the neck. Pain may be exacerbated with neck motion (flexion and extension, lateral bending, or rotation), coughing, or sneezing.

Physical examination of the patient with cervical radiculopathy frequently demonstrates either a decreased range of neck motion or pain with neck motion. Symptoms may be reproduced with axial compression on the patient's head (positive Spurling test). Detailed sensory and motor examination may reveal deficits in the domain of one or more roots.

The occasional simultaneous presentation of cervical radiculopathy with peripheral entrapment neuropathy is termed the *double-crush syndrome*. Whether compression at one level renders a nerve more vulnerable to compressive forces at a second level or whether such cases simply represent two common entities in the same extremity remains the subject of debate.

If a nerve is compressed at more than one location, the more symptomatic area is usually treated first. If both areas are equally symptomatic, the simpler of the two operations is chosen.

Boone S, Gelberman R, Calfee R. The management of cubital tunnel syndrome. *J Hand Surg Am*. 2015;40(9):1897-1904. [PMID: 26243318]

Henning PT, Yang L, Awan T, Lueders D, Pourcho AM. Minimally invasive ultrasound-guided carpal tunnel release: preliminary clinical results. *J Ultrasound Med*. 2018;37(11):2699-2706. [PMID: 29608024]

Peters B, Izadpanah A, Islur A. Analgesic consumption following outpatient carpal tunnel release. *J Hand Surg Am*. 2018;43(2):189.e1-189.e5. [PMID: 29122425]

Tang CQY, Lai SWH, Tay SC. Long-term outcome of carpal tunnel release surgery in patients with severe carpal tunnel syndrome. *Bone Joint J*. 2017;99-B(10):1348-1353. [PMID: 28963157]

Zhang D, Earp BE, Blazar P. Evaluation and management of unsuccessful carpal tunnel release. *J Hand Surg Am*. 2019; 44(9):779-786. [PMID: 31300226]

DISORDERS OF THE FASCIA OF THE HAND

DUPUYTREN DISEASE

Dupuytren disease is a benign proliferative disorder that is characterized by a nodular thickening and contractures of the palmar fascia (Figure 11–24). It is a progressive condition, resulting from pathologic changes mediated by the myofibroblast with predominance of type III collagen. Dupuytren disease occurs most commonly between 40 and 60 years of age. It is observed more often in males than females, with a 2:1 ratio, and it appears earlier and is often more aggressive in males as well. Flexion contractures most frequently occur at the MCP joints but may also tether the PIP joint and, less commonly, the DIP joint. The little and ring fingers are the most commonly involved areas, with the thumb less commonly involved. Patients with generalized diathesis for contractures present with ectopic deposits in the dorsum of

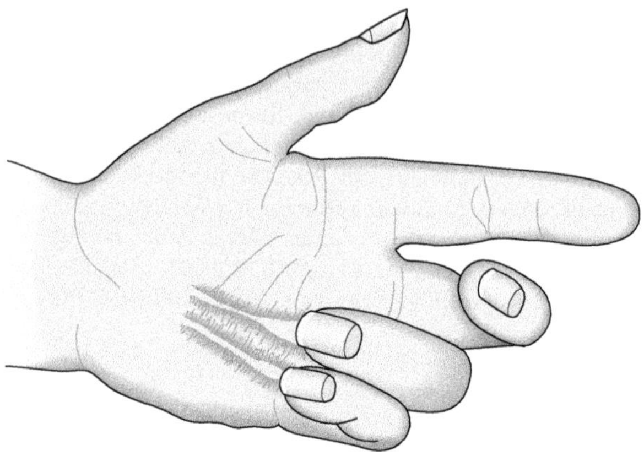

▲ **Figure 11–24. Dupuytren contracture.** (Reprinted with permission, from American Society for Surgery of the Hand. *The Hand: Examination and Diagnosis*, 2nd ed. Philadelphia: Churchill Livingstone; 1983.)

the PIP joint (Garrod's pads), the dorsum of the penis (Peyronie disease), and the plantar fascia of the foot (Ledderhose disease).

Epidemiologic Factors

A number of risk factors are identified. The disease most commonly appears in patients of northern European ancestry and is very rare in Africa or China. Dupuytren disease is associated with epilepsy medications taken for seizure disorders and with alcoholism, HIV, and diabetes. The relationship of work and trauma to the development of the disease remains controversial. The most aggressive disease occurs in patients who have a family history of disease and in those who have onset of disease prior to 40 years of age. More severely involved patients may have extensive bilateral involvement and ectopic deposits on the dorsum of the hands and the feet. Although these patients often undergo surgery at an early age, both extension and recurrence of the disease are common.

Anatomy and Clinical Findings

Dupuytren contracture distorts the anatomy of the palmar fascia. Normal anatomic structures are called bands, and contractures are called cords. Flexion contractures of the MCP joint are caused by pathologic contracture of the pretendinous bands, called central cords. Contracture of the natatory ligaments that normally travel between the digits gives rise to natatory cords that produce web space contractures and scissoring of the fingers. In the fingers, the spiral cord, derived from contracture of the spiral band that merges with the lateral digital sheath, and the Grayson ligaments result in flexion contracture of the PIP joint. When a spiral band contracts, the digital nerve is often displaced palmarly to the band from proximal lateral to distal central in the region of the proximal phalanx. Last, the retrovascular cord is the usual cause for DIP joint contracture.

Treatment

Indications for intervention include a fixed contracture of more than 30 degrees at the MCP and any degree of flexion contracture at the PIP joint. At early stages, ROM exercises may be useful. Enzymatic fasciotomy with *Clostridium histolyticum* collagenase is an alternative to surgery for less severe forms of the disease. This enzyme mainly attacks the collagen type that predominates in the contracted fascial structures (type III collagen). This selectivity is important because the enzyme preferentially hydrolyzes diseased tissue, whereas the connective tissue of the vessels, nerves, and tendons is largely spared since it consists of collagen types I and IV. Stretch manipulation within 24 to 48 hours after injection of the collagenase into the diseased cord is performed. Generally, it is more successful in correction of mild MCP joint contractures, compared to PIP joint contractures, and there is a risk for complications such as pain, skin tear, and flexor tendon rupture.

Nonsurgical treatment is usually ineffective in more severe cases, in which case partial fasciectomy should be performed. Surgical exposure is usually achieved through Brunner zigzag incisions or through longitudinal incisions that are modified for closure by a series of Z-plasty flap transpositions. If there is excessive tension, a transverse incision in the distal palmar crease can be left open to heal by secondary intention (McCash technique).

Severe or recurrent PIP joint disease may occasionally be best treated with a salvage procedure, usually PIP joint arthrodesis. Amputation may be considered when profound stiffness or neurovascular compromise is present in patients with recurrent disease.

Complications

The most common postoperative complication is hematoma, which may expand and compromise skin flaps, leading to skin necrosis. To diminish the possibility of postoperative hematoma, the tourniquet should be released and meticulous hemostasis obtained prior to wound closure. Tight skin closure should be avoided. If limited flap necrosis occurs, the affected regions should be treated by open dressing changes. If skin loss is extensive, skin graft application may be necessary to gain early wound closure.

Joint stiffness may occur, particularly after extensive surgical release of the long-standing fixed PIP joint. Extensive therapy is often necessary, consisting of both active and passive exercises and splinting.

Neurovascular injuries are common in the proximal phalangeal area, as the neurovascular bundle is displaced medial and superficial by the spiral cord. Great attention is needed during dissection, and the bundle should be identified prior to resection of the spiral cord. In case of nerve injury, immediate neurorrhaphy should be performed.

Mild sympathetically mediated pain (reflex sympathetic dystrophy) is not uncommon. For patients who have a more severe form, hospitalization with elevation, sympathetic blocking agents, oral steroids, and intensive therapy may be necessary.

Prognosis

At 2 years, less than 50% of patients have palpable cords following needle aponeurotomy or enzymatic fasciotomy. The recurrence rate at 5 years is 5.3% for open fasciectomy, approximately 22% for needle aponeurotomy, and significantly higher for enzymatic fasciotomy (39.5% for the MCP joint and 65.7% for the PIP joint; Table 11–3). Contracture correction is usually maintained at the MCP joints. Recurrence is more common at the PIP joint, usually due to contractures of other structures such as the volar plate, the collateral ligaments, and the flexor sheath.

Selles RW, Zhou C, Kan HJ, Wouters RM, van Nieuwenhoven CA, Hovius SER. Percutaneous aponeurotomy and lipofilling versus limited fasciectomy for Dupuytren's contracture: 5-year results from a randomized clinical trial. *Plast Reconstr Surg.* 2018;142(6):1523-1531. [PMID: 30489526]

Strömberg J, Ibsen Sörensen A, Fridén J. Percutaneous needle fasciotomy versus collagenase treatment for dupuytren contracture: a randomized controlled trial with a two-year follow-up. *J Bone Joint Surg Am.* 2018;100(13):1079-1086. [PMID: 29975270]

COMPARTMENT SYNDROME

Compartment syndromes result from increased pressure within a closed osseofascial space, compromising the microcirculation and decreasing perfusion of the tissue. The usual pathophysiological mechanism involves trauma that leads to bleeding and edema, increased interstitial pressure, and finally to vascular occlusion and ischemia.

The Volkmann ischemic contracture is the result of an acute compartment syndrome in which fibrous tissue has replaced dead muscle. This can happen to the muscles of the forearm from injuries around the elbow resulting in a

Table 11–3. Contracture recurrence rate[a] at 5 years.

	MCP Joint Recurrence	PIP Joint Recurrence
Open fasciectomy	5.3%	5.3%
Enzymatic fasciotomy	39.5%	65.7%
Needle aponeurotomy	21.8%	23.5%

MCP, metacarpophalangeal; PIP, proximal interphalangeal.
[a]Defined as a 20-degree or greater increase in joint contracture along with palpable cord.

contracture position with elbow flexion, forearm pronation, wrist flexion, MCP joint extension, and interphalangeal joint flexion. Because nerve injury is not always associated with this condition, sensation and intrinsic muscle function may be normal distal to the involved compartment. Because of this, there may be no sensory deficit or loss of motor function in the nerve distal to the involved compartment.

Etiologic Factors

The most common cause of acute compartment syndrome is trauma, including fractures, soft-tissue crush injuries, contusions, gunshot injuries, or arterial injuries. Tight casts and external wrapping can act as an inflexible constraint that can result in compartment syndrome. Postischemic swelling, bleeding disorders, burns, snake bites, and infection can also cause a compartment syndrome. In most cases, fractures are closed or, if open, are grade 1 injuries with only limited disruption of the soft-tissue envelopes of the compartments. Chronic compartment syndrome, also called exertional compartment syndrome, from intensive use of muscles, as can happen with demanding exercise, is less common in the upper than the lower extremity. It has been reported in throwing athletes.

Clinical Findings

The diagnosis of compartment syndrome is established predominantly based on clinical findings. The clinician must always be aware of the potential for bleeding or swelling that can lead to a compartment syndrome, such as following a crush injury. Compartment syndromes are characterized by pain out of proportion to the initial injury. Pain is often persistent, progressive, and unrelieved by immobilization. Aggravation of pain with passive stretching of the involved muscles (eg, finger extension results in stretching of the finger flexors) is the most sensitive finding. Another consistent finding with compartment syndromes is tenseness of the compartment on palpation. Diminished sensation may be noted in the distribution of the nerve whose compartment is being compressed. This phenomenon is believed to be secondary to nerve ischemia. Paralysis of muscles within the compartment is a late finding indicating that full recovery is highly unlikely. Because the elevated pressure within the compartment is not high enough to occlude major arteries completely as they pass through the compartment, distal pulses usually remain strong despite increasing tissue ischemia in the affected soft-tissue compartment. Unless there is a vascular injury, distal pulses are preserved in compartment syndrome. In children, anxiety associated with an increasing analgesic requirement is an indicator of compartment syndrome.

If the diagnosis of compartment syndrome is in question, the clinician is required to measure the pressure within the potential affected compartments. Pressure measurements are very helpful in cases of intubated patients with a concerning history and a palpably tense compartment. Various methods are available to measure compartment pressures, including a portable hand-held pressure monitor or a simple modification of a mercury manometer connected to tubing and a three-way stopcock. Normal intracompartmental pressure is 0 to 8 mm Hg, and the critical pressure is greater than 30 or 40 mm Hg. Although the exact pressure threshold for requiring fasciotomy is debatable, fasciotomy should be strongly considered whenever the compartment pressure is within 30 mm Hg of the diastolic pressure (delta pressure <30 mm Hg) in the forearm. It should be noted that intraoperatively the diastolic pressure is decreased; therefore, the preoperative diastolic pressure should be compared with the compartment pressure. Pressure measurements of the compartments of the hand are difficult to interpret. The decision to perform a fasciotomy of the hand or finger is based solely on clinical judgment.

Treatment

Once the diagnosis of compartment syndrome is established, fasciotomy of the involved compartment should be performed as soon as possible. Elevation of compartment pressure that leads to decreased perfusion for more than 8 hours is associated with irreversible tissue death. Prophylactic fasciotomy at the time of the initial surgical procedure is mandatory with forearm or arm replantation.

There are three compartments in the forearm: the volar compartment, the dorsal compartment, and the mobile wad that includes three muscles (brachioradialis, extensor carpi radialis longus, and extensor carpi radialis brevis). When isolated, the volar compartment of the forearm is most commonly affected and requires release (Figure 11–25A). This should always address both the deep and the superficial components of the volar compartment. The deep flexor muscles of the volar compartment are especially prone to ischemia and susceptible to damage due to the limited vascular supply. The investing fascia that individually confines the flexor digitorum superficialis, the flexor digitorum profundus, and the pronator quadratus should always be incised. The skin incision should extend from the elbow to the carpal tunnel. The preferred skin incision extends from the lateral side of the biceps and swings ulnarly toward the medial epicondyle. The incision may be extended in a radial direction to allow decompression of the mobile wad. In the distal half of the forearm, the incision runs along the ulnar border. The flap is designed to allow coverage of the median nerve in the distal forearm when the wounds are left open at the conclusion of the procedure. The incision is extended obliquely across the wrist to provide exposure of the carpal tunnel in the proximal palm. In some cases, the dorsal compartment of the forearm also needs decompression. For the dorsal decompression, a dorsal longitudinal incision is used (Figure 11–25B).

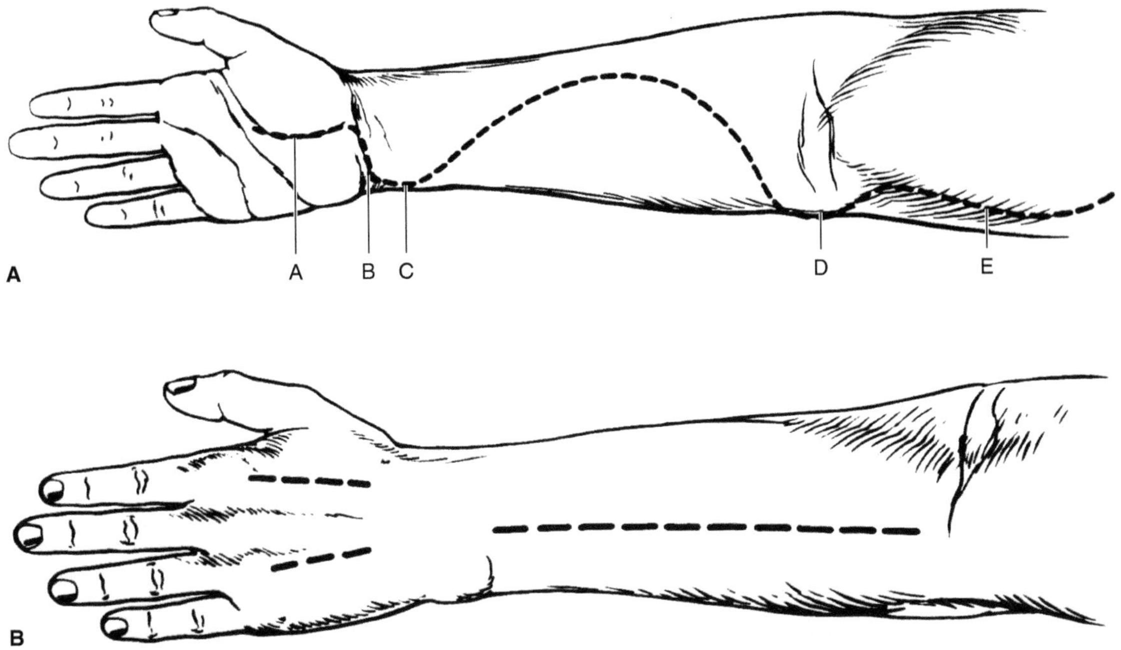

▲ **Figure 11–25. A:** Various skin incisions used for performing a volar arm fasciotomy. **B:** To decompress the dorsal and mobile wad compartments, straight incisions are preferred because fewer veins are damaged. (Reprinted with permission, from Green DP, ed. *Operative Hand Surgery*, 2nd ed. Philadelphia: Churchill Livingstone; 1988.)

During the volar decompression, care must be taken to incise the lacertus fibrosus at the elbow. Care should be also taken to ensure that the deep fascia is incised and the deep muscles of the volar compartment, the flexor pollicis longus and flexor digitorum profundus muscles, are completely decompressed. An epimysiotomy of the individual superficial and deep compartment muscle bellies should be performed as needed. The skin incision should be partially closed over the median nerve in the hand and distal forearm. The proximal wound over muscle should be left open. The open wound can be addressed with wound vacuum-assisted closure or sterile wet-to-dry dressings. The patient should be returned to the operating room within 48 to 72 hours for reevaluation. At the second surgery, dressings are changed, and secondary debridement of any devitalized tissue is performed. Although it is possible in some cases to close the wound, split-thickness skin grafting at a later time is usually required.

There are 10 compartments in the hand: hypothenar, thenar, flexor pollicis adductor, four dorsal interossei, and three volar interossei. Compartment decompression in the hand is achieved through two longitudinal dorsal incisions over the index and ring metacarpals. Through these incisions, each of the interosseous compartments can be entered on both the radial and ulnar sides of each metacarpal. Separate volar incisions are needed for decompression of the thenar (over the radial side of first metacarpal) and hypothenar (over the ulnar side of fifth metacarpal) compartments.

In the finger, fasciotomy may be required for treatment of either severe trauma or snake bite injuries. Because compartment pressures in the finger are impossible to measure accurately, the indications for finger fasciotomy are based on the degree of swelling. Midaxial incisions along the ulnar side of the index, middle, and ring fingers and the radial side of the little finger and thumb allow satisfactory digital decompression. Care is taken to retract the neurovascular bundle palmarward, and the fascia between the neurovascular bundle and the flexor tendon sheath are then incised. Digital wounds are left open postoperatively, and wound closure is achieved either secondarily or with a split-thickness skin graft.

Liu B, Barrazueta G, Ruchelsman DE. Chronic exertional compartment syndrome in athletes. *J Hand Surg Am.* 2017; 42(11):917-923. [PMID: 29101975]

Stewart SK, Singleton JA. Spontaneous extensor carpi ulnaris compartment syndrome. *J Hand Surg Am.* 2016;41(6):e143-e145. [PMID: 27118391]

Turkula SC, Fuller DA. Extensile fasciotomy for compartment syndrome of the forearm and hand. *J Orthop Trauma.* 2017;31(suppl 3):S50-S51. [PMID: 28697090]

FRACTURES AND DISLOCATIONS OF THE HAND

Fractures of the metacarpals and phalanges are very common. Phalangeal fractures account for approximately 10% of all fractures, with the distal phalanx fracture being the most common. More than half of all hand fractures are work related. Fractures of the border digits (the thumb and little finger) are most common.

Clinical Findings

Description of a phalangeal or metacarpal fracture should include the location of the fracture along the bone (base, shaft, or neck) and whether the fracture is open or closed. Further description should include the displacement of the fracture (displaced or nondisplaced), if it has an intraarticular component, and whether rotational or angular deformity is present.

Because rotational malalignment of a metacarpal or phalangeal fracture is difficult to evaluate from a radiograph, physical examination is essential. The patient is asked to actively flex the fingers individually and together. Nail rotation, finger orientation, and overlapping of the fingers are assessed. Associated vascular, nerve, and tendon injuries, as well as the adequacy of soft-tissue coverage, also should be evaluated.

Treatment

In cases of nondisplaced fractures, the goal of conservative treatment is sufficient immobilization to maintain the proper alignment of the fragments, with early motion of the uninvolved fingers to prevent stiffness. Regardless of the type of immobilization, the hand has to be placed in an intrinsic plus or safe position to avoid secondary joint contracture (see Figure 11–10). The immobilization method that is required to maintain fracture reduction depends on the fracture location and characteristics. Stable phalanx fractures may be treated by either buddy taping the affected finger to an adjacent finger and allowing early motion or with a brief period of splint immobilization. Metacarpal fractures are treated with cast, splint, or brace immobilization and radiographs repeated at 7 to 10 days to assess maintenance of the fracture reduction. Immobilization should rarely exceed 3 weeks for phalangeal fractures or 4 weeks for metacarpal fractures. Because radiologic union usually lags behind clinical union in the hand, initiation of digital motion should not be delayed until radiologic union is visible. Prolonged immobilization increases the likelihood of residual stiffness.

When conservative treatment is unlikely to maintain fracture reduction, internal fixation is required. There are numerous internal fixation techniques for hand fractures, including Kirschner (K)-wire fixation, interosseous wiring, tension band wiring, interfragmentary screw fixation, or fixation with plates and screws. K-wire fixation is versatile but lacks the rigidity of other techniques. Additional stability may be achieved by combining K-wire fixation with tension band wires. Interfragmentary screws provide ideal fixation for long oblique fractures, in which the obliquity of the fracture is more than two times the diameter of the fractured bone. Plates and screws in the hand are particularly helpful in open metacarpal fractures with bone loss. When segmental bone loss occurs, initial treatment includes debridement of an associated open wound and maintenance of skeletal length with either internal or external fixation. After the soft-tissue coverage is established, bony graft reconstruction may be coupled with definitive internal fixation.

PHALANGEAL FRACTURES

1. Distal Phalanx Fractures

Distal phalangeal fractures occur most often in the middle finger and the thumb. These fractures usually result from a crushing injury, such as occurs with a misdirected hammer striking a thumb holding a nail or a protruding middle finger distal phalanx caught in a closing door. They are classified into tuft fractures, shaft fractures, and base fractures.

Tuft fractures do not require manipulation because the nail plate dorsally and the pulp volarly provide stability. Treatment generally consists of 3 to 4 weeks of splinting, without immobilizing the DIP joint. Shaft fractures may be transverse or longitudinal, and they are usually conservatively treated, whereas severely displaced and unstable shaft fractures can be treated with closed reduction and percutaneous pinning. Base fractures are usually unstable and often involve extensor or flexor tendon disruption.

Nail bed injuries are often associated with distal phalanx fractures and are discussed later in this chapter.

2. Proximal and Middle Phalanx Fractures

Angulation of fractures of the proximal and middle phalanges results from the forces of tendons inserting on the bone. The middle phalanx has an extensor force transmitted to it by the central slip attaching dorsally and proximally. The terminal extensor tendon inserts dorsally and distally into the terminal phalanx, providing a secondary dorsiflexion force. The flexor digitorum superficialis inserts volarly over the middle three-fifths of the middle phalanx. Therefore, middle phalanx fractures that occur proximal to the flexor digitorum superficialis insertion angulate with the fracture apex dorsally; fractures that occur distal to the superficialis insertion angulate with the apex palmarly. Proximal phalangeal fractures tend to angulate with the apex palmarly because of the force of lateral bands that pass palmarward to the axis of the MCP joint and dorsalward to the axis of the PIP joint.

Adhesions involving the flexor or extensor tendons are a major complication of proximal and middle phalangeal fractures. Fracture displacement increases the likelihood of tendon adherence and limitation of joint motion. Malunion including malrotation of these fractures may require secondary correction.

Conservative treatment with splinting or buddy tape immobilization for 3 to 4 weeks followed by ROM exercises is recommended for nondisplaced or minimally displaced shaft fractures that have no rotational deformity, less than 2 mm of shortening, and less than 10 degrees of angulation. In case of displaced fractures, operative fixation in the form of percutaneous pinning, ORIF, or external fixation is required. In addition, long oblique, comminuted, or displaced intraarticular fractures should be treated surgically.

METACARPAL FRACTURES

1. Metacarpal Head Fractures

Intraarticular fractures of the metacarpal head are difficult to treat and usually result in some degree of stiffness. Because greater than 1 mm of articular step-off is unacceptable, the majority of these fractures require ORIF. Fixation options include K-wire, screws, or a plate. Fractures with marked comminution of the metacarpal head that are not amenable to internal fixation can be treated with joint-spanning external fixation or arthroplasty.

2. Metacarpal Neck Fractures

The neck is the weakest part of the metacarpal. The fifth and fourth metacarpals are most frequently involved. The fifth metacarpal neck fracture is commonly known as boxer's fracture and almost always results from a direct blow, either delivered to the hand or by the hand striking a solid object. Comminution of the volar cortex results in collapse deformity with apex dorsal angulation (Figure 11–26). Greater residual fracture angulation may be accepted in the ring and little fingers because of the increased mobility of the CMC joints of these fingers, allowing for greater compensatory motion. The flexion and extension arc is 15 degrees in the ring finger CMC joint and 30 degrees in the little finger.

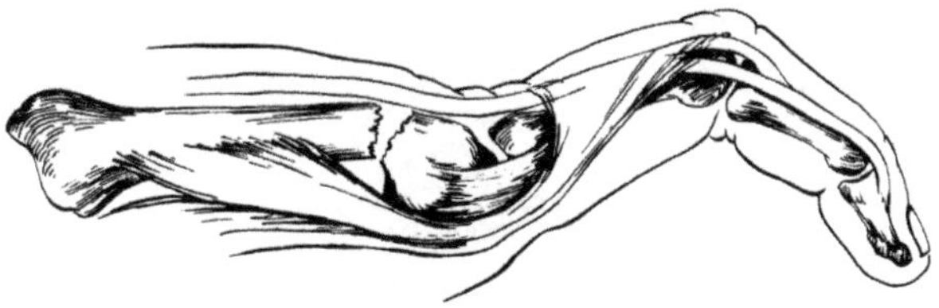

▲ **Figure 11–26.** Boxer's fracture. If the angulation in a metacarpal neck fracture is severe, clawing may result when the patient attempts to extend the finger. This is a good clinical test to supplement the evaluation of the severity of the angulation as seen radiographically. (Reprinted with permission, from Bucholz RW, Green DP, Rockwood CA, eds. Rockwood and Green's fractures in adults, 3rd ed. Philadelphia: Lippincott; 1991.)

Fracture angulation of more than 15 to 20 degrees should not be accepted in the index and middle fingers and should be properly aligned surgically. The acceptable angulation for the ring finger is 30 to 40 degrees, whereas for the small finger, it is 50 to 60 degrees. Rotational deformity is also unacceptable. Immobilization for 3 to 4 weeks with an ulnar gutter splint for the ring and small fingers and with a volar wrist splint including the middle or index fingers is recommended for nondisplaced fractures. When angulation exceeds the acceptable criteria, extensor lag may be noted at the PIP joint, and the patient may complain of a "marble" in the palm when making a fist. Displaced fractures can be treated with closed reduction and percutaneous pinning (antegrade through the metacarpal base or retrograde through the collateral recess) or with ORIF.

3. Metacarpal Shaft Fractures

Metacarpal shaft fractures result from a direct blow or crushing injury. Dorsal angulation of the fracture fragments is secondary to the interosseous muscle forces. The closer the fracture is to the CMC joints, the greater is the lever arm and, hence, the less angulation that can be tolerated. Less shortening occurs in isolated fractures of the middle and ring metacarpals than in the index or little fingers because the deep intermetacarpal ligaments of two adjacent rays tether the fractured metacarpal distally. Nondisplaced metacarpal fractures can be treated with cast or splint immobilization for 4 to 6 weeks. Displaced metacarpal shaft fractures can be fixed with percutaneous pinning, ORIF, or external fixation. The criteria for displacement are based on three parameters: angulation, rotation, and shortening. Fractures that should be considered for reduction and fixation are those with rotational deformities leading to digital overlap and with shortening of more than 5 mm, whereas acceptable angulation varies by location: less than 20 degrees for index and long fingers, less than 30 degrees for ring finger, and less than 40 degrees for small finger. Percutaneous pinning with intramedullary K-wires can be antegrade through the base or retrograde through the collateral recess. Lag interfragmentary screw fixations can be used for long oblique fractures when the fracture length is at least twice the bone diameter, whereas plate fixation is recommended for transverse fractures when the overlying soft tissues are intact.

JOINT INJURIES

1. Distal Interphalangeal Joint Fracture and Fracture-Dislocation

The most common intraarticular fracture of the DIP joint is a bony mallet finger, in which a portion of the dorsal articular surface is avulsed by the extensor tendon. Most bony mallet injuries can be treated with splinting in extension for 6 weeks. Indications for fixation of these fractures are controversial. It is usually recommended to fix bony mallet fingers if there is DIP joint subluxation or if the fracture fragment is more than 50% of the articular surface. Surgical treatment includes pinning or mini-fragment screw fixation.

As opposed to bony mallet fingers that involve the dorsal aspect of the distal phalanx, fractures involving the volar aspect of the articular surface are often flexor digitorum profundus avulsion fractures (jersey finger). These are treated with bone or tendon reattachment to the distal phalanx.

2. Condylar Fractures

Condylar fractures may occur in either the proximal or middle phalanges. These fractures are most often athletic injuries. Anteroposterior, lateral, and oblique radiographs are necessary to identify the fracture fragments. They carry the worst prognosis since the rates of flexion contracture and post-traumatic arthritis are high. Regardless of the form of treatment, anatomic reduction of the fracture is critical because joint incongruity may lead to stiffness, deformity, and early degenerative arthritis. Nondisplaced condylar fractures can be treated with digital splinting for 7 to 10 days, followed by buddy taping and early motion. However, close radiographic follow-up is important. Displaced fractures require internal fixation with K-wires, mini-fragment screws, or mini-plates for anatomic reduction and early motion. The collateral ligament insertion to the condyle must be preserved because it is the only blood supply to the fragment.

3. Proximal Interphalangeal Joint Dislocation and Fracture-Dislocation

Dorsal dislocations of the PIP joint are more common than palmar or lateral dislocations. Dorsal dislocations may be separated into three types (Figure 11–27). The mechanism for volar base fractures (dorsal fracture-dislocations) involves hyperextension during which the volar plate is avulsed, whereas the mechanism for dorsal base fractures (volar fracture-dislocations) involves hyperflexion during which the central tendon is avulsed. The lateral base fracture (lateral dislocations) represents avulsion of the collateral ligaments. Pilon fractures are complete articular fractures that are highly unstable.

Stable fracture-dislocations are associated with fractures in which less than 40% of the middle phalanx base is fractured. These fractures can be treated with extension block splinting for dorsal fracture dislocations or extension splinting for volar dislocations for 3 to 4 weeks, followed by ROM exercises. Unstable fracture-dislocations (>40% bone fracture involvement) need surgical fixation.

When a single large articular fragment is present, internal fixation with screws or mini-plates should be attempted. If the fragments are small and comminuted, a hemihamate arthroplasty can be performed to restore stability, utilizing an autologous osteochondral graft harvested from the dorsal lip of the hamate in order to reconstruct the volar buttress of the middle phalanx. Alternatively, in cases of comminuted fractures involving less than 50% to 60% of the articular base of the middle phalanx, the volar plate can be drawn into the joint with sutures to create a volar soft-tissue buttress to the dorsally unstable joint (volar plate arthroplasty). Highly comminuted fractures can also be treated with static digital external fixators or with dynamic traction external systems. These external fixators can be used either as an isolated procedure or in combination with any of the previous procedures. Several different configurations with K-wires and rubber bands have been described for the dynamic traction systems, or a commercially available dynamic traction system can be used. The basic concept of the dynamic systems involves prevention of dorsal subluxation of the middle phalanx through the pins, while the articular surface is offloaded with constant longitudinal traction through the rubber bands.

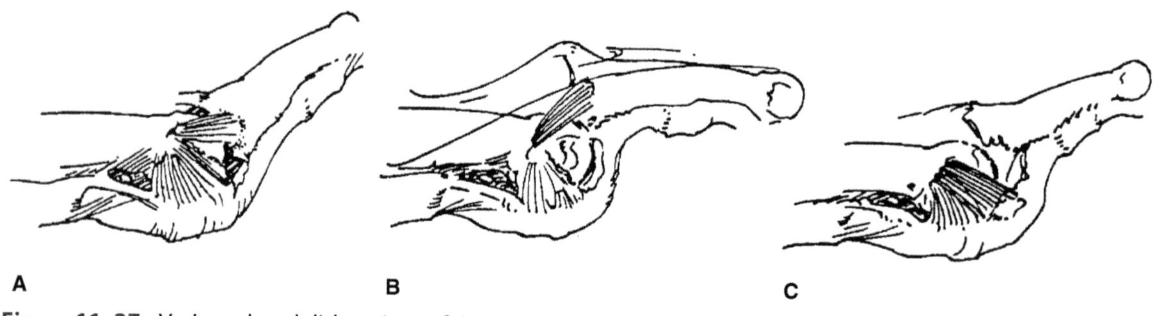

▲ **Figure 11–27.** Various dorsal dislocations of the proximal interphalangeal joint. **A:** Type 1 (hyperextension). The volar plate is avulsed, and an incomplete longitudinal split occurs in the collateral ligaments. The articular surfaces maintain congruous contact. **B:** Type 2 (dorsal dislocation). There is complete rupture of the volar plate and a complete split in the collateral ligaments, with the middle phalanx resting on the dorsum of the proximal phalanx. The proximal and middle phalanges lie in almost parallel alignment. **C:** Type 3 (fracture-dislocation). The insertion of the volar plate, including a portion of the volar base of the middle phalanx, is disrupted. The major portion of the collateral ligaments remains with the volar plate and flexor sheath. A major articular defect may be present.

Volar PIP dislocations are unusual. The condyle of the proximal phalanx may buttonhole between the central slip and the lateral bands. Closed reduction may be attempted by applying traction to the fingers after flexing both the MCP and PIP joints. If closed reduction is successful, the digit should be splinted in extension for 3 to 6 weeks to allow healing of the extensor mechanism. If closed reduction is unsuccessful, open reduction is necessary to free the condyle from the rent in the extensor mechanism.

Radial lateral PIP dislocation is six times more common than ulnar lateral PIP dislocation. These dislocations are associated with avulsion of the volar plate, extensor mechanism, or a portion of the phalangeal base. After the joint is reduced, the residual joint stability should be assessed by observing the active ROM. Stable fracture-dislocations are immobilized at 5 to 10 degrees of flexion for 3 weeks, and then active ROM activities are allowed.

4. Metacarpophalangeal Joint Dislocation

MCP joint dislocations are usually dorsal and most commonly involve either the index finger or the thumb. They are usually caused by a hyperextension injury during which the volar plate is ruptured proximally from the metacarpal. If the joint is subluxed and the volar plate has not yet become interposed in the joint, closed reduction may be achieved by flexion of the joint. Traction across the subluxated MCP joint can transform a reducible joint into an irreducible one. When the joint dislocates, the volar plate may interpose between the dislocated articular surfaces. This injury, termed complex as opposed to simple dislocation where no volar plate interposition occurs, requires open reduction to extract the volar plate from being between the articular surfaces (Figure 11–28).

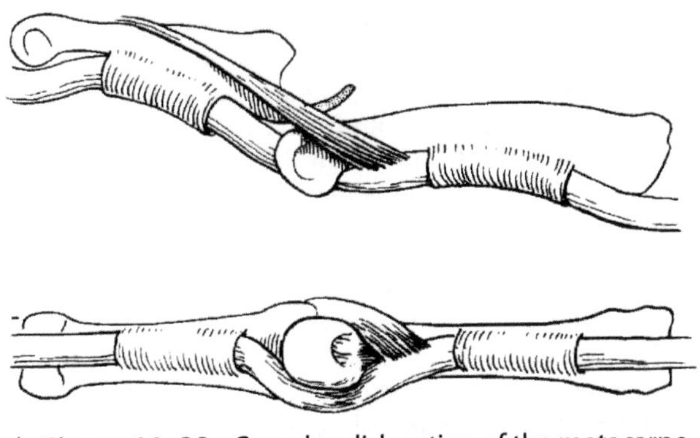

▲ **Figure 11–28.** Complex dislocation of the metacarpophalangeal joint. In the upper lateral diagram, the palmar plate is locked between the head of the metacarpal and the base of the proximal phalanx. In the lower diagram, an anterior view, the head of the metacarpal can be seen trapped between the flexor digitorum profundus on one aspect and the lumbrical on the other. (Reprinted with permission, from Lister G. *The Hand: Diagnosis and Indications*, 3rd ed. Philadelphia: Churchill Livingstone; 1993.)

Open reduction may be accomplished through either a volar or dorsal approach. If the volar approach is used, care should be taken to avoid injury to the neurovascular bundles. The A1 pulley is incised to expose the volar plate, and the volar plate is pushed out of the joint. If the dorsal approach is used, the extensor tendon is incised longitudinally, and the volar plate is split to facilitate reduction. Postoperatively, the MCP joint is immobilized in approximately 30 degrees of flexion for 3 to 5 days. Splinting that allows active motion is maintained for 3 weeks.

Although lateral dislocations of the MCP joint are rare, isolated radial collateral ligament ruptures may occur. These injuries should also be immobilized in approximately 30 degrees of flexion for 3 weeks. The fingers should be protected from ulnar stress for an additional 3 weeks. Unstable index and middle finger radial collateral ligament tears may be surgically repaired.

5. Carpometacarpal Joint Fractures and Fracture-Dislocations

Sprains and fracture-dislocations may involve any of the CMC joints. Sprains of the index and middle finger CMC joints may occur with palmar flexion and torsion. If tenderness is localized to the CMC joint and careful radiographs fail to demonstrate fracture, a sprain may be diagnosed.

Treatment of acute sprain injuries consists of 3 to 6 weeks of immobilization. If localized pain persists, steroid injection may be considered. CMC fracture-dislocations of the ring and little fingers are usually secondary to direct or longitudinal blows. Dorsal dislocations are more common than volar dislocations. A reversed Bennett fracture is a fifth metacarpal base fracture that most commonly occurs with a volar-radial articular fragment left in situ, while the remainder of the metacarpal is dislocated dorsal due to the force exerted by the extensor carpi ulnaris tendon.

Oblique views with partial pronation and supination may be required to visualize the CMC joint clearly. Closed reduction may be achieved with longitudinal distraction. The reduction may be maintained by percutaneous K-wire fixation. When fracture-dislocation of the little finger metacarpal articular surface results in a fragment of the hamate being sheared off, displacement of the metacarpal shaft is likely. Because of forces from the extensor carpi ulnaris and the hypothenar muscles, the metacarpal shaft tends to displace proximally and angulate palmarly. Longitudinal traction and percutaneous K-wire fixation of the ring and little finger metacarpals stabilize these fractures. Open reduction is necessary for an irreducible dislocation or for chronic fracture-dislocations. If the patient develops degenerative arthritis of the hamate metacarpal joint, arthrodesis of the ring or small finger CMC joint (or both) is well tolerated.

6. Thumb Carpometacarpal Joint

Thumb base fractures account for 80% of all thumb fractures. They can be either extraarticular or intraarticular. Two patterns of intraarticular fractures are most commonly encountered—Bennett and Rolando fractures—or the fracture can be extraarticular.

Bennett Fracture

Bennett fracture is a fracture-dislocation of the thumb basal joint in which the small volar ulnar fragment of the metacarpal articular surface remains attached to the anterior oblique ligament and the remainder of the metacarpal articular surface and shaft is displaced proximally, radially, and into adduction in response to the force of the adductor pollicis and abductor pollicis longus muscles insertion on the metacarpal (Figure 11–29). These two forces contribute to combined supination, adduction, and flexion of the metacarpal shaft. Acute Bennett fractures may often be reduced by traction, abduction, and pressure on the proximal metacarpal, with slight pronation. The reduction may then be stabilized by percutaneous pin fixation through the metacarpal shaft and across the fracture site, toward either the trapezium (transarticular K-wire fixation) or the index metacarpal (intermetacarpal K-wire fixation). If satisfactory reduction cannot be achieved by closed means, ORIF is required. Fixation can be achieved with K-wires or mini-fragment screws and sometimes a plate.

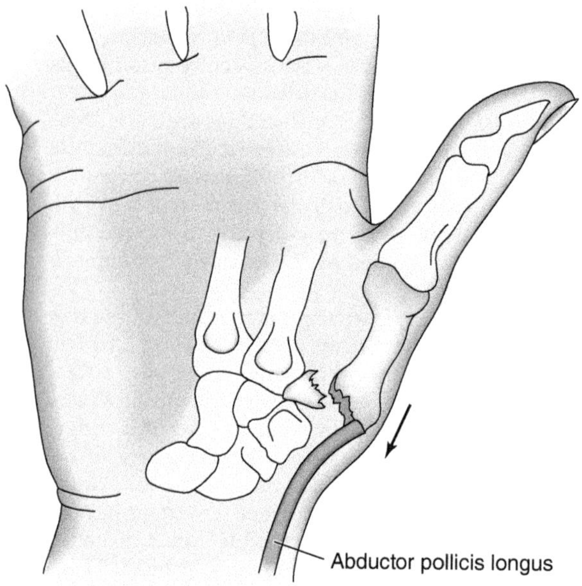

▲ **Figure 11–29.** **Bennett fracture. The first metacarpal shaft is displaced by the pull of the muscle.** (Reprinted with permission, from American Society for Surgery of the Hand. *The Hand: Examination and Diagnosis*, 2nd ed. Philadelphia: Churchill Livingstone; 1983.)

Rolando Fracture

The Rolando fracture is a comminuted T or Y intraarticular fracture of the base of the thumb metacarpal. When large fragments are present, ORIF is possible. When the joint is highly comminuted, percutaneous pinning (fragments too small and not amenable to screw fixation) or distraction and external fixation can be employed.

Extraarticular Fracture

Extraarticular fractures are less likely to develop traumatic arthritis than intraarticular fractures. Because of the mobility of the CMC joint of the thumb, up to 30 degrees of angulation can be accepted without functional loss. These fractures are treated with immobilization in a thumb spica cast for 3 to 4 weeks. Otherwise, percutaneous pinning or internal fixation is required for displaced fractures.

7. Thumb Ulnar Collateral Ligament Injury

The most common injury to the MCP joint is sprain of the ulnar collateral ligament of the thumb. The term *skier's thumb* is used for acute injuries, and the term *gamekeeper's thumb* is used for chronic injuries. This injury occurs when the thumb is forced into radial deviation, stressing the ulnar collateral ligament. The ulnar collateral ligament is composed of the proper and accessory ligaments. When the ulnar collateral ligament is torn from its phalangeal insertion, a Stener lesion may occur; the adductor aponeurosis is interposed between the retracted ligament and bone, preventing healing of the ligament to the proximal phalanx with closed treatment. Evaluation of the integrity of the ligament may be made by stressing the flexed MCP joint in abduction. Deviation more than 30 degrees in both flexion and extension of the MCP joint is diagnostic of a totally disrupted, incompetent ligament. When deviation is more than 30 degrees in only flexion or extension of the MCP joint, a partial rupture is diagnosed. MRI has 100% sensitivity and specificity in diagnosis of this injury. A tear with 3 mm or more of separation on the MRI leads to MCP joint instability if treated conservatively; therefore, surgical treatment is recommended, even in the absence of a Stener lesion.

Closed treatment of a partial ligament tear may be accomplished with a thumb spica splint for 3 to 4 weeks. Complete displaced tears require surgical exploration and reattachment to the metacarpal base usually with one suture anchor. Recent data have shown that a two-anchor repair or augmentation of the repair with suture tape may mitigate the need for postoperative immobilization. Avulsion of the ulnar collateral ligament may also occur with a bony fragment. If the fragment is greater than 15% of the articular surface or if the avulsed fragment is displaced more than 5 mm, open repair of the ligament is recommended.

Chronic symptomatic ulnar collateral ligament injuries may be repaired if the residual ligament is of sufficient quality. Supplementation of the repair with either tendon transfer or tendon grafting may be useful. In patients who develop traumatic arthritis or if ligament reconstruction is not deemed feasible, arthrodesis of the MCP joint is preferred.

Caggiano NM, Harper CM, Rozental TD. Management of proximal interphalangeal joint fracture dislocations. *Hand Clin.* 2018;34(2):149-165. [PMID: 29625635]

Khurana S, Chen Z, Dowdle J. Perihamate-peripisiform-transtriquetrum axial ulnar fracture dislocation of the hand with an associated perilunate injury. *J Hand Surg Am.* 2018;43(3):292.e1-292.e6. [PMID: 28985977]

Pundkare GT, Patil AM. Carpometacarpal joint fracture dislocation of second to fifth finger. *Clin Orthop Surg.* 2015;7(4):430-435. [PMID: 26640624]

SPECIAL TREATMENT PROCEDURES OF THE HAND

REPLANTATION

Replantation is the reattachment of a body part that was totally severed from the body, without any residual soft-tissue continuity. Revascularization is the reconstruction of damaged blood vessels to prevent an attached but ischemic body part from becoming necrotic.

Initial Care of Patient

Effective treatment of the patient and the ischemic or detached body part requires appropriate initial care and prompt referral to a surgeon at a center capable of mobilizing resources for early surgical care. The initial treating physician should place the amputated part in gauze soaked with either normal saline or Ringer's lactate solution. The wrapped part should then be placed into a plastic bag, which is sealed and immersed in an ice-water solution. Under no circumstances should the amputated part be placed directly into ice water or exposed to dry ice.

A tourniquet is usually not required to control bleeding. A compressive dressing should be applied to the amputation stump. No attempt should be made to ligate bleeding vessels because it might compromise subsequent neurovascular repair. If the amputated part is not cooled, ischemia is poorly tolerated and successful revascularization is unlikely after 12 hours for finger amputations and 6 hours for more proximal amputations. Cooled parts may be replanted up to 24 hours after injury for finger amputations and up to 12 hours after injury for more proximal amputations.

Indications and Contraindications

Replantation is indicated for severed thumbs or multiple digits, transmetacarpal hand amputations, wrist- or distal forearm–level amputations, and amputations of almost any body part in a child. For more proximal levels of amputation, only sharp or moderately avulsed parts can be considered for replantation. The more proximal the amputation, the greater is the amount of ischemic muscle mass and the more urgent the need for revascularization.

Contraindications to replantation include severely crushed or mangled parts; multilevel amputation; amputations in patients with arteriosclerotic vessels; amputations in patients with other serious injuries or diseases; and amputations with prolonged warm ischemic times, particularly at proximal levels.

In adults, replantation of a single finger proximal to the insertion of the flexor digitorum superficialis is usually contraindicated because of the poor functional outcome due to stiffness. Limited motion in these replanted fingers is caused by simultaneous zone 2 flexor digitorum superficialis and profundus tendon disruption, phalangeal fracture, and extensor tendon disruption. Replantation at this level may be considered in children or for aesthetic reasons.

Surgical Procedure

The preferred method of anesthesia is axillary or supraclavicular block because it provides a sympathetic block resulting in vasodilation. The surgical sequence of replantation begins with a wide surgical exposure that allows identification and isolation of arteries, veins, and nerves. The soft tissue is then meticulously debrided. The bone is shortened and securely internally fixed with K-wires, screws, or plates with sufficient stability to allow early postoperative motion.

The extensor tendons are repaired first, and then anastomosis of one or preferably two arteries is performed, followed by venous anastomoses. Two veins should be repaired for each artery repaired. Last, repair of the flexor tendons and of the nerves is carried out. Skin should be closed loosely, with care taken to approximate soft tissue over repaired vessels and nerves.

In replantations proximal to the distal forearm, fasciotomies of all muscle compartments should be performed at the time of replantation. The patient undergoing proximal replantation should be returned to the operating room in 48 to 72 hours so the wound may be reevaluated and any additional necrotic tissue debrided.

Postoperative Care

Postoperatively, the hand is protected in a loose, bulky dressing, and the patient must be kept in a warm room (>80°F). Anticoagulation should be given in the perioperative period to diminish the likelihood of anastomosis thrombosis. Low-molecular-weight heparin and aspirin for 5 to 7 days are among the recommended regimens. However, there is no well-established anticoagulation protocol. Some patients, particularly children, may require sedative medications such as chlorpromazine (Thorazine) to decrease early postoperative arterial spasm for the first 5 to 7 days. The duration of postoperative anticoagulation also highly varies. Ideally, anticoagulation should last until complete endothelium healing. However, this is a matter of debate because there are contradicting studies reporting that endothelium healing lasts from 7 up to 21 days. Vasospastic agents such as nicotine, caffeine, theophylline, and theobromine should be restricted for the first few weeks after replantation or revascularization. The patient should be placed on a broad-spectrum antibiotic for 5 to 7 days. Clinical monitoring of the replanted or revascularized part may be supplemented with a pulse oximeter, laser Doppler, or temperature probe. Oxygen saturation less than 94%, skin temperature less than 30°C, and skin temperature decrease of more than 2°C in less than 1 hour are indicative of imminent failure.

In those replanted or revascularized parts with impending failure by change in color, capillary refill, or tissue turgor, the dressing should be loosened, hand position should be changed to relieve pressure on the part, and a heparin bolus of 3000 to 5000 U may be given. The patient must be kept well hydrated and the room warm.

If no improvement is seen after 4 to 6 hours, the patient may be returned to the operating room for exploration of the anastomoses. Vascular revision is most successful when carried out within 48 hours of injury. Technical problems involving vascular anastomoses are most often caused by thrombosis, an ill-placed suture occluding the lumen, poor proximal flow secondary to spasm, or undetected intimal vessel damage. If vascular damage is found, a larger segment of the vessel should be resected and a vein graft interposed.

If failure appears secondary to poor venous outflow, extremity elevation and intermittent application of leeches (*Hirudo* species for 1-5 days) may provide transient venous drainage while adequate venous drainage is reestablished. Leeches release hirudin, a powerful anticoagulant, and they have been used with great success for many years in cases of venous congestion. However, they have been linked with infections from *Aeromonas hydrophila*; therefore, antibiotic prophylaxis with ciprofloxacin is recommended. If leeches are unavailable, heparin-soaked pledgets or gauzes can be used.

Prognosis

Approximately 85% of replanted parts remain viable. Sensory recovery with two-point discrimination of 10 mm or less occurs in approximately 50% of adults. Patients with viable replanted or revascularized parts often complain of cold intolerance during the first 2 or 3 years after replantation. ROM in replanted digits largely depends on the level of injury and averages approximately 50% of the normal side. Tenolysis is the most common secondary procedure following replantations.

In most children, normal sensation is regained after digital replantation, and the epiphyseal plates remain open and achieve approximately 80% of normal longitudinal growth. Although the functional results are more promising in children, the viability rate is lower in children because of the greater technical demands of the small-vessel anastomoses and the greater sympathetic tone.

Because nerves transected in the proximal arm must regenerate over the considerable length of the limb, only limited motor return is seen in the forearm and hand in proximal limb replantations in adults. One potential benefit of a proximal upper limb replantation may be converting a traumatic above-elbow amputation to an assistive limb with elbow control. Replantation may provide dramatic restoration of hand function when the level of initial amputation is either in the distal forearm or at the wrist level (Figure 11–30).

AMPUTATION

The purpose of amputation is to preserve maximal function consistent with bone loss and to achieve an aesthetically acceptable appearance. Due to the common muscle belly of the flexor digitorum profundus muscles, functional shortening of one tendon due to adhesions or overadvancement during tendon repair can result in flexion lag of other digits—the quadriga effect. Amputation of a stiff and insensate finger can improve function of the entire hand. Priority should be given to preserving functional length, minimizing scar and joint contractures, and preventing the development of symptomatic neuromas.

1. Phalangeal Amputation

Digital amputation may be carried out through a phalanx or an interphalangeal joint. If the amputation is through the PIP or DIP joint, the remaining articular surface is reshaped to remove the palmar condylar prominences. If the normal insertion of a tendon was amputated, the tendon should be pulled distally, severed proximally, and allowed to retract. The flexor and extensor tendons should never be sewn over the amputation bone end to provide soft-tissue coverage. Nerves should be identified, gently drawn distally, and transected proximally. The nerve ends should be cauterized to prevent the development of a neuroma adherent to the skin scar. If possible, the thick well-padded skin of the palmar surface of the finger should be used to cover the amputation stump. A nontender, shortened, well-padded digit is preferable to a poorly covered, slightly longer, tender digit.

2. Ray Resection

Amputations through the proximal portion of the proximal phalanx or at the MCP joint of the index or little finger

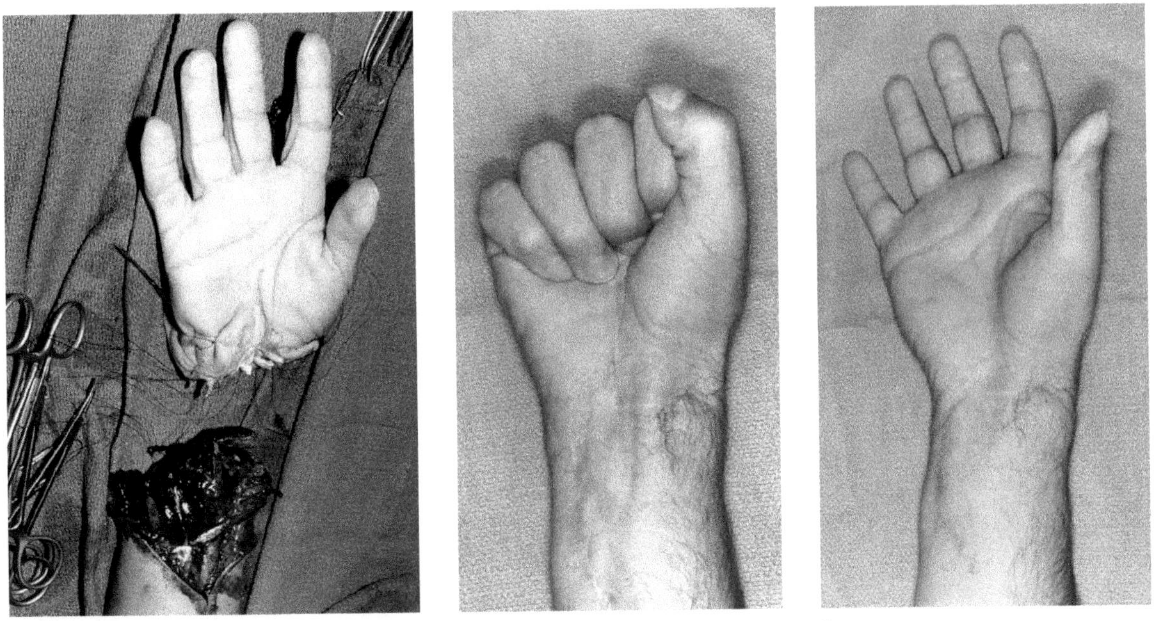
A B C

▲ **Figure 11–30.** Replantation of hand. Intraoperative view **(A)**. Following operation, flexion **(B)** and extension **(C)** are restored.

may leave an unsightly bony prominence on the border of the palm, and amputations at a similar level in the middle or ring finger may create an awkward interdigital gap that allows small objects to fall through the palm. Ray resection of a digit's phalanges and metacarpal may be employed to close traumatic wounds, remove dysfunctional or dysesthetic digits, or treat malignant tumors. The aesthetic and functional advantages of ray resection must be balanced against the loss of palm breadth and, hence, diminution of grip strength.

Index ray resection creates a normal-appearing web between the middle finger and the thumb. Similarly, resection of the little finger metacarpal leaves a smooth ulnar contour. Little finger ray resection is contraindicated in patients who prefer maximal grip strength over cosmesis. Resection of the middle or ring finger ray should be accompanied by either soft-tissue coaptation or metacarpal transposition for gap closure. Bony transposition consists of osteotomy and transposition of the corresponding distal portion of the index ray to the middle-ray position (Figure 11–31) or osteotomy of the little finger metacarpal and transposition to the ring finger ray. However, bony transpositions following central ray resections for gap closure have been linked with several complications such as malunion and nonunion; therefore, shortening of the transverse metacarpal ligament may be a better, alternative option. Although gap closure through shortening of the transverse metacarpal ligament was initially criticized for inadequate gap closure, proper shortening of the deep transverse metacarpal ligament has been found to lead to favorable results.

Charpentier K, Loisel F, Menu G, Feuvrier D, Obert L, Pluvy I. Long-term functional results of digital replantation: a survey of 28 patients. *Hand Surg Rehabil.* 2019;38(6):375-380. [PMID: 31521798]

Ono S, Chung KC. Efficiency in digital and hand replantation. *Clin Plast Surg.* 2019;46(3):359-370. [PMID: 31103081]

Papadopoulos D, Gkiatas I, Batistatou A, et al. Antithrombotic efficacy of direct oral anticoagulants on patency rate following microsurgical anastomosis in crushed rat arteries. *J Orthop Sci.* 2019;24(3):552-557. [PMID: 30392716]

Papadopoulos DV, Kostas-Agnantis I, Gkiatas I, Tsantes AG, Ziara P, Korompilias AV. The role of new oral anticoagulants in orthopaedics: an update of recent evidence. *Eur J Orthop Surg Traumatol.* 2017;27(5):573-582. [PMID: 28314985]

Sotereanos DG, Schmidt CC. Hand and digital amputations. In: Peimer CA, ed. *Surgery of the Hand and Upper Extremity.* McGraw-Hill; 1996:999-1018.

WRIST INJURIES

Anatomy

The wrist is composed of the eight carpal bones, the radiocarpal joint, the distal parts of the bones of the forearm, including the distal radioulnar joint, and the proximal parts of the five metacarpal bones and the joints between these bones.

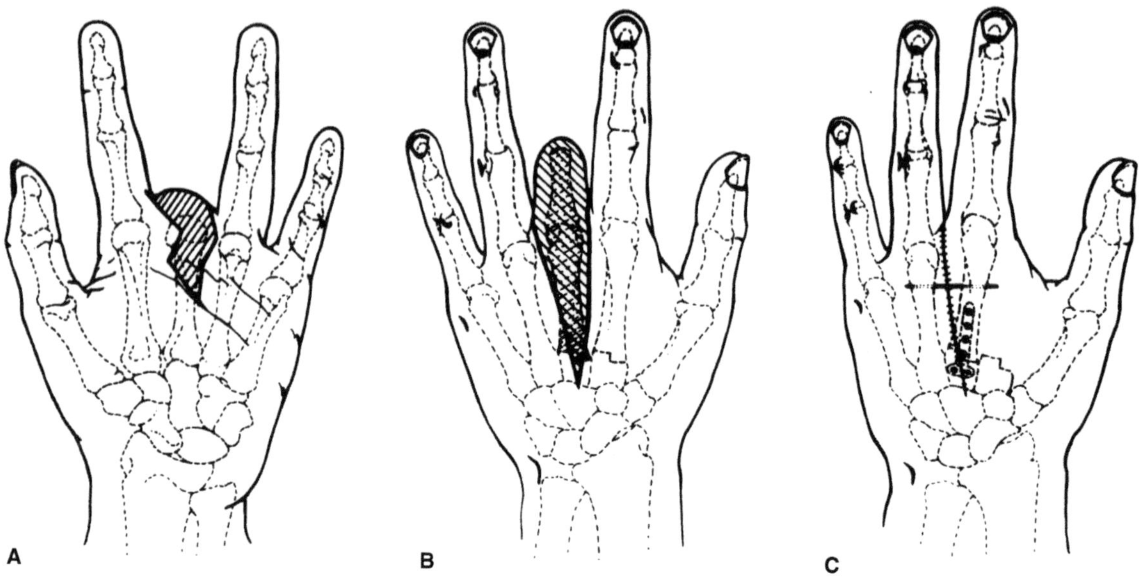

▲ **Figure 11–31.** Middle-ray resection and index-ray transposition. **A:** Converging chevron incisions reduce palmar skin and soft-tissue redundancy. **B:** Corresponding step-cut osteotomies are fashioned in both the index and middle metacarpal proximal metaphyses. **C:** The transposed index finger is fixed to the middle finger with a plate and further stabilized with K-wire into the ring-finger metacarpal. (Reprinted with permission, from Bucholz RW, Green DP, Rockwood CA, eds. Rockwood and Green's fractures in adults, 3rd ed. Philadelphia: J.B. Lippincott; 2001.)

The carpal bones are the scaphoid, lunate, triquetrum, and pisiform in the proximal row and the trapezium, trapezoid, capitate, and hamate in the distal row. These bones are stabilized by the intrinsic ligaments, attaching only to the carpal bones, including the scapholunate ligament, the lunotriquetral ligament, and the TFCCs. The extrinsic ligaments also attach to bones other than the carpal bones; on the dorsum of the wrist, these include the dorsal intercarpal, the dorsal radiotriquetral, and the dorsal radioulnar ligaments, and on the volar wrist, these include the volar radioscaphocapitate, the volar radiotriquetral, the volar ulnolunate, the volar ulnotriquetral, and the volar radioulnar ligaments. The thumb ligaments are the superficial anterior oblique, the deep anterior oblique, and the dorsoradial ligaments.

The CMC joints are five joints that articulate the distal row of carpal bones and the proximal bases of the five metacarpal bones. The CMC joint of the thumb or the first CMC joint, also known as the trapeziometacarpal joint, differs significantly from the other four CMC joints. The palmar CMC ligaments are similar in arrangement to the dorsal CMC ligaments, with the exception of those to the third metacarpal, which are three in number: a lateral one from the trapezium, situated superficial to the sheath of the tendon of the flexor carpi radialis, an intermediate one from the capitate, and a medial one from the hamate.

The distal radioulnar joint is a pivot-joint formed between the ulnar head and the ulnar notch on the distal radius. The dorsal and volar radioulnar ligaments originate on the corresponding margins of the ulnar notch on the distal radius and insert on the ulnar head.

Scaphoid Injuries

The scaphoid is the most commonly fractured bone in the carpus, composing 15% of all wrist injuries. The vascular supply to the scaphoid comes through a narrow nonarticular region at its waist. Most of the blood supply to the scaphoid tuberosity enters distally. In approximately a third of fractures at the waist level, there is diminished flow to the proximal pole, which may result in ischemic necrosis of the proximal pole of the scaphoid. Almost 100% of proximal pole fractures develop ischemic or aseptic necrosis.

Fracture of the scaphoid waist is the most common location (65%), whereas proximal third fractures are the second most common (25%), and distal third fractures occur in only 10%.

Cast immobilization is recommended in the treatment of all stable and nondisplaced scaphoid fractures. Inclusion of the thumb in cast immobilization is not necessary for nondisplaced waist fractures. Criteria for instability include fracture displacement greater than 1 mm, scapholunate angle greater than 60 degrees, flexion (humpback) deformity greater than 15 degrees, intrascaphoid angle greater than 35 degrees, unstable vertical or oblique fractures, comminuted fractures, proximal pole fractures, and fractures with perilunate dislocation. In unstable and displaced fractures, surgical treatment with ORIF with a compression screw is required. Closed reduction and percutaneous fixation with compression screw is an alternative method in cases without gross displacement. Unrestricted activity is allowed following fixation with a compression screw if 50% or more of cortical bridging is evident on CT evaluation.

Treatment of nonunions depends on two factors: presence of humpback deformity and the vascular status of the proximal pole. The vascularity of the proximal pole can be assessed preoperatively with MRI or intraoperatively by assessing the presence of punctate bleeding from the proximal pole. The recommended treatment for nonunions without humpback deformity is debridement of the nonunion site and placement of a narrow rectangular corticocancellous graft (Matti-Russe technique), whereas for humpback deformities, corticocancellous trapezoidal wedge grafts are recommended to correct the deformity (Fisk-Fernandez technique). However, when the proximal and distal poles are large enough to allow for screw purchase, structural corticocancellous grafts are not required and cancellous bone graft alone is a viable graft alternative. Although vascularized bone grafts were traditionally recommended for nonunions with avascular necrosis of the proximal pole, nonvascularized bone grafts may yield similar outcomes in terms of union rates. The vascularized bone grafts can be either local pedicled grafts harvested from the distal radius or distant free grafts from the medial femoral condyle.

Once degenerative arthritis is evident at the radiocarpal joint, salvage procedures include proximal row carpectomy, scaphoid excision and midcarpal arthrodesis, and total wrist arthrodesis.

Lunate and Perilunate Dislocations

Lunate and perilunate dislocations are high-energy injuries with poor outcomes that can commonly be missed on the initial examination. The mechanism of these injuries is usually dorsiflexion, ulnar deviation, and intercarpal supination. In 25% of these cases, signs of median nerve compression may be present. When the entire carpus except the lunate dislocates and the lunate remains normally seated in the lunate fossa of the radius, the abnormality is termed *perilunate dislocation* (Figure 11–32). When the relationship between the carpus and the radius is maintained but the lunate is dislocated palmarward into the carpal tunnel, the condition is termed *lunate dislocation*. The traumatic disruption can go through the greater arc, when ligamentous disruptions are associated with fractures of adjacent bones, or through the lesser arc, when the dislocation is purely ligamentous. Although the lunate is bound to the scaphoid by the scapholunate ligament and to the triquetrum through the lunotriquetral ligament, the interval between the lunate and the capitate, known as the space of Poirier, lacks direct ligamentous connection. The most common types of greater arc disruption include transscaphoid-perilunate, transradial-styloid, and transscaphoid-transcapitate-perilunar.

Mayfield defined four stages of disruption. Stage 1 injuries are disruptions of the scapholunate ligament. Stage 2 injuries also include disruption of the capitolunate articulation. In stage 3 injuries, the arc of disruption extends across the lunotriquetral ligament. In stage 4 injuries, there is total disruption of the entire lunate ligamentous support, and the lunate is dislocated from the lunate fossa of the radius.

Emergent closed reduction and splinting should never be used as a sole treatment, and surgical repair should always follow. Open reduction is achieved through a dorsal or volar approach, whereas in some cases, a combined dorsal and volar approach is required. Then, through the dorsal approach, the intercarpal alignment is visualized, adjusted, and stabilized, and the palmar approach is used to release the transverse carpal ligament, expose the median nerve, and repair the rent in the space of Poirier. Any associated fractures must be fixed, and ligamentous repair especially of the scapholunate ligament is necessary for secure, anatomic reduction. The scapholunate joint can be pinned for further stability

Buijze G, Goslings J, Rhemrev S, et al. Cast immobilization with and without immobilization of the thumb for nondisplaced and minimally displaced scaphoid waist fractures: a multicenter, randomized, controlled trial. *J Hand Surg Am.* 2014;39(4):621-627. [PMID: 24582846]

Chang M, Bishop A, Moran S, Shin A. The outcomes and complications of 1,2-intercompartmental supraretinacular artery pedicled vascularized bone grafting of scaphoid nonunions. *J Hand Surg Am.* 2006;31(3):387-396. [PMID: 16516732]

Cohen M, Jupiter J, Fallahi K, Shukla S. Scaphoid waist nonunion with humpback deformity treated without structural bone graft. *J Hand Surg Am.* 2013;38(4):701-705. [PMID: 23415167]

Dean BJF, Riley ND, McCulloch ER, Lane JCE, Touzell AB, Graham AJ. A new acute scaphoid fracture assessment method: a reliability study of the "long axis" measurement. *BMC Musculoskelet Disord.* 2018;19(1):310. [PMID: 30157835]

Goodman AD, Harris AP, Gil JA, Park J, Raducha J, Got CJ. Evaluation, management, and outcomes of lunate and perilunate dislocations. *Orthopedics.* 2019;42(1):e1-e6. [PMID: 30403823]

Huang HK, Tsai TY, Wang JP. Reduction and association of the lunotriquetral ligament for reverse perilunate dislocation. *J Wrist Surg.* 2019;8(6):508-512. [PMID: 31815067]

Janowski J, Coady C, Catalano LW 3rd. Scaphoid fractures: nonunion and malunion. *J Hand Surg Am.* 2016;41(11):1087-1092. [PMID: 27671767]

Ko JH, Pet MA, Khouri JS, Hammert WC. Management of scaphoid fractures. *Plast Reconstr Surg.* 2017;140(2):333e-346e. [PMID: 2874628]

Sotereanos D, Darlis N, Dailiana Z, Sarris I, Malizos K. A capsular-based vascularized distal radius graft for proximal pole scaphoid pseudarthrosis. *J Hand Surg Am.* 2006;31(4):580-587. [PMID: 16632051]

Tsantes AG, Papadopoulos DV, Gelalis ID, Vekris MD, Pakos EE, Korompilias AV. The efficacy of vascularized bone grafts in the treatment of scaphoid nonunions and Kienbock disease: a systematic review in 917 patients. *J Hand Microsurg.* 2019;11:6-13. [PMID: 30911206]

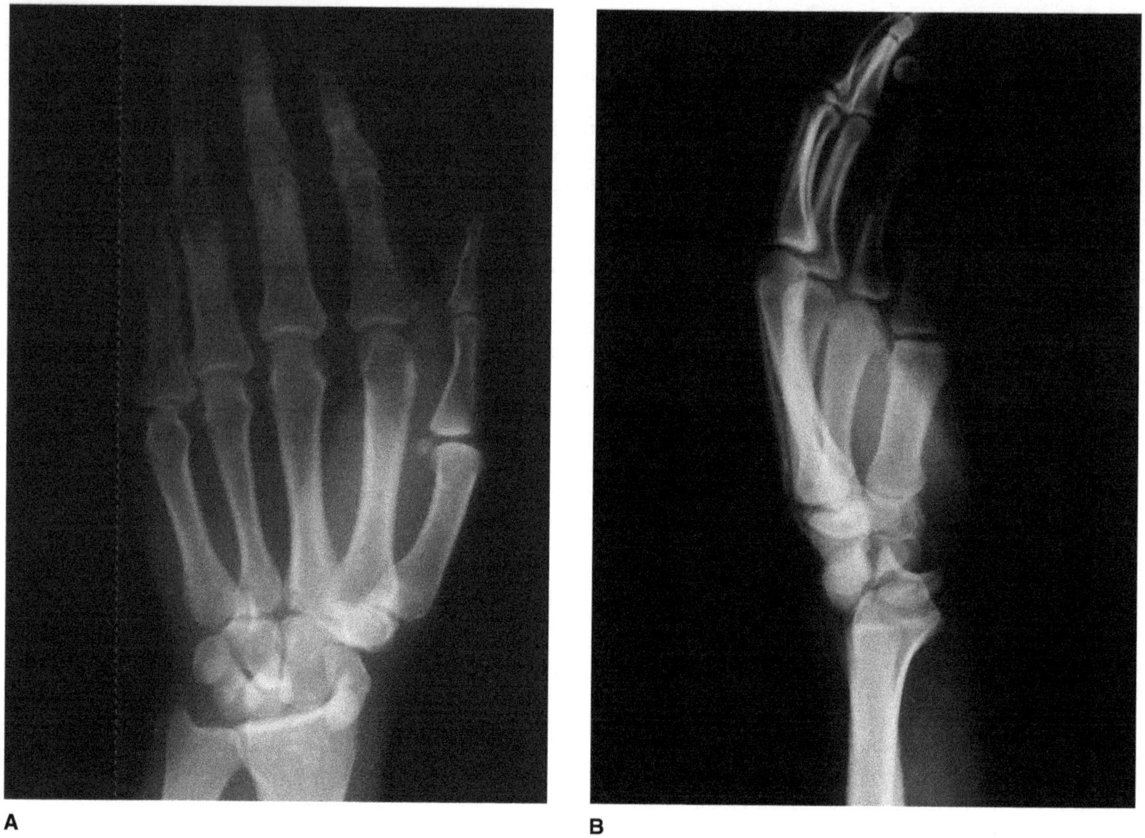

▲ **Figure 11–32.** Perilunate dislocation: Anteroposterior view **(A)**; lateral view **(B)**.

Kienböck Disease

Kienböck disease results from ischemic necrosis of the lunate, most commonly in males aged 20 to 40 years. The cause of the condition is the subject of extensive debate. Biomechanically, a negative ulnar variance and a decreased radial inclination may increase the force transmitted to the lunate through the lunate fossa of the radius. Repetitive trauma may further increase this force, leading to development of this condition. Additionally, anatomic variations in the shape of the lunate and in the vascular supply of the lunate may predispose to Kienböck disease. Patients present with dorsal wrist pain, swelling, and tenderness over the radiocarpal joint, while grip strength may also be decreased.

Kienböck disease may be classified based on the extent of collapse (Figure 11–33). Stage I disease demonstrates a linear compression fracture but an otherwise normal-appearing architecture and density. MRI studies show poor vascularity of the lunate in stage I (Figure 11–34). In stage II disease, there is sclerosis of the lunate on plain films. By stage III, lunate collapse is present. Stage III disease is subdivided into stage IIIA, in which the lunate is collapsed but carpal height remains normal and thus there is no scaphoid rotation, and stage IIIB, in which the lunate is collapsed and carpal height reduced and the scaphoid is rotated volar. In stage IV wrists, extensive osteoarthritic changes are present.

The current recommendations for the treatment of Kienböck disease include joint-level procedure in stages I, II, and IIIA of radial shortening osteotomy for ulnar-negative variance, whereas radial wedge osteotomy or capitate shortening osteotomy is performed for neutral or positive variance. Other options for patients with up to stage IIIA disease include vascularized bone grafts or distal core decompression. In stage IIIB and IV wrists, consideration is given to either proximal row carpectomy or wrist arthrodesis.

Salt Ö, Sayhan MB. Avascular necrosis of lunate bone: Kienböck disease. *Am J Emerg Med.* 2016;34(6):1185.e5-6. [PMID: 26682674]

Carpal Instability

Carpal instability can be broadly classified as dissociative when instability occurs between bones of the same carpal row (scapholunate or lunotriquetral) and nondissociative when instability occurs between different carpal rows (radiocarpal

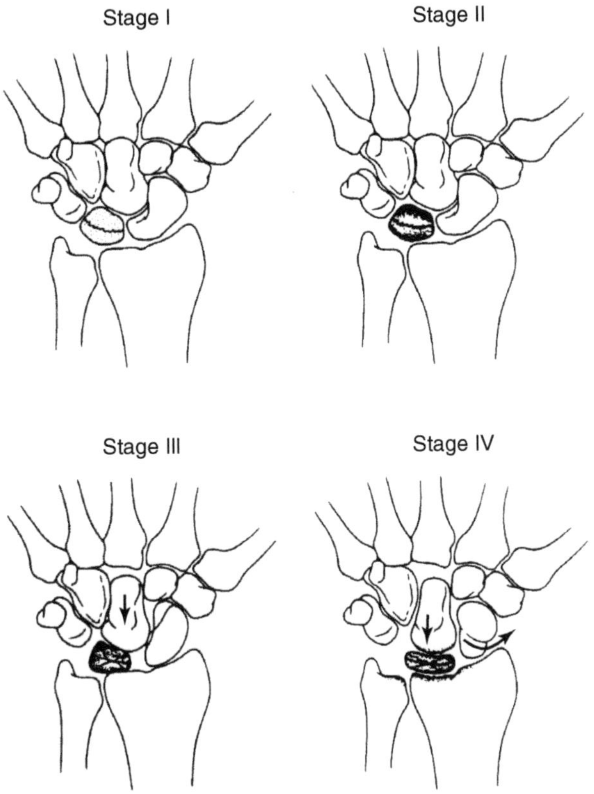

▲ **Figure 11–33.** Staging of Kienböck disease (after Lichtman). Stage I: Routine radiographs (posteroanterior, lateral) are normal, but tomography may show a linear fracture, usually transverse through the body of the lunate. MRI confirms avascular changes. Stage II: Bone density increase (sclerosis) and a fracture line are usually evident on the posteroanterior radiograph. Posteroanterior and lateral tomograms demonstrate sclerosis, cystic changes, and often a clear fracture. There is no collapse deformity. Stage III: Advanced bone density changes are present, with fragmentation, cystic resorption, and collapse. The diagnosis is evident from posteroanterior radiograph. Tomograms (posteroanterior and lateral) show the degree of lunate infractionation and amount of fracture displacement. Proximal migration of the capitate is present, and there is mild to moderate rotary alignment of the scaphoid. Stage IV: Perilunate arthritic changes are present, with complete collapse and fragmentation of the lunate. Carpal instability is evident, with scaphoid malalignment and capitate displacement into the lunate space. (Reprinted with permission, from Bucholz RW, Green DP, Rockwood CA, eds. Rockwood and Green's fractures in adults, 3rd ed. Philadelphia: Lippincott; 1991.)

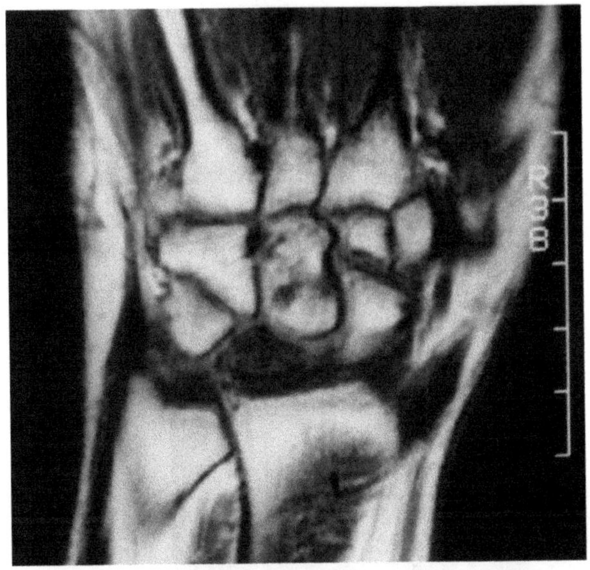

▲ **Figure 11–34.** MRI showing Kienböck disease.

or midcarpal). Combined carpal instability is instability both between bones of the same row and between the carpal rows, as in cases of perilunate dislocations. Patients present with wrist pain located over the dissociation area, clicking or catching sensation in the wrist, and decreased grip strength. On physical examination, inspection may reveal swelling and abnormal shift during wrist movements. On palpation, there is tenderness over the wrist, depending on the location of the dissociated bones.

To evaluate the orientation of the carpus properly, true PA and lateral radiographs are required, and a clenched fist view should also be obtained. Finally, PA views with radial and ulnar wrist deviation are useful to evaluate nondissociative carpal instability. Several radiologic parameters and angles should be evaluated on these views. A gap between the scaphoid and lunate greater than 3 mm on a clenched view indicates scapholunate dissociation (Figure 11–35). A cortical ring sign on the PA view also indicates an abnormally flexed scaphoid as in cases of scapholunate dissociation. In case of radiocarpal nondissociative instability, greater than 50% of lunate width is ulnarly translated off the lunate fossa of the radius with ulnar deviation of the wrist.

On the lateral view with the wrist in a neutral position, the middle metacarpal, capitate, lunate, and radius are collinear. The radioscaphoid angle (Figure 11–36) is usually 40 to 60 degrees. An angle greater than 60 degrees indicates that the scaphoid is abnormally flexed. The orientation of the lunate seen on the lateral radiograph normally reflects a ligamentous balancing of the influences of the adjacent scaphoid and triquetrum. The scaphoid tends to tether the lunate into flexion through the scapholunate ligament, whereas the triquetrum tends to tether the lunate into extension (dorsiflexion)

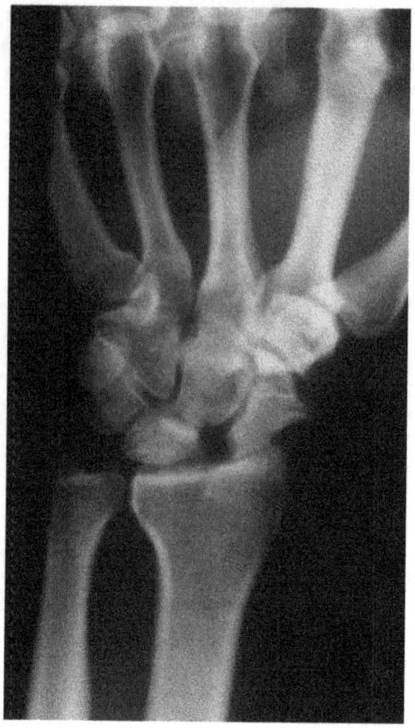

▲ **Figure 11–35.** Anteroposterior view of static scapholunate dissociation.

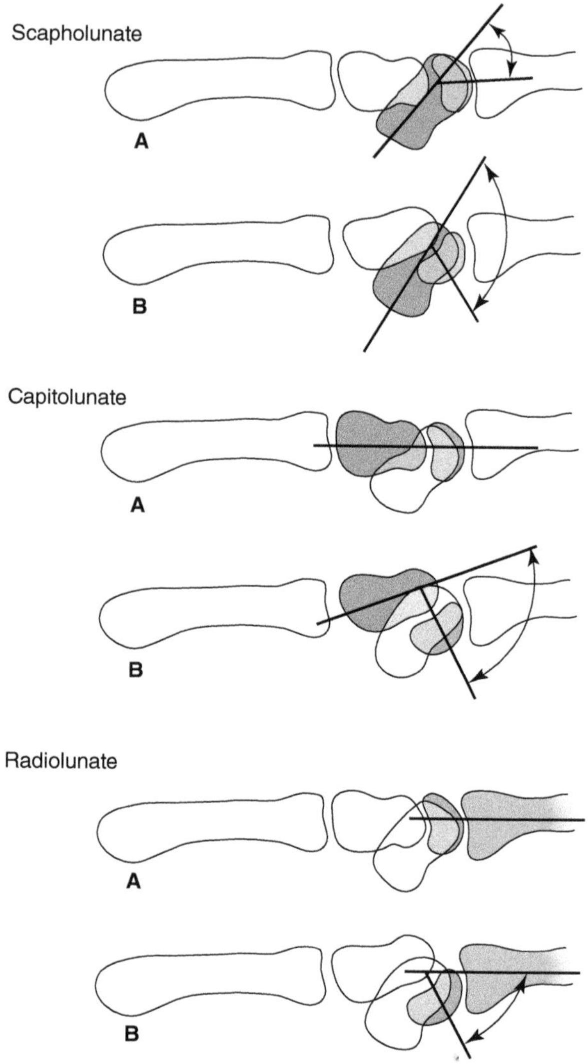

▲ **Figure 11–36.** Carpal angle measurements are of considerable aid in identifying carpal instability patterns. A, normal angle; B, abnormal angle seen in dorsiflexion instability. The capitolunate angle should theoretically be 0 degrees with the wrist in neutral position, but the range of normal probably extends to as much as 15 degrees. The scapholunate angle may be the most helpful; an angle of greater than 80 degrees is definite evidence of dorsiflexion instability. The radiolunate angle is abnormal if it exceeds 15 degrees. (Reprinted with permission, from Green DP, ed. *Operative Hand Surgery*, 2nd ed. Philadelphia: Churchill Livingstone; 1988.)

through the lunotriquetral ligament. When the scapholunate ligament is disrupted, the scaphoid tends to flex excessively, and the lunate, under the unopposed influence of the triquetrum, dorsiflexes (dorsal intercalated segment instability) (Figure 11–37). When the lunotriquetral ligament is disrupted, the lunate, under the unopposed influence of the scaphoid, is flexed (volar intercalated segment instability). An angle between the radial and lunate axes (radiolunate angle) greater than 70 degrees indicates scapholunate dissociation, whereas an angle less than 30 degrees indicates lunotriquetral dissociation.

The optimal treatment for scapholunate dissociation is an area of intense interest. Acute ligamentous disruption is usually treated with direct ligamentous repair and K-wire pinning. When ligamentous repair is not possible, the articular surfaces are undamaged, and the dissociation is reducible, ligamentous reconstruction or dorsal capsular ligamentodesis is recommended. In cases of nonreducible dissocciation or in cases of arthritis, an intercapal fusion may be considered (Figure 11–38).

Treatment of lunotriquetral dissociation has poor results; therefore, observation is usually indicated. In acute injuries, ligamentous repair with further K-wire pinning may be attempted. In chronic cases, lunotriquetral fusion is recommended, but the nonunion rate is high.

In cases of nondissociative instability (radiocarpal or midcarpal instability), treatment depends on whether the instability results from a fracture or malunion or from soft-tissue incompetence. When radiocarpal instability results from distal radius malunion, a corrective osteotomy is recommended, and when it is the result of styloid fractures, fixation of the fractures is required. When all these treatments fail, or in severe cases with soft-tissue incompetence, a

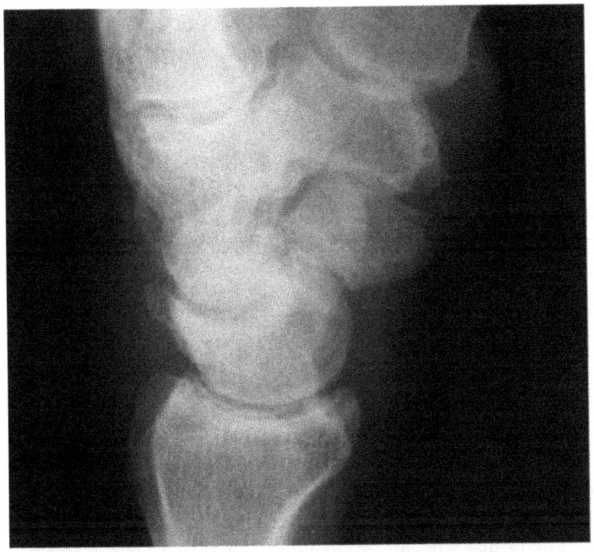

▲ **Figure 11–37.** Lateral radiograph of dorsal intercalated segment instability.

wrist fusion is the final step. In cases of midcarpal instability, immobilization with splinting is initially recommended, and when nonoperative treatment has failed, midcarpal fusion may be attempted.

Garcia-Elias M, Puig de la Bellacasa I, Schouten C. Carpal ligaments: a functional classification. *Hand Clin.* 2017;33(3):511-520. [PMID: 28673627]

TFCC Tears and Ulnar Impaction Syndrome

The ulna also articulates with the ulnar carpus through the TFCC. Approximately 20% of the load from the hand to the forearm passes through the ulnocarpal joint. TFCC tears cause ulnar-sided wrist pain, especially with activities that require forearm rotation, like turning keys or opening bottles. On physical examination, there is tenderness over the soft spot between the ulnar styloid and the pisiform (fovea sign), and the pain is aggravated with ulnar deviation (TFCC compression) or radial deviation (TFCC tension). TFCC lesions are divided into degenerative and traumatic types. Degenerative tears are usually related to ulnocarpal impaction. Traumatic tears usually occur after a twisting injury of the wrist. Central tears and tears near the attachment of the TFCC to the radius are usually treated with an arthroscopic debridement. Tears in the well-vascularized periphery of the TFCC are treated with either arthroscopic or open repair. After repair, patients are maintained in a long arm cast for 6 weeks to allow fibrocartilage healing.

Ulnocarpal impaction syndrome also presents with ulnar side wrist pain, particularly with ulnar deviation, caused by excessive ulnar positive variance. Radiographs may demonstrate degenerative changes of the distal ulna and cysts in the lunate. Treatment consists of shortening the ulna. When 2 to 3 mm of shortening is required, ulnar shortening can be performed arthroscopically by removing the cartilage and the bone under the TFCC (wafer procedure). Otherwise, when more excessive shortening is required, an open ulnar-shortening osteotomy should be performed in the diaphyseal ulna, fixed with a plate and screws. After the wafer procedure, patients often complain of ulnar pain for a prolonged period of 3 to 6 months. Approximately 50% of patients who have an ulnar shortening osteotomy require plate removal after osteotomy healing.

Distal Radioulnar Joint Instability-Arthritis

Instability of the distal radioulnar joint is difficult to treat. Instability is usually the result of trauma, but it may occur after an excessive distal ulna resection. Treatment requires detection and correction of any malunions in the radius or ulna. A number of soft-tissue operations are designed to stabilize the distal ulna, all with varying degrees of success.

Arthritis between the distal radius and ulna can be caused by traumatic, degenerative, or inflammatory disorders. Treatment consists of hemiresection or complete excision of the ulnar head (Darrach procedure). An alternative treatment, the Suave-Kapandji procedure, fuses the distal radioulnar joint and creates a pseudarthrosis of the distal ulna. This is particularly useful in the presence of ulnar translocation of the carpus.

Papatheodorou L, Sotereanos D. Step-cut ulnar shortening osteotomy for ulnar impaction syndrome. *JBJS Essent Surg Tech.* 2017;7(1):e3. [PMID: 30233938]

Tan DMK, Lim JX. Treatment of carpal instability and distal radioulnar joint instability. *Clin Plast Surg.* 2019;46(3):451-468. [PMID: 31103089]

FINGERTIP INJURIES

SOFT-TISSUE DEFECTS

The skin of the fingertips is the contact surface for sensate prehension; therefore, injuries to the fingertips may compromise our interaction with the environment. The pulp of the fingertip is normally covered by tough, highly innervated skin, anchored to the phalanx by fibrous septa. The dorsum of the fingertip is composed of the nail and nail bed.

Treatment

The goals in treatment of fingertip injuries are to provide adequate sensation with minimal tenderness, a durable tip, and a bone support for nail growth. Preservation of bone length should be balanced with the other goals.

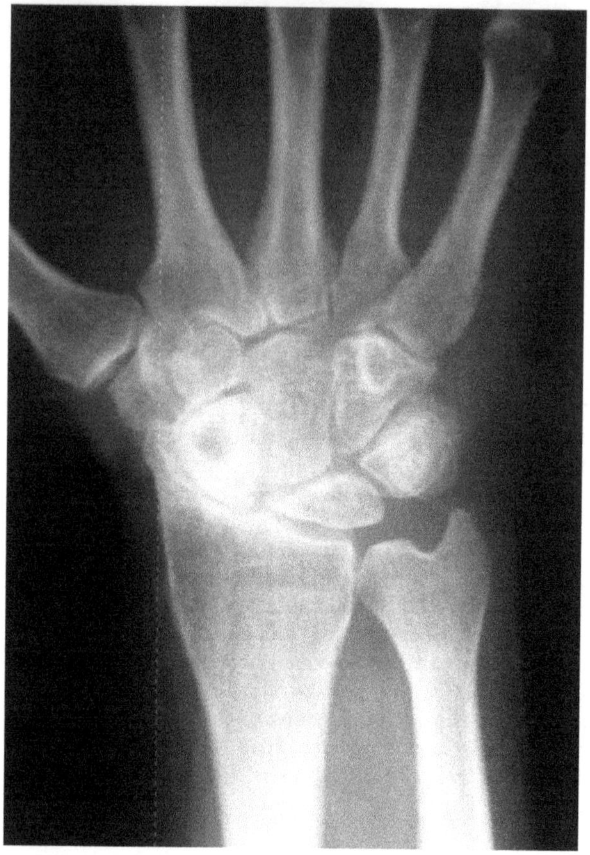

▲ **Figure 11–38.** Scapholunate advanced collapse pattern.

The choice of treatment depends on the size and location of the defect. The mechanism of injury (sharp laceration, crushing, or avulsion), the presence of exposed bone, and the angle of soft-tissue loss are considered in planning treatment.

A. Open Wound Care and Secondary Healing

Open wound care and healing by secondary intention are indicated for most injuries in children even with bone exposure and in defects less than 2 cm^2 in adults with no bone or tendon exposed. The wound is thoroughly cleansed, and soft dressings are applied. Initial dressings are changed on the seventh to tenth day, and soaks in peroxide with soft dressings afterward are performed daily until wound healing, usually at 3 to 5 weeks. Although secondary healing is a simple method that allows early movement, it may result in stump tenderness.

B. Primary Shortening and Closure

Primary bone shortening and closure are indicated when more than 50% of the distal phalanx is lost or the nail matrix is irreparably damaged. This one-stage procedure allows for immediate mobilization. In performing the procedure, the end of the distal phalanx bone should be trimmed to provide a tension-free soft-tissue closure. The remaining nail matrix should be ablated to prevent nail deformities such as a hook-shaped nail. Neurectomy of digital nerves under traction allows the nerve ends to retract into soft tissue proximal to the ultimate scar. If insertions of the extensor or flexor tendon cannot be preserved, disarticulation is preferred.

C. Skin Grafting

Larger skin defects (>2 cm^2) without bone or tendon exposure require coverage with skin grafts. Full-thickness skin grafts provide more durable coverage and better appearance, whereas split-thickness grafts contract more and are less durable. However, full-thickness grafts require a better vascularized bed compared to split-thickness grafts. Full-thickness grafts are usually harvested from the hypothenar region. The donor site can be closed primarily, and the graft is sutured over the defect. A cotton ball can be tied down over the graft to facilitate incorporation with the underlying tissue. The cotton ball is removed after 7 days.

D. Skin Flaps

The most commonly used flaps that are used in the treatment of fingertip injuries include the following

1. V-Y advancement skin flaps—V-Y advancement skin flaps may advance palmar tissue or unite two lateral skin flaps. These skin flaps are helpful in the management of transverse or dorsal oblique amputations in which soft-tissue tip coverage is needed and further skeletal shortening is deemed undesirable. Complete separation of the vertical septa between the skin and the bone is required to mobilize skin flaps for advancement. The septa between the flap and the proximal skin must then be divided. Traction on the flap helps differentiate the septa from vessels and nerves.

2. Cross-finger flap—The cross-finger flap is useful for the management of volar oblique lacerations. Skin is elevated from the dorsum of the adjacent finger, with care taken not to incise the extensor paratenon. The skin is then rotated palmarward and sewn to the palmar defect of the involved fingertip. The donor region on the donor finger is skin grafted. The transposed flap is divided from the donor finger after 2 weeks. Joint stiffness is a potential complication in both the donor and recipient digits. The creation of a defect on a normal digit is another disadvantage.

3. Thenar flap—This flap is also useful for volar oblique lacerations. The thenar flap may be used in children and young (<30 years) adults in whom the potential for joint stiffness is less. A flap of palmar skin is raised at the base of the thumb and applied to the injured tip of the flexed injured finger. More subcutaneous fat is transferred with a thenar flap than with a cross-finger flap. Thenar skin flaps usually result in good matching of color and texture with the pulp.

4. Moberg palmar advancement flap—This palmar advancement flap is useful for volar thumb defects up to 2 cm^2. Bilateral midlateral incisions dorsal to the neurovascular bundles of the thumb allow mobilization of the flap from the flexor tendon sheath. The flap may be maximally advanced by flexion of the thumb interphalangeal joint. When additional coverage is required, the skin of the flap may be transversely divided at the MCP crease while the neurovascular bundles are preserved, the distal portion of the flap may be advanced further, and a skin graft may be placed between the distal flap and the proximal flap. Disadvantages of this flap include the possibility of interphalangeal joint flexion contracture and the potential for dorsal tip necrosis if dorsal vascular branches to the digit are injured.

NAIL BED INJURIES

Clinical Findings

Nail bed injuries, often neglected, should be carefully attended to because the nail enhances sensibility, provides protection and fine manipulation of the finger, and gives the finger a normal appearance. The nail bed may be injured by subungual hematoma, nail matrix laceration, avulsion of the nail matrix from the nail fold, or complete loss of the nail matrix.

Treatment

When a subungual hematoma involves more than 50% of the subungual area (under the nail plate), the nail should be removed and irrigated and the nail bed laceration repaired under digital block anesthesia with fine, 6-0 or 7-0 absorbable suture or skin glue. The nail plate is washed and placed back into the nail fold to act as a biologic splint. Otherwise, a dressing, a piece of aluminum from a suture package, or a piece of gauze can be interposed between the nail roof and the nail bed to prevent synechia (adhesions) with resultant splitting of the nail. Nail bed defects are treated with split-thickness nail bed grafts taken from either an adjacent uninjured fingernail or a toenail. When nail bed injuries occur with an open distal phalangeal fracture, pin fixation of the fracture may be considered because it stabilizes the nail bed repair.

Caution is required in the treatment of nail bed injuries in children from having a fingertip slammed in a door. The nail often lies dorsal to the nail fold, and there is a small subungual hematoma. If a radiograph is obtained, there is usually a physeal fracture of the distal phalanx. Because the nail bed laceration communicates with the physeal fracture, this injury is an open fracture and must be treated appropriately. The nail should be removed and the fracture site irrigated. An interposed portion of the nail bed often must be extracted from between the fragments of the physeal fracture. If the fracture is unstable, pin fixation facilitates nail bed repair. Failure to appreciate the open nature of this pediatric injury may result in osteomyelitis and physeal arrest of the distal phalanx.

Elliot D, Adani R, Hyun Woo S, Tang JB. Repair of soft tissue defects in finger, thumb and forearm: less invasive methods with similar outcomes. *J Hand Surg Eur Vol.* 2018;43(10):1019-1029. [PMID: 30451629]

Gunasagaran J, Sian KS, Ahmad TS. Nail bed and flap reconstructions for acute fingertip injuries: a case review and report of a chemical burn injury. *J Orthop Surg (Hong Kong).* 2019;27(2):2309499019839278. [PMID: 30943852]

Yannascoli SM, Thibaudeau S, Levin LS. Management of soft tissue defects of the hand. *J Hand Surg Am.* 2015;40(6):1237-1245. [PMID: 25936734]

THERMAL INJURY

ACUTE BURN INJURY

Degree of Injury

Burns are characterized and treated according to the depth of skin injury and are classified as first, second, third, and fourth degree. Determination of the skin depth is based on clinical examination, although some centers have implemented ultrasound for evaluation of the burn depth.

A. First-Degree Burns

First-degree burns involve only the epidermis. Patients usually present with painful red areas and blanchable skin when pressure is applied. Care is symptomatic.

B. Second-Degree Burns

Second-degree burns involve both the epidermis and the superficial portion of the dermis. These burns are identified by skin blistering and blanching of the skin. Treatment consists of daily nonadhesive dressing changes, extremity elevation, and hand splinting in the intrinsic plus position. Silver sulfadiazine ointment is also commonly used. The thumb should be maintained in an abducted position to prevent contracture of the first web space. The patient should begin a vigorous therapy program emphasizing active ROM as soon as it is tolerated. Compression garments may reduce swelling and scar hypertrophy after reepithelialization.

C. Third-Degree Burns

Third-degree burns involve the entire epidermis and dermis and a portion of the subcutaneous region. These burns are not painful, and the skin is soft but not blanchable. Third-degree burns should be treated with debridement within the first 7 days and coverage with a full-thickness or split-thickness skin graft. Dermal substitutes can also be used to cover areas with exposed tendons or bones, and subsequent skin grafting can be performed at the same time or as a two-stage procedure.

D. Fourth-Degree Burns

In addition to involvement of the skin, fourth-degree burns involve deep tissues including muscle, tendon, and bone. These burns are also not painful, but the skin is dry and hard. Treatment of these burns is similar to that of third-degree burns. However, in many cases, the only effective treatment for these burns is amputation of the involved part, with appropriate soft-tissue coverage of the residual stump.

Complications

A. Neurovascular Complications

The neurovascular status of the burned hand should be carefully monitored. Massive swelling necessitates release of compartments of the hand and forearm. Digital releases are best performed by longitudinal releases along the ulnar border of the index, middle, and ring fingers and along the radial border of the thumb and little finger. Longitudinal incisions on the dorsal hand allow decompression of interosseous muscle compartments. Incisions are made along the medial and lateral aspects of the arm and forearm.

B. Joint Contractures

Joint contractures are the most common complications of upper extremity burns. Flexion contractures are likely to develop at the elbow. Treatment consists of soft-tissue release and coverage with either skin grafting or local flaps. When there is heterotopic ossification, excision is recommended after it matures, and although the best time for excision is debatable, marked decrease in bone scan activity and normalization of alkaline phosphate may be used as markers of bone maturation. Usually, excision is performed at 1.5 to 2 years after the burn injury. Because the area of most intense heterotopic ossification is posteromedial, care must be taken to define and protect the ulnar nerve during elbow release surgery.

Wrist contracture may tether the hand into either a flexed or extended position, depending on the location of the burn. In the fingers, burns usually involve the thin skin on the dorsum of the finger, often disrupting the central slip insertion onto the middle phalanx. The loss of active PIP joint extension combined with dorsal hand burns may result in development of a clawlike deformity, with flexion contractures of the PIP joints and hyperextension contracture at the MCP joint.

Treatment of MCP joint extension contracture usually requires release of the dorsal scar, addition of a dorsal skin graft, and dorsal metatarsophalangeal joint capsular release. PIP flexion contractures may also occur secondary to scarred volar skin. In such cases, soft-tissue release may be accomplished with either Z-plasty flap transposition or by palmar scar excision and full-thickness skin graft application. The most predictable treatment of severe PIP joint contracture in the burn patient is arthrodesis of the PIP joint.

Adduction contracture of the thumb due to first web contracture is a common deformity. The extent of release required depends on the degree of contracture. A modest adduction contracture that involves only the skin and the underlying fat tissue may be effectively treated with Z-plasty or other types of transposition skin flaps to regain adequate abduction of the thumb. With more severe contracture, release of the adductor pollicis from its origin or at its insertion and release of the first dorsal interosseous muscle origin from the thumb metacarpal may be required. If web space skin coverage is inadequate after muscle release, full-thickness skin grafting or local or distant skin flaps may be needed.

ELECTRICAL BURNS

The extent of injury in electrical burns is proportional to the amount of current that passes through the involved portion of the body. The Ohm law states that the amount of current is equal to the voltage divided by the resistance. Therefore, for a given voltage, those structures that have a lower resistance conduct a greater amount of current. The relative resistance of structures in the arm from least resistance to greatest resistance is as follows: nerve, vessel, muscle, skin, tendon, fat, and bone. Alternating current is more injurious than direct current. Because of its frequency, alternating current produces muscle tetany in the finger flexors, which may prevent the patient from releasing the grasped current source. The duration of contact plays a direct role in the severity of injury because a longer contact period results in more electrical energy passing through the body.

Clinical Findings

The greatest current density occurs at the entrance and exit wounds, usually apparent as charred areas that are blackened and surrounded by a gray-white zone, an area of tissue necrosis in which the tissue is still intact but will die. These areas are surrounded by a red zone, in which there is a variable extent of vessel thrombosis, coagulation, and necrosis.

High-voltage, or arc, burns produce a greater thermal than electric injury. Arc burns may extend across flexor surfaces from the hand to the wrist or from the forearm to the arm. Arc burns are usually associated with a high temperature of 3000 to 5000°C.

It is difficult to assess precisely the extent of tissue necrosis in burn wounds at the time of initial presentation. All burn patients should be examined for fractures, particularly cervical spine fractures, because electrical burn patients were possibly thrown a distance by the current. The possibility of either compartment syndrome or concomitant peripheral nerve injury must also be considered. Patients should be admitted to an intensive care unit and monitored for cardiac arrhythmia, renal failure, sepsis, secondary hemorrhage, and neurologic complications to the brain, spinal cord, or peripheral nerves.

Treatment

Treatment for upper extremity burns consists of initially debriding clearly nonviable tissue. The decision to carry out fasciotomy and nerve decompression should be guided by examination. A second debridement is performed 48 to 72 hours later for tissue in the gray-white zones. Debridement should be continued every 48 to 72 hours until a stable viable wound is achieved. The extent of necrosis often appears to increase with each successive debridement. This phenomenon reflects both an underestimation of the extent of initial injury and progressive vascular thrombosis. After all necrotic tissue is debrided, reconstruction is accomplished with either local or distant skin flaps or amputation.

CHEMICAL BURNS

The severity of chemical burns is directly proportional to the concentration and penetrability of the offending agent, the duration of skin exposure, and the mechanism of contact. Tissue destruction continues until either the chemical combines with tissue or the agent is neutralized by an applied secondary agent or washed from the skin surface. The mainstay of treatment of chemical burns of the skin is irrigation with water.

Two notable exceptions are burns resulting from hydrofluoric acid and from white phosphorous. Because hydrofluoric acid cannot be removed with water, calcium gluconate 10%, either applied to the skin as a gel or injected subcutaneously, is required to neutralize the acid. Patients with hydrofluoride burns experience severe pain that is seemingly out of proportion to the injury. White phosphorus burns, also refractory to water irrigation, are treated with 1% copper sulfate solution.

Iatrogenic chemical burns may occur with extravasation of chemotherapeutic agents administered intravenously. Chemotherapeutic agents are classified as vesicants, which include doxorubicin and vincristine and have a high probability of causing skin necrosis, and nonvesicants, which include cyclophosphamide. Management of both types of injury requires early surgical debridement of the region of extravasation. Secondary wound coverage may be obtained by either split-thickness skin grafting or skin flap coverage.

COLD INJURY (FROSTBITE)

Clinical Findings

With hypothermia, circulation is shunted from the periphery to the core of the body to maintain temperature to the vital body organs, and patients develop severe vasoconstriction as a result of increased sympathetic tone. Frostbite results from extracellular and intracellular crystal formation. Intracellular ice crystals cause cellular injury due to cell membrane damage. With the formation of extracellular ice crystals, osmotic gradients develop, leading to cell dehydration and electrolyte disturbances

Frostbite injuries may be classified as either superficial or deep. Superficial frostbite involves only the skin and usually heals spontaneously, whereas deep frostbite damages both the skin and subcutaneous structures (Figure 11–39). As with burn injuries, the depth of the area of necrosis is difficult to determine initially.

Treatment

Initial resuscitation includes restoration of the core body temperature. The initial treatment of frostbite consists of rapid rewarming of the limb and analgesia, often with intravenous analgesics. Rapid rewarming consists of a water

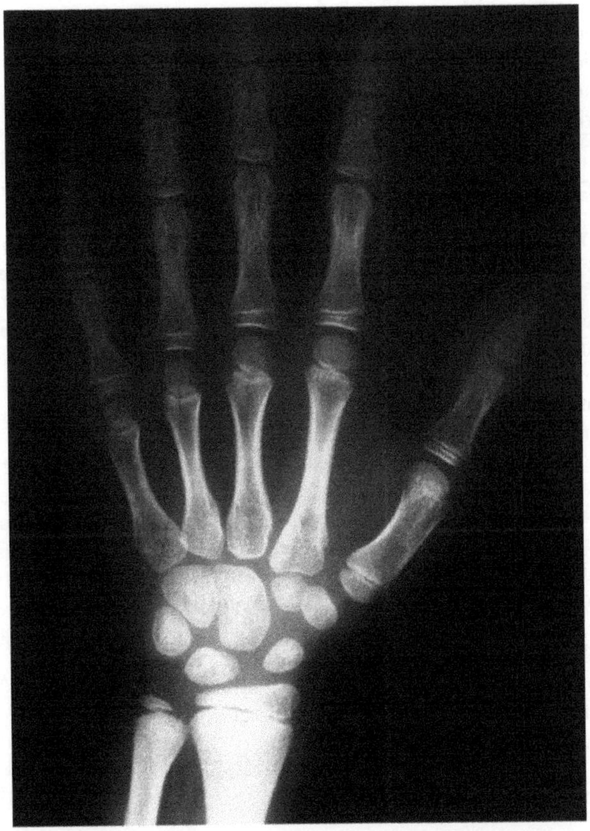

▲ **Figure 11–39.** Radiograph of deformities of the fingers of the left hand in a 12-year-old girl caused by frostbite incurred at 2 years of age. Note the destruction of epiphyses of middle and distal phalanges of all fingers and deformity of epiphysis of proximal phalanx of the little finger. Osseous changes in right hand were similar.

bath at 40 to 42°C. Because rapid rewarming induces severe pain, it should be delayed until adequate analgesia can be administered. Application of silver sulfadiazine ointment or topical antibiotics is recommended for open wounds. After rewarming, treatment should include elevation of the hand, local wound care, and dressing changes. Frequent whirlpool debridement and active ROM exercises should be instituted. In cases of deep frostbites, administration of intravenous TPA within 24 hours has been shown to reduce the rate of digital amputation.

Germann G. Hand reconstruction after burn injury: functional results. *Clin Plast Surg.* 2017;44(4):833-844. [PMID: 28888308]

Ko JH, Levi B. Optimizing the treatment of burn injuries of the upper extremity. *Hand Clin.* 2017;33(2):xiii. [PMID: 28363305]

HIGH-PRESSURE INJECTION INJURY

Injection machinery used in industry may create pressures of 3000 to 10,000 psi. The amount of pressure reflects both the design of the nozzle aperture and the distance between the nozzle and the finger. Virtually all patients who sustain injuries with pressures of over 7000 psi require amputation.

Clinical Findings

Injection injuries usually puncture the palmar digital pulp, track to the flexor tendon sheath, and fill the tendon sheath with the injected material. These injuries have a poor prognosis. Injections into the palm have a somewhat better prognosis because the site of the material is unconfined by fascial planes. Prognostic factors include the time interval from injury to treatment, as well as the amount and type of material injected. Whereas paint injection may cause more necrosis of the finger, grease injection more often leads to fibrosis of the finger. The amputation rate for paint injection injuries is approximately 60%; the rate for grease injection injuries is 20%.

The examiner must be wary of an innocuous-appearing entrance wound at the time of presentation. Initial pain may be modest but increases with time as more distal swelling and early necrosis occur.

Radiographic evaluation may be helpful if defining the extent of soft-tissue infiltration with identification of air within soft-tissue planes or if the material injected is radio-opaque such as lead-based paint.

Treatment

The effectiveness of corticosteroids administered every 6 hours remains controversial in the treatment of injection injuries. Patients should be operatively treated soon after the injury occurs. Thorough debridement of all injected material is easier when the injected material is pigmented. Nonpigmented materials such as kerosene or turpentine are considerably more difficult to remove thoroughly. The hand should be splinted in the safe position. Sympathetic blocks may be helpful in managing pain. Repeat debridement should be done if there is doubt about the adequacy of the initial procedure.

Although injection injuries may appear simple, they are more often severe injuries that compromise function and can result in amputation. The seriousness of these injuries should be recognized at the time of presentation.

Bean B, Cook S, Loeffler BJ, Gaston RG. High-pressure water injection injuries of the hand may not be trivial. *Orthopedics.* 2018;41(2):e245-e251. [PMID: 29377050]

INFECTIONS OF THE HAND

Felon

A felon is a subcutaneous abscess of the fingertip pulp most commonly caused by *Staphylococcus aureus,* gram-negative organisms, or *Eikenella corrodens* in diabetics who bite their nails. Vertical septa between the skin and the bone create small closed mini-compartments within the pulp space. Infection in this region produces localized erythema, swelling, and throbbing pain.

In early cases, treatment consists of oral antibiotics. In more severe cases, treatment of these infections is incision and drainage, with release of the vertical septa to decompress the pulp space completely through a mid-lateral or volar incision (Figure 11–40). A drain is placed in the wound, the hand is elevated, and intravenous antibiotics are administered.

Paronychia

Paronychia is the most common digital infection. The paronychium is the lateral skin fold along both the radial and ulnar borders of the fingernail. The eponychium is the proximal roof of the nail over the nail lunula. Paronychial infections may be classified as acute or chronic.

A. Acute Infection

Acute infections are most often caused by *S aureus* in adults, whereas in children, multiple microorganisms of the oropharyngeal flora are usually isolated. These infections begin as a localized cellulitis, with erythema around the nail. Untreated, this cellulitis may progress to an abscess at the nail margin.

Treatment of early infection with no fluctuance includes warm soaks, oral antibiotics, and avoidance of nail biting. Once an abscess forms, irrigation and debridement are required, followed by oral antibiotics and routine dressing changes. To debride the region adequately, either an incision is made in the abscess and the abscess is packed or a portion of the lateral nail is removed and the abscess is decompressed.

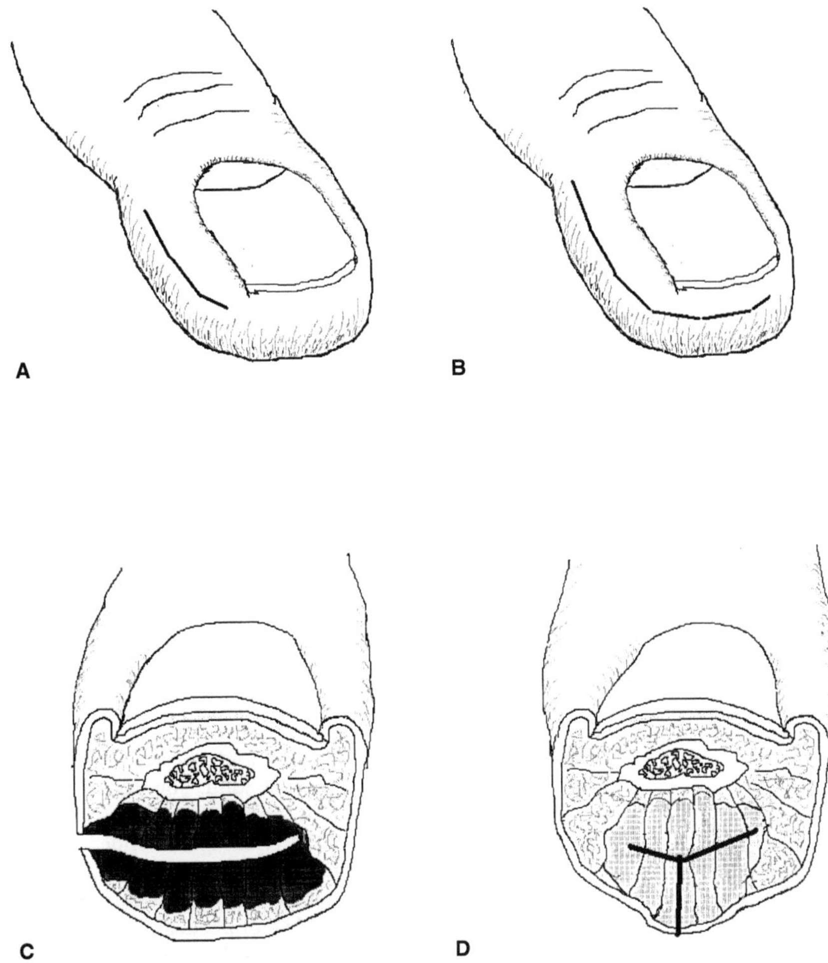

▲ **Figure 11–40.** Incisions for drainage of felons. **A:** Unilateral longitudinal approach that should be used for most felons. It is generally made on the ulnar side of the finger, unless it is the little finger, to preserve sensation. **B:** The hockey stick, or J, incision should be reserved for extensive or severe abscess or felon. **C:** The incision must decompress the longitudinal septa but should not go through and through. **D:** The felon that points volarly may be decompressed through a longitudinal midline incision, which is preferable because of less risk to sensory nerves. A transverse incision may also be made, but there is risk of damage to the digital nerves. (Courtesy of HB Skinner, © 2002.)

B. Chronic Infection

Chronic paronychial infections are most often caused by *Candida* species. These occur in patients who work with their hands in water, such as bartenders or dishwashers. Patients may have repeated episodes of acute infection in addition to chronic infection.

Treatment of chronic infection may be accomplished by eponychial marsupialization, excision of a segment of the eponychia without incision of the nail roof. Simultaneous nail removal may increase the effectiveness of marsupialization.

Web Space Abscess

Web space abscesses most often occur after palmar puncture wounds. The infection spreads from the palm along the path of least resistance to the dorsal web space. Treatment requires dorsal and palmar incision, drain placement, open wound care, and appropriate antibiotic coverage.

Flexor Suppurative Tenosynovitis

Kanavel described four cardinal signs of acute suppurative tenosynovitis: (1) pain with passive digital extension;

(2) semiflexed posture of the digit; (3) fusiform swelling of the digit, which may include the palm; and (4) tenderness along the flexor tendon sheath. Acute suppurative tenosynovitis of the flexor pollicis longus sheath may extend into the thenar space. Likewise, infections in the flexor sheath of the little finger may extend into the ulnar bursa. In some patients, coalescence between the radial and ulnar bursas may allow infection to track in a horseshoe pattern, extending from the thumb to the little finger.

A course of intravenous antibiotics, hand immobilization, and monitoring at the hospital may be considered for early infections with mild signs. However, there should be a low threshold for operative treatment with irrigation and debridement. Although a long mid-axial or Bruner incision may be used, limited incisions are preferred. Short incisions proximal over the MCP joint region at the A1 pulley and distally over the DIP region at the A4 pulley allow thorough sheath irrigation (Figure 11–41). A small angiocatheter (16-gauge catheter) is inserted into the tendon sheath through the distal incision, and a drain is placed in the flexor sheath through the proximal wound. Irrigation can be done in the operating room alone or can be performed intermittently with 5 mL of saline injected every 2 hours. Intravenous antibiotics are administered, and the hand is elevated. Two days after surgery, the dressing is changed. Swelling should be significantly decreased. The catheter is removed, and the patient is encouraged to begin active ROM exercises.

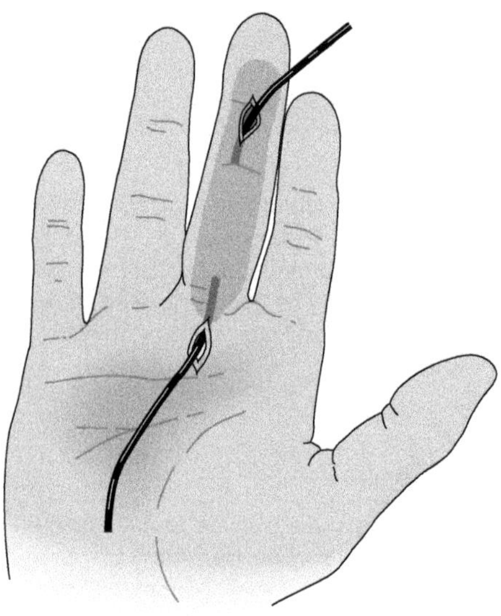

▲ **Figure 11–41. Drainage and closed irrigation for flexor sheath infection. The antibiotic solution drips in through the distal catheter and drains out through the proximal one.** (Reprinted with permission, from Way LW, ed. *Current Surgical Diagnosis and Treatment*, 10th ed. Stamford, CT: Appleton & Lange; 1994.)

Bite Injuries

Bite injuries may inoculate oral flora into the small hand joints through a traumatic arthrotomy. Although bite wounds initially appear harmless, they may have detrimental consequences.

A. Cat and Dog Bites

Cat bites cause small puncture wounds that seal immediately; therefore, they have a higher risk of infection and are more likely to be disregarded than the large tearing wounds of dog bites. Late sequelae are more common after cat bites. Cat and dog bites frequently harbor *Pasteurella multocida* (70%-80% in cat bite infections and 50% in dog bite infections), and the lab should be informed about the potential for this organism because cultures require specific growth media. This organism is best treated with amoxicillin/clavulanic acid or with cephalosporins such as cefuroxime or ceftriaxone. Acute animal bites may be treated with incision and drainage and intravenous antibiotics in the emergency room followed by oral antibiotics.

B. Human Bites

Most human bite wounds result from a fist striking a tooth, which readily penetrates the skin, subcutaneous tissue, extensor tendon, and capsule of the MCP joint (Figure 11–42). They are most commonly located in the dorsal aspect of the third or fourth MCP joint. The most common bacteria with human bites are *S aureus*, *Streptococcus viridans*, and *E corrodens* (7%-29%). The recommended antibiotic treatments for these infections include amoxicillin/clavulanic acid or intravenous ampicillin/sulbactam. Human bite wounds should be debrided, drained, and irrigated with repair of the extensor tendon and arthrotomy of the MCP joint if they are involved and treatment with intravenous antibiotics.

C. Spider Bites

Although most spider bites are innocuous, the bite of a brown recluse spider requires early wide excision to control the locally injected toxin.

Infection Caused by Unusual Organisms

A. Atypical Mycobacterial Infection

Mycobacterium marinum infection is associated with occupational exposure to a marine environment and presents as a chronically inflamed finger. The microorganism is usually inoculated through a puncture wound by the spine or fin of a saltwater fish. Successful culture of the organism is difficult (40% positive cultures) but is most likely at a temperature of 30 to 32°C. Antitubercular drug therapy such as ethambutol with rifampicin is the recommended treatment for eradication of these infections.

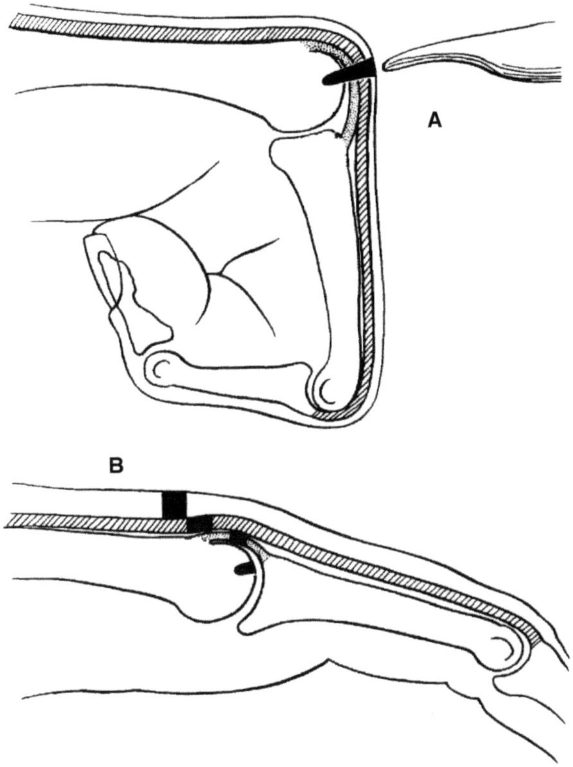

▲ **Figure 11–42.** Human bite wound of metacarpophalangeal joint. **A:** The tooth pierces the clenched fist of the attacker, penetrating skin, tendon, joint capsule, and metacarpal head. **B:** When the finger is extended by swelling and at surgery, the four puncture wounds do not correspond. (Reprinted with permission, from Lister G. *The Hand: Diagnosis and Indications*, 3rd ed. Philadelphia: Churchill Livingstone; 1993.)

B. Gram-Negative Infection

Because of the risk of a gram-negative infection following mutilating farm injuries or injuries with possible fecal contamination, these patients should be treated with broad-spectrum antibiotics.

C. Anaerobic Infection

When *Clostridium perfringens* infection occurs after hand injury, immediate wide fasciotomy and intravenous penicillin should be instituted. Hyperbaric oxygen therapy may be helpful. If infection cannot be adequately controlled, amputation may be necessary to avoid death.

The possibility of *Clostridium tetani* contamination must be remembered with any puncture wound. Initial evaluation of all patients with penetrating wounds must include questioning about tetanus inoculation. If inoculation is not up to date, antitoxin should be administered.

D. Gonorrhea

A patient who presents with an isolated septic joint or tenosynovitis without a history of puncture wound may have a hematogenous gonorrheal infection. Treatment consists of culturing the involved organism on the appropriate media and treatment with penicillin or tetracycline.

E. Necrotizing Fasciitis

The causative agent in necrotizing fasciitis is most commonly group A *Streptococcus* and can occur after a minor cut or abrasion. Patients with this infection are systemically very ill, and the infection spreads rapidly along fascial planes. Treatment consists of emergent wide surgical debridement to the fascia and appropriate antibiotics. Rates of amputation and mortality are high (20%-30%) for necrotizing fasciitis.

F. Herpetic Whitlow

Herpes simplex infections may involve the fingertips. They are most common in medical or dental personnel who care for the oral tracheal area and are also seen in small children. It may be difficult to distinguish herpetic lesions from acute bacterial infections of the fingers. Close examination reveals the presence of groups (crops) of vesicles, with surrounding erythema. Aspiration of a vesicle yields clear fluid. Serial viral titers confirm the diagnosis. Unlike bacterial infections, herpetic whitlow should not be incised but simply treated with splinting and elevation.

Boles SD, Schmidt CC. Pyogenic flexor tenosynovitis. *Hand Clin.* 1999;14(4):567-578. [PMID: 9884895]

Jagodzinski NA, Ibish S, Furniss D. Surgical site infection after hand surgery outside the operating theatre: a systematic review. *J Hand Surg Eur Vol.* 2017;42(3):289-294. [PMID: 28196439]

Lekic N, Rosenberg AE, Askari M. *Mycobacterium longobardum* infection in the hand. *J Hand Surg Am.* 2018;43(5):491.e1-491.e4. [PMID: 29032284]

Li K, Sambare TD, Jiang SY, Shearer EJ, Douglass NP, Kamal RN. Effectiveness of preoperative antibiotics in preventing surgical site infection after common soft tissue procedures of the hand. *Clin Orthop Relat Res.* 2018;476(4):664-673. [PMID: 29432267]

ARTHRITIS OF THE HAND

OSTEOARTHRITIS

Primary osteoarthritis is an idiopathic degenerative disease, predominantly affecting the DIP joints and the trapeziometacarpal joint of the thumb. On the contrary, osteoarthritis of the wrist is usually posttraumatic. Other causes of secondary osteoarthritis in the hand include trauma such as fractures

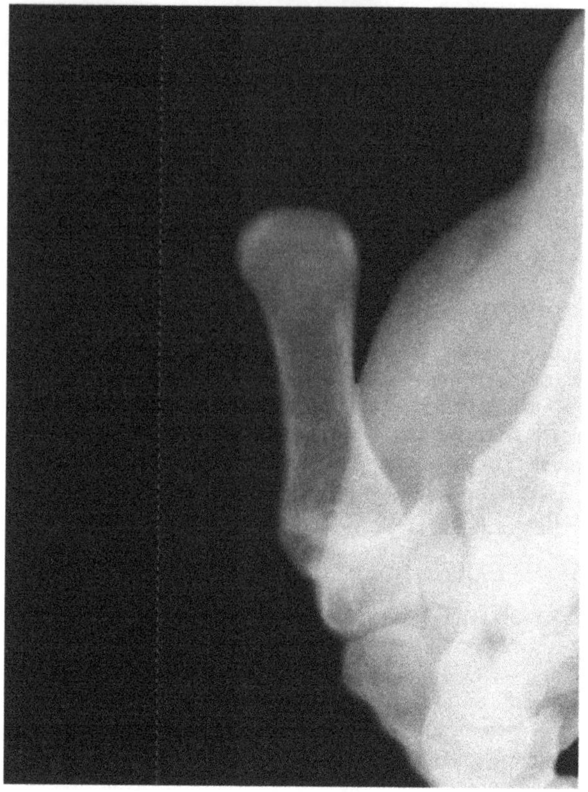

▲ **Figure 11–43.** Osteoarthritis of the carpometacarpal joint of the thumb.

and ligament injuries, avascular necrosis, or metabolic disorders. Osteoarthritis is characterized by pain, deformity, and stiffness, whereas typical radiographic signs include articular cartilage space loss, subchondral sclerosis, subchondral cysts, and peripheral joint osteophytes.

Epidemiologic Factors

The disease occurs commonly in older individuals, with approximately 80% to 90% of adults older than 75 years having radiographic evidence of osteoarthritis (Figure 11–43). The strongest predictors of developing osteoarthritis of the hand are female gender, increasing age, and a family history.

Clinical Findings

Patients with osteoarthritis of the hand often complain of activity-induced or work-related pain and deformity. The bony enlargements commonly seen in the osteoarthritic DIP joints are referred to as Heberden nodes, whereas osteoarthritic enlargements at the PIP joint are known as Bouchard nodes. Most patients experience periods of exacerbation and remission. Functional limitations result from pain, weakness, loss of motion, and deformity. Tenderness and enlargement of the DIP and PIP joints are noted on examination. Axial compression of the thumb trapeziometacarpal with a circumduction motion (grind test) reproduces pain. As the disease progresses, radial subluxation of the thumb metacarpal on the trapezium may develop, leading to adduction deformity of the metacarpal.

Treatment

Nonoperative treatment includes oral NSAIDs, long-acting intraarticular steroid injection, and splint immobilization.

The primary indications for surgery are debilitating pain unresponsive to conservative measures, instability, and deformity. Mucous cyst excision and osteophyte resection are indicated in cases of impending cyst rupture. DIP arthrodesis relieves pain, corrects deformity, and resolves joint instability. Because the severely arthritic DIP joint is often stiff, the additional loss of motion occasioned by arthrodesis is usually tolerated well. The DIP joint is fused in 10 to 15 degrees of flexion, a position in which the fingernail is parallel with the axis of the middle phalanx. Fusion with a headless screw has the lowest rate of nonunions (10%).

At the PIP joint, surgical options include arthroplasty and arthrodesis. Indications for surgery include pain not responding to conservative treatment, instability, and deformity. Implant arthroplasty may be helpful in relieving pain and retaining motion in the ring and little fingers. The motion attained from implant arthroplasty is less in the PIP joints than in the MCP joints. Implant arthroplasty is usually avoided in the index or small finger PIP joint. The radial collateral ligament should be preserved to maintain pinch strength.

Arthrodesis effectively relieves pain at the PIP joint and provides pinch stability. The ideal position of arthrodesis varies from the radial to the ulnar digits. The index finger PIP joint is usually fused at 40 degrees of flexion, the middle finger at 45 degrees, the ring finger at 50 degrees, and the little finger at 55 degrees.

At the trapeziometacarpal joint, conservative treatment includes a hand-based thumb spica splint with the interphalangeal joint left free, cortisone injections, and NSAIDs. Many patients with advanced degenerative changes on radiographs obtain good pain relief with conservative therapy.

The primary indication for surgery is persistent pain that is nonresponsive to conservative treatment. At early stages, first metacarpal dorsal extension osteotomy may result in pain relief as it redirects the forces to the dorsal, uninvolved part of the joint. Trapezium resection arthroplasty relieves pain at the trapeziometacarpal joint and allows retention of full metacarpal base motion. Usually the entire trapezium is resected. A tendon interposition and sling are created using the flexor carpi radialis, a slip of the abductor pollicis longus, or allografts. Although the cost is higher for allografts, they eliminate the negative functional and cosmetic outcomes that are associated with the use of tendon autografts.

Experimental studies have shown that the tendon allografts undergo several changes demonstrating signs of revascularization and repopulation by nitrium cells. Therefore, the interposed allografts act more as viable biologic spacers rather than as dead interposed tissue. The tendon may be threaded through a drill hole in the articular surface of the thumb metacarpal to suspend the thumb metacarpal. The remaining tendon is rolled into a so-called anchovy and placed in the space of the excised trapezium. In 60% of the cases, there is concomitant scaphotrapezoidal arthritis; therefore, resection of the proximal part of the trapezoid is indicated. After surgery, the thumb is immobilized in a cast or splint for 6 weeks. Although the reoperation rate following trapeziometacarpal arthroplasty is low, common reasons for revision surgery include metacarpal subsidence, scaphotrapezoidal arthritis, and MCP deformity.

Arthrodesis of the thumb CMC joint is an alternative to trapeziectomy. With the joint fused, residual motion occurs at the scaphotrapezial joint, but notably patients are unable to lay their hand flat on a table. However, pain relief is excellent, and it may be the procedure of choice for a young laborer.

Lans J, Machol JA 4th, Deml C, Chen NC, Jupiter JB. Nonrheumatoid arthritis of the hand. *J Hand Surg Am.* 2018;43(1):61-67. [PMID: 29132785]

Papatheodorou L, Winston J, Bielicka D, Rogozinski B, Lourie G, Sotereanos D. Revision of the failed thumb carpometacarpal arthroplasty. *J Hand Surg Am.* 2017;42(12):1032.e1-1032.e7. [PMID: 28888570]

RHEUMATOID ARTHRITIS

RA is a chronic systemic disease that affects connective tissue and results in chronic inflammatory synovitis usually with bilateral joint involvement. It is discussed in Chapter 7, so only the aspects pertinent to the hand are described here. RA commonly affects the small joints initially, such as the hand and wrist. RA affects 0.3% to 1.5% of the population. Women are two to three times more commonly affected than men. Arthritis of hand joints that lasts for more than 6 weeks is one of seven diagnostic criteria used by the American College of Rheumatology for diagnosis of the disease. Progressive joint destruction and deformity are less common than in the past, as are surgical procedures for RA, because of the success of the medications used for its treatment, including suppressive or disease-modifying antirheumatic drugs and biologics. Aspirin, NSAIDs, corticosteroids, and immunosuppressive drugs are also used in treatment of RA.

Clinical Findings

The goal in treating the patient's hand with RA is to determine which of the patient's many problems—pain, weakness, or mechanical dysfunction—is most problematic. Tendon rupture, tenosynovitis causing pain, triggering, and nerve compression symptoms occur with RA. The most common nerve compression syndromes are compression of the median nerve at the wrist and compression of the radial nerve at the elbow. The appearance of rheumatoid nodules and ulnar drift deformity at the MCP joint may be disturbing aesthetically. Rheumatoid nodules, occurring in 20% to 25% of patients with RA, are not treated unless associated with erosion, pain, or infection.

Treatment

The shoulder, elbow, forearm, wrist, and hand should be examined individually, as should the cervical spine. Indications for surgical intervention include relieving pain, slowing the progression of disease, improving function, and improving appearance.

Surgical treatment may be classified as either preventive or corrective. Preventive options include tenosynovectomy and synovectomy. Corrective procedures include tendon transfers, nerve decompression, soft-tissue reconstruction, and arthrodesis.

Synovectomy is considered in patients who have pauciarticular persistent synovitis while under good medical control. Contraindications to synovectomy include rapidly progressive disease, multiple joint involvement, and underlying joint destruction.

A. Elbow Reconstruction

Synovitis of the elbow joint may cause pain, joint destruction, and radial nerve compression. Nodules or bursas are common over the olecranon. Surgical treatment of the rheumatoid elbow includes radial head excision and synovectomy. When the disease worsens, total elbow arthroplasty is a consideration.

B. Wrist Reconstruction

RA frequently involves the wrist, sometimes is the first joint involved, and occurs in a predictable pattern. The joint capsule and the periarticular ligaments become attenuated by the extensive synovitis and the pannus formation, resulting in destabilization of the radiocarpal joint and of the distal radioulnar joint. On the radial side of the wrist, the radioscaphocapitate and the radiolunotriquetral ligaments are attenuated, permitting rotatory displacement of the scaphoid. Scapholunate dissociation is followed by radiocarpal collapse.

On the ulnar side of the wrist, the ulnar carpal ligaments become attenuated, allowing the carpus to translate ulnarward along the inclined radius. Attenuation of the distal radioulnar joint allows the head of the ulna to displace dorsally, producing caput-ulnae syndrome. The extensor carpi ulnaris tendon displaces volarly. Attritional rupture of extensor tendons (Vaughn-Jackson syndrome) may occur. These changes lead to supination of the carpus on the radius, ulnar

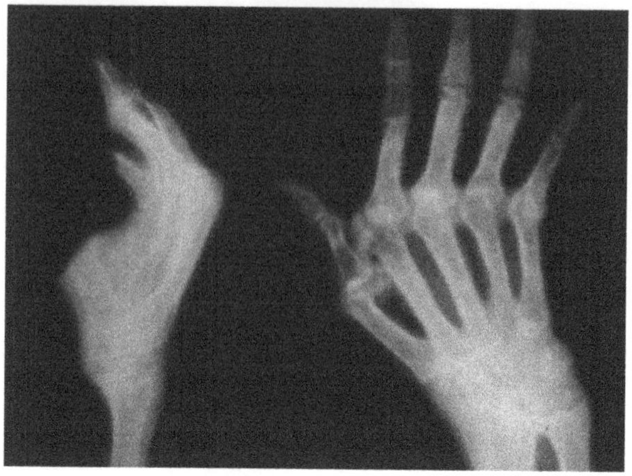

▲ **Figure 11–44.** Radialward displacement of the metacarpals in rheumatoid arthritis.

translocation of the carpus, and a concomitant radialward displacement of the metacarpals (Figure 11–44). Eventually, the carpus may dislocate volarly beneath the radius.

Surgical treatment consists of extensor tenosynovectomy, with transposition of the dorsal retinaculum over the wrist joint to reinforce the capsule, and wrist synovectomy. The extensor carpi ulnaris tendon can be relocated from a volar to a dorsal position.

If pain is present over the distal ulna or if rupture of the little or ring finger extensor tendon results from a sharp prominence of the distal ulna, then resection of the distal ulna is performed. Fusion of the rheumatoid wrist provides stability and may increase function. Either a total wrist arthrodesis or a radiolunate arthrodesis may be elected, depending on the extent of midcarpal joint involvement. With bilateral wrist involvement, replacement of one wrist and fusion of the other should be considered for best function.

C. Hand Reconstruction

Triggering of the digits is a common problem caused by flexor tenosynovitis. In patients with RA, the entire annular pulley system should be preserved to minimize further ulnar drift of the fingers at the MCP joint. Triggering is treated by tenosynovectomy and excision of the ulnar slip of the flexor digitorum superficialis.

If flexor tendon rupture occurs, treatment may include tendon transfer, bridge grafting, or joint fusion. The flexor tendon that most commonly ruptures is the flexor pollicis longus because it rubs over an osteophyte on the volar aspect of the scaphotrapezial joint (Mannerfelt lesion). Extensor tendon ruptures are caused by attrition of the common extensor tendon of the ring and little fingers over the distal ulna (Vaughn-Johnson syndrome).

Treatment of the arthritic hand depends on the joints involved. The DIP joint is usually best treated by arthrodesis. At the PIP joint, synovectomy may be performed if synovitis is isolated to the PIP joint without multiple joint involvement. Alternatives for the more involved joint are arthroplasty or arthrodesis.

At the MCP joint, inflammation of the synovium may cause the extensor mechanism to sublux ulnarly because of attenuation of the radial sagittal band. The mechanism may be relocated to improve function of the joint. For isolated joints without significant destruction, synovectomy may be performed. With more severe joint destruction, resection implant arthroplasty is required (Figure 11–45). Subluxation and ulnar drift alone are not absolute indications for arthroplasty if satisfactory function of the hand remains. Arthroplasty does not increase the ROM of the metaphalangeal joints, but it changes its arc. Because most patients have severe flexion and ulnar deviation of the joints, arthroplasty provides a more functional ROM, especially for grasping large objects. Because the implants fail with extensive use, arthroplasty is indicated only in the low-demand hand and is therefore better suited to rheumatoid than osteoarthritic patients.

1. Boutonnière deformity—Boutonnière deformity is a flexion contracture at the PIP joint along with hyperextension at the DIP joint. Synovitis of the PIP joint results in elongation of the central extensor slip, flexion of the PIP joint, and subsequent volar subluxation of the lateral bands. The lateral bands migrate volar to the center of rotation of the PIP joint, and they become an active flexor force. As the deformity progresses, tightening of the lateral bands leads to DIP joint hyperextension as well. If synovitis persists for greater than 3 months despite maximal medical management, synovectomy is the recommended treatment in order to prevent attenuation of the supporting ligament and of the central tendon. In mild deformities that are passively correctable, lateral band dorsal relocation and tightening of the stretched central tendon are usually performed, although the outcomes of this procedure are unpredictable. In more severe deformities of the PIP joint that are still flexible, consideration may be given to reconstruction of the central slip along with the lateral band dorsal relocation. In the final stage of boutonnière deformity, the joint deformity becomes fixed, and the best form of treatment is arthroplasty or fusion.

2. Swan-neck deformity—Swan-neck deformities consist of hyperextension at the PIP joint and flexion at the DIP joint. The cause of swan-neck deformity in a rheumatic hand may be located in the DIP joint (terminal tendon attenuation), in the PIP joint (volar plate attenuation), or in the MCP joint (volar subluxation of the metacarpal heads leading to relative intrinsic tightness). The surgeons should address the pathology that causes the deformity.

Treatment of swan-neck deformities depends on whether they are flexible or fixed deformities. In case of a flexible deformity, soft-tissue reconstruction includes release of the tight intrinsic tendon, volar plate advancement, or flexor

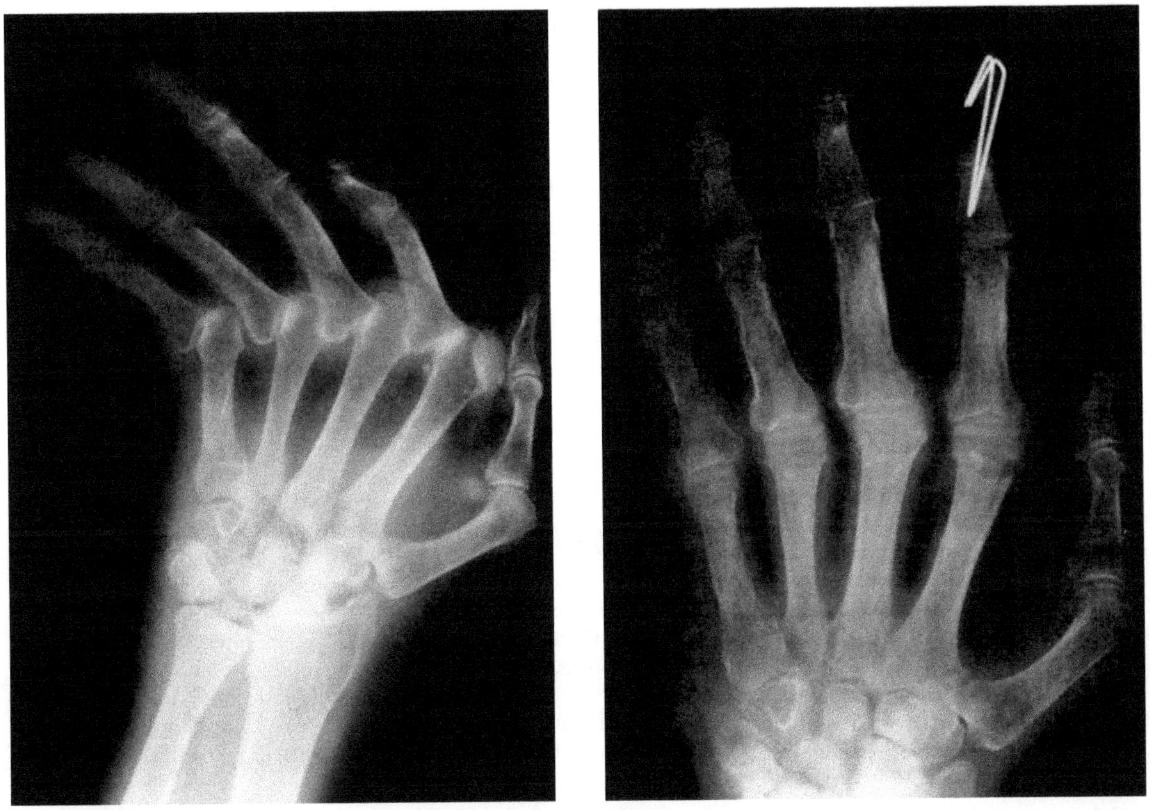

A B

▲ **Figure 11–45.** **A:** Preoperative view of metacarpophalangeal joint in rheumatoid arthritis. **B:** Following resection arthroplasty.

digitorum superficialis tenodesis. Another option in case of supple joints is the Littler oblique retinacular ligament reconstruction where the ulnar lateral band is incised proximally, is rerouted volar to the axis of the PIP joint to act as a flexion force, and is sutured into the bone at the proximal phalanx. If the deformity is fixed, fusion or arthroplasty is recommended.

3. Synovitic MCP joint deformity—The MCP joints subluxes volarly and ulnarly in RA. This deformity results from synovial invasion of the collateral ligaments with secondary laxity, volar and ulnar forces that are normally present on the joint, augmentation of these forces by radial deviation of the wrist, attenuation of the radial sagittal band (allowing ulnar subluxation of the extensor tendon), and contracture of the intrinsic muscles. Treatment of the synovitic MCP joint consists of medical management and splinting. When the joint space is preserved, surgical synovectomy may provide symptomatic relief. Once moderate joint destruction or volar subluxation and ulnar deviation occurs, the decision about surgery is based on the function of the hand. When the patient is still able to use the hand for activities of daily living, splinting and other assistive aids are provided. Once loss of function is noted, MCP arthroplasty is considered. In performing MCP arthroplasty, the wrist deformity should first be corrected, and all soft-tissue releases required to relieve the subluxing forces should be performed. The radial collateral ligament of the index finger should be reconstructed, and the extensor tendon should be relocated. Postoperatively, extensive splinting and therapy are required to hold the hand in proper position. Therapy utilizes an outrigger splint holding the wrist in dorsiflexion and the metaphalangeal joints in full extension and neutral radial-ulnar alignment. The splint is worn full time for 6 weeks and part time for 3 months. The patient wears a splint that holds the hand in the intrinsic plus position at night for 1 year.

D. Thumb Reconstruction

Three patterns of rheumatoid thumb deformities are defined. In type 1 deformity, the MCP joint is flexed while the interphalangeal joint is hyperextended and the thumb metacarpal is secondarily abducted. In type 2 and 3 deformities, CMC subluxation leads to metacarpal adduction.

In type 2 deformities, interphalangeal joint hyperextension develops with MCP flexion, and in type 3 deformities, the MCP joint is hyperextended and the interphalangeal joint is flexed. Type 2 deformities are unusual. Type 1 deformities are usually initiated by synovitis of the MCP joint, leading to attenuation of the extensor pollicis brevis tendon, intrinsic muscle tightness, and ulnar and volar displacement of the extensor pollicis longus.

Treatment is based on the degree of progression. In type 1 deformities, if the MCP and interphalangeal joints are passively correctable, synovectomy and extensor reconstruction may be performed. If the MCP joint flexion deformity is fixed, arthrodesis or arthroplasty of the joint is considered. When fixed MCP flexion and interphalangeal extension deformities are present simultaneously, the interphalangeal joint is fused and the MCP joint is replaced with an arthroplasty or also undergoes arthrodesis.

Type 3 deformities are analogous to swan-neck deformities of the fingers. The CMC joint disease allows dorsal and radial subluxation of the joint, with secondary adduction contraction of the metacarpal and hyperextension of the MCP joint. Treatment with minimal MCP deformity (stage 1) or passively correctable MCP deformity (stage 2) consists of splinting and CMC arthroplasty or fusion. Once the MCP deformity becomes fixed (stage 3), first web release and CMC arthroplasty are required.

E. Surgical Priorities

When multilevel deformity is present, consideration should be given to combined procedures. If wrist and MCP deformities are both present, the wrist should be fused prior to or simultaneously with MCP joint reconstruction. When both MCP and PIP joint deformities are present, motion-preserving procedures such as arthroplasty should be carried out at the MCP joint. Treatment of concomitant PIP joint involvement depends on the stage of deformity. Mild to moderate PIP joint deformities can either be ignored or treated by closed manipulation and pin fixation. With severe deformity, arthrodesis of the PIP joint should be performed.

In all cases, attempts should be made to perform multiple procedures under a single anesthetic. These patients often require numerous operations for multiple joints of the upper and lower extremities, and surgical and rehabilitation time must be used judiciously.

Other Inflammatory Arthropathies

Other inflammatory conditions related to RA may affect the hand, producing joint destruction and deformity.

A. Juvenile Idiopathic Arthritis

Juvenile idiopathic arthritis is a group of heterogenous inflammatory disorders (eg, systemic, oligoarticular, polyarticular, enthesitis-related) that affects children less than 16 years old, with symptoms of arthritis for at least 6 weeks. Early epiphyseal closure occurs as a result of synovitis and increased periarticular blood flow. Narrowing of phalangeal and metacarpal medullary canals makes implant arthroplasty difficult. The MCP joints may deviate radially rather than ulnarly.

B. Psoriatic Arthritis

Psoriatic arthritis is a seronegative inflammatory arthropathy that predominantly involves the DIP joints, although the PIP joints or the MCP joints can be affected as well. Skin manifestations usually include silvery plaques over extensor surfaces. The classic finding in radiographs is the pencil-in-cup deformity of the DIP joints. In arthritis mutilans, the most severe form of psoriatic arthritis, axial shortening because of marked bone loss occurs while the soft-tissue envelope is preserved. Early joint fusions are required to avoid progressive bone loss.

C. Systemic Lupus Erythematosus

SLE affects periarticular soft tissue, resulting in joint laxity with secondary dysfunction. Synovitis is minimal in lupus, and therefore, the articular cartilage is preserved. Soft-tissue reconstruction is ineffective, and joint fusions are preferable to restore stability and function. The exception to this is the MCP joints, where implant arthroplasty may be appropriate, even though normal articular cartilage is sacrificed.

Chung K, Pushman A. Current concepts in the management of the rheumatoid hand. *J Hand Surg Am.* 2011;36(4):736-747. [PMID: 21463736]

O'Sullivan MB, Singh H, Wolf JM. Tendon transfers in the rheumatoid hand for reconstruction. *Hand Clin.* 2016;32(3): 407-416. [PMID: 27387084]

HAND TUMORS

Although hand tumors can be benign or malignant, most mass lesions in the hand and wrist are benign. Benign lesions include ganglions, lipomas, epidermoid inclusion cysts, giant cell tumors, nerve tumors (neurofibroma or neurilemmoma), glomus tumors, vascular tumors (hemangiomas), and pyogenic granulomas. Soft-tissue malignant tumors include epithelioid sarcomas, synovial sarcomas, and squamous cell carcinomas. The most common benign bone tumors are enchondromas and osteoid osteomas. The most common bone malignant tumors are chondrosarcomas, osteosarcomas, Ewing sarcomas, and metastatic lung tumors.

GANGLION

Ganglions are the most common soft-tissue masses of the hand and wrist, accounting for about 60% to 70%. They are cystic structures filled with a mucinous fluid but without a synovial or epithelial lining. They contain joint or tendon sheath fluid. In most cases, a stalk can be identified communicating between the cyst and an adjacent joint or tendon sheath. The most common locations for ganglions are the wrist, digital flexor sheath, and DIP joint (Figure 11–46). Ganglions are usually firm, are well circumscribed, and can transilluminate. These lesions often fluctuate in size, and they may be barely palpable but highly symptomatic, whereas large ganglions are often soft and only mildly symptomatic

Dorsal Wrist Ganglion

In 70% of cases, ganglions are located at the dorsal wrist. Dorsal wrist ganglions arise from the dorsal capsule of the scapholunate joint. Although aspiration of the ganglion may provide transient symptomatic relief, the risk of recurrence is very high (59%), whereas open surgical excision has a significantly lower recurrence rate (21%). To prevent recurrence, adequate exposure is required so the origin is clearly identified and the stalk is resected. Because these lesions arise from the dorsal portion of the scapholunate ligament, care must be taken to preserve the ligament's integrity to avoid iatrogenic scapholunate dissociation. Alternatively, arthroscopic techniques can be used and are especially helpful for small ganglions that may be easier to locate inside than outside the wrist joint.

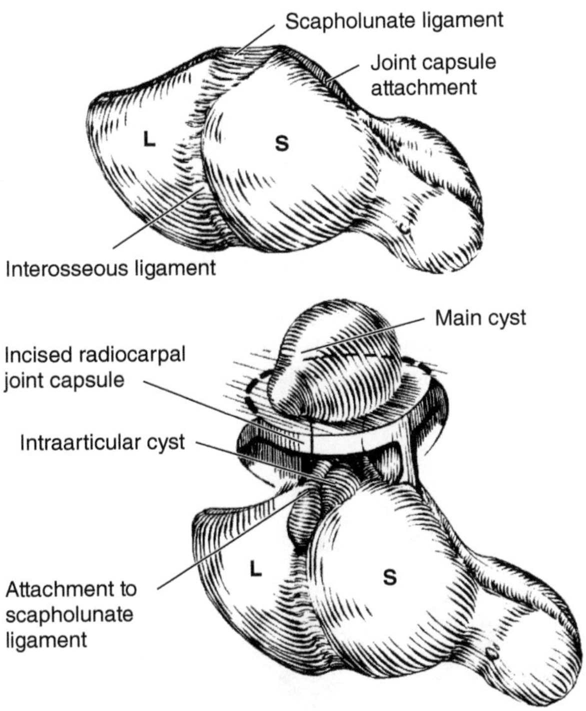

▲ **Figure 11–46. The ganglion and scapholunate attachments are isolated from the remaining uninvolved joint capsule (not shown).** (Reprinted with permission, from Green DP, ed. *Operative Hand Surgery*, 2nd ed. Philadelphia: Churchill Livingstone; 1988.)

Palmar Wrist Ganglion

Palmar wrist ganglions present as swellings on the palmar and radial wrist, adjacent to the radial artery. These lesions arise from either the radioscaphoid or scaphotrapezial joint. The treatment is similar to dorsal ganglions, and the adjacent radial artery must be mobilized and protected. Palmar ganglions have a higher tendency to recur than dorsal ganglions.

Mucous Cyst

Mucous cysts are ganglions arising from the DIP joint in patients with osteoarthritis. Surgical treatment should address the joint osteophyte as well. A retinacular cyst is a similar lesion in the DIP joint, but these arise from the sheath of the terminal extensor tendon. If the skin is thinned, a local rotation flap is required for soft-tissue coverage after excision.

Giant Cell Tumor

Giant cell tumors of tendon sheath, also known as fibroxanthomas, are slow-growing, firm, and usually nontender lesions that often arise from the joint or from the flexor tendon sheath. They are usually fixed to deep tissues, more often on the palmar aspect of the hand or finger. Surgical resection requires delineation of the entire mass and protection of digital nerves that may be displaced, compressed, or encircled by the tumor.

Epidermoid Inclusion Cyst

Epidermoid inclusion cysts are usually the result of penetrating trauma that drives keratinizing epithelium into the subcutaneous tissue. They gradually enlarge into pearlike masses filled with toothpaste-like keratin. Eventually, the mass becomes noticeable, particularly when it is located over the palmar aspect of the pulp. Surgical treatment is excision of the mass without rupture.

Foreign Bodies

Foreign bodies may act as a nidus, inciting the development of a surrounding granuloma. This may be associated with a local inflammatory reaction or infection. Treatment is excision of the foreign body.

Nerve Tumors

The most common nerve tumors in hand include neurofibroma and neurolemmoma also known as Schwannoma. Neurolemmomas originate from the myelin-forming Schwan cells and are more common than neurofibromas. Usually these tumors are painless and have a positive Tinel sign. Nerve injury during marginal excision of these tumors is uncommon because they are encapsulated; therefore, they can be easily shelled out without disruption of the nerve fibers.

Neurofibromas are slow-growing and painless masses that arise from nerve fascicles. Due to their origin, excisions of neurofibromas require resection of a portion of the nerve and bridging with nerve grafts.

Head L, Gencarelli J, Allen M, Boyd K. Wrist ganglion treatment: systematic review and meta-analysis. *J Hand Surg Am.* 2015;40(3):546-553. [PMID: 25708437]

Lubahn JD, Bachoura A. Enchondroma of the hand: evaluation and management. *J Am Acad Orthop Surg.* 2016;24(9):625-633. [PMID: 27454024]

Ulas ST, Diekhoff T, Hermann KGA, Poddubnyy D, Hamm B, Makowski MR. Susceptibility-weighted MR imaging to improve the specificity of erosion detection: a prospective feasibility study in hand arthritis. *Skeletal Radiol.* 2019;48(5): 721-728. [PMID: 30564856]

Yamamoto M, Natsume T, Kurimoto S, et al. Patients with benign hand tumors are indicated for surgery according to patient-rated outcome measures. *J Plast Reconstr Aesthet Surg.* 2017;70(4):487-494. [PMID: 28153429]

CONGENITAL DIFFERENCES

The incidence of congenital hand differences is approximately 1 in 600 live births. The Oberg, Manske, and Tonkin (OMT) classification that was proposed in 2010 was adopted by the International Federation of Societies for Surgery of the Hand (IFSSH) in 2014 and has been updated many times. The OMT classification broadly divides congenital differences into four main categories, and each category is further subdivided. The four main categories include malformations (abnormal formation of a body part), deformations (alternation of a body part after normal formation), dysplasia (abnormality in size, shape, and organization of cells), and syndromes. Most anomalies of the upper extremity are malformations. However, because many congenital hand differences are part of a well-delineated association or syndrome, initial examination of an infant with a congenital hand anomaly should include evaluation of other regions of the body and other organ systems as well. When an infant is seen with bilateral total absence of the radius and normal or very mildly hypoplastic thumbs, the possibility of thrombocytopenia with absent radius (TAR) syndrome should be considered and a platelet count obtained. Radial absence may also be associated with the VATER association, children with abnormalities that may include *v*ertebral, *a*nal, *t*racheal, *e*sophageal, and *r*enal defects.

A number of frequently encountered conditions such as cleft hand are inherited as autosomal dominant traits. The expertise of an experienced geneticist is invaluable in providing counsel to families considering additional children and to patients wishing to know the likelihood that their offspring would be affected by the disorder.

The two most commonly encountered conditions are syndactyly (1 in 2000 births) and polydactyly (1 in 600 births).

Syndactyly

Syndactyly is a hand plate malformation in which two or more digits remain fused together after birth due to a failure of apoptosis. It is classified as cutaneous (simple) syndactyly if soft tissue alone is involved and osseous (complex) syndactyly if bony connections are present (Figure 11–47). Most commonly, the long and ring fingers are involved (50%). Surgery is usually recommended at 12 months of age, although rays of unequal length should be released before 6 months. Surgical release of syndactyly requires the use of local flaps to create a floor for the interdigital web space and to partially surface the adjacent sides of the separated digits. Residual defects along the sides of the separated fingers are covered with full-thickness skin grafts. Surgery is indicated when the webbing occurs distal to the usual point of separation of the fingers and the webbing prohibits full use of the fingers.

Polydactyly

Radial polydactyly is another hand plate malformation that manifests as thumb duplication. When two thumbs are present in the same hand, they are rarely both normal in size, alignment, and mobility (Figure 11–48). The level of bifurcation varies from a bifid distal phalanx with one wide nail to fully formed duplicated metacarpals. The most common form of thumb duplication is characterized by duplicated proximal phalanx (43%). The more ulnar thumb component is usually better developed than the more radial thumb component. Optimal reconstruction of the best possible thumb utilizes the available anatomic structures and often requires merging of components of both digits. If the duplication occurs at the MCP joint, the radial collateral ligament is

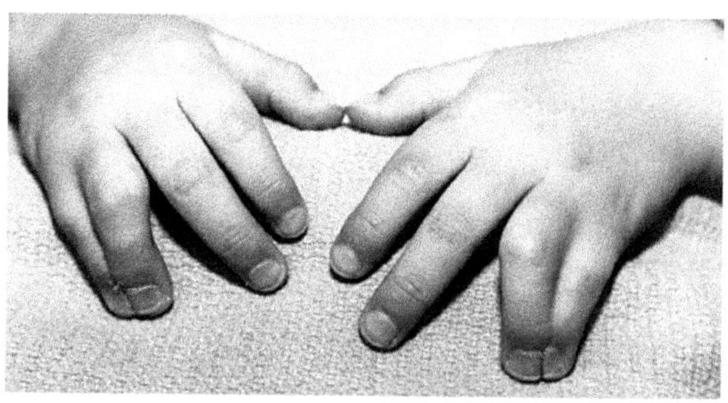

▲ **Figure 11–47.** Bilateral complex syndactyly of the ring and little fingers.

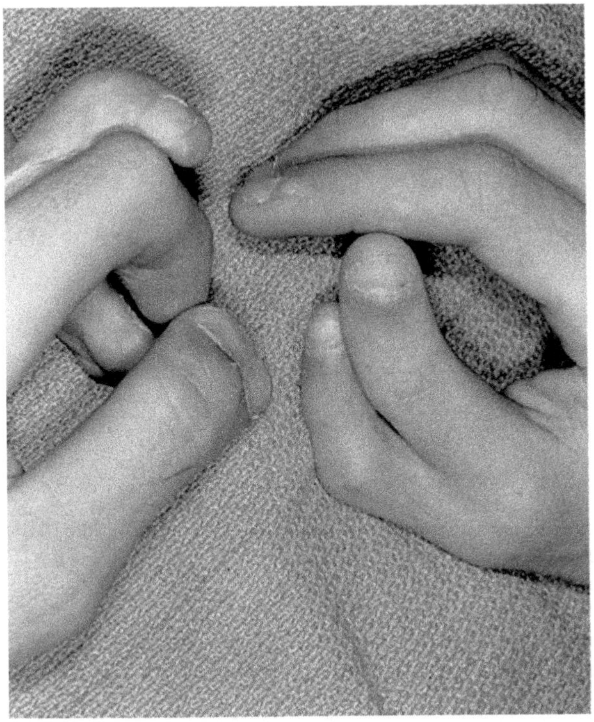

▲ **Figure 11–48.** Thumb polydactyly.

preserved with the metacarpal and attached to the proximal phalanx of the ulnar thumb. Surgery is usually performed at 6 to 12 months of age.

Ulnar polydactyly (small finger polydactyly) is 10 times more frequent in African American children than others. The duplicated small finger can be tied off shortly after birth if it is just a rudimentary skin tag, or it can be excised if it is a well-formed duplicated digit.

Partial or Absent Structures

Absence or partial deficiency of the radius results in inadequate support of the hand and carpus. The unsupported hand angulates radially. Stretching of contracted radial soft-tissue structures is accomplished through repeat manipulation, casting, splinting, or distraction lengthening. The hand is then surgically reoriented onto the end of the ulna by a centralization procedure.

Mild hypoplasia of the thumb is treated by release of the first web space, MCP joint collateral reconstruction, and opponensplasty tendon transfer. More severe hypoplasia or absence of the thumb may be treated by pollicization of the index finger. This procedure shifts the index finger to the thumb position and repositions the index finger extrinsic extensor tendons as well as the dorsal and palmar interosseous tendons to provide balanced control of the shifted digit.

Goldfarb C. Congenital hand anomalies: a review of the literature, 2009–2012. *J Hand Surg Am.* 2013;38(9):1854-1859. [PMID: 23683863]

Goldfarb C, Ezaki M, Wall L, Lam W, Oberg K. The Oberg-Manske-Tonkin (OMT) classification of congenital upper extremities: update for 2020. *J Hand Surg Am.* 2020;45(6):542-547. [PMID: 32093994]

12 Pediatric Orthopedic Surgery

Patrick Bosch, MD
George T. Rab, MD

The scope of pediatric orthopedics ranges from congenital anomalies to injuries in the adolescent. The pathophysiologic manifestations of many of these disorders differ from analogous adult problems because of the added dimension of growth. The physician's relationship with the pediatric patient generally occurs in the context of a protective family environment, in contrast to the more independent relationship the physician may form with an adult. The natural tendency for children to be active and the remarkable regenerative processes of the immature skeleton frequently make formal rehabilitation unnecessary following surgery or serious injury.

Guidelines for Pediatric Orthopedics

The following rules may be helpful when applying general orthopedic principles to the child:

1. A growing bone normally tends to remodel itself toward the adult configuration. A healthy physis or growth plate can remodel even significant deformities, especially in younger children, near the ends of bone, or in the plane of motion of the nearest joint.
2. Injuries to the physis, however, worsen as abnormal growth continues (eg, following permanent damage to the growth plate), especially near rapidly growing areas such as the knee. This characteristic is exaggerated in younger children.
3. Children tolerate long-term immobilization better than adults and tend to recover soft-tissue mobility spontaneously following most injuries.
4. Fracture healing is usually more rapid and predictable in the actively growing skeleton than in the adult skeleton.
5. Many so-called deformities, such as metatarsus adductus, internal tibial torsion, genu valgum (knock-knee), and bowed legs, are actually physiologic variations that correct spontaneously with growth. For example, physiologic bowing is common and benign. It is typically symmetric, involves both the femur and tibia, and is most prominent in toddlers. It usually resolves by 2 years of age, but there is great variability. By age 36 months, almost all children will correct spontaneously. The clinician must distinguish between conditions that need no treatment and those requiring early intervention.

GROWTH DISORDERS

General skeletal growth is discussed in detail in Chapter 1.

1. Limb-Length Inequality

Essentials of Diagnosis

- *Commonly asymptomatic difference in limb length must be detected to plan for appropriate treatment.*
- *Congenital anomalies may lead to significant inequality.*
- *Proper evaluation and planning allow optimal treatment during growth.*

General Considerations

Limb-length inequality may reflect either a congenital deficiency or any of a wide variety of acquired conditions (Table 12–1). Posttraumatic physeal arrest occurs most commonly after injury in the distal medial tibia. Injuries of the distal femoral physis have a high incidence of growth arrest and greater effect on leg length. Upper extremities of unequal length are usually only of cosmetic interest and can easily be compensated for by modifying clothing. In the lower extremities, however, length discrepancies may be severe enough—greater than 3 cm—to limit function and require treatment. Lesser discrepancies can be managed with a shoe lift.

Table 12–1. Causes of limb-length inequality.

Infectious causes
Osteomyelitis
Septic arthritis
Neoplastic causes
Arteriovenous malformations
Hemangioma
Neuromuscular causes
Cerebral palsy
Isolated limb paralysis
Poliomyelitis
Traumatic causes
Malunion of long bones
Physeal injury
Other causes
Avascular necrosis of femoral head (and physis)
Congenital amputations
Legg-Calvé-Perthes disease

Clinical Findings

A. Symptoms and Signs

Most limb inequality in children is asymptomatic, even when severe. Adaptive changes like long leg crouch and short leg equinus must be sought. Marked deformity may cause a painless limp.

Clinical limb measurement is usually possible by checking for a level pelvis with the child standing on calibrated blocks under the short leg. Severe inequality may require alternate exam techniques.

B. Imaging Studies

All children should have an x-ray of the entire limb at initial visit to screen for anomalies and deformities. Full-length long cassette films and new low-radiation films (EOS) are the standard for accurate measurement of inequality, but they can be inaccurate if the child moves. An option in older children is an anteroposterior (AP) pelvis with the child standing on clinically appropriate blocks under the short leg. Skeletal maturity is measured from wrist bone age films.

C. Calculation of Limb Length at Maturity

Clinical management of limb-length inequality in pediatric patients should include calculation of projected lengths at maturity. Several mathematical methods, based on skeletal age, gender, and normal growth rates, are available. The following general rule can be used to estimate the extent of future growth: The average growth rates of the distal femur and proximal tibia are 10 to 12 mm/year and 5 to 6 mm/year, respectively, with growth continuing until bone age 14 in females and 16 in males.

Treatment

A. Shoe Lift

A lift is rarely required in children, but adolescents may desire a lift. It generally will be 1 cm less than the measured difference in limb length.

B. Epiphysiodesis

The simplest surgical procedure to treat pediatric bone-length discrepancies is epiphysiodesis (surgical closure of the growth plate). Physeal closure can be accomplished by disruption of the growth cells (drill or curettage) or spanning the growth plate with implants (tension plate or threaded screw). Epiphysiodesis is usually performed at the distal femoral physis, proximal tibial physis, or both (pan genu), because they are rapidly growing and easily accessible surgically. The exact timing of epiphysiodesis is crucial to attaining equal limb lengths at skeletal maturity. Timing is calculated by various methods. The "growth remaining" and "multiplier methods" use historic growth data and apply the patient's growth rate. The White-Menelaus predictions are based on assumptions of growth: the distal femur contributes 9 mm and the proximal tibia 6 mm per year; and males grow until 16 years of age, whereas females grow until 14 years of age. The effectiveness of epiphysiodesis requires that bone still be growing and that accurate data be collected on this growth.

C. Femoral Shortening

If a child reaches the age when bone growth is insufficient to make epiphysiodesis practical, the long leg may be shortened at skeletal maturity by femoral shortening. This may be performed as an open procedure by removing a segment of femur and fixing the bone with a plate and screws. It may also be done as a closed procedure, using an intramedullary femoral rod introduced through a buttock incision for fixation. A cylindrical segment of femur is cut out of the bone using intramedullary saws, and the bone is pushed aside to allow the femur to shorten over the rod. The excised bone segment eventually resorbs.

D. Other Techniques

Leg-length inequalities projected to be 6 cm or more generally do not respond well to the previously described treatments, which in these cases may lead to unacceptably short stature or limb segments. Although some discrepancies are so severe that amputation of the foot and prosthetic fitting are required, techniques of bone lengthening can be successful in treating these children (see Chapter 1). Improved results are being realized with intramedullary lengthening techniques.

Birch JG, Makarov MA, Jackson TJ, Jo CH. Comparison of Anderson-Green growth remaining graphs and White-Menelaus predictions of growth remaining in the distal femoral and proximal tibial physis. *J Bone Joint Surg Am.* 2019;101(11):1016-1022. [PMID: 31169579]

Birch JG, Samchukov ML. Use of the Ilizarov method to correct lower limb deformities in children and adolescents. *J Am Acad Orthop Surg.* 2004;12:144-154. [PMID: 15161167]

Gordon JE, Davis LE. Leg length discrepancy: the natural history. *J Pediatr Orthop.* 2019;6(suppl 1):S10-S13. [PMID: 31169640]

Paley D, Bhave A, Herzenberg JE, Bowen JR. Multiplier method for predicting limb-length discrepancy. *J Bone Joint Surg Am.* 2000;82(10):1432-1446. [PMID: 11057472]

2. Small Stature and Other Disorders of Growth

Orthopedic disorders (achondroplasia, multiple epiphyseal dysplasia) or other syndromes (Down syndrome, Marfan syndrome) often accompany dwarfism. The classification of skeletal syndromes and dysplasias is undergoing rapid change as knowledge is gained using molecular, biologic, and genetic techniques. In general, autosomal recessive genes code for enzymatic and biochemical defects and autosomal dominant gene defects cause structural deformities. An example of the latter is achondroplasia that results from mutation of fibroblast growth factor receptor 3 (FGFR3), a structural protein that results in the quantitative decrease in cartilage formation. The gene defects are inherited from one of the parents or are sporadic mutations. A detailed review of skeletal syndromes and dysplasias is outside the scope of this text; Table 12–2 lists some of these conditions and the major orthopedic problems associated with them.

Table 12–2. Orthopedic involvement in selected syndromes and dwarfing conditions.

Condition	Orthopedic involvement
Achondroplasia	Short limbs; genu varum; exaggerated lumbar lordosis; spinal stenosis; ligamentous laxity
Apert syndrome	Foot deformities; hand and foot polydactyly
Arthrogryposis	Severe joint stiffness, contractures, and dislocations; resistant clubfoot
Cleidocranial dysplasia	Absent clavicles; coxa vara
Diastrophic dysplasia	Severe clubfoot; joint dislocations; joint stiffness; cervical kyphosis; scoliosis
Down syndrome	Cervical (C1-C2) instability; hip dislocation; ankle valgus; ligamentous laxity
Enchondromatosis	Asymmetric multiple enchondromas in long bones; limb-length inequality; angulation of long bones
Fibrous dysplasia	Multiple fibrous lesions in bone; limb bowing or shortening; occasional endocrine disorders
Larsen syndrome	Hip, knee, and radial head dislocations; severe cervical kyphosis and instability; scoliosis
Marfan syndrome	Scoliosis
Metaphyseal chondrodysplasia	Moderate dwarfing; genu varum; ligamentous laxity; cervical instability
Multiple epiphyseal dysplasia	Mild dwarfism; joint surface deformities with premature osteoarthritis; angular limb deformities
Multiple hereditary exostoses	Mild dwarfing; osteochondroma (external enlargements) at all long bone ends
Osteogenesis imperfecta	Bone fragility and multiple fractures; bowing of bones; scoliosis; mild to moderate dwarfing
Spondyloepiphyseal dysplasia	Severe dwarfing; coxa vara; genu valgum; scoliosis; odontoid hypoplasia, instability, and deformity

INFECTIOUS PROCESSES

1. Hematogenous Osteomyelitis

Essentials of Diagnosis

- *Limp, bone pain, fever, leukocytosis, and elevation of erythrocyte sedimentation rate (ESR) and C-reactive protein (CRP) characterize osteomyelitis.*
- *Methicillin-resistant Staphylococcus aureus (MRSA) osteomyelitis is increasingly common and may include serious life- and limb-threatening complications.*

General Considerations

Osteomyelitis, an infection of bone tissue, usually occurs in the marrow cavity but sometimes affects the cortex as well. There is a predilection for metaphyseal involvement of long bones.

Pathogenesis

In children, osteomyelitis is most commonly caused by hematogenous bacterial spread, frequently following an upper respiratory infection or partially treated distant infection. Direct inoculation of bacteria into an open fracture or

Table 12–3. Common pathogens in pediatric bone and joint infections.

Osteomyelitis
Group A *Streptococcus*
Salmonella (with sickle cell)
Staphylococcus aureus
Septic joint
Escherichia coli (neonatal)
Group A *Streptococcus*
Haemophilus influenzae (age 6-24 months) in non–HIB-immunized patients
Neisseria gonorrhoeae (adolescent)
Pneumococcus
Proteus (neonatal)
Staphylococcus aureus
Streptococcus faecalis (neonatal)
Soft-tissue infection
Escherichia coli (neonatal)
Group A *Streptococcus*
Proteus
Pseudomonas
Staphylococcus aureus
Streptococcus faecalis (neonatal)
Kingella kingae

HIB, *Haemophilus influenzae* type B.

penetrating wound can also lead to infection and may resemble other serious bacterial infections in children (Table 12–3).

Acute bacterial hematogenous osteomyelitis usually occurs in the metaphysis following sludging of bacteria-laden blood in the venous sinusoids. The majority of cases are caused by *S aureus*. As the infection progresses, edema fluid and infected purulent tissue invade the porous cortex and elevate the periosteum, which is highly resistant to infection because of its extreme vascularity. The pressure of the pus beneath the richly innervated periosteum causes localized pain. Eventually, if the infection is untreated, the periosteum itself ruptures, and infected tissue spills into the surrounding soft tissue or ruptures the skin (Figure 12–1).

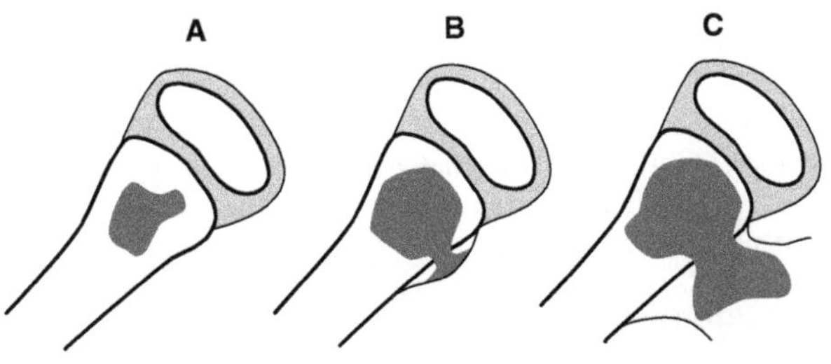

▲ **Figure 12–1.** Hematogenous osteomyelitis in children. Cellulitic phase **(A)** can exude through the cortex, raising periosteum **(B)**. Late rupture into soft tissues **(C)** is rare, unless infection is untreated.

The accumulated purulence in the marrow cavity and under the periosteum creates an efficient avascular culture medium in the cortex between them. This dead cortex is called a *sequestrum*, and, if it is large, surgical removal may be required to control the infection.

The elevated periosteum responds to infection by producing a shell of periosteal new bone called *involucrum*, which provides some stability to the infected bone and rarely becomes infected itself.

Clinical Findings

Pain and tenderness at the infection site are universal signs, limping is common, and frequently the child is irritable. Fever and leukocytosis are common but not universal, and the ESR is almost always elevated, usually to 50 mm/hour or more. CRP is elevated. Children with MRSA infections may present with severe systemic illness and multisystem involvement. Although the diagnosis is usually clear, osteomyelitis should be suspected if a child has bone pain in the absence of other systemic signs but has recently received antibiotic treatment for other conditions.

Imaging Studies

Clinical examination and routine x-rays are usually sufficient to make the diagnosis; occasionally, bone scans or magnetic resonance imaging (MRI) may be required to help localize lesions.

Laboratory Findings

Elevations of ESR (>50 mm/hour) and CRP are typical of osteomyelitis.

Treatment

A. Early Treatment

Treatment depends on the duration of symptoms, radiographic findings, and suspected or cultured organism. If the infection is detected early, no visible radiograph changes usually are apparent except for soft-tissue swelling. In that case, intravenous and, later, oral antibiotics may resolve the infection. Aspiration of the metaphysis can be done for culture before beginning antibiotic therapy. Up to 30% to 40% of cultures may be negative despite other clear evidence of bacterial infection; in that case, empirical treatment (usually with antistaphylococcal antibiotics) is appropriate.

B. Treatment for Advanced Infection or MRSA

In advanced cases, lytic defects or osteoporosis may be present, and periosteal reaction may be visible on radiograph; such cases can benefit from open drainage and debridement of the infected metaphysis. Antibiotic treatment must be continued until there is no evidence of residual infection because bacteria can survive in bone tissue that is not well perfused with antibiotic. In such cases, a prolonged regimen of oral antibiotics (often 3 months) minimizes the possibility of chronic osteomyelitis.

MRSA infections are more likely to require surgical drainage for metaphyseal or subperiosteal abscesses, and multiple operative debridements may be necessary.

2. Septic Joint

Essentials of Diagnosis

- *Septic joints cause pain, limp, and refusal to move a joint.*
- *Aspiration of joint for culture, surgical drainage, and antibiotics is generally successful.*
- *Septic hip is a unique surgical emergency requiring urgent surgery.*

General Considerations

Septic arthritis in children, like osteomyelitis, usually is hematogenous in origin. The bacterial complications are similar to those seen in bone infections (see Table 12–3). Septic joints frequently follow upper respiratory infections; they may be delayed in onset by a week or more and may present in an attenuated form when a previous infection was partially treated.

Clinical Findings

The classic septic joint in a child presents a dramatic picture: The joint is splinted by muscle spasm, and motion of even a few degrees causes extreme pain. There may be effusion, but findings may be less striking if antibiotics were used in the recent past. During this acute inflammatory phase, children are more comfortable if the involved joint is immobilized.

Laboratory Findings

Although white blood cell counts and the ESR are usually elevated, the definitive diagnosis of septic joint requires aspiration and synovial fluid analysis. Sterile aspiration does not harm the joint and should be done immediately when the diagnosis is suspected. Aspiration of deep joints such as the hip may require radiographic control.

Synovial white blood cell counts range from 50,000/μL (in nonpyogenic infections such as *Neisseria gonorrhoeae*) to over 250,000/μL (*S aureus*). This white cell response, with the concomitant high level of lysosomal enzyme release, is most destructive of articular cartilage in septic joints. Although synovial fluid cultures give definitive guidance for therapy, antibiotic treatment can initially be based on results of Gram staining. In addition, immunochemical tests may offer rapid identification of certain pathogens.

Imaging Studies

Most septic joints have normal radiographic findings or nonspecific signs of effusion or local tissue swelling. Late radiographic findings include subluxation, narrowing of joint space, and subchondral bone irregularity. MRI will demonstrate effusion or concurrent osteomyelitis or pyomyositis if present (see later discussion).

Differential Diagnosis

Like osteomyelitis, septic joint may be mimicked by septic pyomyositis (almost always MRSA), with involvement of periarticular tissues with or without actual joint involvement. In some regions, Lyme arthritis can have significantly overlapping signs and symptoms.

Treatment

Treatment always includes drainage of the joint. In easily accessible joints, such as the finger or knee, certain low-grade infections may respond well to repeated aspirations. In most cases, however, surgical drainage by arthrotomy or arthroscopy is preferable.

Antibiotics easily cross the synovial membrane and are continued until the joint inflammation is resolved, usually for at least 3 weeks. Intravenous administration is used initially but may often be followed by oral medication once the temperature, ESR, and leukocyte count return to normal.

Dart AH, Michelson KA, Aronson PL, et al. Hip synovial fluid cell count in children from a Lyme disease endemic area. *Pediatrics.* 2018;141(5):e20173810. [PMID: 29669751]

Hensinger RN. Impending danger: community-acquired methicillin-resistant *Staphylococcus aureus*. *J Pediatr Orthop* 2006;26:701-702. [PMID: 17065929]

Jagodzinski NA, Kanwar R, Graham K, Bache CE. Prospective evaluation of a shortened regimen of treatment for acute osteomyelitis and septic arthritis in children. *J Pediatr Orthop.* 2009;29:518-525. [PMID: 19568027]

Kaplan SL. Acute hematogenous osteomyelitis in children: differences in clinical manifestations and management. *Pediatr Infect Dis J.* 2010;29:1128-1129. [PMID: 21099652]

3. Septic Hip

Septic hip is one of the true surgical emergencies in pediatric orthopedics. It must be differentiated from transient synovitis of the hip, which is a benign condition (see the section on transient synovitis of the hip).

Pathogenesis

Because of the unique structure and blood supply of the proximal femur (Figure 12–2), purulence within the joint capsule can cause thrombosis of epiphyseal vessels and necrosis of the proximal femoral epiphysis. Neglected septic hips may

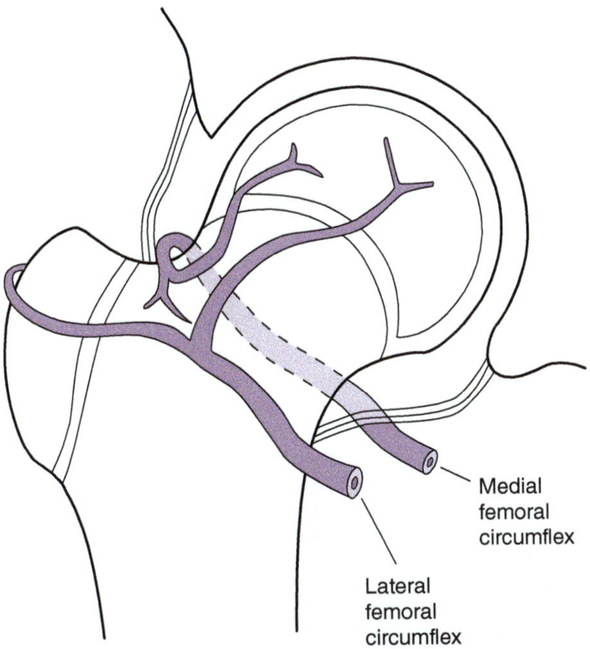

▲ **Figure 12–2.** The blood supply of the proximal femur is unusual because the capsule interferes with the direct routing of blood vessels. The epiphyseal vessels emerge distal to the capsule and course up the surface of the femoral neck, rendering them susceptible to injury, thrombosis, or blockage by increased intraarticular pressure.

subluxate or dislocate because of effusion and laxity caused by hyperemia. Finally, purulence will do irreversible damage to articular cartilage. For these reasons, septic hip (or osteomyelitis of the proximal femur) always requires urgent surgical drainage. An anterior approach is preferred to reduce the risk of vascular injury and subluxation. Some surgeons are reporting successful experience with arthroscopic techniques as well.

Septic hip in a growing child is also a special orthopedic case because the femoral neck (which is intraarticular) is actually the anatomic metaphysis of the proximal femur. It is thus susceptible to hematogenous osteomyelitis, which may rupture into the hip joint and cause sepsis.

Differential Diagnosis

A common clinical problem is the differentiation between septic hip and transient synovitis of the hip. Juvenile arthritis may occasionally be included in the differential. Table 12–4 highlights differences in the conditions.

Treatment

Traditional and current standard treatment for a septic hip is arthrotomy and irrigation through an anterior approach. Irrigation via arthroscopy, as is done is the knee, is being investigated in some centers with experience in hip arthroscopy in pediatric populations.

Caird MS, Flynn JM, Leung YL, Millman JE, D'Italia JG, Dormans JP. Factors distinguishing septic arthritis from transient synovitis of the hip in children. *J Bone Joint Surg Am.* 2006;88(6):1251-1257. [PMID: 16757758]

Edmonds EW, Lin C, Farnsworth CL, Bomar JD, Upasani VV. A medial portal for hip arthroscopy in children with septic arthritis: a safety study. *J Pediatr Orthop.* 2018;38(10):527-531. [PMID: 27603192]

Heyworth BE, Shore BJ, Donohue KS, Miller PE, Kocher MS, Glotzbecker MP. Management of pediatric patients with synovial fluid white blood-cell counts of 25,000 to 75,000 cells/mm^3 after aspiration of the hip. *J Bone Joint Surg Am.* 2015;97(5):389-395. [PMID: 25740029]

Sultan J, Hughes PJ. Septic arthritis or transient synovitis of the hip in children: the value of clinical prediction algorithms. *J Bone Joint Surg Br.* 2010;92:1289-1293. [PMID: 20798450]

Table 12–4. Clinical differential diagnosis of inflammatory hip conditions.

	Septic Hip	Transient Synovitis of Hip	Juvenile Arthritis of Hip
Pain	Severe	Moderate to severe	Moderate
Gait	Cannot walk	Limp or cannot walk	Limp
Fever	Common	No	No or low grade
Radiograph	Negative	Negative	Joint narrowing
WBC	Elevated	Normal	Normal-elevated
Aspirate	Turbid; 5000-250,000 WBC; bacteria present	Normal	25,000-50,000 WBC with monocytes
Treatment	Urgent surgical drainage; antibiotics	Symptomatic	Salicylates, rest, physical therapy

WBC, white blood cells.

4. Puncture Wounds of the Foot

Sneakers and tennis shoes offer little protection from nail punctures of the plantar surface of the foot. The penetrating nail may carry *Pseudomonas* bacteria (which contaminate the soles of tennis shoes) into the plantar fascia, although one series found *S aureus* or group A *Streptococcus* to be most common.

The symptoms of infection include redness, swelling, and pain that persist longer than 1 week. Surgical incision and drainage of the abscess and foreign body excision, when present (approximately one-sixth of cases), are usually curative. Interestingly, prophylactic use of antibiotics does not seem to lessen the chance of developing late abscess. Late presentation is a marker for deep infection.

Eidelman M, Bialik V, Miller Y, Kassis I. Plantar puncture wounds in children: analysis of 80 hospitalized patients and late sequelae. *Isr Med Assoc J*. 2003;5:268-271. [PMID: 14509132]

Schwab RA, Powers RD. Conservative therapy of plantar puncture wounds. *J Emerg Med*. 1995;13:291-295. [PMID: 7673617]

5. Diskitis in Children

Diskitis is a low-grade inflammatory process involving the intervertebral disk, usually in the lumbar spine. It affects children at any age, although it is most frequent between 2 and 6 years of age. The disorder is caused by hematogenous bacterial seeding, with the most common cultures growing *S aureus* from the disk aspirate. The classic presentation in a toddler is refusal to walk; pain is not a prominent symptom in this age group. Older children (up to early teen years) may have either back or abdominal pain.

Clinical Findings

Small children may have limitation of passive hyperextension of the spine (in the prone position) with no other findings. Older children have splinting of the paraspinous muscles and pain with percussion.

Laboratory Findings

The ESR may be normal or elevated; patients with an elevated ESR are more likely to have bacterial growth if cultures are done. Aspirate cultures may be negative in 40% of patients, and even computed tomography (CT)-guided biopsy cultures often fail to yield positive pathologic microbes.

Imaging Studies

Radiographs at first are normal but eventually demonstrate disk space narrowing with sclerosis of adjoining endplates, best visualized on spot lateral views. MRI demonstrates characteristic changes including edema surrounding the involved disk.

Treatment

Management depends on the severity of clinical findings because a large number of diskitis patients have self-limited disease and improve spontaneously. Children with sepsis or elevated ESR may benefit from disk aspiration and culture. Less ill children are usually treated with empirical antistaphylococcal oral antibiotics for 6 weeks. Pantaloon spica cast may occasionally be required for symptom relief. Long-term outcome is universally favorable, although occasional spontaneous fusion of the disk space occurs.

Czuczman GJ, Marrero DE, Huang AJ, Mandell JC, Ghazikhanian V, Simeone FJ. Diagnostic yield of repeat CT-guided biopsy for suspected infectious spondylodiscitis. *Skeletal Radiol*. 2018;47(10):1403-1420. [PMID: 29777259]

Early SD, Kay RM, Tolo VT. Childhood diskitis. *J Am Acad Orthop Surg*. 2003;11:413-420. [PMID: 14686826]

Hamdy RC, Lawton L, Carey T, et al. Subacute hematogenous osteomyelitis: are biopsy and surgery always necessary? *J Pediatr Orthop*. 1996;16:220-223. [PMID: 8742289]

Scott RJ, Christofersen MR, Robertson WW Jr, et al. Acute osteomyelitis in children: a review of 116 cases. *J Pediatr Orthop*. 1990;5:649-652. [PMID: 2203820]

METABOLIC DISORDERS

Essentials of Diagnosis

- *There is growth abnormality and weakening or bowing of long bones in children.*
- *There is widening, bowing, and cupping of the physes.*
- *Serum calcium, phosphorus, alkaline phosphate, blood urea nitrogen, and endocrine studies usually confirm the diagnosis.*

1. Rickets and Rickets-Like Conditions

Nutritional rickets is a dietary deficiency of vitamin D that interferes with skeletal ossification. Although vitamin supplementation of food and milk has virtually eliminated the dietary form of rickets, there is still an increased frequency of nutritional rickets in the United States in children with dark skin pigmentation who are breast fed past 6 months of age without vitamin D supplementation. Nutritional rickets is rare in light-skinned children or those who are formula fed. Numerous rickets-like metabolic conditions persist with orthopedic consequences, however.

Renal Osteodystrophy

Renal osteodystrophy, a disorder of calcium, phosphorus, vitamin D, and parathyroid function in children with chronic renal disease, has potentially serious skeletal manifestations. In transplantation patients, the condition can be aggravated by chronic illness and antimetabolite or steroid usage.

Osteoporosis, leading to compression fractures of the spine, is a common complication. Delayed healing of fractures is also common. Inadequate metaphyseal ossification during skeletal growth results in wide, irregular cartilaginous growth plates, which tend to slip slowly, sometimes producing grotesque hip, knee, and ankle deformities. Such deformities are usually best treated only after transplantation or other improvement in renal status. Occasionally, severe functional disabilities may require osteotomy to correct deformity before renal transplantation. Healing may be delayed, however, and the condition may recur.

Santos F, Carbajo-Pérez E, Rodríguez J, et al. Alterations of the growth plate in chronic renal failure. *Pediatr Nephrol.* 2004;20:330-334. [PMID: 15549411]

Hypophosphatemic Rickets

Hypophosphatemic rickets (vitamin D–resistant rickets) is a dominant X-linked condition in which vitamin D production and metabolism are normal but renal tubular loss of phosphate interferes with skeletal ossification. The major manifestations are a mild-to-moderate decrease in stature and bowing of the lower extremities. The medical history usually discloses a parent or sibling with short stature and bowlegs.

A. Laboratory Findings

Serum phosphorus is reduced, and serum calcium is *normal*. This is because the disorder is caused by phosphorus excretion in the urine (detectible in 24-hour urine sample). Vitamin D levels are normal.

B. Imaging Studies

Characteristic widening of growth plates, funnel-like beaking of the metaphyses, and curvature of the femoral and tibial shafts, which are normally straight (Figure 12–3), are typical.

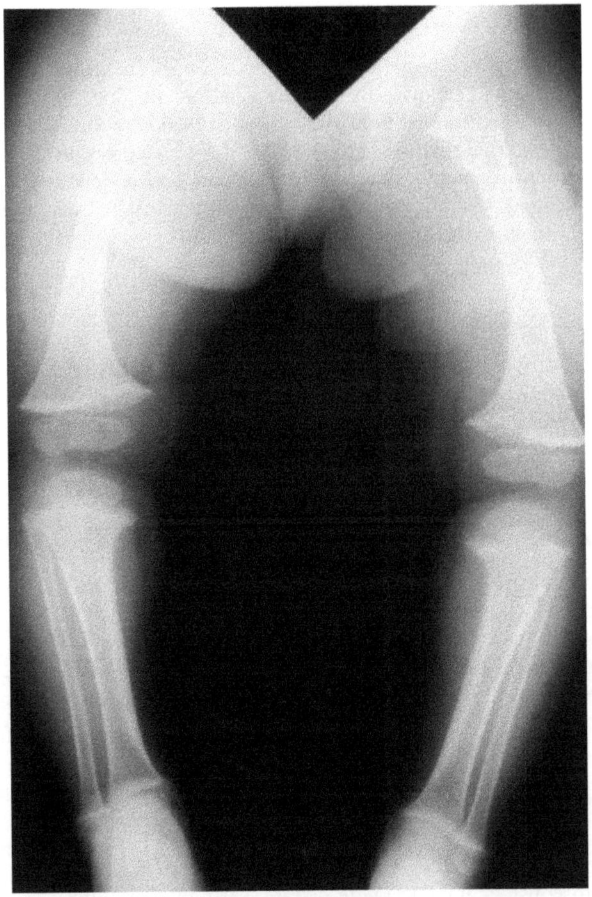

▲ **Figure 12–3.** Hypophosphatemic rickets. Radiographs demonstrate bowing of long bones and flared, irregular physes (see text).

C. Treatment

Medical treatment with megadoses of vitamin D and phosphorus supplementation may not be curative. Functionally disabling deformities can be corrected by growth plate manipulation using hemiepiphyseodesis in younger children, or by multiple-level osteotomies, which usually require bilateral surgery. Because postosteotomy healing is delayed and recurrence of deformity is common during growth, such surgery should be postponed until adolescence, if possible.

Kocaoglu M, Bilen FE, Sen C, Eralp L, Balci HI. Combined technique for the correction of lower-limb deformities resulting from metabolic bone disease. *J Bone Joint Surg Br.* 2011;93:52-56. [PMID: 21196543]

Novais E, Stevens PM. Hypophosphatemic rickets: the role of hemiepiphysiodesis. *J Pediatr Orthop.* 2006;26:238-244. [PMID: 16557142]

Saland JM. Osseous complications of pediatric transplantation. *Pediatr Transplant.* 2004;8:400-415. [PMID: 15265169]

HIP DISORDERS

1. Transient Synovitis of the Hip

Transient synovitis of the hip is a benign, nontraumatic, self-limited disorder that mimics septic hip in clinical presentation. The physician confronting this condition must exclude septic hip, which is a surgical emergency.

Although the cause of transient synovitis is unclear, evidence suggests it is associated with immune responses to viral or bacterial antigens, mediated through the synovial membrane. Aseptic synovial fluid rapidly accumulates under pressure in the hip joint, and there may be severe pain from capsular distension. The fluid is resorbed within 3 to 7 days, with no long-term sequelae.

Clinical Findings

As with septic hip, upper respiratory tract infections often precede transient synovitis by a few days to 2 weeks. The hip contains excess synovial fluid and is held in flexion, abduction, and external rotation because this is the joint's position of maximum capacity. The joint may be sore and resistant to movement, but subluxation does not occur. Usually, the patient allows careful passive movement, and some remain able to bear weight.

Laboratory Findings

Inflammatory labs are useful to workup the atraumatic irritable hip. Generally, transient synovitis has less inflammatory changes in regard to ESR or CRP. Synovial fluid does not show elevation of the white blood cell count, and bacterial cultures are negative.

Imaging Studies

Radiographs reveal only capsular swelling, and effusion may be detected on ultrasound. Although experienced physicians frequently suspect transient synovitis based only on clinical examination, aspiration of the hip following confirmation of needle position by radiograph or ultrasound is the safest approach.

Differential Diagnosis

The most important differential diagnosis is septic hip, which must be excluded. Other atraumatic causes of hip pain to consider include Lyme disease, early juvenile idiopathic arthritis, and Legg-Calvé-Perthes disease. Legg-Calvé-Perthes disease (see section on Legg-Calvé-Perthes disease) may include a synovitic stage that, until the development of characteristic radiograph findings, is indistinguishable from transient synovitis. No evidence indicates that transient synovitis leads to Legg-Calvé-Perthes disease itself. Typically, the pain is less severe than in transient synovitis, the children are a bit older (older than 4-5 years), and there is no history of recent illness.

Treatment

Treatment of transient synovitis includes simple analgesics and activity modification, until symptoms resolve.

Cruz AL, Anari JB, Ramirez JM, Sankar WN, Baldwin KD. Distinguishing pediatric Lyme arthritis of the hip from transient synovitis and acute bacterial septic arthritis: a systematic review and meta-analysis. *Cureus.* 2018;10(1):e2112. [PMID: 29581924]

Nouri A, Walmsley D, Pruszczynski B, Snyder M. Transient synovitis of the hip: a comprehensive review. *J Pediatr Orthop B.* 2014;23(1):32-36. [PMID: 23812087]

2. Developmental Dysplasia of the Hip

Essentials of Diagnosis

- *Certain infants (breech positioning, first born, positive family history, and females) are at higher risk for developmental dysplasia of the hip.*
- *Diagnosis is made clinically or by ultrasound.*
- *Early treatment gives the best results.*

Developmental dysplasia of the hip is one of the most serious problems in pediatric orthopedics. The neonatal hip is a relatively unstable joint because the muscle is undeveloped, the soft cartilaginous surfaces are easily deformed, and the ligaments are lax. Exaggerated positioning in acute flexion and adduction in utero may occur, especially in breech presentation. This situation may cause excess stretching of the posterior hip capsule, which renders the joint unstable after delivery. Laxity may reflect family history or the presence of maternal relaxin hormone in the fetal circulatory system.

This relative instability may lead to asymptomatic subluxation (partial displacement) or dislocation (complete displacement) of the hip joint. Displacement of the femoral head in the infant is proximal (posterior and superior) because of the pull of the gluteal and hip flexor muscles. In the subluxated hip, asymmetric pressure causes progressive flattening of the posterior and superior acetabular rim and medial femoral head (*dysplasia* is the term to describe these structural deviations from normal).

In the completely dislocated hip, dysplasia also occurs because normal joint development requires concentric motion with normally mated joint surfaces. The shallow, deformed dysplastic joint surfaces predispose to further mechanical instability and the inexorable progression of the disorder.

Developmental dysplasia of the hip (DDH) occurs in approximately 1 in 1000 live births in whites, is less common in blacks, and may be more common in certain ethnic groups. It is more likely if certain risk factors are present, such as positive family history, ligamentous laxity, breech presentation (and, by association, cesarean delivery), female gender, large fetal size, and first-born status. Dislocations may be bilateral but are more often unilateral and on the left side.

Clinical Findings

Reversal of dysplasia and subsequent normal hip development depend on early detection of DDH. Early detection is made more challenging by lack of a definitive test or finding on examination. Moreover, because this disorder is painless, there are no symptoms in the infant. Detection of bilateral dislocations may be particularly difficult.

Radiographs are usually not useful in newborn infants because the femoral head is composed of radiolucent cartilage. Ultrasound examination has become the standard of care.

Technologist or surgeon experience with the technique can affect results. Careful physical examination at birth that is repeated at each well-infant check until the child is walking normally should detect most cases. A high index of suspicion is mandatory, especially if risk factors are present.

A. Tests for Dysplasia

Several examination maneuvers require a quiet, relaxed infant and commonly produce false-negative findings. Although it is imperative to detect subluxated or dislocated hips, it is also helpful to identify the very lax (unstable) but still located hip. This type of joint may either dislocate later or exhibit subtle dysplasia during growth that can cause premature osteoarthritis.

1. Asymmetric skin folds—A dislocated hip displaces proximally, causing the leg to be marginally shorter. This occasionally leads to the accordion phenomenon, with wrinkling of thigh skin folds. The most significant fold is between the genitals and gluteus maximus region. This test is not very reliable, frequently producing false-positive and false-negative results (Figure 12–4A).

2. Galeazzi test—With the child lying on a flat surface, flex the hips and knees so the heels rest flat on the table, just distal to the buttock (Figure 12–4B). A dislocated hip is signaled by relative shortening of the thigh compared with the normal leg, as shown by the difference in knee height level. This test is almost always useless in children younger than 1 year old and is negative if dislocation is bilateral.

3. Passive hip abduction—The flexed hips are gently abducted as far as possible (Figure 12–4C). If one or both hips are dislocated, the femoral head (the pivot point during abduction) is posterior, causing relative tightness of the adductor muscles. Asymmetric abduction or limited abduction (usually <70 degrees from the midline) is a positive finding. When the hip is lax (dislocatable but not dislocated), the abduction test is normal despite the presence of subluxation or dislocation.

4. Barlow test—A provocative test that picks up an unstable but located hip, the Barlow test is unsuitable for a dislocated hip. The flexed calf and knee are gently grasped in the hand, with the thumb at the lesser trochanter and fingers at the greater trochanter (knee flexion relaxes the hamstrings). The hip is adducted slightly and gently pushed posteriorly and laterally with the palm (Figure 12–4D, F). Detection of so-called pistoning, or the sensation of the femoral head subluxating over the posterior rim of the acetabulum, is a positive finding.

5. Ortolani test—This test detects hips that are already dislocated. The flexed limb is grasped as in the Barlow test. The hip is abducted while the femur is gently lifted with the fingers at the greater trochanter (Figure 12–4D, E). In a positive test, there is a sensation of the hip reducing back into the acetabulum. Reduction is felt but not heard: The old concept of a so-called hip click is incorrect. The Ortolani test may be negative at 2 to 3 months of age, even when the hip is dislocated, because of the development of soft-tissue contracture.

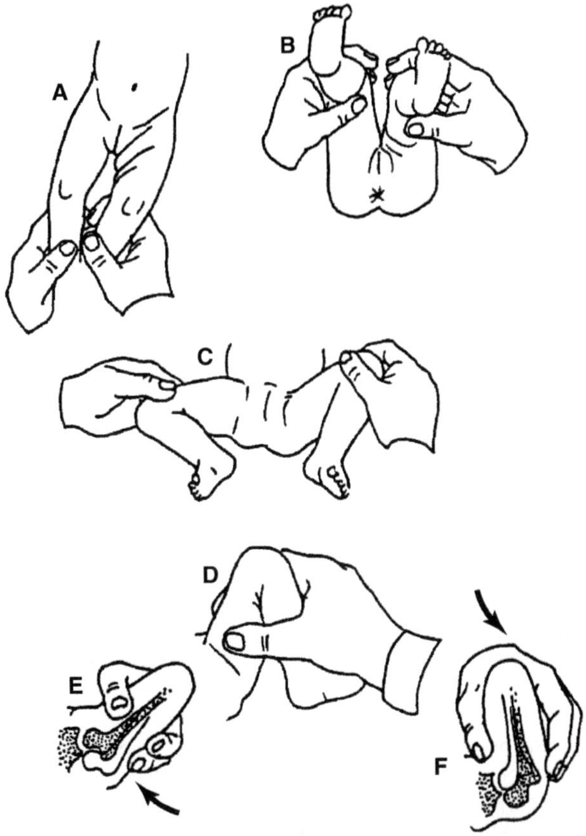

▲ **Figure 12–4.** Clinical examination of developmental dislocation of the hip. In all pictures, the child's left hip is the abnormal side. **A:** Asymmetric skin folds. **B:** Galeazzi test. **C:** Limitation of abduction. **D, E, F:** Ortolani and Barlow tests (see text).

B. Imaging Studies

In the infant, diagnosis is made by physical examination alone, and radiographs are generally unnecessary. Dysplasia, instability, and dislocation may appear on ultrasound studies, which can allow visualization of hip contour and stability before ossification is present. Sonography is a dynamic examination that requires an experienced interpreter, and there can be false positives prior to 6 to 10 weeks of age. Radiographs may be used at any age, but the absence of ossified structures renders them inaccurate in the newborn. After 4 to 6 months, when the ossific nucleus appears in the femoral head, radiographs are more helpful. Because much of the skeleton is cartilaginous at this age, certain lines and angles may be drawn on radiographs to allow estimates of

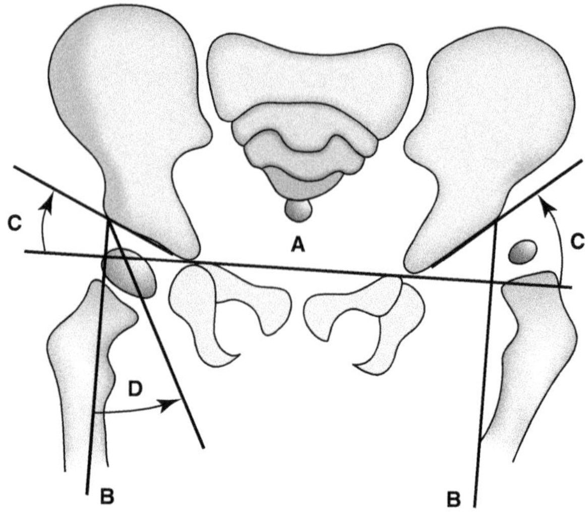

▲ **Figure 12–5.** Lines drawn for measurement in developmental dysplasia of the hip. In the figure, the patient's left hip (on the right of the figure) is the subluxated one. **A:** Hilgenreiner line is a horizontal line of the pelvis, drawn between the triradiate cartilages. The proximal femoral ossification center should be below this line. **B:** Perkin's line is a vertical line (perpendicular to Hilgenreiner line) drawn down from the lateral edge of the acetabulum. The femoral head ossification center, as well as the medial beak of the proximal metaphysis, should fall medial to this line. **C:** The acetabular index is the angle between Hilgenreiner line and a line joining the acetabular center (triradiate) with the acetabular edge as it intersects Perkin's line. It measures acetabular depth and should be below 30 degrees by 1 year of age and below 25 degrees by 2 years of age. **D:** The center-edge angle is the angle between Perkin's line and a line joining the lateral edge of the acetabulum with the center of the femoral head. It is a measure of lateral subluxation that becomes smaller as the hip subluxates laterally. Normal is 20 degrees or greater. Sheldon's line is the smooth curved line drawn from the top of the obturator foramen and along the inferomedial femoral neck of the normal hip.

geometric parameters (Figure 12–5). These may suggest evidence of acetabular dysplasia (a more vertical slope of the acetabular roof, measured as the acetabular index), femoral dysplasia (small or absent ossification center in the femoral head), or lateral superior displacement of the femoral head.

Increased femoral anteversion (external rotation of the femoral head and neck) is often present in DDH but not visible. Increased anteversion may be seen as an increase in relative femoral neck valgus in the older child.

C. Detection of Dysplasia in the Older Child

As the infant grows older, many diagnostic maneuvers that are positive in a young infant become negative because soft-tissue changes accommodate the displaced structures. Thus, the Ortolani and Barlow signs can be negative, even in the face of grossly abnormal hip development, making detection particularly difficult (especially between 4 and 15 months of age). The first signs of developmental dysplasia may then not be recognized until the child begins to walk and demonstrates a waddling gait with excessive lumbar lordosis. Radiographs at this age are diagnostic.

Treatment

Treatment of DDH should be initiated as soon as the diagnosis is suspected. Early treatment is generally successful, whereas a delay in treatment may result in permanent dysplastic changes. Exact treatment depends on patient age at presentation and degree of involvement. Regardless of age, treatment may fail, and the physician may need to institute a more complex treatment plan. The current recommendations are described next.

A. Age 0 to 6 Months

A dislocated hip at this age may spontaneously reduce over 2 to 3 weeks if the hip is held in a position of flexion. This is best accomplished with the Pavlik harness (Figure 12–6), a canvas device that holds the hips flexed at 100 degrees and prevents adduction but does not limit further flexion. Movement in the harness is beneficial for the joint and helps achieve gradual spontaneous reduction and stabilization of the hip. Treatment with a Pavlik harness has a low risk of avascular necrosis (see section on avascular necrosis of the hip). This treatment should not be continued beyond 3 to 4 weeks if there is no improvement. The failure rate of the Pavlik harness is approximately 10%, necessitating more invasive treatment, such as closed or open reduction.

B. Age 6 to 12 Months (Before Walking)

Gentle manipulative reduction of the dislocation under a general anesthetic and maintenance of a located position for 2 to 3 months in a spica cast usually stabilize the joint. Even after the hip is stable, any residual dysplasia must be treated by bracing or surgery. In the past, prereduction skin traction was thought to reduce the risk of avascular necrosis. It is now believed that adequate hip flexion and limited abduction in the spica cast are the most important safety factors, and most surgeons no longer use traction.

C. Age 12 Months to 2 Years

In walking-age children or in those who failed closed reduction, open reduction of the hip is required. Severe flattening of the acetabulum with distortion of the normal spherical femoral head shape is found on opening the hip. The limbus (acetabular rim) may be flattened and inverted, and the ligamentum teres is always hypertrophic. Fibrofatty tissue occupying the center of the acetabulum must be removed.

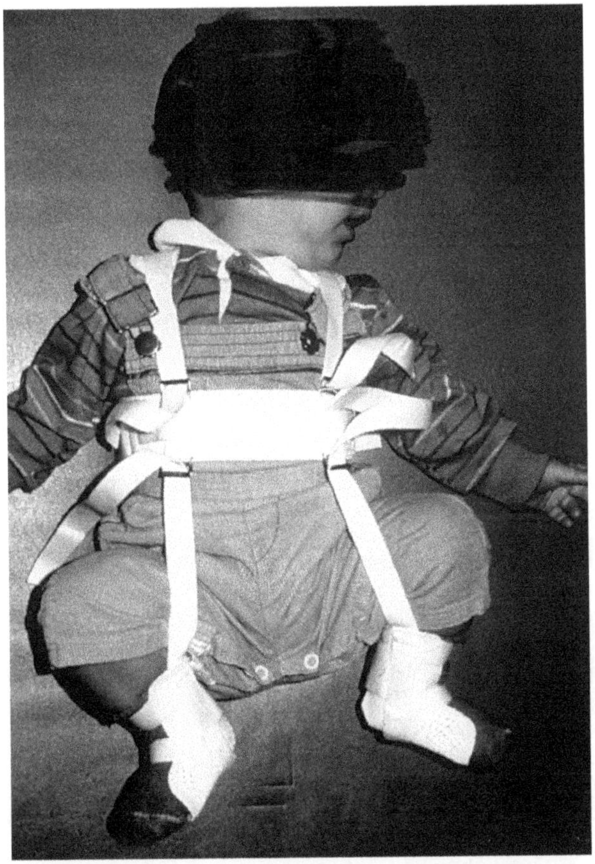

▲ **Figure 12–6.** The Pavlik harness, a device used for treatment of hip dislocation, subluxation, and dysplasia.

Femoral shortening osteotomy may be required at the time of open reduction to reduce soft-tissue tension and minimize the risk of avascular necrosis. After reduction, the position is maintained by capsular repair (capsulorrhaphy) and a cast, until stability is achieved. Prolonged bracing or surgery is often required to resolve the residual dysplasia that accompanies untreated dysplasia in this group of children.

D. Age Older Than 2 Years

Significant residual dysplasia is present in children with DDH who are untreated at this age. Dysplasia may also persist despite successful reduction performed by any method at an earlier age. The dysplasia may be accompanied by a limp, and radiographs show a high acetabular index (more vertical acetabular roof), increased valgus of the femoral neck, and subluxation of the femoral head.

Surgical correction of dysplasia creates a stable mechanical environment that permits remodeling to a more normal joint during growth. Treatment requires bony procedures, either on the acetabular or femoral sides of the joint, or on both sides. Acetabular procedures, such as the Salter, Pemberton, or Dega osteotomies, improve the acetabular index and increase the mechanical stability of the joint.

Femoral osteotomy corrects the anteversion and femoral neck valgus that characterize femoral dysplasia. The exact selection of osteotomy site may be based on maximum radiographic dysplasia or on the individual surgeon's preference. All of the osteotomies require that the femoral head be spherical and the hip joint concentrically reduced before an attempt can be made to correct the dysplasia. In general, the osteotomy should address the site of dysplasia, that is, acetabular dysplasia is not ideally treated with femoral osteotomy. Nevertheless, femoral osteotomy, if performed before 4 years of age, stimulates a dysplastic shallow acetabulum to remodel into a more normal shape. This occurs because the femoral osteotomy renders the hip joint more stable, thus allowing the normal mechanisms of growth to take over. Similarly, patients exhibit a progressive decrease in femoral dysplasia following successful acetabular osteotomy.

1. Salter osteotomy—Salter osteotomy is a surgical procedure to redirect the acetabulum in DDH (Figure 12–7). Animal models demonstrate that residual hip dysplasia is accompanied by acetabular malrotation and deficiency in the anterolateral acetabular rim. Salter osteotomy corrects this deficiency by rotating the acetabular region anteriorly and laterally.

The procedure is indicated in children 18 months to 10 years of age in whom concentric reduction of the hip was achieved. It is used to correct moderate acetabular dysplasia and can improve the acetabular index by 15 degrees. It may also be used to stabilize the hip at the time of open reduction. The pelvis above the hip joint is exposed subperiosteally. A transverse cut is made, using a wire saw, from the sciatic notch to the anteroinferior iliac spine, and the entire distal

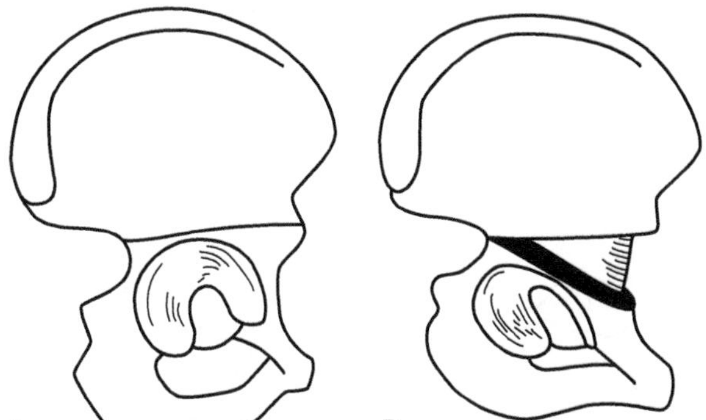

▲ **Figure 12–7.** Salter innominate osteotomy, used for managing acetabular dysplasia. After a transverse cut is made above the acetabulum **(A)**, the acetabular fragment is rotated forward and outward **(B)** to improve acetabular coverage.

fragment (including the acetabulum) is spun on the pivot points of the notch and the pubic symphysis. This redirects the entire dysplastic acetabulum to a more horizontal stable position. A bone graft and pins hold the osteotomy open until it heals. A spica cast is used for 6 weeks to protect the graft during healing.

Salter osteotomy requires a second operation to remove the fixation pins. Because the geometric reorientation afforded is limited, there may be residual dysplasia. In addition, failure to achieve a concentric reduction before pelvic osteotomy usually renders the procedure ineffective.

2. Acetabuloplasty, pelvic osteotomy—Most surgeons perform a form of acetabuloplasty, such as a Dega or Pemberton (Figure 12–8), rather than Salter. The indications are similar: a concentrically reducible hip with relative undercoverage. Unlike a redirectional osteotomy (Salter), an acetabuloplasty is particularly suited for correction of the long stretched-out dysplastic acetabulum because it reduces the capacity of an overly spacious acetabulum. This is done by cutting above the acetabular roof, near to the flexible triradiate cartilage (the growth plate of the center of the acetabulum) and redirecting the supra-acetabular segment. The roof fragment is then pried down to a more horizontal position and held in place by wedging a bone graft into the resulting defect. Coverage can be emphasized more posteriorly or anteriorly depending on graft placement.

Rarely, early extrusion or graft collapse occurs, and transient stiffness may be seen in older children. Because there is no internal fixation, a second procedure is unnecessary.

3. Femoral osteotomy—Femoral osteotomy (Figure 12–9) may be used to correct severe increased femoral anteversion or coxa valga (a high neck-shaft angle), conditions that are sometimes seen in residual DDH.

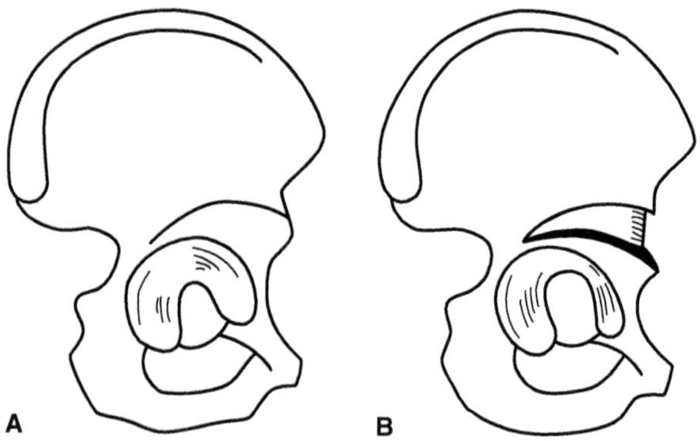

▲ **Figure 12–8.** Pemberton pericapsular iliac osteotomy. An osteotomy cut is made above the acetabulum down to the flexible triradiate cartilage **(A)**. The fragment is pried down to improve acetabular coverage and held with a bone graft **(B)**.

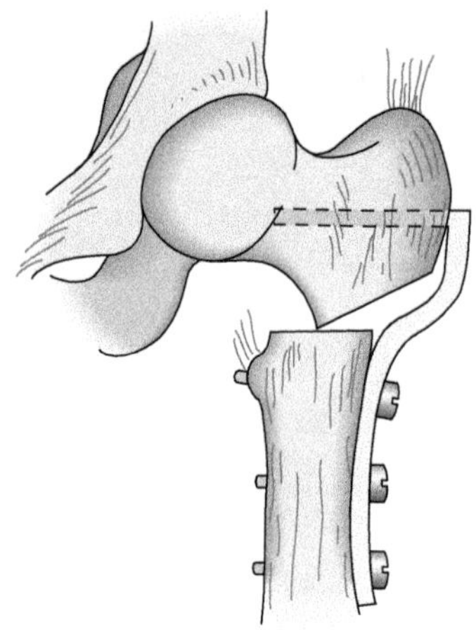

▲ **Figure 12–9.** Femoral osteotomy is performed at the intertrochanteric level and fixed with a plate and screws.

The procedure is particularly indicated when radiographs taken with the hip in abduction and internal rotation show improvement in the overall congruency of the hip. Redirection of an anteverted, valgus hip stimulates spontaneous improvement in dysplastic acetabula in children younger than 4 years.

Femoral osteotomy is performed using a lateral approach, with the cut made across the intertrochanteric region of the femur. This site is chosen both because it is distal to the blood supply of the femoral head and because the cancellous bone heals easily. A metal blade-plate or joint-specific locking plate is placed in the proximal (femoral neck) fragment, usually after positioning with a provisional guidewire. The femoral neck fragment is rotated into a more horizontal position (varus) and is then internally rotated to correct excessive anteversion. The exact degree of correction is determined by preoperative radiograph positioning to achieve maximum congruence and correction of radiographic dysplasia. The plate portion is then clamped to the shaft of the bone and fixed with screws. A spica cast is usually used to supplement fixation.

After healing (6 weeks), the patient may resume walking. A Trendelenburg limp is common for 1 to 2 years after femoral osteotomy because of the geometric distortion of the relationship between the joint and insertion of the abductor muscles. This resolves as the femur remodels with growth and does not present a long-term problem.

4. Late salvage operations—After age 6 to 10 years, reduction and reconstruction of severely dysplastic or dislocated hips may be impossible. If acetabular coverage is poor but the joint is concentric, major reorientation of the acetabulum may be indicated. Salter osteotomy (see earlier discussion) may be inadequate for this degree of reorientation, necessitating the addition of osteotomy cuts in the pubis and ischium to allow more aggressive repositioning of the joint surface (triple innominate osteotomy). Once the triradiate cartilage is closed a periacetabular osteotomy (Bernese or Ganz osteotomy) can be performed in these cases.

For children older than 10 years with hip pain and non-reconstructable joints, Chiari osteotomy reliably improves pain. After a slightly upwardly angled cut is made through the ilium just at the proximal edge of the hip capsule, the hip joint is medially displaced half the width of the iliac cut. After healing, the lateral protruding shelf of the ilium blends with the hip capsule to create a functional equivalent of an augmented hip socket, lined with the smooth capsule, which serves as part of the joint surface.

E. Complications of Surgery for DDH

1. Avascular necrosis of the hip—If a reduction maneuver for DDH was forceful or if there is tension in the soft tissues around the hip, the resulting compression of the joint may cause transient blockage of the blood supply to the femoral head. The subsequent death of the ossific nucleus and proximal growth plate of the femur (avascular necrosis) is a complication of treatment rather than of the disorder itself. A well-recognized cause of avascular necrosis is exaggerated forced abduction in the spica cast used after closed or open reduction. Avascular necrosis may be mild (involving a small fraction of the ossific nucleus), in which case it may go undetected and be of little significance. At the other extreme, avascular necrosis may lead to complete femoral head death and loss of future growth at the proximal physis. As it revascularizes, a dead femoral head may deform significantly, subluxate further, and require abduction bracing or osteotomy. Thus, it can cause leg-length inequality or early osteoarthritis of the hip. The best treatment for avascular necrosis is prevention.

2. Residual dysplasia and degenerative arthritis—No form of treatment uniformly resolves hip dysplasia, and residual dysplasia is common. It may lead to resubluxation or cause failure of remodeling. Older children are more prone to residual problems and may require repeat surgery to help resolve them. Dysplasia is a major cause of premature osteoarthritis of the hip.

Grudziak JS, Ward WT. Dega osteotomy for the treatment of congenital dysplasia of the hip. *J Bone Joint Surg Am.* 2001;83(6):845-854. [PMID: 11407792]

Lehmann HP, Hinton R, Morello P, et al. Developmental dysplasia of the hip practice guideline: technical report. Committee on Quality Improvement, and Subcommittee on Developmental Dysplasia of the Hip. *Pediatrics.* 2000;105:E57. [PMID: 10742378]

Rejholec M. Combined pelvic osteotomy for the bipartite acetabulum in late developmental dysplasia of the hip: a ten-year prospective study. *J Bone Joint Surg Br.* 2011;93:257-261. [PMID: 21282768]

Thomas SRYW. A review of long-term outcomes for late presenting developmental hip dysplasia. *Bone Joint J.* 2015;97-B(6):729-733. [PMID: 26033050]

Walton MJ, Isaacson Z, McMillan D, Hawkes R, Atherton WG. The success of management with the Pavlik harness for developmental dysplasia of the hip using a United Kingdom screening programme and ultrasound-guided supervision. *J Bone Joint Surg Br.* 2010;92:1013-1016. [PMID: 20595124]

Weinstein SL, Mubarak SJ, Wenger DR. Developmental hip dysplasia and dislocation: part II. *Instr Course Lect.* 2004;53:531-542. [PMID: 15116642]

3. Legg-Calvé-Perthes Disease

Essentials of Diagnosis

- *Legg-Calvé-Perthes disease is most common in children age 4 to 8 years and is largely self-healing.*
- *Flexion contracture and loss of abduction are uniform and characteristic.*
- *There may be a small subgroup of patients with Legg-Calvé-Perthes disease who benefit from surgical treatment.*

Legg-Calvé-Perthes disease (LCP; Perthes disease) is a serious but mostly self-limited pediatric hip disorder. Although its cause is unknown, the disease is thought to be related to avascular necrosis of the hip. It affects children between 4 and 10 years of age and is somewhat more common in boys. Children with the disease are often small for their age and have retarded bone age. The disease is generally unilateral. Although bilateral LCP of the hips occurs in about 10% of cases, in patients with symmetric changes/stages, other conditions such as Gaucher disease or multiple epiphyseal dysplasia must be considered. Multiple epiphyseal dysplasia is most readily diagnosed by evaluation of other radiographs, in particular of the knee and, if confirmatory, of the spine to assess for spondyloepiphyseal dysplasia. Patients with multiple epiphyseal dysplasia generally have heights in the fifth percentile or below. Newer investigations suggesting that some cases of LCP might be related to a variety of transient or permanent hypercoagulation states are intriguing but not confirmed in multiple centers. Surprisingly, trauma is not considered a causative factor in LCP.

Although early radiographs may be negative, they eventually show fragmentation, irregularity, and collapse of part or the entire femoral head ossification center (Figure 12–10). The few pathologic specimens that were examined suggest that multiple rather than single episodes of avascular necrosis occur over a period of months. Early bone scans may show a filling defect corresponding to areas of necrosis, and MRI is typical of avascular necrosis. The disease has a characteristic course (see Figure 12–10). Initially, the avascular episodes are silent and the child is asymptomatic. As the disease progresses, the necrotic femoral epiphysis is revascularized. Osteoclasts remove dead bone, while osteoblasts simultaneously lay down new bone on the dead trabeculae (a process known as creeping substitution). During this phase, the femoral head is mechanically weak. Fragmentation and collapse

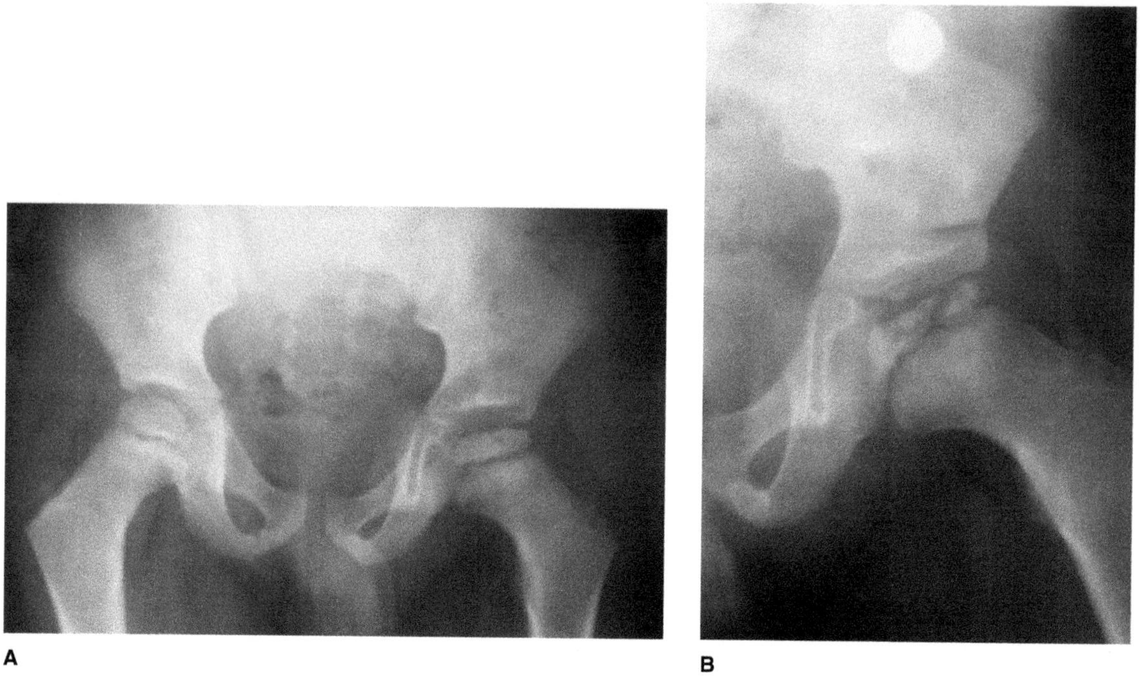

▲ **Figure 12–10.** Legg-Calvé-Perthes disease. **A:** Central necrotic fragment with collapse. **B:** Same patient after healing and partial remodeling.

of the bony structure may then occur, causing geometric flattening and deformity of the ossific nucleus and femoral head. The newly replaced bone takes the shape of the collapsed head. At this point, continued growth may allow gradual remodeling and improvement of the femoral head shape until maturity. The symptomatic collapse phase rarely exceeds 1 to 1.5 years, but full revascularization and remodeling may continue silently for several years thereafter. Although cartilage is not specifically injured by the avascular events, hyperemia can cause articular cartilage thickening, ectopic ossification, and physeal damage that affects femoral neck growth.

Clinical Findings and Classification

A. Symptoms and Signs

The initial presentation of LCP is usually a painless limp, with aching pain in older children. If pain is present, it may be mild and referred to the thigh or knee. Physical examination discloses atrophy of the thigh on the affected side and, usually, limited hip motion. The typical patient has a flexion contracture of 0 to 30 degrees, loss of abduction compared with the opposite side (in severe cases, no abduction beyond 0 degrees), and loss of internal rotation of the hip.

B. Imaging Studies

Radiographs may be negative at first, probably because the initial softening of the femoral head is sufficient to cause symptoms but insufficient to change the radiographic appearance of the femoral head. The eventual characteristic collapse of portions of the femoral head is diagnostic of the disease, however.

The exact extent of necrosis, which is estimated in fourths of the head using the Catterall classification (Figure 12–11), is helpful in determining whom to treat. This may require additional radiographs.

An alternative radiograph classification uses the lateral third of the femoral epiphysis (the so-called lateral pillar). Collapse of this structure suggests a poor prognosis for late deformity (class C), whereas maintenance of pillar height correlates with good long-term results (class A). Partial collapse suggests an intermediate prognosis (class B). The difficulty with all classification systems is their reproducibility and the need to delay until the collapse phase before the exact extent of involvement is clear.

MRI will show changes prior to plain radiograph in early disease. It will also typically demonstrate greater femoral head involvement than what is seen on plain radiography.

Treatment Options

A. No Treatment

Age at presentation and range of motion (ROM) of the hip are the two most significant predictors of long-term outcome. Children with bone age less than 5 years and children

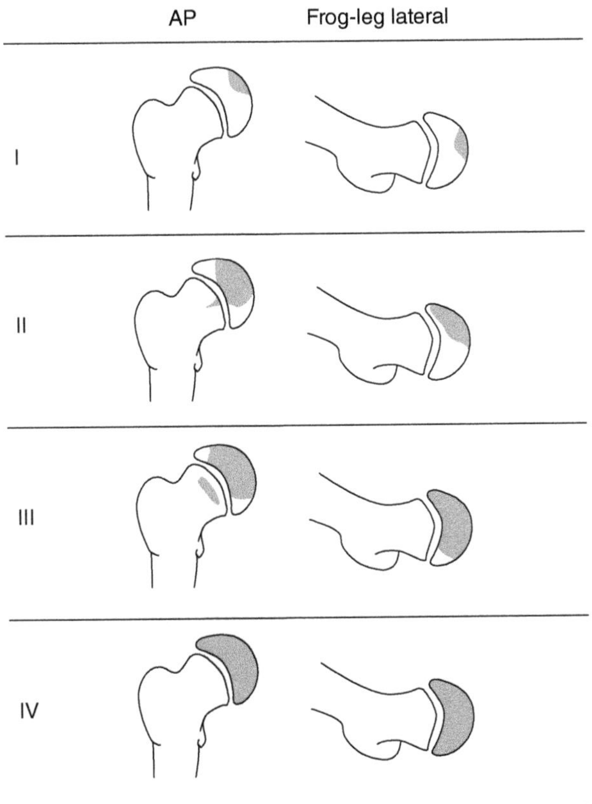

▲ **Figure 12–11.** The Catterall classification is used to determine probable course and prognosis of Legg-Calvé-Perthes disease. It is based on progressive involvement of approximate fourths of the femoral head. AP, anteroposterior.

who exhibit relatively minor involvement (less than half of the femoral head) rarely need treatment. In these children, so much of the femoral head is cartilage, and therefore unaffected by necrosis, that mechanical collapse does not markedly decrease sphericity. Also, younger children have tremendous remodeling potential, and minor collapse can be outgrown before maturity. Limited hip ROM may be due to muscle spasm early on or synovitis; but in late disease, it may reflect incongruity of the joint. Older children who exhibit some radiographic changes but have excellent ROM may require only observation and serial reexamination.

B. Nonoperative and Operative Treatment

The issues surrounding selection of patients with LCP who need treatment are as highly controversial as the treatment itself. Most experts agree that children who maintain excellent motion (particularly abduction greater than 30 degrees in the absence of flexion contracture) may not require intervention. In children older than 4 to 5 years with significant collapse or progressive loss of abduction, treatment is frequently recommended.

No evidence indicates that use of crutches or relief of weight bearing has any effect on femoral head collapse in this disease. For those children requiring it, however, treatment should minimize the effects of collapse and subluxation that often occur when the femoral head deforms. This is best achieved by abduction of the hip until subluxation resolves. The molding action of the acetabular shape is thought to help improve the contour of the collapsing femoral head. Abduction can be accomplished nonoperatively by holding the legs in abduction (Petrie) casts or using an ambulatory brace (Figure 12–12).

Operative procedures are advocated by some and include varus femoral osteotomy and Salter osteotomy, which were adapted from hip dysplasia treatment to control the subluxation seen in some cases of LCP. Healing usually occurs within 18 months. The best current investigations suggest that children over 8 years who have partial head collapse (lateral pillar B-C or Catterall III) may ultimately have better radiographic outcome if treated by surgery.

Despite many studies, there is still no consensus for the best method of treatment; some patients do well without treatment, whereas others have a poor result after aggressive treatment. Prognosis can often be predicted from the knowledge of certain factors (Table 12–5), with age being the most important. Self-reported outcome measures are being applied to this population and may provide better information in the future.

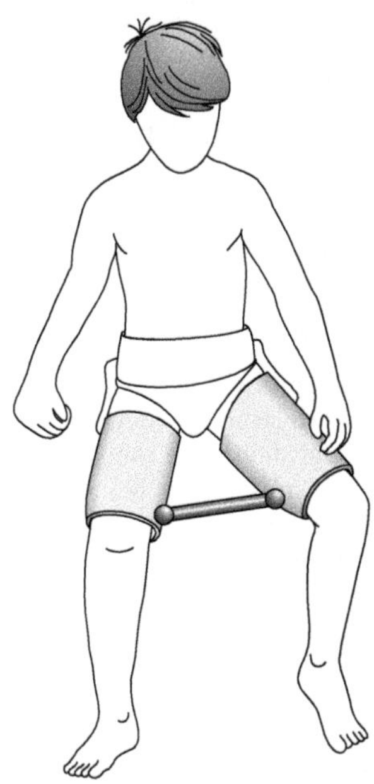

▲ **Figure 12–12.** Abduction bracing is one method used for ambulatory treatment of Legg-Calvé-Perthes disease.

Table 12–5. Factors in long-term prognosis for patients with Legg-Calvé-Perthes disease.

Relative Prognosis	Good	Poor
Age at diagnosis	<5 years	>8-9 years
Hip motion[a]	Maintained (abduction >30 degrees)	Stiff (abduction <15 degrees)
Extent of involvement	<50% of femoral head	>50% or total femoral head
Radiograph features	Little or no subluxation	Subluxation, lateral calcification

[a]During first year of treatment.

Herring JA, Kim HT, Browne R. Legg-Calvé-Perthes disease. Part II: prospective multicenter study of the effect of treatment on outcome. *J Bone Joint Surg Am.* 2004;86(10):2121. [PMID: 15466720]

Karol LA. Legg-Calvé-Perthes disease 100 years on: what have we learned? *J Am Acad Orthop Surg.* 2010;18:643-644. [PMID: 21041798]

Kim HK. Legg-Calvé-Perthes disease. *J Am Acad Orthop Surg.* 2010;18:676-686. [PMID: 21041802]

Matsumoto H, Hyman JE, Shah HH, et al. Validation of pediatric self-reported outcomes measurement information system (PROMIS) measures in different stages of Legg-Calve-Perthes disease. *J Pediatr Orthop.* 2020;40(5):235-240. [PMID: 31318732]

Terjesen T, Wiig O, Svenningsen S. The natural history of Perthes' disease. *Acta Orthop.* 2010;81:708-714. [PMID: 21067434]

4. Slipped Capital Femoral Epiphysis

Essentials of Diagnosis

- *Slipped capital femoral epiphysis is most common in overweight children entering puberty.*
- *Early diagnosis and surgical management give the best results.*

Slipped capital femoral epiphysis is an adolescent hip disorder characterized by displacement of the femoral head on the femoral neck through failure of the proximal femoral physis (growth plate). Displacement changes the geometry of the upper end of the femur and hinders hip function (Figure 12–13). This disorder is one of the main causes of premature osteoarthritis in young adults.

Slipped capital femoral epiphysis affects both male and female adolescents 11 to 13 years of age. In 30% to 40% of patients, the condition is bilateral, although both legs are not always affected simultaneously. The typical patient is overweight—often markedly so—and is in either late prepuberty or early puberty. Rarely, the patient is tall, asthenic, and rapidly growing.

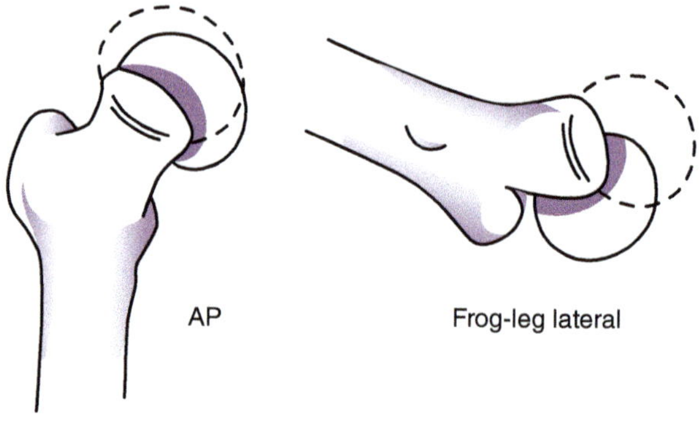

▲ **Figure 12–13.** Anteroposterior (AP) and frog-leg views of a slipped epiphysis. The dotted lines show the normal position of the femoral head.

This disorder occurs at a time when the cartilage physis of the proximal femur is thickening rapidly under the influence of growth hormone. The vigorous secretion of sex hormone has not yet begun, however, the biological effect of sex hormones on closure and stabilization of the growth plate is absent. This combination of thick growth plate cartilage (weaker than bone and subject to shear), lack of sexual maturity (which would stabilize the physis), mechanical stress (caused by obesity), and the peculiar anatomic mechanics of the hip joint renders the growth plate susceptible to slippage.

The direction of the slip is always posterior and often medial, and the mechanical bases of chronic and acute disorders are the same. In chronic slipped capital femoral epiphysis, the most common form (90% of patients), the femoral head slips insidiously at the growth plate over the course of several months. In the acute form, the femoral head is suddenly displaced, a condition that can be superimposed on chronic changes. Displacement may occur during normal activity or following minor trauma.

Because slipped capital femoral epiphysis is a progressive disorder and the prognosis depends on the severity of the slippage, early detection and prompt treatment are imperative.

Clinical Findings

A. Symptoms and Signs

There are two forms of the disorder: chronic and acute. The onset of chronic slipped capital femoral epiphysis is usually insidious, with a history of a painful limp for 1 to several months prior. The pain is characteristically aching and located in the thigh or knee rather than the hip. This referred pain to the knee is responsible for many misdiagnoses. Patients may be seen for knee pain and dismissed as normal after a negative knee examination and radiographs. A high index of suspicion is required to detect slipped capital femoral epiphysis in the obese limping adolescent complaining of knee pain. The change in hip ROM is usually diagnostic: loss of abduction and internal rotation of the hip are evident, although these may be difficult to identify in the grossly overweight child. There is almost always a characteristic obligatory external rotation of the hip when it is flexed because of the distorted hip anatomy caused by the disorder. The femoral head is posterior to its normal position, so the flexed hip must externally rotate to keep the head within the acetabulum.

Acute slipped capital femoral epiphysis is accompanied by severe pain and limping, which may render the patient immobile. The onset is sudden, following little or no trauma, and examination discloses a painful, guarded, restricted range of hip motion. An acute slip is analogous to an epiphyseal fracture. In its unstable form, the patient is unable to bear weight, and there is a high rate of avascular necrosis. In its stable form, the sudden increase in displacement is painful, but limited weight bearing is possible and the risk of avascular necrosis appears to be lower.

B. Imaging Studies

Slipped capital femoral epiphysis can be difficult to detect on standard AP radiographs (Figure 12–14). A frog-leg lateral view is the best for detecting mild forms because slippage is always posterior. A radiograph also shows changes suggesting acute or chronic forms, information that may be critical to management of the disorder.

Establishing the severity of slippage is important in determining treatment and prognosis. Severity is estimated by the percentage of femoral neck left exposed. Slippage of less than 25% of neck width is mild; 25% to 50% is moderate; and more than 50% is severe.

The role of MRI for early detection of slip and to assess vascularity of the epiphysis are areas of interest. CT scan can also be helpful in surgical planning for more complex reconstructions.

Treatment

Slipped capital femoral epiphysis is usually a progressive disease that requires prompt surgical treatment. Because the changes in the chronic form occur so slowly, it is impossible to manipulate the femoral head into a better position. Treatment consists of fixing the slip in its current position and preventing progression. This is done by inserting one or more screws or pins across the growth plate, regardless of the severity of the slip (pinning in situ). Following surgery, aching rapidly resolves, and during the remaining 2 to 3 years of skeletal growth, the extent of remodeling of the distorted proximal femur may be considerable, leading to an improved ROM.

Because of bilateral involvement, some surgeons recommend prophylactic screw fixation of the normal side at the time of initial treatment. This is particularly indicated in children ages 10 years and under.

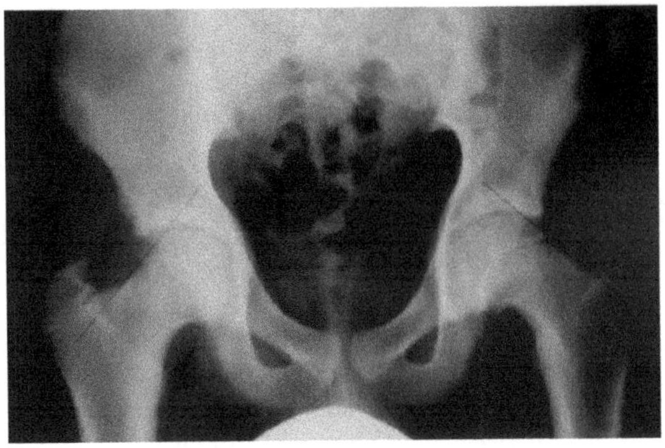

A

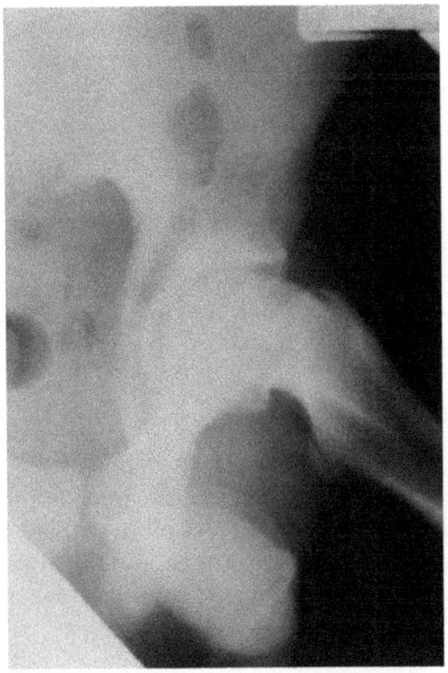

B

▲ **Figure 12–14.** Radiograph diagnosis of left slipped capital femoral epiphysis. **A:** Anteroposterior film shows subtle medial displacement of left epiphysis, best appreciated by drawing a line (Klein line) along the lateral side of the normal and abnormal femoral neck. The slipped epiphysis does not protrude lateral to this line. **B:** Frog-leg lateral radiograph clearly demonstrates posterior displacement.

Acute slips, if unstable, may be gently reduced before fixation, but the risk of further damage to the tenuous blood supply of the proximal femur and subsequent avascular necrosis is always significant. For this reason, many surgeons accept the position of an acute slip and pin it in situ. However, especially in the cases with significant deformity, many centers favor a surgical dislocation of the hip with direct repair including take down of callus (modified Dunn technique). Removing callus that has formed on the slipping femoral neck is hoped to remove an impediment to reduction and decrease the risk of further damage to the blood supply of the femoral head.

Complications

A. Femoral Acetabular Impingement

In situ fixation often leaves deformity of the femoral head that does not remodel. This has been termed a "pistol-grip" deformity, and it results in altered hip biomechanics. The cam shape or prominent anterolateral metaphyseal area abuts against the acetabulum. Symptoms can include pain and altered ROM and can lead to joint deterioration.

Treatment for this has been realignment through osteotomy. Osteotomies have been described as through the femoral neck (Dunn or Fish), basicervical, or intertrochanteric (Imhauser, Southwick). The osteotomy site may be at the level of the slip, which is mechanically effective but relatively risky for the blood supply. Alternatively, osteotomy can be performed at the trochanteric level; this is a safer procedure for correction of the functional deformity but does not resolve the exact anatomic deformity.

Surgical hip dislocation can also supplement an osteotomy with the opportunity to directly reshape the femoral head by performing an osteoplasty.

B. Chondrolysis

In addition to the problems of impingement of the anterior metaphyseal prominence, which can impede motion, patients with slipped capital femoral epiphysis may rarely develop chondrolysis, a poorly understood degeneration of the hip articular cartilage. It may be painful and may progress to severe joint narrowing and degenerative changes within 6 months.

During chondrolysis, cartilage is replaced by fibrous tissue, the joint capsule thickens and contracts, and joint motion is lost. Typically, the joint stiffens in flexion, abduction, and external rotation. Radiographs reveal joint narrowing, irregularity, and subchondral sclerosis, as well as regional osteoporosis from disuse.

Chondrolysis can result from iatrogenic malposition (permanent penetration) of pins or screws used for fixation of slipped capital femoral epiphysis. Although brief penetrations during surgery are probably common and cause no complications, unrecognized permanent pin penetration is disastrous. Chondrolysis also appears without obvious penetration and occasionally is detected in patients before treatment begins.

Chondrolysis is treated by nonsteroidal anti-inflammatory drugs (NSAIDs), aggressive physical therapy and ROM exercises, and observation. Capsular release is sometimes useful in resistant cases. Approximately half of patients eventually recover satisfactory painless motion. The other half may require hip fusion for symptomatic relief.

C. Avascular Necrosis

Patients with an acutely slipped capital femoral epiphysis can develop avascular necrosis of the femoral head (see section on developmental dysplasia of the hip). These patients are usually teenagers so their hips lack potential for remodeling, and the prognosis is therefore poor. Yet, some patients with partial head involvement regain a painless hip after 1 to 2 years of symptoms. Some patients with painless but abnormal ROM may be treatable by intertrochanteric osteotomy to reorient the arc of motion. Long-term pain following avascular necrosis is treated by hip fusion.

Prognosis

Slipped epiphysis is a major cause of early osteoarthritis. In general, the higher the degree of slip, the earlier the degenerative changes begin. In fact, a statistical increase in degenerative arthritis is evident even in the radiographically normal hip of patients with a contralateral slipped epiphysis. This suggests that subclinical bilateral involvement is more common than recognized.

Loder RT, Greenfield ML. Clinical characteristics of children with atypical and idiopathic slipped capital femoral epiphysis: description of the age-weight test and implications for further diagnostic investigation. *J Pediatr Orthop.* 2001;21:481-487. [PMID: 11433161]

Peck D. Slipped capital femoral epiphysis: diagnosis and management. *Am Fam Physician.* 2010;82:258-262. [PMID: 20672790]

Sankar WN, McPartland TG, Millis MB, Kim YJ. The unstable slipped capital femoral epiphysis: risk factors for osteonecrosis. *J Pediatr Orthop.* 2010;30:544-548. [PMID: 20733417]

Sankar WN, Vanderhave KL, Matheney T, Herrera-Soto JA, Karlen JW. The modified Dunn procedure for unstable slipped capital femoral epiphysis: a multicenter perspective. *J Bone Joint Surg Am.* 2013;95(7):585-591. [PMID: 23553292]

Ziebarth K, Zilkens C, Spencer S, Leunig M, Ganz R, Kim YJ. Capital realignment for moderate and severe SCFE using a modified Dunn procedure. *Clin Orthop Relat Res.* 2009;467(3):704-716. [PMID: 19142692]

FOOT DISORDERS

1. Metatarsus Adductus

Metatarsus adductus (metatarsus varus) is the most common foot deformity in the newborn infant, occurring in 5 in 1000 live births, frequently bilaterally. Although it is usually isolated, several apparently unrelated deformities (such as DDH) are statistically more likely to occur in the presence of this disorder. The cause is unknown but might be related to so-called uterine packing.

Clinical Findings

The hallmark of metatarsus adductus is medial deviation of the forefoot, with the apex of the deformity at the midtarsal region. The hindfoot is normal. A deep skin crease frequently is evident at the medial border of the foot, suggesting the deformity has been present for some time. The adducted forefoot usually can be passively corrected to a neutral position but occasionally is fairly rigid. Ankle motion is normal, without contracture of the gastrocnemius-soleus muscles. This normal dorsiflexion helps differentiate metatarsus adductus from more serious deformity.

Treatment

Metatarsus adductus tends to be self-correcting. Even severe cases generally resolve by 12 to 18 months of age without treatment. Nevertheless, many orthopedists use passive stretching to reassure parents the child is being treated. There is no scientific evidence that passive correction and serial plaster casting will speed resolution of the disorder.

2. Congenital Clubfoot

Essentials of Diagnosis

- *Clubfoot is characterized by equinovarus, midfoot supination, and forefoot adductus. Smaller foot size, smaller calf muscles, and decreased ankle dorsiflexion are common.*
- *Treatment with casting and minor surgical tenotomy is usually successful but technique dependent. The most common technique is based on Dr. Ignacio Ponseti's teaching.*
- *Bracing for 1 to 4 years after cast correction improves the ultimate outcome.*

Congenital clubfoot (equinovarus foot; talipes equinovarus) is a severe fixed deformity of the foot (Figure 12–15). It is characterized by fixed ankle plantar flexion (equinus), inversion and axial internal rotation of the subtalar (talocalcaneal) joint (varus), and medial subluxation of the talonavicular and calcaneocuboid joints (adductus). Severe cavus may be present, with a medial and plantar midfoot crease. Calf atrophy, while variable, is always present.

The incidence in the newborn population is 1 in 1000, with increased risk for families in which even distant members have the deformity. There is considerable evidence that clubfoot is an inherited trait, but the disorder appears to reflect polygenetic expression, and exact inheritance patterns are unclear. Although most are isolated deformities and considered idiopathic, clubfoot may be present in association with a wide variety of syndromes that affect the musculoskeletal system, such as arthrogryposis or myelomeningocele.

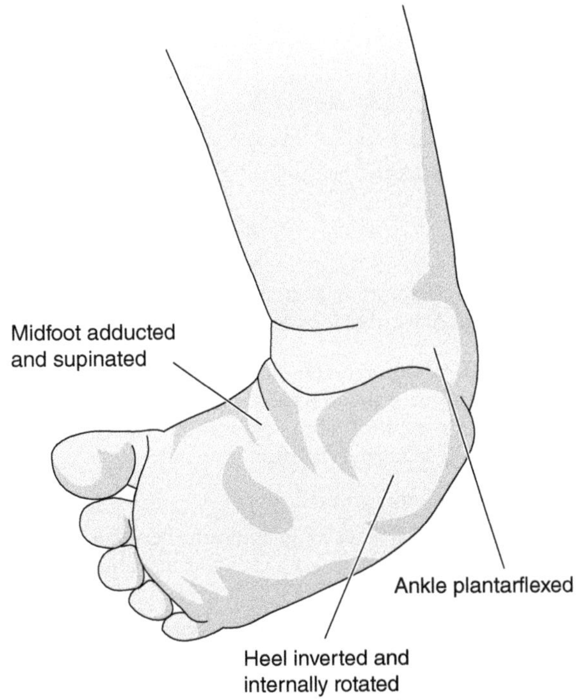

▲ **Figure 12–15.** Clinical appearance of congenital right clubfoot.

Clinical Findings

A. Symptoms and Signs

Clinical diagnosis of clubfoot is straightforward. Because it is a rigid deformity, clubfoot cannot be passively corrected the way metatarsus adductus can. Frequently, the foot is so severely internally rotated and inverted that the sole faces superiorly. Occasionally, the plantar flexion of the ankle is not obvious because the posterior tip of the calcaneus is small, high, and difficult to palpate. Clubfoot is associated with a permanent decrease in calf circumference related to fibrosis of the calf musculature. This may not be obvious at birth but becomes more apparent after the child begins to walk.

Special attention should be paid to the presence of spine deformity, caudal dimpling, or midline spinal hairy patches, all of which may imply a neurogenic component. Thus, the examining physician should carefully search for features of other deformities or syndromes.

B. Imaging Studies

Increasingly, clubfoot is suspected from prenatal ultrasound examination. Radiographs are rarely of value in the initial clubfoot evaluation because the bones of the foot are minimally ossified at birth. Radiographs become more important if the physician is considering surgical intervention or if the

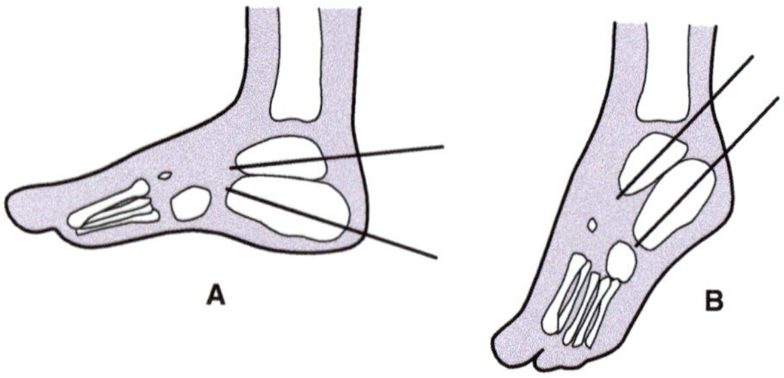

▲ **Figure 12–16.** Diagrammatic appearance of radiograph in clubfoot. **A:** Normal foot. **B:** Clubfoot.

child has reached walking age, and radiographs can quantify the completeness of correction achieved by casting or surgery.

The typical radiographic findings of incompletely treated clubfoot include the following features:

1. Presence of hindfoot plantar flexion
2. Lack of the normal angular relationship between the talus and calcaneus (so-called parallelism of talus and calcaneus)
3. Residual medial or dorsal subluxation of the navicular on the talus and the cuboid on the calcaneus (Figure 12–16)

Treatment

A. Manipulative Treatment

Clubfoot always requires treatment, which should begin at birth. The initial approach is passive manipulation and positioning to the corrected position. In the United States, the majority of orthopedists use serial manipulation and casting, usually at 1-week intervals in the first month of life, and at 1- to 2-week intervals thereafter if required. In other parts of the world, strapping (with adhesive tape) and splinting with a variety of braces are popular methods (in addition to serial casting) for maintaining the manipulated correction. When casting is performed, there is agreement that specific techniques are more likely to be successful. Even when the deformity responds to casting, there is usually sufficient Achilles tightness that a heel cord lengthening needs to be done once the other components of the deformity have been corrected.

The Ponseti method of casting has been widely adopted in many parts of the world as an effective cast protocol. In this method, a specific sequence of casts is applied weekly for 3 to 5 weeks, followed by early percutaneous Achilles tenotomy. After a brief additional period of casting, the foot position is maintained by use of a brace for up to 3 years, worn at nights and during naps.

B. Management of Relapse

Although the Ponseti technique is effective to correct of deformity in over 90% of cases, relapses are a common problem. Most relapses of deformity occur when a child is young, especially if abduction bracing protocols are not adhered to. Failure to tolerate or comply with bracing has been seen in as many as 40% of patients.

Relapses can be managed by restarting serial casting and reintroduction of abduction bracing. In most cases, bracing tolerance does not improve, so alternative strategies are needed. Anterior tibialis tendon transfer can be done to rebalance one of the major deforming forces causing relapse of clubfoot deformity. Often, a repeat Achilles lengthening or limited posterior release is added.

C. Surgical Treatment

Most clubfeet are successfully treated with casting and limited release, but severe clubfeet (often associated with syndromes) may require more extensive surgery. Surgical correction of all clubfoot deformities is generally performed in one stage. At times, the casting corrects most of the midfoot deformity, and simple posterior release (ankle capsulotomy and Achilles tendon lengthening) are all that is required. Frequently, the surgeon must consider correction of the entire group of deformities through a comprehensive, extensive surgical approach.

One common approach uses the so-called Cincinnati incision, which extends from the navicular bone medially, around the superior portion of the heel, to the cuboid bone laterally (Figure 12–17). During surgery, the medial posterior tibial neurovascular bundle must be identified and protected. The tendons of the posterior tibialis, flexor digitorum longus, flexor hallucis longus, and Achilles tendon are Z-lengthened. The capsules of the talonavicular joint, subtalar (talocalcaneal) joint, and posterior ankle joint are

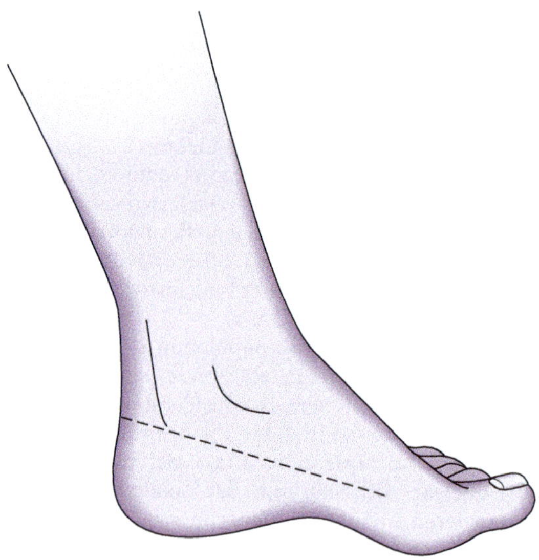

▲ **Figure 12–17.** Cincinnati incision used for surgical correction of clubfoot.

released to allow repositioning of the bones of the hindfoot and midfoot.

The navicular is usually subluxated medially on the head of the talus and must be repositioned onto its normal location. The calcaneus is both inverted and internally rotated on the talus. This is corrected by manually derotating the subtalar joint and tilting the calcaneus back into a neutral position. These corrections are usually held in place after reduction by inserting small K-wires, which are removed after 4 to 6 weeks.

The ankle is repositioned by dorsiflexion to neutral prior to repair of the lengthened Achilles tendon. Postoperative casting allows the gaping capsule to re-form with the bones of the clubfoot in their appropriate, corrected position.

D. Complications

Early complications of clubfoot surgery are rare, but the rate of recurrence within 3 years is 5% to 10%. Mild recurrence of deformity is fairly common, and even when deformity is permanently corrected, the foot always remains smaller and stiffer than normal and calf circumference is reduced. Families must be informed of this possibility early in treatment so they have realistic expectations about the outcome.

If surgical release is too aggressive, overcorrection with late heel valgus and an overlengthened heel cord can occur. There is broad agreement that a slightly underreleased clubfoot is much more functional than an overreleased one, and the trend to less surgery and more conservative treatment is currently strong.

Avilucea FR, Szalay EA, Bosch PP, Sweet KR, Schwend RM. Effect of cultural factors on outcome of Ponseti treatment of clubfeet in rural America. *J Bone Joint Surg Am.* 2009;91(3):530-540. [PMID: 19255212]

Dobbs MB, Morcuende JA, Gurnett CA, et al. Treatment of idiopathic clubfoot: an historical review. *Iowa Orthop J.* 2000;20: 59-64. [PMID: 10934626]

Herzenberg JE, Radler C, Bor N. Ponseti versus traditional methods of casting for idiopathic clubfoot. *J Pediatr Orthop.* 2002;22:517-521. [PMID: 12131451]

Matos MA, de Oliveira LA. Comparison between Ponseti's and Kite's clubfoot treatment methods: a meta-analysis. *J Foot Ankle Surg.* 2010;49:395-397. [PMID: 20610205]

Richards BS, Faulks S, Rathjen KE, Karol LA, Johnston CE, Jones SA. A comparison of two nonoperative methods of idiopathic clubfoot correction: the Ponseti method and the French functional (physiotherapy) method. *J Bone Joint Surg Am.* 2008;90:2313-2321. [PMID: 18978399]

Zionts LE, Dietz FR. Bracing following correction of idiopathic clubfoot using the Ponseti method. *J Am Acad Orthop Surg.* 2010;18:486-493. [PMID: 20675641]

Zionts LE, Zhao G, Hitchcock K, Maewal J, Ebramzadeh E. Has the rate of extensive surgery to treat idiopathic clubfoot declined in the United States? *J Bone Joint Surg Am.* 2010;92:882-889. [PMID: 20360511]

3. Calcaneovalgus Foot

Calcaneovalgus foot is generally considered a uterine-packing problem in which the foot is markedly dorsiflexed at birth so the dorsum of the foot sits against the anterior surface of the tibia (Figure 12–18). The hindfoot is usually in moderate eversion (valgus) as well. Although some flexibility is present with the deformity, there is resistance to full motion, and most cases do not allow ankle plantar flexion beyond a right angle.

Despite its dramatic appearance, calcaneovalgus foot corrects spontaneously within 2 to 3 months. Although some orthopedists brace or apply serial casts and many recommend stretching exercises, all true calcaneovalgus feet resolve without treatment.

Congenital Vertical Talus

Calcaneovalgus foot must be differentiated from a much rarer condition known as congenital vertical talus (congenital rocker-bottom foot, congenital complex pes valgus). In this deformity, although the foot appears to lie against the anterior tibia, the hindfoot is actually plantar flexed (positioned in equinus) because of contracture of the posterior calf muscles. To accommodate plantarflexion of the hindfoot and dorsiflexion of the forefoot, the midfoot joints (talonavicular and calcaneocuboid joints) must subluxate or dislocate dorsally.

Congenital vertical talus often accompanies genetic disorders, syndromes such as arthrogryposis, or neuromuscular disorders such as spina bifida. It is occasionally found in otherwise normal infants, however. Treatment is usually surgical, and casting frequently does not resolve the disorder.

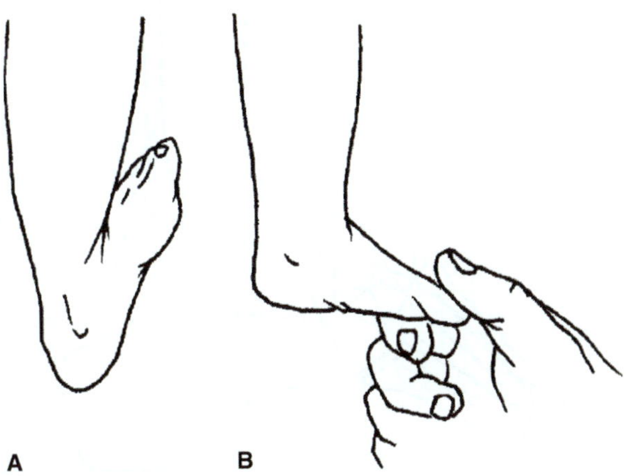

▲ **Figure 12–18.** Calcaneovalgus foot as it appears in relaxed position **(A)** and maximally plantar flexed **(B)**.

4. Cavus Foot

Cavus foot is a foot with an abnormally high arch. Although it is difficult to ascribe a particular threshold of arching beyond which treatment is necessary, most deformities are dramatic enough to make diagnosis straightforward (Figure 12–19).

Cavus foot frequently accompanies hindfoot varus deformity (cavovarus foot), and there may be clawing of the toes and demonstrable weakness of ankle or foot muscles. In addition, calluses beneath the metatarsal heads and heel skin are common. Hindfoot varus in individuals with a cavovarus deformity is nonstructural if it can be corrected with the "block test," and surgical procedures directed at correcting the hindfoot deformity are not necessary. If the patient is symptomatic, the treatment of choice is plantar release with first metatarsal osteotomy and possible tendon transfers.

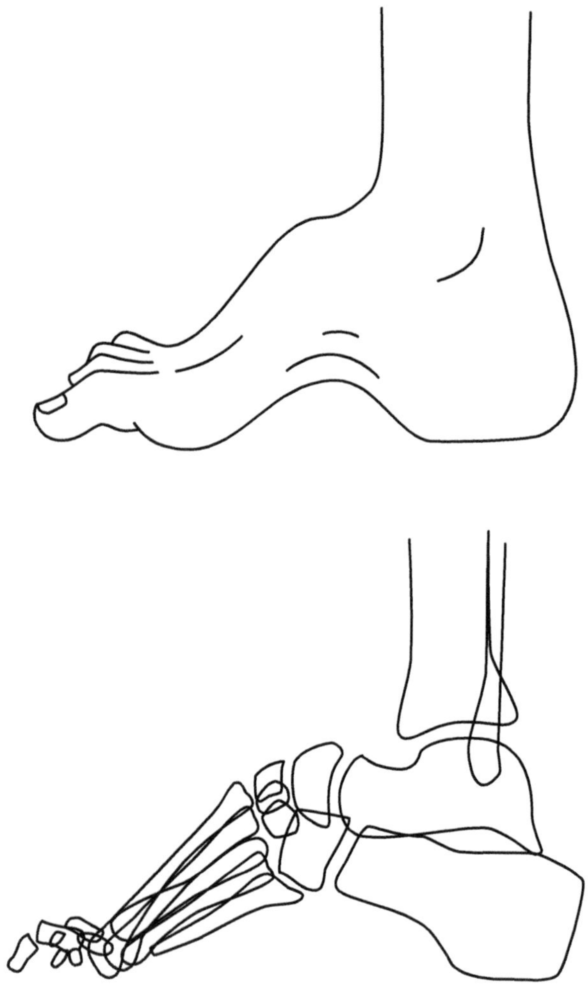

▲ **Figure 12–19.** Cavus foot: clinical appearance and radiographic appearance.

Clinical Findings

One of the most common symptoms of cavus foot is anterior ankle pain, sometimes associated with toe walking. This paradoxical situation occurs because of the pathologic anatomy of the cavus foot. The forefoot is severely plantar flexed on the hindfoot, requiring marked ankle dorsiflexion to compensate. When the cavus becomes too severe, ankle dorsiflexion is blocked, leading to anterior ankle impingement and pain. The inability to dorsiflex further compromises forefoot clearance, and eventually, only the metatarsals can contact the floor. This can be misinterpreted as ankle plantarflexion contracture, leading to unnecessary (and possibly harmful) heel cord release.

Pathogenesis

The cause of cavus foot is usually muscle imbalance in a growing foot. Thus, cavus is rarely found in early childhood but is fairly frequent after 8 to 10 years of age. Although intrinsic muscle weakness is a major cause of cavus foot, weakness of the peroneal or anterior tibialis muscles is also implicated. Cavus foot is rarely found in the absence of an underlying neuromuscular condition.

Cavus foot is a marker for neuromuscular disease. Diagnosis requires a thorough search for the underlying cause and may require neurologic consultation, spinal MRI, and electromyographic (EMG) studies. Table 12–6 lists common neuromuscular causes of cavus foot.

Treatment

Conservative treatment of cavus foot includes accommodation by shoe modifications or inserts. These modalities do not actually correct the condition; severe deformity requires surgical correction by tendon transfers to restore muscle balance, by midfoot wedge osteotomy to correct bony deformity, or by triple arthrodesis (hindfoot fusion in a corrected position).

Schwend RM, Drennan JC. Cavus foot deformity in children. *J Am Acad Orthop Surg.* 2003;11:201-211. [PMID: 12828450]

5. Pes Planus (Flatfoot)

Flatfoot refers to loss of the normal longitudinal arch of the medial foot. Many cases of flatfoot are inherited, and a careful family history may uncover other persons with the condition. The foot is usually flexible, so the arch appears when the foot is not bearing weight. Hindfoot valgus (heel eversion) is often present. In severe cases, flatfoot may be painful, but this aspect of the deformity is often overemphasized.

Clinical Findings

Physical determination of the flexibility of the flatfoot requires careful examination. Subtalar motion is usually normal. In

Table 12–6. Common neuromuscular causes of cavus foot.

Cerebral palsy
Charcot-Marie-Tooth disease
Compartment syndrome
Diastematomyelia
Friedrich ataxia
Muscular dystrophy
Spinal cord tumor
Spinal dysraphism (spina bifida)

feet that exhibit a flat arch and valgus heel while standing, examination from the posterior aspect frequently discloses a normal arch and varus heel by muscle action when the patient stands on tiptoe. If these signs of a flexible flatfoot are not present, alternative diagnoses such as tarsal coalition (see section on tarsal coalition) should be considered. The physician should also look for painful plantar calluses.

Imaging Studies

Standing radiographs disclose loss of the normal medial longitudinal arch and may show mild lateral subluxation of the talonavicular joint as well. In severe chronic cases, degenerative talonavicular spurring may be present.

Treatment

Symptomatic treatment (shoe modifications, arch supports, and plantar inserts) is appropriate because no long-term treatment can alter the anatomic features of the disorder. Posterior tibial advancement, subtalar joint elevation or fusion, and elongation osteotomy of the lateral calcaneal neck are surgical options, but they may not provide reproducible, predictable resolution of the problem.

6. Tarsal Coalition

Tarsal coalition is a congenital connection between two or more tarsal bones. Coalitions may be fibrous, cartilaginous, or bony. Coalitions usually occur between two bones and are cartilaginous in early life but eventually ossify (or nearly ossify) as the foot matures. Frequently bilateral, coalitions often follow an autosomal dominant inheritance pattern.

The most common sites for tarsal coalition are between the calcaneus and the navicular laterally (Figure 12–20) and between the talus and the calcaneus medially.

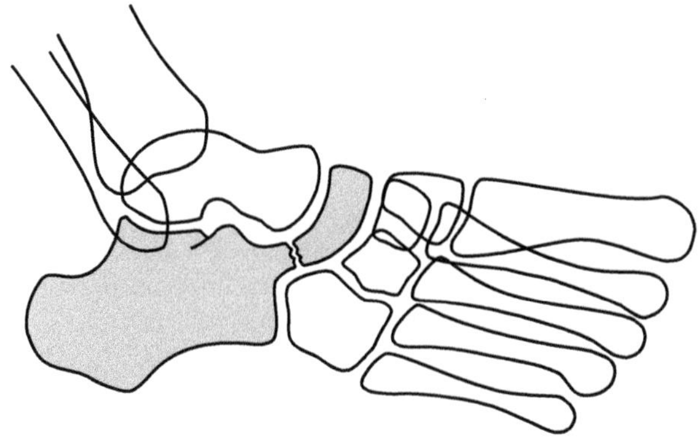

▲ **Figure 12–20.** Calcaneonavicular tarsal coalition is best seen on oblique radiograph projection.

Clinical Findings

Symptoms of tarsal coalition may include foot pain and stiffness as the lesion begins to ossify during early adolescence. The resulting stiffness and abnormal intertarsal movement patterns in the hindfoot lead to progressive loss of subtalar motion and fixed valgus (eversion) of the heel. Tarsal coalition is often called peroneal spastic flatfoot because the peroneals appear to be protectively overactive. As the lesion matures, pain may diminish but stiffness increases, and the abnormal valgus posture persists. These patients commonly cannot walk on the lateral border of the involved foot.

This diagnosis should be suspected in adolescents with foot pain, valgus heel, and decreased subtalar motion.

Imaging Studies

Lateral, AP, and oblique radiographs of the foot confirm the diagnosis of calcaneonavicular coalition, but special subtalar radiographs (Harris views), CT scan, or MRI may be necessary to delineate medial talocalcaneal lesions.

Treatment

Not all coalitions require treatment. The decision to initiate treatment depends on the severity of pain, stiffness, and fixed valgus deformity. Conservative treatment consists of casting to reduce pain and peroneal spasm. If this fails, the coalition can be surgically resected and the resultant space filled with autologous fat or muscle to prevent recurrence. In late or neglected cases with pain or deformity, hindfoot fusion by triple arthrodesis is effective treatment for both symptoms.

Bauer K, Mosca VS, Zionts LE. What's new in pediatric flatfoot? *J Pediatr Orthop*. 2016;36(8):865-869. [PMID: 26296215]

Sankar WN, Weiss J, Skaggs DL. Orthopaedic conditions in the newborn. *J Am Acad Orthop Surg*. 2009;17:112-122. [PMID: 19202124]

Yeagerman SE, Cross MB, Positano R, Doyle SM. Evaluation and treatment of symptomatic pes planus. *Curr Opin Pediatr.* 2011;23:60-67. [PMID: 21169838]

7. Toe Deformities

Toe deformities occur as isolated conditions, in association with similar hand deformities, and as part of other syndromes. The more commonly found deformities are presented here, with mention of associated hand problems.

Simple Syndactyly

Simple syndactyly, a connection of two or more toes, is the most common toe deformity. It is most common between the second and third toes. The webbing is usually complete. This disorder demonstrates a strongly familial inheritance pattern and causes no symptoms. It is rarely treated in the foot. In the hand, however, surgical separation is required to restore normal finger function.

Polydactyly

Polydactyly is the presence of more than five digits on either the hands or the feet. It is frequently hereditary and often bilateral. Duplication of the thumbs may mirror duplication of the great toes, and both generally require surgical treatment. Both preaxial (duplication of medial toes and radial digits) and postaxial polydactyly (duplication of the lateral toes or ulnar digits) often accompany genetic syndromes and should prompt the physician to look for other symptoms. Treatment is by surgical excision at about 1 year of age; the actual surgery, particularly for medial duplications, may be complex.

8. Constriction Bands (Amniotic Bands) and Acrosyndactyly

During gestation, protein-laden amniotic material can condense around limb segments. These amniotic bands may indent delicate embryonic tissues, causing constriction rings or even necrosis and resorption of the distal segment (congenital amputation). Constriction bands may be isolated or associated with Streeter dysplasia. The syndactyly of Streeter dysplasia differs from simple syndactyly in that the distal, rather than proximal, web is obliterated (acrosyndactyly). It is thought to be an acquired, rather than hereditary, condition, caused by shearing of the delicate tips of the embryonic digits, followed by conjoined healing of distal digits. Although acrosyndactyly of the fingers must be released to allow independent function, acrosyndactyly of the toes is rarely symptomatic and does not need treatment.

Constriction bands may be very deep and circumferential and occasionally must be released surgically by Z-plasty immediately after birth to avoid postnatal necrosis. Usually, only half of the circumference of a band is released at one time, to protect any remaining blood supply in the other half. Reports of successful one-stage resection and Z-plasty of constriction bands suggest that the remaining blood supply is probably subfascial and interosseous.

9. Adolescent Bunions (Hallux Valgus)

Although bunion (prominence of the medial metatarsophalangeal joint of the great toe) is rare in children, this troublesome deformity often requires treatment. It is frequently hereditary, usually seen in early adolescence, and almost always found in conjunction with a wide forefoot caused by varus (medial deviation) of the first metatarsal shaft (metatarsus primus varus). The wide forefoot allows severe lateral deviation of the great toe (hallux valgus), causing the prominent base of the great toe to rub against the inside of the shoe and create a painful bunion (Figure 12–21).

Although conservative measures may relieve discomfort, many adolescent bunions are progressive and require surgical management. Surgery must address each aspect of the deformity. The surgeon must trim the bunion, correct the varus angulation of the first metatarsal by osteotomy, and centralize and balance the hallux valgus by lengthening the adductor hallucis muscle. There is a fairly high incidence of recurrence of the deformity following surgery.

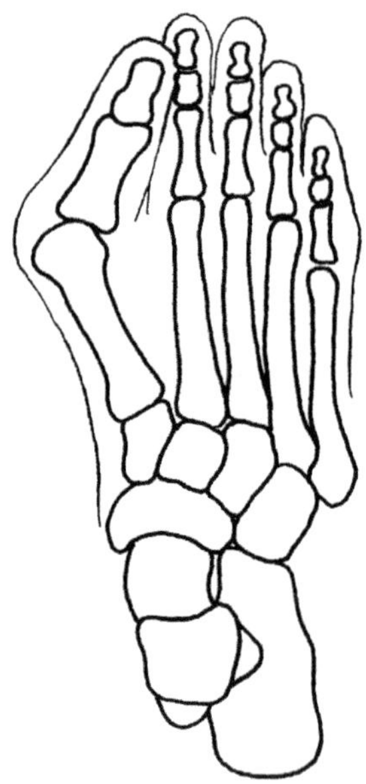

▲ **Figure 12–21.** Adolescent bunion (hallux valgus) is generally accompanied by a wide forefoot with splaying of the first metatarsal (metatarsus primus varus).

Johnson AE, Georgopoulos G, Erickson MA, et al. Treatment of adolescent hallux valgus with the first metatarsal double osteotomy: the Denver experience. *J Pediatr Orthop*. 2004;24: 358-362. [PMID: 15205615]

TORSIONAL AND ANGULAR DEFORMITIES OF THE KNEE AND LEG

Essentials of Diagnosis

- *Most torsional deformities are benign and self-correcting with growth.*
- *Angular deformities at the knee, particularly genu varum, must be distinguished from more common physiologic variants, since they often need early treatment.*

Torsional (rotational) and angular deformities are a major source of referrals to pediatric orthopedic surgeons (Figure 12–22). Most of these patients are young (<5 years) and have internal rotational deformities resulting in a so-called pigeon-toed gait.

The internal rotation, which can occur at the level of the thigh, leg (shin), or foot, is a cosmetic problem. Little evidence indicates that any of the so-called torsional deformities are harmful to the child or cause significant disability in the adult. Angular deformities (usually varus or valgus at the knee) are also usually benign, although careful evaluation and workup, including radiographic or other imaging modalities, occasionally disclose conditions requiring treatment. Nevertheless, most torsional and angular deformities are physiologic variations of normal anatomy, and they correct spontaneously over time.

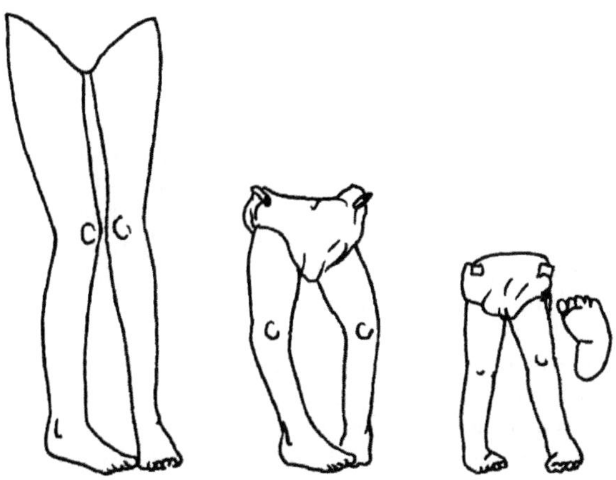

▲ **Figure 12–22.** The major causes of clinical in-toeing include increased femoral anteversion **(A)**, internal tibial torsion **(B)**, and metatarsus adductus **(C)**.

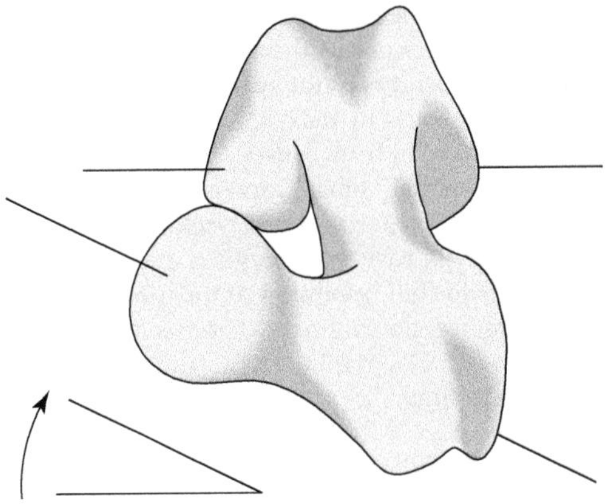

▲ **Figure 12–23.** The angle of anteversion describes the inclination of the femoral neck forward of (anterior to) the frontal plane.

Increased Femoral Anteversion

The normal femoral neck does not lie exactly in the frontal (coronal) plane but rather projects anteriorly from the plane at an angle called the angle of anteversion (Figure 12–23). Infants have anteversion of as much as 40 degrees, but this angle gradually reduces with growth, so normal adult femurs exhibit anteversion of 15 degrees. In some children, this gradual regression is slow or incomplete, causing the child to have excessive anteversion compared with an average child of the same age. This excessive anteversion produces a relative increase in internal femoral rotation, since the hip joint seeks to center itself regardless of the rotational profile of the femur. The clinical manifestation of this increased internal rotation and decreased external rotation of the hip is in-toeing during walking.

Observation of the walking child discloses internal rotation of the entire femur by the medial position of the patella. Although parents may consider this pigeon-toed gait unsightly, increased femoral anteversion is a normal variant that has no effect on function.

Increased femoral anteversion gradually decreases, with improvement in in-toeing, until 9 to 11 years of age. Subsequently, persistent in-toeing in the adult becomes more likely. Increased femoral anteversion requires no treatment.

Internal Tibial Torsion

Some infants are born with a relatively dramatic internal twisting (torsion) of the tibia that makes the foot and ankle appear markedly rotated inward, relative to the axis of the knee. This internal tibial torsion is usually bilateral, frequently familial, and inevitably a normal variant in the wide torsional range seen in infants.

Internal tibial torsion can be clinically measured by comparing the bimalleolar axis (imaginary line connecting the medial and lateral malleoli of the ankle) with the frontal plane of the knee as determined by the position of the patella.

Torsion of 30 to 40 degrees is not uncommon in the newborn. When the child starts to walk, torsion can cause significant in-toeing, which, in turn, causes excessive tripping.

With growth, internal tibial torsion spontaneously resolves, and normal foot position and walking eventually occur. Some children improve by 24 months of age but may require up to 4 years for full resolution of the torsion. Internal tibial torsion requires no treatment. There is no scientific evidence that braces or shoe modifications alter the natural correction of the deformity.

Metatarsus Adductus

Metatarsus adductus may cause apparent in-toeing in the young child, leading to its inclusion as a torsional deformity. It is described in the previous section on the foot (Table 12–7).

Staheli LT, Corbett M, Wyss C, King H. Lower-extremity rotational problems in children. Normal values to guide management. *J Bone Joint Surg Am.* 1985;67:39-47. [PMID: 3968103]

Bowlegs, Knock-Knee, and Genu Varum

Many infants have bilateral symmetric bowing of the legs, which may persist in the first 1 to 2 years of walking before developing into an exaggerated knock-kneed condition. The knock-knee is most dramatic at 3 to 6 years of age when it is known as physiologic genu valgum. At this time, the anatomic angle may be as high as 15 to 20 degrees of valgus. The genu valgum then gradually remodels spontaneously to the adult average value of 5 to 7 degrees of valgus.

Bowing of the legs in infants and excessive valgus of the knees in children 6 years of age are normal phenomena that require no treatment, although parents may have to be reassured that the condition is benign. The rare case of bowing that persists beyond 3 years of age may require further evaluation or treatment. Following are disorders that cause bowing.

Table 12–7. In-toeing summary.

	Metatarsus Adductus	Internal Tibial Torsion	Internal Femoral Torsion (Increased Femoral Anteversion)
Age at resolution	12 months	3-4 years	9-10 years
Leg position	Femur and tibia normal	Patella forward; foot/ankle internally rotated	Patella internally rotated
Hip examination	Normal	Normal	Internal rotation exceeds external rotation

A. Internal Tibial Torsion

Internal tibial torsion may masquerade as bowing when the child walks with the feet forward and the knees rotated externally rather than internally. As the laterally facing knees flex, they give the appearance of bowlegs. Careful physical examination discloses internal tibial torsion, which spontaneously resolves by 4 years of age. As the torsion corrects, the apparent bowlegs disappear.

B. Blount Disease

Also known as tibia vara, Blount disease is a poorly understood loss of medial tibial physeal growth that causes progressive bowing of the leg (Figure 12–24). It may occur as early as 3 years of age and can be bilateral or unilateral. If unilateral, the condition may be suspected earlier because it is obvious by comparison with the other leg. Excessive loading of the knee by early walking in heavy children with physiologic bowing of the legs may contribute to the development of Blount disease, but this is not proven. It occurs in all racial groups but is particularly common in black and Hispanic children.

Diagnosis of Blount disease is based on radiographic evidence of decreased medial tibial physeal growth. Later, the medial articular surface is distorted and the medial physis fuses. This causes progressive angular deformity to develop as the lateral growth plate continues elongating while the medial side is tethered.

Spontaneous resolution of adolescent tibia vara is uncommon but can occur in mild cases. Although some orthopedists recommend bracing to assist the process, there is no consensus that this is necessary or effective.

Severe or progressive cases of Blount disease require surgical correction by tibial osteotomy to regain the normal physiologic valgus angle of the knee. Surgery reduces the physiologic load on the medial tibial plateau and may allow normal growth. Slight overcorrection of the bowing often ensures load reduction, and the resulting valgus slowly resolves as the child grows. A role for guided growth with tension techniques in cases without a medial bar has been established in the literature as well.

Surgical treatment early in life is now popular, and many orthopedists recommend osteotomy after 3 to 4 years of age if radiographic changes are present. In early cases, surgical correction may cause reversal before there is permanent growth arrest that would require physeal bridge resection and/or repeated osteotomies. Once physeal bridging occurs, however, there is no alternative to repeated surgical correction of angular deformity and leg-length inequality until growth ceases at maturity. Surgical elevation of the medial tibial plateau is a procedure that is occasionally necessary in

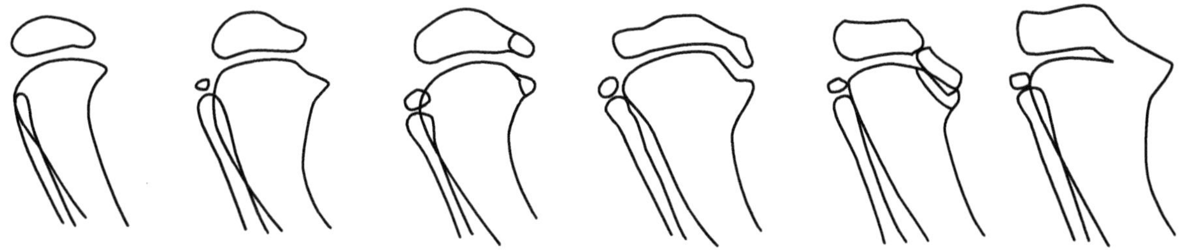

▲ **Figure 12–24.** The Langenskiöld diagrammatic classification of radiographic changes in Blount disease (infantile tibia vara). The higher grades are associated with permanent closure of the medial tibial physis, which leads to progressive varus and internal rotation deformity with growth.

individuals with early-onset Blount disease but is not indicated for individuals with late-onset Blount disease. Distal femoral varus deformity is commonly present and must be addressed as well. Controlled studies of the issues involved in treatment of Blount disease by bracing and surgery are not available.

C. Rickets

Metabolic disorders of calcium intake (nutritional rickets) can decrease the rate of calcification and ossification of physeal cartilage, causing the development of softer bones that are prone to bowing. Vitamin and calcium dietary supplements have virtually eliminated nutritional rickets in the United States. Hypophosphatemic rickets was discussed earlier in the section on metabolic bone disease.

Jain MJ, Inneh IA, Zhu H, Phillips WA. Tension band plate (TBP)-guided hemiepiphysiodesis in Blount disease: 10 year single-center experience with a systematic review of literature. *J Pediatr Orthop.* 2020;40(2):e138-e143. [PMID: 31022017]

Jones JK, Gill L, John M, Goddard M, Hambleton IR. Outcome analysis of surgery for Blount disease. *J Pediatr Orthop.* 2009;29:730-735. [PMID: 20104154]

Rab GT. Oblique tibial osteotomy revisited. *J Child Orthop.* 2010; 4:169-172. [PMID: 20234769]

Tibial Bowing and Pseudarthrosis

The tibia has a propensity to exhibit congenital angular deformities (bowing of the tibial shaft), which, although rare, are significant. The direction of the bowing is important in both diagnosis and prognosis and usually detectable at birth. Bowing direction is described by the apex of the bow, not the direction of displacement of the distal part (Figure 12–25).

A. Congenital Posteromedial Bowing of Tibia

Congenital posteromedial bowing of the tibia is a unilateral birth deformity of the distal fourth of the tibia. The apex of the bow is posteromedial, and often a skin dimple is present over the area. Because of the angle of bowing (often approximately 50 degrees) and the proximity to the ankle joint, the clinical appearance often mimics calcaneovalgus foot. The spatial position of the ankle joint, however, not the foot itself, is responsible for the deformity. Radiographs of posteromedial bowing disclose the curvature of the distal tibia, often with sclerosis in the underlying section of bone.

Despite its dramatic appearance, posteromedial tibial bowing corrects spontaneously in all cases. Some recommend casting to bring the dorsiflexed foot down to plantigrade position, but because the actual deformity is not related to the foot, this advice is not logical: Patients who are never casted resolve as quickly as those who are.

The tibial curvature remodels enough by 3 years of age that the limb appears cosmetically straight, although some bowing may be evident on radiograph for 5 to 8 years. All patients with posteromedial bowing are left with a leg-length discrepancy. At maturity, the involved limb is relatively as much shorter than the longer limb as it was at birth, usually

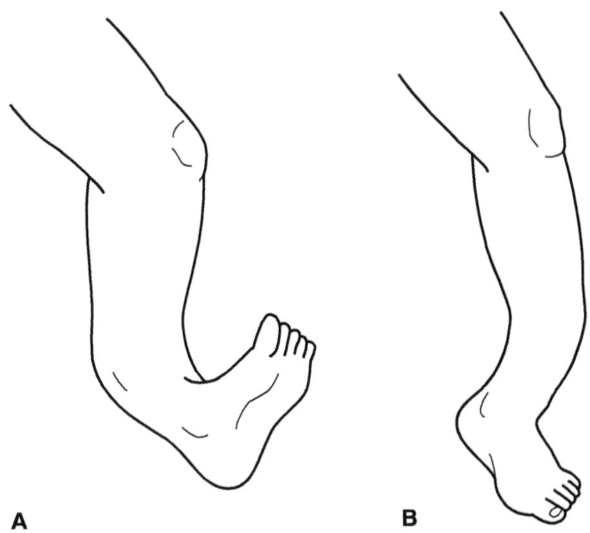

▲ **Figure 12–25.** The major types of tibial bowing. **A:** Posteromedial bowing. The angulation spontaneously corrects, but with limb-length inequality. **B:** Anterolateral bowing. This disorder eventually progresses to spontaneous tibial fracture with resistant pseudarthrosis (see text).

in the range of 4 cm. The residual limb-length discrepancy presents the greatest challenge but can usually be handled with limb-lengthening techniques. Therefore, although the angular deformity needs no treatment, long-term follow-up and treatment of limb inequality are necessary.

B. Congenital Anterolateral Bowing of Tibia and Congenital Pseudarthrosis of the Tibia

Congenital anterolateral bowing of the tibia and congenital pseudarthrosis of the tibia represent the other extreme of tibial bowing. For reasons not understood, anterolateral bowing in the tibia and fibula is associated with inevitable progressive sclerosis and atrophy of the tibial shaft underlying the deformity. The ultimate fate of this atrophic abnormal bone is spontaneous fracture, which does not heal readily as most fractures in children do (ie, pseudarthrosis). Some children with this condition are born with a tibial fracture, whereas others simply have anterolateral bowing and sclerosis at birth, with fractures occurring up to 8 to 10 years of age. In approximately 50% of cases, confirmed neurofibromatosis is present.

All children with variations of this disorder require treatment. Because the prognosis is worse for those whose fracture occurs at a younger age, treatment methods vary. If anterolateral bowing is present but fracture has not occurred, protective bracing may be helpful. The fracture may heal in children whose first fracture occurs at 8 years or older, using prolonged casting or surgical bone grafting (with or without internal fixation).

Bone grafting in children whose fracture occurs before 3 years of age almost always fails, although repeated attempts to graft show some success.

The dismal results with conventional treatment of congenital pseudarthrosis of the tibia in younger patients prompted some surgeons to try innovative treatments. Electrical stimulation, free microvascular transfer of the fibula, and Ilizarov transport of normal bone to the defect are all reported to improve the success of treatment. So much surgery may be required to achieve a functional result, however, that many patients eventually undergo amputation to achieve rapid return to the normal functional activities of childhood.

Feldman DS, Jordan C, Fonseca L. Orthopaedic manifestations of neurofibromatosis type 1. *J Am Acad Orthop Surg.* 2010;18: 346-357. [PMID: 20511440]

Paley D. Congenital psuedoarthrosis of the tibia: biological and biomechanical considerations to achieve union and prevent refracture. *J Child Orthop.* 2019;13(2):120-133. [PMID: 30996736]

Tudisco C, Bollini G, Dungl P, et al. Functional results at the end of skeletal growth in 30 patients affected by congenital pseudarthrosis of the tibia. *J Pediatr Orthop B.* 2000;9:94-102. [PMID: 10868385]

Vander Have KL, Hensinger RN, Caird M, Johnston C, Farley FA. Congenital pseudarthrosis of the tibia. *J Am Acad Orthop Surg.* 2008;16:228-236. [PMID: 18390485]

KNEE DISORDERS

1. Discoid Meniscus

The normal menisci of the knee are semilunar in shape and wedge shaped in cross section. They deepen the flat tibial articular surface to allow cupping of the rounded femoral condyles. The medial meniscus is longer and narrower than the lateral meniscus.

Rarely, the lateral meniscus remains congenitally round (or discoid) instead of acquiring its normal semilunar shape (Figure 12–26). This reduces its cupping function and may cause some instability of either the lateral compartment of the knee or of the lateral meniscus itself.

Clinical Findings

The classic physical finding of discoid meniscus is loud clicking over the lateral meniscus during flexion and extension of the knee. This clicking is usually painless but may be accompanied by aching or effusion. Physical exam may demonstrate an extension block. Discoid meniscus may be suspected on radiograph by widening of the lateral knee compartment, a subtle increase in subchondral sclerosis laterally, and convexity of the lateral tibial articular surface. Confirmation is attained on arthrography or MRI. The abnormal mechanical function of discoid lateral meniscus makes it susceptible to tears, particularly in children older than 10 years.

Treatment

In the past, symptomatic discoid menisci were treated by total lateral meniscectomy, but the resultant late degenerative knee changes dictate a far more conservative course. Current practice is to perform "saucerization." If treatment is required, the safest approach appears to be arthroscopic removal of the central portion of the discoid shape, thus sculpting the lateral meniscus into a roughly semilunar form. Long-term results remain guarded with high rates of re-tears and lateral compartment arthritis reported.

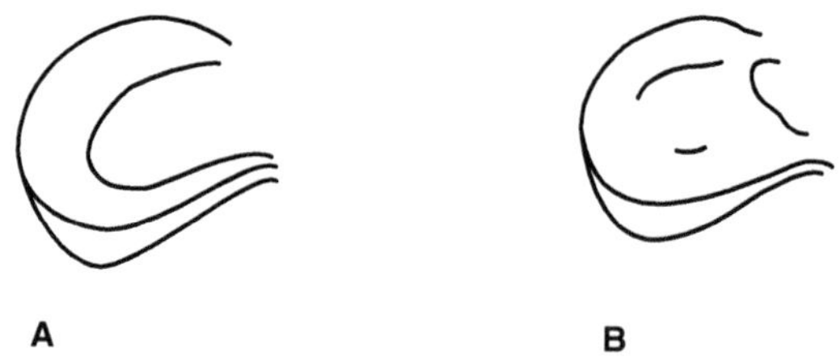

▲ **Figure 12–26. A:** Normal lateral meniscus. **B:** Discoid lateral meniscus, which may cause clicking, effusion, or pain.

Good CR, Green DW, Griffith MH, Valen AW, Widmann RF, Rodeo SA. Arthroscopic treatment of symptomatic discoid meniscus in children: classification, technique, and results. *Arthroscopy.* 2007;23:157-163. [PMID: 17276223]

Kramer DE, Micheli LJ. Meniscal tears and discoid meniscus in children: diagnosis and treatment. *J Am Acad Orthop Surg.* 2009;17:698-707. [PMID: 19880680]

Sabbag OD, Hevesi M, Sanders TL, et al. High rate of recurrent meniscal tear and lateral compartment osteoarthritis in patients treated for symptomatic lateral discoid meniscus: a population-based study. *Orthop J Sports Med.* 2019;7(7):2325967119856284. [PMID: 31367646]

2. Chondromalacia and Internal Derangements of the Knee

Patellar chondromalacia and patellar subluxation are common in active adolescents, particularly in females who have small patellas and a slight exaggeration of knee valgus and quadriceps (Q) angle. Meniscal and ligament injuries are managed similarly to the adults, although these injuries are not as common in children. Some ligamentous reconstructions, however, are modified to avoid injury to an open physis (eg, medial patellofemoral ligament and anterior cruciate ligament reconstructions).

These disorders are described in Chapter 2, "Musculoskeletal Trauma Surgery," and Chapter 4, "Sports Medicine: Lower Extremity."

3. Osteochondritis Dissecans

Osteochondritis dissecans is a poorly understood disorder most commonly of the distal femoral condyle ossification center, although other joints (talus, elbow) can be affected. A portion of the joint surface softens, shears, or separates through the articular cartilage and underlying bone (Figure 12–27). This disorder is common, but not exclusive, in children 8 to 14 years of age; however, it is an infrequent problem in the adult.

The disease appears to be caused by a combination of two factors: (1) mechanical shearing or injury from activity and

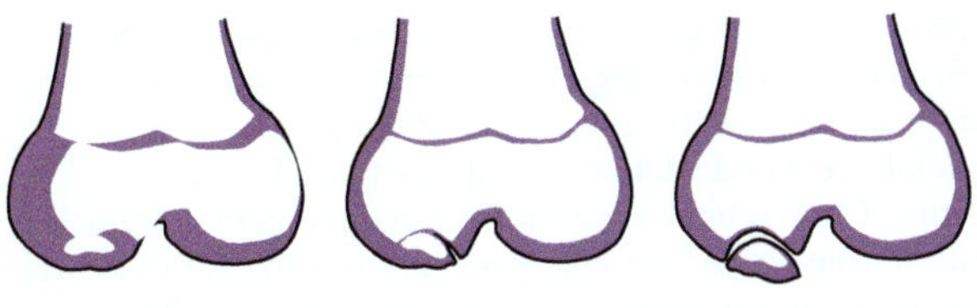

▲ **Figure 12–27.** Various forms of the osteochondritis dissecans lesion found in children. **A:** Defect in ossification center without cartilage defect. **B:** Lesion with a hinged flap. **C:** Complete separation of bone and cartilage, which can lead to loose body in the knee joint.

(2) femoral condyle susceptibility (fragility) resulting from immature ossification of the femoral condyle (which can be quite irregular in children). The importance of each factor depends on age. Athletic trauma seems more important in older children and adults, whereas in younger children, ossification defects render the femoral condyle more susceptible to minor repetitive injury.

Clinical Findings

A. Symptoms and Signs

Symptoms and physical findings can be highly variable. Younger children may have an asymptomatic radiographic abnormality of condylar fragmentation or may simply have a vague aching after strenuous activity. Older children and adults may have pain, effusion, and locking or catching if the affected fragment actually separates and becomes a loose body in the knee joint.

B. Imaging Studies

Plain radiographs show an irregular fragment of the surface that is usually sclerotic but may be osteopenic and is usually on the lateral side of the medial condyle. It is often necessary to obtain tangential views of the condyle such as notch views. Occasionally, the defect is visible only on lateral projection. Contralateral comparison views should always be obtained. So-called ossification defects that mimic osteochondritis dissecans may be normal ossification fronts, seen to be bilateral and symmetric.

In children older than 11 to 12 years, MRI or arthrography is used to determine whether the underlying bone alone is involved or whether there is an actual separation of overlying cartilage. A fragment with cartilage separation and motion is termed unstable. This has significant implications for prognosis and treatment.

Treatment

Young children with asymptomatic osteochondritis dissecans need not be treated because most of these lesions heal spontaneously. In preadolescents with symptomatic lesions seen on radiographs, conservative treatment with weight bearing and activity restriction may heal the defect and eliminates symptoms. The time frame for relative rest is in the 3- to 6-month range; it is difficult for most overuse-prone young athletes to adhere to such recommendations.

If the lesion is large and accompanied by cartilage separation or displacement, if the skeleton has reached maturity, or if the symptoms persist despite conservative measures, treatment may be the same as in the adult. This includes arthroscopic debridement and stabilization of the loose fragment using internal fixation. Excision is less likely to result in a good result. The presence of open physes may necessitate modifications of standard adult techniques.

Grimm NL, Weiss JM, Kessler JI, Aoki SK. Osteochondritis dissecans of the knee: pathoanatomy, epidemiology, and diagnosis. *Clin Sports Med.* 2014;33(2):181-188. [PMID: 24698037]

Gudas R, Simonaityte R, Cekanauskas E, Tamosiūnas R. A prospective, randomized clinical study of osteochondral autologous transplantation versus microfracture for the treatment of osteochondritis dissecans in the knee joint in children. *J Pediatr Orthop.* 2009;29:741-748. [PMID: 20104156]

Kocher MS, DiCanzio J, Zurakowski D, Micheli LJ. Diagnostic performance of clinical examination and selective magnetic resonance imaging in the evaluation of intraarticular knee disorders in children and adolescents. *Am J Sports Med.* 2001;29:292-296. [PMID: 11394597]

Weiss JM, Nikizad H, Shea KG, et al. The incidence of surgery in osteochondritis dissecans in children and adolescents. *Orthop J Sports Med.* 2016;4(3):2325967116635515. [PMID: 27047984]

4. Ligament and Epiphyseal Injury

Children who have not reached skeletal maturity have far fewer major ligament injuries of the knee than do older children and adults. Smaller children tend to participate in lower impact activities and sports, and their lack of muscle bulk (which increases during adolescence) limits body acceleration and the force of collision. In addition, ligaments are relatively strong in the immature skeleton compared with bone or cartilaginous physes. Therefore, physeal fractures and bony avulsions of ligament attachments are more likely than traumatic ruptures of the ligaments themselves.

Residual instability may occur in the child's knee after varus or valgus injury. In the adult, such instability is considered clinical evidence of ligament injury. In children, however, the physis rather than the ligament may be the site of failure. Instability can be caused by a physeal fracture that hinges open rather than the joint opening (Figure 12–28). It is usually clinically obvious that fracture is present, although stress radiographs may help in questionable cases.

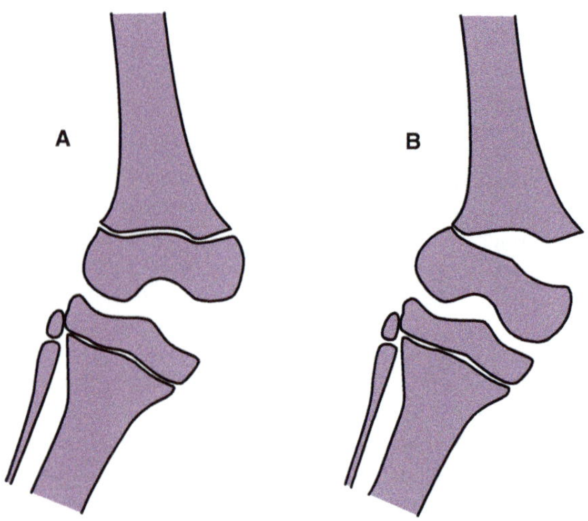

▲ **Figure 12–28.** Stress radiograph of the unstable knee in an immature patient may reveal ligament rupture **(A)** or separation of the femoral physis **(B)**.

Major intraarticular disruptions of the knee joint (meniscal tear or cruciate ligament injury) are rare in children. Detection may be delayed because symptoms may be less severe than in the adult and their presence not given as much weight in the differential diagnosis. Meniscus injury, particularly when peripheral, may lend itself to arthroscopic repair because of the excellent blood supply in children. The femoral and tibial physes represent anatomic challenges to anterior cruciate ligament reconstruction. However, with modifications of techniques, an open physis is not a contraindication for reconstruction, and the bulk of research indicates worse outcomes with delay.

With the exception of cruciate injuries, most childhood knee ligament injuries are treatable by 2 to 4 weeks of splinting and return to function, as tolerated by pain. Physical therapy is rarely necessary in children younger than 15 years. A review of the major signs, symptoms, diagnostic procedures, and treatment options can be found in Chapter 4, "Sports Medicine: Lower Extremity."

Differential Diagnosis

Not all effusions in the knee are traumatic, particularly in younger children. Because children at play are always suffering minor injuries, a history of injury may be inaccurate. The physician must remember to consider septic arthritis and pauciarticular juvenile rheumatoid arthritis in the differential diagnosis of effusion.

Beasley LS, Chudik SC. Anterior cruciate ligament injury in children: update of current treatment options. *Curr Opin Pediatr.* 2003;15:45-52. [PMID: 12544271]

Dingel A, Aoyama J, Ganley T, Shea K. Pediatric ACL tears: natural history. *J Pediatr Orthop.* 2019;39(6, suppl 1):S47-S49. [PMID: 31169648]

Luhmann SJ. Acute traumatic knee effusions in children and adolescents. *J Pediatr Orthop.* 2003;23:199-202. [PMID: 12649021]

OSGOOD-SCHLATTER DISEASE

The proximal tibial physis contains a transverse component that contributes to longitudinal growth and an anterior tongue that contains the attachment of the patellar tendon. In preadolescent and adolescent children (usually boys), the distal tip of this tongue may undergo fragmentation from chronic tensile stress and enlargement from the resultant hyperemic response, which is known as Osgood-Schlatter disease. As the tibial tubercle becomes increasingly prominent, a painful bursa can form over it.

Clinical Findings

Symptoms vary from mild aching at the tubercle to severe pain with patellar function and exaggerated bursal

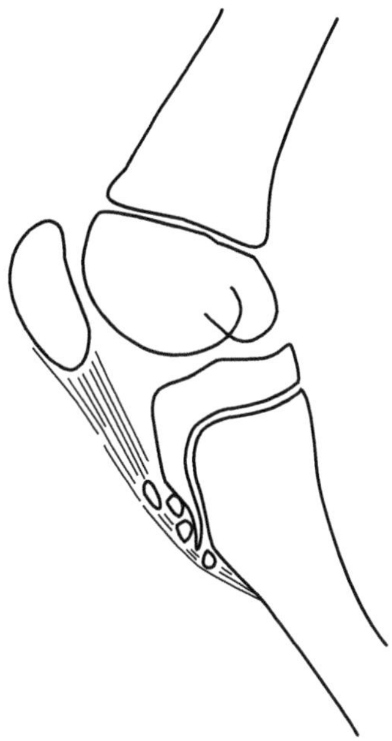

▲ **Figure 12–29.** Osgood-Schlatter disease. The radiographs would show characteristic fragmentation of the tibial tubercle apophysis, similar to diagram.

tenderness. Radiographs of the lateral proximal tibia show the characteristic fragmentation (Figure 12–29).

Treatment

Treatment is symptomatic, including analgesics, knee pads to avert direct pressure, quadriceps stretching, avoidance of sports activities, and brief casting or splinting for painful cases. The disorder resolves spontaneously when the physis closes at skeletal maturity. No evidence indicates that physical activity within the limits of pain is harmful to the child with Osgood-Schlatter disease.

Adirim TA, Cheng TL. Overview of injuries in the young athlete. *Sports Med.* 2003;33:75-81. [PMID: 12477379]

Krause BL, Williams JP, Catterall A. Natural history of Osgood-Schlatter disease. *J Pediatr Orthop.* 1990;10:65-68. [PMID: 2298897]

SPINAL CURVATURE

Spinal curvature may occur in any age group and present with variable findings. Curvatures may be idiopathic, congenital, or accompany a wide variety of neuromuscular disorders, tumors, and infections. Curvatures may be small and nonprogressive or may worsen and require aggressive treatment. Sometimes, spinal curvature is the first clue to important underlying disease. Figure 12–30 shows the different types of spinal deformities.

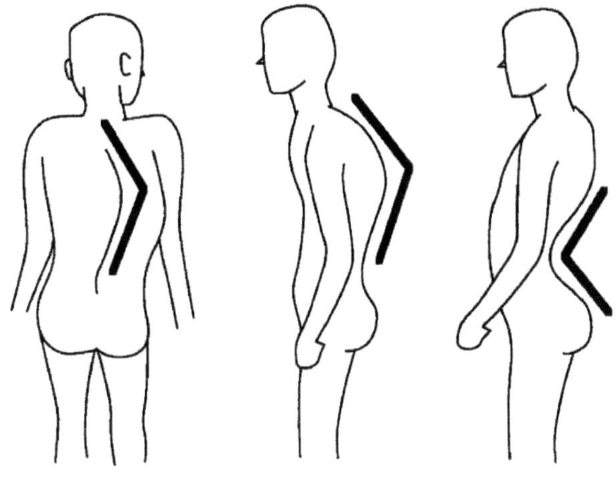

▲ **Figure 12–30.** Definitions of spinal deformities. **A:** Scoliosis. **B:** Kyphosis. **C:** Lordosis. Frequently, a combination of deformities occurs in individual patients (ie, kyphoscoliosis).

Types of Curvatures

A. Scoliosis

Scoliosis is a lateral spinal curvature in the frontal plane, best appreciated by physical examination from the patient's back and by AP radiographs. Curvatures, which may be single or multiple, are described by the direction of their convexity. In a flexible spine, the presence of a single (more rigid) curvature can lead to physiologic compensatory curvatures in the opposite direction, above and below the primary curvature. True scoliosis always includes a rotational component that may not be fully appreciated on radiograph and generally includes a lordotic component as well (see section on lordosis). Surprisingly, lateral curvature is often undetected externally. The rotation of vertebrae that accompanies scoliosis is the physical feature that allows clinical detection.

B. Kyphosis

Kyphosis is a forward (flexed) curvature of the spine in the sagittal plane, best appreciated from the side and by lateral radiographs. If kyphosis is acutely angular, a posterior prominence called a gibbus may be evident in the sagittal plane.

C. Lordosis

Lordosis is a hyperextension deformity of the spine, most common in the lumbar spine but also often accompanying scoliosis. Lumbar lordosis may be secondary to flexion contracture of the hip.

Detection of Curvature

Although spinal curvatures may be detected first during routine radiograph, most lesions are best diagnosed by physical examination. Spinal examination should proceed according to the following specific protocol:

1. Place the patient in the standing position (Figure 12–31).
2. Check the level of the pelvis and look for obvious asymmetry of the rib, scapula, neck, and shoulder height (leg-length inequality can cause apparent scoliosis, which disappears when the short leg is elevated on blocks).
3. Level the pelvis by seating the child on a firm surface if the pelvis cannot be leveled while standing. This is the case in children with hip contracture from neuromuscular disease.
4. Have the child bend forward, carefully noting any asymmetric prominence of the lumbar paraspinous muscle, rib cage, or scapula, which suggests the rotational portion of scoliosis. The magnitude of asymmetry corresponds to the severity of the curvature, with convexity of the curvature directed toward the most prominent side.
5. From the side, check for prominence of the spine that might indicate kyphosis, both in the upright and forward-bending position.
6. Perform a careful neurologic exam, including upper extremity reflexes and abdominal reflexes in addition to thorough lower extremity neurologic examination.
7. Use radiographs to assess type, severity, and location of the curvature and to look for underlying lesions. Because primary scoliosis and kyphosis curvatures are always stiffer than uninvolved spine segments, bending radiographs may reveal which curvatures are "structural" and which are more flexible compensations (secondary curvature). The Cobb method is usually used to measure curvatures (Figure 12–32). The degree of tilt between the most affected vertebral endplates describes curvature magnitude.

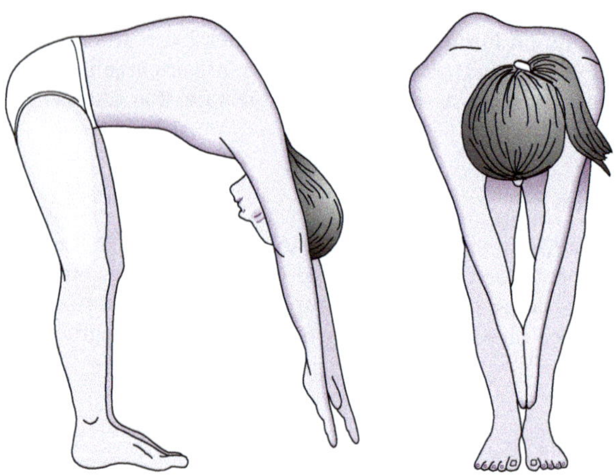

▲ **Figure 12–31.** Examination of the spine for deformity is best carried out by observing for asymmetry and deformity as the patient bends forward (see text).

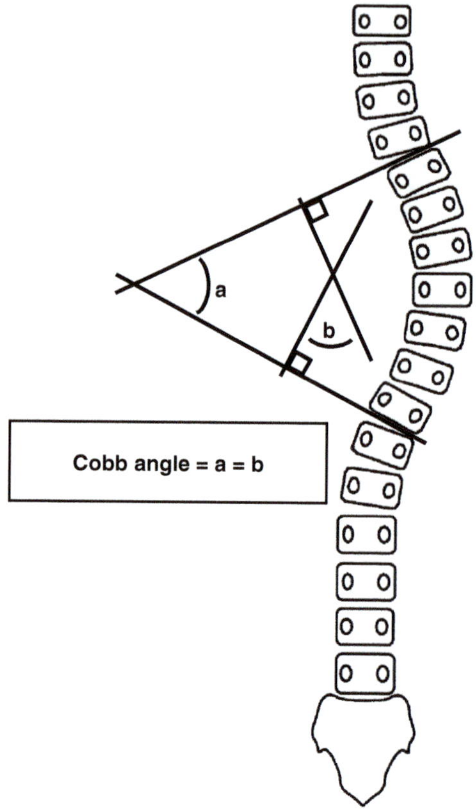

▲ **Figure 12–32.** The Cobb method of measurement is commonly used to assess spinal curvature. It measures the angle between the far (top and bottom) endplates of the most inclined vertebrae. To allow the measurement lines to fit on the radiograph, lines at 90-degree angles to the endplates are often drawn, and their relative angles measured. Geometrically, these angles are the same.

Scoliosis

A. Idiopathic Scoliosis

Idiopathic scoliosis has no apparent underlying cause and can be separated into adolescent (>10 years), juvenile (3-10 years), and infantile (<3 years). Adolescent idiopathic scoliosis accounts for 80% of all idiopathic scoliosis and is found most commonly in early adolescent girls, although it can be found in either gender at any age. There is typically a convex curvature to the right in the thoracic portion of the spine (right thoracic curve pattern). Patients with atypical curvature patterns, such as left thoracic curves and idiopathic curvature in younger children, may require more extensive testing (eg, MRI) before the cause can be definitively designated idiopathic.

Many idiopathic curvatures progress in magnitude with growth and continue to do so until skeletal maturity. Therefore, the clinician must determine if the curvature is progressing and if the spine is still growing. Radiographs document progression, and observations of the ossification pattern of the iliac crest apophysis (Risser sign) and menarchal status are used to estimate skeletal maturity. This ossification pattern begins laterally at puberty and spreads medially across the ilium, capping and fusing with the bone at maturity. Progressive curves in children with substantial growth potential (Risser 2 or less), any curve of greater than 25 degrees, or patients with a curve of greater than 20 degrees with more than 5 degrees of documented progression should be treated. Treatment with bracing to control curve progression during growth has been established as the standard of care. The role of physical therapy (Schroth technique) and manipulative treatments remain unproven. Bracing success is typically defined as preventing progression or keeping a curve less than 45 degrees at maturity.

Children who mature with small or moderate curves have no symptoms and should not progress in adulthood. However, a curve that progresses beyond 45 degrees, even at maturity, is at risk for continued progression in adulthood. Continued progression, or the risk of it, is the main indication for surgical treatment. The long-term natural history for idiopathic scoliosis does not lead to neurologic or significant cardiopulmonary issues.

B. Early-Onset Scoliosis

Idiopathic scoliosis in children less than 10 years of age bears additional mention. Onset at age 3 to 10 years is defined as juvenile onset. It can be considered a more concerning type of scoliosis since these patients have more remaining growth and therefore a worse prognosis in regard to curve progression. In those with juvenile scoliosis with more than a 20-degree Cobb angle, there is about a 20% prevalence of a neurologic abnormality. Therefore, workup in these children should include an MRI of the entire spine.

Infantile idiopathic scoliosis diagnosed in children under 3 years of age appears to be different than juvenile or adolescent scoliosis. Infantile idiopathic scoliosis occurs more commonly in boys, with a 3:1 male-to-female ratio. Spontaneous correction occurs in some individuals. Gender, family history, and age at presentation have not been found to be risk factors for progression. If progression occurs, infantile scoliosis can also have far greater overall health implications: Interference with normal pulmonary development can lead to thoracic insufficiency syndrome.

C. Congenital Scoliosis

Congenital scoliosis is caused by malformations of vertebral shape. It does not refer to the age of the patient: Newborns can have idiopathic scoliosis, despite being born with spinal curvatures. Congenital vertebral malformations generally occur in early embryonic life (before 7 weeks) and are thought to represent errors in formation or segmentation of the spinal segments that originate from primitive mesenchymal condensations of embryonic cells (Figure 12–33).

Curvatures can originate when vertebral parts fail to form (eg, hemivertebrae, wedge vertebrae, butterfly vertebrae) or when embryonic somites fail to segment properly into individual vertebrae (eg, block vertebrae, unilateral unsegmented bar). Because of the embryonic timing of this process, children with congenital scoliosis frequently have abnormalities of other organ systems that form during the same embryonic period. About 60% of patients with congenital anomalies of the spine have other associated findings. The spine develops around the same time as the cardiovascular system, the genitourinary system, and the musculoskeletal system. Around 20% of patients with congenital scoliosis have an associated urologic abnormality. Approximately 25% of patients with congenital scoliosis have an associated cardiac defect. Diagnosis of congenital scoliosis must be followed by a careful cardiac examination and by ultrasound or intravenous pyelography evaluation of the kidneys. Spinal cord abnormalities may be present in as many as 30%, so evaluation of the spinal canal (MRI, EMG) may be required, especially if surgery is contemplated.

Congenital scoliosis may encompass one or many deformed vertebrae, and different types of vertebral abnormalities are often seen in the same patient. Sometimes, two deforming vertebrae “cancel each other out” and no curvature is visible. For this reason, prediction of progression of the scoliosis depends on serial radiographs. If progression occurs, bracing is often attempted as the first treatment, although surgery is indicated if progression is not halted by external means. Curvatures caused by unilateral

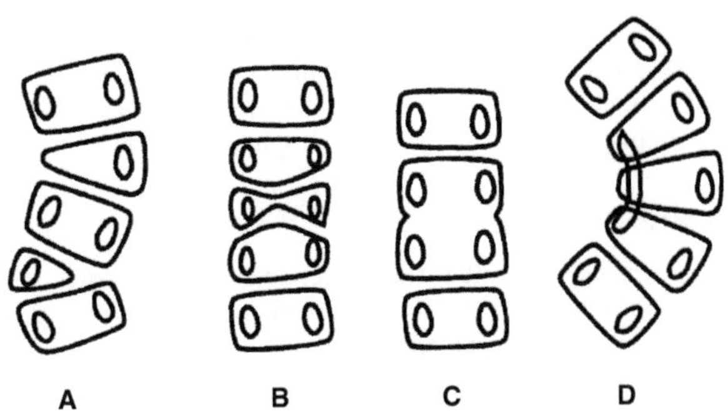

▲ **Figure 12–33.** Vertebral anomalies of congenital scoliosis. **A:** Hemivertebra. **B:** Butterfly vertebra. **C:** Block vertebra. **D:** Unilateral unsegmented bar.

unsegmented bars or fully segmented hemivertebra have a strong tendency to progress and need close follow-up and possible earlier stabilization.

D. Neuromuscular Scoliosis

Neuromuscular scoliosis includes a diverse group of curvature patterns that occur in association with various neuromuscular diseases. The cause varies with the disease. For example, scoliosis in children with cerebral palsy is usually caused by a combination of spasticity (overactivity of muscle) and weakness. Scoliosis in children with muscular dystrophy is the result of severe progressive muscle weakness that eliminates the paraspinous stability of the spinal column. Scoliosis in infants with spina bifida (myelomeningocele) is frequently congenital (see previous discussion), related to loss of posterior elements, or associated with the development of a syrinx (central cystic fluid collection) in the spinal cord, a process similar to hydrocephalus.

Patients with neuromuscular scoliosis often develop curvatures at an early age, when surgical treatment is either impossible or would result in severe stunting of spinal growth. It is common to treat such children by daytime bracing, despite the fact that bracing alone is rarely sufficient to eliminate progression or the need for later surgery. In such cases, some surgeons feel that bracing may slow progression enough to allow additional skeletal growth, and spinal correction and fusion are postponed until puberty. Bracing may simply play a role in postural control to manage sitting balance.

E. Other Scolioses

Childhood scoliosis can be associated with benign tumors of the spine, usually osteoid osteoma and osteoblastoma. Treatment of the tumor is usually curative, although long-standing lesions may require fusion as well.

Neurofibromatosis is associated with both scoliosis and kyphosis and characteristically leads to short high-grade curvatures requiring surgical treatment. Anterior and posterior spinal fusion is required to achieve correction and fusion in neurofibromatosis.

More than 90% of preadolescent children who sustain a significant spinal cord injury subsequently develop scoliosis. Bracing has not been shown to be effective in the prevention of scoliosis in the preadolescent patient with spinal cord injury.

Kyphosis

Kyphosis may be congenital, traumatic, or acquired. Some patients with kyphosis need no treatment, whereas others require immediate surgical attention.

A. Postural Kyphosis (Postural Roundback)

Postural kyphosis, a variation of normal posture, is a cosmetic problem. There is no associated underlying disease, and the spine is flexible and capable of hyperextension. Although it may be worrisome to parents, little scientific evidence indicates that it requires, or responds to, treatment.

B. Scheuermann Kyphosis

Scheuermann kyphosis is a disorder of growth of the vertebral endplates that affects adolescents, particularly boys, and produces a progressive rigid forward curvature of the thoracic spine. Less commonly, it involves the lumbar spine, causing decreased lumbar lordosis (relative kyphosis). It is often moderately painful. Radiographs show wedging of vertebral bodies, irregularity of the endplates with radiographic lucent pits known as Schmörl's nodes, and kyphosis (Figure 12–34).

Lumbar Scheuermann kyphosis responds to symptomatic treatment with nonnarcotic pain medications or a supportive lumbar corset. Thoracic involvement with pain or kyphosis of 15 to 20 degrees greater than normal can be managed with an extension-type thoracolumbosacral orthosis. Brace treatment is usually effective in controlling pain

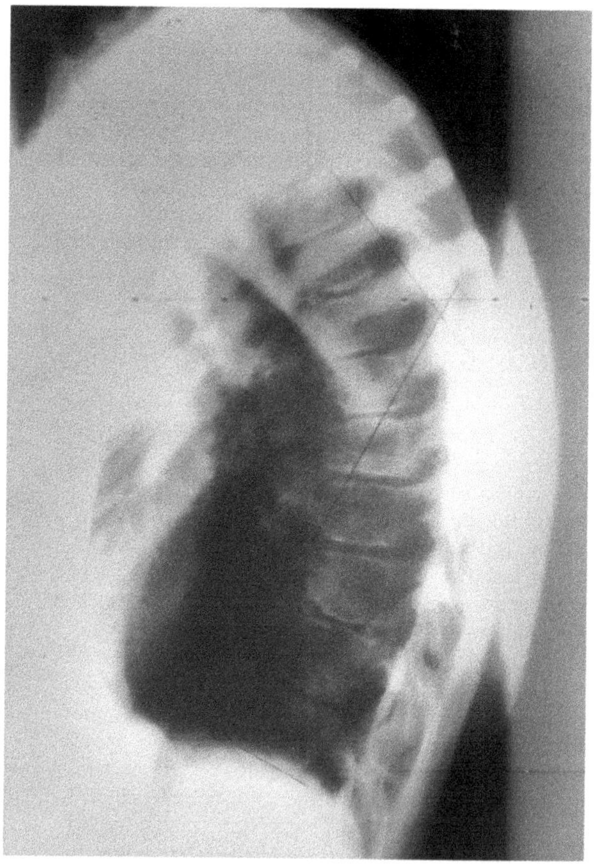

▲ **Figure 12–34.** Scheuermann kyphosis is characterized by vertebral wedging, endplate changes, and kyphosis.

and can produce structural correction of the kyphosis, but it is very unpopular with adolescents.

Scheuermann disease is the exception to the general rule that spinal bracing must be done during the active growth phase to improve deformity. Patients as old as 18 years of age show improvement with the Milwaukee brace. Severe cases (40 degrees of excessive kyphosis) may require surgical correction by spinal instrumentation and fusion.

C. Congenital Kyphosis

Congenital kyphosis is a rare but important group of diseases, which, like congenital scoliosis, may be caused by failure of formation of vertebrae (hemivertebrae) or failure of embryonic segmentation (anterior unsegmented bar). In most cases, the lesion tends to cause uneven growth, so kyphosis gradually increases as the spine elongates. The risk of neurologic compromise associated with congenital kyphosis is normally secondary to risk of progression. The combination of an anterolateral bar with contralateral quadrant vertebrae has the greatest risk. Bowstringing of the spinal cord over the kyphotic prominence can occur and eventually cause paraplegia. Any progressive congenital kyphosis must be fused to prevent neurologic complications, regardless of the child's age.

D. Traumatic Kyphosis

Traumatic kyphosis is a traumatic compression of vertebrae that may lead to either cosmetic or symptomatic kyphosis. This may be prevented by early surgical stabilization of high-grade unstable traumatic spinal injuries.

E. Infectious Kyphosis

Infectious kyphosis refers to septic destruction of vertebral bodies, which can lead to severe kyphosis. In particular, tuberculous vertebral osteomyelitis can produce soft-tissue abscess, high-grade kyphosis, a sharp gibbus, and paraplegia. Bacterial infection can mimic this, although dramatic deformities are far more unusual.

Treatment includes antibiotics, surgical debridement and drainage, decompression of the spinal cord, and spinal fusion to prevent further deformity.

Treatment

A. Bracing

Bracing can be used to slow progression of spinal curvatures, prevent progression, or improve underlying structural deformities. Many different types of braces are available, each with its own advocates and specific applications (Figure 12–35). When the goal is to provide postural support, slow progression, or postpone (but not prevent) surgery, a polypropylene body jacket, or so-called clamshell brace, may suffice for waking or sitting hours.

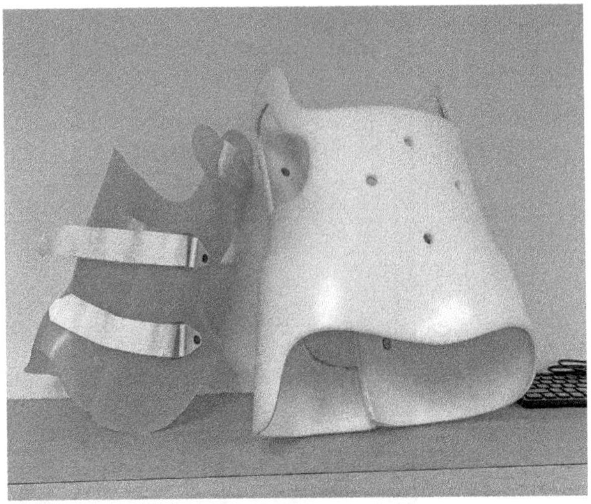

▲ **Figure 12–35.** Two popular brace styles used for the treatment of spinal deformity are the Milwaukee brace **(A)** and the low-profile (Boston-type) brace **(B)**.

Long-term braces designed to arrest progression must be custom molded for the patient, with pads placed to exert appropriate pressure to reduce deformity. Depending on the anatomic level of the curvature, most may be positioned under the arm and should be worn 16 to 18 hours a day.

All braces must be modified or replaced to accommodate growth. In general, bracing is only effective with flexible curvatures in growing children.

B. Surgical Treatment

The basic principles of spinal deformity surgery have not changed: loosen the spine to obtain correction, induce fusion with decortication and bone graft, and hold the correction. Implants have evolved over the years, and currently, most surgeons utilize posterior pedicle screws and hooks affixed to rods. Pedicle screws provide more rigid, three-column fixation of the spine and have demonstrated better three-dimensional correction than past hook-and-wire constructs. Improved stability of these constructs has allowed more posterior-only approaches, and allograft bone has also supplanted iliac crest graft since fusion has been more assured.

1. Surgical stages—Surgery involves two separate stages: correction and stabilization. After posterior exposure of the spine, correction is achieved with a variety of mechanical internal fixation devices. These are usually rods with hooks, screws, wires, or other mechanisms to distract, compress, or bend spinal segments. Correction is rarely complete because mechanical and safety considerations limit the force that can be applied. Once correction is obtained, the cortex of spine is removed and bone graft (autograft or allograft) is placed over the raw bone. Subsequently, solid fusion occurs within 6 months, permanently stabilizing the spine (Figure 12–36).

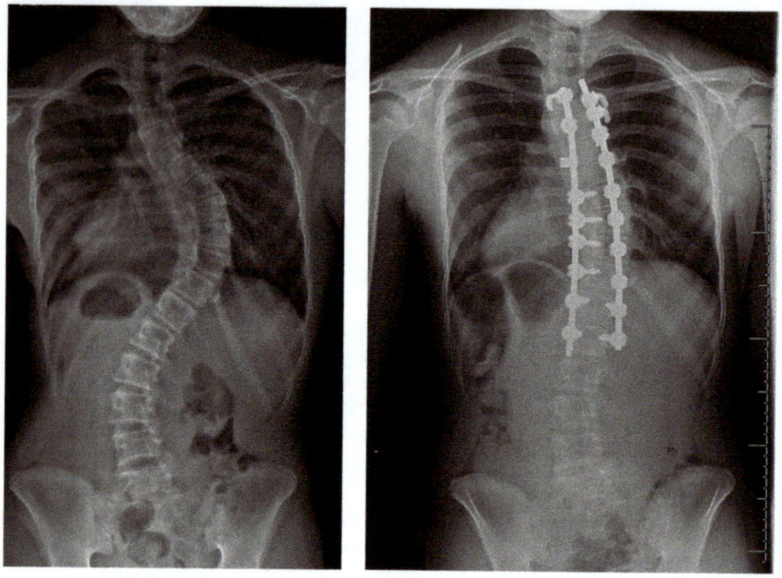

▲ **Figure 12–36.** Example of posterior spinal fusion: 16-year-old female with progressive idiopathic scoliosis underwent instrumented posterior spinal fusion with implants.

2. Treatment of severe curvatures—Some large idiopathic curves and neuromuscular curves require anterior release and bone grafting to render enough acute flexibility for curvature correction and enough late stability for dependable fusion. Occasionally, fusion may fail, causing a pseudarthrosis that may be painful or may allow progression of a previously corrected curvature. In this case, fusion must be repeated.

Belmont PJ Jr, Kuklo TR, Taylor KF, et al. Intraspinal anomalies associated with isolated congenital hemivertebrae: the role of routine magnetic resonance imaging. *J Bone Joint Surg.* 2004: 86(8):1704-1710. [PMID: 15292418]

Bosch P, McIntosh A, Pediatric Spine. Orthopedic Knowledge Update, 11th edition. Cannada L (ed.) AAOS, Rosemont, IL, 2014.

Danielsson AJ, Nachemson AL. Radiologic findings and curve progression 22 years after treatment for adolescent idiopathic scoliosis: comparison of brace and surgical treatment with matching control group of straight individuals. *Spine.* 2001;26:516-525. [PMID: 11242379]

Dobbs MB, Lenke LG, Szymanski DA, et al. Prevalence of neural axis abnormalities in patients with infantile idiopathic scoliosis. *J Bone Joint Surg Am.* 2002;84:2230-2234. [PMID: 12473713]

Dobbs MB, Weinstein SL. Infantile and juvenile scoliosis. *Orthop Clin North Am.* 1999;30:331-341. [PMID: 10393759]

Feldman DS, Jordan C, Fonseca L. Orthopaedic manifestations of neurofibromatosis type 1. *J Am Acad Orthop Surg.* 2010;18: 346-357. [PMID: 20511440]

Nakahara D, Yonezawa I, Kobanawa K, et al. Magnetic resonance imaging evaluation of patient with idiopathic scoliosis: a prospective study of four hundred seventy-two outpatients. *Spine.* 2011;36:E482. [PMID: 20479697]

Negrini S, Negrini F, Fusco C, Zaina F. Idiopathic scoliosis patients with curves more than 45 Cobb degrees refusing surgery can be effectively treated through bracing with curve improvements. *Spine J.* 2011;11:369-380. [PMID: 21292562]

Richards BS, Vitale MG. Screening for idiopathic scoliosis in adolescents. An information statement. *J Bone Joint Surg Am.* 2008;90:195-198. [PMID: 18171974]

Suh SW, Modi HN, Yang JH, Hong JY. Idiopathic scoliosis in Korean schoolchildren: a prospective screening study of over 1 million children. *Eur Spine J.* 2011;20:1087-1094. [PMID: 21274729]

Ueno M, Takaso M, Nakazawa T, et al. A 5-year epidemiological study on the prevalence rate of idiopathic scoliosis in Tokyo: school screening of more than 250,000 children. *J Orthop Sci.* 2011;16:1-6. [PMID: 21293892]

Weinstein SL, Dolan AL, Wright JG, Dobbs MB. Effects of bracing in adolescents with idiopathic scoliosis. *N Engl J Med.* 2013;369(16):1512-1521. [PMID: 24047455]

NEUROMUSCULAR DISORDERS

Essentials of Diagnosis

- *Neuromuscular diseases may cause significant deformities (especially of feet, hips, and spine) due to muscle imbalance during growth.*
- *There is considerable overlap in clinical appearance associated with different diagnoses, so accurate assessment is essential.*
- *Treatment should be influenced by function as well as deformity.*

Because muscle weakness or imbalance changes the underlying structure of a growing skeleton, neuromuscular diseases of children often require orthopedic evaluation. Treatment may be required to reverse skeletal deformity and contracture or to effect functional improvement.

Many childhood neuromuscular diseases require coordinating the services of the pediatrician, neurologist, radiologist, physiatrist, therapist, educator, social worker, nurse, and parent.

1. Cerebral Palsy

Cerebral palsy is a static encephalopathy in a growing child. Although it is often birth related, the term also includes childhood head injury, stroke, metabolic brain conditions, and degenerative neurologic conditions.

The challenges to physicians evaluating cerebral palsy are making an accurate diagnosis and detecting correctable conditions. It is essential that functional evaluation of the child's condition take into account the need for education, communication, socialization, and mobility.

Types of Cerebral Palsy

The hallmark of most cases of cerebral palsy is alteration in motor tone (spasticity or dystonia). Spasticity is increased tone associated with stretching of muscle; dystonia is present without changing muscle length. Diagnosis of spasticity can be direct (increased tone, increased deep tendon reflexes, clasp-knife rigidity, and clonus) or inferred (shortening of muscles, contractures of joints, joint dislocations, and scoliosis). Dystonia can be confused with spasticity, but it does not generally lead to contractures.

A. Hemiplegia

Hemiplegia is spasticity involving only one side of the body. Most hemiplegia involves the pyramidal tract, especially at the cerebral cortex. It may be mild or severe and typically is more pronounced in the distal skeleton (hand and foot-ankle). Hemiplegia is usually caused by congenital loss of portions of the parietal, contralateral cerebral cortex. This loss may reflect vascular insufficiency, trauma, or porencephalic cysts.

Many patients with hemiplegia have normal development and intelligence. Children with hemiplegia frequently walk at a normal age, although sometimes with marked posturing of the involved side. Right hemiplegia (left cerebral cortex) may involve the Broca area and thus cause speech deficits. Because sensory and motor cortex areas are contiguous, hemiplegia is strongly associated with abnormalities of sensation and proprioception in the affected limbs, and particularly in the hand. This may prove more disabling than the spasticity because a child may not appreciate an insensate limb as part of overall body image.

B. Diplegia

Diplegia, or diplegic cerebral palsy, is an encephalopathy usually associated with prematurity. It is characterized by relatively symmetric involvement of the lower extremities and lesser involvement of the upper extremities. Prematurity is often accompanied by intracerebral hemorrhage and periventricular leukomalacia, which lead to edema and necrosis in the region of the trigone. This involvement of the pyramidal tract and associated basal ganglia is the main cause of diplegia.

Most diplegic children exhibit mixed patterns of spasticity with a variety of less obvious neurologic symptoms, including ataxia, rigidity, and athetosis (dystonia). Many have normal intelligence (if the cortex is spared) but may suffer developmental delays caused by damage to associative fibers in the brain. Although they may initially be hypotonic ("floppy"), most diplegic patients develop high tone (spasticity and/or dystonic rigidity) by 12 to 18 months of age.

Diplegia is relatively symmetric and usually more severe in the lower extremities. Many children with diplegia eventually walk, exhibiting a crouching gait characterized by flexed, internally rotated hips, flexed knees, and plantar-flexed ankles.

C. Quadriplegia

Quadriplegia (total body involvement) often occurs in children who suffer birth asphyxia, metabolic encephalopathy, or encephalitis. Severe spasticity, seizures, intellectual disability, joint contractures, and scoliosis are typical but not always individually present in this type of cerebral palsy. Children with quadriplegia are particularly susceptible to spontaneous hip dislocations (because of hip muscle imbalance) and high-grade scoliosis. Both of these conditions interfere with sitting and may require surgery. Most quadriplegic patients require wheelchair assistance and do not walk.

D. Mixed Neurologic Involvement

Mixed neurologic involvement of extrapyramidal portions of the brain can cause athetosis, dystonia, ballismus, and ataxia. Many children with cerebral palsy exhibit subtle signs of some of these disorders, in addition to spasticity. In some children, one of these signs may predominate, but spasticity is absent. In general, prognosis varies with the anatomy of involvement.

Treatment

Before treating cerebral palsy, specific goals should be set for the patient. Although many important goals are not orthopedic, the surgeon may help the patient achieve them. Increased mobility, for instance, may facilitate achieving a variety of nonorthopedic goals. Especially urgent are the patient's ability to communicate, move independently, and socialize. Orthopedic treatment may improve sitting position in the wheelchair or improve walking by releasing muscles or joints.

Many children benefit from physical or occupational therapy during the first few years of life. Although the exact role of such therapy in cerebral palsy remains undefined, therapists often help parents and children deal more effectively with the complex problems presented by the disease. Therapists also help parents and children set optimistic and realistic goals for the future.

Bracing or surgery may be required to control effects of spasticity on individual joints and to decrease spasticity, correct dislocation or contracture, or control scoliosis. Surgery is ineffective in the case of extrapyramidal neurologic symptoms. A variety of nonorthopedic treatments are also used for cerebral palsy. Selective dorsal rhizotomy, a neurosurgical procedure to cut a portion of the posterior roots of the lumbar spinal cord, may reduce spasticity in selected patients by interrupting the reflex arc. Botulinum toxin injection (or phenol injection) into the motor endplate region of a muscle temporarily interrupts the myoneural junction, relaxing a spastic muscle for several months and allowing therapy or other evaluation. Oral baclofen can reduce overall spasticity. Intrathecal baclofen, delivered by a subcutaneous pump, may offer relaxation of troublesome lower extremity muscle tension in both dystonic and spastic patients.

Hip subluxation is common in quadriplegia, and pelvic radiographs in young quadriplegic patients are needed to detect early, reversible involvement. Subluxation may be treated in children younger than 3 years by adductor muscle release, which improves abduction. Rarely, the anterior obturator nerve (which innervates the adductor longus muscle) is resected to weaken the adductors. In older children, bony reconstruction by varus-derotation osteotomy and acetabular reorientation or supplementation may be necessary to correct the bone malformation that results from the force of spastic muscles on the growing skeleton. Children who develop hip subluxation often develop scoliosis as well (see section on scoliosis).

A. Adductor Release

Adductor release may be done as an open procedure (usually by myotomy or transverse sectioning of the adductor longus and a portion of the adductor brevis) or by percutaneous adductor tenotomy (section of the tendon origin of the adductor longus at the pelvis). The exact technique and amount of release is dictated by the severity of contracture and other factors. When done for hip subluxation, adductor release is most effective before 3 years of age. Release should be sufficient to allow hip abduction of 70 to 80 degrees on the operating table. When frank subluxation is present, some surgeons perform an anterior obturator neurectomy in addition to the adductor myotomy. This open procedure removes a segment of the obturator nerve that supplies the released adductor longus muscle, so the muscle remains loose after spontaneously reattaching after surgery.

Obturator neurectomy must be used carefully because it can cause excessive weakening of the adductors and, subsequently, late hip abduction contracture. After each of these procedures, the patient is casted in abduction for 3 to 4 weeks to allow muscle healing in the new elongated position.

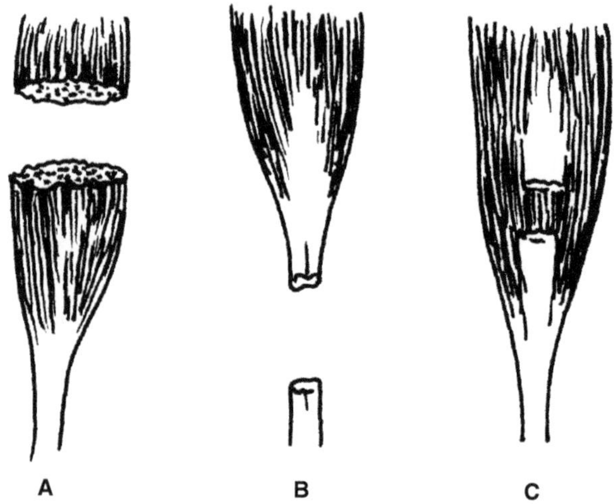

▲ **Figure 12–37.** Schematic representation of surgical options for muscle release or lengthening in cerebral palsy. **A:** Myotomy; **B:** tenotomy; **C:** aponeurotomy.

Dynamic spasticity or joint contracture (the result of chronic spasticity) can interfere with walking in children with hemiplegia or diplegia. This may be treated by bracing involved joints in a functional position or by surgical lengthening of the muscle–tendon unit. Such muscle releases can be done by complete tenotomy, tendon Z-lengthening (common at the Achilles tendon), or lengthening of the aponeurosis of a muscle, which is often done for the iliopsoas or hamstrings (Figure 12–37).

It is convenient to combine multiple procedures for children with cerebral palsy. For example, a typical hemiplegic with a tiptoe (equinus) gait may benefit from lengthening the Achilles tendon to make the foot plantargrade. A typical diplegic patient with a crouching gait may benefit from hip flexor, hamstring, and Achilles tendon lengthenings performed bilaterally during a single operation. The exact timing and extent of surgery are controversial among experts in cerebral palsy. Three-dimensional computerized gait analysis, performed in motion laboratories, can guide the surgeon.

B. Muscle Release for Dynamic Deformity

Muscle releases for dynamic deformity may be done in several ways, depending on the specific muscle, the presence of contracture, and the surgeon's preference. The goal is to weaken spastic muscles to reduce their abnormal influence while not lengthening them so much that the opposite deformity occurs. The more common procedures are described here.

1. Achilles tendon lengthening—Achilles tendon lengthening is usually done by Z-lengthening of the distal tendon.

Cuts for Z-lengthening can be either open or percutaneous. The ankle is carefully dorsiflexed just beyond neutral to allow the tendon fibers to slide into an elongated position. The surgeon must avoid overlengthening (a matter of judgment) because an excessively weakened gastrocnemius-soleus group hinders walking and can actually encourage a deeper crouching gait.

2. Gastrocnemius lengthening—Gastrocnemius lengthening is required in patients whose gastrocnemius is considerably more spastic than the soleus. In such cases, ankle dorsiflexion is limited and ankle clonus occurs when the knee is extended, but free dorsiflexion occurs when the knee is flexed. In such patients, the gastrocnemius alone may be released by approaching the musculotendinous junction in the calf and sectioning the aponeurosis or by release of the insertion of the gastrocnemius where it attaches to the soleus and Achilles tendon. This effectively recesses the muscle, selectively weakening it while retaining soleus strength for pushoff during walking.

3. Hamstring lengthening—Hamstring lengthening is indicated when the hamstrings are tight (limited straight-leg raising) and knee flexion is persistent during the stance phase of gait (crouching gait). Usually, the distal medial and lateral hamstrings are released, but procedures vary widely among surgeons. On the medial side, the gracilis and semitendinosus tendons are usually Z-lengthened or tenotomized (transversely released). The semimembranosus is lengthened by transverse incision of its aponeurosis, which allows the interior muscle fibers to stretch and lengthen. Laterally, both heads of the biceps femoris can be managed by aponeurotic lengthening as well. The procedure must be done carefully to avoid cutting or stretching the sciatic or peroneal nerves. The leg is splinted or casted in extension for 3 to 4 weeks to allow soft-tissue healing.

4. Iliopsoas lengthening—The hip flexors (psoas and iliacus) may be released at the insertion of the conjoined tendon into the lesser trochanter, usually done in sitters also undergoing adductor release for spastic hip subluxation. If the child is walking and less weakening of hip flexion is desired, the psoas tendon alone can be sectioned at the level of the pelvic brim, retaining the iliacus portion of the muscle for strength.

Davids JR. Management of neuromuscular hip dysplasia in children with cerebral palsy. *J Pediatr Orthop.* 2018;38 (suppl 6):S21-S27. [PMID: 29877942]

Gordon GS, Simkiss DE. A systematic review of the evidence for hip surveillance in children with cerebral palsy. *J Bone Joint Surg Br.* 2006;88:1492-1496. [PMID: 17075096]

Muthusamy K, Chu HY, Friesen RM, Chou PC, Eilert RE, Chang FM. Femoral head resection as a salvage procedure for the severely dysplastic hip in nonambulatory children with cerebral palsy. *J Pediatr Orthop.* 2008;28:884-889. [PMID: 19034183]

Rutz E, Vavken P, Camathias C, Haase C, Jünemann S, Brunner R. Long-term outcome predictors in one-stage hip reconstruction in children with cerebral palsy. *J Bone Joint Surg Am.* 2015;97:500-506. [PMID: 25788307

Schwartz MH, Viehweger E, Stout J, Novacheck TF, Gage JR. Comprehensive treatment of ambulatory children with cerebral palsy: an outcome assessment. *J Pediatr Orthop.* 2004;24:45-53. [PMID: 14676533]

2. Myelomeningocele (Spina Bifida)

Myelomeningocele (or meningomyelocele) is a complex birth defect affecting the spinal cord and central nervous system. Although the cause is not fully understood, there is a hereditary component. Lack of maternal folic acid is identified as a causative factor in an estimated 50% to 70% of cases.

Embryologic Defect

The basic embryologic defect is a failure of complete tubulation and dorsal closure of the embryonic neural tube and placode, including incomplete closure of the skin over the spinal cord, resulting from lack of induction. In its mildest form, this spinal dysraphism consists of a simple spina bifida occulta or isolated meningocele (protrusion of spinal membranes, but not nerve, outside of the spinal canal, without neurologic deficit). The more severe varieties include herniation of membranes and nervous tissue through large dorsal bony and skin defects at birth and hydrocephalus with cerebral malformations (Figure 12–38).

Myelomeningocele can occur at any spinal level but usually is seen between levels T12 and S2. Because neural tissue

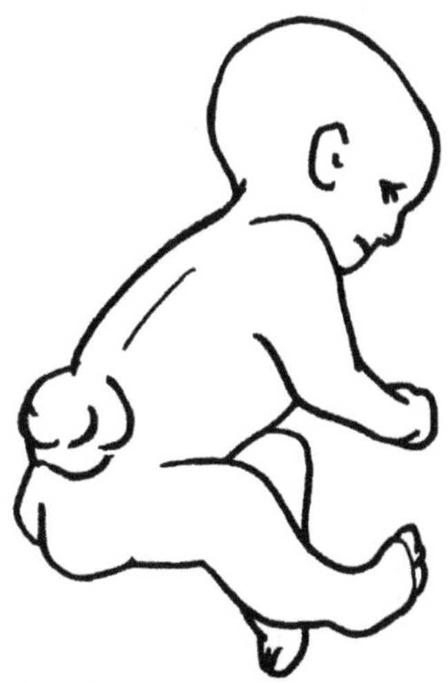

▲ **Figure 12–38.** Spina bifida (myelomeningocele). The sac includes dysplastic spinal cord and membrane elements, and it must be surgically closed in the first days of life. Hydrocephalus and congenital scoliosis are commonly associated.

Table 12–8. Muscle function at neurologic levels in myelomeningocele (spina bifida).

Neurologic Level	Functions	Muscles Active
T12	Hip flexion (weak)	Iliopsoas (weak)
L1	Hip flexion	Iliopsoas
L2	Hip adduction (weak)	Adductor longus, brevis (weak)
L3	Hip adduction Knee extension (weak)	Adductors Quadriceps (weak)
L4	Knee extension Ankle dorsiflexion	Quadriceps Anterior tibialis (variable)
L5	Knee flexion Hip abduction	Medial hamstring Tensor fascia lata
S1	Knee flexion Ankle plantar flexion	All hamstrings Gastrocnemius-soleus
S2	Toe flexion	Flexor digitorum longus

fails to form properly, the child is paraplegic and insensate below the level of the dysraphism. The clinical determination of neurologic level is most easily accomplished by describing the last muscles contracting under active voluntary motor control (Table 12–8). This may be difficult because of anatomic variability, the age of the child, and other central nervous system involvement.

Treatment of Orthopedic Problems

Orthopedic problems associated with myelomeningocele include clubfoot or congenital vertical talus, torsional deformities of the legs, contractures, hip dislocations, and scoliosis. The lack of sensation may allow extensive pressure sores to develop, or painless fractures may go undetected by patients. The health defects of children with spina bifida, in addition to their paralysis, usually include nonmusculoskeletal organ system problems such as hydrocephalus or Arnold-Chiari malformation (brain), syrinx formation or tethering (spinal cord), and neurogenic bladder or hydronephrosis (renal system). Early in life, most of these are more important than the orthopedic manifestations, and a team approach is needed to decide when and how best to coordinate management. The most pressing needs of the infant born with spina bifida are usually neural defect closure and ventricular shunting.

Orthopedic management depends on the deformities and the long-term mobility goals for the child. The level of paralysis often is helpful in determining whether the child will ultimately be able to walk (L5 or S1 function usually required) or will require a wheelchair (because of function only proximal to L4 or L5). Foot deformities such as clubfoot or congenital vertical talus usually require surgery. If foot deformities recur or progress, tethered cord should be suspected.

Spina bifida is theoretically a static neurologic disease, but many children exhibit a drifting deterioration of neurologic function as they grow; progression of foot deformities, especially during growth spurts, suggests tethering (and therefore stretching) of the cord. Hip dislocations, although dramatic on radiograph, frequently require no treatment; they are painless and tend to occur in children with neurologic involvement at L2 to L4, which precludes long-term walking.

A young child with scoliosis may require bracing until the thorax is long enough for spinal fusion. Scoliosis surgery is complicated by absent posterior neural arches. Some scoliosis seen with spina bifida is congenital (see section on scoliosis). If rapidly progressive scoliosis occurs, the physician should suspect a neurologic cause such as syrinx. Because of chronic exposure to latex materials in contact with mucous membranes and internal tissues (shunts, catheters), children with spina bifida are exceedingly susceptible to latex allergy, which can be fatal. Steps to limit latex exposure are essential in this population and must be observed by medical personnel working with them.

Bartonek A, Saraste H. Factors influencing ambulation in myelomeningocele: a cross-sectional study. *Dev Med Child Neurol.* 2001;43:253-260. [PMID: 11305403]

Centers for Disease Control and Prevention. Spina bifida and anencephaly before and after folic acid mandate—United States, 1995–1996 and 1999–2000. *MMWR Morb Mortal Wkly Rep.* 2004;53:362-365. [PMID: 15129193]

3. Muscular Dystrophy

Duchenne muscular dystrophy is an X-linked disorder that presents in boys 6 to 9 years of age. The disorder is one of progressive muscle weakness, usually first involving more proximal muscles of the limb girdles. Pseudohypertrophy caused by replacement of gastrocnemius muscles (or other muscles) with fat is a classic finding, as is Gower sign (an inability to rise from the floor without using the hands to "walk up" the body and legs). As the muscles weaken, imbalance can cause fixed flexion contractures of the hip, knee, and ankle plantar flexors, which limits walking ability. Because weakness eventually forces patients into a wheelchair, a decision to brace or correct these contractures surgically depends on estimates of remaining strength and likely duration of ambulation after treatment. Most often, progressive foot deformities (usually equinovarus) require muscle release and correction (including bracing) because use of the wheelchair also requires relatively well-positioned feet.

As weakness progresses, the child requires an electric wheelchair for mobility. At this point, scoliosis begins to appear and is usually relentlessly progressive. Attempts to control the scoliosis of muscular dystrophy by wheelchair inserts and braces are ineffective. Early surgery (before cardiorespiratory status deteriorates) is often the best answer. Chapter 13, "Rehabilitation," provides more information. Medical management of Duchenne muscular dystrophy has changed the orthopedic issues, and patients are living longer and with greater preservation of function.

4. Myotonic Dystrophy

Myotonic dystrophy is a genetic muscle disease whose name reflects the hallmark of the disease: myotonic EMG potentials. The disease is often associated with mild-to-moderate intellectual disability, obesity, and foot deformities. Initial diagnosis is made by identifying the characteristic myotonic face (weak perioral muscles with a distinctive pyramidal mouth), confirmed by EMG. Myotonic dystrophy worsens with each succeeding generation; genetic markers are available for diagnosis.

The most frequent foot deformity is equinovarus, often with weakness of the anterior tibialis and overactivity of the posterior tibialis. Surgery is often required, and recurrence requiring additional surgery is common. Surgical treatment of myotonic dystrophy foot deformities includes joint release (for passive correction of the deformity) and muscle transfers (for rebalancing muscle forces).

5. Spinal Muscular Atrophy

This heterogeneous group of disorders includes static and degenerative lesions of the anterior horn cell population in the spinal cord. These disorders all involve muscle weakness caused by a lower motor neuron lesion, that is, flaccid paralysis. Sensation is intact, and the major goals are mobility (with electric wheelchair), adaptive devices to aid in daily living (eg, feeding devices), and control of scoliosis, which is similar to management of scoliosis in advanced muscular dystrophy (see section on muscular dystrophy).

Apkon SD, Alman B, Birnkrant DJ, et al. Orthopedic and surgical management of the patient with Duchenne muscular dystrophy. *Pediatrics.* 2018;142(suppl 2):S82-S89. [PMID: 30275252]

King WM, Ruttencutter R, Nagaraja HN, et al. Orthopedic outcomes of long-term daily corticosteroid treatment in Duchenne muscular dystrophy. *Neurology.* 2007;68:1607-1613. [PMID: 17485648]

Mercado E, Alman B, Wright JG. Does spinal fusion influence quality of life in neuromuscular scoliosis? *Spine (Phila Pa 1976)* 2007;32(suppl 19):S120. [PMID: 17728678]

Voisin V, de la Porte S. Therapeutic strategies for Duchenne and Becker dystrophies. *Int Rev Cytol.* 2004;240:1-30. [PMID: 15548414]

6. Arthrogryposis (Arthrogryposis Multiplex Congenita)

Arthrogryposis is not a disease per se but rather a symptom complex that includes joint contractures or dislocations, rigid skeletal deformities (especially clubfoot), shiny skin with decreased wrinkling and subcutaneous tissue, weakness, and muscle wasting. Although many factors contribute to arthrogryposis, the common link among the symptoms appears to be decreased fetal movement during a critical period in limb development. This can be caused by neurologic lesions (congenital absence of anterior horn cells, Werdnig-Hoffman spinal muscular atrophy, myelomeningocele), myopathic lesions (myotonic dystrophy, congenital myopathies), various syndromes (Moebius syndrome), or physical restriction associated with oligohydramnios.

Arthrogrypotic infants frequently have extension or flexion contractures of knees and elbows, dislocated hips, and severe clubfeet. The contractures may partially resolve with passive ROM therapy in the first 6 to 12 months of life; however, they must be released surgically after that if they interfere with walking or arm use. Hip dislocations may not limit function and often are not treated. Clubfeet require surgery, which is often of limited success; multiple operations are frequently necessary. Arthrogrypotic children are generally highly resourceful in achieving mobility, and they care for themselves completely independently, despite seemingly overwhelming skeletal problems.

Bernstein RM. Arthrogryposis and amyoplasia. *J Am Acad Orthop Surg.* 2002;10:417-424. [PMID: 12470044]

Fassier A, Wicart P, Dubousset J, Seringe R. Arthrogryposis multiplex congenita. Long-term follow-up from birth until skeletal maturity. *J Child Orthop.* 2009;3:383-390. [PMID: 19669823]

Van Bosse HJP. Challenging clubfeet: the arthrogrypotic clubfoot and the complex clubfoot. *J Child Orthop.* 2019;13(3):271-278. [PMID: 31312267]

TUMORS

Skeletal neoplasms, particularly benign ones, are fairly common in children. Common benign bone lesions of childhood include osteochondroma, osteoid osteoma, unicameral (simple) bone cysts, chondroblastoma, hemangioma, histiocytosis X (eosinophilic granuloma), and fibrous dysplasia. Malignant tumors, which are usually seen after 10 years of age, include Ewing sarcoma and osteosarcoma. Certain systemic diseases can be manifested in childhood as apparent bone tumors (hyperparathyroidism, renal disease, leukemia). Chapter 5 offers a detailed discussion of bone tumors.

AMPUTATIONS

Congenital Amputations and Absence of Segments

Congenital absence of limb segments at birth can occur sporadically, as part of a syndrome (Streeter dysplasia) or as a result of mutagens (eg, thalidomide). Absence may be terminal (eg, congenital below-knee amputation) or intercalary (eg, congenital shortening or absence of the humerus).

Although congenital amputations can be dramatic in appearance, the missing limb is not part of the child's body image. Thus, the child has a natural instinct to be mobile. Children with severe limb deficiencies at birth are almost always able to be completely independent and functional. They accept prostheses quite readily but only if the device truly improves their efficiency. For example, nearly all congenital above-elbow amputees reject artificial limbs, opting for function over appearance. Parents may harbor strong feelings of guilt over the child's condition, so the psychological issues associated with the condition are more those of the adults than the child.

It is not unusual for congenital amputations to require conversion to a level more easily fitted with a prosthesis. For example, fibular hemimelia (severe shortening of the tibia with absent fibula and foot deformity) sometimes can be most effectively treated by removing the foot and converting the limb to an ankle disarticulation level. This facilitates prosthetic fitting and simplifies management of the leg-length discrepancy, thus permitting normal function.

Boostra AM, Rijnders LJ, Groothoff JW, et al. Children with congenital deficiencies or acquired amputations of the lower limbs: functional aspects. *Prosthet Orthot Int.* 2000;24:19-27. [PMID: 10855435]

Ephraim PL, Dillingham TR, Sector M, et al. Epidemiology of limb loss and congenital limb deficiency: a review of the literature. *Arch Phys Med Rehabil.* 2003;84:747-761. [PMID: 12736892]

Fixsen JA. Major lower limb congenital shortening: a mini review. *J Pediatr Orthop B.* 2003;12:1-12. [PMID: 12488764]

Klaassen Z, Shoja MM, Tubbs RS, Loukas M. Supernumerary and absent limbs and digits of the lower limb: a review of the literature. *Clin Anat.* 2011;24:570-575. [PMID: 21647959]

Traumatic Amputation

In contrast to the congenital amputee, the child with a traumatic amputation is particularly likely to be male, adolescent, rebellious, and troubled. Although pediatric traumatic amputations are often caused by inadvertent incidents, many result from high-risk behavior. These factors must be taken into account when dealing with the psychological issues of the patient and family; social, as well as medical, intervention is often appropriate.

The orthopedic management of traumatic amputees is modified in children by the presence of growth plates and the remarkable healing and rehabilitation powers of children. This must be considered during surgical completion of amputations because injury to the physis may cause severe shortening or angulation of a stump, rendering the amputation far less satisfactory than a similar amputation in the adult. The child amputee rarely has vascular problems, however, and the use of split-thickness skin grafting may allow preservation of length that would be impossible in most adults.

Overgrowth of Amputation Stump

Amputations through the long bones of children exhibit the unique phenomenon of terminal overgrowth. Eventually, the distal end of the stump may develop a long, thin, sometimes painful bony prominence. Overgrowth is not physeal in origin (ie, closure of the physis by epiphysiodesis does not eliminate its formation), and it appears to be related to aggressive bone formation associated with the periosteal membrane.

Although overgrowth can occur in any bone, it is most troublesome in the tibia, fibula, and humerus. When symptomatic, overgrowth is treated by resecting the spike of bone (revision of the amputation), but the process does continue, and recurrence is common. Some pediatric amputees require two or more surgical revisions during growth. Overgrowth ceases at skeletal maturity. Various attempts at capping the overgrowing bone end (using foreign materials or free epiphyseal grafts) have met with inconsistent success.

Jeans KA, Browne RH, Karol LA. Effect of amputation level on energy expenditure during overground walking by children with an amputation. *J Bone Joint Surg Am.* 2011;93:49-56. [PMID: 21209268]

Tenholder M, Davids JR, Gruber HE, et al. Surgical management of juvenile amputation overgrowth with a synthetic cap. *J Pediatr Orthop.* 2004;24:218-226. [PMID: 15076611]

FRACTURES

Common Pediatric Fracture Patterns

Many fractures in children are similar to their counterparts in adults. However, the added factor of growth contributes to the unique issues of fracture care in children. Pediatric bone is softer and more easily broken than adult cortical bone. Thus, the amount of energy required to produce a fracture is less in the child, even as soft-tissue injury is frequently less severe in the child than in the adult. In addition, the periosteal membrane in children is far thicker and more osteogenic than in adults. The periosteum is so leathery in immature humans that it frequently holds bone ends together, contributing greatly to stability and ease of manipulative reduction. The excellent osteogenic potential of pediatric periosteum permits rapid, aggressive fracture healing, so nonunions are extremely rare in children.

Less brittle pediatric bone is subject to fracture patterns unique to children (Figure 12–39). A greenstick fracture is a transverse crack that retains its continuity, just as a small moist twig breaks without actually snapping apart.

A torus fracture is a small buckle or impaction of one cortex with a slight bend on the opposite cortex. Plastic deformation is a change in the natural shape of a bone without a detectable fracture line.

Remodeling (gradual correction in alignment or size of a fractured bone back to normal) is generally far more rapid in children than in adults. Remodeling of angular deformities is particularly rapid when the deformity is in the same plane of motion as the nearest joint (Figure 12–40) or when the deformity is near a rapidly growing physis. Remodeling

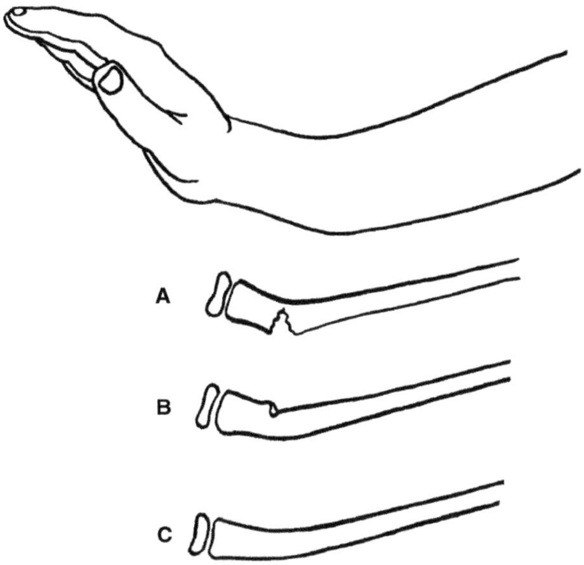

▲ **Figure 12–39.** Softer bone in children can lead to unique fracture behavior (in addition to the fracture patterns seen in adults). **A:** Greenstick fracture; **B:** torus fracture; **C:** plastic deformation.

of rotational deformities is less reliable. Overgrowth is a singular feature of remodeling that occurs in certain fractures of the long bones, particularly the femur. It is a product of physeal stimulation by the hyperemic response to fracture and healing and may increase the length of a bone by 2 cm or more over the course of a year.

The combination of low-energy injury, rapid bone healing, and dependable remodeling of angular deformity makes it possible to treat many pediatric fractures by simple closed reduction (often incomplete) and casting. Surgical management of children's fractures is rarely required. The surgeon may accept a less-than-perfect reduction if the fracture is known to remodel into satisfactory alignment.

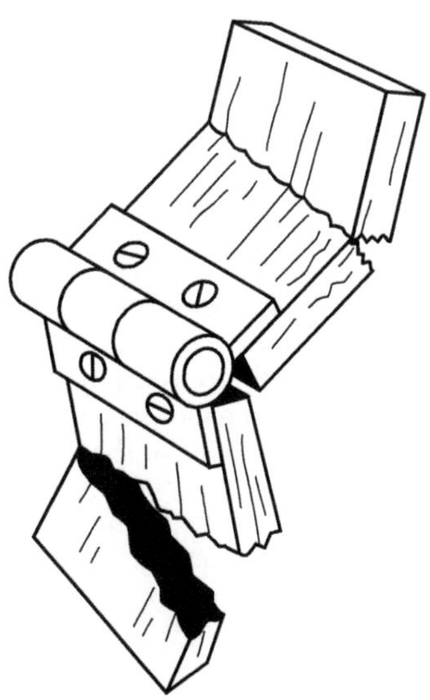

▲ **Figure 12–40.** Remodeling of bone after fracture is most rapid when it is in the plane of a nearby joint. Schematically, if the joint is thought of as a hinge, the fracture above (in the plane of the hinge) is likely to remodel faster than the fracture below the hinge (out of plane).

1. Epiphyseal Fracture

The cartilage physeal plates are a region of low strength relative to the surrounding bone and are susceptible to fracture in the child. They are analogous to a scratch on a pane of glass, in which concentrated force facilitates damage. Once injury occurs, the physis usually is able to recover and resume growth. But if an offset occurs in the physeal substance, bone may grow across it (from epiphyseal bone to metaphyseal bone), forming a bridge that anchors further growth and leads to either progressive shortening or a worsening angulation (Figure 12–41).

Because physes are near joints and physeal fractures are common, children may suffer injuries to joint surfaces that require careful surgical repair and realignment. Thus, open reduction is more likely in fractures involving physes and joints than in other pediatric fractures.

Most physeal fractures propagate through the weakest region of the cartilage. Physeal cartilage begins in a dense resting zone on the epiphyseal side, and chondrocytes gradually multiply, elongate, and arrange into longitudinal columns that produce longitudinal growth. Hypertrophic, balloon-like chondrocyte columns then undergo cell death, and the remaining cell walls are calcified and eventually ossify to form metaphyseal bone.

The weakest spot is usually the interface between hypertrophic dying columns of cells and the stiff calcified cell walls beneath them; this area is highly susceptible to shearing forces. So, physeal fractures (eg, Salter-Harris fractures) typically occur through the zone of hypertrophy. Fortunately, the region also represents the boundary between the process

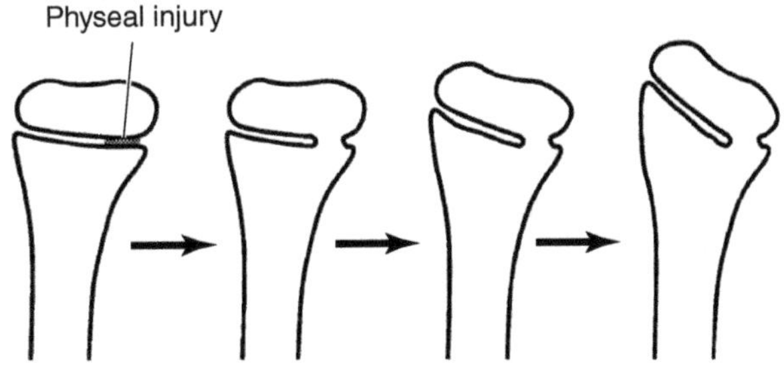

▲ **Figure 12–41.** Progressive angular deformity can occur if there is asymmetric closure of the physis after fracture.

of epiphyseal elongation (supported by the epiphyseal blood supply) and metaphyseal ossification (supported by the metaphyseal blood supply). Thus, physeal fractures do not often damage the growth potential of the physis because they do not interrupt its critical blood supply. An exception to the usual location of these fractures is the growth plate in the distal femur. It has an undulating topography, with prominences called mammillary bodies that interdigitate with other portions of the physis to provide stability at the distal femur. A typical distal femoral physeal fracture propagates through multiple layers of the growth plate. This results in displaced physeal fractures of the distal femur being at high risk for causing premature growth arrest of the involved physis and subsequent deformity.

Although physeal fractures can occur in a wide variety of configurations, certain patterns are seen frequently enough that a descriptive classification aids in understanding physeal injury (Figure 12–42). Fractures that either cross the joint or result in spatial malalignment of portions of the physis have the worst prognosis.

Physeal fractures heal rapidly, usually within 4 weeks. Careful monitoring is required to detect early posttraumatic closure of the growth plate. Occasionally, an epiphyseal-metaphyseal bony bridge forms and tethers growth. If this growth is minor, surgical removal of the bridge (epiphyseal bar resection) may successfully restore physeal growth. Otherwise, the procedures for evaluation and treatment of limb-length inequality should be followed (see previous section on limb-length inequality).

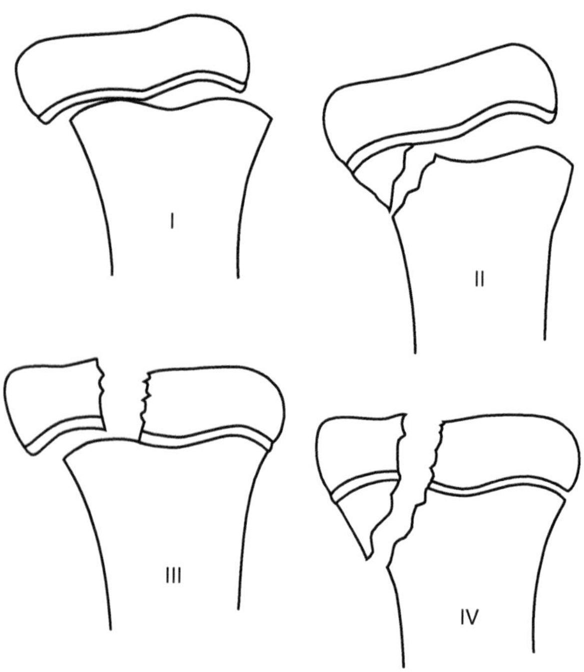

▲ **Figure 12–42.** The Salter-Harris classification of physeal fractures is widely used to describe such injuries. With some exceptions, the potential for problems with growth arrest is greater in the higher numbered patterns.

Salter RB, Harris WR. Injuries involving the growth plate. *J Bone Joint Surg Am.* 1963;45:587-622. [No PMID]

2. Upper Extremity Fractures

Clavicle Fracture

Clavicle fractures are among the most common injuries in children. They are usually closed and may be treated with a simple sling. Healing occurs rapidly with abundant callus, which leaves a lump that may concern parents. This enlargement remodels over several years of growth.

Clavicle fractures can occur at birth and heal rapidly but are sometimes accompanied by neurologic injury. Then, return of active biceps before 3 months and preservation of full passive shoulder ROM are predictors of a good outcome. Breech delivery is usually associated with preganglionic injury. Preganglionic injury can result in a Horner sign, which includes ptosis, miosis, and anhidrosis. Preganglionic injuries are unlikely to recover. The Moro reflex is elicited by dropping a baby's head a short distance and observing active elbow extension and fanning of the fingers, followed by elbow flexion and crying. Absence of the Moro reflex suggests a poor prognosis.

An extremely rare condition, atraumatic congenital pseudarthrosis of the clavicle can mimic the radiographic appearance of fracture. It may be right sided or bilateral, with little or no pain and no history of trauma. Treatment is generally unnecessary.

Proximal Humerus Fracture

Proximal humerus fractures are usually epiphyseal injuries (usually Salter-Harris type II injuries) that may progress into significant varus angulation (medial deviation). Fortunately, the proximal humerus is a rapidly growing physis and shoulder motion is full in all planes, so remodeling is rapid. These fractures generally require only a sling or shoulder immobilization for 3 to 4 weeks, without reduction. A hanging arm cast can be a form of portable gentle traction for fractures with moderate deformity or shortening. Rarely, fractures with extreme angulation (>90 degrees) may require surgical reduction and fixation.

Elbow Region Fracture

Most elbow region fractures are indirect injuries caused by a fall on the outstretched hand. Both diagnosis and treatment can be difficult in this serious group of injuries. Epiphyseal ossification is incomplete in the group that is susceptible

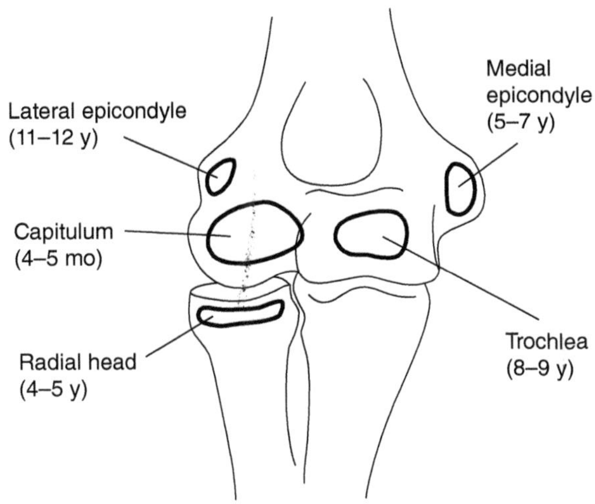

▲ **Figure 12–43.** Ages of appearance of ossification centers. The ossification centers of the elbow region emerge at different ages as indicated and can complicate the interpretation of radiographs. It is often advisable to obtain comparison radiographs of the opposite elbow if injury is suspected.

to falls (2-10 years of age), making radiographs difficult to interpret (Figure 12–43). Swelling, if severe, can block venous or arterial structures and lead to forearm compartment syndromes. Reductions are often unstable, and operative intervention may be required. Most surgeons immobilize pediatric elbow fractures for 4 weeks after treatment. The most important fractures are listed next.

A. Supracondylar Fracture of Humerus

Supracondylar fracture of the humerus occurs at the metaphyseal bone, proximal to the elbow joint, and does not involve the growth plate (Figure 12–44). Displacement may be severe, and nerve injury, usually caused by stretching, is common. If swelling is marked, there may be interruption of the blood supply; it is not uncommon for such a distal extremity to lack a pulse.

The most appropriate treatment is rapid anatomic reduction under general anesthesia. Because the reduction is highly unstable, most surgeons prefer to fix the fracture after reduction with percutaneous wires. Once the fracture is reduced, the swelling recedes rapidly and the pulse returns. On rare occasions, the surgeon must perform vascular or nerve exploration or repair.

Some displaced supracondylar humerus fractures are incompletely reduced or lose position because of fracture instability after apparently adequate initial reduction. This progresses to a characteristic malunion with an apex-lateral angular deformity of the elbow (known as cubitus varus or so-called gunstock deformity). Although cosmetically unsightly, cubitus varus rarely has any significant functional consequences. If desired, it may be corrected by valgus osteotomy at the old fracture site.

B. Lateral Condyle Fracture

The lateral condyle fracture is an oblique shearing fracture of the lateral portion of the joint surface that occurs when the radial head drives into the capitulum of the humerus during a fall. The lack of significant ossification may obscure the fracture or give the false appearance of a benign Salter-Harris II fracture pattern, but most lateral condyle fractures are highly unstable Salter-Harris IV fractures (Figure 12–45). Because both the joint surface and the physis are displaced, they usually require open reduction and fixation using pins.

C. Radial Neck Fracture

Fracture of the radial neck is similar to a lateral condyle fracture. The radial neck just distal to the joint may angulate up to 70 to 80 degrees, although lesser angulation is more common (Figure 12–46). It is important to determine the location of the radial head despite traumatic angulation of the radial neck. Surprisingly, angulation of 45 degrees or less usually remodels spontaneously and requires only symptomatic treatment that permits early return to activity. Larger degrees of angulation can often respond to closed manipulation.

D. Forearm Fracture

Forearm fractures are a common result of falls. If they involve both bones, one bone may be completely displaced while the other only bends or suffers a greenstick fracture. In children, most forearm fractures that involve both bones can be treated successfully by closed reduction and casting; minor angular malalignment can easily be tolerated if rotational alignment of the bone ends is accurate. In addition, the ends of fractured bones often overlap. This is not necessarily of concern if alignment is satisfactory because side-to-side bone healing and remodeling are rapid in children.

E. Monteggia Fracture

Monteggia fracture is fracture of the ulna only, with the radius remaining intact. Because two-bone systems generally must fail in two spots if they break at all, the radial head dislocates from the capitulum. In such cases, reduction must include the elbow component. As with other pediatric forearm fractures, closed reduction is usually successful, although some Monteggia fractures require open reduction. The physician should be alert to the possibility of Monteggia fracture because the fracture can lead to chronic loss of elbow motion if it is not properly reduced.

In children, Galeazzi fracture of the radius, in which the distal radioulnar joint is dislocated, is far less common than the analogous Monteggia fracture.

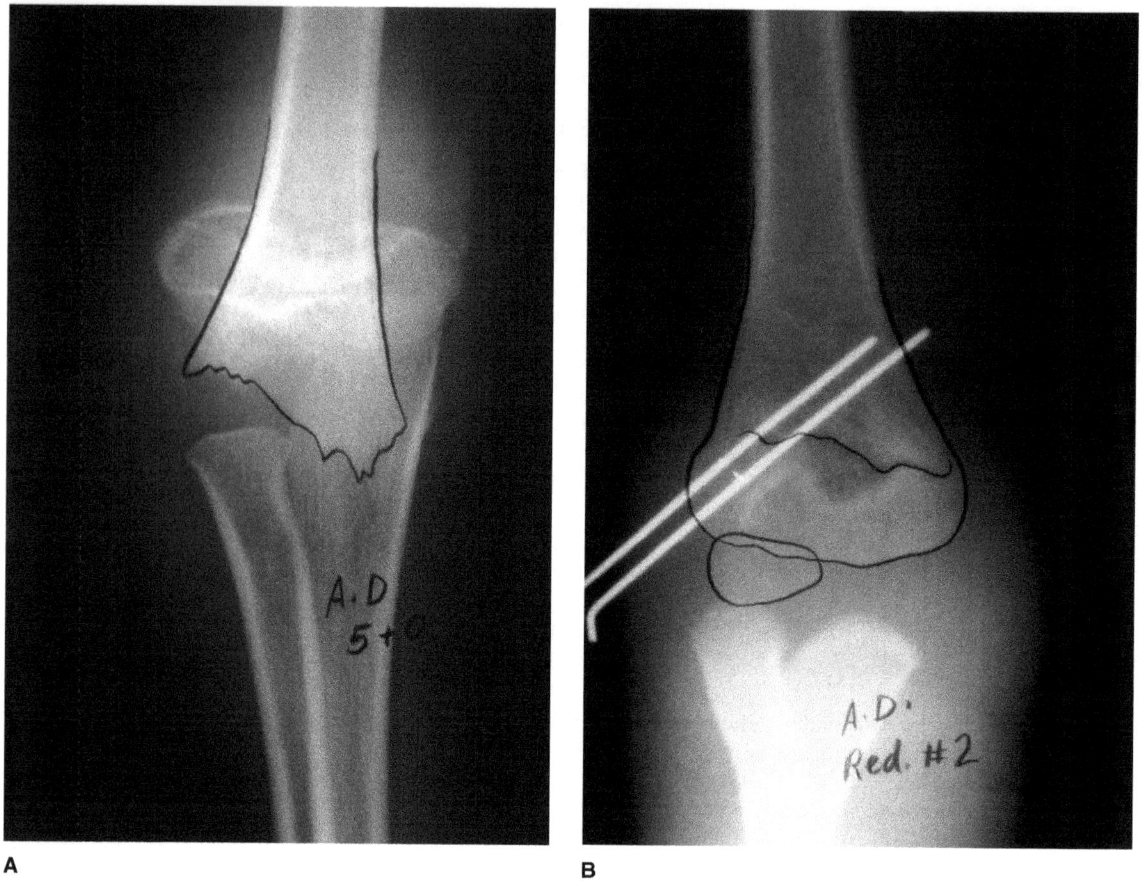

▲ **Figure 12–44.** Displaced supracondylar fracture of the humerus. Injury film **(A)**; after closed reduction and internal fixation using percutaneous pins **(B)**.

F. Torus Fracture of Radius

Torus fracture of the radius is a minor buckle of the dorsal cortex of the distal radius, usually 1 to 2 cm proximal to the distal radial physis. It occurs after a minor fall on the hand. Many torus fractures are mistaken for wrist sprains because they are stable and not as painful as unstable fractures. They heal uneventfully in 3 to 4 weeks, with excellent long-term results.

Crawford SN, Lee LSK, Izuka BH. Closed treatment of overriding distal radial fractures without reduction in children. *J Bone Joint Surg Am.* 2012;94(3):246-252. [PMID: 22298057]

Larson L, Firoozbakhsh K, Passarelli R, Bosch P. Biomechanical analysis of pinning techniques for pediatric supracondylar humerus fractures. *J Pediatr Orthop.* 2006;26(5):573-578. [PMID: 16932093]

Mirsky EC, Karas EH, Weiner LS. Lateral condyle fractures in children: evaluation of classification and treatment. *J Orthop Trauma.* 1997;11:117-120. [PMID: 9057147]

Price CT. The treatment of displaced fractures of the lateral humeral condyle in children. *J Orthop Trauma.* 2010;24:439. [PMID: 20577076]

Wattenbarger JM, Gerardi J, Johnston CE. Late open reduction internal fixation of lateral condyle fractures. *J Pediatr Orthop.* 2002;22:394-398. [PMID: 11961463]

Weiss JM, Graves S, Yang S, Mendelsohn E, Kay RM, Skaggs DL. A new classification system predictive of complications in surgically treated pediatric humeral lateral condyle fractures. *J Pediatr Orthop.* 2009;29:602-605. [PMID: 19700990]

▶ Metacarpal and Phalangeal Fractures

Fractures of the metacarpals and phalanges commonly occur from crush injuries in children (eg, catching a hand or finger in a door) and are generally quite stable because the periosteum remains intact. Rarely severely angulated or rotationally malaligned, they can usually be managed by immobilization for 2 to 3 weeks.

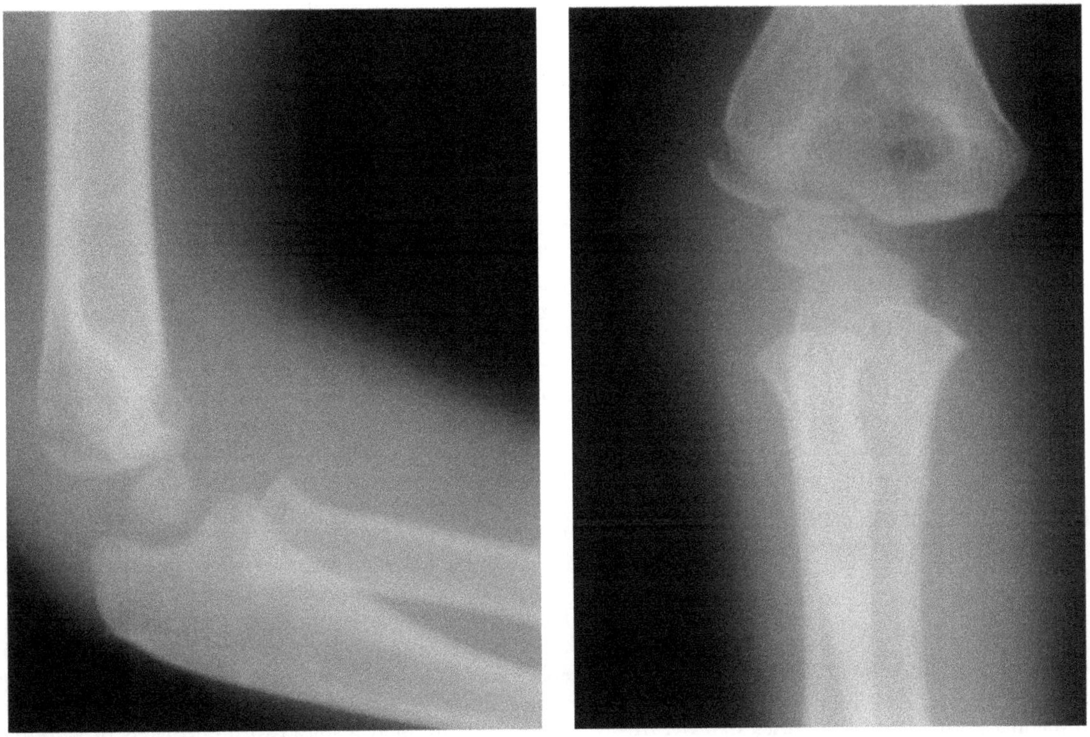

A

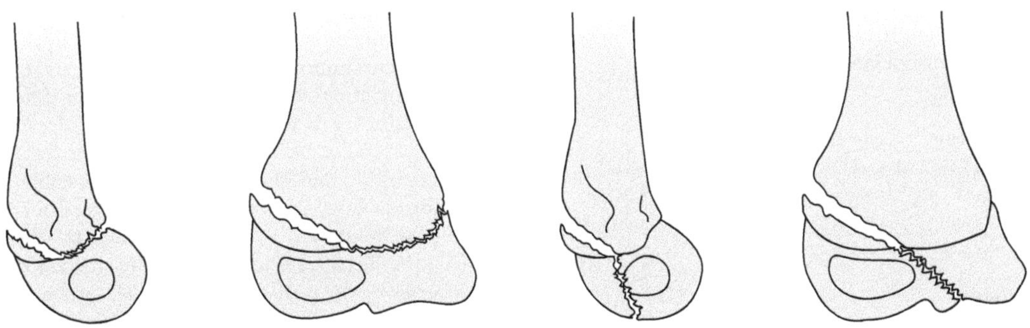

B C

▲ **Figure 12–45.** Lateral condyle fracture of the humerus **(A)** can easily be mistaken for a relatively simple Salter-Harris type II injury, which carries a good prognosis **(B)**. In reality, however, it is almost always a Salter-Harris type IV injury, with a fracture pattern crossing both the joint surface and the physis **(C)**; unless it is not displaced, it requires open reduction.

3. Lower Extremity Fractures

Pelvic Fracture

Pelvic fractures in children are usually seen in conjunction with major blunt trauma. Gross displacement is fairly uncommon and usually can be treated symptomatically because the intact periosteum stabilizes the large flat bones. The patient should be carefully evaluated for intraabdominal and other injuries. Properly treated pelvic fractures in an immature skeleton resolve satisfactorily.

Adolescents exhibit a special type of avulsion fracture of apophyses because aggressive pulling of muscles during sports can detach an apophysis from its parent bone. These avulsion fractures are sometimes called transitional fractures because the physes are in transition within 2 years of skeletal maturity. During this time, relatively weak cartilage physes may not be strong enough to withstand the

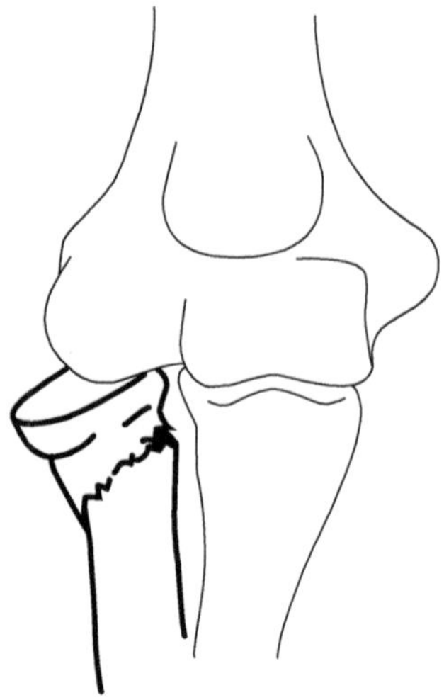

▲ **Figure 12–46.** Fracture of the radial neck may angulate greatly yet still remodel spontaneously in the younger child.

pull of growing muscles suddenly grown powerful under the influence of hormones. Transitional avulsion fractures may occur at the iliac crest (abdominal muscles), lesser trochanter of the femur (iliopsoas muscle), or ischial tuberosity (hamstring muscle). Transitional fractures of the pelvis and femur are treated symptomatically. Although these fractures do not require reduction, they may heal with a significant bump that requires excision later.

Tsirikos AI, Spiegel PG, Laros GS. Transepiphyseal fracture-dislocation of the femoral neck: a case report and review of the literature. *J Orthop Trauma.* 2003;17:648-653. [PMID: 14574194]

Hip Fracture

Pediatric hip fractures are rare but may be serious because trauma to this area may produce significant injury. As in the adult, the fracture pattern may disrupt the blood supply of the proximal femoral head and lead to avascular necrosis of the proximal femoral epiphysis, femoral neck, or both. In older children, this can be a devastating complication; it is treated like LCP but may result in such severe collapse that hip fusion is required.

Femoral neck fractures in children are highly unstable and treated by reduction and internal fixation. The mechanical fixation may be imperfect because the surgeon must avoid injury to the proximal femoral physis. For this reason, a spica cast (body and legs) is generally used as well.

Odent T, Glorion C, Pannier S, et al. Traumatic dislocation of the hip with separation of the capital epiphysis: 5 adolescent patients with 3–9 years of follow-up. *Acta Orthop Scand.* 2003;74:49-52. [PMID: 12635793]

Femoral Shaft Fracture

Fractures of the femoral shaft are common injuries caused by falls as well as bicycle and motor vehicle accidents. In young children, they may be the result of child abuse. Although most are closed injuries, blood loss can be significant because of bleeding into the soft tissues of the thigh. Nerve injury is rare, and the fact that the fracture is surrounded by richly nourished muscle ensures rapid solid union (usually within 6 weeks).

Longitudinal muscle pull and spasm cause femoral shaft fractures to shorten and angulate. Initial treatment requires longitudinal traction (skin traction in younger children, skeletal traction in older children) to restore length and alignment. At this point, treatment largely depends on the patient's age.

Femur fractures in children 4 years of age have a strong tendency to exhibit overgrowth of 1 to 2.5 cm because of fracture hyperemia. In this age group, therefore, it may be desirable to use a cast and allow some shortening to occur. Rapid remodeling of the bone makes perfect reduction unnecessary. Most surgeons apply a spica cast immediately or within the first week.

Most children between 4 and 10 years of age are no longer managed in spica cast or skeletal traction. Intramedullary fixation with flexible nails that avoid the femoral physes is most common. Open fixation with plates and screws, often so-called "bridge plating" with locking plates, is used for length unstable fractures. Fractures near the ends of the diaphysis or with long spiral or butterfly components are less optimal for flexible nailing and considered length unstable. Adult-type, piriformis entry nails are usually reserved for mature adolescents without even a femoral physeal scar. The medial femoral circumflex artery supplies blood to the femoral head. Its position along the posterior-superior femoral neck places this structure at risk with intramedullary nailing of the femur. Therefore, lateral entry through the greater trochanter is preferred when intramedullary fixation is performed.

After healing or cast removal, the child may begin walking. Limping is common in the first month after fracture because the hip girdle musculature regains its strength only slowly. No physical therapy is required, however, because normal walking permits spontaneous recovery, and long-term results of pediatric femur fractures are excellent.

Epiphyseal Separation

Epiphyseal separations (fracture) of the distal femoral physis are usually Salter-Harris type I or II injuries. All are caused by significant trauma, and injury to the growth mechanism of the plate is common. As many as 50% of cases exhibit subsequent growth arrest. Major neurovascular injury can occur, as with knee dislocations. Displaced epiphyseal separations require gentle reduction under general anesthesia. Some are so unstable, however, that they require percutaneous pin fixation for several weeks until the fracture is sticky, as it were, or healed enough so displacement does not occur. If physeal closure occurs, the treatment depends on age and remaining growth potential. (See earlier discussion of limb-length inequality.)

Tibial Eminence Injury

The tibial eminence (spine), located entirely on the proximal tibial epiphysis, is the site of attachment of the anterior cruciate ligament. Twisting injuries of the knee can shear off the eminence and may displace it within the joint. Most fractures occur in children ages 8 to 14 years, and they typically present with a painful hemarthrosis and refusal to bear weight. A type I fracture is minimally displaced, type II is anteriorly displaced with an intact posterior hinge, and type III is completely displaced. Long leg casting for 6 weeks, until the bone heals (Figure 12–47), is advocated for type I fractures, although there is debate about whether the knee should be maintained in full extension or in 10 to 20 degrees of flexion. Management of type II and III fractures is much more controversial. Type II fractures can be treated closed if adequate reduction can be achieved, but if not, surgical management is indicated. Surgery is also indicated for type III fractures. In these displaced injuries, the medial meniscus can be trapped under the fragment and/or the lateral meniscus; if the anterior cruciate ligament is still attached to the avulsed fracture fragment, this may cause pulling on the fragment and therefore block reduction. Unlike many other pediatric fractures, tibial eminence injuries often lead to mild long-term knee symptoms, especially during athletic activities.

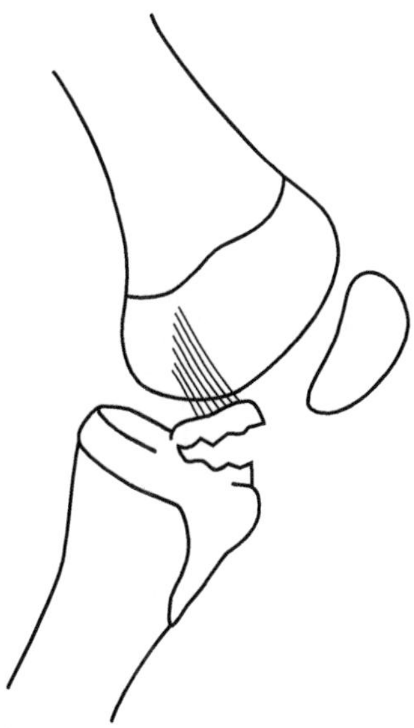

▲ **Figure 12–47.** Tibial eminence fracture usually includes an anterior cruciate avulsion component. It can be treated nonoperatively if the fragment reduces with extension of the knee.

Tibial Tubercle Avulsion Fracture

Tibial tubercle avulsion fractures are most often seen in adolescent males (13-14 years of age) who suffer sports-related injuries. The anterior tongue of the proximal tibial epiphysis is the site of attachment of the patellar tendon. During strenuous jumping, as in basketball, the tongue may avulse and displace. Tibial tubercle avulsions are transitional fractures in that they occur immediately before physeal closure and are not seen in younger children. They are classified as follows: type I, a small fragment of the tuberosity is avulsed and is displaced upward; type II, the whole tongue formed by the anterior aspect of the tibial epiphysis is hinged upward without being completely fractured at its base; and type III, the entire tibial tuberosity is fractured at its base, with the line of fracture directed proximally and posteriorly into the articular surface. Nearly all these fractures require open reduction and internal fixation, although the surgeon need not take the usual precautions when operating near the physis because maturity follows too rapidly to permit deformity. There is a high incidence of compartment syndrome seen in type III tibial tubercle fractures. Fasciotomy should be considered at the time of initial repair. Type III tibial tubercle fractures extending through the joint are often associated with meniscal injuries, which must be repaired. Delayed complications included recurvatum and refracture.

Proximal Tibial Metaphyseal Fracture

Proximal tibial metaphyseal fractures are usually undisplaced or minimally displaced. In the absence of fibular overgrowth (Figure 12–48), they can exhibit troublesome late angular deformity (valgus) caused by tibial overgrowth after fracture. The phenomenon is most pronounced at the age of maximum physiologic valgus (3-6 years). Over a number of years, the valgus has a tendency to remodel, so the best approach is observation.

Tibial Shaft Fracture

Tibial shaft fractures, which are usually accompanied by fibula fractures, generally result from major trauma. An exception is the nondisplaced, isolated spiral tibial fracture often seen after minor trauma in children just learning to

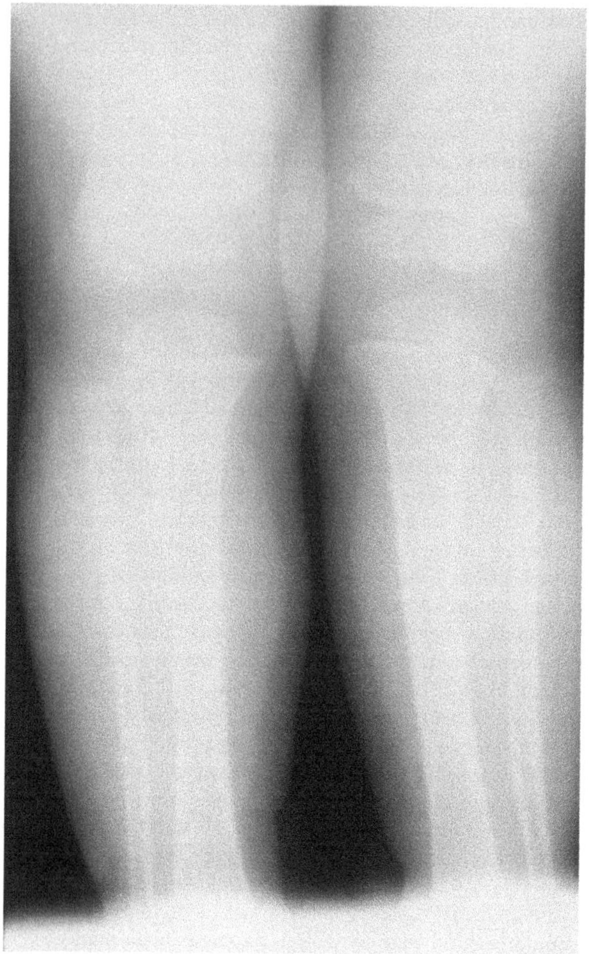

▲ **Figure 12–48.** Even when not displaced, fracture of the proximal tibial metaphysis can stimulate the tibial physis and cause progressive valgus deformity, especially in patients younger than 6 years. Long-term observation indicates that slow remodeling eventually occurs.

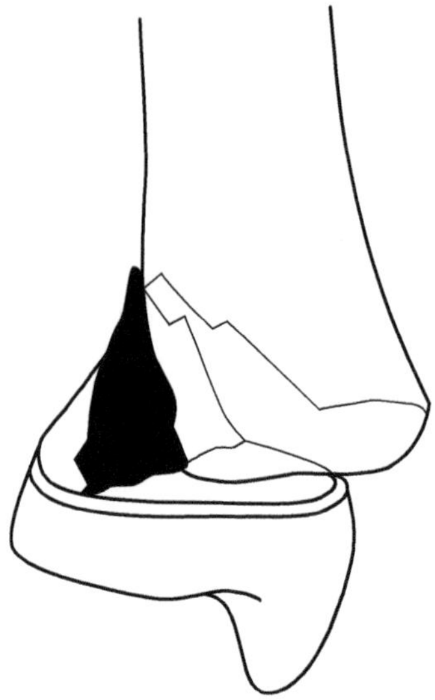

▲ **Figure 12–49.** Simple fracture of the distal tibia (and fibula) at the ankle is usually a Salter-Harris type II pattern in patients younger than 10 years.

walk (toddler's fracture). In the pediatric population, open tibia fractures are fairly common. As in the adult, injury to neurovascular structures and compartment syndromes are major risks (see Chapter 2, "Musculoskeletal Trauma Surgery"). Open fractures of the tibia and fibula require surgical debridement, but because skin loss is less likely than in the adult, they can often be managed the same way as closed fractures, following lavage.

Most tibial fractures in children can be adequately aligned and immobilized in above-knee casts. Rare, unstable cases, some open fractures, or fractures in older children also may require external fixation or other devices to maintain reduction and alignment. As in the adult, pediatric tibia fractures are relatively slow to heal, frequently requiring 10 to 12 weeks; nonunion is rare, however.

Ankle Fracture and Distal Tibial Fracture

Ankle fractures and distal tibial fractures in younger children are often either metaphyseal or Salter-Harris type II distal tibial physeal injuries that heal rapidly. These fractures have very little tendency to suffer growth arrest or other serious consequences (Figure 12–49). Posttraumatic physeal arrest occurs most commonly after injury in the distal medial tibia. In children 8 to 11 years of age, inversion injuries can push off the medial malleolus, causing an oblique Salter-Harris type IV fracture that disrupts both the joint and the growth plate. These fractures generally require open reduction for accurate realignment of the physis and articular surface. Subsequent growth arrest can cause a medial physeal bridge and produce a progressive varus deformity of the distal tibial articular surface as the lateral physis continues untethered elongation. If this occurs, either epiphyseal bar resection or corrective tibial osteotomy should be considered.

The distal tibia is the site of several distinct transitional fracture patterns. These physeal injuries occur only at the end of growth, shortly before complete distal tibial physeal closure at maturity. The distal physis begins early closure medially, with gradual lateral closure over the next year. The exact fracture pattern depends on how much of the plate is still open and on the force applied (ie, mechanism of injury).

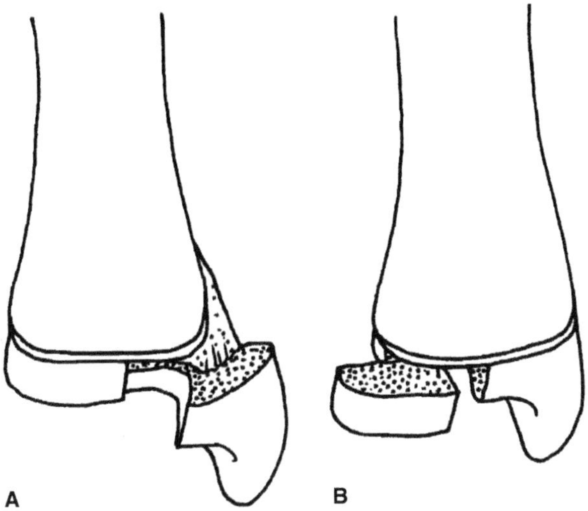

▲ **Figure 12–50.** The triplane **(A)** and juvenile Tillaux **(B)** fractures are variations of ankle fracture that occur in the adolescent shortly before physeal closure. Because they involve the joint surface, such fractures may require open reduction.

When just the medial physis is closed, a triplane fracture (ie, sagittal, transverse, and frontal) of the distal tibia occurs (Figure 12–50). This fracture contains a complex of fracture lines and crosses the growth plate. Triplane fractures usually require open reduction, although minimally displaced injuries can be managed nonoperatively. CT scans may be necessary to define the exact fracture configuration for accurate treatment.

In slightly older patients, when only a small anterolateral segment of the physis remains open, this anterolateral fragment can be avulsed by fibers of the distal tibiofibular syndesmosis (juvenile Tillaux fracture). This is a Salter-Harris type III fracture involving the articular surface and frequently requires open reduction to restore perfect joint anatomy.

Leary JT, Handling M, Talerico M, Yong L, Bowe JA. Physeal fractures of the distal tibia: predictive factors of premature physeal closure and growth arrest. *J Pediatr Orthop*. 2009;29:356-361. [PMID: 19461377]

Sink F, Faro F, Polousky J, Flynn K, Gralla J. Decreased complications of pediatric femur fractures with a change in management. *J Pediatr Orthop*. 2010;30(7):633-637. [PMID: 20864844]

Spiegel PG, Cooperman DR, Laros GS. Epiphyseal fractures of the distal ends of the tibia and fibula: a retrospective study of two hundred and thirty-seven cases in children. *J Bone Joint Surg Am*. 1978;60:1046-1050. [PMID: 721852]

INJURIES RELATED TO CHILD ABUSE

Child abuse crosses all socioeconomic boundaries and takes many forms. The musculoskeletal system is frequently the site of abuse-related injuries, but findings may be subtle or misleading. The most critical issue to consider in suspected abuse is whether the history can explain the injury adequately and believably.

The classic radiographic picture of abuse is the presence of multiple healing fractures of various ages; in the absence of a bone fragility syndrome, the diagnosis may thus be obvious (Figure 12–51). Soft-tissue injuries were found in 92% of children suspected of having been physically abused, with ecchymosis as the most common finding, increasing in incidence with age. Long bones (femur or humerus) are the

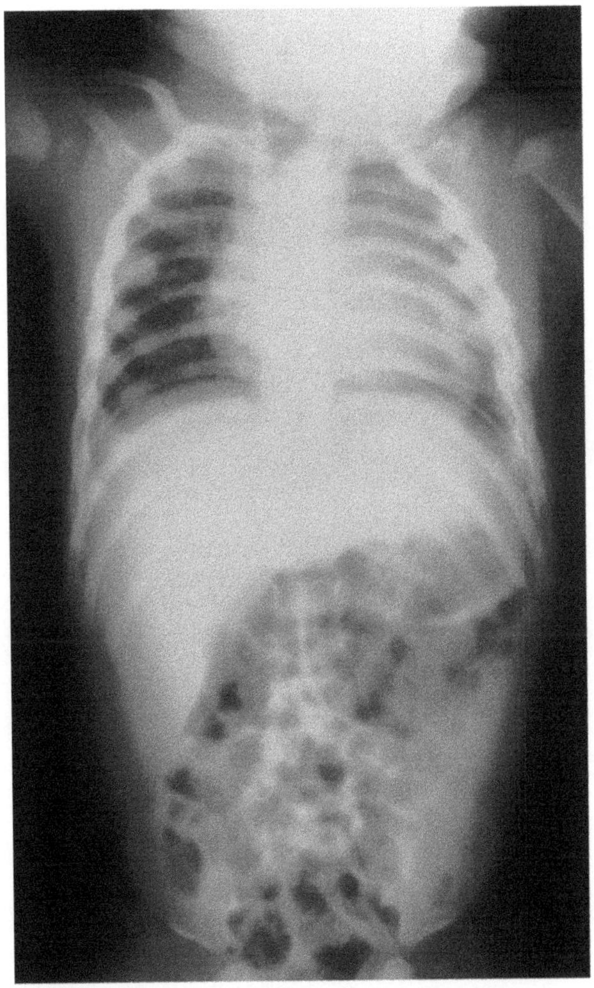

▲ **Figure 12–51.** The presence of multiple fractures of various ages as well as unexplained long-bone fracture in a young child should suggest the diagnosis of child abuse.

bones most commonly fractured during child abuse. These fractures are transverse or oblique shaft injuries, a common pattern that is not by itself diagnostic. The history is often one of a minor fall or a limb "catching" in the side of the crib. But studies of fractures in young children disclosed that injury mechanisms of this type are almost never the cause of serious skeletal injury, and the dichotomy between story and findings is highly suggestive of abuse. A good rule of thumb is to consider any long bone fracture in a child younger than 3 years as abuse until proved otherwise.

The orthopedic management of abuse fractures is rarely complex, and simple closed methods usually suffice. Nearly all such fractures carry an excellent prognosis and heal or remodel rapidly. It is the detection of the abuse, and its subsequent social management, that are the main determinants of outcome.

McMahon P, Grossman W, Gaffney M, et al. Soft-tissue injury as an indication of child abuse. *J Bone Joint Surg Am.* 1995;77:1179-1183. [PMID: 7642662]

Oral R, Blum KL, Johnson C. Fractures in young children: are physicians in the emergency department and orthopedic clinics adequately screening for possible abuse? *Pediatr Emerg Care.* 2003;19:148-153. [PMID: 12813297]

Rehabilitation

13

Mary Ann E. Keenan, MD
Patrick J. McMahon, MD

GENERAL PRINCIPLES OF REHABILITATION

Rehabilitation involves care of the injured person with either neurologic or musculoskeletal problems. It focuses on improving function through surgical and nonsurgical management and is recognized as an important part of the care of both acute and chronic problems. Rehabilitation programs address a variety of problems, including congenital or acquired musculoskeletal problems (eg, bone deformities, arthritis, or fractures) as well as neurologic trauma or diseases that affect limb function (eg, spinal cord injury [SCI], stroke, or poliomyelitis). Rehabilitation in these patients frequently involves increasing range of motion (ROM) and muscle strength, maximizing motor control, training individuals to make the most effective use of residual function, and providing adaptive equipment to minimize limb deformities.

The most successful model for rehabilitation addresses all the needs of the patient, including physical and emotional needs, and is based on a team approach. Among those frequently included in the team are physicians and nurses from various medical specialties, physical and occupational therapists, speech therapists, psychologists, orthotists, and social workers as well as patients and their family members. The shared goal of team members is to prevent barriers to rehabilitation by (1) diagnosing all current problems, (2) treating the problems adequately, (3) establishing adequate nutrition, (4) monitoring the patient for any complications that might impede progress in recovery, (5) mobilizing the patient as soon as possible, and (6) restoring function or helping the patient adjust to an altered lifestyle.

Management of Common Problems in Rehabilitation

Inadequate nutrition, decubitus ulcers, urinary tract infections, impaired bladder control, spasticity, contractures, acquired musculoskeletal deformities, muscle weakness, and physiologic deconditioning are common complications that can obstruct rehabilitation efforts and cause further loss of function in an already compromised patient. Because these problems are costly in both human and financial terms, every effort should be made to prevent them.

A. Inadequate Nutrition

Good nutritional status is a basis for avoiding many complications. After trauma, a patient's nutritional requirements are markedly increased from the normal maintenance requirement of 30 kcal/kg/day. Most trauma patients had been receiving intravenous fluids with minimal nutritional benefit and so arrive at the rehabilitation center in various degrees of malnutrition. Patients with chronic illnesses commonly have poor appetites. Physically handicapped people expend much of their energy performing simple activities of daily living (ADLs) and may also have difficulty in obtaining and preparing adequate amounts of food. Poor nutrition is often overlooked in obese patients. Individuals with high body mass index (BMI) can become malnourished after trauma. In addition, inactivity leads to diminished calorie needs, but boredom may result in increased consumption of an unbalanced diet in which certain nutrients are lacking.

B. Decubitus Ulcers (Pressure Sores)

The combination of poor nutritional status, lack of sensation at pressure points of the body, and decreased ability to move can cause decubitus ulcers (Figure 13–1) and greatly add to a patient's discomfort and the length and cost of their hospital stay. The ulcer is a potential source of sepsis in an already compromised individual. And for a severe sacral decubitus ulcer, for example, it may be necessary to have surgery to rotate a flap graft to cover the defect. This in turn requires the patient to remain prone until the graft heals and significantly hampers the patient's participation in a rehabilitation program because mobility and ability to interact with others are hindered. Prevention is the best treatment. The clinical rule

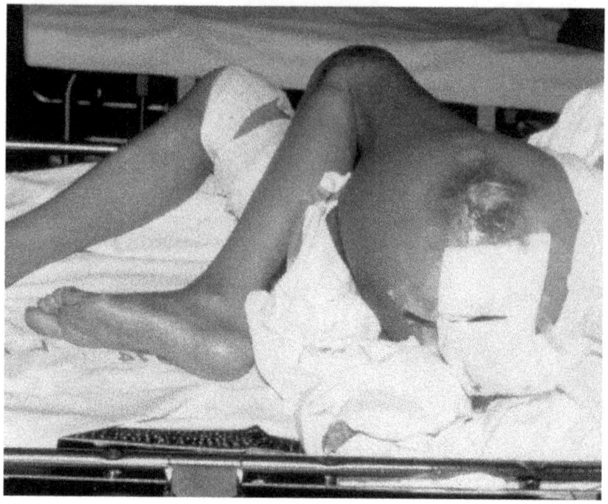

▲ **Figure 13–1.** Patient with contractures and a decubitus ulcer over the greater trochanter of the femur.

of protecting the patient's skin is to change position every 2 hours. No cushion alone can prevent decubitus ulcers.

C. Urinary Tract Infections and Impaired Bladder Control

Urinary tract infections are a common source of sepsis and prolonged illness. An indwelling catheter is the most frequent source. In an acutely ill or multiply injured patient, an indwelling catheter may be necessary for medical reasons but should be removed as soon as possible. Urinary incontinence is not sufficient reason for continued use of an indwelling catheter. In male patients, incontinence can be managed with a carefully applied condom catheter. Care must be taken to inspect the penis frequently for signs of skin maceration or pressure. In female patients, diapering and frequent linen changes suffice.

Restoring bladder function to achieve adequate reflex voiding or a balanced bladder may require the use of an intermittent catheterization program. The basis of a balanced bladder program is that the volume of residual urine not exceed a third of the volume of voided urine. In general, an intermittent catheterization program is initiated if the residual volume is greater than 100 mL or if the voided volume exceeds 400 mL. The patient is catheterized every 4 hours initially and then every 6 hours for 24 hours, and the patient is reassessed. Good records are necessary throughout the program.

D. Muscle Weakness and Physiologic Deconditioning

During sustained exercise, the metabolism is mainly aerobic. The principal fuels for aerobic metabolism are carbohydrates and fats. In aerobic oxidation, the substrates are oxidized through a series of enzymatic reactions that lead to the production of adenosine triphosphate (ATP) for muscular contraction. A physical conditioning program can increase the aerobic capacity by improving cardiac output, increasing hemoglobin levels, enhancing the capacity of cells to extract oxygen from the blood, and increasing the muscle mass by hypertrophy.

Prolonged immobilization of extremities, bed rest, and inactivity lead to pronounced muscle wasting and physiologic deconditioning in a short time. Because disabled patients generally expend more energy than normal individuals in performing routine ADLs, they must be mobilized as quickly as possible to prevent unnecessary physiologic decline and subsequent decline in abilities. They should also be placed on a daily exercise program to maximize muscle strength and aerobic capacity.

E. Spasticity

Patients with spasticity exhibit an excessive response to the quick stretch of a muscle, which leads to hyperactive deep tendon reflexes and clonus. Spasticity must be managed aggressively to prevent permanent deformities and joint contractures.

1. Spasmolytic drugs—Drugs can be of some assistance in controlling spasticity associated with upper motor neuron diseases. Drugs are used when spasticity affects multiple large muscle groups in the body and when the spasticity is not severe.

Baclofen (Lioresal) can inhibit both polysynaptic and monosynaptic reflexes at the spinal cord level. It does, however, depress general central nervous system function. Use of oral baclofen should be avoided in traumatic brain-injured patients, when possible, because it may cause sedation and impede cognitive recovery. Patients with attention deficits or memory disorders may be compromised by antispastic agents, such as diazepam and clonidine, which, like baclofen, have sedating properties. Tizanidine (Zanaflex) affects the central nervous system less than other agents and may be useful.

Baclofen pump technology has an advantage over oral drug therapy because of the small concentrations that can be introduced intrathecally. The small intrathecal doses control spasticity effectively while minimizing central nervous system side effects. The pump is placed in a subcutaneous pocket in the abdominal wall. A catheter is routed subcutaneously from the intrathecal space to the pump. The pump can be refilled by injection into the reservoir chamber. The dosage and rate of administration can be easily adjusted by using a laptop computer that sends radio signals to the pump.

Dantrolene (Dantrium), another drug that can be used to control spasticity, is the drug of choice for treating clonus. Dantrolene produces relaxation by directly affecting the contractile response of skeletal muscle at a site beyond the myoneural junction. It causes dissociation of the excitation–contraction coupling probably by interfering with the release of calcium from the sarcoplasmic reticulum. Although it does not affect the central nervous system directly, it does cause drowsiness, dizziness, and generalized weakness, which may interfere with the patient's overall function. Use of dantrolene for the control of spasticity is indicated in upper motor neuron diseases, such as SCI, cerebral palsy, stroke, or multiple sclerosis. The most serious problem with use of dantrolene is hepatotoxicity. The risk appears greatest in females, in patients older than 35 years, and in patients taking other medications. When using dantrolene, the lowest effective dose should be used, and liver enzyme functions should be monitored closely. If no effect is noted after 45 days of use, the drug should be stopped.

2. Casts—Casting temporarily reduces muscle tone and is frequently used to correct a contracture. The cast is changed weekly until the problem is corrected. If a cast must be used for a prolonged period, the patient should be placed on anticoagulant therapy to prevent deep venous thrombosis.

3. Splints—Anterior and posterior clamshell splints can be used to control joint position and still allow for active and passive ROM of the joints in therapy. A splint applied to only one side of an extremity is not sufficient to control excessive spasticity and may result in skin breakdown from motion against the splint. A splint can also obscure an early contracture.

4. Phenol and botulinum blocks—Ultrasound can be used to more accurately locate the nerves for injection.

A. Nerve-blocking agents—Anesthetic and phenol nerve blocks are often combined with a casting or splinting program. Anesthetic nerve blocks are commonly used to eliminate muscle tone temporarily. They can be used diagnostically to evaluate what portion of a deformity is dynamic (occurring because of muscle spasticity) and what portion is static, secondary to myostatic contracture. The block can also be prognostic of the likely results of surgical neurectomy or tendon lengthening. Repeated blocks of local anesthetics have a carryover effect to decrease muscle tone.

When muscle spasticity requires control for an extended period of time but the patient still has potential for spontaneous improvement, a phenol nerve block may be indicated. Phenol exerts two actions on the nerves. The first is a short-term effect, similar to the effect produced by a local anesthetic and directly proportional to the thickness of the nerve fibers. The second is a long-term effect that results from protein denaturation. Although this leads to wallerian degeneration of the axons, experimental studies in animals show that the nerves regenerate with time. In patients, the direct injection of a nerve with a 3% to 5% solution of phenol after surgical exposure gives relief of spasticity for up to 6 months. Mixed nerves containing sensory fibers should not be injected because it could cause unwanted sensory loss or painful dysesthesia. Reduction of spasticity for up to 3 months can also be achieved by the percutaneous injection of muscle motor points with an aqueous solution of phenol after localization using a needle and nerve stimulator (Figure 13–2).

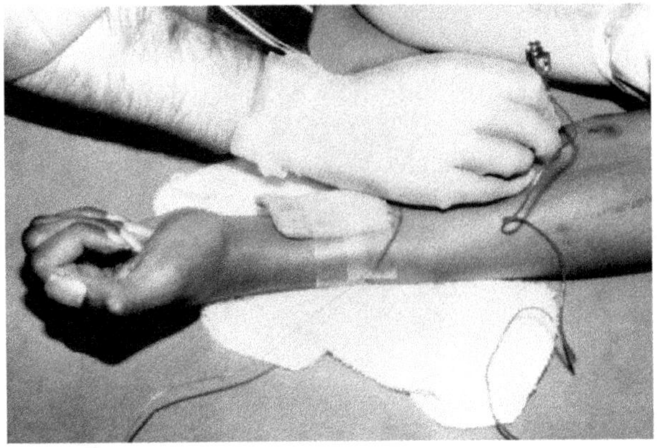

▲ **Figure 13–2.** Use of a Teflon-coated needle and nerve stimulator to locate the motor points of spastic forearm muscles for phenol injection.

B. Botulinum toxin—Ordinarily, an action potential propagating down a motor nerve to the neuromuscular junction triggers the release of acetylcholine (ACh) into the synaptic space. The released ACh causes depolarization of muscle membrane. Botulinum toxin type A is a protein produced by *Clostridium botulinum* that attaches to the presynaptic nerve terminal and inhibits the release of ACh at the neuromuscular junction. Botulinum toxin A is injected directly into a spastic muscle with clinical benefit of 3 to 5 months. Current practice is to avoid administering a total of more than 400 U in a single treatment session to avoid excessive weakness or paralysis. This upper limit of 400 U may be reached rather quickly when injecting a few large muscles. A delay of 3 to 7 days between injection and the onset of clinical effect is typical. Because the patient does not see effects immediately, a follow-up visit is usually arranged to check the result. Because botulinum toxin A is the most potent biologic toxin known and the cost is relatively high, the smallest possible dose should be used to achieve results. Most studies report side effects in 20% to 30% of patients per treatment cycle. The incidence of adverse effects varies based on the dosage used (ie, the higher the dose, the more frequent the adverse effects); however, the incidence of complications is not related to the total dose of botulinum toxin used. Local pain at the injection site is the most commonly reported side effect. Other adverse effects such as local hematoma, generalized fatigue, lethargy, dizziness, flulike syndrome, and pain in neighboring muscles are also reported.

5. Surgical procedures—If muscle spasticity is permanent and no change in muscle tone is anticipated, definitive procedures such as dorsal rhizotomy, peripheral neurectomy, tendon lengthening or release, and tendon transfer should be considered.

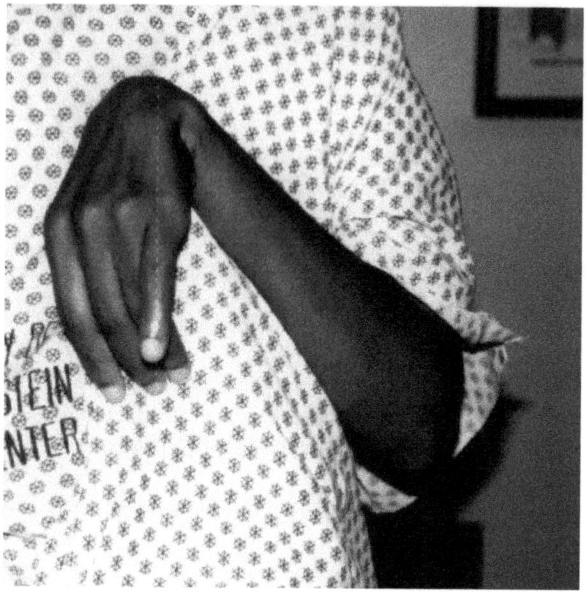

▲ **Figure 13–3.** Upper extremity contractures in a patient with untreated spasticity.

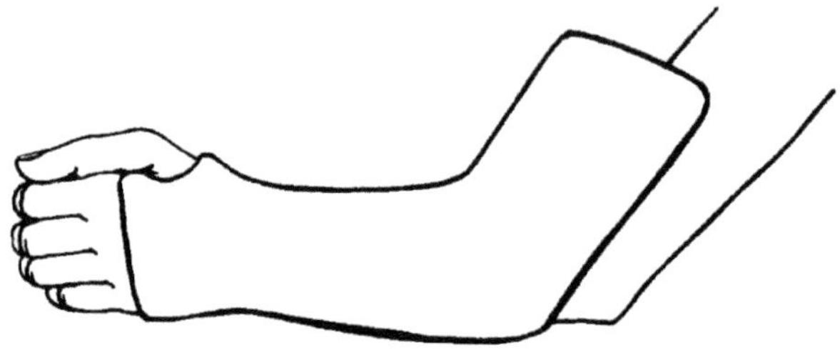

▲ **Figure 13–4.** An elbow dropout cast used to increase elbow extension while preventing flexion.

F. Joint Contractures

Inactivity and uncontrolled spasticity often lead to joint contractures (Figure 13–3), which are difficult to correct and greatly extend the needed rehabilitation program. Contractures may cause difficulties in positioning in a bed or chair or problems in using orthotic devices. They can also cause difficulties with hygiene and skin care and increase the risk of decubitus ulcers. Shoe wear may be rendered impossible because of foot deformities.

Muscle weakness is accentuated by contractures and malalignment, which cause the muscle to function at a mechanical disadvantage. Sitting and standing balance are compromised when contractures abnormally displace the center of gravity relative to the base of support. Functional use of the extremities is severely limited by lack of adequate joint motion. Joint contractures may require surgical release, which could further decrease function in an already compromised individual. Moreover, in children, joint contractures can lead to structural changes in the skeleton. Muscle growth lags behind skeletal growth, and this discrepancy in growth rates can cause increasing deformity with time.

To prevent contractures, exercises to maintain ROM must be performed several times daily. The patient, family members, therapists, and nursing personnel should all participate in this task.

Splinting can help maintain joints in a functional position when motor control is lacking. Splints should be removed regularly to inspect the skin condition and reassess their efficacy in maintaining the desired position.

Treatment of established contractures can be time consuming and expensive. In general, if a contracture is present for less than 3 months, it may be amenable to nonsurgical methods of correction such as serial casting or electrical stimulation of the antagonist muscles. Excessive muscle tone must be treated aggressively if present because it accentuates the tendency to form contractures. An anesthetic nerve block can be given to eliminate excessive tone temporarily and provide analgesia prior to manipulation of the joint and application of a cast. Each week, the cast is removed, a nerve block is given, and a new cast is applied. When the desired limb position is obtained, a holding cast is used to maintain the position for an additional week. The cast can then be bivalved and made into anterior and posterior clamshell splints, which can be removed for ROM or other activities. Another useful technique is the application of a dropout cast (Figure 13–4), which allows for further correction of the contracture while preventing the original deformity from recurring.

When contractural deformities are long standing and fixed, surgical release is indicated. Tendons, ligaments, and joint capsules are all involved. If the deformity is severe, complete correction at the time of surgery may be impossible. Neurovascular structures must be protected from excessive traction. Serial casts or dropout casts may be necessary following surgery to gain the desired limb position.

G. Other Acquired Musculoskeletal Deformities

Paralysis or weakness of trunk muscles can lead to scoliotic deformities of the spine. When severe, these deformities can impair respiratory function and tend to cause balance problems with walking and sitting. External support in the form of bracing or seating modifications can minimize or eliminate this.

Disuse and lack of muscle tone lead to osteoporosis, which in turn predisposes patients to fractures. The fractures should be treated aggressively and in a manner that maximizes function rather than prolongs immobilization.

Peripheral nerve palsy can result from pressure secondary to decreased mobility in patients confined to a bed or chair. Pressure can also result from braces, splints, and casts, and these require careful monitoring. In patients who form heterotopic ossification (HO), which is the presence of lamellar bone in nonskeletal tissue, the new bone formation and the accompanying inflammation may impinge on peripheral nerves, thereby causing nerve palsy.

Evaluation of Impairment

A. Nerves

Many disabilities requiring rehabilitation result from diseases affecting the nervous system. The location and the extent of the primary lesion determine not only the degree of injury but also the extent to which motor control is impaired and spasticity is present. In injuries or diseases of the peripheral nerves, the damage is confined to the lower motor neurons. Normal motor control is preserved, spasticity is absent, and the magnitude of disability depends on the extent of paralysis and weakness (paresis). In pathologic conditions of the brain or spinal cord, the upper motor neurons are affected, which not only causes muscular weakness but also impairs motor control.

Motor activity can be considered as a hierarchic system of voluntary and involuntary neurologic mechanisms.

1. Voluntary muscle activity—Two types of voluntary muscle activity are clinically identifiable: selective and patterned movements. The highest level of motor activity, selective movement, depends on the integrity of the cerebral cortex. Selective movement is the ability to flex or extend one joint preferentially without initiating a mass flexor or extensor motion at other joints of the limb. Patterned movement (synergy) at a joint refers to the ability to move one joint by invoking a mass flexion or extension synergy involving movement at other joints of the limb. Patients with central nervous system disorders may have voluntary patterned movement but lack selective movement. Because most patients have mixtures of selective and patterned movement at different joints, however, the strength of each type of activity must be assessed at each joint. Patterned flexion and extension movements of the lower limb can provide sufficient motor control for ambulation, but patterned motion does not provide sufficient fine control for upper extremity function.

2. Involuntary muscle activity—Spasticity relates to two types of involuntary muscle activity: clonic and tonic responses. Each type depends on the sensitivity of the muscle spindle to the rate of stretch. If a muscle is quickly extended above the threshold of the velocity-sensitive receptors of the spindle, a phasic response may be elicited. If spasticity is severe, sudden stretch may trigger clonus, which consists of repeated bursts of phasic activity at 6 to 8 cycles per second. The phasic stretch response has practical clinical significance. For example, if an ankle equinus deformity is present and spasticity is severe, clonus of the triceps surae may be triggered in the stance phase each time the patient takes a step. A rigid ankle-foot orthosis (AFO) that blocks ankle motion and prevents the triceps surae from stretching may inhibit clonus, enabling the foot to be held in a neutral position. An articulated or flexible AFO that allows the ankle to move and the triceps surae to stretch may not prevent clonus from being elicited and may be less effective.

If the muscle is stretched slowly below the threshold of the velocity components of the spindle, a phasic response is not triggered, but the spindle is still capable of detecting changes in length that may generate a tonic response consisting of continuous muscle hypertonus. The tonic muscle activity during slow stretch is called **clasp-knife resistance**. This tonic activity is also of practical significance. Even if the ankle is slowly dorsiflexed for a prolonged time, hypertonus may persist in the triceps surae and restrict normal motion. Consequently, it may be necessary to differentiate spasticity from myostatic contracture by performing peripheral nerve blocks.

Patients with injury involving the brainstem may exhibit severe hypertonus that is continuously present and is called either **decerebrate rigidity** or **decorticate rigidity**, depending on the posture of the limbs. In decerebrate posturing, the patient's arms are held tightly flexed while the legs are held in extension. In decorticate posturing, both the upper and lower extremities are in rigid extension. Patients with severe muscular rigidity are at extreme risk of developing contractural deformities.

When a spastic patient is sitting or standing, labyrinthine activation increases tone in the extensor muscles of the lower extremity and also increases upper limb flexion. Consequently, patients who are examined for spasticity should be evaluated in the upright rather than supine position to elicit the maximal stretch response. Conversely, patients who are examined for maximal ROM should be evaluated in the supine position to minimize muscle tone and enable maximal joint range. The limb posture of patients also influences the intensity of reflex and voluntary activity.

3. Sensory perception—The final steps of sensory integration occur in the cerebral cortex, where basic sensory data are integrated into the more complex sensory phenomena. When central nervous system injury involves the cerebral cortex, the patient responds to basic modalities of touch and pain. Responses to tests of more complex aspects of sensation (eg, shape, texture, and proprioception) and two-point discrimination may be impaired, however. These simple tests quickly determine the patient's ability to interpret basic sensory information. Patients with absent proprioception across the major lower joints have balance abnormalities or are unable to walk. Most patients do not routinely use an affected hand unless proprioception is intact. Patients without lesions of the cerebral cortex can generally discriminate between two points less than 10 mm apart applied simultaneously to the fingers.

B. Muscles

Manual muscle testing is often useful for evaluating an individual's ability to perform functional tasks and also

Table 13–1. Muscle strength.

Grade	Strength	Description
0	Absent	Muscle does not contract.
1	Trace	Muscle contracts, but no motion is generated.
2	Poor	Muscle contraction produces movement, but muscle cannot function against gravity.
3	Fair	Muscle functions against gravity.
4	Good	Muscle can overcome some outside resistance as well as gravity.
5	Normal	Muscle can overcome resistance to motion.

documents progress made in the rehabilitation program. Several systems are currently used, but all are based on the grading system introduced by Robert Lovett in 1932. The evaluation is subjective, but the use of gravity resistance provides a measure of objective standardization (Table 13–1). A normal muscle grade as determined by manual testing does not always imply normal strength. A significant amount of weakness (a 25%-30% loss of strength) must be present to be detected by this method.

C. Gait

1. Normal gait—Normal gait is the combination of postures and muscle activities that produce forward motion with minimal energy expenditure (Figure 13–5).

A. SWING PHASE—The swing phase (Figures 13–5 and 13–6) is divided into three equal periods: initial swing, midswing, and terminal swing. During the three-part phase, the pelvis rotates from backward to forward and the hip flexes 20 to 30 degrees. The knee flexes to 60 degrees initially and then extends in preparation for contact with the ground. The knee flexion is largely responsible for the foot clearing the ground during swing. Knee flexion occurs as the result of the forward momentum of the limb swinging and not as a result of hamstring contraction. The ankle joint initially plantarflexes 10 degrees and then assumes a neutral position during terminal swing so that the heel normally contacts the floor first.

The hip flexor muscles provide the power for advancing the limb and are active during the initial two-thirds of the swing phase. The ankle dorsiflexors become active during the latter two-thirds of the phase to ensure foot clearance as the knee begins to extend. The hamstring muscles decelerate the forward motion of the thigh during the terminal period of the swing phase.

B. STANCE PHASE—The stance phase (Figures 13–5 and 13–7) accounts for 60% of the gait cycle and can be divided into five distinct activities: initial contact, the loading response, midstance, terminal stance, and preswing. At initial ground contact, the ankle is in neutral position, the knee is extended, and the hip is flexed. The hip extensor muscles contract to stabilize the hip because the body's mass is behind the hip joint. During the loading response, the knee flexes to 15 degrees, and the ankle plantarflexes to absorb the downward force and conserve energy by minimizing the up-and-down movement of the body's center of gravity. As the knee flexes and the stance leg accepts the weight of the body, the quadriceps muscle becomes active to stabilize the knee. In midstance, the knee is extended, and the ankle is in a neutral position. As the body's mass moves forward of the ankle joint, the calf muscles become active to stabilize the ankle and allow the heel to rise from the floor. In terminal stance, the heel leaves the floor, and the knee begins to flex as momentum carries the body forward. In the final portion of terminal stance, as the body rolls forward over the forefoot, the toes dorsiflex at the metatarsophalangeal joints. During preswing, the knee is flexed to 35 degrees and the ankle plantarflexes to 20 degrees. Because the opposite extremity is also in contact with the floor, the preswing is called the time of double-limb support.

Throughout the stance phase, the hip gradually extends and the pelvis rotates backward. During the first portion of the stance phase, the ankle dorsiflexors and hamstring muscles remain active. During the loading response and early midstance, the gluteus and quadriceps muscles become active to provide hip and knee stability. In midstance, the gastrocnemius and soleus muscles become active to stabilize the ankle joint and control the forward advancement of the tibia. This allows the heel to rise from the floor and the body weight to roll forward over the forefoot.

2. Abnormal gait—The study of movement (kinesiology) provides many important tools for evaluating patients with gait abnormalities. Among the areas of study are stride analysis, motion analysis (kinematics), force analysis (kinetics), and muscle activity analysis.

Three of the many specialized tools used in these studies are dynamic electromyography (EMG), force plate studies, and motion analysis. Dynamic EMG, which records the electrical activity in multiple muscles simultaneously during functional activities, elucidates the patterns of motor control in both the upper and the lower extremities and helps in the management of spasticity and gait abnormalities. Force plate studies, which measure ground reaction forces and the fluctuations of the center of pressure, can be used to analyze gait problems and quantify balance reactions in impaired patients. Motion analysis uses multiple cameras located at different positions around the room. The cameras detect sensors placed on the patient and create a three-dimensional model of the patient moving through space.

Muscle strength can be accurately measured using torque, which can be correlated with joint position. Joint stiffness can also be assessed by measuring torque while moving the joint through a passive arc of motion. Joint powers can be calculated by multiplying joint moment times angular velocity.

	SWING 40%			STANCE 60%				
	Initial swing	Mid-swing	Terminal swing	Initial contact	Loading response	Mid-stance	Terminal stance	Pre-swing
	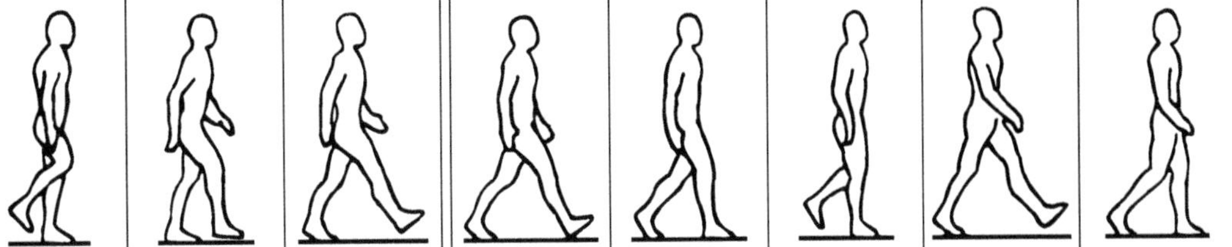							
TRUNK	Erect neutral	Erect neutral	Erect neutral	Erect neutral	Erect neutral	Erect neutral	Erect neutral	Erect neutral
PELVIS	Level: backward rotation 5 degree	Level: neutral rotation	Level: forward rotation 5 degree	Level: maintains forward rotation	Level: less forward rotation	Level: neutral rotation	Level: backward rotation 5 degree	Level: backward rotation 5 degree
HIP	Flexion 20 degree Neutral rotation abduction adduction	Flexion 20 degree-30 degree Neutral rotation abduction adduction	Flexion 30 degree Neutral rotation abduction adduction	Flexion 30 degree Neutral rotation abduction adduction	Flexion 30 degree Neutral rotation abduction adduction	Extending to neutral Neutral rotation abduction adduction	Apparent hyperext 10 degree Neutral rotation abduction adduction	Neutral extension Neutral rotation abduction adduction
KNEE	Flexion 60 degree	Flexion 60 degree-30 degree	Extension to 0 degree	Full extension	Flexion 15 degree	Extending to neutral	Full extension	Flexion 35 degree
ANKLE	Plantar-flexion 10 degree	Neutral	Neutral	Neutral heel first	Plantar-flexion 15 degree	From plantar-flexion to 10 degree dorsiflexion	Neutral with tibia stable and heel off prior to initial contact opposite foot	Plantar-flexion 20 degree
TOES	Neutral	Neutral	Neutral	Neutral	Neutral	Neutral	Neutral IP extended MP	Neutral IP extended MP

▲ **Figure 13–5. The normal gait cycle.** (Reproduced, with permission, from American Academy of Orthopaedic Surgeons. Home study syllabus. In Heckman JD, ed. *Orthopaedic Knowledge Update*, I. Rosemont, IL: American Academy of Orthopaedic Surgeons; 1984.)

Measurement of velocity, stride length, cadence, and single- and double-limb support times can be combined with dynamic EMG, force plate studies, and joint goniometric recordings to present a complete analysis of gait dysfunction. These studies can also be used to assess the influence of surgery, orthotic corrections, or prosthetic design on gait characteristics.

D. Oxygen Consumption and Aerobic Capacity

Perhaps the most important measurement for understanding the difficulties faced by disabled people comes from oxygen consumption studies. Oxygen consumption indicates the energy required to perform an activity. Measuring an individual's maximal aerobic capacity is the single best indicator of the level of physical fitness.

1. Effects of disease and aging on energy expenditure— Cardiorespiratory disease, anemia, muscle atrophy, and any other condition that restricts oxygen uptake cause a decrease in the maximal aerobic capacity. Even in a healthy person, 3 weeks of bed rest decreases maximal aerobic capacity by up to 30%.

During normal walking, the rate of energy expenditure by adults varies from approximately 30% to 45% of the maximal

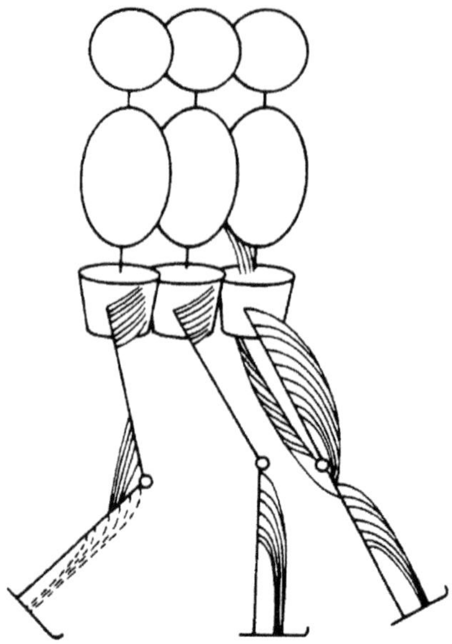

▲ **Figure 13–6.** Swing phase of gait. (Reproduced, with permission, from American Academy of Orthopaedic Surgeons. Home study syllabus. In Heckman JD, ed. *Orthopaedic Knowledge Update*, I. Rosemont, IL: American Academy of Orthopaedic Surgeons; 1984.)

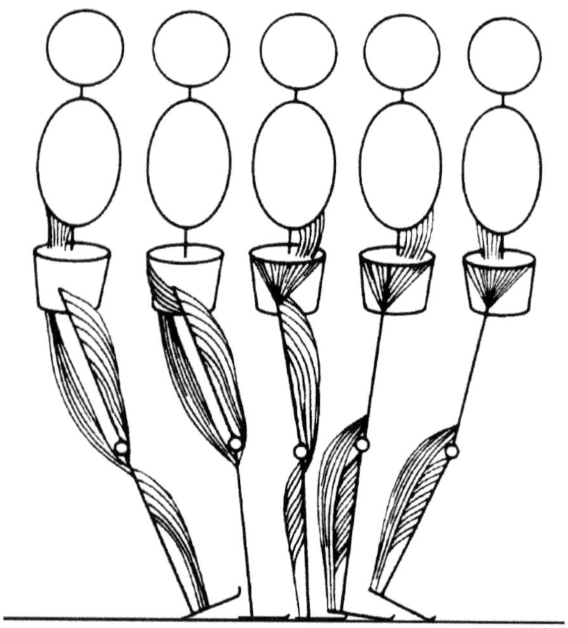

▲ **Figure 13–7.** Stance phase of gait. (Reproduced, with permission, from American Academy of Orthopaedic Surgeons. Home study syllabus. In Heckman JD, ed. *Orthopaedic Knowledge Update*, I. Rosemont, IL: American Academy of Orthopaedic Surgeons; 1984.)

aerobic capacity, with the higher percentage being in people over 60 years. Because of the decline in maximal aerobic capacity with age, an older person is more susceptible than a person under 50 to 60 years of age to the penalties of a gait disability.

2. Effects of exercise on energy expenditure—When exercise is performed at less than 50% of an individual's maximal aerobic capacity, the exercise can be continued for prolonged periods because the ATP needed for muscle contraction is provided by aerobic pathways. Anaerobic pathways of ATP production, which do not use oxygen, increasingly come into play when exercise is performed at work rates exceeding approximately 50% of maximal aerobic capacity. The amount of energy that can be delivered by anaerobic metabolism is limited, and fatigue ensues because of the accumulation of lactate in the muscle. Consequently, the normal ADLs and work that must be performed throughout an 8-hour day, including walking, are performed below anaerobic threshold.

3. Effects of musculoskeletal impairment on energy expenditure—Gait abnormalities that interfere with efficient, coordinated limb movement can increase energy demand. Some affected patients respond to this increased demand by working harder, which increases the output of physiologic energy and is reflected in the higher-than-normal heart rate and oxygen consumption rate. Rather than increasing the rate of energy expenditure, however, most patients slow their gait velocity in an effort to keep the power requirement from exceeding normal limits.

Among amputees, patients progressively walk slower at increasingly more proximal amputation levels. Younger patients with traumatic or congenital amputations walk faster than older dysvascular amputees because of their greater maximal aerobic capacity. Children with a Syme amputation, transtibial amputation, or knee disarticulation walk with the same speed and energy expenditure as control children. Children with bilateral amputations, unilateral transfemoral amputation, or unilateral hip disarticulation walk at a lower speed, higher heart rate, and higher energy expenditure. Patients with limited joint movement or with arthritis and painful joints also reduce their gait velocity. The heart rate and energy expenditure rate do not exceed normal in any of these groups of patients if crutches are not required.

Patients requiring crutches and exerting considerable force to support the body often have high heart rates and energy expenditure rates. A swing-through, crutch-assisted gait in a paraplegic or a patient who has a fracture and is unable to bear weight on one leg requires strenuous physical exertion, which is why few paraplegics use swing-through gait and why older patients with fractures can ambulate for only short distances. Even patients who use a reciprocal gait pattern, such as patients with low lumbar paraplegia resulting from SCI or myelodysplasia, use their arms for considerable exertion. Consequently, these types of patients may also be restricted ambulators in the community.

Patients with hip and knee flexion deformities caused by fixed or dynamic contractures require increasing muscle effort not only to walk but also to maintain an upright posture because the center of gravity during stance passes farther away from the axis of rotation of the joint. The fact that knee flexion greater than 30 degrees significantly increases the energy expenditure rate points to the importance of preventing and correcting contractures.

Children who have cerebral palsy and diplegia and who walk in a crouch gait may have energy expenditure rates that are above the anaerobic threshold. This is why these children are restricted ambulators who frequently discontinue walking when they mature and their maximal aerobic capacities decrease.

Use of Orthoses

Orthotic (brace) prescription plays a vital role in rehabilitation. The clinician must understand the functional needs of the patient and provide the orthotist with an exact prescription that specifies the materials, type of joints, joint position, and ROM. Brace prescriptions should not be left to the discretion of the patient and orthotist.

A temporary orthosis may be used in an early stage of illness until a definitive, custom-fitted orthosis is fabricated. Definitive orthoses for the lower extremity are the below-knee AFO and the above-knee knee-ankle-foot orthosis (KAFO).

The bichannel adjustable ankle-locking (BiCAAL) type of AFO may be used as the first orthosis following stroke, head trauma, spinal injury, or other condition that causes extensive muscle imbalance about the foot and ankle (Figure 13–8). A rigid ankle is useful in controlling plantarflexion spasticity, stabilizing the ankle in a flaccid limb, and correcting a dynamic varus deformity (inversion of the foot). The adjustable ankle joint mechanism enables the clinician to determine the optimal ankle position in the acute period following onset of illness when the neurologic picture and orthotic requirement are changing. The use of plastic materials in lower extremity orthotics is now widespread. Orthoses fabricated from plastics are light, comfortable, and attractive. A plastic AFO can be rigid or can be flexible allowing motion at the ankle. Polypropylene is presently the most practical plastic material. Skillful fitting is critical because of the close skin and bone contact. A moderately flexible carbon fiber AFO (Figure 13–9A) is lighter weight and is used more often than a plastic (polypropylene) orthosis (Figure 13–9B) once neurologic recovery stabilizes.

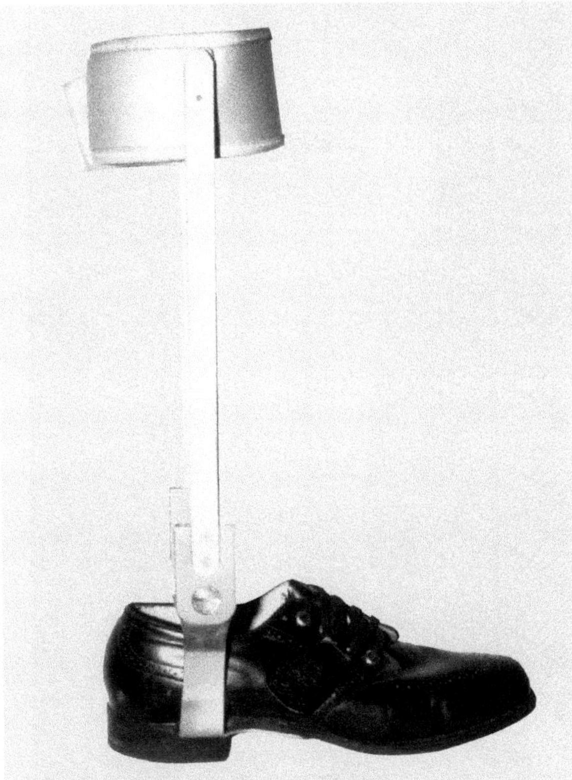

▲ **Figure 13–8.** The bichannel adjustable ankle-locking (BiCAAL) type of ankle-foot orthosis.

A. Ankle-Foot Orthosis

1. Types—Of several currently available orthoses classified as limited-motion ankle joint orthoses, two are commonly used: the conventional metal, double-upright, single-adjustable ankle joint with dorsiflexion spring assist (Klenzak) and the molded plastic posterior shells made from 116-inch polypropylene. The use of plastic materials makes the latter design preferable for most patients. When a greater restriction of ankle motion is desired, rigidity can be attained in several ways: by using a thicker sheet of polypropylene, by extending the lateral trim lines farther anteriorly at the ankle to serve as side struts, by adding an anterior shell to the posterior shell and totally enveloping the ankle, or by stiffening the posterior shell with the use of carbon fiber or lamination techniques. The trim lines may be reinforced with metal or additional layers of plastic. The foot plate of the orthosis extends just proximal to the metatarsal heads. Total circumferential orthoses combining anterior and posterior shells require exceptionally careful fitting to avoid excessive skin pressure over bony prominences. They are not recommended for routine use.

Insertion of a polypropylene or carbon fiber orthosis inside a shoe generally requires a shoe size that is a half size larger and wider than that previously worn by the patient. To eliminate the need to purchase two pairs of shoes of different sizes, an inlay can be inserted in the shoe of the sound limb to prevent excessive looseness once a shoe is fitted on the polypropylene side. The ankle position of the polypropylene orthosis should be assessed with the patient wearing his or her shoe with the normal heel height.

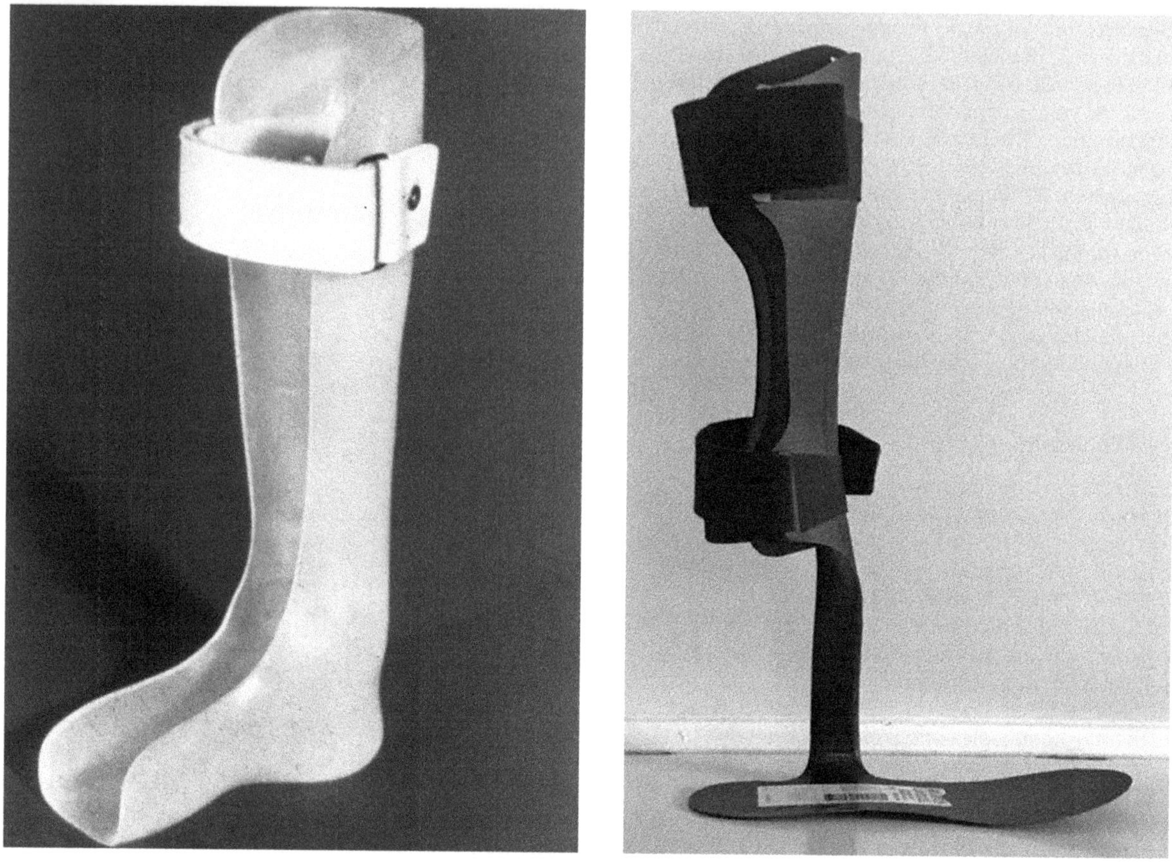

▲ **Figure 13–9. A:** A moderately flexible ankle-foot. **B:** The molded polypropylene ankle-foot orthosis.

2. Indications—The primary requirement for orthotic support is that all joints must be passively capable of being positioned in adequate alignment. An orthosis cannot correct a fixed bony deformity or fixed joint contracture.

a. Inadequate dorsiflexion for foot clearance during swing—An AFO is indicated for inadequate toe clearance (footdrop) during the midswing phase of gait. This problem may result from inadequate ankle dorsiflexion caused by weakness of the dorsiflexors or by the inability of dorsiflexors to overcome spasticity of the triceps surae. A lightweight, flexible polypropylene orthosis is indicated if inadequate dorsiflexion is the only problem at the ankle. A flexible orthosis can also be used for a mild swing-phase varus deformity (foot inversion). A rigid orthosis is needed in patients who have excessive plantarflexion resulting from severe spasticity and in patients who initiate a strong extensor pattern activity prior to heel strike.

b. Inadequate dorsiflexion for initial contact—A patient with inadequate dorsiflexion, from any cause, contacts the ground with the forefoot or with the foot flat and the tibia extended backward. This problem is commonly combined with varus deformity, and weight bearing is on the lateral edge of the foot. The results are a backward thrust to the limb, which decreases forward momentum and produces excessive hyperextension forces on the knee, which leads to knee instability in the patient who is a functional walker. A rigid AFO in the neutral position results in heel strike for the patient who has full-knee extension and allows the tibia to rotate forward during stance.

c. Medial-lateral subtalar instability during stance—Varus deformity is more common than valgus deformity. The patient walks on the lateral border of the foot and is hesitant to accept weight on the leg. A rigid orthosis can correct the varus deformity unless spasticity is severe. To correct a mild varus deformity, a limited ankle orthosis may be used. No orthosis is effective in controlling the severe spastic varus deformity.

d. Inadequate tibial stability during stance—Some patients have inadequate strength or control of the plantarflexors for maintenance of normal tibial position and alignment during stance. Early after midstance, this problem is manifested by excessive dorsiflexion and accompanying knee flexion. Whether or not the limb collapses during weight bearing depends on the amount of quadriceps muscle control and strength. Patients with sufficient proprioception learn to compensate by locking the knee in hyperextension as the foot contacts the floor, which keeps the knee from buckling. A rigid orthosis that prevents both dorsiflexion and plantarflexion is indicated to provide vertical tibial alignment during midstance. Its use prevents tibial collapse during terminal stance as a substitution for adequate calf control.

A knee extension thrust, caused by inadequate calf control as described earlier, may result also from severe plantarflexion tone or fixed equinus deformity resulting from contracture. At foot strike, the forefoot strikes the floor first, resulting in a knee extension or hyperextension thrust. A rigid AFO with a plantarflexion block prevents the development of knee instability and pain.

A T-strap (a leather T-shaped strap attached to the brace at the ankle and applied around the ankle to hold the foot from either an inverted or everted position) is usually not desirable for correction of severe varus deformity in patients fitted with metal orthoses. If a T-strap is applied with sufficient force to provide significant control to prevent foot twisting, it usually causes excessive pressure over the lateral malleolus in the patient with severe spasticity. This problem can be treated better by the use of a split anterior tibial tendon transfer or by the addition of a lateral wedge and flare to the shoe of the nonsurgical candidate.

B. Knee-Ankle-Foot Orthosis

A KAFO may be used if quadriceps muscle weakness or hamstring muscle spasticity is present. A knee immobilizer may be used as a training aid before having a KAFO fabricated. A KAFO is more difficult to don than a below-knee brace, and most patients with a central nervous system disease such as stroke or cerebral palsy have difficulty walking with a KAFO. Consequently, if hamstring spasticity rather than quadriceps spasticity necessitates external support to align the knee in extension, it is preferable to perform hamstring tenotomy or tendon lengthening, thereby eliminating the need for knee support.

Most patients with lower extremity quadriceps paresis resulting from SCI lack sufficient proprioception to walk with a free-knee mechanism (unlocked knee joint mechanism) when a KAFO is prescribed for quadriceps paresis. Then, it is necessary to determine if the knee will be locked while walking or if it will be freely movable to allow knee flexion in swing. When a KAFO is prescribed because of knee instability or because of varus or valgus instability, a polycentric joint (a joint in which the center of rotation moves following the anatomic instantaneous center of rotation) permits flexion extension movement but blocks medial and lateral angulation. A posterior stop added to the knee mechanism prevents excessive hyperextension.

If proprioception is intact, as is the case with poliomyelitis, even patients with considerable quadriceps weakness may be able to walk with an unlocked knee using an offset knee joint. This is accomplished by careful orthotic alignment. The center of rotation of the orthosis is positioned anterior to the center of rotation of the knee. As long as the patient can fully extend the knee in the swing stage preparatory to limb loading, the resulting movement caused by vertical loading acts to extend the knee against the posterior stop, thereby locking the knee in extension. This requires at least fair (grade 3) hip flexor strength (see Table 13–1) to provide sufficient forward momentum of the leg to position the knee in full extension.

The substitution of plastic components, such as a pretibial shell, has led to significantly improved fit and reduced weight in KAFOs.

Buyukavci R, Akturk S, Ersoy Y. Evaluating the functional outcomes of ultrasound-guided botulinum toxin type A injections using the Euro-musculus approach for upper limb spasticity treatment in post-stroke patients: an observational study. *Eur J Phys Rehabil Med.* 2018;54(5):738-744. [PMID: 29422486]

Cleland TL, Wilson R, Kim C, Jain NB. What's new in orthopaedic rehabilitation. *J Bone Joint Surg Am.* 2019;101(22):1983-1989. [PMID: 31764360]

Loveless MS, Fry AL. Pharmacologic therapies in musculoskeletal conditions. *Med Clin North Am.* 2016;100(4):869-890. [PMID: 27235619]

McCormick ZL, Chu SK, Binler D, et al. Intrathecal versus oral baclofen: a matched cohort study of spasticity, pain, sleep, fatigue, and quality of life. *PM R.* 2016;8(6):553-562. [PMID: 26498518]

Paparella G, Vavla M, Bernardi L, Girardi G, Stefan C, Martinuzzi A. Efficacy of a combined treatment of botulinum toxin and intensive physiotherapy in hereditary spastic paraplegia. *Front Neurosci.* 2020;14:111. [PMID: 32153352]

Potter BK, Sheu RG, Stinner D, et al. Multisite evaluation of a custom energy-storing carbon fiber orthosis for patients with residual disability after lower-limb trauma. *J Bone Joint Surg Am.* 2018;100(20):1781-1789. [PMID: 30334889]

SPINAL CORD INJURY

Trauma to the spinal cord causes dysfunction of the cord, with nonprogressive loss of sensory and motor function distal to the injury. Approximately 400,000 people have spinal cord damage in the United States, and the incidence is about 10,000 per year. The leading causes of SCI are motor vehicle accidents, gunshot wounds, falls, sports injuries, and water (especially diving) injuries.

Patients are generally categorized into three groups. The first consists predominantly of younger individuals who sustained their injury from a motor vehicle collision or other high-energy traumatic accident. The second consists of individuals over 50 years of age with cervical spinal stenosis caused by congenital narrowing or spondylosis. Patients in this second group often sustained their injury from minor trauma and commonly have no vertebral fracture. The third group consists of people with gunshot wounds, which are now the leading cause of spinal injury in many urban centers in the United States. With the benefits of an organized program of medical care, the life expectancy of survivors of SCI is now approaching normal.

Terminology

A. Tetraplegia

The term *tetraplegia* (preferred to *quadriplegia*) refers to loss or impairment of motor or sensory function (or both) in the cervical segments of the spinal cord with resulting impairment of function in the arms, trunk, legs, and pelvic organs.

B. Paraplegia

Paraplegia refers to loss or impairment of motor or sensory function (or both) in the thoracic, lumbar, or sacral segments of the spinal cord. Arm function is intact but, depending on the level of the cord injured, impairment in the trunk, legs, and pelvic organs may be present.

C. Complete Injury

The term *complete injury* refers to an injury with no spared motor or sensory function in the lowest sacral segments.

D. Incomplete Injury

Incomplete injury refers to an injury with partial preservation of sensory or motor function (or both) below the neurologic level and includes the lowest sacral segments.

Neurologic Impairment and Recovery

A. Neurologic Examination

The neurologic examination is critical to the classification and treatment of spinal injuries because it determines the patient's potential level of recovery. The neurologic level of the lesion refers to the highest neural segment having normal motor and sensory function. Patients are further subdivided according to whether they have complete or incomplete spinal cord function. This is determined by the absence or presence of motor or sensory function in the most distal part of the spinal cord innervating the sacral nerves. The presence of sacral nerve function is critical because patients with incomplete injuries have the potential to recover normal neurologic function over a time span of up to 2 years even if paralysis is initially complete.

1. Spinal shock—The diagnosis of complete SCI cannot be made until the period of spinal shock is over, as evidenced by the return of the bulbocavernosus reflex. To elicit this reflex, the clinician examines the patient's rectum digitally, feeling for contraction of the anal sphincter while squeezing the glans penis or clitoris. The concept of spinal shock is important and can be understood on the basis of the monosynaptic stretch reflex. At a given neural segment of the spinal cord, afferent sensory fibers enter the spinal cord and anastomose with the anterior motor neurons at the same level. If trauma to the spinal cord causes complete injury, reflex activity at the site of injury will not return because the reflex arc is permanently interrupted. When spinal shock disappears, however, reflex activity does return in the distal segments below the level of injury. In a patient with complete SCI, spinal shock may last for as little as several hours or as long as several months. Patients with complete SCI who have recovered from spinal shock have a negligible chance for any useful motor return.

2. Sacral reflexes—The presence or absence of sacral function determines the completeness of the injury. Sacral motor function is assessed by testing contraction of the external anal sphincter (graded as present or absent). Sacral sensation is tested at the anal mucocutaneous junction. Additionally, testing of the external anal sphincter is performed by assessing perceived deep sensation as present or absent when the examiner's finger is inserted.

B. Spinal Cord Syndromes

1. Anterior cord syndrome—Anterior cord syndrome commonly results from direct contusion to the anterior cord by bone fragments or from damage to the anterior spinal artery. Depending on the extent of cord involvement, only posterior column function (proprioception and light touch) may be present. The ability to respond to pain (tested by discriminating sharp and dull) and to light touch (tested with a wisp of cotton) signifies that the entire posterior half of the cord has some intact function and thus offers a better prognosis for motor recovery. If there is no recovery of motor function and pain sensation 4 weeks after injury, the prognosis for significant motor return is poor.

2. Central cord syndrome—Central cord syndrome can be understood on the basis of the spinal cord anatomy. The gray matter in the spinal cord contains nerve cell bodies and is surrounded by white matter consisting primarily of ascending and descending myelinated tracts. The central gray matter has a higher metabolic requirement and is therefore more susceptible to the effects of trauma and ischemia. Central cord syndrome often results from a minor injury such as a fall in an older patient with cervical spinal canal stenosis. The overall prognosis for patients with central cord syndrome is variable. Most patients are able to walk despite severe paralysis of the upper extremity.

3. Brown-Séquard syndrome—Brown-Séquard syndrome is caused by a complete hemisection of the spinal cord, resulting in a greater ipsilateral proprioceptive motor loss and a greater contralateral loss of pain and temperature sensation. Affected patients have an excellent prognosis and can usually ambulate.

4. Mixed syndrome—Mixed syndrome is characterized by a diffuse involvement of the entire spinal cord. Affected patients have a good prognosis for recovery. As with all incomplete SCI syndromes, early motor recovery is the best prognostic indicator.

Management

A. Acute Management

Most patients with SCIs have associated injuries. In this setting, assessment and treatment of airway, breathing, and circulation take precedence. The patient is best treated initially in the supine position.

Airway management in the setting of SCI, with or without a cervical spine injury, is complex and difficult. The cervical spine must be maintained in neutral alignment. Clearing of oral secretions and/or debris is essential to maintain airway patency and to prevent aspiration. Failure to intubate emergently when indicated for respiration, because of concerns regarding the instability of the patient's cervical spine, is a potential pitfall.

Hypotension may be hemorrhagic and/or neurogenic in acute SCI. Hemorrhagic hypotension is associated with tachycardia and neurogenic with bradycardia. Because of vital sign confusion in acute SCI and the high incidence of associated injuries, a diligent search for occult sources of hemorrhage must be made. The most common causes of occult hemorrhage are chest, intraabdominal, or retroperitoneal injuries and pelvic or long bone fractures. Appropriate investigations, including radiography or computed tomography (CT) scanning, are required.

Once occult sources of hemorrhage are excluded, initial treatment of neurogenic shock focuses on fluid resuscitation. Judicious fluid replacement with isotonic crystalloid solution to a maximum of 2 L is the initial treatment of choice.

Associated head injury occurs in approximately 25% of SCI patients. A careful neurologic assessment for associated head injury is compulsory. The presence of amnesia, external signs of head injury or basilar skull fracture, focal neurologic deficits, associated alcohol intoxication or drug abuse, and a history of loss of consciousness mandate a thorough evaluation for intracranial injury, starting with a noncontrast CT scan of the head.

Ileus is common. Placement of a nasogastric tube is essential. Aspiration pneumonitis is a serious complication in the SCI patient with compromised respiratory function. Antiemetics should be used aggressively.

Current neuroprotective drugs for SCI remain controversial. Some think there is improvement in motor function and sensation in patients with complete or incomplete SCIs treated with high doses of methylprednisolone within 8 hours of injury. The treatment protocol is to start steroids within 3 hours as follows: methylprednisolone 30 mg/kg bolus over 15 minutes and an infusion of methylprednisolone at 5.4 mg/kg/h for 23 hours beginning 45 minutes after the bolus. A National Acute Spinal Cord Injury Study (NASCIS III) evaluated methylprednisolone 5.4 mg/kg/h for 24 or 48 hours versus tirilazad 2.5 mg/kg every 6 hours for 48 hours. Tirilazad is a potent lipid preoxidation inhibitor. High doses of steroids or tirilazad are thought to minimize the secondary effects of acute SCI. All patients received a 30 mg/kg bolus of methylprednisolone intravenously. The study found that in patients treated earlier than 3 hours after injury, the administration of methylprednisolone for 24 hours was best. In patients treated 3 to 8 hours after injury, the use of methylprednisolone for 48 hours was best. Tirilazad was equivalent to methylprednisolone for 24 hours. However, others have found no benefit, and the risks of steroid therapy are not inconsequential as there is increased incidence of avascular necrosis and infectious complications such as pneumonia, urinary tract infections, and wound infections.

B. Lower Extremities

Prevention of contractures and maintenance of ROM are important in all patients with SCI and should begin immediately following the injury. Teaching the patient to sleep in the prone position is the most effective means of preventing hip and knee flexion contractures. Passive stretching of the hamstring muscles with the knee extended is initiated to prevent shortening of these muscles secondary to spasticity. For patients to be able to dress the lower parts of their body independently, they must be able to flex the lumbar spine and hip 120 degrees with the knee extended.

Patients with extensive paralysis of the lower extremity need strength in both arms to manipulate crutches and bring the body to a standing position. Patients who lack at least fair (grade 3) strength in their quadriceps muscles (see Table 13–1) require KAFOs to stabilize the knee and also require the knee to be locked in extension while walking. Patients who have bilateral KAFOs commonly use a swing-through, crutch-assisted gait rather than a reciprocal gait. Because strenuous upper extremity exertion is required and the rate of energy expenditure is extremely high when crutches are used, nearly all patients prefer to use a wheelchair. In contrast, patients who have fair (grade 3) or greater strength in their hip flexors and knee extensors are able to walk with unlocked (free) knees and only require AFOs to stabilize their feet and ankles. These patients also usually require crutches because of absent or impaired hip extensor and adductor muscles, but they are able to achieve a reciprocal gait pattern and can walk for a limited duration outside the home. Most of them prefer a wheelchair when they must ambulate over long distances.

Because most ambulatory patients with SCI have impaired hip extensor support, they learn to hyperextend the lumbar spine so the center of gravity of the trunk is posterior to the hip joint in the stance phase of gait. This prevents forward collapse and decreases the demand on the arms during crutch use. Spine stabilization procedures that decrease the flexibility of the lower lumbar spine or reduce the amount of lordosis deprive the patient of an important gait maneuver.

C. Upper Body and Extremities

1. C4 level function—Patients with cervical lesions above C4 may have impairment of respiratory function, depending on the extent of injury, and may require a tracheostomy and mechanical ventilatory assistance.

Phrenic nerve stimulation via implanted surgical electrodes enables patients to use their own diaphragm and ventilate without mechanical assistance if the cause of their diaphragm paralysis is upper motor neuron injury. With training, these patients should be able to achieve a vital capacity that is 50% to 60% of normal using only the diaphragm.

Patients with high tetraplegia can use chin or tongue controls to operate an electric wheelchair with attached respiratory equipment. Mouth sticks that are lightweight rods attached to a dental bite plate enable patients to perform desktop skills, operate push-button equipment, and pursue vocational and recreational activities.

2. C5 level function—At the C5 level, the key muscles are the deltoid and biceps muscles, which are used for shoulder abduction and elbow flexion. If these muscles are weak, the patient benefits from mobile arm supports attached to the wheelchair and balanced to exert a vertical force to counteract gravity. This enables the patient with poor muscle strength to feed independently and perform other functional tasks with the hands. A ratchet wrist-hand orthosis (WHO) with a fixed wrist joint and a passively closing mechanism attached to the thumb and fingers enables the patient to grasp objects between the thumb and fingers.

Surgery can further enhance upper extremity function. The goals of surgery are to provide active elbow and wrist extension and to restore the ability to pinch the thumb against the index finger (key pinch or lateral pinch). Transferring the posterior deltoid to the triceps muscle provides active elbow extension, and another option is to transfer the biceps to the triceps. One option is to transfer the brachioradialis to the extensor carpi radialis brevis to provide active wrist extension and attach the flexor pollicis longus tendon to the distal radius and fuse the interphalangeal joint of the thumb to provide for key pinch by tenodesis when the wrist is extended.

3. C6 level function—At the C6 level, the key muscles are the wrist extensors, which enable the patient to propel a wheelchair manually, transfer from one position to another, and even live independently.

If wrist extensor strength is poor, an orthosis is indicated. A WHO with a free wrist joint and a rubber-band extensor-assist mechanism enables the patient to complete wrist extension. A wrist-driven WHO with a flexor hinge mechanism that causes the metacarpophalangeal joint to flex when the wrist is extended enables the patient to grasp actively between the fingers and thumb. Some patients develop a natural tenodesis of their thumb and finger flexor muscles because of myostatic contracture or spasticity, and this tenodesis enables them to grasp without an orthosis.

Most patients with good wrist extensor strength are able to operate a manual wheelchair but may require an electric wheelchair for long distances. These patients may also be able to transfer independently if they have no elbow flexion contractures and they can lock their elbows passively in extension while transferring.

The goals of surgery in the C6 patient are the restoration of lateral pinch and active grasp. Lateral pinch can be restored either by tenodesis of the thumb flexor or by transfer of the brachioradialis to the flexor pollicis longus. Active grasp can be restored by transfer of the pronator teres to the flexor digitorum profundus.

4. C7 level function—At the C7 level, the key muscle is the triceps. All patients with intact triceps function should be able to transfer and live independently if no other complications are present. Despite their ability to extend the fingers, these patients may also require a WHO with a flexor hinge mechanism.

The goals of surgery in the C7 tetraplegic patient are active thumb flexion for pinch, active finger flexion for grasp, and hand opening by extensor tenodesis. Transfer of the brachioradialis to the flexor pollicis longus provides active pinch. Transfer of the pronator teres to the flexor digitorum profundus allows for active finger flexion and grasp. If the finger extensors are weak, tenodesis of these tendons to the radius provides hand opening with wrist flexion.

5. C8 level function—At the C8 level, the key muscles are the finger and thumb flexors, which enable a gross grasp. The functioning flexor pollicis longus enables patients to obtain lateral pinch between the thumb and the side of the index finger. Intrinsic muscle function is lacking, and clawing of the fingers is usually present. A capsulodesis of the metacarpophalangeal joints corrects the clawing and improves hand function. Active intrinsic function can be gained by splitting the superficial finger flexor tendon of the ring finger into four slips and transferring these tendons to the lumbrical insertions of each finger.

D. Skin

Maintaining skin integrity is crucial to spinal injury care. From the moment the patient enters the emergency room, preventive measures are instituted to avoid skin breakdown even while critical diagnostic procedures and lifesaving measures are performed. Only 4 hours of continuous pressure on the sacrum are sufficient to cause full-thickness skin necrosis. Turning the patient from side to back to side every 2 hours diminishes risk of skin ulceration, a problem that greatly prolongs the cost and length of rehabilitation. Following the simple procedures outlined here usually obviates the need for flotation devices, cyclically rotating beds, and similar equipment.

Once the patient is allowed to sit, a progressive program to increase the time of sitting tolerance is undertaken. Paraplegics with normal upper extremity function are taught to perform raises automatically in the wheelchair and decompress the skin for approximately 15 seconds every 15 minutes. Tetraplegics who are unable to perform raises can lean to either side or lean forward for 1-minute intervals every hour. Those patients unable to perform decompressive maneuvers require assistance from another person or may use an electric wheelchair with a powered recliner that enables them to assume a supine posture every hour.

All patients must be taught to inspect their skin at least twice a day, when dressing and undressing. Mirrors attached to a rod enable paraplegics to examine their skin over the sacrum and ischia independently. Tetraplegics usually require assistance with skin inspection.

If there is evidence of chronic skin inflammation over bony prominences or if redness persists 30 minutes after removal of pressure, action must be taken to avoid incipient pressure necrosis. Pressure transducers placed under the bony prominences determine if pressure exceeds acceptable levels. Up to 40 mm Hg is well tolerated by most patients. If pressures exceed this amount, a custom-fitted foam cushion with appropriate cutouts is prescribed.

Development of any open areas in the skin over the ischia or sacrum, even superficial areas, is an indication to discontinue sitting temporarily. The patient must remain in a prone or side-lying position to avoid pressure until the lesion is healed. Failure to take aggressive steps to eliminate pressure and allow healing leads to chronic inflammation, scarring, and a loss of elasticity, creating a vicious cycle that further increases susceptibility to pressure necrosis.

Excessive hip and knee flexor spasticity that prevents patients from assuming the prone position or lying supine and requires them constantly to assume a side-lying posture when in bed can lead to excessive pressure over the greater trochanters. Flexor spasticity or contracture that prevents continuous turning should be corrected medically prior to development of pressure sores and must be performed before a skin flap. Failure to correct flexion deformities inevitably decreases the likelihood of successful skin closure. Surgical tenotomy and myotomy of hip and knee flexors is the most effective surgical method for correcting the problem when nonoperative measures fail. Neurosurgical procedures such as myelotomy or rhizotomy are usually less effective and run the risk of interfering with reflex bladder emptying and penile erections.

In the neglected patient with a full-thickness pressure sore, surgery is necessary. The initial phase consists of debridement of all infected soft tissue and bone as well as treatment of spasticity and contractures that may have predisposed the patient to pressure sores. Once all wounds have a clean granulating base and the patient is able to remain prone 24 hours a day, he or she becomes a candidate for a rotational flap. The gluteus maximus, the tensor fasciae latae, and other types of musculocutaneous flaps give the surgeon a superior and reliable method of providing skin coverage. Sitting tolerance must be carefully reestablished following skin flap surgery. Because most pressure sores in patients with chronic SCI are the result of failure to relieve pressure by appropriate measures, patient education is the key element of a successful rehabilitation outcome.

Ischial or trochanteric pressure sores commonly lead to septic arthritis of the hip. In such cases, femoral head and neck resection is required. In the paraplegic with an intact hip joint, the passive weight of the limbs cantilevered about the posterior thigh exerts an upward force on the pelvis, which decompresses the ischia. Consequently, approximately 30% of the body weight is supported on the thigh. Femoral head and neck resection disrupts results in greater pressure on the ischia, thereby increasing the chance of recurrence even after successful flap closure.

Pressure sores affecting the ankle commonly occur over the heel or malleolus. After initial debridement, wound healing can nearly always be obtained by placing the patient in a short leg cast that protects the wound from any external pressure. The cast is changed every 1 or 2 weeks until healing occurs. Rotational flaps are rarely needed.

E. Bladder Function

Intermittent catheterization has allowed for a nearly normal life span of those with SCIs. In this group, urinary tract infection is no longer the leading cause of death. Most patients who have intact sacral reflex activity following complete injury are able to obtain reflex bladder emptying. Some patients with complete SCI are able to trigger reflex bladder emptying by tapping the suprapubic area, stroking the thighs, or using the Credé method (applying external pressure on the bladder to induce emptying) or the Valsalva maneuver (forcibly exhaling against the closed glottis). These patients require an external condom catheter for men or diapering for women. Patients with nonreflex bladders void by the application of pressure on the bladder by the Valsalva maneuver or Credé method. Not all so-called reflex bladders empty reflexively, and some, despite reflex emptying, have an excessive amount of residual urine. Anticholinergic medications to decrease bladder neck spasm of the smooth muscle of the internal sphincter or spasmolytic medications to decrease tone in the striated muscle of the external sphincter may improve bladder emptying. Some patients require surgical sphincterotomy.

Bladder diversion using an ileal conduit as a primary means of achieving bladder drainage is contraindicated. This procedure leads to a chronic acid–base imbalance, osteoporosis, and, ultimately, renal failure from secondary infection. The suprapubic catheter also is to be avoided as a means of primary treatment for the same reasons that permanent indwelling catheters are contraindicated. The constant presence of an indwelling catheter leads to bladder constriction and increases the risks of renal calculi, infection, and death from renal failure. For male patients, the external condom catheter is the treatment of choice. For female patients, padding or diapering is the preferred treatment, although some women prefer an indwelling catheter despite the risks of a shortened life span.

F. Sexual Function

Women with or without intact reflex activity can perform coitus and deliver normal children. Approximately 90% of men with complete SCI and sacral reflex activity can be expected to have reflex erections. Most of these men are able to perform coitus; however, fewer than half can ejaculate. Sacral sparing plays a great role in prognosticating sexual potential in the male patient. Those able to distinguish pain (discrimination of sharp and dull) are usually able to achieve psychogenic erections.

G. Autonomic Dysreflexia

Splanchnic outflow conveying sympathetic fibers to the lower body exits at the T8 region. Patients with lesions above T8 are prone to autonomic dysreflexia. They are subject to bouts of hypertension that may be heralded by dizziness, sweating, and headaches. A plugged catheter is the most common precipitating cause of dysreflexia. The catheter should be carefully checked and the bladder irrigated. Other frequent causes of dysreflexia include calculi or infections in any portion of the urinary system, fecal impaction, and pressure sores. If the patient's blood pressure does not lower in response to treatment of the causative agent, management with antihypertensive medication is begun.

Recovery

The *International Standards for Neurological and Functional Classification of Spinal Cord Injury*, published by the American Spinal Injury Association (ASIA) and the International Medical Society of Paraplegia (IMSOP), represent the most reliable instrument for assessing neurologic status in SCI. These standards provide a quantitative measure of sensory and motor function.

Neurologic recovery is assessed by determining the change in ASIA Motor Score (AMS) between successive neurologic examinations. The AMS is the sum of strength grades for each of the 10 key muscles tested bilaterally that represent neurologic segments from C5 to T1 and L2 to S1. In a neurologically intact individual, the total possible AMS is 100 points.

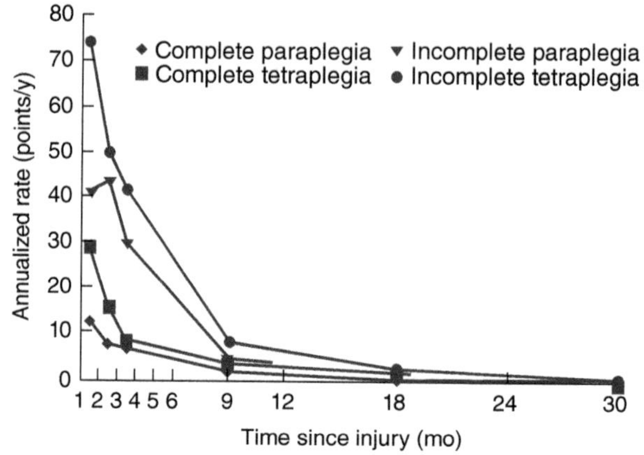

▲ **Figure 13–10. Recovery rates of American Spinal Injury Association (ASIA) Motor Score for persons with incomplete and complete paraplegia and tetraplegia.** (Reproduced, with permission, from Waters RL, Adkins R, Yakura J, Sie I. Functional and neurological recovery following acute SCI. *J Spinal Cord Med.* 1998;21:195-199.)

The most important prognostic indicator of recovery is completeness of injury using the sacral-sparing definition. Using completeness and level of injury (tetraplegia or paraplegia), patients are divided into four groups: complete tetraplegia, incomplete tetraplegia, complete paraplegia, and incomplete paraplegia. The rate of motor recovery in all groups declines rapidly in the first 6 months following injury with minimal further changes after this time (Figure 13–10).

A. Complete Paraplegia

Patients with paraplegia that remains complete 1 month after injury have a 96% chance of remaining complete. Thirty-eight percent of those with injuries at or below T9 recover some lower extremity function. No patients with a neurologic level above T9 regain volitional lower extremity motor function. Only 5% of muscles with a strength of 0/5 at 1 month recover to 3/5 or greater strength 1 year after injury. Furthermore, only 5% of individuals become independent community ambulators at 1 year.

B. Incomplete Paraplegia

Motor recovery is better in individuals with incomplete injuries. Between 1 month and 1 year after injury, the AMS increases by an average of 12 points regardless of the level of injury. Additionally, these patients have a 76% chance of becoming community ambulators.

C. Complete Tetraplegia

Ninety percent of individuals with complete tetraplegia 1 month after injury remain complete. Among the 10% who undergo late conversion to incomplete status, lower extremity motor recovery is minimal and inadequate for ambulation. Recovery of AMS points is independent of neurologic level. Waters and colleagues reported that with the exception of the triceps muscle, all upper extremity muscles with a grade of at least 1/5 1 month after injury recover to at least 3/5 1 year after injury.

D. Incomplete Tetraplegia

In patients with incomplete tetraplegia, motor recovery of upper and lower extremity muscles occurs concurrently. Nearly all muscles with at least 1/5 strength 1 month after injury recover to at least 3/5 1 year after injury. Forty-six percent of the patients examined by Waters and colleagues attained independent community ambulation status 1 year after injury. The number of individuals with incomplete tetraplegia who can attain independent community ambulation is less than for individuals with incomplete paraplegia and comparable lower extremity function. This is because upper extremity function may be insufficient to allow crutch-assisted ambulation in the former group, whereas those with incomplete paraplegia have normal upper extremity strength. Regaining hand and arm function is a high priority for those with tetraplegia, and this requires adequate shoulder ROM and strength. Patients do better when they participate in a rehabilitation program focused on shoulder stretching and strengthening as well as training in optimizing transfers, raises from a sitting position, and wheelchair propulsion.

Taken as a whole, a minority of individuals with SCI can ambulate independently after injury. The proportion of patients who can ambulate does, however, vary with the level and completeness of the injury. The lower extremity motor score (LEMS), which is the sum of the strength grades of the bilateral key lower extremity muscles, can be used to predict successful ambulation (Table 13–2). The motor groups are as follows: L2, hip flexors (iliopsoas); L3, knee extensors (quadriceps); L4, ankle dorsiflexors (tibialis anterior); L5, long toe extensors (extensor hallucis longus); and S1, ankle plantarflexors (gastrocnemius, soleus). In an individual with no deficit, the total possible LEMS is 50 points. The LEMS at 30 days is used to predict the chance of successful ambulation in incomplete tetraplegics, incomplete paraplegics, and complete paraplegics. All individuals with an LEMS of at least 20 and an incomplete injury are expected to be community ambulators 1 year after injury.

Table 13–2. Community ambulators at 1 year after injury.

ASIA Lower Extremity Motor Score[a] (at 30 days after injury)	Complete Paraplegia (%)	Incomplete Paraplegia (%)	Incomplete Tetraplegia (%)
0	<1	33	0
1-9	45	70	2
10-19		100	63
20 or greater		100	100
Total	5	76	46

[a]Score based on five key muscles.
Total possible 50 points for both lower extremities for normals.
Reprinted, with permission, from Waters RL, Adkins R, Yakura J, et al. Functional and neurological recovery following acute SCI. *J Spinal Cord Med.* 1998;21:195-199.

Bracken MB, Shepard MJ, Holford TR, et al. Administration of methylprednisolone for 24 or 48 hours or tirilazad mesylate for 48 hours in the treatment of acute spinal cord injury. Results of the Third National Acute Spinal Cord Injury Randomized Controlled Trial. National Acute Spinal Cord Injury Study. *JAMA.* 1997;277(20):1597-1604. [PMID: 9168289]

Canton J, Moutel L, Berrut G, Perrouin-Verbe B. Elderly and spinal cord injury: a cohort study, neurological, functional recovery and outcomes. *Geriatr Psychol Neuropsychiatr Vieil.* 2019;17(2):129-136. [PMID: 31010800]

Fehlings MG, Wilson JR, Harrop JS, et al. Efficacy and safety of methylprednisolone sodium succinate in acute spinal cord injury: a systematic review. *Global Spine J.* 2017;7(3 suppl): 116S-137S. [PMID: 29164020]

Liu Z, Yang Y, He L, et al. High-dose methylprednisolone for acute traumatic spinal cord injury: a meta-analysis. *Neurology.* 2019;93(9):e841-e850. [PMID: 31358617]

Pattanakuhar S, Kammuang-Lue P, Kovindha A, Komaratat N, Mahachai R, Chotiyarnwong C. Is admission to an SCI specialized rehabilitation facility associated with better functional outcomes? Analysis of data from the Thai Spinal Cord Injury Registry. *Spinal Cord.* 2019;57(8):684-691. [PMID: 30842632]

Sultan I, Lamba N, Liew A, et al. The safety and efficacy of steroid treatment for acute spinal cord injury: a systematic review and meta-analysis. *Heliyon.* 2020;6(2):e03414. [PMID: 32095652]

STROKE

Stroke (cerebrovascular accident or brain attack) occurs when thrombosis, embolism, or hemorrhage interrupts cerebral oxygenation and causes the death of neurons in the brain. This leads to deficits in cognition and in motor and sensory function.

In the United States, where cerebrovascular accidents are the leading cause of hemiplegia in adults and the third leading cause of death, two million people have permanent neurologic deficits from stroke. The annual incidence of stroke is 1 in 1000, with cerebral thrombosis causing nearly three-fourths of the cases. More than half of stroke victims survive and have an average life expectancy of approximately 6 years. Most survivors have the potential for significant function and useful lives if they receive the benefits of rehabilitation.

Neurologic Impairment and Recovery

Infarction of the cerebral cortex in the region of the brain supplied by the middle cerebral artery (MCA) or one of its branches is most commonly responsible for stroke. It supplies

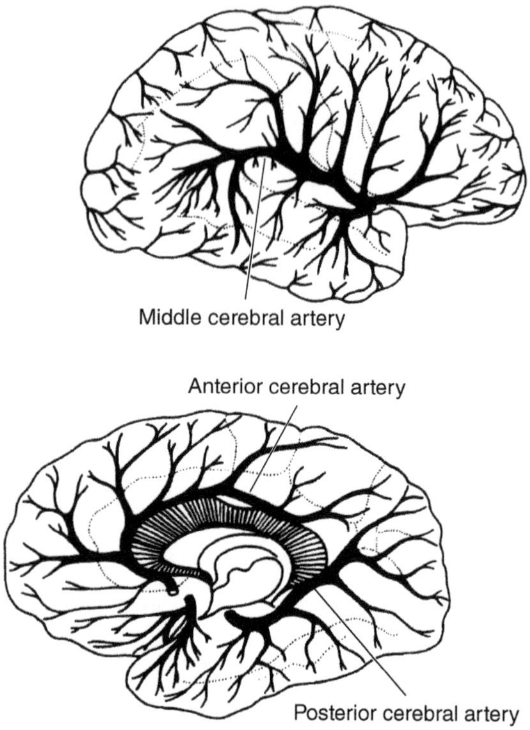

▲ **Figure 13–11.** Cerebral artery circulation.

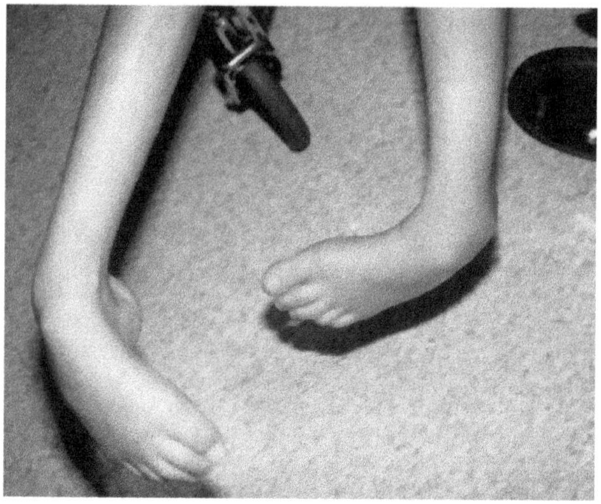

▲ **Figure 13–12.** Equinovarus deformities of the feet in a patient with spasticity.

the area of the cerebral cortex responsible for hand function; the anterior cerebral artery supplies the area responsible for lower extremity motion (Figure 13–11). The typical clinical picture following MCA stroke is contralateral hemianesthesia (decreased sensation), homonymous hemianopia (visual field deficit), and spastic hemiplegia with more paralysis in the upper extremity than in the lower extremity. Because hand function requires relatively precise motor control, even for activities with assistive equipment, the prognosis for the functional use of the hand and arm is considerably worse than for the leg. Return of even gross motor control in the lower extremity may be sufficient for walking.

Infarction in the region of the anterior cerebral artery causes paralysis and sensory loss of the opposite lower limb and, to a lesser degree, the arm.

Patients who have cerebral arteriosclerosis and suffer repeated bilateral infarctions are likely to have severe cognitive impairment that limits their general ability to function even when motor function is good.

After stroke, motor recovery follows a fairly typical pattern. The size of the lesion and the amount of collateral circulation determine the amount of permanent damage. Most recovery occurs within 6 months, although functional improvement may continue as the patient receives further sensorimotor reeducation and learns to cope with disability.

Initially after a stroke, the affected limbs are completely flaccid. Over the next few weeks, muscle tone and spasticity gradually increase in the adductor muscles of the shoulder and in the flexor muscles of the elbow, wrist, and fingers. Spasticity also develops in the lower extremity muscles. Most commonly, there is an extensor pattern of spasticity in the leg, characterized by hip adduction, knee extension, and equinovarus deformities of the foot and ankle (Figure 13–12). In some cases, however, a flexion pattern of spasticity occurs, characterized by hip and knee flexion.

Whether the patient recovers the ability to move one joint independently of the others (selective movement) depends on the extent of the cerebral cortical damage. Dependence on the more neurologically primitive patterned movement (synergy) decreases as selective control improves. The extent to which motor impairment restricts function varies in the upper and lower extremities. Patterned movement is not functional in the upper extremity, but it may be useful in the lower extremity, where the patient uses the flexion synergy to advance the limb forward and the mass extension synergy for limb stability during standing.

The final processes in sensory perception occur in the cerebral cortex, where basic sensory information is integrated to complex sensory phenomena such as vision, proprioception, and perception of spatial relationships, shape, and texture. Patients with severe parietal dysfunction and sensory loss may lack sufficient perception of space and awareness of the involved segment of their body to ambulate. Patients with severe perceptual loss may lack balance to sit, stand, or walk. A visual field deficit further interferes with limb use and may cause patients to be unaware of their own limbs.

Management

A. Acute Management

Medical intervention in the treatment of a stroke is most effective when initiated early, within hours after the onset of symptoms. However, it may be beneficial, although usually less so, if administered at longer times, up to 24 hours after onset.

1. Thrombolytics

A. Tissue plasminogen activator (t-PA) (also known as recombinant t-PA or recombinant tissue-type plasminogen activator [rt-PA])—Treatment with t-PA results, more often, in resolved or diminished symptoms compared to those who did not receive it. There is increased risk of intracerebral hemorrhage but little or no difference in mortality.

Key points about the administration of thrombolytic agents include the following:

1. They must be administered soon, preferably within 3 hours of symptom onset. The time of onset in patients who wake up with symptoms or those who cannot describe accurately the time of their symptom onset is when they were last known to be well.
2. An imaging study of the head (CT scan or magnetic resonance imaging [MRI]) must be performed prior to treatment to rule out hemorrhage as a cause of symptoms.
3. Blood pressure should be lower than 185 mm Hg systolic and 110 mm Hg diastolic. Agents such as labetalol may be used to lower the blood pressure for the purposes of treatment.
4. Blood must be tested for platelet count (should be >100,000), international normalized ratio (INR) (many recommend it be <1.6), partial thromboplastin time (PTT) (many recommend <40), and glucose (should be 50-400). INR has particular relevance because individuals properly treated with warfarin to diminish the incidence of stroke (eg, those with atrial fibrillation) may not be candidates for thrombolytic treatments.

B. Prourokinase (also known as recombinant prourokinase, or r-pro-UK)—This intraarterial therapy requires the involvement of a skilled interventionist. The time window is 6 hours from symptom onset. Patients with a CT scan showing over a third involvement of the MCA territory as seen on CT scan are not eligible for treatment. Treatment with r-pro-UK results, more often, in resolved or diminished symptoms compared to those who did not receive it. There is increased risk of intracerebral hemorrhage but little or no difference in mortality.

This therapy may be useful for patients who arrive more than 3 hours after symptom onset and who have less than a third involvement of the MCA territory on initial scan.

2. Antiplatelet agents

A. Aspirin—The Chinese Acute Stroke Trial (CAST) (160 mg/day) and the International Stroke Trial (IST) (300 mg/day) are two large studies evaluating the use of acetylsalicylic acid, otherwise known as aspirin, within 48 hours of ischemic stroke symptom onset. A combined analysis of 40,000 patients randomized in these two trials revealed a net decrease of 9 per 1000 treated in the risk of further stroke or death in hospital. Because higher doses are associated with more gastric problems, 75 to 150 mg/d may be the optimal dose range for aspirin. This strong benefit for acute initiation of aspirin after ischemic stroke has been largely superseded by better benefit from the combination of aspirin and clopidogrel.

B. Clopidogrel—Clopidogrel 75 mg/day reduces the risk of recurrent stroke similar to aspirin and the complication of intracranial hemorrhage is similar, but there are fewer gastric problems. Aspirin and clopidogrel reduce recurrent stroke compared with aspirin alone in patients with transient ischemic attack (TIA) or minor stroke in the short term when the risk of recurrent stroke is highest, within the first 90 days after an acute ischemic stroke or TIA. There is less benefit in the longer term from combination therapy and probable harm from hemorrhage.

C. Dipyridamole—Dipyridamole is usually given in combination with aspirin and has similar benefit to aspirin and clopidogrel. The clinician should be aware that aspirin-dipyridamole has higher rates of discontinuation and noncompliance because of headaches and should watch for them.

D. Ticagrelor—Ticagrelor (90 mg) is reversible and short acting, so it must be given twice daily. It has a similar or possibly lower stroke rate than aspirin in the acute setting, and this may be more pronounced in those with large artery disease and atherosclerotic stroke. However, dyspnea and minor bleeding may lead to discontinuations of ticagrelor.

3. Anticoagulants

A. Warfarin—No studies have evaluated use of warfarin for the acute treatment of stroke. It is used to diminish stroke and recurrence in those with conditions associated with stroke, such as atrial fibrillation.

B. Heparin and heparinoids—There may be benefit at 6 months for heparins or heparinoids in acute ischemic stroke.

C. Direct oral anticoagulants—Direct oral anticoagulants (DOACs), including dabigatran, rivaroxaban, and apixaban, are used to diminish stroke and recurrence in those with conditions associated with stroke, such as atrial fibrillation. They may have better long-term outcomes than warfarin in older patients with ischemic stroke and a history of atrial fibrillation. Patients who receive DOACs are less likely to experience major adverse cardiovascular events, death, all-cause readmissions, cardiovascular readmissions, hospitalizations with bleeding, and hemorrhagic strokes but have a higher risk of gastrointestinal bleeding.

B. Mechanical Thrombectomy

Mechanical thrombectomy is a minimally invasive treatment for ischemic stroke that removes clots that block large blood vessels using a combination of catheterization, angiogram, and a device that grabs clots and removes them to reestablish blood flow to the brain. Over three-quarters of strokes are ischemic strokes, and up to one-quarter of ischemic strokes are caused by large-vessel blockages. Thrombolytics are more effective in resolving small than large thrombi. Mechanical thrombectomy should be initiated soon, within 6 hours of onset of acute stroke symptoms, but can benefit patients under certain conditions if done even within 24 hours of onset and should include t-PA treatment in eligible patients. Patients who receive mechanical thrombectomy more often have resolved or diminished symptoms compared to those who did not receive it. Complications include conversion of an ischemic to a hemorrhagic stroke, incomplete recanalization, secondary embolism, and access site complications.

C. Lower Extremities

1. Hemiplegia—To walk independently, the hemiplegic patient requires intact balance reactions, hip flexion to advance the limb, and stability of the limb for standing. If a patient meets these criteria and has acceptable cognition, the clinician can restore ambulation in most cases by prescribing an appropriate lower extremity orthosis and an upper extremity assistive device such as a cane. Orthopedic surgery to rebalance the muscle forces in the leg can greatly enhance ambulation.

Except for the correction of severe contractures in nonambulatory patients, surgical procedures should be delayed for at least 6 months to allow spontaneous neurologic recovery to occur and the patient to learn how to cope with the disability. After this time, surgery may safely be performed to improve usage in the functional limb.

In the nonfunctional limb, surgery may be performed to relieve pain or correct severe hip and knee flexion contractures caused by spasticity. Most severe contractural deformities in the nonfunctional limb, however, are the result of an ineffective program of daily passive ROM, splinting, and limb positioning.

Most hemiplegics with motor impairment have hip abductor and extensor weakness. A quad cane (cane with four feet to provide more stability) or a hemiwalker is prescribed to provide better balance. Because of paralysis in the upper extremity, the hemiplegic patient is unable to use a conventional walker.

2. Limb scissoring—Scissoring of the legs caused by overactive hip adductor muscles is a common problem. This gives the patient an extremely narrow base of support while standing and causes balance problems. When no fixed contracture of the hip adductor muscles is present, transection of the anterior branches of the obturator nerve denervates the adductors and allows the patient to stand with a broader base of support. If a contracture of the adductors occurs, surgical release of the adductor longus, adductor brevis, and gracilis muscles should be performed (Figure 13–13).

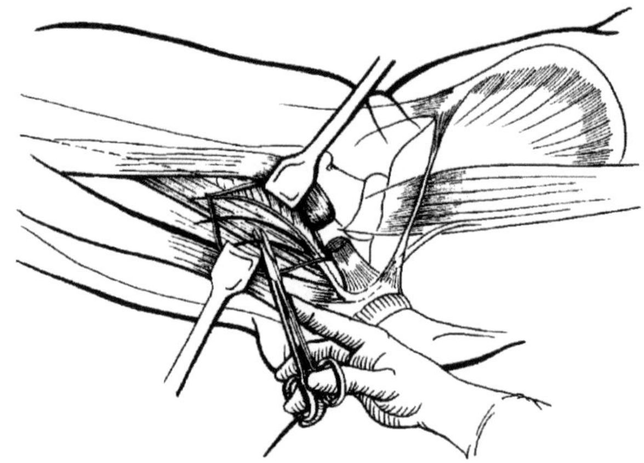

▲ **Figure 13–13.** Release of the hip adductor tendons and neurectomy of the anterior branches of the obturator nerve to correct the problem of limb scissoring. (Illustration by Anthony C. Berlet. Reproduced, with permission, from Keenan MAE, Kozin SH, Berlet AC. *Manual of Orthopaedic Surgery for Spasticity*. Philadelphia, PA: Raven; 1993.)

3. Stiff-knee gait—Patients with a stiff-knee gait are unable to flex the knee during the swing phase of gait. The deformity is a dynamic one, meaning that it only occurs during walking. Passive knee motion is not restricted, and the patient does not have difficulty sitting. Usually the knee is maintained in extension throughout the gait cycle. Toe drag, which is likely in the early swing phase, may cause the patient to trip. Thus, balance and stability are also affected. The limb seems to be longer than the other side, but this is only functional. Circumduction of the involved limb, hiking of the pelvis, or contralateral limb vaulting may occur as compensatory maneuvers.

A gait study with dynamic EMG should be done preoperatively to document the activity of the individual muscles of the quadriceps. Dyssynergic activity is commonly seen in the rectus femoris from preswing through terminal swing throughout the gait cycle. Abnormal activity is also common in the vastus intermedius, vastus medialis, and vastus lateralis muscles. If knee flexion is improved with a block of the femoral nerve or with botulinum toxin injection of the quadriceps, the rationale for surgical intervention is strengthened. Any equinus deformity of the foot should be corrected prior to evaluation of a stiff-knee gait because equinus causes a knee extension force during stance. Because the amount of knee flexion during swing is directly related to the speed of walking, the patient should be able to ambulate with a reasonable velocity to benefit from surgery. Hip flexion strength is also needed for a good result because the forward momentum of the leg normally provides the inertial force to flex the knee. In the past, a selective release of the rectus femoris or both the rectus femoris and vastus intermedius was done to remove their inhibiting knee flexion. On average, a 15-degree improvement in peak knee flexion is seen after surgery. Transfer of the rectus femoris to a hamstring tendon not only removes it as a deforming muscle force but also converts the rectus into a corrective flexion force. This procedure provides improved knee flexion over selective release. When any of the vasti muscles are involved, they can be selectively lengthened at their myotendinous junction (Figure 13–14), and knee flexion improves.

4. Knee flexion deformity—A knee flexion deformity increases the physical demand on the quadriceps muscle, which must continually fire to hold the patient upright. Knee flexion often leads to knee instability and causes falls. It is most often caused by spasticity of the hamstring muscles. A KAFO can be used to hold the knee in extension on a temporary basis as a training aid in physical therapy. Such an orthosis, however, is difficult for the stroke patient to don and wear for permanent usage.

Surgical correction of the knee flexion deformity is the most desirable treatment. Hamstring tenotomy (Figure 13–15) eliminates the dynamic component of the deformity and generally results in a 50% correction of the contracture at the time of surgery. The residual joint contracture is then corrected by serial casting done weekly after surgery. Hamstring function posterior to the knee joint is not necessary for ambulation. In fact, ambulation may only be feasible

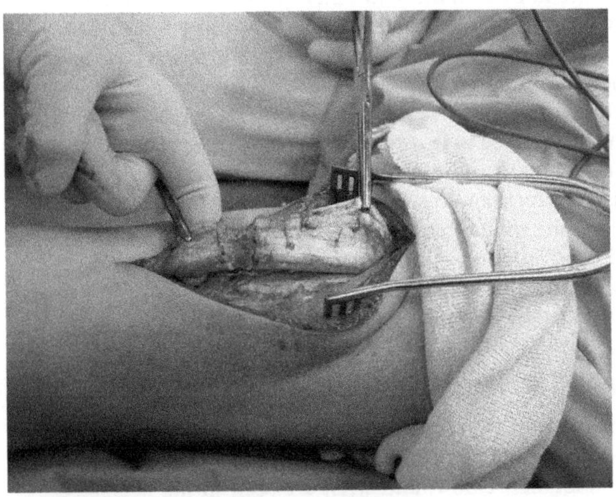

▲ **Figure 13–14.** Selective lengthening of the rectus femoris tendon to correct a stiff-knee gait abnormality.

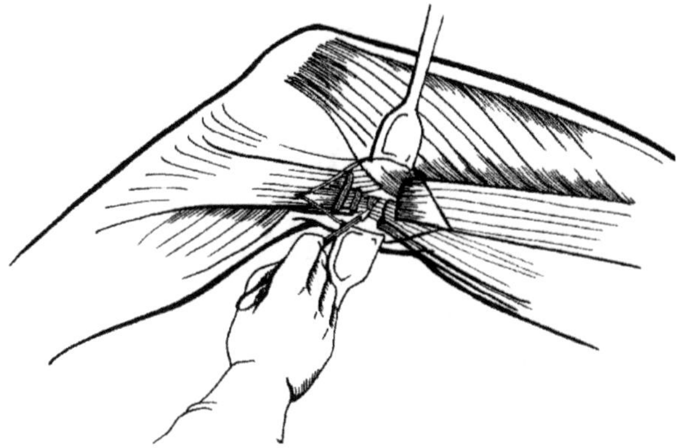

▲ **Figure 13–15.** Distal release of the hamstring tendons to correct a knee flexion contracture. (Illustration by Anthony C. Berlet. Reproduced, with permission, from Keenan MAE, Kozin SH, Berlet AC. *Manual of Orthopaedic Surgery for Spasticity*. Philadelphia, PA: Raven; 1993.)

in patients with knee flexion deformities of greater than 30 degrees if a hamstring release is done.

5. Equinus or equinovarus foot deformity—Surgical correction of an equinus deformity is indicated when the foot cannot be maintained in the neutral position with the heel in firm contact with the sole of the shoe in a well-fitted, rigid AFO. Despite a wide variety of surgical methods designed to decrease the triceps surae spasticity, none is more effective than Achilles tendon lengthening. In this procedure, triple hemisection tenotomy is performed via three stab incisions, with the most distal cut based medially to alleviate varus pull of the soleus muscle (Figure 13–16).

An anesthetic block of the posterior tibial nerve can be a valuable tool in preoperative assessment of the patient with equinus deformity because it demonstrates the potential benefits of Achilles tendon lengthening if the deformity is a result of increased muscle tone.

Surgical release of the flexor digitorum longus and brevis tendons at the base of each toe (Figure 13–17) is done prophylactically at the time of Achilles tendon lengthening because increased ankle dorsiflexion following heel cord tenotomy increases tension on the long toe flexor and commonly leads to excessive toe flexion (toe curling). The flexor hallucis longus and flexor digitorum longus tendons can be transferred to the os calcis to provide additional support to the weakened calf muscles.

Surgical correction of varus deformity is indicated when the problem is not corrected by a well-fitted orthosis. It is also indicated to enable the patient to walk without an orthosis when varus deformity is the only significant problem. The tibialis anterior, tibialis posterior, extensor hallucis longus, flexor hallucis longus, flexor digitorum, and soleus pass medial to the axis of the subtalar joint and are potentially responsible for varus deformity. EMG studies demonstrate

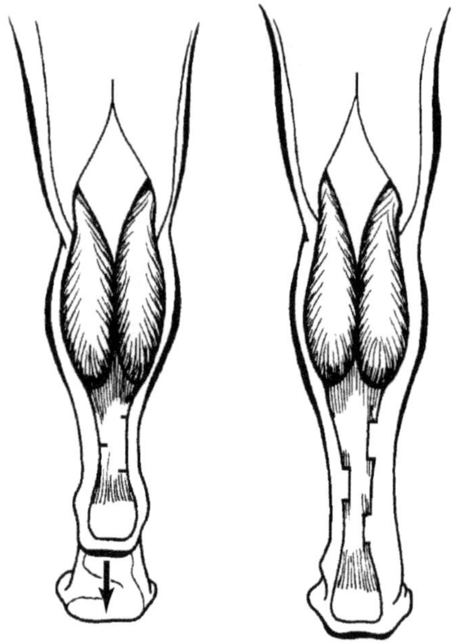

▲ **Figure 13–16. Hoke triple hemisection Achilles tendon lengthening to correct an equinus foot deformity.** (Illustration by Anthony C. Berlet. Reproduced, with permission, from Keenan MAE, Kozin SH, Berlet AC. *Manual of Orthopaedic Surgery for Spasticity*. Philadelphia, PA: Raven; 1993.)

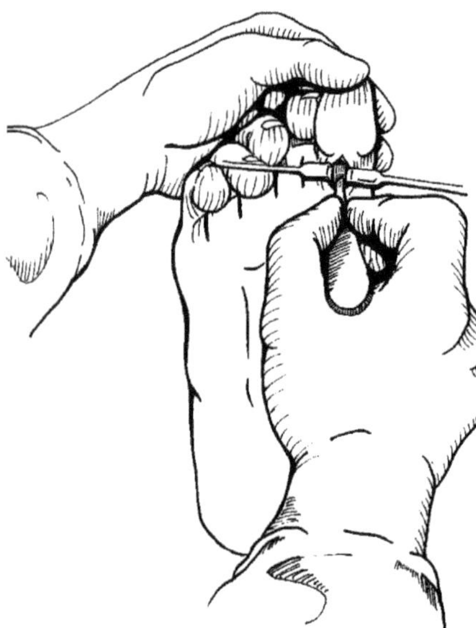

▲ **Figure 13–17. Release of the flexor digitorum longus and brevis tendons to correct the problem of toe curling.** (Illustration by Anthony C. Berlet. Reproduced, with permission, from Keenan MAE, Kozin SH, Berlet AC. *Manual of Orthopaedic Surgery for Spasticity*. Philadelphia, PA: Raven; 1993.)

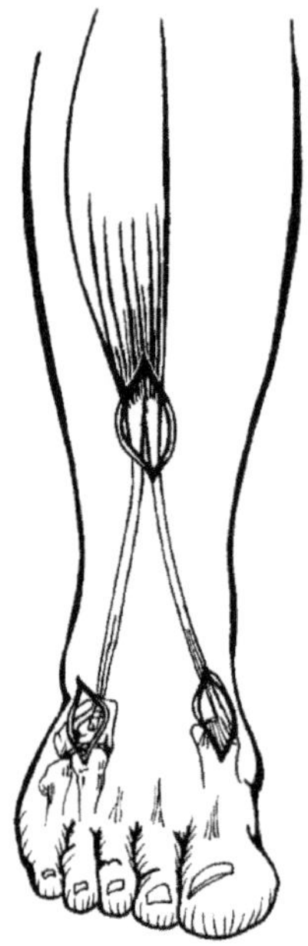

▲ **Figure 13–18. Split anterior tibial tendon transfer to correct a spastic varus foot deformity.** (Illustration by Anthony C. Berlet. Reproduced, with permission, from Keenan MAE, Kozin SH, Berlet AC. *Manual of Orthopaedic Surgery for Spasticity*. Philadelphia, PA: Raven; 1993.)

that the peroneus longus and peroneus brevis are generally inactive, and the tibialis posterior is also usually inactive or minimally active.

The tibialis anterior is the key muscle responsible for varus deformity, and in most patients, this can be confirmed by visual examination or palpation while the patient walks. A procedure known as the split anterior tibial tendon transfer (Figure 13–18) diverts the inverting deforming force of the tibialis anterior to a corrective force. In this procedure, half of the tendon is transferred laterally to the os cuboideum. When the extensor hallucis longus muscle is overactive, it can be transferred to the middorsum of the foot as well.

Treatment of equinovarus deformity consists of simultaneously performing the Achilles tendon lengthening procedure and the split anterior tibial tendon transfer. At surgery, the tibialis anterior is secured and held sufficiently taut to maintain the foot in a neutral position. After healing, 70% of patients are able to walk without an orthosis.

D. Upper Extremities

1. Spasticity—The first objective in treating the spastic upper extremity is to prevent contracture. Severe deformities at the shoulder, elbow, and wrist are seen in the neglected or noncompliant patient. Assistive equipment can be used to position the upper extremity, to aid in prevention of contractures, and to support the shoulder. Positioning extends spastic muscles but does not subject them to sudden postural changes that trigger the stretch reflex and aggravate spasticity. Brief periods should be scheduled when the upper extremity is not suspended and time can be devoted to ROM therapy and hygiene.

Most hemiplegics do not use their hand unless some selective motion is present at the fingers or thumb. Thumb opposition begins with opposition of the thumb to the side of the index finger (lateral or key pinch) and proceeds by circumduction to oppose each fingertip. In most stroke patients with selective thumb–finger extension, proximal muscle function is comparatively intact. Hence, orthotic stabilization of proximal joints is rarely necessary in the patient with a functional hand.

An overhead suspension sling attached to the wheelchair is used for patients with adductor or internal rotator spasticity of the shoulder. An alternative is an arm trough attached to the wheelchair.

It is usually not possible to maintain the wrist in neutral position with a WHO when wrist flexion spasticity is severe or when the wrist is flaccid. With minimal to moderate spasticity, either a volar or dorsal splint can be used. The splint should not extend to the fingers if the finger flexor spasticity is severe because slight motion and sensory contact of the fingers or palm may elicit the stretch reflex or grasp response, causing the fingers to jack-knife out of the splint.

2. Shoulder or arm pain—The hemiplegic shoulder deserves special attention because it is a common source of pain. A variety of different factors contribute to the painful shoulder: reflex sympathetic dystrophy, inferior subluxation, spasticity with internal rotation contracture, adhesive capsulitis, and degenerative changes about the shoulder. If early ROM exercises are performed and the extremity is properly positioned with a sling to reduce subluxation, severe or chronic pain at the shoulder can usually be prevented or minimized.

The classic clinical signs of reflex sympathetic dystrophy (swelling and skin changes) may not be apparent in the hemiplegic patient. If the patient complains that the arm is painful and no cause is apparent, a technetium bone scan assists in establishing the diagnosis (Figure 13–19). Treatment should be instituted immediately, and the patient should be given positive psychological reinforcement. The use of narcotics must be avoided. Treatment options include the use of medications, such as corticosteroids, amitriptyline, or gabapentin (Neurontin), physical therapy, or nerve blocks (stellate ganglion blocks, brachial plexus blocks, or Bier IV regional blocks). Each of these techniques is successful with some patients; however, none is reliable for all patients.

3. Shoulder contracture—Contracture of the shoulder can cause pain, hygiene problems in the axilla, and difficulty in dressing and positioning. Shoulder adduction and internal rotation are caused by spasticity and myostatic contracture

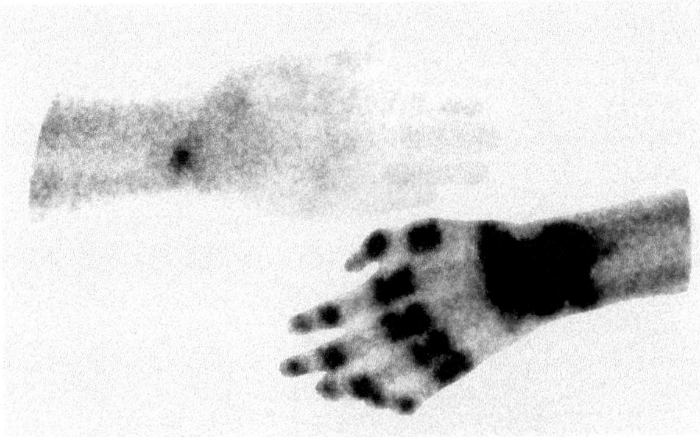

▲ **Figure 13–19.** Technetium bone scan showing the periarticular increase in activity characteristic of reflex sympathetic dystrophy.

of four muscles: the pectoralis major, the subscapularis, the latissimus dorsi, and the teres major.

When the deformity is not fixed, lengthening of the pectoralis major, latissimus, and teres major at their myotendinous junction provides satisfactory correction of the deformity. In a nonfunctional extremity, surgical release of all four muscles (Figure 13–20) is usually necessary to resolve the deformity. Release of the subscapularis muscle is performed without violating the glenohumeral joint capsule. The joint capsule should not be opened because instability or intraarticular adhesions may result. A Z-plasty of the axilla may be needed if the skin is contracted. After the wound heals, an aggressive mobilization program is instituted. Gentle ROM exercises are employed to correct any remaining contracture. Careful positioning of the limb in abduction and external rotation is necessary for several months to prevent recurrence.

4. Inferior subluxation of the shoulder—This is common in people with flaccid paralysis of the shoulder girdle after stroke or brain injury. Often a sling or orthosis fails to reduce the subluxation. If the shoulder is chronically subluxated and painful, biceps suspension surgery can be done with tenotomy and transferring the distal biceps tendon to the proximal humerus to diminish the pain and hold the joint reduced.

5. Elbow flexion contracture—Persistent spasticity of the elbow flexors causes a myostatic contracture and flexion deformity of the elbow. Frequent accompanying problems include skin maceration, breakdown of the antecubital space, and compression neuropathy of the ulnar nerve.

Surgical release of the contracted muscles and gradual extension of the elbow correct the deformity and decrease the ulnar nerve compression. The brachioradialis muscle and biceps tendon are transected. The brachialis muscle is fractionally lengthened at its myotendinous junction by transecting the tendinous fibers on the anterior surface of the muscle while leaving the underlying muscle intact (Figure 13–21).

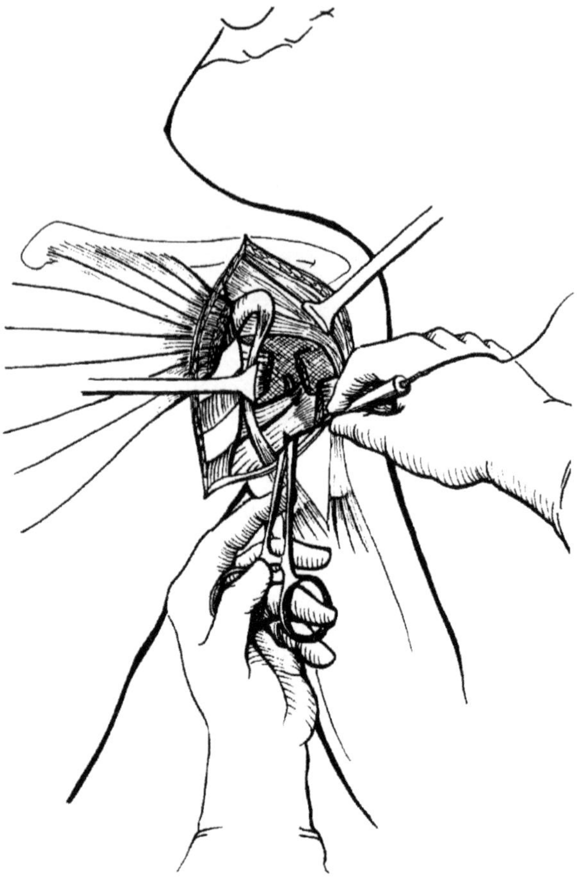

▲ **Figure 13–20. Release of the pectoralis major, subscapularis, latissimus dorsi, and teres major to correct an internal rotation and adduction contracture of the shoulder.** (Illustration by Anthony C. Berlet. Reproduced, with permission, from Keenan MAE, Kozin SH, Berlet AC. *Manual of Orthopaedic Surgery for Spasticity.* Philadelphia, PA: Raven; 1993.)

Complete release of the brachialis muscle is not performed unless a severe contracture was present for several years. An anterior capsulectomy is not needed and should be avoided because of the associated increased stiffness and intraarticular adhesions that occur postoperatively. Anterior transposition of the ulnar nerve may be necessary to further improve ulnar nerve function.

Approximately 50% correction of the deformity can be expected at surgery without causing excessive tension on the contracted neurovascular structures. Serial casts or dropout casts can be used to obtain further correction over the ensuing weeks.

6. Clenched-fist deformity—A spastic clenched-fist deformity in a nonfunctional hand causes palmar skin breakdown and hygiene problems. Recurrent infections of the fingernail beds are also common.

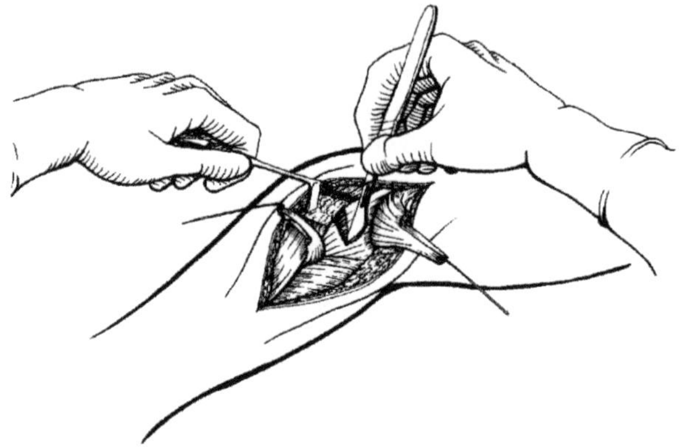

▲ **Figure 13–21. Surgery of the brachioradialis muscle, biceps tendon, and brachialis muscle to correct an elbow flexion contracture in a nonfunctional arm.** (Illustration by Anthony C. Berlet. Reproduced, with permission, from Keenan MAE, Kozin SH, Berlet AC. *Manual of Orthopaedic Surgery for Spasticity.* Philadelphia, PA: Raven; 1993.)

Adequate flexor tendon lengthening to correct the deformity cannot be attained by fractional or myotendinous lengthening without causing discontinuity at the musculotendinous junction. Transection of the flexor tendons is not recommended because any remaining extensor muscle tone may result in an unopposed hyperextension deformity of the wrist and digits. The recommended procedure is a superficialis-to-profundus tendon transfer (Figure 13–22), which provides sufficient flexor tendon lengthening with preservation of a passive tether to prevent a hyperextension deformity. The wrist deformity is corrected by release of the wrist flexors. A wrist arthrodesis is done to maintain the hand in

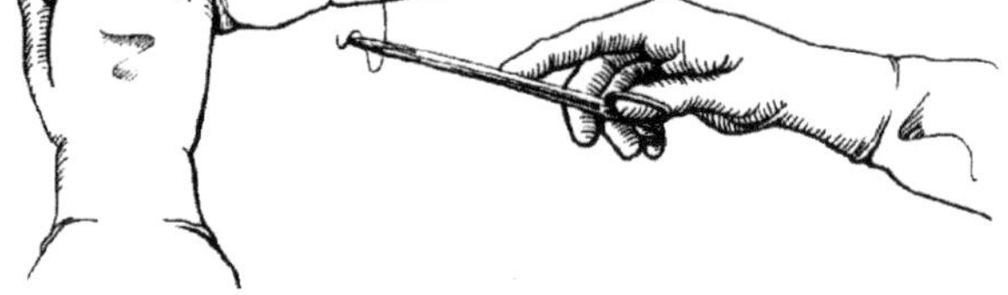

▲ **Figure 13–22. The superficialis-to-profundus tendon transfer to correct a severe clenched-fist deformity in a nonfunctional hand.** (Illustration by Anthony C. Berlet. Reproduced, with permission, from Keenan MAE, Kozin SH, Berlet AC. *Manual of Orthopaedic Surgery for Spasticity.* Philadelphia, PA: Raven; 1993.)

a neutral position and to eliminate the need for a permanent splint. Because intrinsic muscle spasticity is always present in conjunction with severe spasticity of the extrinsic flexors, a neurectomy of the motor branches of the ulnar nerve in the Guyon canal should be routinely performed along with the superficialis-to-profundus tendon transfer to prevent the postsurgical development of an intrinsic plus deformity.

After surgery, the wrist and digits are immobilized for 4 weeks in a short arm cast extended to the fingertips.

Namdari S, Keenan MA. Outcomes of the biceps suspension procedure for painful inferior glenohumeral subluxation in hemiplegic patients. *J Bone Joint Surg Am.* 2010;92(15):2589-2597. [PMID: 21048178]

Saber H, Narayanan S, Palla M, et al. Mechanical thrombectomy for acute ischemic stroke with occlusion of the M2 segment of the middle cerebral artery: a meta-analysis. *J Neurointerv Surg.* 2018;10(7):620-624. [PMID: 29127196]

Tilson JK, Wu SS, Cen SY, et al. Characterizing and identifying risk for falls in the LEAPS study: a randomized clinical trial of interventions to improve walking poststroke. *Stroke* 2012;43:446-452. [PMID: 22246687]

Tsivgoulis G, Goyal N, Katsanos AH, et al. Intravenous thrombolysis for large vessel or distal occlusions presenting with mild stroke severity. *Eur J Neurol.* 2020;27(6):1039-1047. [PMID: 32149450]

Tsivgoulis G, Saqqur M, Sharma VK, et al. Timing of recanalization and functional recovery in acute ischemic stroke. *J Stroke.* 2020;22(1):130-140. [PMID: 32027798]

Viña Soria L, Martín Iglesias L, López Amor L, et al. Results and functional outcomes of acute ischemic stroke patients who underwent mechanical thrombectomy admitted to intensive care unit. *Med Intensiva.* 2018;42(5):274-282. [PMID: 29137863]

Xian Y, Xu H, O'Brien EC, et al. Clinical effectiveness of direct oral anticoagulants vs warfarin in older patients with atrial fibrillation and ischemic stroke: findings from the Patient-Centered Research Into Outcomes Stroke Patients Prefer and Effectiveness Research (PROSPER) study. *JAMA Neurol.* 2019;76(10):1192-1202. [PMID: 31329212]

GERIATRIC ORTHOPEDICS

General Principles

A major challenge facing society is the aging of the population. There are over 50 million Americans older than 65 years, making up about 12% of the population. By 2040, 68 million people will be older than 65 years. Both the absolute numbers and proportion of elderly people is increasing dramatically. People are living longer and have higher expectations for a good quality of life. Despite this trend, proportionally less disability occurs among the elderly now than in the past.

Although the passage of time, chronological age, is the convenient measure used, it is not necessarily the most precise marker of aging. A more sensitive marker would be to consider the person's functional age, but this is often difficult to define and measure. Age 65 is generally considered the beginning of old age. The young elderly are those individuals 65 to 75 years of age. These people are generally healthy and functional. They may have isolated orthopedic problems, such as mild osteoporosis, osteoarthrosis, overuse injuries (sports), and occasionally cancer.

The frail, very elderly are generally those persons older than 80 years. These people may have multiple musculoskeletal impairments such as advanced osteoporosis, generalized muscle weakness, multiple organ diseases, neurological problems, and dementia.

1. Disability

The leading causes of death in the elderly are heart disease, malignant neoplasms, and cerebrovascular disease. The overall leading causes of disability in the elderly are cancer, heart disease, neurological problems, dementia, and musculoskeletal disorders. The leading causes of disease-related disability before death are arthritis, hypertension, hearing impairment, heart disease, and orthopedic conditions. Despite the increasing incidence of disability with aging, only slightly over 5% of Americans aged 65 and older live in nursing homes, assisted living, and board-and-care homes.

When evaluating the elderly, five functional domains of disability need to be considered:

1. *Physical ADLs* include activities such as bathing, dressing, eating, and walking.
2. *Instrumental ADLs* are home management tasks such as shopping, meal preparation, money management, using the telephone, and performing light housework.
3. *Cognitive functioning* is particularly important in the elderly. Dementia is one of the four leading causes of disability in the elderly and a principal reason for institutionalization.
4. *Affective function* is important. Secondary depressions are common in the elderly, and suicide is a more frequent cause of death in the elderly than in the young and has a male bias.
5. *Social functioning* is less of a problem. Only 1% of the elderly rate their social interactions as inadequate.

Disability in basic ADLs is common among community-dwelling older persons, with prevalence rates ranging from 7% in those 65 to 74 years of age to 24% in those 85 years of age or older. Restricted activity, defined as staying in bed for at least half a day and/or cutting down on usual activities because of an illness, injury, or other problem, is common among community-living older persons, regardless of risk for disability, and it is usually attributable to several concurrent health-related problems. Although disability in older persons is often thought to be progressive or permanent, previous research shows it is a dynamic process, with individuals moving in and out of states of disability.

To set realistic goals and plan for appropriate care, disabled older persons, along with their families and clinicians, need accurate information about the likelihood and time course of recovery. Prevention of functional decline and disability includes not only management of acute episodes of disability and promotion of recovery, but also ongoing evaluation and management of key risk factors for disability and use of preventive interventions. The high likelihood of recurrent disability among older persons suggests that those who recently recovered from an episode of disability are an important target population for preventive interventions. Although some interventions designed to prevent recurrent disability may be disease specific (eg, anticoagulation after embolic stroke), others may be broadly applicable regardless of the specific precipitant of disability (eg, exercise-based programs).

2. Challenges for the Clinician

When working with the elderly, the orthopedic surgeon becomes a member of a multidisciplinary team. The people making up this team include orthopedic surgeons, internists, geriatricians, psychiatrists, psychologists, social workers, nutritionists, skin care specialists, rehabilitation specialists including physical and occupational therapists, and friends and relatives including so-called young elderly children. Osteoporosis, fractures, arthritis, foot disorders, stroke, and amputations are the most frequent causes of musculoskeletal impairment.

3. Osteoporosis

Osteoporosis is an age-related disorder characterized by decreased bone mass and increased fracture risk in the absence of other recognizable causes of bone loss. Osteoporosis can occur either as a primary disorder or secondary to other diseases.

A. Primary Osteoporosis

Primary osteoporosis, the most common form of the disease, occurs in people from 51 to 65 years of age with a female-to-male ratio of 6:1. Primary osteoporosis can be further subdivided into two types. Type I, postmenopausal osteoporosis, results from decreased circulating levels of estrogen. It is seen in postmenopausal women and affects the majority of persons older than 70 years. Bone loss is rapid. There is swift trabecular bone loss up to 8% per year. Type I osteoporosis causes primarily trabecular bone loss with only 0.5% cortical bone loss per year. Fractures occur in locations of trabecular bone loss such as the distal radius and vertebrae. The cause of primary osteoporosis is a changing hormonal milieu. Type II, senile osteoporosis, is a consequence of aging. It causes a more global bone loss affecting cortical and cancellous bone such as in the femoral neck. Type II osteoporosis is seen in persons older than 70 years. The female-to-male ratio is 2:1. The bone loss occurs in both the trabecular and cortical bone and averages 0.3% to 0.5% per year. Fractures occurring as the result of type II osteoporosis typically involve the hip, pelvis, humerus, tibia, and vertebral bodies. The causes of senile osteoporosis are those seen with aging and include calcium deficiency, decreased vitamin D, and increased parathormone activity.

B. Secondary Osteoporosis

Secondary osteoporosis results from a variety of causes. The most common are chronic or prolonged corticosteroid use, endocrine disorders, and hypogonadism. The endocrine disorders associated with osteoporosis include hyperthyroidism, hyperparathyroidism, diabetes, Cushing disease, and euplastic disorders. The hypogonadal states associated with osteoporosis include Tuner syndrome, Klinefelter syndrome, anorexia nervosa, early menopause, and bilateral oophorectomy or testiculectomy.

Prevention Strategies

Restoration of bone is difficult. It is therefore imperative to maximize peak bone mass during skeletal growth and then to maintain it during maturity. This requires adequate dietary calcium and vitamin D intake. The recommended amounts for adults are 1200 mg/day of calcium and 400 mg of vitamin D. For postmenopausal women, 1500 mg/day of calcium is recommended. Impact exercise is effective in maintaining bone mass. It is also important to avoid those factors that promote osteoporosis such as the use of tobacco products and excessive alcohol consumption.

Diagnosis

Osteoporosis is a clinical diagnosis often made following a fracture. Radiographic findings include osteopenia (seen with >30% mineral loss); loss of horizontal trabeculae in vertebral bodies; thoracic wedge fractures; lumbar spine endplate fractures; stress fractures of the pelvis; and fractures of humerus, wrist, hip, supracondylar femur, and tibial plateau. Quantification of bone mass is done for confirmation and follow-up. Dual-energy x-ray absorptiometry (DEXA) is used to quantify bone mass. The following criteria for diagnosis are based on the DEXA scan:

Normal: within 1 standard deviation (SD) of young adult reference

Osteopenia: between 1.0 and 2.4 SDs below reference

Osteoporosis: 2.5 or more SDs below reference

Severe osteoporosis: 2.5 plus one or more fragility fractures

Treatment

Weight-bearing exercise is useful in maintaining bone mass. Adequate daily calcium replacement is also helpful.

Calcium and vitamin D alone do not prevent bone loss but may reduce the risk of hip fractures if given in combination. In late menopause (>6 years), calcium replacement does reduce bone loss.

Hormone therapy in postmenopausal women has been controversial. Current evidence supports the use of hormone therapy to prevent osteoporosis in women at high risk of fracture. Estrogen therapy has a more favorable benefit-risk profile for long-term use compared to estrogen-progestogen therapy, which has increased breast cancer risk.

Bisphosphonates, teriparatide, and denosumab have been shown to be effective in reducing the risk of fragility fractures. These osteoporosis treatments generally maintain bone mineral density over time and have relatively few side effects including stomach upset, heartburn, musculoskeletal aches, and, with long-term bisphosphonate use, low-impact atypical femoral fractures such as subtrochanteric fractures and osteonecrosis of the jaw.

Bisphosphonates are a class of compounds similar to pyrophosphate that are readily adsorbed by bone mineral surfaces. Once bound, they inhibit the bone absorption activity of osteoclasts. Bisphosphonates currently available for clinical use include alendronate, risedronate, ibandronate, and zoledronic acid. Teriparatide is a recombinant form of parathyroid hormone, a primary regulator of calcium and phosphate metabolism in bone and kidney. Intermittent exposure to parathyroid hormone activates osteoblasts more than osteoclasts, and once-daily injections of teriparatide are thought to have a net effect of stimulating new bone formation, leading to increased bone mineral density. Denosumab is a human monoclonal antibody that targets RANKL, a protein that acts as the primary signal to promote bone removal. Raloxifene is a selective estrogen receptor modulator that has estrogenic effects on bone and thus is used in prevention of osteoporosis in women. Romosozumab is a humanized monoclonal antibody that targets sclerostin, a glycoprotein produced by the osteocyte that has antianabolic effects on bone formation.

Exercise

The ability to walk safely is vital for independent living. Both strength and endurance determine the capacity for independent movement. Muscle strength is associated with the capacity to perform ADLs. A reduction in strength with age is attributed to the following factors:

1. A loss of muscle mass because of smaller and fewer fibers
2. A loss of motor neurons (anterior horn cells)
3. Changes in muscle architecture
4. A defect in the excitation-contraction mechanism
5. Psychosocial changes leading to reduced capacity to activate motor units

Strength training can lead to major functional improvements in the elderly. The plasticity of the motor system to adapt to a training load appears to be maintained into the 10th decade of life. Strength training has no effect on the central determinants of aerobic capacity such as maximum heart rate, blood pressure, hemoglobin concentration, and blood volume.

Aerobic exercise does lead to increased endurance and functional capacity. Endurance is the time a person can maintain either a static force or a power level involving a combination of concentric or eccentric muscular contractions. The stress that exercise imposes on a person and the tolerance or endurance for that exercise intensity depends on how much energy is needed to perform the task in relation to the person's maximal capacity. With training, activities become easier to perform. The person has increased endurance for submaximal exercise. Improvements in movement can lower the energy cost of an activity.

4. Arthritis

Osteoarthritis is very prevalent in the elderly. Total joint arthroplasty has dramatically improved the mobility and quality of life for the elderly. A variety of studies confirm the appropriateness and effectiveness of both total hip and total knee arthroplasty in the elderly with low complication rates. The elderly patient is more likely to require the use of an upper extremity assistive device for ambulation following joint replacement.

5. Fractures

A. General Considerations

One of the most compelling reasons to determine the etiology of a fracture and provide appropriate treatment is that a previous low-energy fracture is one of the strongest risk factors for new fractures. Specifically, patients with a low-energy fracture of the wrist, hip, proximal humerus, or ankle have nearly a two- to four-fold greater risk for future fractures than individuals who have never experienced a fracture. Furthermore, up to half of the patients with a prior vertebral fracture experience additional vertebral fractures within 3 years, many within the first year. Indeed, compared to individuals with no history of fracture, a patient with a prior vertebral fracture has nearly a five-fold increased risk of future vertebral fractures and up to a six-fold increased risk of hip and other nonvertebral fractures. Taken together, these data indicate that patients with a history of any type of prior fracture have a two- to six-fold increased risk of subsequent fractures compared to those without a previous fracture.

These findings emphasize that optimal care of fragility fracture patients includes not only management of the presenting fracture, but also evaluation, diagnosis, and treatment of the underlying cause(s) of the fracture, including low bone density or other medical conditions. In this regard, supplementation with calcium and vitamin D lowers fracture risk in the elderly. In addition, several pharmacologic agents reduce the risk of future fracture by as much as 50% in patients with existing fractures. Nonpharmacologic interventions, such as fall prevention programs and individually tailored exercise programs, reduce falls among the elderly, which may decrease the incidence of fractures. In addition, trochanteric padding dramatically reduces hip fractures among those at highest risk. Thus, initiating interventions soon after a fragility fracture occurs may significantly reduce the incidence and severity of subsequent fractures.

In the elderly, fractures result from low-energy injuries. Falls in the home most frequently result in fractures of the hip, distal radius, pelvis, proximal humerus, and ribs. Approximately 90% of fractures of the pelvis, hip, and forearm result from a fall. Only 3% to 5% of falls result in fractures.

Many of the risk factors for fracture are also risk factors for falls. Risk factors can be divided into categories. Risk factors associated with aspects of aging include primary osteoporosis, impaired vision or balance, gait abnormalities, and loss of muscle and fat padding the bones. Environmental risk factors consist of uneven surfaces; slippery surfaces; obstacles such as throw rugs, pets, and steps; poor lighting; and lack of railings or other supports for balance. Fall prevention programs include home safety measures such as the installation of safety bars in the bathtub and shower, elimination of heavily waxed floors and slippery rugs, and the use of rubber sole shoes with low wide heels that provide more stability.

Genetic factors are seen in both gender and race. Women sustain more fractures than men. Whites have more fractures than African Americans. Illnesses commonly associated with fractures include stroke, syncope, hypotension, secondary osteoporosis, Parkinson disease, dementia, and paraparesis. The use of medications such as benzodiazepines, tricyclic antidepressants, antipsychotics, corticosteroids, and barbiturates is connected with fractures. Lifestyle factors include exercise, nutrition, alcohol or other substance abuse, immobilization, and shoe style.

Other factors contribute to the risk of traumatic fractures occurring in falls. The first is the orientation of the fall. A fall that happens while standing still or walking very slowly imparts little or no forward momentum, so the point of impact is near the hip. Gait velocity slows with aging, putting the hip more at risk of injury in a fall. Protective responses during a fall decrease with age. Local shock absorbers, muscle and fat, that surround the bone decrease with age. Bone strength is less secondary to the osteoporosis associated with aging.

B. Hip Fractures

Fractures of the hip are classified by location and severity. The basic considerations are whether the fracture occurs in the intracapsular or extracapsular area and the stability of the fracture pattern. Intracapsular fractures occur along the neck of the femur. When they are displaced, the blood supply to the femoral head is likely disrupted, which increases the possibility of osteonecrosis.

Treatment of hip fractures is operative whenever possible because nonoperative treatments involve months of bed rest and sometimes traction. It requires excellent nursing care to avoid decubitus ulcers and respiratory dysfunction. Fracture malunion, limb-length inequality, pain, and higher mortality rates are common with nonoperative care. The chances for eventual ambulation are only 55% compared with 76% for patients treated operatively. Nonoperative treatment of hip fractures is very occasionally chosen for patients at high medical risk and is also sometimes recommended for demented nonambulatory patients.

The basic principles of treatment of hip fractures are well established. Nondisplaced fractures of the femoral neck are usually treated with multiple pins or screws. Displaced fractures of the femoral neck are usually treated with a hemiarthroplasty because of the high incidence of avascular necrosis. Intertrochanteric fractures are generally treated with a sliding screw and either a side plate or intramedullary rod. In very osteoporotic bone, it may be necessary to add methyl methacrylate bone cement to gain sufficient fixation and stability. A patient with prior hip arthritis may be treated with a total hip arthroplasty.

The postoperative rehabilitation of the elderly patient is critical to a successful outcome. Non–weight-bearing ambulation is extremely difficult and more often impossible for elderly patients. Every effort should be made in the operative treatment to gain enough stability of the fracture to allow weight bearing as tolerated. The patient should be mobilized on the first or second day after surgery to prevent the many complications of immobility. Pain management is important to allow mobilization while minimizing oversedation. After arthroplasty, dislocation must be avoided. The elderly patient may not remember the precautions. Use of elevated chairs and toilet seats helps avoid the excessive hip flexion associated with posterior dislocation. A knee immobilizer splint while in bed prevents knee flexion that in turn also prevents flexion of the hip. It is sometimes prudent to place the patient in a hip brace, which limits flexion and adduction while soft-tissue healing occurs.

C. Fractures of the Pelvis

A common pelvic classification is based on whether or not the ring of the pelvis is disrupted because this indicates the amount of energy involved with the initial trauma. A fracture that does not disrupt the pelvic ring such as a pubic ramus fracture is a low-energy injury. Formerly, pelvic fractures were associated with high-energy trauma, were displaced, and occurred in patients less than 40 years old. With the aging of America, now more than 50% of fractures occur in those older than 60 years, with a preponderance occurring in women. The majority of pelvis fractures in the elderly are low-energy injuries and can be treated nonoperatively with analgesia and bed rest. Early mobilization is desirable to prevent the complications of immobility. Full weight bearing is allowed. A walker or other assistive device is useful to decrease pain and increase stability during walking. Stool softeners are often helpful. Fractures of the coccyx and sacrum are treated in a similar manner.

D. Fractures of the Distal Femur

The management of distal femur fractures in elderly patients must be individualized. Advanced age in itself is not a contraindication to surgery. The objects of surgical treatment of the distal femur are anatomic reduction and stable fixation. In the presence of severe osteopenia, stable fixation is difficult. The addition of methyl methacrylate or long-stem knee replacement can help with stability. Occasionally, a postoperative cast brace is needed to supplement the internal fixation.

E. Fractures of the Forearm

Most fractures of the distal radius (Colles fracture) can be treated by closed reduction and casting. Significant loss of radial height and dorsal comminution can occur in osteoporotic bone even after lower energy injuries. In this situation, most surgeons would agree that external fixation and bone grafting of the fracture are warranted to obtain and maintain a more anatomic reduction. Early ROM exercises for both the shoulder and the fingers should be encouraged to avoid stiffness.

F. Fractures of the Proximal Humerus

Fractures of the proximal humerus account for 4% to 5% of all fractures and occur most commonly in the elderly. Humeral fractures in the elderly are minimally displaced 80% of the time. In these cases, sling immobilization is used to control pain. Pendulum exercises are begun within 2 weeks after injury to prevent excessive stiffness. Limited external rotation of the shoulder predisposes to a future spiral fracture of the humerus while dressing. Unstable, displaced fractures are best treated with open reduction and internal fixation, and those involving the humeral head and/or prone to avascular necrosis are best treated with hemiarthroplasty. In the frail elderly, a reverse total shoulder arthroplasty is also an option.

6. Stroke

As detailed earlier, stroke is a common cause of disability in the elderly.

7. Foot Disorders

The foot tends to widen with age as the transverse arch support weakens and abnormal bony alignments of the foot become common. Surgical reconstruction of foot deformities may be contraindicated in the frail elderly patient, particularly because of peripheral vascular disease. Nonoperative treatment consists of active and passive ROM exercises of the foot to maximize flexibility. Strengthening exercises of the lower extremity can be useful to improve the overall gait pattern. The patient should try to optimize body weight to eliminate excessive forces on the foot. Functional orthoses of a semirigid material with little or no posting may improve the foot position and provide symptomatic relief. Accommodative orthoses of a soft material may also be used. These soft orthoses are designed to control foot posture and eliminate areas of pressure, but they are not intended to correct the foot position. Orthoses are used in combination with soft extra-depth shoes that provide more clearance for deformities of the toes. Flat shoes are helpful for forefoot deformities because they prevent the foot sliding forward in the shoe. A shoe with a low heel is desirable for patients with a severe pronation deformity because the Achilles tendon is commonly tight. Placing the heel cord on stretch only increases the pronation forces on the foot.

8. Amputation

The majority of all amputations done in a civilian population are of the lower extremity. Most amputations are done in the sixth decade of life or later and are the result of vascular insufficiency. Posttraumatic amputations largely result from blunt trauma, with motor vehicle collisions and machinery accidents being the most common etiologies. Most are of the lower extremity, and about two thirds are amputations of one or more digits. In these patients, multiple limb amputation is an independent risk factor for death, whereas a single limb amputation is not.

The issues associated with amputation are discussed in Chapter 11.

Conley RB, Adib G, Adler RA, et al. Secondary fracture prevention: consensus clinical recommendations from a multistakeholder coalition. *J Bone Miner Res*. 2020;35(1):36-52. [PMID: 31538675]

Curtis EM, Woolford S, Holmes C, Cooper C, Harvey NC. General and specific considerations as to why osteoporosis-related care is often suboptimal. *Curr Osteoporos Rep*. 2020;18(1):38-46. [PMID: 32103393]

Dirschl DR, Rustom H. Practice patterns and performance in U.S. fracture liaison programs: an analysis of >32,000 patients from the own the bone program. *J Bone Joint Surg Am*. 2018;100(8):680-685. [PMID: 29664856]

Hiligsmann M, Cornelissen D, Vrijens B, et al. Determinants, consequences and potential solutions to poor adherence to anti-osteoporosis treatment: results of an expert group meeting organized by the European Society for Clinical and Economic Aspects of Osteoporosis, Osteoarthritis and Musculoskeletal Diseases (ESCEO) and the International Osteoporosis Foundation (IOF). *Osteoporos Int*. 2019;30(11):2155-2165. [PMID: 31388696]

Hiligsmann M, Williams SA, Fitzpatrick LA, Silverman SS, Weiss R, Reginster JY. Cost-effectiveness of sequential treatment with abaloparatide followed by alendronate vs. alendronate monotherapy in women at increased risk of fracture: a US payer perspective. *Semin Arthritis Rheum.* 2020;50(3):394-400. [PMID: 32160943]

Lim SJ, Yeo I, Yoon PW, et al. Incidence, risk factors, and fracture healing of atypical femoral fractures: a multicenter case-control study. *Osteoporos Int.* 2018;29(11):2427-2435. [PMID: 30039251]

Yang FZ, Jehu DAM, Ouyang H, Lam FMH, Pang MYC. The impact of stroke on bone properties and muscle-bone relationship: a systematic review and meta-analysis. *Osteoporos Int.* 2020;31(2):211-224. [PMID: 31720713]

TRAUMATIC BRAIN INJURY

Traumatic brain injury (TBI) is a leading cause of death and disability. Millions of Americans suffer a TBI each year. Most are mild, causing a brief change in mental status; these are commonly called concussions. But TBIs can be severe (coma), presenting a challenge to the team of health care providers involved in providing emergency treatment and long-term management. TBIs have many etiologies including falls, being struck by an object, sporting injuries, and motor vehicle accidents.

Neurologic Impairment and Recovery

The Glasgow Coma Score (Table 13–3) is frequently used to evaluate eye opening, motor response, and verbal response of patients with impaired consciousness. Approximately 50% of patients with impaired consciousness survive. Six months after injury, moderate or good neurologic recovery was seen in about 82% of patients with initial (24-hour) Glasgow scores of 11 or higher, 68% of patients with initial scores of 8 to 10, 34% with initial scores of 5 to 7, and 7% with initial scores of 3 or 4. Age was an important factor related to neurologic outcome, with 62% of patients younger than 20 years and 46% of patients between 20 and 29 years of age showing moderate or good recovery.

Table 13–3. The Glasgow Coma Score.

Response	Description	Numerical Value
Eye opening	Spontaneous response	4
	Response to speech	3
	Response to pain	2
	No response	1
Motor response	Obeying response	6
	Localized response	5
	Withdrawal	4
	Abnormal flexion	3
	Extension	2
	No response	1
Verbal response	Oriented conversation	5
	Confused conversation	4
	Inappropriate words	3
	Incomprehensible sounds	2
	No response	1

Adapted, with permission, from Teasdale G, Jennett B. Assessment of coma and impaired consciousness. A practical scale. *Lancet.* 1974;2:81-84.

The incidence of good recovery declines not only with advancing age but also with advancing duration of coma. Patients recovering from coma within the first 2 weeks of injury have a 70% chance of good recovery. The recovery rate drops to 39% in the third week and to 17% in the fourth week. Decerebrate or decorticate posturing indicates a brainstem injury and is indicative of a poor prognosis.

Management

The rehabilitation process has three distinct phases: the acute injury period, the subacute period of neurologic recovery, and the residual period of functional adaptation. Health care workers from a variety of disciplines are involved in each phase.

A. Phases of Patient Care and Rehabilitation for Severe Traumatic Brain Injury

1. Acute injury phase—The initial phase of rehabilitation begins as soon as the patient reaches the acute-care hospital. Severe TBI is frequently the result of a high-velocity accident. Diagnosis is problematic because multiple injuries are common, resuscitation and other lifesaving efforts make a complete examination difficult, and the patient who is comatose or disoriented cannot assist in the history or physical examination.

Under the circumstances, three important principles should be followed. The first is to make an accurate diagnosis based on a thorough examination. Fractures or dislocations are missed in 11% of patients, and peripheral nerve injuries are missed in 34%. The second is to assume that the patient will make a good neurologic recovery. Basic treatment principles should not be ignored on the erroneous assumption that the patient will not survive. The third principle is to anticipate uncontrolled limb motion and lack of patient cooperation. The patient often goes through a period of agitation as neurologic recovery progresses. Traction and external fixation devices are best avoided for extremity injuries. Open reduction and internal fixation of fractures and dislocations diminishes complications, requires less nursing care, allows for earlier mobilization, and results in fewer residual deformities.

2. Subacute phase of neurologic recovery—During the subacute phase, when the patient is generally in a rehabilitation facility, spontaneous neurologic recovery occurs. During this recovery period, which may last from 12 to 18 months, spasticity is frequently present, and HO may develop. Management is aimed at preventing limb deformities, maintaining a functional arc of motion in the joints, and meeting both the physical and the psychological needs of the patient.

3. Residual phase or period of functional adaptation—When neurologic recovery reaches a plateau, the third phase of rehabilitation begins. Medical and surgical management is aimed at correction of residual limb deformities and excision of HO while specialists from various disciplines continue moving toward the goals planned for the individual patient.

B. The Team Approach to Patient Care and Rehabilitation

Members of the rehabilitation team are involved in setting short-term goals, which are meant to be accomplished by the time of discharge from the rehabilitation program, and long-term goals, which will take an extended period of time to achieve. The identification of needs and the setting of goals are performed independently by health care workers from each discipline. The team members then meet to discuss their goals and draw up a coordinated plan.

1. Medical management—General medical goals are usually straightforward. Because most patients with TBIs are younger persons, chronic premorbid illnesses are uncommon. Prevention and treatment of infections are important goals, especially while shunts, tubes, and catheters are in place. If seizures are present, controlling them without causing sedation is vital.

In patients with decreased ROM in a joint, the cause of the problem should be explored. Possible causes include increased muscle tone, pain, myostatic contracture, periarticular HO, an undetected fracture or dislocation, and lack of patient cooperation secondary to diminished cognition. Peripheral nerve blocks with local anesthetics are useful in distinguishing between severe spasticity and fixed contractures.

Phenol blocks or botulinum toxin injections may be used to decrease spasticity only during the period of potential neurologic recovery. The rationale for phenol injection is that by the time the nerve regenerates, the patient will have recovered more control of the affected muscle. Phenol blocks and botulinum toxin injections can be done using ultrasound guidance to increase the accuracy of locating the precise anatomical structures.

The technique for administering the phenol block depends on the anatomic accessibility and composition of the nerve; the direct injection of a peripheral nerve gives the most complete and long-lasting block. If a peripheral nerve has a large sensory component, however, direct injection is not recommended because loss of sensation is undesirable and some patients may develop painful hyperesthesia. In some cases, it is necessary to dissect surgically the individual motor branches of a nerve that runs to a muscle and inject each branch separately. In other cases, the motor points of the muscles can be localized using a needle electrode and nerve stimulator and then injected. Motor point injections do not completely relieve spasticity but can be helpful in reducing muscle tone. The duration of motor point blocks is approximately 2 months, and the blocks can be repeated as necessary.

Botulinum toxin is injected directly into the muscle belly. The onset of action is delayed but lasts for approximately 3 months. The injections can be repeated as needed and do not result in scarring of the muscle. The limitation of botulinum toxin is the total dose tolerated at a given time and its high cost relative to phenol.

2. Nursing care—Nursing goals concentrate on basic bodily needs such as nutrition, hygiene, and handling of secretions. Removal of tubes at the earliest possible time is a desirable goal.

Tracheostomy tubes are commonly used in patients with TBI. General principles of care include changing an uncuffed tube as soon as possible to prevent pressure necrosis of the trachea, adding mist if necessary to provide moisture to the artificial airway, establishing suctioning procedures to prevent trauma and infection, and eliminating the dressing once the tracheostomy incision is healed because the dressing can be a source of infection. The size of the tube is gradually reduced, and the tube is then plugged to tolerance. When continual plugging is tolerated for 3 consecutive days, the tube can be removed.

Feeding tubes are also commonly used. If oral feeding is not anticipated in the near future, a percutaneous endoscopic gastrostomy tube is recommended. If oral feeding is anticipated soon, a nasogastric tube is inserted, cleaned daily, and changed once a week. Instituting and carrying out an oral feeding program requires the combined efforts of the nursing and physical therapy staffs. Head and trunk control are necessary to provide alignment of swallowing structures. The presence of a cough reflex indicates some measure of laryngeal control and the ability to clear the airway. The presence of a swallowing reflex indicates inherent coordination of swallowing structures. The gag reflex, although protective, is not necessary for functional swallowing. Oral feeding should be started with thickened liquids and pureed foods, which provide more oral stimulus and allow time to initiate swallowing. Thin liquids are more difficult to swallow and can be easily aspirated.

The ability to inhibit voiding is generally a cognitive function. Restoring continence in the TBI patient requires a consistent routine with repeated instructions and positive feedback. Bowel programs should be initiated as soon as the patient begins taking nourishment via the gastrointestinal tract. Again, a consistent routine is most successful.

3. Cognitive and neuropsychological management—The return of cognitive abilities follows the same sequence of stages that normal cognitive development follows, with each

Table 13–4. Cognitive function.

Level	Description
I	No response
II	Generalized response
III	Localized response
IV	Confused, agitated response
V	Confused, inappropriate response
VI	Confused, appropriate response
VII	Automatic, appropriate response
VIII	Purposeful, appropriate response

Adapted from Malkmus D. *Rehabilitation of the Head-Injured Adult. Comprehensive Cognitive Management.* Downey, CA: Professional Staff Association of Rancho Los Amigos Hospital; 1980.

new level of cognitive function stemming from the previous level. Table 13–4 shows the eight levels. Cognitive and behavioral management focuses on providing stimulation for patients with a level II or III response; providing structure for patients with a level IV, V, or VI response; and encouraging community activities for patients with a level VII or VIII response.

Memory loss and diminished cognitive function are frequently the most pervasive limitations to overall function. Cognitive retraining is an essential part of the rehabilitation process at every stage. As cognition increases and the patient becomes more aware of the TBI, increasing awareness of the possible consequences requires counseling and psychological support.

4. Speech therapy—After TBI, patients may have temporary or permanent physical handicaps that prevent them from communicating effectively. In communicating with nonverbal patients, a variety of methods and devices can be used, ranging from yes-and-no signals to communication boards and electronic devices. Patients need to acquire at least a minimal level of attention, memory, and organizational skills to facilitate use of such communication devices. In verbal patients, language disorders may be present because of an underlying cognitive disruption following TBI. The most frequent residual language disorders are those seen in the areas of work retrieval and auditory processing. Language therapy in patients with these long-term disorders should be directed toward reorganization of the cognitive process.

5. Physical therapy—Areas of concern in physical therapy include patient positioning, mobility, and performance of daily activities. Making it possible for bedridden patients to sit can significantly improve the quality of life and greatly enhance the opportunities to interact with other people. In some patients, casts or orthotic devices may be required to maintain the desired limb positions. Aggressive joint ROM exercises are necessary to prevent contractures.

Among the factors that influence whether a patient can walk are limb stability, motor control, good balance reactions, and adequate proprioception. Equipment and devices to aid in movement (eg, canes, walkers, wheelchairs) should always be of the least complex design to accomplish the goal and should be chosen on the basis of the individual patient's cognitive and physical level of function.

In developing appropriate exercises and activities for a patient, the physical therapist should consider factors such as the joint ROM, muscle tone, motor control, and cognitive functions of the patient. Even the confused and agitated patient may respond to simple, familiar functional activities such as washing the face and brushing the teeth. Patients with higher cognitive function should be encouraged to carry out hygiene, grooming, dressing, and feeding activities.

6. Surgical management of residual musculoskeletal problems—After neurologic recovery stabilizes, surgical procedures may be indicated to correct residual limb deformities and to excise HO.

Surgical correction of limb deformities has traditionally been done with tendon lengthening, but surgical hyperselective neurectomies can be performed as an alternative to tendon lengthening. Here the motor nerves are identified and transected as they enter the muscle. This procedure does not correct any significant shortening of the muscle. When there is little or no muscle contracture, the ROM can be improved with postoperative therapy.

A. Correction of limb deformities in the lower extremities—In functional lower limbs, surgery is most often directed at correcting the equinovarus deformity of the foot (see Figure 13–12). The procedures needed for correction of the deformity are determined by clinical evaluation combined with laboratory assessment using dynamic polyelectromyography (poly-EMG). Commonly, several procedures are done simultaneously: lengthening of the Achilles tendon (see Figure 13–16); release of the flexor digitorum longus, flexor hallucis longus, and flexor brevis tendons (see Figure 13–17); a split anterior tibial tendon transfer (see Figure 13–18); and transfer of the flexor digitorum longus tendon to the heel. The object of surgery is to provide a plantigrade foot for standing and walking, and the surgery is highly successful in this goal. Seventy percent of patients are able to ambulate without a brace after surgery.

A stiff-knee gait is a common deformity that causes the patient to hike the pelvis and circumduct the leg for clearance of the foot during the swing phase of walking. Inappropriate activity in the quadriceps muscle at this time prevents knee flexion. If the vasti muscles of the quadriceps muscle are firing out of phase, the affected head or heads can be lengthened surgically (see Figure 13–14) to allow knee flexion while retaining quadriceps function. Transfer of the rectus femoris muscle to the sartorius or gracilis muscle provides active knee flexion during swing.

In nonfunctional lower limbs, surgery commonly consists of releasing contractures of the hips and knees.

B. Correction of limb deformities in the upper extremities—In functional upper limbs, surgery is frequently needed to correct problems of the wrist, fingers, and thumbs. If active hand opening is restricted by flexor spasticity, lengthening of the extrinsic finger flexors (Figure 13–23) weakens the overactive flexors and improves hand function while preserving the ability of the patient to grasp objects. In cases in which spastic thenar muscles cause thumb-in-palm deformity, a procedure consisting of proximal release of the thenar muscles (Figure 13–24) corrects the problem while preserving function of the thumb. In some patients, adequate placement of the hand for functional activities is impaired by elbow spasticity, although triceps function is generally normal. In these patients, lengthening the elbow flexors (Figure 13–25) enhances the ability to extend the elbow smoothly while preserving active flexion.

In nonfunctional upper limbs, common procedures consist of releasing various contractures and performing neurectomies to eliminate muscle spasticity. The problems of shoulder contracture, elbow contracture, and clenched-fist deformity are discussed earlier in this chapter in the section on stroke, and the surgical procedures used in their treatment are shown in Figures 13–20 to 13–22.

C. Excision of heterotopic ossification—Surgical measures for treatment of this problem are discussed later in this chapter.

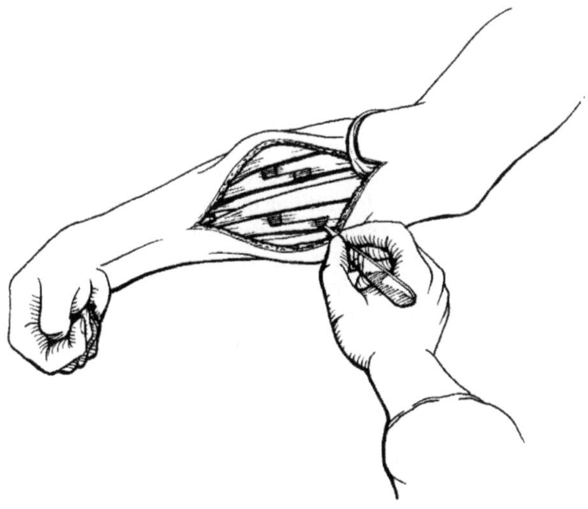

▲ **Figure 13–23. Lengthening of the extrinsic finger flexors to correct the problem of flexor spasticity and improve hand function while preserving the ability to grasp objects.** (Illustration by Anthony C. Berlet. Reproduced, with permission, from Keenan MAE, Kozin SH, Berlet AC. *Manual of Orthopaedic Surgery for Spasticity*. Philadelphia, PA: Raven; 1993.)

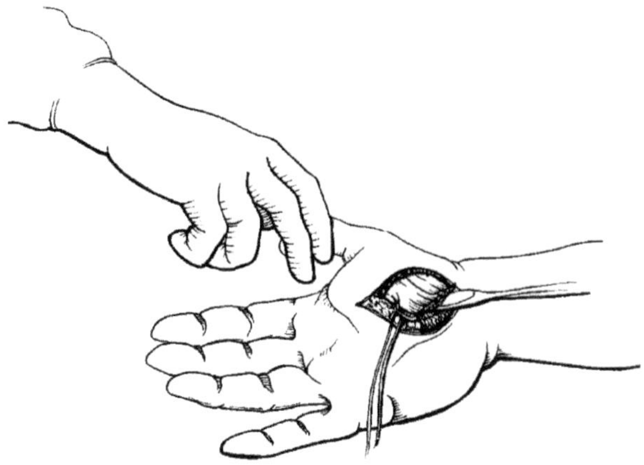

▲ **Figure 13–24. Proximal release of the thenar muscles to correct a thumb-in-palm deformity while preserving function of the thumb.** (Illustration by Anthony C. Berlet. Reproduced, with permission, from Keenan MAE, Kozin SH, Berlet AC. *Manual of Orthopaedic Surgery for Spasticity*. Philadelphia, PA: Raven; 1993.)

D. Occupational therapy and social services—Before patients are released from the hospital or rehabilitation facility, both they and their families must be informed about social service agencies, support groups, and special programs that can be of help. Social adjustment and the resumption of occupational pursuits and leisure activities depend on the recovery of mental factors first, personality status second, and physical factors third. Physical factors are more responsive to rehabilitation than are mental, personality, or social factors. Mental impairment, however, interferes the most with independence in ADLs.

7. Inpatient rehabilitation—Changes in the rules governing inpatient rehabilitation hospitals and units, particularly

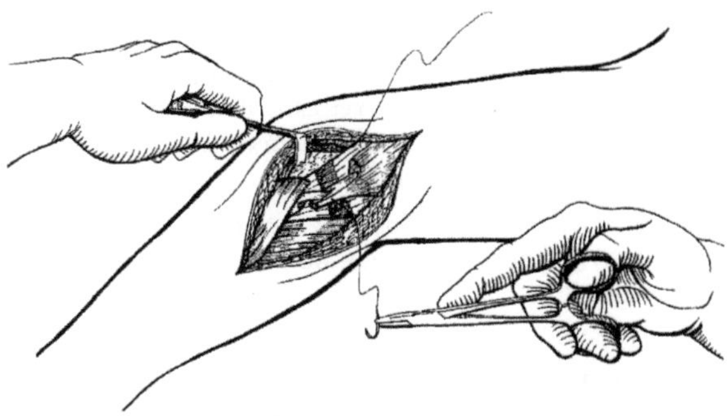

▲ **Figure 13–25. Lengthening of the elbow flexors to correct flexor spasticity and improve movement of the elbow.** (Illustration by Anthony C. Berlet. Reproduced, with permission, from Keenan MAE, Kozin SH, Berlet AC. *Manual of Orthopaedic Surgery for Spasticity*. Philadelphia, PA: Raven; 1993.)

the implementation of the new prospective payment system for inpatient rehabilitation facilities by the Centers for Medicare and Medicaid Services, complicate the admission of patients with rehabilitation goals to an inpatient setting.

Physicians generally agree on the circumstances that justify a medical or surgical patient's hospitalization. In addition, in some cases, an admission to a rehabilitation hospital or to the rehabilitation service of a short-term hospital can be justified on essentially the same medical or surgical grounds. In other cases, however, a patient's medical or surgical needs alone may not warrant inpatient hospital care, but hospitalization may nevertheless be necessary because of the patient's need for rehabilitative services.

Patients needing rehabilitative services require a hospital level of care if they need a relatively intense rehabilitation program that requires a multidisciplinary coordinated team approach to upgrade their ability to function (eg, patients with TBI or SCI after corrective extremity surgery). Two basic requirements must be met for inpatient hospital stays for rehabilitation care to be covered:

1. The services must be reasonable and necessary (in terms of efficacy, duration, frequency, and amount) for the treatment of the patient's condition.
2. It must be reasonable and necessary to furnish the care on an inpatient hospital basis, rather than in a less intensive facility such as a skilled nursing facility, or on an outpatient basis.

To meet the requirements just cited, the following basic components must be met:

1. The patient needs close medical supervision by a physician with specialized training or experience in rehabilitation.
2. The patient requires the 24-hour availability of a registered nurse with specialized training or experience in rehabilitation.
3. The general threshold for establishing the need for inpatient hospital rehabilitation services is that the patient must require and receive at least 3 hours a day of physical and/or occupational therapy.
4. A multidisciplinary team (usually including, at minimum, a physician, rehabilitation nurse, and one therapist) is needed.

Andelic N, Forslund MV, Perrin PB, et al. Long-term follow-up of use of therapy services for patients with moderate-to-severe traumatic brain injury. *J Rehabil Med.* 2020;52(3):jrm00034. [PMID: 32179933]

de Franca SA, Tavares WM, Salinet ASM, Paiva WS, Teixeira MJ. Early tracheostomy in severe traumatic brain injury patients: a meta-analysis and comparison with late tracheostomy. *Crit Care Med.* 2020;48(4):e325-e331. [PMID: 32205623]

Downing M, Hicks A, Braaf S, et al. Factors facilitating recovery following severe traumatic brain injury: a qualitative study. *Neuropsychol Rehabil.* 2020;23:1-25. [PMID: 32200692]

Leclercq C. Selective neurectomy for the spastic upper extremity. *Hand Clin.* 2018;34(4):537-545. [PMID: 30286968]

Namdari S, Alosh H, Baldwin K, Mehta S, Keenan MA. Shoulder tenotomies to improve passive motion and relieve pain in patients with spastic hemiplegia after upper motor neuron injury. *J Shoulder Elbow Surg.* 2011;20(5):802-806. [PMID: 21232986]

HETEROTOPIC OSSIFICATION

HO is commonly detected 2 months after TBI or SCI and is characterized by increasing pain and decreasing ROM about a joint. The problem affects adults but is virtually unheard of in children. Although the cause of HO is unknown, a genetic predisposition is suspected. Unidentified humoral factors that enhance osteogenesis are demonstrated in the sera of patients with TBI. Other contributing factors include soft-tissue trauma and spasticity.

Clinical Findings

Clinically significant HO is seen in 20% of adults with TBIs or SCIs and may affect one joint or multiple joints. The overall rate of joint ankylosis is about 15%. In affected patients, the bone forms in association with spastic muscles, and the alkaline phosphatase level is elevated. Bone scans may aid in early diagnosis, and the diagnosis is most commonly confirmed by radiographs.

In 27% of patients with HO, shoulder involvement is found inferomedial to the glenohumeral joint. Although ankylosis of the joint in these cases is unusual, motion may be sufficiently restricted to require surgical resection. Elbow involvement is seen in a quarter of patients with HO and in 90% of those who suffer a fracture or dislocation about the elbow. When HO forms posterior to the elbow joint, pressure neuritis of the ulnar nerve is common. Anterior transposition of the ulnar nerve is frequently required to prevent entrapment, and this procedure also facilitates later bone resection. Joint ankylosis is a common complication in patients with elbow involvement. Hip involvement is seen in 44% of patients who form ectopic bone. Bilateral hip involvement and joint ankylosis are common in these patients. HO of the knee joint is less common but significantly impedes both flexion and extension of the joint.

Management

A. Early Measures

Aggressive treatment of spasticity is necessary because this problem appears to play an etiologic role in mechanically stimulating bone formation. To diminish spasticity in the muscle groups adjacent to the bone formation, phenol blocks may be administered, and etidronate may be given to diminish deposition of calcium crystals in the collagen matrix of the periarticular connective tissue. When the HO is detected very early, the use of intravenous etidronate, 300 mg for 3 days, followed by oral therapy is very effective. The recommended dosage is 20 mg/kg/day orally in a single dose, and the drug should be taken on an empty stomach for proper absorption. Anti-inflammatory medications are also used to control the intense inflammatory reaction that occurs during the formation of HO. The most commonly documented medication is indomethacin, 75 to 150 mg daily, but other nonsteroidal anti-inflammatory drugs (NSAIDs) are equally effective. Physical therapy is aimed at providing gentle ROM to the joint to prevent ankylosis. Forceful joint manipulation is not advised because it can cause fractures or soft-tissue damage with subsequent contracture.

Surgical excision is also treatment for HO. Following surgery, physical therapy and NSAIDs or low-dose radiation therapy should be used to diminish recurrence.

Bachman DR, Fitzsimmons JS, O'Driscoll SW. Safety of arthroscopic versus open or combined heterotopic ossification removal around the elbow. *Arthroscopy.* 2020;36(2):422-430. [PMID: 31870750]

Behery OA, Dai AZ, McLaurin TM. Posttraumatic heterotopic ossification of the hip. *J Orthop Trauma.* 2018;32(suppl 1): S18-S19. [PMID: 29985897]

Cirino CM, Chan JJ, Patterson DC, et al. Risk factors for heterotopic ossification in operatively treated proximal humeral fractures. *Bone Joint J.* 2020;102-B(4):539-544. [PMID: 32228071]

Yolcu YU, Wahood W, Goyal A, et al. Pharmacologic prophylaxis for heterotopic ossification following spinal cord injury: a systematic review and meta-analysis. *Clin Neurol Neurosurg.* 2020;193:105737. [PMID: 32169744]

Zhu XT, Chen L, Lin JH. Selective COX-2 inhibitor versus nonselective COX-2 inhibitor for the prevention of heterotopic ossification after total hip arthroplasty: a meta-analysis. *Medicine (Baltimore).* 2018;97(31):e11649. [PMID: 30075549]

RHEUMATOID ARTHRITIS

Rheumatoid arthritis (RA) is a chronic systemic disease that affects connective tissue and results in chronic inflammatory synovitis, usually with bilateral joint involvement. It is discussed in Chapter 7, so only the aspects pertinent to rehabilitation are described here.

The systemic nature of RA and its variable clinical pattern make it difficult to devise a precise system for describing the overall functional ability of the patient. The most commonly employed scale is the functional classification devised by the American Rheumatism Association (Table 13–5). In addition, patient-reported outcome measures are effective in rating disease activity.

Table 13–5. American Rheumatism Association classification of function in patients with rheumatoid arthritis.

Class	Description
I	Complete function; able to perform usual duties without handicap.
II	Adequate function for normal activities, despite handicap of pain or limited range of motion in one or more joints.
III	Limited function; able to perform few or none of the duties of usual occupation or self-care.
IV	Largely or wholly incapacitated; bedridden or confined to a wheelchair; able to perform little or no self-care.

Management

A. The Team Approach to Patient Care and Treatment

Optimal management requires an interdisciplinary team approach involving many specialists, including a liaison nurse, rheumatologist, orthopedic surgeon, physical therapist, occupational therapist, psychologist, and social worker. The patient and family are also important members of the team. Because the disease is an ongoing and progressive process, the goal of management is to prevent deformities and maintain function for the patient over a lifetime.

1. Nursing care and patient education—The liaison nurse functions as the coordinator of the team. The nurse provides the critical link between the inpatient medical and surgical management of the disease and the continuation of treatment in the outpatient environment.

Much of the responsibility for patient education in the daily care of the disease rests with the nurse, who explains the techniques for protecting joints; advises patients about the need to perform exercises for maintaining joint ROM and optimizing failing muscle strength; cautions patients that exercising too vigorously can damage weakened joints and ligaments; and reminds patients that because the disease tends to decrease their physical activity, they will need regular periods of rest during the day and good nutrition to maximize their general health and to prevent obesity.

2. Medical and surgical management—The rheumatologist is commonly the team leader and in charge of medical management, which is directed toward the control of synovitis, the relief of pain, and the prevention or treatment of other organ involvement by the disease. The medications used for treatment include aspirin, NSAIDs, corticosteroids, suppressive or disease-modifying antirheumatic drugs (DMARDs), immunosuppressive drugs, and biologics. A local injection of corticosteroids can be useful in controlling an acute inflammatory process in a specific joint.

The orthopedic surgeon should be involved early in the course of the patient's disease and not merely be called on when medical management fails to be effective. Knowledge of biomechanics, gait dynamics, and energy requirements can be useful in preserving function for the patient. The orthopedist can often recommend orthotic supports, walking aids, and shoe wear that minimize unwanted stress on joints and maximize strength.

In selected situations, early surgical intervention may prevent excessive deterioration of joint structure and function. Because of advances in medical treatment, synovectomy is rarely done today, but it remains effective in preventing tendon rupture in the hand, whereas arthroscopic synovectomy of the knee and shoulder aid in diminishing symptoms and joint destruction. Fusion of an unstable cervical spine can prevent the disastrous effect of an SCI.

Most surgical procedures are reconstructive. Because diminishing pain is the most consistent result, pain is the primary indication for surgery. Correction of deformity of the large joints is generally effective as well. Restoration of function is more difficult to achieve as persistent loss of motion and mild weakness are common. Preoperative assessment is a painstaking process. In addition to performing a physical examination and reviewing radiographic findings, the surgeon must attempt to elicit sufficient information from the patient, family, and therapists to ascertain which deformities are causing the greatest functional losses. The patient can only tolerate a finite number of surgical procedures, and these must be carefully staged to obtain the maximal result.

3. Physical therapy—The physical therapist uses modalities such as heat and ultrasound to decrease joint stiffness and relieve pain. An exercise program is essential for preserving the functional abilities of the patient. The exercise should gently put all joints through their full arc of motion to maintain this range.

Patients with joint effusions and synovitis automatically assume positions that minimize intraarticular pressure and therefore minimize pain. These positions are usually not optimal for function and can result in flexion deformities. An abnormal position may be reversible if discovered early. Daily joint ROM exercises are central to preventing unwanted contractures.

Muscles weakened by the concomitant myopathy need strengthening but are susceptible to damage from overuse or from an excessively vigorous exercise program. Orthotics may be indicated to support weakened ligaments and provide a means of joint protection and support for functional activities such as walking. Upper extremity walking aids may be useful to give the patients additional support. These aids often require modification to meet the specific needs of the individual. Forearm troughs allow the patient to use the entire arm for support when the hands and wrists are weak or deformed. They are also useful for protecting the hands from excessive stress. A rolling walker, which does not require the patient to lift the walker for advancement, may be useful in patients with limited strength.

4. Occupational therapy—The occupational therapist evaluates and instructs the patient in modified techniques for performing ADLs, such as grooming, dressing, and meal preparation. Because of the weakness and deformities imposed by the arthritis, adaptive equipment and alternative methods are commonly needed. Modifications in clothing, such as larger fasteners for ease of manipulation, Velcro strips at seams or on shoes, and front openings, can all facilitate dressing. Upper extremity splints can be used to provide joint protection and stabilization and to prevent further deformity from occurring. The splints must be lightweight and easily donned by the patient.

5. Psychological counseling—It is not uncommon for patients or their family members to have feelings of anxiety, denial, anger, or depression. The psychologist provides assistance in dealing with these feelings and coping with alterations in lifestyle and self-image. Comprehensive care involves an understanding of how patients respond to weakness, fatigue, altered physical appearance, progressive disability, diminished independence, and the financial burdens of chronic illness. Coping skills are needed to deal with these problems as well as with pain, which becomes an everyday occurrence and may interfere with both intellectual and emotional functioning.

6. Social services—A variety of modifications in lifestyle accompany chronic illness with RA. Occupational changes may be necessary, or the patient may no longer be able to work at all. Additional assistance may be needed in the home for housework and the preparation of meals. In more advanced stages, the patient may require help for personal care. Transportation needs become more complex, and the patient finds it increasingly difficult to leave the home. The social worker becomes an invaluable team member in helping families with the numerous practical arrangements required for everyday existence and for locating financial aid to help defray the mounting costs.

Küçükdeveci AA. Nonpharmacological treatment in established rheumatoid arthritis. *Best Pract Res Clin Rheumatol.* 2020;5:101482. [PMID: 31987686]

POLIOMYELITIS

Poliomyelitis is caused by an enterovirus that attacks the anterior horn cells of the spinal cord. Infection can lead to a variety of clinical findings, ranging from minor symptoms to paralysis. The last major epidemics in the United States occurred during the early 1950s. Immunization programs are effective and safe, but parental concerns persist and ought to be acknowledged. Acute poliomyelitis is now rare in the United States and other developed nations of the world.

Nevertheless, orthopedic surgeons today may be called on to treat patients with postpoliomyelitis syndrome.

Classification

Four stages of poliomyelitis are recognized.

A. Acute Poliomyelitis

All of the anterior horn cells are attacked during the acute stage, which accounts for the diffuse and severe paralysis seen with the initial infection. The anterior horn cells control the skeletal muscle cells of the trunk and limbs. Clinically, the infection is characterized by the sudden onset of paralysis and the presence of fever and acute muscle pain, often accompanied by stiff neck. Paralysis of the respiratory muscles is life-threatening in the acute stage. When the shoulder muscles are involved, respiratory compromise should be suspected because of the close proximity of the anterior horn cells controlling each in the spinal cord. Mechanical support of ventilation may be required.

A variable number of anterior horn cells survive the initial infection. The treatment in the acute stage of the disease consists of providing the needed respiratory support, decreasing muscle pain, and performing regular ROM exercises to prevent the formation of joint contractures.

B. Subacute Poliomyelitis

Anterior horn cell survival, axon sprouting, and muscle hypertrophy occur in the subacute phase and provide three mechanisms for regaining strength. An average of 47% (range of 12%-94%) of the anterior horn cells in the spinal cord survive the initial attack. Because cell survival occurs in a random fashion, the distribution of paralysis is variable and depends on which anterior horn cells were destroyed. Each anterior horn cell innervates a group of muscle cells. When a group of muscle cells is orphaned, as it were, by the death of the anterior horn cell that supports it, a nearby nerve cell can sprout additional axons and adopt some of the orphaned cells. By means of this process, a motor unit (defined as a nerve cell and the muscle cells it innervates) can expand greatly. Moreover, muscle cells in the unit enlarge, and this hypertrophy provides additional strength for the patient.

C. Residual Poliomyelitis

It is only after 16 to 24 months following onset that the ultimate extent of poliomyelitis can be determined and procedures to restore lost function and provide structural stability can be instituted.

D. Postpoliomyelitis Syndrome

Patients who had acute poliomyelitis during childhood often complain of increased muscle weakness 30 to 40 years later. This weakness is not a result of infectious spread of the earlier disease but, rather, is caused by the overuse of muscles that were originally affected, whether or not they were known to have been affected at the onset of the disease. Studies show that a muscle must lose from 30% to 40% of its strength for weakness to be detected using manual muscle testing. Studies of gait also demonstrate that the ADLs require more muscle strength and stamina than were previously appreciated. The traditional program, which encouraged patients to work harder to regain strength and was based on the concept of "no pain, no gain," proved detrimental because it encouraged chronic overuse of muscles and resulted in further deterioration of function.

The diagnosis of postpoliomyelitis syndrome is based on a history of poliomyelitis; a pattern of increased muscle weakness that is random and does not follow any nerve root or peripheral nerve distribution; and the presence of additional symptoms such as muscle pain, severe fatigue, muscle cramping or fasciculations, joint pain or instability, sleep apnea, intolerance to cold, and depression. No pathognomonic tests for the syndrome are currently available. Electromyography can demonstrate the presence of large motor units resulting from the previous axon sprouting. This finding is supportive but not diagnostic of poliomyelitis.

Management

A. Acute Poliomyelitis

When the shoulder muscles are involved, respiratory compromise should be suspected, and mechanical support of ventilation should be instituted. Other measures are aimed at decreasing muscle pain and preventing complications. Regular ROM exercises prevent the formation of joint contractures.

B. Subacute Poliomyelitis

During the subacute stage, which may last as long as 24 months, the emphasis is on preventing deformities and preserving function. Splints and braces are often helpful for maintaining joint position and supplementing function.

C. Residual Poliomyelitis

Patients with compromised function of the diaphragm can be taught glossopharyngeal breathing. This method, in which air is swallowed into the lungs, provides sufficient air exchange for the patient to perform light activities in the sitting position. Mechanical support of ventilation may still need to be continued while the patient sleeps. It is during the residual stage that orthopedic surgery is commonly performed to restore lost function and provide structural stability. If the patient is still growing, it is important to prevent the formation of skeletal deformities that result from muscle imbalance. Before any surgery that requires general anesthesia or significant sedation is performed, the vital capacity should be assessed to determine the patient's need for respiratory support.

D. Postpoliomyelitis Syndrome

Treatment is directed at preserving current muscle strength and preventing further weakness from occurring. Generally, strength cannot be restored in a muscle that was weakened by poliomyelitis. Some gain in strength can be seen, however, when chronic overuse is corrected.

General management strategies consist of modifying lifestyle to prevent chronic overuse of weak muscles; instituting a limited exercise program that incorporates frequent rest periods to prevent disuse atrophy and weakness; providing lightweight orthotic support of the limbs to protect joints and substitute for muscle function; and performing orthopedic surgery to correct limb or trunk deformities.

Specific management strategies depend on the areas of disease involvement.

1. Spine—Back pain is a common complaint and usually results from postural strain caused by excessive lumbar extension in patients who have weak or paralyzed hip extensor muscles. Neck pain, like back pain, is a common complaint associated with slowly increasing weakness. Both complaints can be treated by the use of external supports. Patient education is imperative because many patients are reluctant to don braces again, after having passed decades without using them. Patients should be instructed in methods to relieve excess strain on the neck muscles and prevent further deterioration. Tilting the chair seat 10 degrees backward is often sufficient to relieve the fatigue of the posterior cervical muscles from supporting the head.

Paralysis of the cervical spine musculature can result in the inability to maintain the head erect and can interfere with the performance of a vast number of functions, including ambulation. Surgical fusion of the cervical spine corrects the problem.

Scoliosis is common in patients with muscle imbalance caused by paralysis. The condition is particularly pronounced in patients with leg-length discrepancies. External supports can be used to hold the spine in position, but these often interfere with respiration if the patient depends on the use of accessory muscles for breathing. Posterior spinal fusion may be needed to control the spine adequately. After fusion is performed, prolonged immobilization must be avoided. Segmental spine fixation may be helpful.

2. Lower extremities—Full ROM of the hip and knee joints is needed for function. Contractures should be corrected when possible to permit more effective bracing. In iliotibial band contractures, which are common deformities, the hip assumes a position of flexion, external rotation, and abduction; the knee assumes a valgus alignment; and the tibia is externally rotated on the femur. Release or lengthening of the iliotibial band corrects the deformity.

A patient with flailing lower extremities can stand using crutches and a KAFO with the knees locked in extension and the ankles in slight dorsiflexion by hyperextending the hips and using the strong anterior hip capsule for support. Flexion contractures of the hips or knees prevent this alignment. If trunk support and upper extremity strength are adequate, the patient could ambulate with a swing-through gait for short distances. This gait has high-energy demands. With time, the posterior knee joint capsule becomes stretched, and the knee develops a recurvatum deformity that is painful and can lead to arthritic degeneration of the knee. A KAFO protects the knee and provides improved stability for walking. If there is fair (grade 3) strength in the hip flexor muscles (see Table 13–1) and passive full-knee extension, then the knee joints can be left unlocked for walking. In this case, a posteriorly offset knee joint is used to stabilize the knee, and ankle dorsiflexion is limited to minus 3 degrees of neutral dorsiflexion to provide a hyperextension moment to the knee for stability. Thus, at stance phase, the net ankle plantarflexion locks the knee in hyperextension, restrained by posterior capsular static structures.

Quadriceps muscle strength is not essential for ambulation. A strong gluteus maximus and good calf strength can substitute by keeping the knee locked in extension. If the calf strength is inadequate to control the forward motion of the tibia in mid to late stance, an AFO is needed. It is not necessary to fix the ankle in mild plantarflexion to provide knee stability, and such a position could cause a recurvatum deformity in any case. An equinus position of the foot inhibits forward momentum and limits step length by preventing body weight from rolling over the forefoot prior to contact of the contralateral extremity with the ground. When good hamstring function is present, the biceps femoris and the semitendinosus can be transferred anteriorly to the quadriceps tendon to provide dynamic knee stability.

Muscle imbalances in the foot can lead to deformity. When muscle imbalances exist, tendon releases or transfers should be considered prior to the development of fixed deformities.

Equinus contracture of the ankle is a common problem and results in genu recurvatum. Accommodating the equinus posture by using an elevated heel places excessive stress on the calf muscles to control the leg. A surgical procedure to lengthen the Achilles tendon is frequently needed to correct the equinus contracture of the ankle and to permit adequate bracing.

A cavus foot deformity causes forefoot equinus, which also limits bracing. If no fixed bony abnormalities are present, then release of the plantar fascia is sufficient to correct the deformity. If the cavus deformity is caused by bony abnormalities, then a closing wedge osteotomy is needed. A triple arthrodesis of the hindfoot can also be used to correct deformities and provide a stable base of support.

The long-standing muscle imbalances, patterns of muscle substitution, and resulting joint and ligament strains often lead to degenerative arthritis. Total joint replacement can be performed, but several special considerations are needed. In patients with postpoliomyelitis syndrome, osteoporosis is common because of prolonged lack of muscle action on the bone. Joint contractures must be corrected at the time of surgery to prevent excessive forces on the prosthetic components because these forces might lead to loosening of the prosthesis. Weak muscles must be supported with the appropriate orthoses after surgery. The rehabilitation program is lengthy because it takes an extended period to regain joint motion and muscle function. Continuous passive motion devices and frequent joint ROM must be used to gain joint mobility after surgery. Because the hip joint is difficult to brace, there must be at least fair (grade 3) strength (see Table 13–1) in the hip extensors, abductors, and flexors to provide stability to the hip after surgery. Surgery can be expected to weaken the surrounding muscles, which must be taken into account before total hip arthroplasty is undertaken to prevent chronic dislocation.

3. Upper extremities

A. Shoulders—The shoulder is important for placing the hand in the desired position for use. The shoulder totally depends on muscle strength for active mobility. In patients who use a wheelchair, weak muscles about the shoulder can be made more functional with the use of mobile arm supports on the wheelchair. These supports allow the patient a greater arc of motion with less muscle strength. Shoulder stability is more important in the ambulatory patient who requires upper extremity aids. A glenohumeral fusion may be helpful if the patient has sufficient strength in the scapulothoracic muscles. When the shoulder is fused, scapulothoracic motion is maintained, allowing use of the extremity for tabletop activities. Glenohumeral fusion does restrict the ability of the patient to position the hand for bathroom hygiene, so it is undesirable to perform the procedure on both shoulders.

Preservation of shoulder strength should be a priority of treatment. Rotator cuff tears are a common problem in postpolio patients. Surgical repair of the torn rotator cuff should be done when possible. In large tears that cannot be repaired, arthroscopic debridement offers significant relief of pain. Shoulder weakness is found in 95% of patients with postpoliomyelitis syndrome and correlates closely with the amount of lower extremity weakness present. Patients with weak legs use their arms to push up from a chair and pull themselves up stairs. They also lean heavily on upper extremity aids while walking. It is therefore important to remove as many unnecessary strains from the shoulders as possible with the use of elevated seats, motorized lift chairs, elevators or motorized stair chair glides, and optimal lower extremity bracing. In minimally ambulatory or nonambulatory patients, an electric wheelchair or motorized scooter should be prescribed to prevent excessive strain on the shoulder muscles caused by propelling a manual wheelchair.

B. Elbows—The elbow requires sufficient flexor strength to lift an object against gravity for function. A mobile arm support can maximize the effectiveness of the muscle strength for the patient. Tendon transfers, such as those involving the deltoid and biceps muscles, may also be useful in restoring active flexion.

C. Wrists and hands—Opponens paralysis is common in the hand and results in a 50% loss of hand function. A splint used during the acute and recovery phases is useful in preventing an adduction contracture. Opponens function can be restored by tendon transfer. The most common muscle transferred is the flexor digitorum superficialis of the ring finger.

Paralysis of the intrinsic muscles of the hand interferes with function. A lumbrical bar orthosis prevents hyperextension of the metacarpophalangeal joints and allows the long extensors to extend the fingers and open the hand. Surgical capsulodesis to limit metacarpophalangeal joint extension accomplishes the same result.

Paralysis of the finger flexors and extensors can be overcome with the use of a flexor hinge orthosis if wrist extensor function is present. Tendon transfers can provide the same result, allowing the tenodesis effect to provide grasp and pinch functions.

Checa Betegón P, Valle Cruz J, García Coiradas J, et al. Fractures in patients with poliomyelitis: past or current challenge? *Injury*. 2020;51(suppl 1):S48-S54. [PMID: 32111460]

Gellman YN, Khoury A, Liebergall M, Mosheiff R, Weil YA. Outcome of femoral fractures in poliomyelitis patients. *Int Orthop*. 2019;43(11):2607-2612. [PMID: 30643935]

Matsuda PN, Eagen T, Hreha KP, Finlayson ML, Molton IR. Relationship between fear of falling and physical activity in people aging with a disability. *PM R*. 2020;12(5):454-461. [PMID: 31736266]

CEREBRAL PALSY (STATIC ENCEPHALOPATHY)

Cerebral palsy is a nonprogressive and nonhereditary disorder of impaired motor function. The onset may be prenatal, perinatal, or postnatal. An exact cause is not always known, but the impairment is sometimes associated with prematurity, perinatal hypoxia, cerebral trauma, infertility treatments, infections or neonatal jaundice. In the United States, more than 500,000 people are affected by cerebral palsy. The degree of neurologic impairment is severe in a third of patients and mild in approximately a sixth.

Classification

Because of the diversity of neurologic findings seen in patients with cerebral palsy, a classification system is essential. The disease can be classified by the types of movement disorder and by the patterns of neurologic deficit.

A. Types of Movement Disorder

Three types of disorder are seen.

1. Spastic disorders—These are characterized by the presence of clonus and hyperactive deep tendon reflexes. Patients with spastic movement can be helped by orthopedic intervention.

2. Dyskinetic disorders—Among the conditions classified as dyskinetic disorders are athetosis, ballismus, chorea, dystonia, and ataxia. For practical purposes, these conditions are grouped together because they are not amenable to surgical correction.

3. Mixed disorders—These usually consist of a combination of spasticity and athetosis with total body involvement.

B. Patterns of Neurologic Involvement

1. Monoplegia—With single-limb involvement, the disorder is usually spastic in nature. Because monoplegia is rare, it is advisable to test the patient before making the diagnosis. The stress of performing an activity such as running at a fast pace often uncovers spasticity in another limb.

2. Hemiplegia—Spasticity affects the upper and lower extremities ipsilaterally. Equinovarus posturing is common in the lower extremity. The upper extremity is usually held with the elbow, wrist, and fingers flexed and the thumb adducted. The major problem interfering with upper extremity function, however, is a loss of proprioception and stereognosis. Surgery for the upper extremity is aimed at making the hand assistive and at improving cosmesis. An arm that is involuntarily held in severe flexion while walking can be a major social disadvantage for the patient.

3. Paraplegia—In paraplegia, neurologic deficits involve only the lower extremities. Because paraplegia is rare in patients with spastic cerebral palsy, the presence of a high spinal cord lesion that could also be responsible for the neurologic findings must be ruled out. Bladder problems coexist with spastic paralysis that affects the lower extremities and is secondary to spinal cord damage.

4. Diplegia—Spastic diplegia, seen in 50% to 60% of cerebral palsy patients in the United States, is the most common neurologic pattern. It is characterized by major involvement in both lower extremities with only minor incoordination in the upper extremities. Findings in the lower extremities include marked spasticity, particularly about the hips, hyperactive deep tendon reflexes, and a positive Babinski sign. The hips are commonly held in a position of flexion, adduction, and internal rotation secondary to the spasticity. The knees are in the valgus position and may have excessive external rotation of the tibia. The ankles are held in the equinus position, with a valgus attitude of the feet. Speech and intellectual functions are usually normal or only slightly impaired. Esotropia and visual perception problems are common.

5. Total-body involvement—Sometimes referred to as quadriplegia, total-body involvement is characterized by impairments affecting all four extremities, the head, and the trunk. Sensory deficits are typical, and speech and swallowing are commonly impaired. The most serious deficit is often the inability to communicate with others. Although mental retardation is found in approximately 45% of patients, intelligence is often masked by communication dysfunction. Ambulation is not usually a goal because the equilibrium reactions of affected patients are severely impaired or absent. Sitting may require braces or adaptive supportive devices. Scoliosis, contractures, and dislocated hips are common orthopedic problems and may interfere with sitting.

Management

Because cerebral palsy in children is discussed elsewhere (see Chapter 12), the following discussion concentrates on the needs of the adult with cerebral palsy.

A. Special Considerations in Adult Patients

1. Musculoskeletal problems—Long-standing deformities may be rigid. Bony deformities are common and may preclude surgery for soft-tissue rebalancing unless concomitant osteotomies are done. In comparison with the young patient, the adult patient has a greater body mass to support and therefore has increased energy demands. Spastic muscles are weak and frequently further compromised by the chronic overuse of muscles to compensate for contractural deformities.

2. Mobility—The patient who can sit independently has good balance and may propel a wheelchair. It may be easier to propel the wheelchair backward, using the feet to push. A self-propped sitter may require some external support to remain erect, whereas a propped sitter needs a straight spine and flexible hips to remain erect with support.

Ambulation can be divided into four categories: community ambulation, household ambulation, physiologic ambulation (exercise), and wheelchair ambulation. A patient categorized as a community ambulator is able to maneuver independently and safely around obstacles normally encountered in the community. Orthotics or upper extremity walking aids may be required. A household ambulator is able to walk independently for short distances but requires assistance to negotiate obstacles such as stairs or curbs and requires a wheelchair for long distances. A physiologic ambulator is someone who is capable of walking for short distances with assistance or walks as a means of exercise but finds it impractical to walk for normal activities. The energy requirements for walking determine the category to which a patient belongs and also determine the types of equipment that are recommended. It is unreasonable to expect patients to expend all their energy in merely transporting themselves from one location to another.

B. Treatment of Patients With Lower Extremity Problems

1. Hips—An adduction and internal rotation deformity of the hip is sometimes seen during ambulation. Release of the hip adductor tendons (see Figure 13–13) may be needed to correct this tendency.

A crouch gait and lumbar lordosis are evidence of hip flexion deformity. In patients with cerebral palsy, gait studies with dynamic poly-EMG demonstrated dysphasic activity of the iliopsoas, which is the main hip flexor muscle. Gait studies with poly-EMG should be undertaken to evaluate the activity of the iliopsoas and pectineus and to aid in surgical decision making. If release of the iliopsoas is indicated, the tendon is cut distally and allowed to retract proximally to the point where it reattaches to the anterior hip capsule (Figure 13–26). Release of the pectineus muscle is often also necessary.

2. Knees—Correction of a knee flexion deformity in a patient with a crouch gait may be necessary. Attention should first be paid to the hip deformity. Weakness of the gastrocnemius and soleus muscles and inability to maintain the position of the tibia may also contribute to a crouch posture and should be considered prior to performing any knee surgery. Gait electromyograms are useful in determining which muscles are responsible for the abnormal posture. Release of the offending hamstring tendons (see Figure 13–15) or hamstring lengthening may be useful.

3. Feet—Equinus posturing of the ankle is common. If no fixed contracture is present, an AFO controls the position of the foot. If the deformity is the result of an equinus contracture, Achilles tendon lengthening (see Figure 13–16) should be performed to bring the foot to a neutral position. The foot should be immobilized for 6 weeks following surgery. An AFO is then used to maintain the position of the foot and support the tibia during walking.

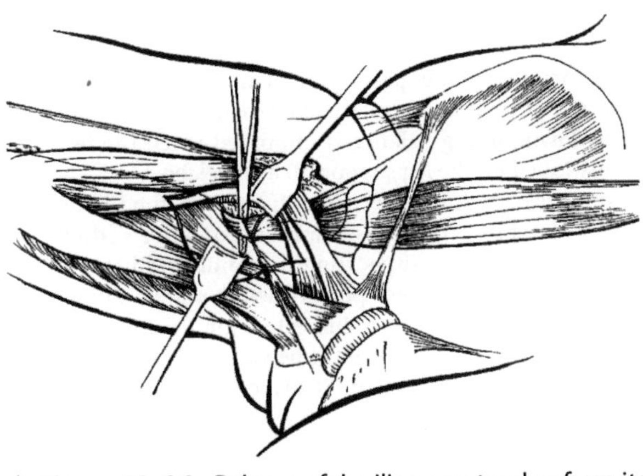

▲ **Figure 13–26. Release of the iliopsoas tendon from its insertion on the lesser trochanter of the femur to correct a hip flexion deformity.** (Illustration by Anthony C. Berlet. Reproduced, with permission, from Keenan MAE, Kozin SH, Berlet AC. *Manual of Orthopaedic Surgery for Spasticity.* Philadelphia, PA: Raven; 1993.)

Equinovarus posturing of the ankle is also common. Although the anterior tibial muscle is the primary varus force in patients with stroke or TBIs, it is equally likely that the posterior tibial muscle may be causing equinovarus posturing in patients with cerebral palsy. Therefore, in order to find the cause and make the correct decision concerning surgery, it is important to make dynamic EMG recordings while the patient walks.

If the anterior tibial muscle is overactive, Achilles tendon lengthening should be accompanied by a split anterior tibial tendon transfer (see Figure 13–18). If the posterior tibial muscle is overactive, it is advisable to lengthen the posterior tendon. If the EMG studies show that the posterior tibial muscle is active only during the swing phase of gait, it may be more logical to transfer the posterior tendon through the interosseous membrane to the dorsum of the foot, rather than performing a split anterior tibial tendon transfer. After surgery is performed, immobilization that allows weight bearing is worn for 6 weeks, and the leg is then supported with an AFO. If hallux valgus subsequently develops, management consists of correcting the subtalar deformity and realigning the first digital ray.

A pes cavus deformity of the foot is occasionally seen in patients with spasticity of the intrinsic muscles. If the problem is detected early, it can be corrected by plantar fasciotomy and release of the flexor origins from the os calcis. If the problem is detected late and a concomitant bony deformity is present, a wedge osteotomy of the midtarsal bones should be performed.

C. Treatment of Patients with Upper Extremity Problems

Function of the upper extremities depends on a variety of factors, including cognition, intact sensation, and the ability to place the hand in space. The amount of spasticity present also affects the ability to control movement of the arm and hand. Surgery can influence hand placement and modify spasticity, but a successful outcome requires the ability to cooperate with postoperative therapy programs. Mental impairment, motion disorders, and poor sensation are relative contraindications to surgery in the functional arm and hand.

1. The functional upper extremity—In patients with problems involving the functional hand, treatment begins with careful clinical evaluation of motor and sensory deficits. Dynamic EMG is extremely useful in determining which muscles should be lengthened or transferred to improve function. The least severely involved hands exhibit a minor degree of spasticity in the flexor carpi ulnaris and a resulting mild flexion deformity of the wrist. In this case, all that is required to improve hand function and position is surgical lengthening of the flexor carpi ulnaris tendon.

In some patients, release of objects from the hand is a problem. In this case, the synergistic action of the finger extensors and wrist flexors causes difficulty with finger extension when the wrist is extended. This resembles the tenodesis effect seen in paralytic hands, but the mechanism is a dynamic one. Selective lengthening of the overactive finger flexors (see Figure 13–23) improves hand function.

Transfer of a wrist flexor to a wrist extensor should be done with caution. Often a patient flexes the wrist to adjust the dynamic balance between the finger flexors and extensors. Holding the wrist in extension can rob the patient of this important method of compensation.

The thumb-in-palm deformity is treated by proximal release of the thenar muscles (see Figure 13–24) and lengthening of the flexor pollicis longus tendon. Distal release of the thenar muscles is not recommended because it may cause a hyperextension deformity of the metacarpophalangeal joint of the thumb.

2. The nonfunctional upper extremity—Surgery may be indicated in the nonfunctional upper extremity to prevent skin breakdown, to improve hygiene or cosmesis, or to make dressing easier. The problems of shoulder contracture and elbow contracture are discussed in the section on stroke, and the surgical procedures used in their treatment are shown in Figures 13–20 and 13–21. Patients who have a flexed wrist with flexed fingers and a thumb-in-palm deformity should be treated because severe wrist flexion can cause median nerve compression against the proximal edge of the transverse carpal ligament. An arthrodesis of the wrist in neutral position, combined with a superficialis-to-profundus tendon transfer (see Figure 13–22), reliably corrects the wrist deformity and also improves skin care. Management of the thumb deformity consists of lengthening the flexor pollicis longus tendon, fusing the interphalangeal joint, and performing a proximal release of the thenar muscles (see Figure 13–24).

D. Treatment of Patients With Total-Body Involvement

Patients with total-body involvement are rarely functional ambulators, although they may transfer from one position to another either independently or with assistance. They frequently have a combination of spasticity and motion disorders such as athetosis, and they spend most of their time in a chair. Flexible hips and a straight spine are needed for functional sitting.

Occasionally, knee flexion deformities require distal hamstring release or lengthening to allow for greater flexibility in positioning the patient. Rigid extension contractures of the knee are sometimes seen and interfere with sitting tolerance. Lengthening of the quadriceps tendon (Figure 13–27) allows the knee to flex.

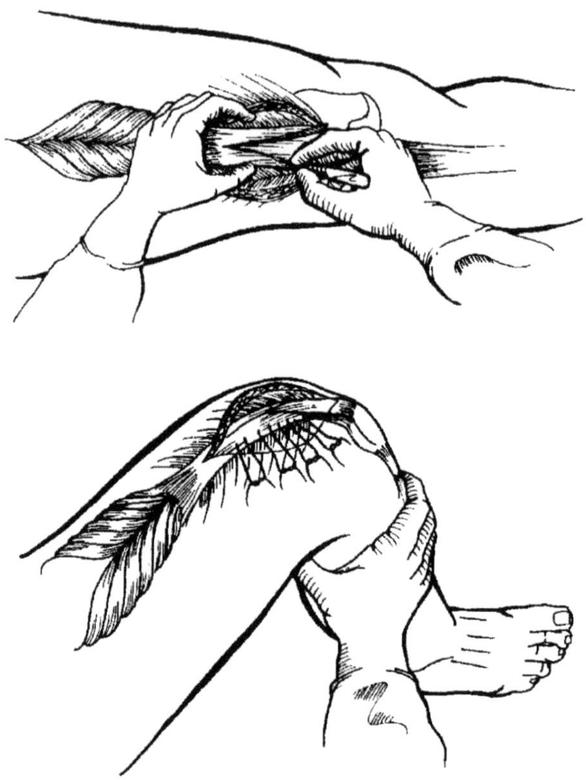

▲ **Figure 13–27.** **The dV-Y incision (*top*) and lengthening (*bottom*) of the quadriceps tendon to correct a rigid extension contracture of the knee and allow improved sitting.** (Illustration by Anthony C. Berlet. Reproduced, with permission, from Keenan MAE, Kozin SH, Berlet AC. *Manual of Orthopaedic Surgery for Spasticity*. Philadelphia, PA: Raven; 1993.)

Foot deformities in the spastic patient are extremely common and require treatment to allow shoe wear and to prevent skin breakdown. Sitting balance is improved when the feet can be positioned on the leg support of a wheelchair.

The spine is of major concern in patients with total-body involvement because scoliosis is common. Adaptive seating or orthotics are useful in supporting the spine and helping the patient maintain an erect posture while seated. Spinal fusion with instrumentation is indicated for treatment of progressive scoliosis. Obliquity of the pelvis greatly interferes with sitting. When this problem is present, fusion should include the sacrum.

Hosseinzadeh P, Baldwin K, Minaie A, Miller F. Management of hip disorders in patients with cerebral palsy. *JBJS Rev.* 2020;8(3):e0148. [PMID: 32224639]

Levin S, Sheiner E, Wainstock T, et al. Infertility treatments and long-term neurologic morbidity of the offspring. *Am J Perinatol.* 2019;36(9):949-954. [PMID: 30452068] van Gorp M, Hilberink SR, Noten S, et al. Epidemiology of cerebral palsy in adulthood: a systematic review and meta-analysis of the most frequently studied outcomes. *Arch Phys Med Rehabil.* 2020;101(6):1041-1052. [PMID: 32059945]

NEUROMUSCULAR DISORDERS

The neuromuscular disorders represent a diverse group of chronic diseases characterized by the progressive degeneration of skeletal musculature, which results in weakness, atrophy, joint contractures, and increasing disability. These disorders are best classified as motor unit diseases because the primary abnormality may involve the motor neuron, the neuromuscular junction, or the muscle fiber. Two broad categories are considered. Myopathies are diseases of the muscle fibers. Neuropathies are disorders in which muscle degeneration is seen secondary to lower motor neuron disease. Most of the neuromuscular disorders are hereditary (Table 13–6), although point mutations may result in spontaneous cases. Early diagnosis is important not only for initiation of appropriate therapy but also for genetic counseling. Treatment programs are aimed at symptomatic and supportive care. Appropriate orthopedic intervention can significantly increase the functional capacity of patients with neuromuscular disorders.

Diagnosis

A. History and Physical Examination

A careful genetic history is important. The clinical history and physical examination delineate the onset and pattern of muscle involvement. Neuropathies generally present with distal involvement. Muscle fasciculation and spasticity are common, and muscle atrophy is in excess of the weakness. Myopathies usually display weakness of the proximal limb musculature initially. Fasciculations and spasticity are not seen. The weakness is more pronounced than the atrophy. Disorders of neuromuscular transmission, such as myasthenia gravis, present with fatigue and ptosis.

Table 13–6. Classification of the more commonly encountered neuromuscular disorders.

Disorder	Inherited	Creatine Phosphokinase Level	Electromyographic Pattern	Nerve Conduction	Biopsy Pattern
Muscular dystrophies					
Duchenne (pseudohypertrophic) type	Yes	Markedly elevated	Myopathic	Normal	Myopathic
Facioscapulohumeral type	Yes	Normal or elevated	Myopathic	Normal	Myopathic
Limb-girdle type	Yes	Elevated	Myopathic	Normal	Myopathic
Spinal muscular atrophy					
Werdnig-Hoffmann and Kugelberg-Welander types	Yes	Normal or slightly elevated	Neuropathic	Normal	Neuropathic
Hereditary motor and sensory neuropathies	Yes	Normal	Neuropathic	Markedly decreased	Neuropathic
Type I (Charcot-Marie-Tooth disease)	Yes	Normal	Neuropathic	Decreased or normal	Neuropathic
Type II	Yes	Normal	Neuropathic	Decreased	Neuropathic
Type III	Yes	Normal	Neuropathic		Neuropathic
Type IV	Yes	Normal	Neuropathic	Normal	Neuropathic
Type V					
Myopathies					
Central core, nemaline, minicore, mitochondrial, myotubular, and other types	Often	Often normal	Normal or mildly myopathic	Usually normal	Myopathic
Poliomyelitis	No		Neuropathic	Normal	Neuropathic
Guillain-Barré syndrome	No	Normal	Neuropathic	Slow in acute phase	Neuropathic
Polymyositis	No	Normal or elevated	Myopathic	Normal	Myopathic
Myotonic diseases	Usually	Usually normal	Diagnostic	Normal	
Myasthenia gravis	Sometimes		Diagnostic		

Data compiled by Irene Gilgoff, MD, Rancho Los Amigos Medical Center, Downey, CA.

B. Muscle Enzyme Studies

Serum levels of muscle enzymes are elevated in myopathies but normal in neuropathies. The enzymes studied include creatine phosphokinase (CPK), lactate dehydrogenase (LDH), aldolase, aspartate aminotransferase (AST, SGOT), and alanine aminotransferase (ALT, SGPT). CPK levels are the most elevated in the Duchenne type of muscular dystrophy and less elevated in the more slowly progressive disease forms. In Duchenne-type muscular dystrophy, the highest enzyme levels are seen at birth and during the first few years of life, before the disease is clinically apparent. As the disease progresses and the muscle mass deteriorates, the enzyme levels decrease.

C. Electromyography and Nerve Conduction Studies

EMG and nerve conduction studies differentiate between primary muscle diseases and neuropathies (see Table 13–6). EMG is useful in differentiating among muscle diseases, peripheral nerve disorders, and anterior horn cell abnormalities. A myopathic pattern on EMG is characterized by (1) increased frequency, (2) decreased duration, and (3) decreased amplitude of action potentials. In addition, increased insertional activity, short polyphasic potentials, and a retained interference pattern are evident. A neuropathic pattern on EMG is characterized by the opposite constellation of findings: (1) decreased frequency, (2) increased duration, and (3) increased amplitude of action potentials. In addition, frequent fibrillation potentials, a group polyphasic potential, and a decreased interference pattern can be seen. In myasthenia gravis and the myotonic diseases, the patterns on EMG are diagnostic. In myasthenia gravis, the fatigue phenomenon is exhibited. In myotonia, the EMG is characterized by positive waves and trains of potentials that fire at high frequency and then wax and wane until they slowly disappear.

D. Muscle Biopsy

To gain the maximal amount of information from muscle biopsy, the clinician should choose a muscle that has mild to moderate involvement and was not recently traumatized by electrodes during EMG. Muscle biopsy can be used to differentiate myopathy, neuropathy, and inflammatory myopathy. The biopsy, however, cannot be used to determine prognosis. Histochemical staining further distinguishes the congenital forms of myopathy.

Histologically, myopathies are characterized by muscle fiber necrosis, fatty degeneration, proliferation of the connective tissue, and an increased number of nuclei, some of which have migrated from their normal peripheral position to the center of the muscle fiber.

Neuropathies display small, angulated muscle fibers. Bundles of atrophic fibers are intermingled with bundles of normal fibers. There is no increase in the amount of connective tissue.

Biopsy findings in polymyositis include prominent collections of inflammatory cells, edema of the tissues, perivasculitis, and segmental necrosis with a mixed pattern of fiber degeneration and regeneration.

1. Duchenne-Type Muscular Dystrophy

Duchenne-type muscular dystrophy, which is also called **pseudohypertrophic muscular dystrophy**, is classically known as a progressive disease that affects males. It results from gene mutations of the *DMD* gene that codes the protein dystrophin, is inherited in an X-linked recessive manner, and has its onset in early childhood. It affects about 1 in 3500 male births. Generally, affected children have a normal birth and developmental history. But by the time they reach 3 to 5 years of age, sufficient muscle mass has been lost to impair function. Female carriers of Duchenne-type muscular dystrophy are usually not affected, but about 10% may have mild muscle weakness, fatigue, or cramping of their muscles, and as many as 15% may have cardiac symptoms.

Up to 10% of female carriers of Duchenne-type muscular dystrophy may be mildly affected with asymmetrical muscle weakness, compensatory movements, or both.

▶ Clinical Findings

Early signs of disease include pseudohypertrophy of the calf, which is the result of the increase in connective tissue; planovalgus deformity of the feet, which is secondary to heel cord contracture; and proximal muscle weakness. Muscle weakness in the hips may be exhibited by the Gower sign, in which the patient uses the arms to support the trunk while attempting to rise from the floor. Other signs are hesitance when climbing stairs, acceleration during the final stage of sitting, and shoulder weakness.

Weakness and contractures prevent independent ambulation in approximately 45% of patients by 9 years of age and in the remainder by 12 years of age. It is common for patients to have difficulty first in rising from the floor, next in ascending the stairs, and then in walking. Cardiac involvement is seen in 80% of patients. Findings generally include posterobasal fibrosis of the ventricle and electrocardiographic changes. In patients with a decreased level of activity, clinical evidence of cardiomyopathy may not be obvious. Pulmonary problems are common in the advanced stages of the disease and are found during periodic evaluations of pulmonary function. Mental retardation, noted in 30% to 50% of patients, is present from birth and not progressive.

▶ Management

Efforts are made to keep patients ambulating for as many years as possible to prevent the complications of obesity, osteoporosis, and scoliosis. The hip flexors, tensor fasciae latae, and triceps surae develop ambulation-limiting contractures. With progressive weakness and contractures, the base of support decreases and the patient cannot use normal mechanisms to maintain upright balance. The patient walks with a wide-based gait, hips flexed and abducted, knees flexed, and the feet in equinus and varus position. Lumbar lordosis becomes exaggerated to compensate for the hip flexion contractures and weak hip extensor musculature.

Equinus contractures of the Achilles tendon occur early and are caused by the muscle imbalance between the calf and pretibial muscles. Initially, this problem can be managed by heel cord stretching exercises and night splints. A KAFO may be needed to control foot position and substitute for weak quadriceps muscles. When contractures are worse, serial casting is often effective. Stretching exercises and pronation can be employed to treat early hip flexion contractures.

Surgical intervention is directed toward the release of ambulation-limiting contractures. Early postoperative mobilization is important to prevent further muscle weakness. Anesthetic risks are increased in these patients because of their limited pulmonary reserve and because the incidence of malignant hyperthermia is higher than normal in patients with muscle disease.

The triceps surae and tibialis posterior are the strongest muscles in the lower extremity of the patient with muscular dystrophy. These muscles are responsible for equinus and varus deformities. Management that consists of releasing the contracted tensor fasciae latae, lengthening the Achilles tendon, and transferring the tibialis posterior muscle anteriorly is indicated and prolongs walking for approximately 3 years. Postoperative bracing is required.

Scoliosis is common in nonambulatory patients confined to a wheelchair. Adaptive seating devices that hold the pelvis level and the spine erect are useful in preventing deformity. Alternatively, a rigid plastic spinal torso orthosis may be used for support. When external support is not effective, scoliosis develops rapidly. Spinal fusion is occasionally indicated. Blood loss during surgery is high, and the incidence of pseudarthrosis is increased. Postoperative immobilization is to be avoided; therefore, segmental spinal stabilization is often the preferred technique of internal stabilization.

Fractures in patients with myopathies occur secondary to osteoporosis from the inactivity and the loss of muscle tension. No abnormalities of bone mineralization are present. The incidence of fracture increases with the severity of the disease. Most fractures are metaphyseal in location, show little displacement, cause minimal pain, and heal in the expected time without complication.

Da Silva THD, Anequini IP, Fávero FM, et al. Functional performance and muscular strength in symptomatic female carriers of Duchenne muscular dystrophy. *Arq Neuropsiquiatr.* 2020;78(3):143-148. [PMID: 32022138]

Ishizaki M, Kobayashi M, Adachi K, Matsumura T, Kimura E. Female dystrophinopathy: review of current literature. *Neuromuscul Disord.* 2018;28(7):572-581. [PMID: 29801751]

Mercuri E, Bönnemann CG, Muntoni F. Muscular dystrophies. *Lancet.* 2019;394(10213):2025-2038. [PMID: 31789220]

Yildiz S, Glanzman AM, Estilow T, et al. Retrospective analysis of fractures and factors causing ambulation loss after lower extremity fractures in Duchenne muscular dystrophy. *Am J Phys Med Rehabil.* 2020;99(9):789-794. [PMID: 32195737]

2. Spinal Muscular Atrophy

Spinal muscular atrophy is a neuromuscular disorder with degeneration of alpha motor neurons leading to progressive muscular weakness and atrophy. The disorder is caused by a deletion or loss-of-function mutations in the *SMN1* gene, which codes for survival of motor neuron (SMN) protein and is inherited in an autosomal recessive pattern. The severe infantile form of the disease is called **Werdnig-Hoffmann paralysis.** Only about 20% of patients with spinal muscular atrophy are ambulatory, and 1% are totally dependent. Fractures are common in these patients, occurring secondary to decreased mobility and function. Nusinersen was approved by the US Food and Drug Administration in December 2016 is and is administered directly to the central nervous system using intrathecal injection. When administered immediately after establishing the genetic diagnosis of SMA in presymptomatic infants and emerging newborns, it diminishes muscle atrophy and weakness, allowing sitting, walking, and freedom from permanent ventilation in children. Among children with later-onset SMA, those who receive nusinersen also have significant and clinically meaningful improvement in motor function.

The goal of orthopedic intervention is to prevent collapse of the spine and contractures. Orthotic support is often needed to stabilize the spine. In the nonambulatory patient, adaptive seating devices or orthotics may be used. If collapse of the spine occurs, spinal fusion is indicated, but progression can occur even with after fusion. Skeletal immaturity and length of posterior instrumentation may influence curve progression and should be considered during preoperative planning.

De Vivo DC, Bertini E, Swoboda KJ, et al. Nusinersen initiated in infants during the presymptomatic stage of spinal muscular atrophy: interim efficacy and safety results from the Phase 2 NURTURE study. *Neuromuscul Disord.* 2019;29(11):842-856. [PMID: 31704158]

Dunaway Young S, Montes J, Salazar R, et al. Scoliosis surgery significantly impacts motor abilities in higher-functioning individuals with spinal muscular atrophy. *J Neuromuscul Dis.* 2020;7(2):183-192. [PMID: 32083590]

Mercuri E, Darras BT, Chiriboga CA, et al. Nusinersen versus sham control in later-onset spinal muscular atrophy. *N Engl J Med.* 2018;378(7):625-635. [PMID: 29443664]

3. Charcot-Marie-Tooth Disease

Charcot-Marie-Tooth (CMT) disease is the most common of the hereditary degenerative myopathies, affecting at least 1 in

2500 persons. CMT is caused by mutations in genes that produce proteins involved in the structure and function of either the peripheral nerve axon or the myelin sheath. The nerves slowly degenerate, resulting in muscle weakness, atrophy, and in some individuals, pain. Different proteins are abnormal in different forms of CMT disease, including CMT1, CMT2, CMT3, CMT4, and CMTX, and more than 30 causative genes have been described. CMT1 is the most common type of CMT, accounting for about two-thirds of all cases and is inherited in an autosomal dominant pattern. Other forms are inherited in an autosomal recessive or an X-linked fashion. EMG studies show a neuropathic pattern, and the nerve conduction velocity of the involved nerves is markedly decreased. Muscle enzyme levels are normal. Clinical onset of the disease is usually between 5 and 15 years of age. The severity of symptoms varies greatly among individuals and even among family members with the disease. Progression of symptoms is gradual.

The peroneal muscles are affected early in the course of the disease. For this reason, CMT disease is sometimes referred to as **progressive peroneal muscular atrophy**. The intrinsic muscles of the feet and hands are affected later. Patients usually present with progressive claw toe and cavus deformities (high arches) of the feet. In the skeletally immature patient, release of the plantar fascia is done to correct the cavus deformity. This is often combined with transfer of the extensor digitorum longus tendon to the neck of the metatarsal and fusion of the proximal interphalangeal joints of the toes to correct the claw toe deformities. If the tibialis posterior muscle is active during swing phase, it can be transferred through the interosseous membrane to the lateral cuneiform bone. Triple arthrodesis is often necessary in the adult to correct the deformity.

The intrinsic minus hand deformity causes difficulty in grasping objects. An orthosis with a lumbrical bar to hold the metacarpophalangeal joints flexed improves hand use. A capsulodesis of the volar portion of the metacarpophalangeal joints accomplishes the same objective. To restore active intrinsic muscle function in the hand, the flexor digitorum superficialis tendon of the ring finger can be divided into four slips and transferred through the lumbrical passages to the proximal phalanx. A specific sign that may be found in people with CMT1 is nerve enlargement that may be felt or even seen through the skin. These enlarged nerves, called hypertrophic nerves, are caused by abnormally thickened myelin sheaths.

Bjelica B, Peric S, Basta I, et al. Neuropathic pain in patients with Charcot-Marie-Tooth type 1A. *Neurol Sci.* 2020;41(3):625-630. [PMID: 31729581]

Louwerens JWK. Operative treatment algorithm for foot deformities in Charcot-Marie-Tooth disease. *Oper Orthop Traumatol.* 2018;30(2):130-146. [PMID: 29417158]

Murakami T, Sunada Y. Schwann cell and the pathogenesis of Charcot-Marie-Tooth disease. *Adv Exp Med Biol.* 2019;1190:301-321. [PMID: 31760652]

PARKINSON DISEASE

A. Epidemiology

Parkinson disease (PD) is a progressive neurodegenerative disorder associated with a loss of dopaminergic nigrostriatal neurons. PD is recognized as one of the most common neurologic disorders, affecting approximately 1% to 2% of individuals older than 65 years. The incidence and prevalence of PD increase with age, and PD affects 4% to 5% of those over 85 years of age. The average age of onset is approximately 60 years. Onset in persons younger than 40 years is relatively uncommon.

B. Pathophysiology

The major neuropathologic findings in PD are a loss of pigmented dopaminergic neurons in the substantia nigra and the presence of Lewy bodies. The loss of dopaminergic neurons occurs most prominently in the ventral lateral substantia nigra. Approximately 60% to 80% of dopaminergic neurons are lost before clinical symptoms of PD emerge.

C. History

Onset of PD is typically asymmetric, with the most common initial finding being an asymmetric resting tremor in an upper extremity. Approximately 20% of patients first experience clumsiness in one hand. Over time, patients notice symptoms related to progressive bradykinesia, rigidity, and gait difficulty. The initial symptoms of PD may be nonspecific and include fatigue and depression.

D. Physical Examination

The three cardinal signs of PD are resting tremor, rigidity, and bradykinesia. Of these cardinal features, two of three are required to make the clinical diagnosis. Postural instability is the fourth cardinal sign, but it emerges late in the disease, usually after 8 years or more.

E. Medical Care

The goal of medical management of PD is to provide control of signs and symptoms for as long as possible while minimizing adverse effects. Medications (eg, levodopa) usually provide good symptomatic control for the first several years, and after this, disability progresses despite best medical management, and many patients develop long-term motor complications including fluctuations (wearing off) and dyskinesia. Additional causes of disability in late disease include postural instability (balance difficulty), difficulty speaking and swallowing, and cognitive problems.

F. Neurosurgical Care

Neurosurgical interventions include ablative surgery (thalamotomy, subthalamotomy, and pallidotomy) and, when medical management has become less effective or to reduce medication, deep brain stimulation, the most commonly performed surgical treatment for PD. Deep brain stimulation typically works best to lessen motor symptoms of stiffness, slowness, and tremor. It does not work as well for imbalance, freezing of gait (sudden inability to move when walking), or nonmotor symptoms.

G. Orthopedic Care

Treatment of orthopedic problems in patients with PD can be problematic because rehabilitation and compliance are often hampered. Despite successful pain relief, the functional results of total joint arthroplasty in patients with PD are less predictable, and complications are more frequent. When symptoms of PD can be managed with appropriate treatments such as medications and deep brain stimulation, the chances of a satisfactory outcome are improved.

Bhidayasiri R, Panyakaew P, Trenkwalder C, et al. Delivering patient-centered care in Parkinson's disease: challenges and consensus from an international panel. *Parkinsonism Relat Disord.* 2020;72:82-87. [PMID: 32146380]

Mansouri A, Taslimi S, Badhiwala JH, et al. Deep brain stimulation for Parkinson's disease: meta-analysis of results of randomized trials at varying lengths of follow-up. *J Neurosurg.* 2018;128(4):1199-1213. [PMID: 28665252]

BURNS

More than 2 million people sustain burns of sufficient severity each year in the United States to require medical attention. Of these, 50,000 individuals remain hospitalized for more than 2 months, attesting to the serious nature of their injuries.

Thermal burns affect the skin most directly but can also involve the underlying muscles, tendons, joints, and bones. Scar contractures cause the greatest limitation to later function and the greatest deformity. Rehabilitation efforts ideally should begin when the patient first enters the hospital, immediately following acute resuscitation and continuing through the reconstruction process.

Classification

Burn wounds are traditionally classified as first, second, or third degree, depending on the depth of the damage. Currently, it is thought to be more useful to simply divide burns into two categories: partial thickness (involving part of the dermis) and full thickness (involving the entire dermis). In children, a burn size of roughly 60% total body surface area is a crucial threshold for postburn morbidity and mortality.

First-degree burns damage only the epidermis. They cause erythema, minor edema, and pain. The skin surface remains intact, and healing occurs uneventfully in 5 to 10 days, without residual scar formation.

Second-degree burns involve the epidermis and a variable amount of the underlying corium. The depth of damage to the corium determines the outcome of healing. In the more superficial second-degree burns, blister formation is prominent and occurs secondary to the osmotic gradient formed by particles in the vesicle fluid. Superficial second-degree burns heal in 10 to 14 days, with minimal scarring. Deep dermal burns are characterized by either a reddish appearance or by the presence of a white tissue that is barely perceptible and adheres to the underlying viable dermis. These wounds may advance to a full-thickness loss if infection occurs. They heal with a fragile epithelial covering. Healing occurs over 25 to 30 days, and dense scar formation is common.

Third-degree burns are full-thickness injuries that damage the epidermis and the entire corium. Because of the loss of pain receptors, which are normally found within the corium, pain is absent. The burns have a thick leathery surface of dead tissue.

Management

A. Techniques for Maintaining Functional Position

Burn scars contract and become rigid, so it is critical to maintain the head, trunk, and extremities in a functional position. Contractures, if allowed to form, severely limit later function. The location of the burns determines which techniques are useful in preventing deformity.

To prevent deformities of the neck and jaw in patients with burns of the neck or upper torso, molded splints should be applied early to maintain the head and neck in a neutral position or in slight extension. Patients with burns in the shoulder region are at risk for contractures characterized by a protracted scapula with an adducted arm. Placing a roll between the scapulae and providing support with a firm mattress help prevent scapula protraction. To keep the arms abducted 75 to 80 degrees and the shoulder flexed 20 to 30 degrees, axillary foam pads are used and can be held in position with a figure-of-eight wrapping, which maintains the glenohumeral joint in a functional position. Untreated contractures not only limit limb motion but also can result in joint subluxation from extremes in positioning.

When the burns involve the torso, the goal is to maintain a straight spine in the face of contracting scar tissue. Burns involving only one side of the trunk sometimes result in scoliosis. This should be corrected by scar excision and splinting. If left uncorrected, the scoliosis becomes structural, with resultant bony changes. Burns in the groin area tend to cause flexion and adduction contractures of the hip. To prevent this, the patient should be positioned with the hips extended and in 15 to 20 degrees of abduction. If the patient is lying on a soft mattress, mild flexion deformities of the hips may be masked. Daily pronation is useful in maintaining the extension range of the hips.

Regardless of the location of burn wounds on the extremities, the knees and elbows tend to develop flexion contractures. Custom-molded thermoplastic splints can be applied over dressings or skin grafts to maintain the extremities in extension. The splints should be removable to allow for daily wound care. Burns in the ankle area result in equinus contractures with inversion of the foot. Splints can be used here also to maintain the foot in a neutral position, but care must be taken to ensure the splint is holding the foot adequately and not merely obscuring a deformity. Custom-molded splints applied to the anterior and posterior surfaces in a clamshell fashion are more effective in maintaining the desired position. They also assist in the control of edema and can be removed for wound care and motion exercises. Burns on the dorsum of the foot cause hyperextension deformities of the toes. Early grafting and toe traction are useful.

Burns of the hands present special problems. Scar contracture results in a flexion deformity of the wrist and a claw hand position similar to that seen with loss of the intrinsic musculature. The hand should be splinted with the wrist in neutral or in a slightly extended position. The metacarpophalangeal joints should be flexed 60 to 75 degrees and the interphalangeal joints extended. The thumb should be held with the metacarpal in abduction and flexion, the metacarpophalangeal joint in mild flexion, and the interphalangeal joint in the extended position.

B. Skeletal Traction and External Suspension

In patients with circumferential burns on an extremity, the use of skeletal traction or external fixators and suspension is efficacious and has several advantages. It permits access to all surfaces, elevates the limb to decrease edema, and maintains the extremity in the desired position while allowing joint motion. Traction can be used to correct contractures. In addition, traction still allows for daily hydrotherapy. Generally, traction is only employed for a 2-week period because longer use may result in a pin tract infection with formation of sequestra.

Special splints are fabricated for use in the hand. The traction frame is secured proximally with a pin inserted through the distal radius. Pins are also placed through the distal phalanges of the fingers and thumb by drilling through the nail bed from the dorsal to the volar surface. Traction is applied to the fingers in the desired direction by attaching rubber bands from the distal pins to the outrigger frame. The frame can be modified for use in the foot to apply traction to the toes. In this case, the traction frame is secured proximally with a pin inserted through the calcaneus.

C. Pressure Dressings

Consistent pressure of 25 torr applied evenly aids in the prevention of hypertrophic scar formation and contracture. Elastic wraps applied over splints are used early after the injury and following grafting because they can be adjusted for changes in the amount of edema present. Later, when the amount of swelling shows little fluctuation, custom elastic garments are employed. Pressure must be continued for as long as the scar tissue is biologically active. When the skin is soft and flat and returns to normal color, the pressure can be discontinued. Pressure dressings should be employed for a minimum of 6 months and may be necessary for as long as a year. The daily application of lanolin relieves the dryness of grafted skin or substitutes for the loss of sebaceous gland secretions in deep burns.

D. Mobilization

Early motion is desirable for burned and uninvolved extremities. Splints should be removed frequently to allow for ROM exercises. If the patient is being treated with skeletal traction, motion exercises can be performed on the extremities. If the patient is receiving hydrotherapy for the burn wounds, the motion exercises are facilitated with the extremities supported in the fluid environment.

Patients with burns of the lower extremities can begin to stand or walk before skin grafts are performed, provided the legs are wrapped with elastic supports to control edema. Ambulation should be resumed after skin grafting as soon as the grafts are stable. Early mobilization not only preserves joint motion but also decreases the incidence of sequelae such as osteoporosis, physiologic deconditioning, muscle atrophy, and HO.

E. Treatment of Special Problems

1. Fractures—If fractures occurred at the time of the burn, they can be treated with the use of skeletal traction or external supports such as splints. Diagnosis may be delayed if the fractures do not result in any obvious deformity. If fractures occur secondary to disuse osteoporosis, they are usually minimally displaced and heal uneventfully. Pathologic fractures are less common with early mobilization.

2. Osteomyelitis—Osteomyelitis is not a common complication, despite the high incidence of sepsis associated with burns. Prolonged exposure of bone sometimes results in the formation of a tangential sequestrum in the devitalized cortex. Exposed bone surfaces can be drilled to promote the formation of a granulation tissue bed for skin grafting without an increased risk of infection. The prolonged use of pins for skeletal traction causes infection in 5% of patients who require traction. The use of threaded traction pins minimizes the motion of the pin in the bone. Pins should be removed as soon as possible.

3. Exposed joints—Children and adolescents with exposed joint surfaces may retain some function after healing, but adults often develop joint ankylosis or deformities that require arthrodesis at a later date. To maintain the joint in the desired position, traction can be used. The joint should be irrigated with hypochlorite solution daily and debrided as necessary. The exposed bone surfaces can be drilled to promote the formation of granulation tissue. When the bed of tissue covers the joint, skin grafting is performed.

4. Heterotopic ossification—HO is the presence of lamellar bone in nonskeletal tissue. Periarticular bone formation is seen in 2% to 3% of patients with severe burns. Although the cause is unknown, predisposing factors include full-thickness burns involving more than 30% of the body surface, prolonged immobilization, and superimposed trauma. The location of the HO is not determined by the distribution of the burns. Ossification can occur in any of the major joints. In adults, the elbow is the joint most frequently affected; the hip is rarely affected. In children, the hip and elbow are common sites; the shoulder is an uncommon site.

HO can continue to form as long as open granulating wounds are present. If joint ankylosis does not occur, the ossification gradually diminishes after the burns heal. In children, it may disappear completely. If joint ankylosis occurs, surgical resection is indicated and usually restores a functional arc of motion, particularly when the articular surface is not damaged. This may be done with multiple small incisions without raising cutaneous flaps. Early mobilization of patients with burns decreases the incidence and severity of HO.

Barrett LW, Fear VS, Waithman JC, Wood FM, Fear MW. Understanding acute burn injury as a chronic disease. *Burns Trauma.* 2019;7:23. [PMID: 31534977]

Lensing J, Wibbenmeyer L, Liao J, et al. Demographic and burn injury-specific variables associated with limited joint mobility at discharge in a multicenter study. *J Burn Care Res.* 2020;41(2):363-370. [PMID: 31895409]

Liu HF, Zhang F, Lineaweaver WC. History and advancement of burn treatments. *Ann Plast Surg.* 2017;78(2 suppl 1):S2-S8. [PMID: 28079548]

Yelvington ML, Godleski M, Lee AF, et al. A comparison of contracture severity at acute discharge in patients with and without heterotopic ossification: a burn model system national database study. *J Burn Care Res.* 2019;40(3):349-354. [PMID: 30838385]

Index

NOTE: Page numbers followed by *f* or *t* indicate figures or tables, respectively.

www.ingramcontent.com/pod-product-compliance
Ingram Content Group UK Ltd.
Pitfield, Milton Keynes, MK11 3LW, UK
UKHW052240160626
472267UK00003B/39

9 781260 135978